Shorter O...
of Psychiatry

D1586622

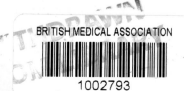

Shorter Oxford Textbook of Psychiatry

SEVENTH EDITION

Paul Harrison
Philip Cowen
Tom Burns
Mina Fazel

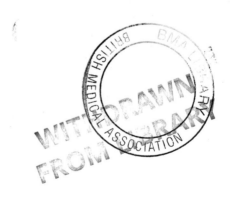

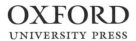

OXFORD
UNIVERSITY PRESS

OXFORD
UNIVERSITY PRESS

Great Clarendon Street, Oxford, OX2 6DP,
United Kingdom

Oxford University Press is a department of the University of Oxford.
It furthers the University's objective of excellence in research, scholarship,
and education by publishing worldwide. Oxford is a registered trade mark of
Oxford University Press in the UK and in certain other countries

First Edition published in 1983
Second Edition published in 1989
Third Edition published in 1996
Fourth Edition published in 2001
Fifth Edition published in 2006
Sixth Edition published in 2012
Seventh Edition published in 2018

Impression: 1

Published in the United States of America by Oxford University Press
198 Madison Avenue, New York, NY 10016, United States of America

British Library Cataloguing in Publication Data

Data available

Library of Congress Control Number: 2017932616

ISBN 978–0–19–874743–7

Printed in Great Britain by
Bell & Bain Ltd., Glasgow

Preface to the seventh edition

In the 5 years since the sixth edition of this book, psychiatry has seen important advances in understanding and treatment of its disorders, as well as the publication of revised diagnostic criteria in DSM-5. These developments have been incorporated into this substantially rewritten edition, which includes a new chapter on global mental health, and division of mood disorders into separate chapters on depression and bipolar disorder.

As in previous editions, we have sought to provide information in a format, and at a level of detail, to assist those training in psychiatry. We hope the book will also continue to be useful to medical students and other health professionals, including those working in primary care, community health, and the many professions and groups contributing to multidisciplinary mental health care. More detailed information can be found in the companion reference textbook, the *New Oxford Textbook of Psychiatry*, the third edition of which is nearing completion.

We welcome Mina Fazel. Mina is the first child psychiatrist, and the first woman, to be an author of the *Shorter Oxford Textbook of Psychiatry* since its inception. We are delighted that both these unfortunate omissions have been corrected, and this edition benefits greatly from her contributions.

We thank Sarah Atkinson, Linda Carter, and Sue Woods-Gantz for secretarial assistance. We are very grateful to Charlotte Allan, Chris Bass, Christopher Fairburn, and Kate Saunders for their expert advice and helpful comments.

PH
PC
TB
MF
Oxford, March 2017

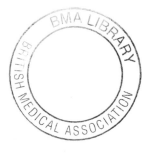

Contents

CHAPTER 1
Signs and symptoms of psychiatric disorders

Introduction

Psychiatrists require two distinct capacities. One is the capacity to collect clinical data objectively and accurately, and to organize and communicate the data in a systematic and balanced way. The other is the capacity for intuitive understanding of each patient as an individual. When the psychiatrist exercises the first capacity, he draws on his skills and knowledge of clinical phenomena; when he exercises the second capacity, he draws on his knowledge of human nature and his experience with former patients to gain insights into the patient he is now seeing. Both capacities can be developed by listening to patients, and by learning from more experienced psychiatrists. A textbook can provide the information and describe the procedures necessary to develop the first capacity. The focus of the chapter on the first capacity does not imply that intuitive understanding is unimportant, but simply that it cannot be learned directly or solely from a textbook.

Skill in examining patients depends on a sound knowledge of how symptoms and signs are defined. Without such knowledge, the psychiatrist is liable to misclassify phenomena and thereby make inaccurate diagnoses. For this reason, this chapter is concerned with the definition of the key symptoms and signs of psychiatric disorders. Having elicited a patient's symptoms and signs, the psychiatrist needs to decide how far these phenomena fall into a pattern that has been observed in other

psychiatric patients. In other words, he decides whether the clinical features conform to a recognized syndrome. He does this by combining observations about the patient's present state with information about the history of the condition. The value of identifying a syndrome is that it helps to predict prognosis and to select an effective treatment. It does this by directing the psychiatrist to the relevant body of accumulated knowledge about the causes, treatment, and outcome in similar patients. Diagnosis and classification are discussed in the next chapter, and also in each of the chapters dealing with the various psychiatric disorders. Chapter 3 discusses how to elicit and interpret the symptoms described in this chapter, and how to integrate the information to arrive at a syndromal diagnosis, since this in turn is the basis for a rational approach to management and prognosis.

As much of the present chapter consists of definitions and descriptions of symptoms and signs, it may be less easy to read than those that follow. It is suggested that the reader might approach it in two stages. The first reading would be applied to the introductory sections and to a general understanding of the more frequently observed phenomena. The second reading would focus on details of definition and the less common symptoms and signs, and might be done best in conjunction with an opportunity to interview a patient exhibiting these.

General issues

Before individual phenomena are described, some general issues will be considered concerning the methods of studying symptoms and signs, and the terms that are used to describe them.

Psychopathology

The study of abnormal states of mind is known as *psychopathology*. The term embraces two distinct approaches to the subject—*descriptive* and *experimental*. This chapter is concerned almost exclusively with the former; the latter is introduced here but is discussed in later chapters.

Descriptive psychopathology

Descriptive psychopathology is the objective description of abnormal states of mind avoiding, as far as possible, preconceived ideas or theories, and limited to the description of conscious experiences and observable behaviour. It is sometimes also called *phenomenology* or *phenomenological psychopathology*, although the terms are not in fact synonymous, and phenomenology has additional meanings (Berrios, 1992). Likewise, descriptive psychopathology is more than just *symptomatology* (Stanghellini and Broome, 2014).

The aim of descriptive psychopathology is to elucidate the essential qualities of morbid mental experiences and to understand each patient's experience of illness. It therefore requires the ability to elicit, identify, and interpret the symptoms of psychiatric disorders, and as such is a key element of clinical practice; indeed, it has been described as 'the fundamental professional skill of the psychiatrist'.

The most important exponent of descriptive psychopathology was the German psychiatrist and philosopher, Karl Jaspers. His classic work, *Allgemeine Psychopathologie* (*General Psychopathology*), first published in 1913, still provides the most complete account of the subject, and the seventh edition is available in an English translation (Jaspers, 1963). A briefer introduction can be found in Jaspers (1968), and Oyebode (2014) has provided a highly readable contemporary text on descriptive psychopathology.

Experimental psychopathology

This approach seeks to explain abnormal mental phenomena, as well as to describe them. One of the first attempts was *psychodynamic psychopathology*, originating in Freud's psychoanalytic investigations (see p. 91). It explains the causes of abnormal mental events in terms of mental processes of which the patient is unaware (i.e. they are 'unconscious'). For example, Freud explained persecutory delusions as being evidence, in the conscious mind, of activities in the unconscious mind, including the mechanisms of repression and projection (see p. 277).

Subsequently, experimental psychopathology has focused on empirically measurable and verifiable conscious psychological processes, using experimental methods such as cognitive and behavioural psychology and functional brain imaging. For example, there are cognitive theories of the origin of delusions, panic attacks, and depression. Although experimental psychopathology is concerned with the causes of symptoms, it is usually conducted in the context of the syndromes in which the symptoms occur. Thus its findings are discussed in the chapter covering the disorder in question.

Terms and concepts used in descriptive psychopathology

Symptoms and signs

In general medicine there is a clear definition of, and separation between, a symptom and a sign. In psychiatry the situation is different. There are few 'signs' in the medical sense (apart from the motor abnormalities of catatonic schizophrenia or the physical manifestations of anorexia nervosa), with most diagnostic information coming from the history and observations of the patient's appearance and behaviour. Use of the word 'sign' in psychiatry is therefore less clear, and two different uses may be encountered. First, it may refer to a feature noted by the observer rather than something spoken by the patient (e.g. a patient who appears to be responding to a hallucination). Secondly, it may refer to a group of symptoms that the observer interprets in aggregation as a sign of a particular disorder. In practice, the phrase 'symptoms and signs' is often used interchangeably with 'symptoms' (as we have done in this chapter) to refer collectively to the phenomena of psychiatric disorders, without a clear distinction being drawn between the two words.

Subjective and objective

In general medicine, the terms *subjective* and *objective* are used as counterparts of symptoms and signs, respectively, with 'objective' being defined as something observed directly by the doctor (e.g. meningism, jaundice)—even though, strictly speaking, it is a subjective judgement on his part as to what has been observed.

In psychiatry, the terms have broadly similar meanings as they do in medicine, although with a blurring between them, just as there is for symptoms and signs. 'Objective' refers to features observed during an interview (i.e. the patient's appearance and behaviour). The term is usually used when the psychiatrist wants to compare this with the patient's description of symptoms. For example, in evaluation of depression, complaints of low mood and tearfulness are subjective features, whereas observations of poor eye contact, psychomotor retardation, and crying are objective ones. If both are present, the psychiatrist might record 'subjective *and* objective evidence of depression', with the combination providing stronger evidence than either alone. However, if the patient's behaviour and manner in the interview appear entirely normal, he records 'not objectively depressed', despite the subjective complaints. It is then incumbent on the psychiatrist to explore the reasons for the discrepancy and to decide what diagnostic conclusions he should draw. As a rule, objective signs are accorded greater weight. Thus he may diagnose a depressive disorder if there is sufficient evidence of this kind, even if the patient denies the subjective experience of feeling depressed. Conversely, the psychiatrist may question the significance of complaints of low mood, however prominent, if there are none of the objective features associated with the diagnosis.

Form and content

When psychiatric symptoms are described, it is useful to distinguish between form and content, a distinction that is best explained by an example. If a patient says that, when he is alone, he hears voices calling him a homosexual, the *form* of the experience is an auditory hallucination (see below), whereas the *content* is the statement that he is homosexual. Another patient might hear voices saying that she is about to be killed. Again the form is an auditory hallucination, but the content is different. A third patient might experience repeated intrusive thoughts that he is homosexual, but he realizes that these are untrue. Here the content is the same as that of the first example, but the form is different.

Form is often critical when making a diagnosis. From the examples given above, the presence of a hallucination indicates (by definition) a psychosis of one kind or another, whereas the third example suggests obsessive–compulsive disorder. Content is less diagnostically useful, but can be very important in management; for example, the content of a delusion may suggest that the patient could attack a supposed persecutor. It is also the content, not the form, that is of concern to the patient, whose priority will be to discuss the persecution and its implications, and who may be irritated by what seem to be irrelevant questions about the form of the belief. The psychiatrist must be sensitive to this difference in emphasis between the two parties.

Primary and secondary

With regard to symptoms, the terms *primary* and *secondary* are often used, but unfortunately with two different meanings. The first meaning is *temporal*, simply referring to which occurred first. The second meaning is *causal*, whereby primary means 'arising directly from the pathological process', and secondary means 'arising as a reaction to a primary symptom'. The two meanings often coincide, as symptoms that arise directly from the pathological process usually appear first. However, although subsequent symptoms are often a reaction to the first symptoms, they are not always of this kind, for they too may arise directly from the pathological process. The terms primary and secondary are used more often in the temporal sense because this usage does not involve an inference about causality. However, many patients cannot say in what order their symptoms appeared. In such cases, when it seems likely that one symptom is a reaction to another—for example, that a delusion of being followed by persecutors is a reaction to hearing accusing voices—it is described as secondary (using the word in the causal sense). The terms primary and secondary are also used in descriptions of syndromes.

Understanding and explanation

Jaspers (1913) contrasted two forms of understanding when applied to symptoms. The first, called *Verstehen* ('understanding'), is the attempt to appreciate the patient's subjective experience: what does it feel like? This important skill requires intuition and empathy. The second approach, called *Erklären* ('explanation'), accounts for events in terms of external factors; for example, the patient's low mood can be 'explained' by his recent redundancy. The latter approach requires knowledge of psychiatric aetiology (Chapter 5).

The significance of individual symptoms

Psychiatric disorders are diagnosed when a defined group of symptoms (a syndrome) is present. Almost any single symptom can be experienced by a healthy person; even hallucinations, often regarded as a hallmark of severe mental disorder, are experienced by some otherwise healthy people. An exception to this is that a delusion, even if isolated, is generally considered to be evidence of psychiatric disorder if it is unequivocal and persistent (see Chapter 11). In general, however, the finding of a single symptom is not evidence of psychiatric disorder, but an indication for a thorough and, if necessary, repeated search for other symptoms and signs of psychiatric disorder. The dangers of not adhering to this principle are exemplified by the well-known study by Rosenhan (1973). Eight 'patients' presented with the complaint that they heard the words 'empty, hollow, thud' being said out loud. All eight individuals were admitted and diagnosed with schizophrenia, despite denying all other symptoms and behaving entirely normally. This study also illustrates the importance of descriptive psychopathology, and of reliable diagnostic criteria (see Chapter 2), as fundamental aspects of psychiatry.

The patient's experience

Symptoms and signs are only part of the subject matter of psychopathology. The latter is also concerned with the patient's experience of illness, and the way in which psychiatric disorder changes his view of himself, his hopes for the future, and his view of the world (Stanghellini and Broome, 2014). This may be seen as one example of the understanding (*verstehen*) mentioned above. A depressive disorder may have a very different effect on a person who has lived a satisfying and happy life and has fulfilled his major ambitions, compared with a person who has had many previous misfortunes but has lived on hopes of future success. To understand this aspect of the patient's experience of psychiatric disorder, the psychiatrist has to understand him in the way that a biographer understands his subject. This way of understanding is sometimes called the life-story approach. It is not something that can be readily assimilated from textbooks; it is best learned by taking time to listen to patients. The psychiatrist may be helped by reading biographies or works of literature that provide insights into the ways in which experiences throughout life shape the personality, and help to explain the diverse ways in which different people respond to the same events.

Cultural variations in psychopathology

The core symptoms of most serious mental disorders are present in culturally diverse individuals. However, there are cultural differences in how these symptoms present in clinical settings and to the meanings that are attributed to them. For example, depression can present with prominent somatic symptoms in many Asian populations, such as those from India and China. The content of symptoms can also differ between cultures. For example, for sub-Saharan African populations, delusions not infrequently centre upon being cursed, a rare delusional theme in Europeans. Cultural differences also affect the person's subjective experience of illness, and therefore influence that person's understanding of it (Fabrega, 2000). In some cultures, the effects of psychiatric disorder are ascribed to witchcraft—a belief that adds to the patient's distress. In many cultures, mental illness is greatly stigmatized, and can, for example, hinder prospects of marriage. In such a culture the effect of illness on the patient's view of himself and his future will be very different from the effect on a patient living in a society that is more tolerant of mental disorder.

Descriptions of symptoms and signs

Disturbances of emotion and mood

Much of psychiatry is concerned with abnormal emotional states, particularly disturbances of mood and other emotions, especially anxiety. Before describing the main symptoms of this kind, it is worth clarifying two areas of terminology that may cause confusion, in part because their usage has changed over the years.

First, the term 'mood' can either be used as a broad term to encompass all emotions (e.g. 'anxious mood'), or in a more restricted sense to mean the emotion that runs from depression at one end to mania at the other.

The former usage is now uncommon. The latter usage is emphasized by the fact that, in current diagnostic systems, 'mood disorders' are those in which depression and mania are the defining characteristics, whereas disorders defined by anxiety or other emotional disturbances are categorized separately. In this section, features common to both 'mood' and 'other emotions' are described first, before the specific features of anxiety, depression, and mania are discussed separately.

The second point concerns the term 'affect'. This is now usually used interchangeably with the term 'mood', in the more limited meaning of the latter word (e.g. 'his affect was normal', 'he has an affective disorder').

However, in the past, these words had different nuances of meaning; mood referred to a prevailing and prolonged state, whereas affect was linked to a particular aspect or object, and was more transitory.

Emotions and mood may be abnormal in three ways:

- Their nature may be altered
- They may fluctuate more or less than usual
- They may be inconsistent with the patient's thoughts or actions, or with his current circumstances.

Changes in the nature of emotions and mood

These can be towards anxiety, depression, elation, or irritability and anger. Any of these changes may be associated with events in the person's life, but they may arise without an apparent reason. They are usually accompanied by other symptoms and signs. For example, an increase in anxiety is accompanied by autonomic overactivity and increased muscle tension, and depression is accompanied by gloomy preoccupations and psychomotor slowness.

Changes in the way that emotions and mood vary

Emotions and mood vary in relation to the person's circumstances and preoccupations. In abnormal states, this variation with circumstances may continue, but the variations may be greater or less than normal. Increased variation is called *lability* of mood; extreme variation is sometimes called *emotional incontinence*.

Reduced variation is called *blunting* or *flattening*. These terms have been used with subtly different meanings, but are now usually used interchangeably. Blunting or flattening usually occurs in depression and schizophrenia. Severe flattening is sometimes called *apathy* (note the difference from the layman's meaning of the word).

Emotion can also vary in a way that is not in keeping with the person's circumstances and thoughts, and this is described as *incongruous* or *inappropriate*. For example, a patient may appear to be in high spirits and laugh when talking about the death of his mother. Such incongruity must be distinguished from the embarrassed laughter which indicates that the person is ill at ease.

Clinical associations of emotional and mood disturbances

Disturbances of emotions and mood are seen in essentially all psychiatric disorders. They are the central feature of the mood disorders and anxiety disorders. They are also common in eating disorders, substance-induced disorders, delirium, dementia, and schizophrenia.

Anxiety

Anxiety is a normal response to danger. Anxiety is abnormal when its severity is out of proportion to the threat of danger, or when it outlasts the threat. Anxious mood is closely coupled with somatic and autonomic components, and with psychological ones. All can be thought of as equivalent to the preparations for dealing with danger seen in other mammals, ready for flight from, avoidance of, or fighting with a predator. Mild-to-moderate anxiety enhances most kinds of performance, but very high levels interfere with it.

The anxiety response is considered further in Chapter 8. Here its main components can be summarized as follows.

- *Psychological.* The essential feelings of dread and apprehension are accompanied by restlessness, narrowing of attention to focus on the source of danger, worrying thoughts, increased alertness (with insomnia), and irritability (that is, a readiness to become angry).
- *Somatic.* Muscle tension and respiration increase. If these changes are not followed by physical activity, they may be experienced as muscle tension tremor, or the effects of hyperventilation (e.g. dizziness).
- *Autonomic.* Heart rate and sweating increase, the mouth becomes dry, and there may be an urge to urinate or defaecate.
- *Avoidance of danger.* A *phobia* is a persistent, irrational fear of a specific object or situation. Usually there is also a marked wish to avoid the object, although this is not always the case—for example, fear of illness (hypochondriasis). The fear is out of proportion to the objective threat, and is recognized as such by the person experiencing it. Phobias include fear of animate objects, natural phenomena, and situations. Phobic people feel anxious not only in the presence of the object or situation, but also when thinking about it (*anticipatory anxiety*). Phobias are discussed further in relation to anxiety disorders in Chapter 5.

Clinical associations

Phobias are common among healthy children, becoming less frequent in adolescence and adult life. Phobic symptoms occur in all kinds of anxiety disorder, but are the major feature in the phobic disorders.

Depression

Depression is a normal response to loss or misfortune, when it may be called grief or mourning. Depression is abnormal when it is out of proportion to the misfortune, or is unduly prolonged. Depressed mood is closely coupled with other changes, notably a lowering of self-esteem, pessimistic or negative thinking, and a reduction in or loss of the experience of pleasure (*anhedonia*). A depressed person has a characteristic expression and appearance, with turned-down corners of the mouth, a furrowed brow, and a hunched, dejected posture. The level of arousal is reduced in some depressed patients (*psychomotor retardation*) but increased in others, with a consequent feeling of restlessness or agitation. The psychopathology of depression is discussed further in Chapter 9.

Clinical associations

Depression can occur in any psychiatric disorder. It is the defining feature of mood disorders, and commonly occurs in schizophrenia, anxiety, obsessive–compulsive disorder, eating disorders, and substance-induced disorders. It can also be a manifestation of an organic disorder.

Elation

Happy moods have been studied less than depressed mood. Elation is an extreme degree of happy mood which, like depression, is coupled with other changes, including increased feelings of self-confidence and well-being, increased activity, and increased arousal. The latter is usually experienced as pleasant, but sometimes as an unpleasant feeling of restlessness. Elation occurs most often in mania and hypomania.

Irritability and anger

Irritability is a state of increased readiness for anger. Both irritability and anger may occur in many kinds of disorder, so they are of little value in diagnosis. However, they are of great importance in risk assessment and risk management, as they may result in harm to others and self (see Chapter 3). Irritability may occur in anxiety disorders, depression, mania, dementia, and drug intoxication.

Disturbances of perception

Specific kinds of perceptual disturbance are symptoms of severe psychiatric disorders. It is therefore important to be able to identify these symptoms and to distinguish them from the other, much less significant, alterations in sensory experience which occur. We shall therefore describe perceptual phenomena in some detail.

Perception and imagery

Perception is the process of becoming aware of what is presented through the sense organs. It is not a direct awareness of data from the sense organs, because these data are acted on by cognitive processes that reassemble them and extract patterns. Perception can be attended to or ignored, but it cannot be terminated by an effort of will.

Imagery is the awareness of a percept that has been generated within the mind. Imagery can be called up and terminated by an effort of will. Images are experienced as lacking the sense of reality that characterizes perception, so that a healthy person can distinguish between images and percepts. A few people experience *eidetic imagery*, which is visual imagery so intense and detailed that it has a 'photographic' quality akin to a percept, although in other ways it differs from a percept. Imagery is generally terminated when perception starts. Occasionally, imagery persists despite the presence of percept (provided this is weak and unstructured). This sort of imagery is called *pareidolia*.

Percepts may alter in intensity and in quality. Anxious people may experience sensations as more intense than usual; for example, they may be unusually sensitive to noise. In mania, perceptions seem more vivid than usual. Depressed patients may experience perceptions as dull and lifeless.

Illusions

Illusions are misperceptions of external stimuli. They occur when the general level of sensory stimulation is reduced and when attention is not focused on the relevant sensory modality. For example, at dusk the outline of a bush may be perceived at first as that of a man, although not when attention is focused on the outline. Illusions are more likely to occur when the level of consciousness is reduced, as in delirium, or when a person is anxious. Illusions have no diagnostic significance, but need to be distinguished from hallucinations.

Hallucinations

A *hallucination* is a percept that is experienced in the absence of an external stimulus to the corresponding sense organ. It differs from an illusion in being experienced as originating in the outside world or from within the person's body (rather than as imagined). Hallucinations cannot be terminated at will.

Hallucinations are generally indications of significant psychiatric disorder, and specific types of hallucination are characteristic of different disorders, as outlined below. However, as noted above, hallucinations do occur in some otherwise healthy people. It is also common to experience them when falling asleep (*hypnagogic hallucinations*) or on waking (*hypnopompic hallucinations*). These two types of hallucination may be either visual or auditory, the latter sometimes as the experience of hearing one's name called. Such hallucinations are common in narcolepsy (see page 327). Some recently bereaved people experience hallucinations of the dead person. Hallucinations can occur after sensory deprivation, in people with blindness or deafness of peripheral origin, occasionally in neurological disorders that affect the visual pathways, in epilepsy (see page 379), and in Charles Bonnet syndrome (see page 555).

Types of hallucination

Hallucinations can be described in terms of their complexity and their sensory modality (see Box 1.1). The term *elementary hallucination* refers to experiences such as bangs, whistles, and flashes of light, whereas the term *complex hallucination* refers to experiences such as hearing voices or music, or seeing faces and scenes.

Auditory hallucinations may be experienced as noises, music, or voices. Voices may be heard clearly or indistinctly; they may seem to speak words, phrases, or sentences. They may seem to address the patient directly (*second-person hallucinations*), or talk to one another, referring to the patient as 'he' or 'she' (*third-person hallucinations*). Sometimes patients say that the voices anticipate what they are about to think a few moments later. Sometimes the voices seem to speak the patient's thoughts as he is thinking them (*Gedankenlautwerden*),

Box 1.1 **Description of hallucinations**

According to complexity
  Elementary
  Complex

According to sensory modality
  Auditory
  Visual
  Olfactory and gustatory
  Somatic (tactile and deep)

According to special features
  Auditory
  Second-person
  Third-person
  Gedankenlautwerden
  Écho de la pensée
  Visual
  Extracampine

Autoscopic hallucinations
  Reflex hallucinations
  Hypnagogic and hypnopompic

or to repeat them immediately after he has thought them (*écho de la pensée*).

Visual hallucinations may also be elementary or complex. The content may appear normal or abnormal in size; hallucinations of dwarf figures are sometimes called *lilliputian*. Occasionally, patients describe the experience of visual hallucinations located outside the field of vision, usually behind the head (*extracampine hallucinations*).

Olfactory hallucinations and *gustatory hallucinations* are frequently experienced together. The smells and tastes are often unpleasant.

Tactile hallucinations, sometimes called *haptic* hallucinations, may be experienced as sensations of being touched, pricked, or strangled. Sometimes they are felt as movements just below the skin, which the patient may attribute to insects, worms, or other small creatures burrowing through the tissues. *Hallucinations of deep sensation* may be experienced as feelings of the viscera being pulled upon or distended, or of sexual stimulation or electric shocks.

An *autoscopic hallucination* is the experience of seeing one's own body projected into external space, usually in front of oneself, for short periods. The experience is reported occasionally by healthy people in situations of sensory deprivation, when it is called an out-of-body experience, or after a near-fatal accident or heart attack, when it has been called a near-death experience. Rarely, the experience is accompanied by the conviction that the person has a double (*Doppelganger*).

Reflex hallucination is a rare phenomenon, in which a stimulus in one sensory modality results in a hallucination in another; for example, music may provoke visual hallucinations.

Clinical associations of hallucinations

Hallucinations occur in diverse disorders, notably schizophrenia, severe mood disorder, organic disorders, and dissociative states. Therefore the finding of hallucinations does not itself help much in diagnosis. However, as with delusions, there are certain kinds of hallucination which do have important implications for diagnosis of schizophrenia and other disorders.

- *Auditory hallucination.* Only clearly heard voices (not noises or music) have diagnostic significance. Third-person hallucinations (introduced above) are strongly associated with schizophrenia. Such voices may be experienced as commenting on the patient's intentions (e.g. 'He wants to make love to her') or actions (e.g. 'She is washing her face'), or may make critical comments. Second-person auditory hallucinations (i.e. those that appear to address the patient) do not point to a particular diagnosis, but their content and the patient's reaction to them may do so. Thus voices with derogatory content (e.g. 'You are a failure, you are wicked') suggest severe depressive disorder, especially when the patient accepts them as justified. In schizophrenia, the patient more often resents such comments. Voices which anticipate, echo, or repeat the patient's thoughts also suggest schizophrenia.

- *Visual hallucinations* should always suggest the possibility of an organic disorder, although they also occur in severe affective disorders, schizophrenia, and dissociative disorder. The content of visual hallucinations is of little significance in diagnosis. Autoscopic hallucinations also raise suspicion of an organic disorder, such as temporal lobe epilepsy.

- *Hallucinations of taste and smell* are infrequent. They may occur in schizophrenia, severe depressive disorders, and temporal lobe epilepsy, and in tumours affecting the olfactory bulb or pathways.

- *Tactile and somatic hallucinations* are suggestive of schizophrenia, especially if they are bizarre in content or interpretation. The sensation of insects moving under the skin (*formication*) occurs in people who abuse cocaine.

Pseudohallucinations

This term refers to experiences that are similar to hallucinations but which do not meet all of the requirements of the definition, nor have the same implications. The word has two distinct meanings, which correspond to two of the ways in which an experience can fail to meet the criteria for a hallucination. In the first meaning, pseudohallucination is a sensory experience that differs from a hallucination in not seeming to the patient to represent external reality, being located within the mind rather than in external space. In this way pseudohallucinations resemble imagery although, unlike imagery, they cannot be dismissed by an effort of will. In the second meaning, the sensory experience appears to originate in the external world, but it seems unreal. For a more detailed discussion, see Hare (1973) and Taylor (1981).

Both definitions of pseudohallucinations are difficult to apply clinically, because patients can seldom describe their experiences in adequate detail. In any event, it is usually sufficient to decide whether a perceptual experience is a 'true' hallucination or not, since it is only the former which carries diagnostic significance. If it is not a hallucination, the experience should be described, but need not be labelled as one kind of pseudohallucination or the other.

Abnormalities in the meaning attached to percepts

A *delusional perception* is a delusion arising directly from a normal percept. This is sometimes erroneously considered to be a perceptual disturbance, but it is really a disorder of thought, and is therefore discussed in the next section.

Disturbances of thoughts

Disturbances of thoughts and thought processes are among the most diagnostically significant symptoms in psychiatry. As with disturbances of perception, therefore, this area of descriptive psychopathology merits relatively detailed description. It covers two kinds of phenomena:

- *Disturbance of thoughts* themselves—that is, a change in the *nature* of individual thoughts. The category of delusion is particularly important. Disturbances of thought are covered in this section.

- *Disturbance of the thinking process* and the linking together of different thoughts; this may affect the speed or the form of the relationship between thoughts. It can occur even if individual thoughts are unremarkable in nature. These phenomena are covered in the next section.

Delusions

A *delusion* is a belief that is firmly held on inadequate grounds, that is not affected by rational argument or evidence to the contrary, and that is not a conventional belief that the person might be expected to hold given their educational, cultural, and religious background. This definition is intended to separate delusions, which are cardinal symptoms of severe psychiatric disorder (and specifically of psychosis), from other kinds of abnormal thoughts and from strongly held beliefs found among healthy people. There are several problems with the definition, which is summarized in Box 1.2, but it suffices as a starting point for more detailed discussion of delusions.

Although not part of the definition, another characteristic feature of delusions is that they have a marked effect on the person's feeling and actions—in the same way that strongly held normal beliefs do. Since the behavioural response to the delusion may itself be out of keeping or even bizarre, it is often this that

Box 1.2 Problems with the definition of delusions

Delusions are firmly held despite evidence to the contrary

The hallmark of a delusion is that it is held with such conviction that it cannot be altered by presenting evidence to the contrary. For example, a patient who holds the delusion that there are persecutors in the adjoining house will not be convinced by evidence that the house is empty. Instead he may suggest that the persecutors left the house shortly before it was searched. The problem with this criterion for delusions is that some of the ideas of normal people are equally impervious to contrary evidence. For example, the beliefs of a convinced spiritualist are not undermined by the counterarguments of a non-believer. Strongly held non-delusional beliefs are called *overvalued ideas* (see page 14).

A further problem with this part of the definition of delusion relates to *partial delusions*. Although delusions are usually held strongly from the start, sometimes they are at first held with a degree of doubt. Also, during recovery it is not uncommon for patients to pass through a stage of increasing doubt about their delusions before finally rejecting them. The term 'partial delusion' refers to both these situations of doubt. It should be used during recovery only when it is known that the beliefs were preceded by a full delusion, and applied to the development of a delusion only when it is known in retrospect that a full delusion developed later. Partial delusions are not, in isolation, helpful in diagnosis—akin to the status of pseudohallucinations mentioned on page 8.

Delusions are held on inadequate grounds

Delusions are not arrived at by the ordinary processes of observation and logic. Some delusions appear suddenly without any previous thinking about the subject (primary delusions). Other delusions appear to be attempts to explain another abnormal experiences—for example, the delusion that hallucinated voices are those of people who are spying on the patient.

Delusions are not beliefs shared by others in the same culture

This criterion is important when the patient is a member of a culture or subculture (including a religious faith), because healthy people in such a group may hold beliefs that are not accepted outside it. Like delusions, such cultural beliefs are generally impervious to contrary evidence and reasoned argument—for example, beliefs in evil spirits. Therefore, before deciding that an idea is delusional, it is important to determine whether other members of the same culture share the belief.

Delusions as false beliefs

Some definitions of delusions indicate that they are false beliefs, but this criterion was not included in the definition given above. This omission is because, in exceptional circumstances, a delusional belief can be true or can subsequently become true. A well-recognized example relates to pathological jealousy (see page 306). It is not falsity that determines whether the belief is delusional, but the nature of the mental processes that led up to it. (The difficulty with this statement is that we cannot define these mental processes precisely.) There is a further practical problem concerning the use of falsity as a criterion for delusion. It is that if the criterion is used, it may be assumed that, because a belief is highly improbable, it is false. This is certainly not a sound assumption, because improbable stories—for example, of persecution by neighbours—sometimes turn out to be true and arrived at through sound observations and logical thought. Therefore ideas should be investigated thoroughly before they are accepted as delusions.

These issues are discussed further in Spitzer (1990) and Butler and Braff (1991). See Garety and Freeman (2013) for a cognitive account of delusions.

---

first brings the person to psychiatric attention, and leads to the delusion being elicited. For example, a man with the delusion that he was being irradiated by sonic waves covered his windows with silver foil and barricaded his door. Occasionally, however, a delusion has little influence on feelings and actions. For example, a patient may believe that he is a member of the royal family while living contentedly in a group home. This separation is called *double orientation*, and usually occurs in chronic schizophrenia.

Types of delusions

Several types of delusions are recognized, and they are categorized either by the characteristics or by the theme of the delusion (see Box 1.3). Many of the terms are simply useful descriptors, but a few of them carry particular diagnostic implications; for example, specific types of delusions are *first rank symptoms* of schizophrenia (see page 255). Most categories of delusions can be diagnosed reliably (Bell *et al.*, 2006). For further descriptions, see also Oyebode (2014).

Primary and secondary delusions

A *primary* or *autochthonous* delusion is one that appears suddenly and with full conviction but without any mental events leading up to it. For example, a schizophrenic patient may be suddenly and completely convinced, for no reason and with no prior thoughts of this kind, that

---

Box 1.3 Descriptions of delusions

According to fixity
  Complete
  Partial
According to onset
  Primary
  Secondary
Other delusional experiences
  Delusional mood
  Delusional perception
  Delusional memory
According to theme
  Persecutory (paranoid)
  Delusions of reference
  Grandiose (expansive)
  Bizarre
  Delusions of guilt
  Nihilistic
  Hypochondriacal
  Religious
  Jealous
  Sexual or amorous
  Delusions of control
  Delusions concerning possession of thought:
  Thought insertion
  Thought withdrawal
  Thought broadcasting
According to other features
  Shared delusions
  Mood congruency

---

he is changing sex. Not all primary delusional experiences start with an idea. Sometimes the first experience is a delusional mood (see below) or a delusional perception (see below). Because patients do not find it easy to remember the exact sequence of such unusual and distressing mental events, it is often difficult to be certain which experience came first. Primary delusions are given considerable weight in the diagnosis of schizophrenia, and they should be recorded only when it is certain that they are present.

Secondary delusions are delusions apparently derived from a preceding morbid experience. The latter may be of several kinds, including hallucinations (e.g. someone who hears voices may believe that he is being followed), low mood (e.g. a profoundly depressed woman may believe people think that she is worthless), or an existing delusion (e.g. a person who is convinced he is being 'framed' may come to believe that he will be imprisoned). Some secondary delusions seem to have an integrative function, making the original experiences more comprehensible to the patient, as in the first example above. Others seem to do the opposite, increasing the sense of persecution or failure, as in the third example. Secondary delusions may accumulate until there is a complicated and stable delusional system. When this happens the delusions are said to be *systematized*.

Delusional mood

When a patient first experiences a delusion, he responds emotionally. For example, a person who believes that a group of people intends to kill him is likely to feel afraid. Occasionally, the change of mood precedes the delusion. This preceding mood is often a feeling of foreboding that some, as yet, unidentified sinister event is about to take place. When the delusion follows, it appears to explain this feeling. In German this antecedent mood is called *Wahnstimmung*. This term is usually translated as *delusional mood*, although it is really the mood from which a delusion arises.

Delusional perception

Sometimes the first abnormal experience is the attaching of a new significance to a familiar percept without any reason to do so. For example, the position of a letter that has been left on the patient's desk may be interpreted as a signal that he is to die. This experience is called *delusional perception*. Note, however, that the perception is normal, and it is the delusional interpretation that is abnormal.

Delusional misidentification

This is the delusional misidentification of oneself or of specific other people. Several eponymous forms are described, and have been considered to be both symptoms and syndromes. In line with the latter view, 'delusional misidentification disorder' is described in Chapter 12.

Delusional memory

In *delusional memory*, a delusional interpretation is attached to past events. Fish (1962) distinguishes two forms of delusional memory. In the commoner form, the past event was genuine, and the term 'delusional' refers to the significance which has now become attached to it. For example, a patient who believes that there is a current plot to poison her may remember (correctly) that she vomited after a meal, eaten long before her psychosis began, and now concludes (incorrectly) that she had been intentionally poisoned. Alternatively, a sudden (autochthonous) delusion arises, which is wrongly dated to a past event. This latter form might be viewed as a true delusional memory (i.e. the memory itself is the delusion), whereas in the first kind described, the memory is normal but a delusional interpretation is placed upon it.

Shared delusions

As a rule, other people recognize delusions as false and argue with the patient in an attempt to correct them. Occasionally, a person who lives with a deluded patient comes to share his delusional beliefs. This condition is known as shared delusions or *folie à deux* (see page 310). Although the second person's delusional conviction is as strong as the partner's while the couple remain together, it often recedes quickly when they are separated.

Delusional themes

For the purposes of clinical work, it is useful to group delusions according to their main themes, since the themes have some diagnostic significance. However, it is first worth considering the word 'paranoid', which is used widely but not always clearly in this context (see Box 1.4).

Persecutory delusions

These are most commonly concerned with persons or organizations that are thought to be trying to inflict harm on the patient, damage his reputation, or make him insane. Such delusions are common but of little help in diagnosis, because they can occur in delusional disorders, organic states, schizophrenia, and severe affective disorders. However, the patient's attitude to the delusion may point to the diagnosis. In a severe depressive disorder, a patient with persecutory delusions characteristically accepts the supposed activities of the persecutors as justified by his own wickedness. In schizophrenia, however, he resents these activities as unwarranted.

Delusions of reference

These are concerned with the idea that objects, events, or people that are unconnected with the patient have a personal significance for him. For example, the patient may believe that an article in a newspaper or a remark on television is directed specifically to him, either as a message to him or to inform others about him. Delusions of reference may also relate to actions or gestures made by other people which are thought to convey a message about the patient. For example, a person who touches his hair may be thought by the patient to be signalling that he, the patient, is turning into a woman. Although most delusions of reference have persecutory associations, some relate to grandiose or reassuring themes.

Delusions of control (passivity phenomena)

A patient who has a delusion of control believes that his actions, impulses, or thoughts are controlled by an outside agency. These are also called *passivity phenomena*. Delusions of control are strongly suggestive of schizophrenia, and have forensic implications, so particular care should be taken when eliciting and recording them. The symptom may be confused with voluntary obedience to commands from hallucinatory voices, with religious beliefs that God controls human actions, or with a metaphorical view of one's free will. By contrast, a patient with a delusion of control firmly believes that his movements or actions are brought about by an outside agency (other than the divine), and are not willed by himself. Moreover, other symptoms of schizophrenia are usually present as well.

Delusions concerning the possession of thought

Healthy people take it for granted that their thoughts are their own. They also know that thoughts are private experiences that become known to other people only if they are spoken aloud, or revealed in writing or through facial expression, gesture, or action. Patients with delusions concerning the possession of thoughts lose these normal convictions in one or more of three ways, all of which are strongly associated with schizophrenia:

- *Thought insertion* is the delusion that certain thoughts are not the patient's own but are implanted by an outside agency. Often there is an associated explanatory delusion—for example, that persecutors have used radio waves to insert the thoughts. This experience must not be confused with that of the obsessional patient, who may be distressed by thoughts that he feels are alien to his nature but who never doubts that these thoughts are his own. The patient with a delusion of thought insertion believes that the thoughts are not his own, but that they have been inserted into his mind.

> ### Box 1.4 The term 'paranoid'
>
> The term 'paranoid' is often used as if it were equivalent to 'persecutory'. Strictly interpreted, however, the word 'paranoid' has a wider meaning (Lewis, 1970). It was used in ancient Greek writings to mean the equivalent of 'out of his mind'. For example, Hippocrates used it to describe patients with febrile delirium. Many later writers applied the term to grandiose, erotic, jealous, and religious delusions, as well as to persecutory delusions. Although for historical reasons it is preferable to retain the broader meaning of the term, the narrower usage is now more common, as sanctioned in the diagnostic category of paranoid personality disorder (see page 301). Because the term 'paranoid' has two possible meanings, the term 'persecutory' is preferable when the narrow sense of paranoid is required. The issue also affects the use of the word to describe syndromes in which such symptoms predominate; the older term 'paranoid psychoses' (or 'paranoid states') is now replaced by 'delusional disorders', in part to avoid the ambiguities (see also Chapter 12).

- *Thought withdrawal* is the delusion that thoughts have been taken out of the mind. The delusion usually accompanies thought blocking, in which the patient experiences a sudden break in the flow of thoughts and believes that the 'missing' thoughts have been taken away by some outside agency. Often there are associated explanatory delusions comparable to those that accompany delusions of thought insertion (see above).
- *Thought broadcasting* is the delusion that unspoken thoughts are known to other people through radio, telepathy, or in some other way. In addition, some patients believe that their thoughts can be heard out loud by other people, a belief that also accompanies the experience of hearing one's own thoughts spoken (*Gedankenlautwerden*), described above in the section on 'Types of hallucination'.

Grandiose delusions

These are beliefs of exaggerated self-importance. The patient may consider himself to be wealthy, endowed with unusual abilities, or a special person. Such expansive ideas occur particularly in mania, and in schizophrenia.

Bizarre delusions

Delusions with highly improbable content (e.g. of control by aliens who communicate via birds) are said to be *bizarre*. They are often given particular weight in the diagnosis of schizophrenia, but the category has problems of reliability and definition (Bell *et al.*, 2006; Cermolacce *et al.*, 2010), and it is not included in current diagnostic criteria.

Delusions of guilt

These beliefs are found most often in depressive illness, and for this reason are sometimes called *depressive delusions*. Typical themes are that a minor infringement of the law in the past will be discovered and bring shame upon the patient, or that his sinfulness will lead to retribution on his family.

Nihilistic delusions

These are beliefs that some person or thing has ceased, or is about to cease, to exist. Examples include a patient's delusion that he has no money, that his career is ruined, or that the world is about to end. Nihilistic delusions are seen in severe depression. Occasionally, nihilistic delusions concern failures of bodily function (often that the bowels are blocked), and are often referred to as *Cotard's syndrome* (see page 196).

Hypochondriacal delusions

These are beliefs concerned with illness. The patient believes, wrongly and in the face of all medical evidence to the contrary, that he is suffering from a disease. Such delusions are more common in the elderly, reflecting the increasing concern with health among people in this age group. Other hypochondriacal delusions are concerned with cancer or venereal disease, or with the appearance of parts of the body, especially the nose. They must be distinguished from the health worries of hypochondriasis (see page 650), which are not delusional.

Mood-congruent and mood-incongruent delusions

If a delusion 'makes sense' in terms of the person's mood, it is said to be mood-congruent. Hypochondriacal and nihilistic delusions in psychotic depression, and grandiose delusions in mania, both fall into this category. In contrast, a delusion that is out of keeping with the prevailing mood is mood-incongruent, and is suggestive of schizophrenia. The concept of congruency can also be applied to hallucinations.

Delusions of jealousy

These are more common among men than women. Not all jealous ideas are delusions; less intense jealous preoccupations and obsessions are common. Jealous delusions are important because they may lead to aggressive behaviour towards the person(s) who is thought to be unfaithful. A patient with delusional jealousy is not satisfied if he fails to find evidence supporting his beliefs; his search will continue. These important and potentially dangerous problems are discussed further in Chapter 12.

Sexual or amorous delusions

These are rare, and are more frequent in women than in men. Sexual delusions are occasionally secondary to somatic hallucinations felt in the genitalia. A person with amorous delusions believes that she is loved by a man who is usually inaccessible to her, and often of higher social status. In many cases she has never spoken to the person. Erotic delusions are the most prominent feature of De Clérambault's syndrome (see page 308).

Obsessional and compulsive symptoms

Obsessions

Obsessions are recurrent persistent thoughts, impulses, or images that enter the mind despite efforts to exclude them. One characteristic feature is the subjective sense of a struggle—the patient resists the obsession, which nevertheless intrudes into awareness. Another characteristic feature is the conviction that to think something is to make it more likely to happen. Obsessions are recognized by the person as his own and not implanted from elsewhere (in contrast to delusions of thought insertion). Another important distinction from delusions is that obsessions are regarded as untrue or senseless. They are generally about matters that the patient finds distressing or otherwise unpleasant. They are often, but not always, accompanied by compulsions (see page 14).

The presence of resistance is important because, together with the lack of persistent or complete conviction about the truth of the idea, it distinguishes obsessions from delusions. However, in practice this distinction can, in isolation, be more difficult, since the resistance tends to diminish when obsessions have been longstanding. Furthermore, when obsessions are very intense, patients may become less certain that they are false. However, a careful history, not only of the symptom but also of other relevant features (e.g. compulsions, other evidence of psychosis) should avoid diagnostic difficulties. It is also necessary to distinguish clinically significant obsessions from similar thoughts that occur in healthy people, especially when they are tired or under stress. This requires evidence of dysfunction and

persistence. Obsessional symptoms are also a trait in anankastic personality disorder (see page 403).

Obsessions can take various forms (see Box 1.5).

- *Obsessional thoughts* are repeated and intrusive words or phrases that are upsetting to the patient—for example, repeated obscenities or blasphemous phrases coming into the awareness of a religious person.
- *Obsessional ruminations* are repeated worrying themes of a more complex kind—for example, about the ending of the world.
- *Obsessional doubts* are repeated themes expressing uncertainty about previous actions—for example, whether or not the person turned off an electrical appliance that might cause a fire. Whatever the nature of the doubt, the person realizes that the degree of uncertainty and consequent distress is unreasonable.
- *Obsessional impulses* are repeated urges to carry out actions, usually ones that are aggressive, dangerous, or socially embarrassing—for example, the urge to pick up a knife and stab another person, to jump in front of a train, or to shout obscenities in church. Whatever the urge, the person has no wish to carry it out, resists it strongly, and does not act on it.
- *Obsessional phobias.* This term denotes an obsessional symptom associated with avoidance as well as anxiety—for example, the obsessional impulse to injure another person with a knife may lead to consequent avoidance of knives. Sometimes obsessional fears of illness are called *illness phobias*.
- *Obsessional slowness.* Many obsessional patients perform actions slowly because their compulsive rituals or repeated doubts take time and distract them from their main purpose. Occasionally, however, the slowness does not seem to be secondary to these other problems, but appears to be a primary feature of unknown origin.

Box 1.5 Obsessional and compulsive symptoms

Obsessions
Thoughts
Ruminations
Doubts
Impulses
Obsessional phobias
Compulsions (rituals)
Obsessional slowness

Although the content (or themes) of obsessions are various, most of them can be grouped into one or other of six categories:

- dirt and contamination
- aggression
- orderliness
- illness
- sex
- religion.

Thoughts about *dirt and contamination* are usually associated with the idea of harm to others or self through the spread of disease. *Aggressive thoughts* may be about striking another person or shouting angry or obscene remarks in public. Thoughts about *orderliness* may be about the way objects are to be arranged or work is to be organized. Thoughts about *illness* are usually of a fearful kind—for example, a dread of cancer. Obsessional ideas about *sex* usually concern practices that the individual would find shameful. Obsessions about *religion* often take the form of doubts about the fundamentals of belief (e.g. 'does God exist?') or repeated doubts about whether sins have been adequately confessed ('scruples').

Compulsions

Compulsions are repetitive and seemingly purposeful behaviours that are performed in a stereotyped way (hence the alternative name, 'compulsive rituals') in response to an obsession. They are accompanied by a subjective sense that the behaviour must be carried out and by an urge to resist it. The compulsion usually makes sense given the content of the obsession. For example, a compulsion to wash the hands repeatedly is usually driven by obsessional thoughts that the hands are contaminated. Sometimes obsessional ideas concern the consequences of failing to carry out the compulsion in the 'correct' way—for example, that another person will suffer an accident. Compulsions may cause problems for several reasons.

- They may cause direct harm (e.g. dermatitis from excessive washing).
- They may interfere with normal life because of the time they require.
- Although the compulsive act transiently reduces the anxiety associated with the obsession, in fact the compulsions help to maintain the condition. Strategies to reduce them are central to behavioural treatments of obsessive–compulsive disorder.

There are many kinds of compulsive acts, but four types are particularly common.

- *Checking rituals* are often concerned with safety—for example, checking over and over again that the fire has been turned off, or that the doors have been locked.
- *Cleaning rituals* often take the form of repeated hand washing, but may involve household cleaning.
- *Counting rituals* usually involve counting in some special way—for example, in threes—and are frequently associated with doubting thoughts such that the count must be repeated to make sure that it was carried out adequately in the first place. The counting is often silent, so an onlooker may be unaware of the ritual.
- In *dressing rituals* the person lays out clothes, or puts them on, in a particular way or order. The ritual is often accompanied by doubting thoughts that lead to seemingly endless repetition.

Overvalued ideas

Overvalued ideas were first described by Wernicke in 1900, and were reviewed by McKenna (1984). An overvalued idea is a comprehensible and understandable idea which is pursued beyond the bounds of reason. It may preoccupy and dominate a person's life for many years, and affect their actions. It therefore shares some characteristics of delusions. However, it is essential to distinguish the two types of belief, as their diagnostic implications are very different. Overvalued ideas differ from delusions in two main ways.

- The content of, and basis for, the overvalued idea is usually understandable when the person's background is known, whereas delusions and the person's explanation of them tend to be bizarre. For example, a person whose mother and sister suffered from cancer one after the other may understandably become convinced that cancer is contagious.
- The theme also tends to be culturally common and acceptable, as in the overvalued ideas about body shape that characterize anorexia nervosa.

With an overvalued idea, there is a small degree of insight and willingness to at least entertain alternative views, even though this is not persistent and the patient always returns to and retains the belief.

Overvalued ideas must also be distinguished from obsessions. This is usually easier than the distinction from delusions, since there is no sense of intrusiveness or senselessness of the thought, nor is there resistance to it. Overvalued ideas differ from normal religious beliefs in that the latter are shared by a wider group, arise from religious instruction, and are subject to periodic doubts. Despite these differences, it can on occasion be difficult to recognize an overvalued idea and distinguish it unequivocally from a delusion, obsession, or normal belief. However, this should rarely lead to practical problems, because diagnosis depends on more than the presence or absence of a single symptom.

The beliefs concerning body shape and weight that are held in anorexia nervosa are perhaps the clearest example of overvalued ideas. According to McKenna (1984), the term also applies to abnormal beliefs in many other conditions, including dysmorphophobia, hypochondriasis, paranoid personality disorder, and morbid jealousy. However, it is important to emphasize that overvalued ideas are defined by their form, not their content, and they have no inviolable relationship with, or implication for, any particular diagnostic category. Thus some cases of morbid jealousy are clearly delusional, whereas in hypochondriasis or dysmorphophobia the belief often has the character of an obsession or a worry, not of an overvalued idea.

Disturbances of thinking processes

Disturbances of the stream of thought

In disturbances of the stream of thought, the amount and speed of thinking are changed. In *pressure of thought*, ideas arise in unusual variety and abundance and pass through the mind rapidly. In *poverty of thought*, the patient has few thoughts, and these lack variety and richness and seem to move slowly through the mind. Pressure of thought occurs in mania; poverty of thought occurs in depressive disorders. Either may be experienced in schizophrenia. Given that the phenomena are recognized through the person's use of language, they are also known as *pressure of speech* or *poverty of speech*.

Thought block

Sometimes the stream of thought is interrupted suddenly. The patient feels that his mind has gone blank, and an observer notices a sudden interruption in the patient's speech. In a minor degree this experience is common, particularly when a person is tired, anxious, or distracted. In thought blocking, the interruptions are sudden, striking, and repeated, and are experienced by the patient as an abrupt and complete emptying of his mind. Thought blocking is an important symptom, as it strongly suggests schizophrenia. The diagnostic association with schizophrenia is stronger when the patient interprets the experience in an unusual way—for example, when he says that another person has removed his thoughts.

Disorders of the form of thought

Disorder of the form of thought (also known as *formal thought disorder*) is usually recognized from speech and writing, but is sometimes evident from the patient's behaviour—for example, he may be unable to file papers under appropriate category headings. Disorders of the form of thought can be divided into several kinds, as described below. Each kind has associations with a particular mental disorder, but none of the associations is strong enough to be diagnostic.

Perseveration

Perseveration is the persistent and inappropriate repetition of the same thoughts. The disorder is detected by examining the person's words or actions. Thus, in response to a series of simple questions, the person may give the correct answer to the first question, but continue to give the same answer inappropriately to subsequent questions. Perseveration occurs in, but is not limited to, dementia and frontal lobe injury.

Flight of ideas

In flight of ideas, thoughts and speech move quickly from one topic to another so that one train of thought is not carried to completion before another takes its place. The normal logical sequence of ideas is generally preserved, although ideas may be linked by distracting cues in the surroundings and by distractions arising from the words that have been spoken. These verbal distractions are of three kinds, namely *clang associations* (a second word with a sound similar to the first), *puns* (a second meaning of the first word), and *rhymes*. In practice, it is difficult to distinguish between flight of ideas and loosening of associations (see below), especially when the patient speaks rapidly. When this happens it is often helpful to record a sample of speech. Flight of ideas is characteristic of mania.

Loosening of associations

This denotes a loss of the normal structure of thinking. To the interviewer the patient's discourse seems muddled, illogical, or tangential to the matter in hand. It does not become clearer when the patient is questioned further; indeed, the interviewer has the experience that the more he tries to clarify the patient's thinking (or the longer he allows the patient to speak without interruption), the less he understands it. Several specific features of this muddled thinking have been described, but they are difficult to identify with certainty, and the most striking clinical impression is often a general lack of clarity, best described by recording an example of the speech and the impression made on the interviewer. This lack of clarity differs from that of people who are anxious or of low intelligence. Anxious people give a more coherent account when they have been put at ease, and people with low intelligence usually express their ideas more clearly when the interviewer simplifies the questions and allows more time for the reply.

Three characteristic kinds of loosening of associations have been described, all of which are seen most often in schizophrenia.

- In *talking past the point* (*Vorbeireden*) the patient seems always about to get to the endpoint of the topic in question, but then skirts round it and never in fact reaches it.
- *Knight's move* or *derailment* refers to a transition from one topic to another, either between sentences or in mid-sentence, with no logical relationship between the two topics and no evidence of the associations described above under flight of ideas.
- *Verbigeration* is said to be present when speech is reduced to the senseless repetition of sounds, words, or phrases. This abnormality can occur with severe expressive aphasia and occasionally in schizophrenia. When this abnormality is extreme, the disorder is called *word salad*.

Other disorders of thinking

Overinclusion refers to a widening of the boundaries of concepts, such that things are grouped together which are not normally regarded as closely connected.

Neologisms are words or phrases invented by the patient, often to describe a morbid experience. Neologisms must be distinguished from incorrect pronunciation, the wrong use of words by people with limited education, dialect words, obscure technical terms, and the 'private words' that some families invent for their own use. Before deciding that a word is a neologism, the interviewer should ask the patient what he means by it. Neologisms occur most often in chronic schizophrenia.

Depersonalization and derealization

Depersonalization is a change of self-awareness such that the person feels unreal, detached from his own experience, and unable to feel emotion (Sierra and David, 2011). *Derealization* is a similar change in relation to the environment, such that objects appear unreal and people appear as lifeless two-dimensional 'cardboard' figures. Despite the complaint of inability to feel emotion, both depersonalization and derealization are described

as highly unpleasant experiences. These central features are often accompanied by other morbid experiences, including changes in the experience of time, changes in the body image (e.g. a feeling that a limb has altered in size or shape), and occasionally a feeling of being outside one's own body and observing one's own actions, often from above.

Because patients find it difficult to describe the feelings of depersonalization and derealization, they often resort to metaphor, and this can lead to confusion between depersonalization and delusional ideas. For example, a patient may say that he feels 'as if part of my brain had stopped working', or 'as if the people I meet are lifeless creatures'. Sometimes careful questioning is required to make the distinction; the 'as if' quality is a useful discriminator.

Depersonalization and derealization are experienced quite commonly by healthy people—especially when they are tired—as transient phenomena of abrupt onset (Sedman, 1970). The symptoms have been reported after sleep deprivation and sensory deprivation, and as an effect of hallucinogenic drugs. They occur in anxiety disorders, post-traumatic stress disorder, depressive disorders, schizophrenia, and temporal lobe epilepsy. There is also a rarely used diagnostic category of depersonalization–derealization syndrome.

Motor symptoms and signs

Abnormalities of social behaviour, facial expression, and posture occur frequently in mental disorders of all kinds; motor symptoms and signs can also be side effects of medication. They are considered in Chapter 3, where the examination of the patient is described. Motor slowing and agitation, which are important features of depressive disorder, are discussed in Chapter 9. With the exception of tics, the specific symptoms listed here are mainly observed in schizophrenia, particularly catatonic schizophrenia (see page 256).

- *Tics* are irregular repeated movements involving a group of muscles—for example, sideways movement of the head or the raising of one shoulder.
- *Mannerisms* are repeated movements that appear to have some functional significance—for example, saluting.
- *Stereotypies* are repeated movements that are regular (unlike tics) and without obvious significance (unlike mannerisms)—for example, rocking to and fro.
- *Catatonia* is a state of increased muscle tone that affects extension and flexion and is abolished by voluntary movement.

- *Catalepsy (waxy flexibility, flexibilitas cerea)* is a term used to describe the tonus in catatonia. It is detected when a patient's limbs can be placed in a position in which they then remain for long periods while at the same time muscle tone is uniformly increased. Patients with this abnormality sometimes maintain the head a little way above the pillow in a position that a healthy person could not maintain without extreme discomfort (*psychological pillow*). Catalepsy should not be confused with *cataplexy* (see page 327).

- *Posturing* is the adoption of unusual bodily postures continuously for a long time. The posture may appear to have a symbolic meaning (e.g. standing with both arms outstretched as if being crucified), or may have no apparent significance (for example, standing on one leg).

- *Grimacing* has the same meaning as in everyday speech. The term *Schnauzkrampf* (snout cramp or spasm) denotes pouting of the lips to bring them closer to the nose.

- *Negativism.* Patients are said to show negativism when they do the opposite of what is asked, and actively resist efforts to persuade them to comply.

- *Echopraxia* occurs when the patient imitates the interviewer's movement automatically, even when asked not to do so.

- *Mitgehen* (going along with) describes another kind of excessive compliance in which the patient's limbs can be moved into any position with the slightest pressure.

- *Ambitendence.* Patients are said to exhibit ambitendence when they alternate between opposite movements—for example, putting out the arm to shake hands, then withdrawing it, extending it again, and so on repeatedly.

Disturbances of the body image

The body image or body schema is a person's subjective representation against which the integrity of their body is judged and the movement and positioning of its parts assessed. Specific abnormalities of the body image arise in neurological disorders. These abnormalities include the awareness of a *phantom limb* after amputation, *unilateral lack of awareness or neglect* (usually following stroke), *hemiasomatognosia* (in which the person feels, incorrectly, that a limb is missing), and *anosognosia* (lack of awareness of loss of function, often of hemiplegia). These abnormalities are described in textbooks of neurology and in David *et al.* (2009a).

Distorted awareness of size and shape of the body occurs occasionally in healthy people when they are tired or falling asleep. The experience, which includes feelings that a limb is enlarging, becoming smaller, or otherwise being distorted, also occurs in migraine, as part of the aura of epilepsy, and after taking LSD. The person is aware that the experience is unreal. However, changes in the shape and size of body parts are described by some schizophrenic patients, and in this instance the symptoms are delusional or hallucinatory and there is no insight. *Coenestopathic states* are localized distortions of body awareness—for example, when the nose feels as if it is made of cotton wool.

A *general distortion of the body image* occurs in anorexia nervosa, where the patient is convinced that they are fat when in fact they are underweight, sometimes to the point of emaciation.

The *reduplication phenomenon* is the experience that the body has doubled, or that part of the body has done so—for example, that there are two left arms. The experience is reported very occasionally in migraine, temporal lobe epilepsy, and schizophrenia. The related experience of *autoscopic hallucinations* was described on page 7.

Disturbances of the self

The experience of self has several aspects. It is more than the awareness of the body; we have a feeling of unity between the various aspects of the self, we recognize our activities as our own, we recognize a boundary between the self and the outside world, and we have a feeling of continuity between our past and present selves. The concept of self is closely related to, but distinct from, that of the *body image*. Although the body image is usually experienced as part of the self, it can also be experienced in a more objective way, as when we say 'my leg hurts'. Some of these aspects of the self are changed in certain psychiatric disorders. The experiences are often associated with other abnormal phenomena, so that the account of abnormalities of the self overlaps with several other parts of this chapter.

Disturbances concerned with activities

We take it for granted that, other than in a metaphorical or religious sense, our actions are our own. Patients with delusions of control (see page 11) lose this awareness. They have the experience that thoughts are not their own and believe instead that these have been inserted from outside. Some patients lose the conviction that their actions are their own, and believe instead that they have been imposed by an outside agency.

Disturbed awareness of the unity of the self

Some patients lose the normal experience of existing as a unified being. Patients with *dissociative identity disorder* (see page 655) have the experience of existing as two or more selves, alternating at different times. In the experience of *autoscopy* and the related experience of the *Doppelganger* (see page 7), the person experiences two selves, present at the same time, but with the conviction that each is a version of the self.

Disturbances of the unity of the self

Although we recognize that we change over time, we retain a conviction of being the same person. Rarely, this feeling of continuity is lost in schizophrenia. For example, a patient may say that he is a different person from the one who existed before the disorder began, or that a new self has taken over from the old one.

Disturbances of the boundaries of the self

This type of disorder is experienced by some people after taking LSD or other drugs, who may report that they felt as if they were dissolving. Hallucinations can be regarded as involving a loss of awareness of what is within the self and what is located outside. The same inability to determine what is part of the self, and what is not, is seen in passivity phenomena, in which actions willed by the patient are experienced as initiated from outside.

Disturbances of memory

The features of memory disturbance and its assessment are discussed in detail in Chapters 3 and 14. In this chapter we introduce some key terms and concepts.

Failure of memory is called *amnesia*. The related term *dysmnesia* is occasionally used. *Paramnesia* is distortion of memory. Several kinds of disturbed memory occur in psychiatric disorders, and it is usual to describe them in terms of the temporal stages that approximate crudely to the scheme of memory derived from psychological research. A discussion of this subject can be found in textbooks of neuropsychology or in David *et al.* (2009a,b).

- *Immediate memory* concerns the retention of information over a short period, measured in minutes. It is tested clinically by asking the patient to remember a novel name and address and to recall it about 5 minutes later.
- *Recent memory* concerns events that have taken place in the past few days. It is tested clinically by asking about events in the patient's daily life which

are known also to the interviewer directly or via an informant (for example, what the patient has eaten) or in the wider environment (for example, well-known news items).

- *Long-term (remote) memory* concerns events that have occurred over longer periods of time. It is tested by asking about events before the presumed onset of memory disorder.

When testing any state of memory, a distinction is made between spontaneous *recall* and *recognition* of information. In some conditions, patients who cannot recall information can recognize it correctly.

Memory loss most commonly occurs in dementia and delirum. It usually affects recall of recent events more than recall of distant ones. In dementia, it usually progresses with time and becomes severe, but is rarely total. Some organic conditions give rise to an interesting partial effect known as *amnestic disorder*, in which the person is unable to remember events that occurred a few minutes earlier, but can recall remote events (see page 354). Total loss of all memory, or selective loss of personal identity, strongly suggests psychogenic causes (see below) or malingering. Some patients with memory disorder recall more when given cues. When this happens, it suggests that the disorder is concerned at least in part with retrieval.

After a period of unconsciousness, memory is impaired for the interval between the ending of complete unconsciousness and the restoration of full consciousness (*anterograde amnesia*). Some causes of unconsciousness (e.g. head injury and electroconvulsive therapy) also lead to inability to recall events before the onset of unconsciousness (*retrograde amnesia*).

Disturbances of recognition

Several *disorders of recognition* occur occasionally in neurological and psychiatric disorders.

- *Jamais vu* is the failure to recognize events that have been encountered before.
- *Déjà vu* is the conviction that an event is repeating one that has been experienced in the past, when in fact it is novel.
- *Confabulation* is the confident recounting of quite false 'memories' for recent events, and is characteristic of amnestic syndrome. For example, a patient with no memory of what they ate for breakfast may confabulate a completely incorrect menu. This is done in a plausible manner without any apparent difficulty, and without any awareness of the falsity of the information.

Recall of events can be biased by the mood at the time of recall. Importantly, in depressive disorders, memories of unhappy events are recalled more readily than other events, a process which adds to the patient's low mood.

Psychogenic amnesia

This is thought to result from an active process of repression which prevents the recall of memories that would otherwise evoke unpleasant emotions. The ideas arose from the study of *dissociative amnesia* (see page 654), but the same factors may play a part in some cases of organic amnesia, helping to explain why the return of some memories is delayed longer than that of others.

False memory syndrome

It is a matter of dispute whether memories can be repressed completely but return many years later. The question arises most often when memories of sexual abuse are reported during psychotherapy by a person who had no recollection of the events before the psychotherapy began, and the events are strongly denied by the alleged abusers. Many clinicians consider that these recollections have been 'implanted' by overzealous questioning, while others contend that they are true memories that have previously been completely repressed. Those who hold the latter opinion point to evidence that memories of events other than child abuse can sometimes be completely lost and then regained, and also that some recovered memories of child abuse are corroborated subsequently by independent evidence (for review, see Brewin, 2000). Although the quality of the evidence has been questioned, the possibility of complete and sustained repression of memories has not been ruled out. However, it seems likely that only a small minority of cases of 'recovered memory syndrome' can be explained in this way.

Disturbances of consciousness

Consciousness is awareness of the self and the environment. The *level* of consciousness can vary between the extremes of alertness and coma. The *quality* of consciousness can also vary: sleep differs from unconsciousness, as does stupor.

- *Coma* is the most extreme form of impaired consciousness. The patient shows no external evidence of mental activity, and little motor activity other than breathing. He does not respond even to strong stimuli. Coma can be graded by the extent of the remaining reflex responses and by the type of EEG activity.

- *Clouding of consciousness* refers to a state that ranges from barely perceptible impairment to definite drowsiness in which the person reacts incompletely to stimuli. Attention, concentration, and memory are impaired to varying degrees, and orientation is disturbed. Thinking appears to be muddled, and events may be interpreted inaccurately. Clouding of consciousness is a defining feature of delirium.

- *Stupor*, in the sense used in psychiatry, refers to a condition in which the patient is immobile, mute, and unresponsive, but appears to be fully conscious in that the eyes are usually open and follow external objects. If the eyes are closed, the patient resists attempts to open them. Reflexes are normal and resting posture is maintained. Stupor may occur in catatonia (see page 16). Note that in neurology the term 'stupor' is used differently and generally implies an impairment of consciousness.

- *Confusion* means an inability to think clearly. It occurs characteristically in states of impaired consciousness, but it can occur when consciousness is normal. In delirium, confusion occurs together with partial impairment (clouding) of consciousness, along with other features. In the past, delirium was called a confusional state, with the result that the term 'confusion' was used to mean impairment of consciousness as well as muddled thinking.

Other terms that are used to describe states of impaired consciousness include the following:

- *oneiroid states*, in which there is dream-like imagery although the person is not asleep; if prolonged, this may be called a *twilight state*

- *torpor*, in which the patient appears drowsy, readily falls asleep, and shows evidence of slow thinking and narrowed range of perception.

In addition, there are sleep–wake disorders that can present with impaired consciousness, such as narcolepsy, in which there are often recurrent, sudden, brief collapses owing to loss of muscle tone (*cataplexy*).

Disturbances of attention and concentration

Attention is the ability to focus on the matter in hand. *Concentration* is the ability to maintain that focus. The ability to focus on a selected part of the information reaching the brain is important in many everyday situations—for example, when conversing in a noisy place. It is also important to be able to attend to more than one source of information at the same time—for example, when conversing while driving a car.

Attention and concentration may be impaired in a wide variety of psychiatric disorders, including depressive disorders, mania, anxiety disorders, schizophrenia, and organic disorders. Therefore the finding of abnormalities of attention and concentration does not assist in diagnosis. Nevertheless, these abnormalities are important in management. For example, they affect patients' ability to give or receive information when interviewed, and can interfere with a patient's ability to work, drive a car, or take part in leisure activities.

Insight

In psychopathology, the term *insight* refers to awareness of morbid change in oneself and a correct attitude to this change, including, in appropriate cases, a realization that it signifies a mental disorder. This awareness is difficult for a patient to achieve, since it involves some knowledge of what are the limits of normal mental functioning and mental experience. Furthermore, insight has to be assessed against the background of knowledge and beliefs about psychiatric disorder—it is not the same as complete agreement with the views of the doctor. Insight is also influenced by cultural and cognitive factors (Saravanan *et al.*, 2004; Nair *et al.*, 2014).

Although, in the past, lack of insight was said to be a feature that distinguishes between psychosis (where it was said to be absent) and neurosis (where it is present), this distinction is no longer thought to be reliable or useful. The 'lack of insight' in psychosis is better conceptualized in terms of 'impaired reality testing' or 'reality distortion' (see Chapter 11).

Insight is not simply present or absent. It has several facets, each being a matter of degree.

- Is the patient aware of phenomena that others have observed (e.g. that he is unusually active and elated)?
- If so, does he recognize the phenomena as abnormal (rather than, for example, maintaining that his unusual activity and cheerfulness are due to normal high spirits)?
- If so, does he consider that the phenomena are caused by mental illness (as opposed to, say, a physical illness or poison administered by enemies)?
- If so, does he think that he needs treatment?

The answers to these questions are more informative and more reliable than those of the single question as to whether insight is present or not. The value of determining the degree of insight is that it helps to predict whether the patient is likely to accept the need for help and treatment.

In discussions of psychotherapy, insight has a different meaning from that considered so far which is used in general psychiatry. In psychotherapy, insight is the capacity to understand one's own motives and to be aware of previously unconscious aspects of mental activity. The term *intellectual insight* is sometimes used to denote the capacity to formulate this understanding, whereas the term *emotional insight* refers to the capacity to feel and respond to the understanding.

For review of insight, see Landi *et al.* (2016).

Further reading

Berrios GE (1996). *The History of Mental Symptoms*. Cambridge University Press, Cambridge. (A fascinating history of descriptive psychopathology.)

Jaspers K (1963). *General Psychopathology* (translated from the 7th German edition by J Hoenig and MW Hamilton). Manchester University Press, Manchester. (The classic work on the subject. Chapter 1 is particularly valuable.)

Oyebode F (2014). *Sims' Symptoms in the Mind: an introduction to descriptive psychopathology*, 5th edn. Saunders, London. (A comprehensive and readable modern text.)

CHAPTER 2
Classification

Introduction

Chapter 1 outlined the symptoms and signs of psychiatric disorder. In Chapter 3 we describe the psychiatric assessment, by which these symptoms and signs are elicited, interpreted, and used as the basis upon which psychiatric diagnoses are made. Before doing so, in this chapter we discuss the principles of psychiatric diagnosis and classification, since this provides the framework within which this clinical process happens. The term *nosology* is sometimes used to refer to classification and its study.

Classification is needed in psychiatry for several purposes:

- to enable clinicians to communicate with one another about the diagnoses given to their patients

- to aid patients and their families, by allowing clinicians to provide a framework for them to understand their symptoms and difficulties, and for proposed treatments

- to understand the implications of these diagnoses in terms of their symptoms, prognosis, and treatment, and sometimes their aetiology

- to relate the findings of clinical research to patients seen in everyday practice

- to facilitate epidemiological studies and the collection of reliable statistics

- to ensure that research can be conducted with comparable groups of subjects.

Of these, the first four are the most relevant to clinical practice. Indeed, it is difficult to imagine, or justify, how psychiatry could be practised in any reasonable or evidence-based manner without the order that classification provides (Craddock and Mynors-Wallis, 2014). In this respect, the position of classification as one of the fundamental and essential 'building blocks' of psychiatry is no different from that in the rest of medicine. However, in other respects psychiatric classification does raise particular challenges and controversies, largely as a consequence of the uncertain aetiology, or independent biological validation, of most disorders, which means that its diagnostic categories are almost entirely *syndromal*—a collection of symptoms and signs. The resulting difficulties are of two kinds. The first is conceptual, relating to the nature of mental illness and the question of what, if anything, should be classified. The second difficulty is a practical one, concerning how categories are defined and organized into a classificatory scheme. In this chapter, the conceptual issues and criticisms are covered first, followed by a historical perspective to classification. We then describe and compare the two schemes in widespread use at present, namely Chapter V of the *International Classification of Diseases, 10th edition* (*ICD-10*; World Health Organization, 1992b), and the *Diagnostic and Statistical Manual of Mental Disorders, 5th edition* (*DSM-5*; American Psychiatric Association, 2013a).

Concepts of mental illness

In everyday speech the word 'illness' is used loosely. Similarly, in psychiatric practice the term 'mental illness' is used with little precision, and often synonymously with 'mental disorder'. In this context, the terms 'mental' and 'psychiatric' are also used interchangeably.

A good definition of mental illness is difficult to achieve, for both practical and philosophical reasons, as outlined here. In routine clinical work the difficulty is important mainly in relation to ethical and legal issues, such as compulsory admission to hospital. In forensic psychiatry the definition of mental illness (by the law) is particularly important in the assessment of issues such as criminal responsibility.

Diverse discussion of the concepts of mental illness can be found in Lazare (1973), Kendell (1975), Zachar and Kendler (2007), and Tyrer (2013).

Definitions of mental illness

Many attempts have been made to define mental illness, none of which is satisfactory or uniformly accepted. A common approach is to examine the concept of illness in general medicine and to identify any similarities or analogies with mental illness. In general medicine there are five types of definition:

- *Absence of health.* This approach changes the emphasis of the problem but does not solve it, because health is even more difficult to define. The World Health Organization, for example, defined health as 'a state of complete physical, mental and social well-being, and not merely the absence of disease or infirmity.' As Lewis (1953) rightly commented, 'a definition could hardly be more comprehensive than that, or more meaningless.' Many other definitions of health have been proposed, all equally unsatisfactory.
- *Disease is what doctors treat.* This definition has the attraction of simplicity, but does not really address the issue. The notion that disease is what doctors *can* treat has somewhat more merit, since there is evidence that, as a medical treatment for a condition becomes available, it becomes more likely that the condition will be regarded as a disease (Campbell *et al.*, 1979).
- *Biological disadvantage.* The idea of defining disease in terms of biological disadvantage was proposed by Scadding (1967), and is the most extreme biomedical view of disease. Scadding never defined biological disadvantage, but the term has been used in psychiatry to include decreased fertility (reproductive fitness) and increased mortality. Viewing disease in terms of 'evolutionary disadvantage' is a similar concept (Wakefield, 1992).
- *Pathological process.* Some extreme theorists, most notably Szasz (1960), take the view that illness can be defined only in terms of *physical* pathology. Since most mental disorders do not have demonstrable physical pathology, according to this view they are not illnesses. Szasz takes the further step of asserting that most mental disorders are therefore not the province of doctors. This kind of argument can be sustained only by taking an extremely narrow view of pathology. It is also arbitrary, based on current knowledge, and is increasingly incompatible with the evidence of a genetic and neurobiological basis to the major psychiatric disorders, and their associated morbidity and mortality.
- *Presence of suffering.* This approach has some practical value because it defines a group of people who are likely to consult doctors. A disadvantage is that the term cannot be applied to everyone who would usually be regarded as ill in everyday terms. For example, patients with mania may feel unusually well and may not experience suffering, although most people would regard them as mentally ill.

Biomedical versus social concepts

The above concepts may be divided into those that view mental illnesses in purely biomedical terms, and those that consider them to be social constructs or value judgements. This debate is still ongoing, and depends in part on one's opinion about their aetiology, but it is now generally accepted that value judgements play a part in all diagnoses, even if the disorders themselves are considered from a biomedical perspective (Fulford, 1989). For example, beliefs and emotions are central to most psychiatric disorders, yet it is a value judgement as to whether a given belief or emotion is 'reasonable' or 'unhelpful' for a given individual in their particular social context, and therefore what, if any, diagnostic significance it has. Would we use 'useful' or 'dysfunctional' to decide whether a belief was 'illness'? Would 'normal' or 'abnormal' be better?

Impairment, disability, and handicap

It is useful in medicine, and particularly in psychiatry, to describe and classify the consequences of a disorder. This approach is related to the concept of disease as involving dysfunction (Wakefield, 1992), as incorporated into the definitions of mental disorder used in ICD-10 and DSM-5 (see below). Three related terms, derived from medical sociology and social psychology, are used to describe the harmful consequences of a disorder.

- *Impairment* refers to a pathological defect—for example, hemiparesis after a stroke.
- *Disability* is the limitation of physical or psychological function that arises from an impairment—for example, difficulties with self-care that are caused by the hemiparesis.
- *Handicap* refers to the resulting social dysfunction—for example, being unable to work because of the hemiparesis.

Incapacity may be seen as another harmful consequence of illness, although the term usually refers in a legal sense to the effect that illness has on one's competence to make treatment decisions, as enshrined in the United Kingdom by the Mental Capacity Act (see Chapter 4).

Diagnoses, diseases, and disorders

The term 'diagnosis' has two somewhat different meanings. It has the general meaning of 'telling one thing apart from another', but in medicine it has also acquired a more specific meaning of 'knowing the underlying cause' of the symptoms and signs about which the patient is complaining. Underlying causes are expressed in quite different terms from the symptoms. For example, the symptoms of acute appendicitis

are distinct from the idea that will form in the mind of the doctor that the appendix is inflamed and producing peritoneal irritation. To be able to make a diagnosis of this type is, of course, satisfying for the doctor and useful for the patient, since it immediately suggests what investigations and treatment are needed. Its clear utility also makes redundant most theoretical or philosophical concerns about classification. Unfortunately, for most psychiatric patients it is rarely possible to arrive at this type of diagnosis, the only exception to this being, by definition, 'organic' psychiatric disorders (see page 26).

The lack of clear disease categories, in a medical sense, has led to the use of the more general term 'disorder'. The definition of a psychiatric disorder in ICD-10 is:

. . .a clinically recognizable set of symptoms or behaviour associated in most cases with distress and with interference with personal functions. Social deviance or conflict alone, without personal dysfunction, should not be included in mental disorder as defined here.

(World Health Organization, 1992b, p. 5).

The DSM-5 definition of a mental disorder is longer but similar:

. . .a syndrome characterized by clinically significant disturbance in an individual's cognition, emotion regulation, or behavior that reflects a dysfunction in the psychological, biological, or developmental processes underlying mental functioning. Mental disorders are usually associated with significant distress or disability in social, occupational, or other important activities. An expectable or culturally acceptable response to a common stressor or loss, such as the death of a loved one, is not a mental disorder. Socially deviant behavior (e.g. political, religious, or sexual) and conflicts that are primarily between the individual and society are not mental disorders unless the deviance or conflict results from a dysfunction in the individual, as described above.

(American Psychiatric Association, 2013a, p. 20).

Despite the similarity, there is an important difference between the two definitions. 'Interference with personal functions' in ICD-10 refers only to such things as personal care and one's immediate environment, and does not extend to interference with work and other social roles. In DSM-5, as in the extract above, impairment refers to all types of functioning.

Both definitions illustrate that most psychiatric disorders are based not upon theoretical concepts, or presumptions about aetiology, but upon recognizable clusters of symptoms and behaviours. This reliance explains much of the debate about the reliability and validity of the categories being classified, as will be discussed later in this chapter.

Criticisms of classification

In contrast to the view that classification is an essential, albeit insufficient and imperfect, basis for clinical practice (Craddock and Mynors-Wallis, 2014; Tyrer, 2014), the use of psychiatric classification is sometimes criticized as being inappropriate or even harmful. In part, such criticisms arise from the various controversies outlined above: if the concept of mental disorder is itself disputed, then so will any classifications thereof. These criticisms were most prevalent and trenchant at the height of the 'anti-psychiatry' movement in the 1960s, although they continue to be voiced by a vociferous 'critical psychiatry' lobby (Bracken *et al.*, 2012). Three main criticisms of this kind are made.

- *Allocating patients to a diagnostic category distracts from the understanding of their unique personal difficulties.* However, the good clinician always considers and takes into account a patient's unique experiences, qualities, and circumstances when making diagnoses, not least because this contextual information often affects treatment and prognosis.

- *Allocating a person to a diagnostic category is simply to label deviant behaviour as illness.* Some sociologists have argued that such labelling serves only to increase the person's difficulties. There can be no doubt that terms such as epilepsy or schizophrenia attract stigma (see Box 2.1, but this does not lessen the reality of disorders that cause suffering and require treatment. However, it does emphasize that mental illness should not be defined solely in terms of socially deviant behaviour. The presence of the former must be separately established based on the psychiatric history and mental state examination. Moreover, if mental illness is inferred from socially deviant behaviour alone, political abuse may result. A serious example of the latter occurred in the former Soviet Union, where some psychiatrists colluded with the government in being willing to classify political dissent as evidence of mental illness. A further reason for excluding purely social criteria from the definition of mental illness, and from diagnostic criteria, is that many behaviours are appraised differently in different countries and at different times. For example, homosexuality was considered to be a mental disorder in the United Kingdom until the 1970s.

- *Individuals do not fit neatly into the available categories.* Although it is not feasible to classify a minority of disorders (or patients), this is not a reason for abandoning classification for the majority.

It is certainly true that at times classification has been inappropriately used as part of a broader abuse of psychiatry, whether for political, financial, or other reasons. Although such abuses are fortunately rare, they are an extreme illustration of the fact that making diagnoses and classifying patients are not neutral acts, but carry significant ethical and other implications (see Chapter 4). One of these implications concerns *stigma*, which remains a serious problem for patients with mental health problems, even if one does not accept the rest of the sociological thesis outlined above. It is incumbent on all those who use psychiatric diagnostic terms that they do so appropriately and judiciously, paying due attention to their correct usage and purpose, and the context in which they are being applied. Doing so can help to reduce the problem of stigmatization, but cannot solve it, because stigma results from many other factors too (Thornicroft, 2006). The issue of stigma in psychiatry is discussed in Box 2.1.

Although these criticisms are important, they are arguments only against the improper use of, or over-reliance upon, classification. Disorders and their harmful consequences cannot be made to disappear by ceasing to give names to them. ICD-10 and DSM-5, to be discussed later, emphasize that classification is a means of communication and a guide to decision-making, but acknowledge that they are provisional and imperfect schemes. Psychiatrists, other mental health professionals, and researchers must use their clinical experience and common sense, as well as being guided by the descriptions of the disorders that make up the classifications.

Other criticisms of classification in psychiatry are mostly concerned with the specifics rather than the principles—for example, whether a particular diagnostic category is reliable and valid, and the severity threshold at which the diagnosis should be made. These issues are introduced later in this chapter, and at various points throughout the book.

Box 2.1 Stigma

People stigmatize others when they judge them not on their personal qualities but on the basis of a mark or label which assigns them to a feared or unfavoured group. The tendency to stigmatize seems to be deeply rooted in human nature as a way of responding to people who appear or behave differently. Stigmatization is based on fear that those who seem different may behave in threatening or unpredictable ways, and it is reduced when it becomes clear that the stigmatized person is unlikely to behave in these ways.

Stigma in psychiatry

People fear mental illness and they stigmatize those who are affected by it. The reasons for this are complex. They include the notion that people with mental illness cannot control their own behaviour, and that they may act in odd, unpredictable, and possibly violent ways. Thus they are seen as directly threatening, and perhaps also as indirectly threatening because their lack of self-control threatens our belief in our ability to control our actions. Whatever the underlying psychological mechanisms, fear of mental illness makes people react to mentally ill individuals in the same cautious and unfavourable way—that is, to stigmatize them.

Diagnoses, as labels, have the potential to be stigmatizing (e.g. leprosy and AIDS). It has been suggested that the stigma of mental illness would be reduced if diagnoses such as schizophrenia were abandoned. This proposal misses the point that the basis of stigma is fear, and that simply removing the label does not reduce the fear. The mentally ill were stigmatized long before modern diagnostic terms were in use, and people who fear mental illness invent their own labels, such as 'nutter', which are far more stigmatizing than a diagnosis. To reduce stigma it is necessary to reduce fear, and this requires accurate information about mental illness and better understanding of mentally ill people.

Psychiatric stigma arises from a number of false beliefs. For example, concern about dangerousness is a major component of psychiatric stigma. Other important components are ideas that:

- people with mental illness are unpredictable
- people with mental illness feel different from the rest of us
- people with mental illness are hard to talk and relate to
- mental illness cannot be cured, and people with mental illness do not recover.

These beliefs make people draw back from those with mental illness and discourage them from engaging in social relationships. Consequently they do not learn that their assumptions are wrong. In the same way, fear of being stigmatized adds greatly to the problems of people with mental illness. It discourages them from seeking help at an early stage, and from sharing their distress with relatives and friends. Stigma also has wider social effects—for example, it makes it harder for mentally ill people to obtain work. Stigmatization may also affect the allocation of resources for the care of people with mental illness, with a reluctance to fund care in the community or to give appropriate priority to mental health services generally.

Reducing stigma

Campaigns to reduce stigma generally include:

- information about the true nature of mental illness, and about the low frequency of dangerous behaviour
- encouragement to persuade public figures who have had a mental illness to speak out about their experiences
- a focus on young people, whose attitudes may be less fixed than those of their elders.

Although stigma can be reduced, this cannot be done easily or quickly. In the past, people with epilepsy were stigmatized, but as knowledge of the condition spread and as treatment improved, attitudes gradually changed. Changes are now beginning to be seen in the stigma attached to some psychiatric disorders. For example, autism is now generally a much less stigmatizing term than it was previously, whereas schizophrenia is not. Thus there is an ongoing need for public education campaigns to reduce the fear and misunderstanding that perpetuate stigma. However, existing anti-stigma programmes have had only modest benefits (Griffiths et al., 2014). For reviews of stigma and its reduction, see Sartorius et al. (2010) and Henderson et al. (2013).

The history of classification

Efforts to classify abnormal mental states have occurred since antiquity. One reason for including a chronological perspective here is that contemporary psychiatric classifications are, in part, a 'hybrid' of various historical themes and opinions.

The early Greek medical writings contained descriptions of different manifestations of mental disorder—for example, excitement, depression, confusion, and memory loss. This simple classification was adopted by Roman medicine and developed by the Greek physician Galen, whose system of classification remained in use until the eighteenth century.

Interest in the classification of natural phenomena developed in the eighteenth century, partly stimulated by the publication of a classification of plants by Linnaeus, a medically qualified professor of botany who also devised a less well-known classification of diseases in which one major class was mental disorders. Many classifications were proposed, notably one published in 1772 by William Cullen, a Scottish physician. He grouped mental disorders together, apart from delirium, which he classified with febrile conditions. According to his scheme, mental disorders were part of a broad class of 'neuroses', a term that he used to denote diseases which affect the nervous system (Hunter and MacAlpine, 1963). Cullen's classification contained an aetiological principle—that mental illnesses were disorders of the nervous system—as well as a descriptive principle for distinguishing individual clinical syndromes within the neuroses. In Cullen's usage, the term neurosis covered the whole range of mental disorders, as well as many neurological conditions. The modern narrower usage developed later (see page 27).

In the early nineteenth century, several French writers published influential classifications. Pinel's *Treatise on Insanity*, which appeared in English in 1806, divided mental disorders into mania with delirium, mania without delirium, melancholia, dementia, and idiocy. Pinel's compatriot, Esquirol, wrote another widely read textbook, which was published in English in 1845, and added a new category, 'monomania', characterized by 'partial insanity', in which there were fixed false ideas that could not be changed by logical reasoning (i.e. delusions). Like other psychiatrists of the time, Pinel and Esquirol did not discuss neuroses (in the modern sense), because these conditions were generally treated by physicians.

Meanwhile, in Germany, Kahlbaum formulated two requirements for research on nosology, namely that the total clinical picture, and its entire course, were both fundamental to the definition of a mental illness and thus to classification. These ideas were adopted at the end of the nineteenth century by Emil Kraepelin, who used these criteria to make the landmark distinction between manic–depressive psychosis (bipolar disorder) and schizophrenia. Successive editions of Kraepelin's textbook made further refinements to the classification of mental illness, which form the basis of today's systems.

At the same time, separate developments in the emerging specialty of neurology led to decreasing medical interest in the 'nervous patient', a term used throughout the nineteenth century in the United Kingdom and North America to refer to a large group of patients with varied complaints. These were gradually seen as a part of the new specialty of psychiatry alongside the major mental illnesses. The writings of Sigmund Freud and his contemporaries led to greater recognition of the psychological causes of nervous symptoms and 'neurotic' disorders, and to the modern concepts of hysteria and anxiety disorder.

For a review of nosological models in psychiatry, see Pichot (1994) and Zachar and Kendler (2007).

Organizing principles of contemporary classifications

As well as these historical roots, it is worth considering the major issues that contemporary classifications have faced with regard to their organizing principles.

Organic and functional

The first issue concerns the distinction that is conventionally drawn between organic and functional disorders. Organic disorders are those that arise from a demonstrable cerebral or systemic pathological process; the core disorders are dementia, delirium, and the various neuropsychiatric syndromes (David *et al.*, 2009). 'Functional disorder' is consequently an umbrella or default term for all other psychiatric disorders. The organic–functional dichotomy has two main implications for classification.

- It has a philosophical dimension, being inextricably linked to dualism and concepts of mind and body. At its extreme, the implication is that functional disorders have no biological basis, whilst psychological and social factors are irrelevant to organic disorders. This polarization can be reflected in the apparent divide between psychiatry and neurology. The same dualism may also unintentionally encourage psychiatrists to be either 'mindless' or 'brainless', rather than seeing that both aspects of aetiology always make a contribution (Eisenberg, 1986; Anonymous, 1994). Equally, it has led to the suggestion that the two specialties should use a merged classificatory system (White *et al.*, 2012).

- It has practical implications, since the term 'organic' defines disorders aetiologically or pathologically, whereas all other psychiatric disorders are, by default, purely descriptive and based on clusters of symptoms and signs. This is not only unsatisfactory for psychiatry (Arango and Fraguas, 2016) but leads to inconsistencies and difficulties at the intersection; these are currently best illustrated with regard to schizophrenia and organic schizophrenia-like disorders (Chapter 11).

There is general agreement that, for these and other reasons, the organic–functional dichotomy is neither valid nor helpful (Spitzer *et al.*, 1992). However, it has proved difficult to come up with an alternative. The ways in which ICD-10 and DSM-5 deal with the issue are discussed below and in Chapter 14.

Neurosis and psychosis

In the past, the concepts of neurosis and psychosis were important in most systems of classification. Although neither is used as an organizing principle in ICD-10 or DSM-5, in everyday clinical practice these terms are still useful as general descriptors, so it is of relevance to understand their history.

Psychosis

The term *psychosis* was suggested by Feuchtersleben, who in 1845 published a book entitled *Principles of Medical Psychology*. He proposed the use of the term for severe mental disorders, whilst he used the term *neurosis* for mental disorders as a whole. Thus he wrote that 'every psychosis is at the same time a neurosis, but not every neurosis is a psychosis' (Hunter and MacAlpine, 1963, page 950). As the concept of neurosis narrowed, psychosis (also used in the plural, psychoses) came to be regarded as independent. Many of the difficulties encountered today in defining the terms neurosis and psychosis are related to these origins.

In modern usage, the term psychosis refers broadly to severe psychiatric disorders, including schizophrenia, and some organic and affective disorders. Numerous criteria have been proposed to achieve a more precise definition, but there are problems with all of them. Greater severity of illness is a common suggestion, but some cases are relatively mild (and some neuroses are severe and at least as disabling). Lack of insight is often suggested as a criterion, but insight itself is difficult to define (see page 20). A somewhat more straightforward criterion is the inability to distinguish between subjective experience and external reality, as shown by the presence of delusions and hallucinations. Indeed, the presence of a delusion is sometimes regarded as sufficient to diagnose a psychosis. However, as well as the problems involved in fully defining these terms (ICD-10 even avoids defining delusion), the label 'psychosis' is unsatisfactory because the conditions embraced by the term have little in common, and it is usually more informative to classify the particular disorder concerned. For these reasons, the neurosis–psychosis distinction, which was a fundamental organizing principle, was abandoned in ICD-10 and DSM-IV. Nevertheless, psychosis remains a convenient term for disorders that are usually severe, and which feature delusions, hallucinations, or unusual or bizarre behaviour (presumed to be secondary to these phenomena), especially when a more precise diagnosis cannot yet be made. The adjectival form is also useful, and survives in ICD-10 categories such as 'Other nonorganic psychotic disorders'. Another example is the use of the term 'antipsychotic' drugs.

Neurosis

As already noted, the term *neurosis* was introduced by Cullen to denote diseases of the nervous system. Gradually the category of neurosis narrowed, first as neurological disorders with a distinct neuropathology (e.g. epilepsy and stroke) were removed, and later with the development of a separate category of psychosis.

The objections to the term neurosis are similar to the objections to the term psychosis, and explain its removal as an organizing principle in current classification. First, the concept is difficult to define (Gelder, 1986). Second, the conditions that neurosis embraces have little in common. Thirdly, more information can be conveyed by using a more specific and descriptive diagnosis, such as 'anxiety disorder'. A further objection is that the term neurosis has been widely used with the unproven assumption of an aetiological meaning in the psychodynamic literature.

In the same way as for psychosis, the terms 'neurosis' and 'neurotic' remain useful as simple descriptors, especially if the specific disorder cannot yet be determined, to indicate disorders that are often comparatively mild, and usually associated with some form of anxiety. Reflecting its familiarity and utility, ICD-10 retains the adjective in the heading of one group of disorders, namely 'Neurotic, stress-related, and somatoform disorders'. In DSM-5, even the adjectival form is not used.

Categories, dimensions, and axes

Categorical classification

Traditionally, psychiatric disorders have been classified by dividing them into categories that are supposed to represent discrete clinical entities. As already noted, in the absence of knowledge of underlying pathology, these categories can only be defined in terms of symptom patterns and course. Such categorization facilitates the decisions that have to be made in clinical work about treatment and management, but presents two problems.

- Although definitions and descriptions can be agreed upon (to improve *reliability*; see page 29), there is uncertainty about the extent to which these categories represent distinct entities or 'carve Nature at her joints' (*validity*; see page 30).
- A significant proportion of patients do not closely match the descriptions of any disorder, or meet criteria for two or more categories (*comorbidity*; see page 29).

These are all significant points, and they are addressed further in the following sections. However, a more satisfactory and practical alternative system has not yet been devised.

Dimensional classification

Dimensional classification does not use separate categories, but characterizes the subject by means of scores on two or more dimensions. In the past, Kretschmer and several other psychiatrists advocated it, and subsequently it was strongly promoted by the psychologist Hans Eysenck, on the grounds that there is no systematic objective evidence to support the existence of discrete categories. Eysenck (1970b) proposed a system of three dimensions—psychoticism, neuroticism, and introversion–extroversion.

The concept of dimensionality has been revived and advanced by epidemiological surveys that have emphasized that there is a continuum between the healthy population and individuals with diagnosed psychiatric disorders. This applies, for example, to psychotic symptoms, and argues that even a severe disorder such as schizophrenia can be seen as occurring at one end of a dimension of psychotic-like experience (Linscott

and van Os, 2013). The dimensional view of psychiatric disorder is comparable to that of hypertension and other medical diagnoses that are really extremes of a normal distribution, and this view reflects the nature of the underlying genetic predisposition and presumed neurobiology (Cuthbert and Insel, 2013; Owen, 2014) much better than a categorical one. However, the problem with dimensions is that they are not of great value in clinical practice. For most patients, yes–no decisions need to be made, the most critical of these being whether the person has a psychiatric disorder that merits treatment, and, if so, which one. These clinical imperatives strongly favour categorical approaches to classification.

The multiaxial approach

The term *multiaxial* is applied to schemes of classifications in which two or more separate sets of information (such as symptoms, aetiology, and personality type) are coded. Essen-Møller was probably the first to propose such a system for use in psychiatry, using one axis for the clinical syndrome and another for aetiology (Essen-Møller, 1971). Multiaxial classification is available within ICD-10. However, although attractive for several reasons, there is a danger that multiaxial schemes are too complicated and time-consuming to be suitable for everyday use, especially if the clinical utility of each axis has not been demonstrated. Indeed, for these reasons, DSM-5 removed the multiaxial diagnostic classification system used in DSM-IV, replacing it with a simpler approach. A multiaxial scheme remains popular in child and adolescent psychiatry, with the axes describing intellectual level, functional impairment, and psychosocial adversity (Rutter, 2011; see Chapter 16).

Hierarchies of diagnosis

Categorical systems often include an implicit hierarchy of categories. If two or more disorders are present, it has been conventional (although not always made explicit) to assume that one takes precedence and is regarded as the main disorder for the purposes of treatment and recording. For example, organic disorders 'trump' schizophrenia, and schizophrenia takes precedence over affective disorders and anxiety. This type of assumption is justified because there is some clinical evidence for an inbuilt hierarchy of significance between the disorders. For instance, anxiety symptoms occur commonly with depressive disorders, and are sometimes the presenting feature. If the anxiety is treated, there is little response in the depressive symptoms, but if the depressive disorder is treated, there is often improvement in anxiety as well as in the depressive symptoms. These points may be important when making decisions about the order of treatment to be used and when deciding which disorder to record in service statistics if only one is required. Nevertheless, they must not obscure the importance of noting in the case record all disorders and symptoms that are present, and how they change with time and treatment.

Comorbidity

Recently, less emphasis has been placed on hierarchies of diagnosis, with greater weight being placed on comorbidity (also called *dual diagnosis*). This has occurred for three reasons. First, research has shown that comorbidity is very common (Kessler, 2004). For example, about 50% of patients with major depressive disorder also meet the criteria for an anxiety disorder. Secondly, it reminds the clinician to focus on all the various disorders that may be present, and not to assume that the disorder highest in the hierarchy is necessarily the only, or even the most important, target for treatment. The advent of multiaxial systems of classification, mentioned above, in part reflects this

perspective. Thirdly, the diagnostic 'rules' used in current classificatory systems allow, if not encourage, multiple diagnoses to be made, and it has been argued that at least some psychiatric comorbidity is in fact an artefact of this (Maj, 2005), and that a simpler classificatory system which reduced it would be desirable (Goldberg, 2010).

The term *comorbidity* covers two different circumstances:

- *Disorders that are currently considered to be distinct but which are probably causally related.* In other words, there is one disease process, but there are two or more clinical manifestations, which are currently diagnosed separately owing to lack of knowledge or because of clinical convention.
- *Disorders that are causally unrelated.* This refers to the chance co-occurrence of two disorders—for example, the onset of presenile dementia in a person with long-standing panic disorder.

Note that comorbidity applies only when the criteria for two or more diagnoses are met. It should not be used for patients who fall between diagnostic categories but who do not meet the criteria for any one of them.

Reliability and validity

Reliability of psychiatric diagnoses

A prerequisite for any satisfactory classification scheme, whatever its organizing principle, is that the items (diagnoses) that are being classified can be recognized reliably (Kendell, 1975). However, although reliability is now known and is reasonable for most categories, this was not the case until relatively recently, for the reasons described below. Studies conducted in the 1950s and 1960s demonstrated substantial diagnostic disagreement between psychiatrists, which arose for two main reasons (Kreitman, 1961):

- *The interviewing technique and characteristics of the psychiatrist.* This included the way in which symptoms and signs were elicited and interpreted and the weight attached to them. These elements in turn probably reflect many influences, including training, professional culture, etc.
- *The differing use of diagnostic terms and criteria.* At the time, there were no widely accepted glossaries or definitions of key terms. Therefore it was impossible to

ensure that psychiatrists were using the same criteria for symptoms and syndromes. A key study by Stengel (1959) illustrated 'the chaotic state of the classifications in current use' by collecting 28 classifications in a variety of languages. None of the 28 classifications was accompanied by any indication of the meaning of the constituent terms.

Illustrating the importance of these factors, one study concluded that 62% of diagnostic disagreement arose from inadequate use of diagnostic terms, 32% from inadequate interview technique, and only 5% was due to inconsistency in the patient (Ward *et al.*, 1962).

International studies of diagnostic criteria

The increasing concern in the 1960s about the level of diagnostic disagreement between countries heralded international studies intended to identify the source of the variation, and then to improve the reliability. This work adopted the suggestion of the philosopher Carl Hempel that *operational definitions* should be developed—that is, the specification of a category (e.g. a symptom) by a series of precise inclusion and exclusion statements.

A key study was the US–UK Diagnostic Study (Cooper *et al.*, 1972), which followed on from the demonstration that both diagnostic and admission rates for manic depression and schizophrenia differed considerably between the two countries. For example, the rate for manic–depressive illness in the UK was more than 10 times that in equivalent mental hospitals in the USA, whereas the rate for schizophrenia was about twice as high in the USA (and even higher in New York) as it was in the UK. Another seminal study was the International Pilot Study of Schizophrenia (IPSS), a large international collaborative study organized by the World Health Organization, with centres in nine countries taking part. The IPSS first demonstrated clearly that structured interviews could be translated and used in different cultures, enabling it to show that patients with typical symptoms of schizophrenia could be found in all nine countries (World Health Organization, 1973). The IPSS findings are discussed further in Chapter 11.

Standardized interview schedules

A major step towards improving diagnostic reliability came with the development of standardized interview schedules that minimize the variations in interviewing technique and symptom rating between psychiatrists. This development was closely linked with the international studies mentioned above. Thus the US–UK Diagnostic Study used the Present State Examination (PSE), one of the first structured psychiatric interviews (Wing *et al.*, 1974). Standardized interview schedules specify the content and sequence of the interview, and provide scoring rules by which the presence and severity of symptoms are rated. They are now widely used and both specialist and lay forms are available, for use in different settings and with different populations. Further examples are given in Chapter 3.

Diagnosis by computer

The IPSS also revealed that, although a great deal of the variation between psychiatrists in the rating of symptoms could be removed by the use of structured interviews, some variation remained in the resulting diagnoses. This was because of different diagnostic interpretations of the symptoms and behaviours. This led to the development of computer programs such as CATEGO (Wing *et al.*, 1974), which generate a diagnosis using the symptom ratings, eliminating both the personal bias of the diagnosticians and any chance errors made for other reasons. Although computer-generated diagnoses inevitably reflect the diagnostic preferences of whoever wrote the program, they have proved valuable for epidemiological studies, and are widely used in research.

Validity of psychiatric diagnoses

The above discussion has focused upon the reliability of diagnoses, because without a reasonable level of inter-observer reliability it is not possible to test whether or not a concept is valid. Validity is a much more difficult topic. In a general sense, validity refers to the extent to which a concept means what it is supposed to mean. It is also closely connected with usefulness (utility). For a discussion of reliability and validity in psychiatry, see Jablensky (2016).

Three forms of validity are usually recognized.

- *Face validity* is the correspondence with the clinical concepts and descriptions currently accepted in clinical practice. This is fairly easy to achieve by the careful use of glossaries and lists of criteria (illustrating the fact that reliability and validity are not wholly separate).
- *Predictive validity* is the extent to which disorders predict response to treatment and outcome. This has high utility.
- *Construct validity* is the third and most fundamental form of validity, in which there is a demonstrable relationship between a disorder and its underlying aetiology and pathophysiology. Unfortunately, most psychiatric disorders have an unknown and probably low construct validity, reflecting the descriptive criteria upon which most are currently based.

To date, little progress has actually been made towards establishing the validity of the existing schemes of classification.

Current psychiatric classifications

The International Classification of Diseases (ICD), Chapter V

The International Classification of Diseases (ICD) is produced by the World Health Organization (WHO) as an aid to the collection of international statistics about disease. The current version is the 10th edition (ICD-10). Of the 21 chapters, Chapter V is devoted to psychiatry.

Mental disorders were included for the first time in 1948, in the sixth revision (ICD-6), but neither ICD-6 nor

ICD-7 were widely used because they consisted merely of a list of names and code numbers by which national statistics could be tabulated, with no glossary to indicate suggested meanings of the constituent terms. As noted, the survey of Stengel in 1959 was an important first step in much-needed improvements in this regard, setting the stage for an extensive and ongoing WHO programme geared towards achieving a 'common language'. ICD-9, published in 1978, was the first satisfactory and widely used version.

ICD-10

By the time ICD-10 was due, it had become evident that a major process of international collaboration was needed. The objectives of this process were that ICD-10 Chapter V should be:

- suitable for international communication about statistics for morbidity and mortality
- a reference standard for national and other psychiatric classifications
- acceptable and useful to a wide range of users in different cultures
- an aid to education.

The process started in 1982, and included extensive field trials to demonstrate the reliability and utility of the diagnostic categories. The final version, entitled *Clinical Descriptions and Diagnostic Guidelines*, was published as ICD-10 in 1992 (World Health Organization, 1992b). It contains descriptions of each of the disorders, and the diagnostic instructions for users make it clear that these allow some latitude for clinical judgement.

All of the diagnostic codes start with the letter F and, like the other chapters, it has 10 major divisions (Box 2.2), each of which can be divided into 10 subdivisions, and so on. For example, F20, schizophrenia, can be followed by a further number for the category within the group (e.g. F20.1, hebephrenic schizophrenia), and a fourth character if it is necessary to subdivide further. Although ICD-10 is basically a descriptive classification, available knowledge and ingrained clinical practice mean that aetiology is a defining criterion in some of the main categories, notably organic (F0), substance use-related (F1), and stress-related (F4).

Because ICD-10 is used for several purposes, it exists in several forms, each of which is derived from, and compatible with, the core version. For example, the primary healthcare version has only 27 categories, each with reminders about likely management and treatment. There is a research version (DCR-10), which

contains more specific diagnostic criteria, but DSM-5 is much more widely used for research.

ICD-11 is currently expected to be published in 2018 (see page 34).

Diagnostic and Statistical Manual (DSM)

The history of DSM

In 1952 the American Psychiatric Association (APA) published the first edition of the Diagnostic and Statistical Manual (DSM-I) as an alternative to the widely criticized ICD-6. DSM-I was strongly influenced by the views of Adolf Meyer and Karl Menninger, and its simple glossary reflected the prevailing acceptance of psychoanalytic ideas in the USA. DSM-II was published in 1968, and combined psychoanalytic ideas with those of Kraepelin.

DSM-III was published in 1980, and was an important step forward, containing five main innovations.

- Operational criteria were provided for each diagnosis, with explicit rules for inclusion and exclusion (Feighner *et al.*, 1972). This was the first complete classification to do so, and the first to be based on criteria that had been field-tested.

> ### Box 2.2 The main categories of ICD-10 Chapter V (F)
>
> F0 Organic, including symptomatic, mental disorders
>
> F1 Mental and behavioural disorders due to psychoactive substance use
>
> F2 Schizophrenia, schizotypal, and delusional disorders
>
> F3 Mood (affective) disorders
>
> F4 Neurotic, stress-related, and somatoform disorders
>
> F5 Behavioural syndromes associated with physiological disturbances and physical factors
>
> F6 Disorders of adult personality and behaviour
>
> F7 Mental retardation
>
> F8 Disorders of psychological development
>
> F9 Behavioural and emotional disorders with onset usually occurring in childhood or adolescence
>
> Source: data from The ICD-10 classification of mental and behavioural disorders: clinical descriptions and diagnostic guidelines, Copyright (1992), World Health Organization.

- A multiaxial classification was adopted, with five axes (Axis I: Clinical syndromes; Axis II: Personality disorders; Axis III: Physical disorders; Axis IV: Severity of psychosocial stressors; Axis V: Highest level of adaptive functioning in the last year).

- The nomenclature was revised and some syndromes were regrouped. For example, the terms neurosis and hysteria were discarded, and all mood disorders were grouped together.

- Its approach was empirical, and psychodynamic concepts were largely eliminated.

- For some conditions, duration of illness was introduced as a diagnostic criterion.

The next full revision, DSM-IV, followed in 1994. It contained some revisions and additions to diagnostic categories, but retained the basic structures and features from DSM-III.

DSM-5

When planning for DSM-V (later renamed DSM-5) began, it was hoped that the classification could be based on aetiology (including the use of biomarkers) rather than description (Hyman, 2007). It was also intended to make much greater use of dimensions rather than categories. However, it became apparent that for all major disorders both steps were premature, and DSM-5 retains the same key elements as its predecessors, albeit with some new and revised diagnostic criteria and other features that have generated controversy for several reasons, including concerns about specificity and sensitivity, reliability, and conflicts of interest (Frances and Nardo, 2013; Blashfield *et al.*, 2014).

For a history and critique of DSM, see Blashfield *et al.* (2014).

Comparing ICD-10 and DSM-5

ICD-10 and DSM-IV were developed in parallel and, to avoid unnecessary differences, there was close consultation between the working parties preparing the two documents. The efforts were largely successful, with the systems sharing most fundamental concepts and categories, but there were some differences (Table 2.1). The arrival of DSM-5 has slightly increased the differences with ICD-10, but most of these are minor and are discussed as appropriate in later chapters. However, a few are worthy of mention here. See also Tyrer (2014) for a comparison of ICD and DSM classifications.

- The duration of the symptoms required for a diagnosis of schizophrenia. ICD-10 specifies 1 month, whereas DSM-5 requires a duration of 6 months, including a prodromal period (see Chapter 11).

- Terms such as *neurotic, neurasthenia, and mental retardation* are not used in DSM-5.

- Bereavement is an exclusion criterion for a depressive episode in ICD-10 (as it was hitherto in DSM) but this exclusion has been removed in DSM-5.

- Dementia and amnesic syndromes have been combined in DSM-5 in a new category of *major neurocognitive disorder* (see Chapter 14).

It is important to realize that the two classifications are complementary rather than in competition. ICD-10 results from an international effort, and was designed for use in all countries with their varied cultures, professional needs, and traditions. DSM-5 is a national classification, and reflects the professional, educational, and financial priorities of its parent organization, the American Psychiatric Association. Notably, even in the USA, hospital records utilize the ICD system, not DSM.

Current and future issues in psychiatric classification

Many of the issues relating to classification discussed in this chapter continue to be topical and under active debate. This section raises some additional issues, especially those that may influence future developments.

Cultural issues

Although ICD-10 and DSM-5 make national approaches to classification less important (see Box 2.3), local and cultural factors remain important in classification in several respects.

Psychiatrists and physicians in countries that have their own longstanding and comprehensive systems of ideas about health and illness, such as India, Pakistan, and China, sometimes complain that classifications developed in Europe and North America give too much emphasis to separation of mind and body. For example, the concept of somatoform disorders depends on viewing mind and body as alternatives. This approach causes problems in western medicine and is not understood at all elsewhere. Investigation of these issues is difficult, as outsiders may not appreciate

Table 2.1 **Differences between ICD-10 and DSM-5**

	ICD-10	DSM-5
Origin	World Health Organization	American Psychiatric Association
Usage	Official global classification, for use by all health practitioners in all health settings	Mainly American psychiatrists, and psychiatric researchers
Presentation	Different versions for clinical work, research, and use in primary care	A single document
Languages	Available in all widely spoken languages	English version only
Structure	Part of overall ICD framework	Stand alone
Content	Clinical descriptors and guidance used	Operational criteria used
	Guidelines and criteria do not include social consequences of disorders	Diagnostic criteria usually include significant impairment in social functions

important cultural and local factors, or the varying ways in which emotions and behaviour are described in different languages.

A list of so-called 'culture-specific' disorders is provided as appendices to ICD-10. The limited and largely anecdotal information available at present suggests that most of these conditions are culturally influenced varieties of anxiety, depression, and violent behaviour, rather than distinct disorders of different types.

Reflecting an increased focus on culture and health (Napier *et al.*, 2014), DSM-5 pays greater attention to cultural issues than earlier versions, and distinguishes three concepts:

- Cultural syndrome: syndromes characteristically found in one cultural group.
- Cultural idiom of distress: terms, phrases, and ways of communicating suffering that are characteristic of a cultural group.

Box 2.3 Other national systems of classification

The widespread international acceptance of ICD-10 and DSM-5 has diminished the importance of pre-existing national diagnostic traditions. However, the latter are of historical interest and, at times, still have some influence on educational programmes.

The descriptive concepts introduced by Kraepelin and Bleuler have been very influential in most European countries, particularly in Germany, UK, and Scandinavian countries. In Scandinavia, emphasis has also been placed on the concept of psychogenic or reactive psychoses (Strömgren, 1985). In addition, Scandinavia was notable for its early concepts of multidimensional diagnoses.

In France, Kraepelinian views of schizophrenia were less widely accepted, and two other diagnostic categories of psychosis not commonly used elsewhere have persisted, namely *bouffée délirante* and *délires chroniques*. *Bouffée délirante* is the sudden onset of a delusional state with trance-like feelings, of short duration and good prognosis. This disorder is included in ICD-10 within the category of 'acute transient psychotic disorder', which also incorporates features of the Scandinavian concept of reactive psychosis. *Délires chroniques* are conditions that in ICD-10 would be classified as 'persistent delusional disorders', and are subdivided into the 'non-focused', in which several areas of mental activity are affected, and the 'focused', with a single delusional theme, such as erotomania. These disorders are discussed in Chapter 12.

Another example of international variation is the Chinese national classification (*Chinese Classification of Mental Disorders, 3rd edition, CCMD-3*), introduced in 2001. Although largely based upon ICD-10, it excludes almost all of the somatoform disorders, so that particular prominence can be given to the category of *neurasthenia*, which remains one of the most frequent diagnoses in Chinese psychiatry.

- Cultural explanation or perceived cause: a label for, or attribution of, a cause of symptoms or distress that is accepted within a cultural group.

ICD-11

Originally it was intended that DSM-5 and ICD-11 would be contemporaneous, and with greater harmonization than between their predecessors. However, delays to ICD-11 (now scheduled for completion in 2018) prevented the former, and there is ongoing debate about whether ICD-11 should strive for harmonization with DSM-5 in light of concerns with aspects of the latter (Frances and Nardo, 2013).

The main principles and properties of ICD-11 will remain unchanged from ICD-10, including the lack of operationalized criteria, and the intention that it can be used by many professional groups in all cultures and health systems. Although the detailed content of ICD-11 is not finalized, the following are some of the main changes anticipated compared to ICD-10 (Luciano, 2014):

- Sleep–wake disorders and sexuality-related conditions and dysfunctions will have their own chapters.

- For schizophrenia, first-rank symptoms (see page 255) will be of less diagnostic importance, and the subtypes of schizophrenia omitted.

- In mood disorders, bipolar II disorder will become a distinct entity (as it is in DSM). In contrast, unlike DSM-5, reactions to bereavement will continue to be excluded from diagnosis of a depressive episode.

- In eating disorders, criteria for anorexia nervosa will be broadened, and binge eating disorder recognized as a specific category.

- Mental retardation will be renamed 'intellectual development disorders'.

- The problematic areas of somatoform disorders and personality disorder remain under review.

- A goal of these changes is to improve the clinical utility of the classification, especially in lower-income countries.

Research domain criteria

The scientific arguments for a dimensional rather than categorical approach to diagnostic classification have been outlined above. One manifestation of this was the move in 2010 by the United States' National Institute for Mental Health to advocate 'domains', and to require these to be used as the basis for research funding, not DSM-5 (or ICD-10) categories (Cuthbert and Insel, 2013). Such domains may include neuropsychological constructs (such as working memory, or reward sensitivity) or brain systems (e.g. corticostriatal circuits), which underpin—and are thought to cut across—current diagnostic categories. The advent of Research Domain Criteria (RDoC) is having a major, if controversial, impact on psychiatric research. However, it is not of clinical relevance until (and unless) it discovers domains that have the necessary utility and reliability to accompany their greater validity.

Classification in this book

In this book, both ICD-10 and DSM-5 classifications are used, and compared. Where they differ, the ICD-10 approach is usually adopted. As in other textbooks, disorders are grouped in chapters for convenience. The headings of the chapters do not always correspond to the terms used in ICD-10 or DSM-5; any difference means that the heading more appropriately summarizes the scope of the chapter.

Further reading

American Psychiatric Association (2013). *Diagnostic and Statistical Manual of Mental Disorders, Fifth Edition (DSM-5)*. American Psychiatric Association, Washington, DC.

Bolton D (2008). *What is Mental Disorder? An essay in philosophy, science and values*. Oxford University Press, Oxford.

Kendell RE (1975). *The Role of Classification in Psychiatry*. Blackwell Scientific Publications, Oxford.

World Health Organization (1992). *The ICD-10 Classification of Mental and Behavioural Disorders: clinical descriptions and diagnostic guidelines*. 10th edn. World Health Organization, Geneva.

CHAPTER 3
Assessment

Introduction

Psychiatric assessment has three main goals:

- *To make a diagnosis.* Despite its limitations (see Chapter 2), diagnosis is central to the practice of psychiatry, since it provides the basis for rational, evidence-based approaches to treatment and prognosis (Craddock and Mynors-Wallis, 2014). A major goal of most assessments, especially those of new patients, is therefore to allow a diagnosis or differential diagnosis to be made. This in turn requires that the symptoms and signs of psychiatric disorder (see Chapter 1) can be elicited, and their diagnostic significance appreciated.

- *To understand the context of the diagnosis.* The psychiatrist needs to have sufficient information about the patient's life history, current circumstances, and personality. This is necessary to try and understand why the disorder has occurred in this person at this time; it also has a major bearing on decisions about management and prognosis.

- *To establish a therapeutic relationship.* The psychiatrist must ensure that the patient feels able and willing to give an accurate and full history. Without this skill, the necessary diagnostic information is unlikely to be obtained. Thus, establishment of a therapeutic relationship is essential if the patient is to engage fully in

discussions about management, and to adhere to any treatment decisions which are agreed upon.

The *process* of psychiatric assessment, also known as the *psychiatric interview*, can be broken down into the following stages:

- *Preparation.* This includes having the interviewing skills necessary to achieve the above goals, acquiring as much background information as possible (e.g. the reason for referral, and whether informants are available) to help guide the assessment and identify areas for particular focus, and anticipating whether the interview may need to be adapted (e.g. owing to language difficulties, or a shortage of time).

- *Collecting the information.* This is usually addressed by means of a series of headings covering the psychiatric history, mental state examination, and other components, as described below.

- *Evaluating the information* to arrive at a diagnosis or differential diagnosis. This is the hardest part of the process to describe to readers new to psychiatry, as it requires knowledge of the diagnostic significance of particular symptoms and symptom combinations. It is therefore suggested that this chapter should be returned to at regular intervals, to refine how assessments are conducted to match one's developing knowledge and skills.

- *Using the information* to make treatment decisions and form prognostic opinions.
- *Recording and communicating the information collected, and the conclusions drawn.* The information must be shared with other health professionals involved with the care of the patient both now and in the future, and with the patient and their significant others. Various modes of communication are necessary (e.g. with regard to its nature and level of detail) depending on the circumstances of the assessment and the needs of the recipient.

This chapter covers these areas in turn, concentrating on the full initial assessment of a patient by a general adult psychiatrist. It also discusses how this process should be adapted in other circumstances. First, however, the basic process of psychiatric interviewing will be outlined. At the outset, it is worth emphasizing that the description of assessment in textbooks tends to make the process appear to be a passive, even predetermined, one of extensive data collection. In practice, however, assessment is an active, selective process, in which diagnostic clues are pursued, hypotheses tested, and the focus of questioning adapted to the particular circumstances. This 'dynamic' aspect of assessment can only be learned from practical experience. It also requires a working knowledge of the main psychiatric syndromes for the significance of specific symptoms or history items that emerge during the assessment to be appreciated. It was for this reason that the preceding chapter covered psychiatric classification.

It is assumed that the reader is already competent in medical history-taking and physical examination, and these topics are considered only briefly.

Psychiatric interviewing

Preparing for the assessment

Psychiatric assessments are conducted in many settings. The following recommendations should be followed as far as is practicable, but they cannot always be achieved in their entirety. In some locations, such as an Accident and Emergency department, the setting may be far from ideal. Nevertheless, it is important to do what is possible to ensure safety and confidentiality, and to put the patient at ease.

Before starting the interview, it is always worth finding out what is already known about the patient and the circumstances in which the assessment has come about. This will often be in the form of a referral letter from another doctor, or there may be notes available from previous assessments. This information will reveal areas of enquiry that may require particular emphasis, and may modify the diagnosis that is subsequently made. Equally, every assessment should, of course, begin with an open mind (not least since prior diagnoses may be incorrect, or the present presentation may be different).

Only a small minority of patients are potentially dangerous, but the need for precautions should be considered before every interview. The interviewer should always:

- make sure that another person knows where and when the interview is taking place and how long it is expected to last. This is especially relevant to interviews in the community;
- ensure that help can be called if it is needed. In hospital, check for an emergency call button and its position, and otherwise try to arrange for another person to be within earshot;
- ensure that neither the patient nor any obstruction is between you and the exit;
- remove from sight any objects that could be used as weapons.

If the risk is thought to be high, or if these requirements cannot be met, it may be necessary to defer the interview.

Starting the assessment

The psychiatrist should welcome the patient by name, give their own name and status, and explain in a few words the reason for and purpose of the assessment. If the patient is being seen at the request of another doctor, the interviewer should indicate this. If the patient is accompanied, the interviewer should greet the companion(s) and explain how long they should expect to wait and whether they will be interviewed. It is usually better to see the patient alone first, provided that he is able to provide an adequate history. The interviewer should explain that notes will be taken, and that these will be confidential. If the interview is for the purposes of a report to an outside agency (e.g. a medicolegal report), this should be made clear. The general structure of the interview should be explained, and the time available stated; the latter is not only a matter of courtesy but is also valuable if the psychiatrist later needs to interrupt the patient, or ask him to give more concise answers, to ensure the assessment can be completed.

The patient should be comfortable and the interviewer should not face the patient directly but arrange his chair at an angle. If possible, the interviewer should also avoid sitting at a much higher level. Whenever possible, the interviewer should make notes (whether on paper or electronically) during the interview, as writing up an assessment afterwards is time-consuming and not always wholly accurate. However, it is usually better to delay note-taking for some minutes until the patient feels that he has the interviewer's undivided attention. The patient should be placed at the left side of a right-handed interviewer. With this arrangement, the interviewer can attend to the patient and maintain an informal atmosphere while writing.

The following techniques have been shown to improve the results of the interview (Goldberg *et al.*, 1980). The interviewer should:

- adopt a relaxed posture and appear unhurried—even when time is short;
- maintain appropriate eye contact with the patient and not appear engrossed in note-taking;
- be alert to verbal and non-verbal cues of distress as well as to the factual content of the interview;
- maintain control of the interview if the patient is over-talkative or discursive.

Continuing and completing the assessment

The interview should begin with an open question (one that cannot be answered with a simple 'yes' or 'no'), such as 'Tell me about your problems or difficulties'. The patient should be allowed to talk freely for several minutes before further questions are asked. As the patient describes their problems, the interviewer should observe their responses and manner—for example, whether they are reticent or unduly circumstantial.

The first step is to obtain a clear account of the patient's problems. It is important to separate symptoms from their consequences, and from other life problems that the patient may want to discuss. For example, a patient may have low mood, sexual difficulties, or

financial worries as the presenting complaint. In each case the common denominator may prove to be depression, but it will require your assessment to discover this. Your priority at the start is to focus upon the symptoms and signs of psychiatric disorder, leaving the other kinds of problem until later.

From the start, consider the possible diagnoses and, as the interview progresses, select questions to confirm or reject these diagnoses. For example, if the patient mentions hearing voices, this immediately raises the possibility of schizophrenia and requires that, at some stage in the assessment, the other cardinal features of the disorder are sought, and their presence or absence clearly noted. The interviewer also considers what information is relevant to prognosis and treatment. Thus, as noted earlier, interviewing is not simply the asking of a routine set of questions. It is an active and iterative process in which the focus of attention is directed by hypotheses formed from the information already elicited, and modified repeatedly as more information is collected. This active process of interviewing is particularly necessary when time is short and when immediate treatment decisions must be made. Obviously, as the interviewer gains confidence and acquires more psychiatric knowledge, he or she becomes better at thinking of possible diagnoses, and proceeding in a way that rules them in or out more rapidly and convincingly.

It is generally better to establish clearly the nature of the symptoms before asking how and when they developed. If there is any doubt about the nature of the symptoms, the patient should be asked to describe specific examples. When all of the presenting symptoms have been explored sufficiently, direct questions are asked about others that have not come to light but which may be relevant. In doing this, the interviewer uses his knowledge of psychiatric syndromes to decide what further questions to ask. For example, a person who complains of feeling depressed would be asked about thoughts concerning the future, and about suicidal ideas. If suicidal thoughts are acknowledged, further specific questions should be asked. Also ask about the impact that the symptoms have had on the patient's life, looking for evidence of functional impairment.

The onset and course of the symptoms are clarified next, together with their relationship to any stressful events or physical illness. Considerable persistence may be needed to date the onset or an exacerbation of symptoms accurately. It sometimes helps to ask how the onset related to an event that the patient is likely to remember, such as a birthday. The patient's attempts to cope with the symptoms are noted—for example, increased drinking of alcohol to relieve distress. If treatment has already been given, its nature, timing, and effects are noted, together with the patient's concordance with it.

The interviewer completes the relevant parts of the full assessment schedule, which is described in later sections of this chapter. When time is adequate, the mental state is usually examined at the end of the interview, together with any relevant physical examination. If time is short, it may be better to examine the mental state after the presenting complaints have been clarified. This can make it easier to select the key points to be asked about in the rest of the history.

Throughout the interview, allow the patient, as far as possible, to describe their problems spontaneously. In this way, unexpected material may be volunteered that might not be revealed by the answers to questions. However, questions may be needed to bring the patient back to the point after a digression, and to elicit specific information—for example, about the relationship between symptoms and stressful events. Whenever possible, the interviewer should use open rather than leading or closed questions (a leading question suggests the answer, whereas a closed question allows only the answers 'yes' or 'no'). Thus, for example, instead of the closed question 'Are you happily married?' the interviewer might ask 'How do you and your wife get on?' When there is no alternative to a closed question, the answer should be followed by a request for an example.

Before ending the interview, it is good practice to ask a general question such as 'Is there anything that I have not asked you about, that you think I should know?' It is also useful to summarize for the patient what you consider to be the key points, to check for any errors of fact, and to see whether the patient agrees with your initial understanding of events.

Box 3.1 summarizes some techniques that promote effective interviewing.

Interviewing informants

Whenever possible, the patient's history should be supplemented by information from a close relative or another person who knows them well. This is much more important in psychiatry than in the rest of medicine, for several reasons. Some psychiatric patients are unaware of the extent or significance of their symptoms. Others are aware of their problems but do not wish to reveal them—for example, people who misuse alcohol often conceal the extent of their drinking. Patients and relatives may also give quite different accounts of personality characteristics, or have contrasting interpretations of recent events and symptoms. Interviews with a partner or relative are used not only to obtain additional

> ### Box 3.1 Some techniques for effective psychiatric assessments
>
> - Help the patient to talk freely. This can be done using open questions, and by non-verbal cues such as nodding, or saying 'Go on' or 'Tell me more about that'
> - Keep the patient to relevant topics. Again, non-verbal cues are useful, as well as specific interventions such as 'At this point I'd like to ask you more about how you've been feeling. We can return to your money worries later'
> - Make systematic enquiries, but avoid asking so many questions that other, unanticipated issues are not volunteered
> - Check your understanding, and that you have enquired about all of the areas the patient thinks are important, by summarizing the key points of the history back to the patient. This step also helps you to begin to formulate your views on the diagnosis and causes
> - Be flexible in assessments, with regard to both their length and sequence. Select questions according to the emerging possibilities regarding diagnoses, causes, and plans of action

information about the patient's condition, but also to assess their attitudes to the patient and the illness, and often to involve them in the subsequent management plan. In addition, they provide an opportunity to learn what burdens the illness has placed on the partner or relative, and how they have tried to cope. A history from an informant is essential when the patient is unable to give an accurate account of his or her condition (e.g. because of impaired memory). Finally, when it is important to know about the patient's early development or childhood, an interview with a parent is usually the best way to discover the relevant information.

Informants can either be seen separately from the patient, or invited to join the interview. The choice depends on both the assessor's and the patient's preference, but in both instances the patient must give consent. If the patient refuses, explore the reasons for this and explain the difficulties that it will pose. There are a few situations in which the patient's permission is not required before interviewing a relative or other informant—for example, if the patient is a child, or when adult patients are mute or confused. In other cases, the doctor should explain to the patient the reasons for interviewing the informant, while emphasizing that confidential information given by the patient will not be passed on. If any information needs to be given to a relative—for example, about treatment—the patient's permission should be obtained. Questions from relatives should be dealt with in the same way.

The psychiatrist begins by explaining the purpose of the interview, and may need to reassure the informant. For example, a relative may fear that they will be viewed as responsible in some way for the patient's problems. The interviewer should be sensitive to such ideas and, when appropriate, discuss them in a reassuring way, but without colluding or becoming involved in ways that might conflict with their primary duty to the patient. If the informant has been interviewed separately from the patient, the psychiatrist should not tell the patient what has been said unless the informant has given their permission. This is important even when the informant has revealed something that should be discussed with the patient—for example, an account of excessive drinking.

Sometimes it is necessary to speak to employers, educators, friends, police, or others to collect further information. This should be done only with the patient's permission, unless there are legal or safety issues which override this principle—for example, if the patient is in custody, or if there are grounds for concern that the patient may harm a third party.

The psychiatric history

The main parts of a psychiatric assessment are the *psychiatric history* and the *mental state examination.* The latter covers the symptoms and signs present during the interview, and the former deals with everything else. The assessment is then completed by the physical examination, and sometimes by further investigations. This section covers the psychiatric history, followed by the mental state examination, and then the other aspects of the assessment.

A commonly used scheme for history-taking is given below. For ease of reference, the scheme is presented as a list of headings and items. More details, and some background information to the questions, are provided in the subsequent notes. As noted above, much of the interview is designed to elicit diagnostic symptoms, but other questions are intended to obtain information about the patient's life and circumstances, while the interview as a whole must try to establish the rapport needed to achieve these goals and form the basis for a subsequent therapeutic relationship.

The following scheme is comprehensive and systematic, as an ability to conduct this form of assessment is essential before briefer interviews are attempted. Modification of the interview for use in briefer or specific settings is described later. Moreover, although it is neither possible nor necessary to take a full history on every occasion, the information that has been elicited should always be recorded systematically and in a standard order. This practice helps the interviewer to remember all of the potentially important topics and to add further information later. The practice also makes it easier for colleagues who need to refer to the notes in the future. This order can be followed in the written or electronic record, even when it was not possible to elicit the information in the desired sequence. This and all other entries in the notes should be dated and, whenever possible, signed.

A scheme for history-taking

Information is grouped under the headings shown in Box 3.2. For clarity, this section is written in the style of short notes and illustrative questions. The next section explains why these topics are relevant, and some of the problems that may occur when covering them.

Informant(s)

- Usually the principal informant is the patient. If not, state the reason.
- The name(s), relationship to the patient, and length of acquaintance of any other person(s) interviewed.
- The name of the referrer and the reasons for referral.

History of present condition

Also known as the *history of presenting complaint,* this section is in many ways the core of the interview, usually providing most of the key diagnostic information.

- List the symptoms, with the onset, duration, severity, and fluctuation of each. Quantitative information is valuable. For example, a patient can rate their low mood on a 10-point scale.
- Ask about and record symptoms that might have been expected but which are *not* present (e.g. no

> ## Box 3.2 Outline of the psychiatric history
>
> Name, age, and address of the patient
> Name(s) of informant(s) and their relationship to the patient
> History of present condition
> Family history
> Personal history (expanded in Box 3.3)
> Past illness
> Personality (expanded in Box 3.4)

> ## Box 3.3 Outline of the personal history
>
> Mother's pregnancy and the birth
> Early development
> Childhood: separations, emotional problems, illnesses, education
> Occupations
> Relationships and sex
> Children
> Social circumstances
> Substance use
> Forensic history

suicidal ideation in a person with low mood; no first-rank symptoms of schizophrenia in a patient with delusions).

- The temporal relationship between symptoms and any physical disorder, or psychological or social problems.
- The nature and duration of any functional impairment caused by the symptoms.
- Any treatment received, and its effects and side-effects.

Family history

- Parents and siblings—age, current state of health or date and cause of death, occupation, personality, quality of relationship with patient. Psychiatric and medical family history.
- When the family history is complex and relevant, summarize it as a family tree.

Personal history

This is a particularly variable section of the history (see Box 3.3). In the case of a young person with a disorder suspected to have origins early in life, it will be important and extensive; for older patients or some other disorders, only limited questioning may be necessary.

- Pregnancy and birth abnormalities (e.g. infections, prematurity, problems with labour).
- Early developmental milestones—walking, talking, etc.
- Childhood—any prolonged separation from the parents, and the patient's reaction to it. Any emotional problems (age of onset, course, and treatment). Any serious illness in childhood.
- Schooling and higher education—type, courses, qualifications, extracurricular achievements, relationships with teachers and other students. Note any experience

of bullying (nature, duration, and impact) or school exclusions.

- Occupations—present job (dates, duties, performance, and satisfaction), earlier jobs (list them, with reasons for changes).
- Significant relationships —identity and gender of current partner, duration and nature of relationship. Partner's health and attitude to the patient's illness. Nature and number of previous relationships.
- Sexual history—attitude to sex, any sexual difficulties and their relationship to current symptoms. Knowing how, and how far, to enquire about sexual matters is discussed further on page 42.
- Children—identities, date of any abortions or stillbirths, temperament, emotional development, mental and physical health. Who are the child carers.
- Social circumstances—accommodation, household composition, financial situation.
- Use of alcohol, tobacco, illicit drugs—which ones, when, and how much. Problems arising from substance use.
- Forensic history—arrests, convictions, imprisonment. Nature of the offences, especially with regard to dangerousness. For a few patients, the forensic history is a key part of the assessment (see Chapter 18.

Past psychiatric and medical history

- Past psychiatric illnesses—nature and duration, and their similarity to current episode. Include any episodes of self-harm. Date, duration, nature, location, and outcome of any treatment.

- Past medical history—illnesses, operations, accidents, and drug treatments.
- Current medication, including over-the-counter medicines and alternative remedies. Any allergic or other adverse reactions.

Personality

By this stage in the interview, the patient's manner and description of their history will have provided some indication about their personality. However, a specific focus is also necessary, covering the domains noted in Box 3.4. Personality can be a relatively difficult area of the history, as outlined below in the section 'Notes on history-taking'.

- Relationships—friendships (few or many, superficial or close, with own or opposite sex), relationships with work colleagues and superiors.
- Use of leisure time—hobbies and interests.
- Predominant mood and emotional tone (e.g. anxious, despondent, optimistic, pessimistic, self-deprecating, overconfident, stable or fluctuating, controlled or demonstrative).
- Character traits (e.g. perfectionist, obsessional, isolated, impulsive, sensitive, controlling).
- Attitudes and standards (e.g. moral or religious; attitude towards health).
- 'Ultimate concern'—what or who matters most in their life?

Notes on history-taking

The scheme outlined above lists the items to be considered when a full history is taken, but has not indicated why these items are important or what sort of difficulties may arise when eliciting them. These issues are discussed in this section, which is written in the form of notes approximating to the headings used above.

> ### Box 3.4 Assessment of personality
>
> Relationships
> Leisure activities
> Prevailing mood and emotional tone
> Character
> Attitudes and standards
> 'Ultimate concern'

The reason for referral

Only a brief statement need be given—for example, 'severe depression with somatic symptoms'. The reason for referral usually, but not always, proves to be the main focus of the interview. Check that the patient has the same understanding as to why they have been referred. If not, this in itself is useful information. For example, the patient may disagree that they are depressed, believing that their somatic symptoms are due to cancer. This may affect their willingness to engage fully in the assessment or accept the treatment for depression that is subsequently recommended.

History of present condition

Because it is central to the assessment, it is always worth spending sufficient time on this part of the history to identify the key elements. There will often be several such symptoms, and each should be characterized fully to appreciate its diagnostic significance. Record the severity and duration of each symptom, how and when it began, what course it has taken (increasing or decreasing, constant or intermittent), and what factors affect it. Indicate which symptoms co-vary. As noted above, record any symptoms or features that would have diagnostic significance but which are not present (e.g. lack of anhedonia in a person complaining of low mood).

Note any treatments that have been given during this episode, the response, and any adverse effects. If a drug was ineffective, ask whether the patient took it regularly and at the required dosage.

Family history

A family history of psychiatric disorder may indicate genetic or environmental influences. A genetic contribution is more likely for some disorders than for others, and increases as more relatives are affected. Although family environment has, as a rule, proved to be less important than genes in explaining family history (see Chapter 5), knowledge about the family's circumstances remains part of the basic information required for understanding the origin and presentation of the patient's problems.

Recent events in the family may have been stressful to the patient—for example, the serious illness or divorce of a family member. Events in the family may throw light on the patient's concerns. For example, the death of an older sibling from a brain tumour may partly explain a patient's extreme concern about headaches.

Personal history

Pregnancy and birth

Events in pregnancy and delivery are most likely to be relevant when the patient is learning disabled, although they are also risk factors for several psychiatric disorders which have their onset in childhood, adolescence, or early adulthood. An unwanted pregnancy may be followed by a poor relationship between mother and child.

Child development

Few patients know whether they have passed through developmental stages normally. Failure to do so may be a sign of learning disability and also a risk factor for later disorders such as schizophrenia. However, this information is usually more important if the patient is a child or adolescent, in which case the parents are likely to be available for interview. The effects of separation from the mother vary considerably, and depend in part on the age of the child, the duration, and the reason for separation. Questioning about the child's emotional development provides information about early temperament and emerging personality, and abnormalities or delays may serve as risk factors for, or early signs of, later problems. However, childhood behavioural characteristics as a rule are weak predictors of adult disorders, and only require detailed consideration when assessing children and adolescents. Assessment in child psychiatry is covered in Chapter 16.

Education

The school record gives an indication of intelligence, achievements, and social development. Ask whether the patient made friends and got on well with teachers, and about success at games and other activities. Bullying is a risk factor for later psychological difficulties, and other negative events such as exam failures may be important stressful memories. Similar questions are relevant to higher education.

Occupational history

Information about the present job helps the interviewer to understand the patient's current abilities, interests, and financial and social circumstances, and may be a potential source of stress. A list of previous jobs and reasons for leaving is relevant to the assessment of personality. If the status of jobs has declined, this may reflect chronic illness or substance misuse.

Marital history

This heading includes all enduring intimate relationships. Ask about the current and any previous lasting relationships, preferably phrased in a way that does not assume the gender of the partner(s). Frequent broken relationships may reflect abnormalities of personality. The partner's occupation, personality, and state of health are relevant to the patient's circumstances and, like the nature of the relationship itself, will affect the partner's role in the care and management of the patient.

Sexual history

The interviewer should use common sense when deciding how much to ask the individual patient, depending on the response to initial questions, demographic factors (such as age and relationship status), and the nature of the presenting complaint. Usually the interviewer is concerned to establish generally whether the patient's sexual life is in any way involved in their current difficulties, whether as a cause, a correlate, or a consequence. If so, then more detailed enquiry is appropriate.

Judgement must also be used about the optimal timing and amount of detail of questioning about childhood abuse, especially sexual abuse. Unfortunately, such past experiences are sufficiently common to merit enquiry. However, often it may not be appropriate to raise the matter in a first interview, unless prompted by the patient or in the light of background information available to the interviewer. The decision to raise the topic also depends on the clinical suspicion, and the time and expertise available to the interviewer. Sensitivity is also necessary when deciding what information to record and with whom it should be shared.

Assessment of sexual history and sexual disorders is considered further in Chapter 13.

Children

Pregnancy, childbirth, miscarriages, and terminations are events that are sometimes associated with adverse psychological reactions. Information about the patient's children is relevant to present worries and the pattern and characteristics of family life.

Consideration of the welfare and needs of any children is always integral to an assessment, as their health and care may be adversely affected by the parent's illness or its treatment. For example, if a seriously depressed woman has a young baby, due steps to ensure the baby's wellbeing are essential, and the situation may influence decisions about the mother's care (e.g. about medication if she is breastfeeding, and about hospital admission). In turn, any concerns about the care or welfare of children should be clearly recorded, and followed by appropriate discussions and, if necessary, interventions. Such considerations are increasingly covered by guidelines, protocols, and legislation (which differ from country to country), and the reader is advised to keep up to date in this respect.

Social circumstances

Questions about housing, finances, and the composition of the household help the interviewer to understand the patient's circumstances. Assets and resources (including potential carers) are assessed, as well as problems and sources of stress. There can be no general rule about the amount of detail to elicit, and this must be guided by common sense.

Substance use and misuse

This includes past as well as present consumption of alcohol and other substances, and the impact of their use on the patient's health and life. Misuse of prescribed drugs should also be considered. The patient's answers may be evasive or misleading, and may need to be checked with other informants and sources of information (e.g. urine screens, blood tests). See Chapter 20 for further information about interviewing in this area.

Past psychiatric and medical history

In many instances, a patient being assessed will have a past psychiatric history. A previous diagnosis increases the probability that the current diagnosis will prove to be similar, but it is important always to keep an open mind, as the diagnosis may have changed, or the previous diagnosis may have been incorrect. Patients or relatives may be able to recall the general nature of the illness and treatment, but it is nearly always appropriate to request information from others who have treated the patient.

The medical history is also important (Phelan and Blair, 2008). A medical disorder or its treatment may be directly related to the presentation (e.g. a recurrence of hypothyroidism presenting with lethargy, or mania induced by corticosteroids), but may also be indirectly relevant (e.g. via the psychosocial effects of chronic ill health, or as a sign of somatoform disorder).

Assessment of personality

This is important because:

- it helps the interviewer to understand the patient as a person, and to put their current difficulties into context;
- personality traits can be a risk factor for psychiatric disorders (e.g. obsessionality increases the risk of developing a depressive disorder);
- personality traits can colour the presentation of psychiatric disorder;

- personality can be disordered, and personality disorder may be a differential or comorbid diagnosis.

Aspects of personality can be assessed by asking for a self-assessment, by asking others who know the patient well, and by observing behaviour. Good indications of personality can often be obtained by asking how the patient has behaved in particular circumstances, especially at times when social roles are changing, such as when starting work, or becoming a parent. However, mistakes can arise from paying too much attention to the patient's own assessment of their personality, especially during a single interview. Some people give an unduly favourable or unfavourable account. For example, antisocial people may conceal the extent of their aggressive behaviour or dishonesty and, conversely, depressed patients often judge themselves negatively and critically. When assessing personality from behaviour at interview, take into account the artificiality of the situation and the anxiety that it may provoke. These factors mean that it is essential to interview other informants whenever possible, and to avoid drawing premature or unjustified conclusions about personality. Personality tests are now rarely used in clinical practice, but interview schedules for diagnosis of personality disorder are widely used in forensic and other settings (see Chapters 15 and 18).

Relationships

Is the patient shy or do they make friends easily? Are their friendships close and are they lasting? Leisure activities can throw light on personality, by reflecting the patient's interests and preference for company or solitude, as well as their levels of energy and resourcefulness.

Mood and emotional tone

Ask whether the patient is generally cheerful or gloomy and whether they experience marked changes of mood, and, if so, how quickly these moods appear, how long they last, and whether they follow life events. Information about prevailing mood and mood swings may also reveal evidence suggestive of mood disorder, which can be enquired about further.

Character

Common sense and experience will indicate the depth and focus of character assessment that are needed for each patient. If the patient (or informant) has difficulty describing their character with an open question, offer them options—for example, 'Would you call yourself an optimist or a pessimist? A loner or a socialite?' Do not focus entirely on negative attributes, but ask about positive ones, including resilience in the face of adversity.

This is important not just to gain a balanced impression, but because strengths are usually better targets for intervention if personality proves to be therapeutically relevant.

For details on the assessment of personality, see Cloninger (2009). The assessment of personality disorder has been described by Tyrer *et al.* (2015), and is discussed further in Chapter 15.

The mental state examination

The history records symptoms up to the time of the interview. The mental state examination is concerned with symptoms, signs, and behaviour during the interview, and is usually conducted after the history. Although the distinction is traditional, and conceptually useful, in practice the boundary between the history and the mental state examination is somewhat blurred. In particular, very recent symptoms and signs are often recorded in the mental state examination, even if the phenomena are not experienced or elicited during the interview. The mental state examination is also sometimes used to elicit and record symptoms and signs which, for whatever reason, have not been covered previously in the interview (e.g. whether the patient is suicidal). For a history of the mental state examination, see Huline-Dickens (2013).

The mental state examination uses a standard series of headings under which the relevant phenomena, or their absence, are recorded (see Box 3.5). The symptoms and signs referred to in the following account are described in Chapter 1 and, with a few exceptions, are not repeated. Mental state examination is a skill that should be learned by watching experienced interviewers and by practising repeatedly under supervision, as well as by reading. The mental state examination provides, in conjunction with the history of the present condition, most of the key diagnostic information. The ability to carry out and record an accurate and comprehensive mental state examination is therefore a core skill required by all psychiatrists and other mental health professionals. It is also specified by the United Kingdom General Medical Council as a requirement for all newly qualified doctors (General Medical Council, 2009).

Appearance and behaviour

General appearance

Much diagnostically useful information can be obtained from the patient's appearance and behaviour. Indeed, as discussed later, experienced clinicians often make provisional diagnoses within minutes of meeting a patient, relying heavily on this information. The process of observation starts from the first moment you see the patient. For example, what is their manner and behaviour in the waiting room? Are they sitting quietly, pacing around, or laughing to themselves? When greeted, what is their response? As they walk towards the interview room, is there evidence of parkinsonism or ataxia? Note their general attire. A dirty, unkempt appearance may indicate self-neglect. Manic patients often dress brightly or incongruously. Occasionally an oddity of dress may provide the clue to diagnosis—for example, a rainhood worn on a dry day may be the first evidence of a patient's belief that rays are being shone on their head by persecutors. An appearance suggesting recent weight loss should alert the observer to the possibility of depressive disorder, anorexia nervosa, or physical illness.

Facial appearance and emotional expression

The facial appearance provides information about mood. In depression, the corners of the mouth are turned down, and there are vertical furrows on the brow. Anxious patients have horizontal creases on the forehead, widened palpebral fissures, and dilated pupils. Facial expression may reflect elation, irritability, or anger, or the fixed 'wooden' expression due to drugs with parkinsonian side-effects. The facial appearance may also suggest physical disorders (e.g. thyrotoxicosis).

> ## Box 3.5 Mental state examination headings
>
> Appearance and behaviour
> Speech
> Mood
> Thoughts
> Perceptions
> Cognitive function
> Insight

Posture and movement

Posture and movement also reflect mood. A depressed patient characteristically sits with hunched shoulders, with the head and gaze inclined downwards. An anxious patient may sit on the edge of their chair, with their hands gripping its sides. Anxious people and patients with agitated depression may be tremulous and restless—for example, touching their jewellery or picking at their fingernails. Manic patients are overactive and restless. Other abnormalities of movement include tardive dyskinesia (see page 729) and the motor signs seen mainly in catatonic schizophrenia (see page 256).

Social behaviour

The patient's social behaviour and interactions with the interviewer are influenced by their personality and by their attitude to the assessment, as outlined above. However, their behaviour can also be influenced by psychiatric disorder, so it provides another potential source of diagnostic information. Manic patients tend to be unduly familiar or disinhibited, whereas those with dementia may behave as if they were somewhere other than in a medical interview. A person with schizophrenia may be withdrawn and preoccupied, whilst a person with antisocial personality disorder may behave aggressively. If the patient's social behaviour is highly unusual, note what exactly is unusual, rather than simply using imprecise terms such as 'bizarre'.

Speech

Speech and thoughts are recorded in different parts of the mental state examination, even though it is only through speech that thoughts become known to the interviewer. By convention, the 'speech' section covers the rate, quantity, volume, and flow of speech, and any delays in responding to questions or apparent difficulties producing or articulating speech. The content of speech, in the sense that it reveals the patient's thoughts (e.g. preoccupations about death, grandiose delusions) is deferred until the 'Thoughts' section.

Rate and quantity

Speech may be unusually fast and increased in amount, as in mania (*'pressure of speech'*), or slow, sparse, and monotonous, as in depression. Depressed or demented patients may pause for a long time before replying to questions, and then give short answers, producing little spontaneous speech. The same may be observed among shy people or those of low intelligence.

Difficulties with speaking

If the patient is having problems finding or articulating words, consider the possibility of dysphasia or dysarthria. For further details, see Box 3.6 and consult a neurology textbook (e.g. Kaufman and Milstein, 2017).

Neologisms

Neologisms are private words invented by the patient, often to describe morbid experiences. If the interviewer is uncertain whether a word is a neologism, ask the patient to repeat and spell the word, and explain its meaning.

Flow of speech

Abnormalities in the flow of speech may simply reflect an anxious, distracted patient, or one of low intelligence. More significantly, such abnormalities may be evidence of disturbances in the stream or form of thoughts. For example, sudden interruptions may indicate thought blocking, and rapid shifts from one topic to another suggest flight of ideas. For a description of these features, see Chapter 1. It can be difficult to be certain about these abnormalities; if possible, write down a representative example.

Mood

Conventionally, the mood section includes recording of other emotions such as anxiety, and also related phenomena, including suicidal thoughts. The phenomenology of mood and its disorders are discussed in more detail in Chapters 9 and 10.

Depression and mania

The assessment of mood begins with the observations of behaviour described already, and continues with direct questions such as 'What is your mood like?' or 'How are you in your spirits?' To assess depression, questions should be asked about a feeling of being about to cry (actual tearfulness is often denied), pessimistic thoughts about the present, hopelessness about the future, and guilt about the past. Suitable questions are 'What do you think will happen to you in the future?' or 'Have you been blaming yourself for anything?' Questions about elevated mood correspond to those about depression—for example, 'How are you in your spirits?' followed, if necessary, by direct questions such as 'Do you feel in unusually good spirits?' Note that the mood in mania can be irritable as well as cheerful. It can be useful to ask the patient to rate their current mood on a numerical or other scale.

Box 3.6 **The neuropsychiatric examination**

Language abilities

Dysarthria is difficulty in the production of speech by the speech organs. **Dysphasia** is partial failure of language function of cortical origin; it can be receptive or expressive. Testing for dysarthria can be done by giving difficult phrases such as 'West Register Street' or a tongue twister.

Receptive dysphasia can be detected by asking the patient to read a passage of appropriate difficulty or, if they fail in this, individual words or letters. If they can read the passage, they are asked to explain it. Comprehension of spoken language is tested by asking the patient to listen to a spoken passage and explain it (first checking that memory is intact) or to respond to simple commands (e.g. to point at named objects).

Expressive dysphasia is detected by asking the patient to name common objects such as a watch, key, and pen, and some of their parts (e.g. the face of a watch), and parts of the body. The patient is also asked to talk spontaneously (e.g. about hobbies) and to write a brief passage, first to dictation, and then spontaneously, on a familiar topic (e.g. the members of the family). A patient who cannot do these tests should be asked to copy a short passage.

Language disorders point to the left hemisphere in right-handed people. In left-handed patients localization is less certain, but in many it is still the left hemisphere. The type of language disorder gives some further guide to localization. Expressive dysphasia suggests an anterior lesion, receptive dysphasia suggests a posterior lesion, mainly auditory dysphasia suggests a lesion towards the temporal region, and mainly visual dysphasia suggests a more posterior lesion.

Construction abilities

Apraxia is inability to perform a volitional act even though the motor system and sensorium are sufficiently intact for the person to do so. Apraxia can be tested in several ways.

- **Constructional apraxia** is tested by asking the patient to draw simple figures (e.g. a bicycle, house, or clock face).
- **Dressing apraxia** is tested by asking the patient to put on some of their clothes.

- **Ideomotor apraxia** is tested by asking the patient to perform increasingly complicated tasks to command, usually ending with a three-stage sequence such as: (1) touch the right ear with (2) the left middle finger while (3) placing the right thumb on the table.

Apraxia, especially if the patient fails to complete the left side of figures or dressing on the left side, suggests a right-sided lesion in the posterior parietal region. It may be associated with other disorders related to this region, namely sensory inattention and anosognosia.

Agnosia is the inability to understand the significance of sensory stimuli even though the sensory pathways and sensorium are sufficiently intact for the patient to be able to do so. Agnosia cannot be diagnosed until there is good evidence that the sensory pathways are intact and consciousness is not impaired.

- **Astereognosia** is failure to identify three-dimensional form; it is tested by asking the patient to identify objects placed in their hand while their eyes are closed. Suitable items are keys, coins of different sizes, and paper clips.
- **Atopognosia** is inability to locate the position of an object on the skin.
- In **finger agnosia** the patient cannot identify which of their fingers has been touched when their eyes are closed. Right–left confusion is tested by touching one hand or ear and asking the patient which side of the body has been touched.
- **Agraphognosia** is failure to identify letters or numbers 'written' on the skin. It is tested by tracing numbers on the palms with a closed fountain pen or similar object.
- **Anosognosia** is failure to identify functional deficits caused by disease. It is seen most often as unawareness of left-sided weakness and sensory inattention.
- **Agnosias** point to lesions of the parietal association cortex posterior to the primary somatosensory cortex. Lesions of either parietal lobe can cause contralateral astereognosia, agraphognosia, and atopognosia. Sensory inattention and anosognosia are more common with right parietal lesions. Finger agnosia and right–left disorientation are said to be more common with lesions of the dominant parietal region.

A distinction is sometimes drawn between 'objective' and 'subjective' mood. The latter is the patient's view of their own mood; the former refers to the interviewer's conclusion based upon their observation of the patient during the interview and the responses to their questions. On occasion the two may differ—for example, a severely depressed person may deny low mood. It is important therefore to record the presence of the various symptoms and signs of depression (or mania) during the mental state examination.

Both depressed and elevated mood, if clinically significant, are accompanied by other features of depression and mania, respectively—for example, anhedonia, tiredness, or poor concentration in depression. In practice, therefore, it is common to extend this part of the mental state examination to include questioning about other diagnostic features of mood disorder, if these have not been asked about already. Whether the interviewer chooses to record them in the notes under this heading or to insert them into the relevant part of the history is a matter of personal preference and convenience.

Fluctuating and incongruous mood

As well as assessing the prevailing mood, the interviewer should ascertain how mood varies. When mood varies excessively, it is said to be *labile*—for example, the patient appears dejected at one point in the interview but quickly changes to a normal or unduly cheerful mood. Any lack of emotional response, sometimes called blunting or flattening of affect (see page 5), should also be noted.

Normally, mood varies during an interview in parallel with the topics that are being discussed. The patient appears sad while talking about unhappy events, angry while describing things that have irritated them, and so on. When the mood is not suited to the context, it is recorded as *incongruent*—for example, if the patient giggles when describing the death of their mother. Before concluding that such behaviour reflects an incongruous mood, consider whether it could be a sign of embarrassment or an effort to conceal distress.

Suicidal ideation

Some inexperienced interviewers are wary of asking about suicide due to fear that they may suggest it to the patient. There is no evidence to warrant this caution, and an explicit assessment of suicide risk should be part of every mental state examination. Nevertheless, questioning should be handled sensitively and in stages, starting with open questions such as 'Have you ever thought that life is not worth living?' and, if appropriate, going on to ask 'Have you ever wished that you could die?' or

'Have you ever considered any way in which you might end your life?' and then leading on to direct questioning about current suicidal intent or plans. The interviewer may also be concerned that they will not be able to cope if the patient does admit to being suicidal. A basic training in this topic, and knowledge of self-harm and suicide, should preclude these worries. Questions about suicide are considered further on page 615.

Anxiety

Anxiety is assessed both by asking about subjective feelings and by enquiring about the physical symptoms and cognitions associated with anxiety, as well as by observation. For example, the interviewer should start with a general question such as 'Have you noticed any changes in your body when you feel upset?' and then go on to enquire specifically about palpitations, dry mouth, sweating, trembling, and the various other symptoms of autonomic activity and muscle tension. Such features may also be apparent during the interview. To detect anxious thoughts, the interviewer can ask 'What goes through your mind when you are feeling anxious?' Possible replies include thoughts of fainting or losing control. Many of these questions overlap with enquiries about the history of the disorder.

Depersonalization and derealization

These are usually symptoms of anxiety disorders, but occasionally they are diagnosed as a separate disorder (see page 656). Their importance in the mental state examination is largely due to the fact that they are easily mistaken for psychotic symptoms and must be distinguished from them. Patients who have experienced depersonalization and derealization find them difficult to describe, and patients who have not experienced them may say that they have done so because they have misunderstood the questions. Try to obtain specific examples of the patient's experiences. It is useful to begin by asking 'Do you ever feel that things around you are unreal?' and 'Do you ever feel unreal or that part of your body is unreal?' Patients with derealization often describe things in the environment as seeming artificial and lifeless. Patients with depersonalization may say that they feel detached, unable to feel emotion, or as if they are acting a part.

Thoughts

In this section, any predominant *content* of the person's thoughts can first be noted. For example, there may be a preoccupation with persecutory themes, negative or self-deprecating responses to questions, or a repeated return of the conversation to diet and body shape. This information may signify a delusional disorder, depression, and an eating disorder, respectively, and indicate areas for further questioning. However, the main purpose of this section is to determine the *nature* of the patient's thoughts, and in particular to identify obsessions and delusions.

Thinking can also be abnormal in terms of the flow of thoughts, and the links from one topic to another, called *formal thought disorder*. This was introduced in Chapter 1 (see page 15).

Obsessions

Obsessions were described on page 13. An appropriate question is 'Do any thoughts keep coming into your mind, even though you try hard to stop them?' If the patient says 'Yes', they should be asked for an example. Patients may be ashamed of obsessional thoughts, especially those about violence or sexual themes, so persistent but sympathetic questioning may be required. Before recording thoughts as obsessional, the interviewer should be certain that the patient accepts them as their own (and not implanted by an outside agency).

Compulsions

Many obsessional thoughts are accompanied by compulsive acts (see page 14). Some of these can be observed directly (although rarely during the interview), but others are private events (e.g. repeating phrases silently), and are detected only because they interrupt the patient's conversation. Appropriate questions are 'Do you have to keep checking activities that you know you have completed?', 'Do you have to do things over and over again when most people would have done them only once?', and 'Do you have to repeat exactly the same action many times?' If the patient answers 'Yes' to any of these questions, the interviewer should ask for specific examples.

Delusions

A delusion cannot be asked about directly, because the patient does not recognize it as differing from other beliefs. Because of the difficulty that this poses for the interviewer, and the diagnostic significance of delusions, these were described in detail in Chapter 1.

The interviewer may be alerted to the possibility of delusions by information from other people or by events in the history. When searching for delusional ideas, it is useful to begin by asking what might be the reason for other symptoms or unpleasant experiences that the patient has described. For example, a patient who says that life is no longer worth living may be convinced

that he is thoroughly evil and that his internal organs are already rotting away. Some patients hide delusions skilfully, and the interviewer needs to be alert to evasions, changes of topic, or other hints that information is being withheld. However, once the delusion has been uncovered, patients often elaborate on it without much prompting.

When ideas are revealed that could be delusional, the interviewer needs to determine whether they meet the criteria for a delusion (see page 9). First, ascertain how strongly they are held. Achieving this without antagonizing the patient requires patience and tact. The patient should feel that they are having a fair hearing. If the interviewer expresses contrary opinions to test the strength of the patient's beliefs, their manner should be enquiring rather than argumentative. The next step is to decide whether the beliefs are culturally determined convictions rather than delusions. This judgement may be difficult if the patient comes from a culture or religious group whose attitudes and beliefs are not known to the interviewer. In such cases any doubt can usually be resolved by finding an informant from the same country or religion, and by asking this person whether others from the same background share the patient's beliefs.

Some types of delusion, which are characteristic of schizophrenia and included in the list of *first rank symptoms* (see page 255), present particular problems of recognition:

- *Delusions of thought broadcasting* must be distinguished from the belief that other people can infer a person's thoughts from his expression or behaviour. When eliciting such delusions an appropriate question is 'Do you ever feel that other people know what you are thinking, even though you have not spoken your thoughts aloud?' If the patient says 'Yes', the interviewer should ask how other people know this. (Some patients answer 'Yes' when they mean that others can infer their thoughts from their facial expression.)

- *Delusions of thought insertion*. A suitable question is 'Have you ever felt that some of the thoughts in your mind were not your own but were put there from outside?' A corresponding question about *delusions of thought withdrawal* is 'Do you ever feel that thoughts are being taken out of your head?' In each case, if the patient answers 'Yes', detailed examples should be sought.

- *Delusions of control* (passivity of thought) present similar difficulties. It is appropriate to ask 'Do you ever feel that some outside force is trying to take control of you?' or 'Do you ever feel that your actions are controlled by some person or thing outside you?' Some patients misunderstand the question and answer 'Yes' when they mean that they have a religious or philosophical conviction that man is controlled by God or some other agency. Others think that the questions refer to the experience of being 'out of control' during extreme anxiety, while some say 'Yes' when in fact they have experienced auditory hallucinations commanding them to do things. Therefore positive answers should be followed by further questions to eliminate these possibilities.

Finally, the reader is reminded of the various categories of delusion described in Chapter 1 (see page 10). The interviewer should also distinguish between primary and secondary delusions, and be alert for the (rare) experiences of delusional perception and delusional mood. These issues only need to be addressed when there is already clear evidence of a psychosis, when they are useful in distinguishing schizophrenia from other psychotic disorders.

Perceptions

When asking about hallucinations, as with delusions, enquiries should be made tactfully to avoid distressing the patient and to encourage them to elaborate on their experiences without being ridiculed. Questions can be introduced by saying 'Some people find that, when their nerves are upset, they have unusual experiences.' This can be followed by enquiries about hearing sounds or voices when no one else is within earshot. Whenever the history makes it relevant, corresponding questions should be asked about visual hallucinations and those in other modalities. Conversely, in assessments where there has been no previous evidence of psychosis at all, it may be appropriate to omit assessment of them altogether.

Auditory hallucinations

If the patient describes auditory hallucinations, certain further questions are required depending on the type of experience, because of their diagnostic significance. Has the patient heard a single voice or several? If there were several voices, did they appear to talk to the patient or to each other about the patient in the third person? The latter experience must be distinguished from that of hearing actual people talking and believing that they are discussing the patient (an idea or delusion of reference). If the patient says that the voices are speaking to them, the interviewer should find out what the voices say and, if the words are experienced as commands, whether the patient feels that they must be obeyed. Note down examples of the words spoken by hallucinatory voices.

Visual hallucinations

Visual hallucinations must be distinguished from visual illusions. Unless the hallucination is experienced at the time of the interview, this distinction may be difficult because it depends on the presence or absence of a visual stimulus which has been misinterpreted. Ascertaining whether there is an 'as if' quality to the image, or asking if it is seen 'out there, or in your mind's eye' may aid the distinction. The interviewer should also distinguish hallucinations from dissociative experiences. The latter are described by the patient as the feeling of being in the presence of another person or a spirit with whom they can converse. Such experiences are reported by people with histrionic personality, although they are not confined to them, and are encouraged by some religious groups. They have little diagnostic significance.

Cognitive function

Early on in the interview, any significant cognitive difficulties will have already become apparent from the patient's interactions with the interviewer and their responses to questions. If so, the assessment of cognitive function should be brought forward, as the result may lead the interviewer to curtail the rest of the interview or to postpone it until an informant is available. The Mini-Mental State Examination (Folstein *et al.*, 1975) is a widely used cognitive screen in the elderly or where dementia or other organic disorder is suspected; see Chapter 14 for discussion of cognitive assessment in these contexts. Conversely, if the interview is nearing completion and no evidence or suspicion of any difficulties with memory or attention has arisen, cognition can be assessed very briefly.

Orientation

This is assessed by asking about the patient's awareness of time, place, and person. Specific questions begin with the day, month, and year. When assessing the replies, remember that many healthy people do not know the exact date and that, understandably, patients in hospital may be uncertain about the day of the week or their precise location. If the patient cannot answer these basic questions correctly, they should be asked about their own identity; this is preserved except in severe dementia, dissociative disorders, or malingering.

Attention and concentration

While taking the history the interviewer should look out for evidence of attention and concentration. In this way an opinion will already have been formed about these abilities before reaching the mental state examination. Formal tests add to this information, and can provide a semi-quantitative indication of changes between occasions. A useful first test is '*serial sevens*': the patient is asked to subtract 7 from 100 and then to keep subtracting 7 from the remainder until the resulting number is less than 7. The time taken to do this is recorded, together with the number of errors. If poor performance seems to be due to lack of skill in arithmetic, the patient should be asked to do a simpler subtraction, or to state the months of the year in reverse order.

Memory

While taking the history the interviewer should compare the patient's account of past events with those of any other informants, and be alert for gaps or inconsistencies. If memory is impaired, any evidence of confabulation (see page 355) should be noted. During the mental state examination, tests are given of short-term, recent, and remote memory. Since none of these is wholly satisfactory, the results should be assessed alongside other information about memory and, if there is any doubt, supplemented by standardized psychological tests. Objective evidence of memory impairment and its impact on normal activities (e.g. shopping, dressing) is also essential.

Short-term memory can be assessed by asking the patient to memorize a name and a simple address, to repeat it immediately (to make sure that it has been registered correctly), and to retain it. The interview continues on other topics for 5 minutes before recall is tested.

A healthy person of average intelligence should make only minor errors. If recall is imperfect, memory can be prompted (e.g. by saying '35, Juniper . . .' and the patient may then recall 'Street').

Memory for recent events can be assessed by asking about news items from the last few days.

Remote memory can be assessed by asking the patient to recall personal events or well-known items of news from former years. Personal items could be the birth dates of children or the names of grandchildren (provided these are known to the interviewer), and news items could be the names of well-known former political leaders. Awareness of the sequence of events is as important as the recall of individual items.

The reader is again referred to Chapter 14 for detailed assessment of cognitive functioning.

Insight

A note that merely records 'insight present' or 'no insight' is of little value. Instead the interviewer should enquire about the different aspects of insight discussed on page 20. This includes the patient's appraisal of their difficulties and prospects, and whether they ascribe them to illness or to some other cause (e.g. persecution). If the patient recognizes that they are ill, do they think that the illness is physical or mental, and do they think that they need any treatment? If so, what are their views on medication, psychotherapy, or admission, as appropriate? The interviewer should also find out whether the patient thinks that stressful life experiences or their own actions have played a part in causing their illness. The patient's views on these matters are a guide to their likely collaboration with treatment.

Other components of psychiatric assessment

Although the psychiatric history and mental state examination are the main parts of the psychiatric assessment, several other elements may also be necessary as part of the 'work-up' of a patient. This section does not cover more specialized aspects of assessment (e.g. the use of rating scales; see below) or those not directly linked to diagnosis or initial management (e.g. assessment for psychotherapy).

Physical examination

Physical examination provides three kinds of information in the assessment.

- It may reveal diagnostically useful signs (e.g. a goitre or absent reflexes), and it is therefore particularly important in the diagnosis or exclusion of organic disorders (see Chapter 14). Neurological (including cerebrovascular) and endocrine systems most commonly require detailed examination, although other systems should not be neglected. The reader should consult a relevant textbook (e.g. Kaufman and Milstein, 2017) if instruction is required in these aspects of clinical practice.

- Psychotropic drugs may produce physical side-effects, which need to be identified or measured (e.g. hypertension, parkinsonism, or a rash).

- The patient's general health, nutritional status, and self-care may all be affected by psychiatric disorders.

For these reasons, a physical examination is an integral part of the psychiatric assessment. In practice, however, the extent of the physical examination, and the medical responsibility for it, vary. For example, in the United Kingdom, the general practitioner may have recently carried out an appropriate physical examination, and hence the latter is unnecessary for most patients seen in outpatient clinic or the community. In the case of inpatients, the psychiatrist is generally responsible for their physical as well as their mental health, and every newly admitted patient should have a full physical examination. Whatever the circumstances, the psychiatrist should decide what physical examination is relevant, and either carry it out themselves or ensure that this is or has been done by another doctor. Discussion with a neurologist or other physician is appropriate if the initial examination reveals equivocal or complex findings, or if a second opinion is sought. In some cases, more detailed assessment of higher neurological functions is required, as in the neuropsychiatric examination, which is summarized in Box 3.6. This may be a prelude to formal neuropsychological or neurological assessment.

Laboratory and other investigations

These vary according to the nature of the differential diagnosis, the treatments that are being given, the patient's general health, and the resources available. At one extreme, no investigations may be necessary. At the other, extensive brain imaging, genetic testing, and biochemical screening may be needed—for example, if there is a strong suspicion of a treatable organic disorder, a familial dementia, or learning disability. There is no one set of routine investigations that is applicable to every case although, by convention, routine blood tests (full blood count, renal, liver, and thyroid function) are usually carried out on admission to hospital.

Investigations are discussed further in the chapters on individual syndromes and drug treatments.

Psychological assessment

Clinical psychologists and psychological testing can contribute to psychiatric assessment in several ways. However, they are not required in most cases, and their availability is increasingly limited in many settings. We therefore only introduce the topic briefly here,

illustrating the main forms and roles of psychological assessment. For further information, see Powell (2009).

Neuropsychological assessment

There are many psychometric tests available that measure different aspects of neuropsychological performance, ranging from overall intelligence to specific domains of memory, speed of processing, or tests that putatively assess functioning of a particular part of the brain (Lezak *et al.*, 2012). Neuropsychological testing in psychiatry is primarily used in the following areas (Adams and Grant, 2009):

- In learning disability, where IQ defines the severity of the condition.
- In dementia, where tests measure the severity and domains of cognitive impairment.
- If a decline in performance from premorbid abilities is suspected. In this instance, a discrepancy may be seen between verbal and performance IQ.
- To monitor the progress of neuropsychological deficits during the course of illness, by repeated administration of tests.
- To reveal deficits that may be subtle and neglected clinically, but which may be functionally important. For example, in schizophrenia there are persistent impairments in specific domains of memory and attention, and these predict poor outcome (see Chapter 11).
- If an organic cause of psychiatric disorder is suspected, he profile of test results may suggest the location of the lesion. However, this use of neuropsychological testing to localize brain lesions has largely been replaced by neuroimaging.

Cognitive assessment

The term 'cognitive' is sometimes used interchangeably with the term 'neuropsychological'. In the present context, however, cognitive assessment refers to the assessment of a patient's cognitions (thoughts), assumptions, and patterns of thinking. It is used to determine the suitability for, and focus of, cognitive therapy (see Chapter 24).

Behavioural assessment

Observations and ratings of behaviour are useful in everyday clinical practice, especially for inpatients. When no ready-made rating scale is available, ad hoc ratings can be devised. For example, a scale could be devised for the nurses to show how much of the time a patient with depression was active and occupied.

This could be a five-point scale, in which the criteria for each rating refer to behaviour (e.g. playing cards or talking to other people) relevant to the individual patient. As well as providing baseline information, the scale could also help to monitor progress and response to treatment.

Behavioural assessment is also used to evaluate the components of a patient's disorder—for example, in a phobia, the elements of anticipatory anxiety, avoidance, and coping strategies, and their relationship to stimuli in the environment (e.g. heights), more general circumstances (e.g. crowded places), or internal cues (e.g. awareness of heart action). Behavioural assessment is a necessary preliminary to behaviour therapy (see page 683).

Personality assessment

In the past, detailed personality testing, including the use of 'projective' tests such as the Rorschach test, was often part of psychiatric assessment. These tests are now rarely used in psychiatry, as they do not measure aspects of personality that are most relevant to psychiatric disorder, and they have not been shown to be valid predictors of diagnosis or outcome. Instead, personality is assessed descriptively as part of the history (described above), supplemented for research purposes with schedules for diagnosing personality disorders (see Chapter 15).

Risk assessment

Risk assessment is an essential part of psychiatric assessment. Risk in this context refers to risk of harm to others (through violence or neglect) and risk to self (through suicide, deliberate self-harm, or neglect). A failure to carry out and clearly document a risk assessment, and the resulting risk management plan, is a common criticism of enquiries that follow homicides and suicides involving psychiatric patients. All assessments, however brief, should include assessment of risk, and include a statement about the presence and magnitude of any acute risks in the record of the assessment.

Risk to self is covered in Chapter 21. Here we consider assessment of the risk of violence to others. Three kinds of information are used to assess such risks—personal factors, factors related to illness, and factors in the mental state. These factors are summarized in Box 3.7, with the most important ones in each category indicated by means of an asterisk. Further information on

risk assessment, in the context of forensic psychiatry, can be found in Chapter 18.

A history of violence is the best predictor of future violence. Therefore it is important to seek full information on this not only by questioning the patient but, in appropriate cases, from additional sources, including relatives and close acquaintances, previous medical and social services records, and in certain cases the police. Antisocial, impulsive, or irritable features in the personality are a further risk factor. Social circumstances at the time of any previous episodes of violence may reveal provoking factors, and should be compared with the patient's current situation (see below). A parental history of violence, social isolation, and a recent life crisis also increase the risk. Among the illness factors, psychotic disorder and drug or alcohol misuse are important, and the combination of psychosis, substance misuse, and personality disorder is associated with the highest risk of violence.

The mental state factors in Box 3.7 require careful consideration. Thoughts of violence to others are very important, especially if they are concerned with a specific person to whom the patient has access. The entry concerning suicidal ideas refers to the occasional killing, usually of family members, by a patient with severe (usually psychotic) depression. Features of morbid jealousy and other delusional disorders may pose specific risks of harm against a perceived aggressor or rival (see page 307).

Situational factors are extremely important. Actual or perceived confrontational behaviour towards the patient by others may trigger violence, as may a return to situations in which violence has been expressed in the past. Enquiries should always be made about the availability of weapons.

Clinical experience and common sense have to be used to combine the risk factors into an overall assessment. Risk assessment schedules have been developed, but they cannot replace thorough and repeated clinical assessment (Fazel *et al.*, 2011). The assessment of risk should be shared among the members of the team treating the patient or, if the patient is in individual treatment, it may need to be discussed with a colleague. In certain circumstances the assessment may need to be made known to an individual at risk. Risk assessments should be reviewed regularly, combining information from the members of the clinical team. For further information, see Mullen and Ogloff (2009).

Although risk assessment is essential, and can be of value in a number of respects (Abderhalden *et al.*, 2008),

Box 3.7 Risk factors for harm to others

Personal factors

Previous violence to others*

Antisocial, impulsive, or irritable
personality traits

Male and young

Recent life crisis

Poor social network

Divorced or separated

Unemployed

Social instability

Parent with history of violence

Illness-related factors

Pychotic symptoms*

Substance abuse*

Treatment-resistant

Poor compliance with treatment

Stopped medication recently

Factors in the mental state

Irritability, hostility, anger

Suspiciousness

Thoughts of violence towards others

Threats to people to whom patient has access*

Planning of violence*

Persecutory delusions

Delusions of jealousy

Delusions of influence

Hallucinations commanding violence to others

Suicidal ideas with severe depression

Clouding of consciousness

Lack of insight about illness

Situational factors

Confrontation and provocation by others

Situations associated with previous violence

Ready availability of weapons*

Asterisks denote the most important factors in each category.

it is also important to put it in context. First, the vast majority of psychiatric patients pose no risk to others, and are more likely to be the victims than the perpetrators of violence. The assumption that all patients with severe mental illness, especially schizophrenia, are potentially violent, is unwarranted and contributes to the stigma that is attached to all psychiatric patients. Secondly, as the physicist Niels Bohr said, 'Prediction is very difficult, especially about the future.' Even a complete risk assessment provides only a weak guide to future harm to others. Many such acts are carried out by people with no past history of violence, and many of those who have multiple risk factors will never commit further acts of violence (Szmukler, 2001; Fazel *et al.*, 2011c).

Assessment of needs

For patients with severe or enduring mental illness, particularly psychosis, it is important to focus on their needs in the broadest sense (e.g. physical health, hygiene, social isolation, domestic skills, etc.). The concern arises from findings that such needs are often substantial, and are neither well recognized nor met. Although the conceptual status of needs is not as straightforward as is often implied, interest in its measurement is well established. The Camberwell Assessment of Need scale is widely used. This rates 22 domains as absent, present, or modified, has versions for different age and patient groups (e.g. those with learning disability), and is available in several languages (Phelan *et al.*, 1995).

Special kinds of psychiatric assessment

So far this chapter has been concerned with the complete psychiatric assessment as carried out by psychiatrists on patients who are being seen in a psychiatric setting, and for whom sufficient time is available. However, most

assessments do not meet all of these criteria. Many are conducted by non-specialists in non-psychiatric settings, with limited time and imperfect surroundings. Nevertheless, a well-focused interview can often yield a reliable diagnosis and plan of action in a surprisingly short time. This section considers how psychiatric assessment and interviewing are modified in these circumstances.

Interviews in an emergency

In an emergency, the interview has to be brief, focused on the key issues, and effective in leading to a provisional diagnosis and a plan of immediate action. These assessments generally involve acutely distressed or disturbed patients, and often take place in difficult settings, such as a police station or medical ward. The diagnoses that are usually in question are the psychoses (schizophrenia, mania, drug-induced), and delirium and other organic brain disorders. Throughout, the interviewer should consider which questions need to be answered at the time and which can be deferred. The most important issues are those that impact on immediate management decisions. The latter are likely to include whether the patient should be detained, whether laboratory investigations are indicated, whether medication should be given, and whether acute medical treatment is also required.

Because the assessment may be limited by the patient's ability or willingness to participate fully, seek out all available information before commencing the interview. For example, ask whoever is accompanying the person what they know about the patient and the recent events. The patient's belongings may reveal evidence of prior illness or medication. If the patient has a past psychiatric history, strenuous efforts should be made to obtain their case notes or to contact a professional involved in their care. The safety of the patient and those around them must also be actively considered when planning the nature and location of the interview.

An emergency assessment should, wherever possible, include the following core information:

- The presenting problem in terms of symptoms or behaviours, together with their onset, course, and present severity.
- Other relevant symptoms, together with their onset, course, and severity.
- History of psychiatric or medical disorder.
- Current medication.
- Use of alcohol and drugs.
- Recent stressful circumstances and possible precipitants.
- Social circumstances, and the possibilities of support.

- Risk assessment, including the immediate risks of harm to self and others.

Interviews in general practice

In general practice, many presentations are with psychiatric disorders, notably depression and anxiety disorders, as well as substance misuse and somatoform disorders. Such cases commonly present with physical complaints (e.g. chronic pain, fatigue), and the doctor needs to be aware of the possibility that the symptoms reflect an underlying psychiatric disorder. The interplay of physical and psychological factors is emphasized by the finding that general practitioners who diagnose psychiatric disorder accurately, as compared with a standard assessment, have a good knowledge of general medicine (Goldberg and Huxley, 1980). Other patients present in primary care with an explicit psychological complaint (e.g. low mood, panic attacks).

Whether the presentation is physical or psychological, it is a challenge to undertake an effective psychiatric assessment, given the very limited time that is usually available. There are two components to achieving this goal. First, the chances of detecting psychiatric disorder can be increased by attending to the way that the interview is conducted—for example, by being alert to cues in the patient's history, appearance, and behaviour. Secondly, screening questions can be used that detect the common disorders and identify areas that may require more detailed assessment (see Table 3.1).

Goldberg and Huxley (1980) reported the first substantive work in this field, and described how the assessment of a patient in general practice whose complaint may have a psychological cause should cover four areas:

- *General psychological adjustment*: fatigue, irritability, poor concentration, and the feeling of being under stress.
- *Anxiety and worries:* physical symptoms of anxiety and tension, phobias, and persistent worrying thoughts.
- *Symptoms of depression:* persistent depressive mood, tearfulness, crying, hopelessness, self-blame, thoughts that life is unbearable, ideas about suicide, early-morning waking, diurnal mood variation, weight loss, and loss of libido.
- *The psychological context (i.e. the patient's personality and circumstances)*: although often known to the general practitioner from previous contacts, this should be reviewed and brought up to date.

Subsequently, more formalized sets of screening questions for psychiatric disorders were developed which are suitable for brief interviews in primary care, and which focus on the disorders that are commonly encountered in this setting. The questions in Table 3.1 are adapted from Spitzer *et al.* (1994).

If the interview is conducted with psychological issues in mind, and screening questions are used appropriately, then it should be possible to identify many psychiatric disorders in the 10 to 15 minutes that are available in primary care. A preliminary plan can be made, and a further appointment arranged to evaluate the diagnosis and discuss management in more detail.

Interviews in a general hospital

Similar considerations apply to interviews that are conducted in a general medical setting, such as an accident and emergency department or a medical ward (Segal and Ranjith, 2016). In these situations, particular attention again needs to be given to physical symptoms and the possibility of somatoform disorder, and to the assessment of suicidal risk. Delirium and the possibility of other organic disorders is also a common reason for a psychiatric consultation involving a medical or surgical inpatient, and hence a focused assessment of cognitive function is often required.

Interviews in the patient's home

Many services now try to assess a significant proportion of patients at home, particularly in the case of severely ill and disorganized patients who would otherwise fail to attend for assessment. Such a visit often throws new light on the patient's home life and gives a more realistic evaluation of the relationship between family members. Home visits are especially important in the assessment of elderly patients for whom psychiatric and physical difficulties frequently coexist. Before arranging a visit the psychiatrist should, if possible, talk to the general practitioner, who often has first-hand knowledge of the patient and their family. The safety of the interviewer should always be considered before embarking on a domiciliary visit. The interviewer should ensure that another member of the team is aware of the location and time of the visit. If there is any concern about potential risk, a joint assessment should be made.

Interviews with the family

In child and adolescent psychiatry in particular, an interview is usually conducted with several family members together to find out their attitudes to the patient and the illness, and the nature of any conflicts within the family (see Chapter 16). The interviewer should remember that the family has usually tried to help the patient but failed, and may be feeling demoralized, frustrated, or guilty, so they should be careful not to add to these feelings.

The interviewer should ask the following questions:

- How has the illness affected family life, and how has the family tried to cope?
- How do different members of the family perceive the illness and its origins?
- Are the family members willing to try new ways of helping the patient?

For further information about family interviews, see Goldberg (1997). Family interviewing in the context of family therapy is covered in Chapter 16.

Table 3.1 Brief screening questions for psychiatric disorders

During the past month	Screening for
1. Have you felt low in spirits?	Depression
2. Do you enjoy things less than you usually do?	Depression
3. Have you been feeling generally anxious?	Neurosis (anxiety)
4. Are you worried about your health or other specific things?	Neurosis (health anxiety)
5. Has your eating felt out of control?	Eating disorder
6. Do you drink alcohol? If so, ask the FAST or CAGE questions*	Alcohol problem
7. Present three items and ask patient to recall them after 2 minutes	Dementia/delirium

* FAST and CAGE each consist of four questions designed to detect alcohol misuse (see Chapter 20.

Patient characteristics that may affect the interview

Interviews can prove difficult for a variety of reasons. Many of these reflect the situation (e.g. noisy surroundings, lack of time) or interviewer characteristics (e.g. inexperience, tiredness). However, other problems arise from the characteristics of the patient, and these are outlined here. Remember that such problems can be diagnostically useful—for example, a patient may be monosyllabic because of depression, and a disturbed patient may have delirium.

Anxious patients

Although anxiety may be part of the patient's disorder, it may also relate to the interview. If the person seems unduly anxious, the interviewer can say that many people feel anxious when they first take part in a psychiatric interview, and then go on to explore the patient's concerns.

Taciturn patients

Taciturn patients can be encouraged to speak more freely if the interviewer shows non-verbal expressions of concern (e.g. leaning forward a little in the chair with an expression of interest), in addition to verbal expressions that are part of any good interview.

Garrulous patients

It is not easy to curb an over-talkative patient. If efforts to focus the interview are unsuccessful, the interviewer should wait for a natural break in the flow of speech and then explain that, because time is limited, they will need to interrupt from time to time to help the patient to keep focused on the issues that are important for planning treatment. If this proposal is made tactfully, most garrulous patients will accept it.

Overactive patients

Some patients are so active and restless that systematic questioning about their mental state is difficult. The interviewer then has to limit their questions to a few that seem particularly important, and concentrate on observing the patient's behaviour. However, if the patient is being seen in an emergency, some of their overactivity may be a reaction to other people's attempts to restrain them. In such cases a quiet but confident approach by

the interviewer may calm the patient enough to allow more adequate examination.

Confused patients

When the patient gives a history in a muddled way, or appears perplexed, the interviewer should test cognitive functions early in the interview. If there is evidence of impaired cognition or consciousness, the interviewer should try to orientate and reassure the patient, before starting the interview again in a simplified form. In such cases every effort should be made to interview another informant.

Uncooperative or 'difficult' patients

Some patients are reluctant to be interviewed and have come at the insistence of a third party (e.g. their partner). If the patient seems unwilling to collaborate, the interviewer should talk over the circumstances of the referral, and try to persuade them that the interview will be in their own interests. Remember that lack of cooperation may occur because the patient does not realize that they are ill (e.g. some patients with delirium, or with psychosis). In such cases it may be necessary to interview an informant before returning to the patient.

Some patients (or, in the case of a child, their parents) try to dominate the interview, while others adopt an unduly friendly approach that threatens to convert the interview into a social conversation. In either case, the interviewer should explain why he needs to guide the patient towards relevant issues. In the longer term, developing a manner which is confident and assertive, but not domineering, helps to avoid such problems.

Unresponsive patients

If the patient is mute or stuporous, it is essential to interview an informant who can describe the onset and course of the condition. With regard to the mental state, the interviewer can only observe behaviour, but this can be informative. Because some stuporous patients change rapidly from inactivity to violent overactivity, it is wise to have help available when seeing such a patient.

Before deciding that a patient is mute, the interviewer should allow adequate time for reply, and try several topics. If the patient still fails to respond, attempt to persuade them to communicate in writing. Apart from observations of behaviour, the interviewer should note whether the patient's eyes are open or closed. If they are open, note whether they follow objects, move apparently without purpose, or are fixed. If the eyes are closed, find out whether the patient opens them on request and, if not, whether attempts at opening them are resisted. A physical examination, including neurological assessment, is essential in all such cases. In addition, certain signs that are found in catatonia should be sought (see page 16).

Patients with learning disability

When interviewing people with learning disability, certain points should receive particular attention. Questions should be brief and worded in a simple way. It may be difficult to avoid closed questions, but if they are used the answers should be checked. For example, if the question 'Are you sad?' is answered 'Yes', the question 'Are you happy?' should not be answered in the same way. People with learning disability may have difficulty in timing the onset of symptoms or describing their sequence, and to obtain this and other information it is important to interview an informant.

For further discussion of the assessment of patients with learning disability, see Chapter 17.

Patients from another culture

The interviewer may be unfamiliar with the patient's culture and may find it more difficult to ascertain the significance of the patient's manner and appearance.

Certain factors may have different implications for a patient from another culture to those that they would have in the interviewer's culture. The stigma of mental illness may be greater. Priorities within the family may be different, with the wellbeing of the family outweighing that of its individual members. Emotional disorder may be experienced more in terms of physical symptoms than of mental ones. Expectations and fears about treatment may be based on knowledge of health services in the country of origin. Behaviours that suggest illness in

one culture may be socially sanctioned ways of expressing distress in others (e.g. displays of extreme emotion). Ideas about causation may differ, an extreme example being that distress may be ascribed to the actions of evil spirits. It may be particularly difficult to decide whether strongly held ideas are delusional or normal within the culture or subculture. The influence of cultural differences on diagnosis and classification was discussed on page 32.

Patients who do not speak the same language as the interviewer

If the patient and interviewer do not speak the same language, it will need to be decided who the best choice of interpreter is. There are advantages to a family member interpreting, as they are often trusted by the patient and can potentially help the interviewer understand some of the complexities of a different cultural context. However, there are disadvantages, including incorrect translations and possible reluctance of the interviewee to share sensitive information with their relative. If an official interpreter is used, it is valuable if they are also a health care professional as they can then assist in the assessment itself. Whatever interpreter is used, bear in mind gender issues; in particular, women from paternalistic cultures or from some religious groups may be reluctant to describe personal matters to a male interviewer.

The presence of a third person and the process of translation affect the interview and lengthen it considerably. It may therefore be necessary to focus on the essential topics in a first assessment, and complete the process in a second interview.

Children and the elderly

Psychiatric assessment of children and adolescents is described in Chapter 16 and discussed by Bostic and Martin (2009). Assessment in elderly patients is described in Chapter 19 and by Jacoby (2009).

Integrating and evaluating the information

So far this account of assessment has been largely about data gathering. The following section explains how the facts that emerge are evaluated and integrated with

knowledge of psychiatry to arrive at a diagnosis, provide prognostic information, and determine treatment decisions. We emphasize again that, in practice, information is evaluated as it is collected, with hypotheses being tested as they arise during the assessment. Clearly, this skill takes time to learn and also requires a solid foundation of psychiatric knowledge.

Drawing conclusions and making decisions

The areas in which an opinion must be formed, or a decision made, are listed in Box 3.8. It may also be useful to think in terms of a set of rhetorical questions that need to be answered:

- What is the diagnosis?
- What are the effects on the patient's life?
- Are there immediate risks that need to be managed?
- What are the patient's current circumstances?
- Does the patient have any dependants?
- Why has the disorder occurred?
- What treatment is indicated?
- What is the prognosis?
- What other information is needed to answer these questions?
- What does the patient need and want to know?

What is the diagnosis?

The first step is to make a diagnosis using information about the symptoms and signs that have been obtained

---

> #### Box 3.8 Topics to be evaluated in a psychiatric assessment
>
> The patient's problem and its consequences
> - Diagnosis
> - Impact on self and others (dysfunction)
> - Risk to self and others
> - Effects on others
>
> The patient and their circumstances
> - Personal history
> - Current circumstances
> - Personality
>
> Aetiology
>
> The response to the patient's problem
> - Treatment
> - Prognosis
>
> The patient's understanding of the above

---

from the history and mental state examination and, in relevant cases, from the physical examination and any investigations that have been performed. This information is then used to make a diagnosis based upon knowledge of psychiatric classification and the criteria for each diagnostic category. Sometimes a diagnosis has to be provisional, or several diagnostic possibilities entertained, until further information becomes available. The diagnosis of specific psychiatric disorders is discussed in subsequent chapters; here we are concerned with the general approach to assessment. Diagnosis is accompanied by an assessment of the severity of the disorder to determine whether it is mild, moderate, or severe. Remember that the outcome of some assessments is that the patient does not have evidence of any psychiatric disorder.

What are the effects on the patient's life?

When patients describe their problems, they will include both symptoms and other matters. A key purpose of the assessment is to identify and characterize the psychopathology, as it is these that determine which disorder will be diagnosed. However, it is also necessary to enquire about the effects that the patient's symptoms are having on their life, in part since evidence of impaired functioning is relevant to, or an essential part of, most diagnoses. It is therefore helpful to ascertain the patient's usual level of functioning and how far the current state differs from it.

Are there immediate risks that need to be managed?

As we have discussed, risk assessment is a core part of the psychiatric assessment. Once any risks have been identified, they need to be managed. For example, if the patient is at risk of self-neglect or self-harm, this will influence whether compulsory admission is necessary. If a risk of harm to another party has been identified, that individual may need to be warned. Risk management is covered in Chapter 18.

What are the patient's current circumstances?

Knowledge of the patient's accommodation, finances, interests, values, and relationships may influence both management and prognosis. For example, a homeless person will require a different care package from a patient with the same disorder who has a stable home and a carer. The current circumstances may also act as maintaining factors for the disorder, and therefore be a target for intervention.

If the patient has children or other dependants, their welfare must be taken into account. If necessary, more information should be obtained, and a plan developed, to ensure that this duty of care can be discharged.

Why has the disorder occurred?

Aetiology is discussed in Chapter 5. Here we are concerned with how aetiological factors are applied to the individual patient. A useful approach is a chronological one, with causes being divided into those that are *predisposing, precipitating,* and *perpetuating*. Predisposing factors may be genetic or related to temperament, or to damage to the brain in early life. Precipitating factors are often stressful life events. Perpetuating (maintaining) factors may be continuing stressors or be related to the way that the patient attempts to cope with stressors (e.g. avoiding anxiety-provoking situations, misusing alcohol). Perpetuating factors are highly relevant to treatment. Intersecting this chronological approach to causation, one can divide the causal factors into *biological, psychological, and social*.

A comment about personality is appropriate here. Clear appreciation of a patient's personality is part of the full understanding of their life history and their psychiatric disorder. For this reason we emphasize the collection of sufficient and reliable information about personality during the assessment. As well as aiding the aetiological formulation, this knowledge is useful when planning management and predicting outcome. For example, comorbid personality disorder worsens the prognosis of many conditions, and may also influence decisions about psychological treatment.

What treatment is indicated?

A key decision to be made is what, if any, treatment the patient requires. If treatment is indicated, the options should be discussed with the patient, and the evidence for each possible treatment presented in terms of efficacy, side-effects, etc. These issues are discussed in later chapters, especially Chapters 24 and 25.

What is the prognosis?

The prognosis depends primarily on the disorder concerned. It also depends on the individual characteristics of the patient (e.g. their age, severity of symptoms, comorbid conditions, etc.). Not all of this information may be available after an initial assessment. However, it is usually possible to make a cautious prediction about the short-term outcome at this stage, and most patients will expect and appreciate this. The patient can be told that more accurate and longer-term prognostic judgements will be possible as further information is obtained, and the course of the disorder is followed over subsequent weeks and months.

What other information is needed to answer these questions?

For many patients, assessment is not complete after one interview. Assessment should be viewed as an iterative process in which opinions and conclusions undergo continuing review (both within the initial interview and thereafter), as further information about the patient and their illness is obtained. For descriptive purposes, this chapter focuses on the diagnostic purpose of assessment, but in practice there is no firm distinction between this and the other goals of assessment (e.g. to assess risk, or response to treatment). Each interaction between the psychiatrist and the patient contains a mixture of assessment, evaluation, review, and decision-making. Assessment, and its revision, is a process that continues throughout treatment and follow-up.

What does the patient need and want to know?

The guiding principle is that, as a rule, a patient (and their carer) should be given as much information as possible about the diagnosis, and the likely prognosis and presumed causation, and should be fully involved in, and aware of, all decisions that affect them. The practical implications are introduced below, and are discussed in later chapters with regard to specific disorders and treatments.

Other issues that affect how the information is evaluated

Disease and illness

These concepts were introduced in Chapter 2, but a brief mention is required here. *Illness* refers to a patient's experience, and *disease* refers to the pathological cause of this experience. Patients can be diseased without feeling ill, or feel ill without having an identifiable disease. In general medicine, patients tell doctors about their experience of illness, and doctors seek to discover the disease that is causing the illness, as this will guide treatment. Patients and their relatives also want to find a cause and a treatment for their illness, but they do not always understand how a medical diagnosis helps in finding these. Psychiatrists also search for disease as a cause of illness, but should always look for other causes, too. The patient's experience can be understood sometimes as an extreme variation from the norm, sometimes as a reaction to circumstances, and sometimes as a combination of both. Other mental health professionals may emphasize one or other of these factors to a greater extent, depending on their background. For example, psychologists focus on variation from the norm, whereas social workers focus on the role of reaction to circumstances and the place of the patient in a family and social context. These differences in emphasis can lead to apparent disagreements during multidisciplinary assessment. It is important that psychiatrists are aware of this possibility, so that they can help to integrate the social, psychological, and medical approaches, and thereby use the various skills of the multidisciplinary team to best help the patient.

Evaluations by experienced psychiatrists

Throughout this chapter, a systematic and logical approach to assessment has been advocated, in which information is collected carefully and eliciting of symptoms and signs forms the basis of diagnosis. Anyone new to psychiatry should follow this approach closely until they have mastered the process and have a good grounding of psychiatric knowledge. However, studies show that experienced psychiatrists actually carry out assessments rather differently. They make rapid diagnoses, often within the first few minutes of the interview, that presumably reflect the predictive power of the patient's initial appearance, behaviour, and utterances (Gauron and Dickinson, 1966; Kendell, 1975). The psychiatrist may not realize the cues and clues that they are using to form these diagnostic judgements. Schwartz and Wiggins (1987) called this process *typification*. The rest of the interview then functions primarily to confirm and refine this diagnostic opinion. Regardless of their seniority and experience, the interviewer should always ensure that they have not come to premature conclusions about a case, causing them to fail to gather necessary information, to interpret findings in a biased way, or to disregard contrary evidence.

Recording and communicating information

Having completed the assessment, it is necessary to record and communicate your understanding of the patient, their disorder, and its management. These records and communications take a variety of forms (e.g. written, verbal, electronic), and differ according to their source, purpose, and intended recipients. As with assessment itself, it is helpful to learn the 'traditional' and relatively detailed formats for communicating information (e.g. case summaries and formulations), while also appreciating that in practice many other—and briefer—modes of communication are the norm. Regardless of format, all communications should follow certain basic principles.

- Information should be presented clearly and concisely. Include important negatives (e.g. 'He is not suicidal'). Avoid repetition of information that is already known to the recipient. Use subheadings to highlight key points (e.g. 'Diagnosis: . ...', 'Current medication: . ...', 'Acute risks: . ....').
- In many countries, patients are entitled to read what is written about them. This information may also be used for legal purposes. In some countries, including the UK, it is now expected that patients are copied into all correspondence between doctors that concerns them, unless there is a compelling reason not to do so or unless they decline the offer. Ensure that all information is accurate, and that any opinions or inferences you make are reasonable, and avoid unwarranted or unnecessarily personal comments. It is sometimes better to communicate verbally with the doctor or other health professional to expand on some details of the case.
- All communications should be kept confidential.

Here we consider a range of ways in which information is recorded and shared—within the psychiatric team, and between the psychiatrist and other doctors, but first, between the psychiatrist and the patient.

Discussing the diagnosis and management plan with the patient

When discussing the conclusions from your assessment with the patient, and with their relatives, it may be useful to begin by briefly summarizing the key points for them. This helps to ensure that you have understood the history correctly and have not omitted anything which in their opinion is significant. This process is also helpful in that it demonstrates your engagement and empathy with the patient, and sets the scene for discussion about the diagnosis and how you propose to proceed.

When introducing the diagnosis, do not use medical terms without explaining them. The patient may misunderstand their meaning or make incorrect assumptions about their implications. Explain the significance of the diagnosis in terms of cause, prognosis, and treatment options—and any diagnostic uncertainty that remains.

When discussing the proposed plan of management, it is useful to begin by asking what treatment the patient has been expecting, and whether they have strong views—for example, with regard to the use of medication. Whether drug treatment or psychological treatment is planned, there are several relevant issues to raise and discuss (see Chapters 24 and 25). It is important to set aside enough time for this explanation during the interview, as it is likely to improve concordance with the treatment plan. If, after they have been given a full explanation, the patient refuses to accept part of the plan, the interviewer should document this, and try to negotiate an acceptable alternative.

Box 3.9 summarizes the points that should be considered when communicating with patients and their relatives. In the NHS in the UK, this information will usually be recorded on a pro forma as part of the Care Programme Approach (CPA) for any patients who require either prolonged or complex secondary care (see Chapter 26).

The importance of case notes

Good case records, whatever their format, are important in every branch of medicine. In psychiatry they are vital because a large amount of information has to be collected from a variety of sources. It is important to summarize the information in a way that allows essential points to be grasped readily by someone new to the case, especially a colleague who has been called to deal with an emergency. Case notes are not just an aide-mémoire for the writer—they are important for others concerned with the patient. They are also of medicolegal importance. If a psychiatrist is called upon to justify their actions after a serious untoward incident, after a complaint has been made, or in court, he or she will be greatly assisted by notes which are comprehensive but concise, well organized, and legible. Indeed, imagining being in a situation of this kind may help the psychiatrist to judge what constitutes appropriate record-keeping, not just for case notes but for other forms of communication.

Inpatient notes

Admission notes

When a patient is admitted to hospital urgently, the doctor often has only limited time available. The admission note should contain at least the following:

Box 3.9 Communicating with patients and relatives

The diagnosis

- What is the diagnosis? If uncertain, what are the main possibilities?
- What further information or investigations are required?
- What are the implications of the diagnosis for this patient?
- What may have caused the condition?

The care plan

- What is the plan, and how will it help the patient and their family?
- Are there any legal powers to be used? If so, why, and what is their effect?
- What needs to be communicated about medication or psychological treatments?

Who does what?

- What is the role of the psychiatrist, and how often will they see the patient?
- Who is the key worker and what will they do?
- What is the role of the other members of the psychiatric team?
- What is the role of the general practitioner?
- What can the family (or other carers) do to help?

Emergencies

- What are the likely acute risks, and how might they be avoided?
- Are there possible early warning signs?
- Who should be approached in an emergency, and how can they be contacted?

- The reasons for admission.
- Any information that is required for a decision about provisional diagnosis and immediate treatment. This may include a physical examination and laboratory investigations.
- Any other relevant information that will not be available later, such as details of the mental state on admission (and prior to medication), and information from any informant who may not be available again.

If there is time, a systematic history can be added. However, inexperienced interviewers sometimes spend too much time on details that are not essential to the immediate decisions, while failing to record details of the mental state that may be transitory and yet of great importance in diagnosis. The rest of the assessment can always be completed over the next few days. The admission note should end with a brief plan of immediate management, which has been agreed with the senior nurses caring for the patient at the time.

Continuation (progress) notes

Continuation notes for both inpatients and patients in the community need to be succinct, clear, and regularly updated, and to contain specific information if they are to be of value. Instead of recording merely that the patient feels better or is behaving more normally, record in what ways they feel better (e.g. less preoccupied with thoughts of suicide). The notes should also record treatments, including both medication and other interventions, accompanied by a brief explanation of the rationale for the treatment, and the temporal relationship between a change in treatment (e.g. dose of drug) and change in clinical state. A note should be made of any information or advice given by the doctor to the patient or their relatives. This should be sufficient to make it clear whether the patient was appropriately informed when consenting to any new treatment.

Observations of progress are made not only by psychiatrists but also by nurses, occupational therapists, clinical psychologists, and social workers. These other professionals may also keep separate notes, but it is desirable that important items of information are written in the medical record. A note should also be kept of formal discussions between members of the team.

Discharge notes

It is particularly important to set out clearly the plans made for the patient's further care on discharge from hospital, including the identity of the key worker, and how the patient or their carer can contact the team in an emergency. These arrangements are formalized in the UK in the CPA (see above and Chapter 26), in part because it is recognized that the days after discharge are a particularly high-risk period for suicide. A phone call to the patient's general practitioner is desirable if there are any acute concerns about the patient's welfare, or if there is any delay anticipated in production of the discharge letter or case summary. A statement of the diagnosis at the time of discharge is also important, since it may have changed since admission.

Case summaries

Case summaries are generally used for inpatients, but they are valuable for all patients with complex, long-standing, or recurrent disorders. In the inpatient setting they are ideally written in two parts, the first part being written soon after admission, to record the initial presentation, and the second part being written at discharge, filling in the subsequent progress. In practice, however, a single summary covering all of the salient aspects of the case is often produced, not least since inpatient stays are generally much shorter than was the case in the past.

Summaries should be brief but comprehensive, written in telegraphic style using a standard format, to help other people to find particular items of information. A completed summary should seldom need to be any longer than 1–1.5 typewritten pages. An example is given in Box 3.10. The completed summary will provide a valuable record should the patient become ill again, especially if they are under the care of a different team.

Some of the items in the summary call for comment.

- The reason for referral should state the problem rather than anticipate the diagnosis—for example, 'found wandering at night in an agitated state, shouting about the devil', rather than 'schizophrenia.'
- The description of personality is important. The writer should strive to find words and phrases that characterize the person in a non-judgemental way.
- Unless an abnormality has been found, the results of the physical examination and investigations can be summarized briefly.
- When the mental state is recorded, a comment should be made under each heading as to whether or not any abnormality has been found.
- Diagnoses should be made using ICD-10 or DSM-5 criteria. If the diagnosis is uncertain, alternatives can be listed, with an indication of which is judged to be more likely.
- The summary of treatment should include the dosage and duration of any medication. The roles of the mental health team and of the general practitioner and any other agencies in the treatment plan should be made clear.
- The prognosis should be stated briefly but as definitely as possible. Statements such as 'prognosis guarded' are of little help to anyone.

Box 3.10 Example of a case summary

Patient: Mrs AB. *Date of birth:* 7.2.83

Consultant: Dr C. Summary compiled by Dr D (CT2 core trainee)

Admitted: 27.6.17 *Discharged:* 12.8.17

Reason for referral: Attempted suicide by hanging. Continuing suicidal intent and low mood.

Family history: Father, 66, retired gardener, well, mood swings, not close to patient. Mother died from cancer when patient aged 4. Sister, 37, divorced, well. Mental illness: father's brother—'manic depression'; father's sister—depression.

Personal history and current circumstances: Birth and early development normal. Childhood health good. School 6–16, uneventful, 5 GCSEs. Few friends. Worked 16–22, shop assistant. Several boyfriends; married at 22, husband 2 years older, lorry driver. Unhappy in last year after discovering his infidelity. Children: Jane, 7, well; Paul, 4, epileptic. Current financial worries.

Previous illness: Aged 31, (postnatal) depressive illness lasting a few weeks, saw counsellor. Hypothyroidism, on thyroxine.

Previous personality: Cyclothymic, but usually anxious and with low self-esteem. Interested in supernatural phenomena. Drinks occasionally, non-smoker, no illicit drugs.

History of present illness: For 3 months, increasingly low and tearful, waking early, worse in morning. Anhedonic, loss of appetite and weight. Worrying about marriage, and has become preoccupied that she is responsible for her son's epilepsy. Strong suicidal ideation, culminating in abortive attempt to hang herself on night of admission. Getting worse despite venlafaxine 75–150 mg/day for 2 months, taken regularly. On waiting list for CBT.

On examination: Physical: n.a.d., no evidence of myxoedema. Mental state: dishevelled, agitated, psychomotor retardation. Speech: slow, quiet, normal form. Thoughts: the preoccupations noted above are held intensely, and the belief that she caused her son's epilepsy (because she did not take enough care in pregnancy) is delusional in nature. Prominent suicidal ideation, and intent, wishing she were dead. Mood: subjectively and objectively very depressed, with self-blame, hopelessness. Perceptions: imagines she sees and hears her dead grandmother talking to her 'as if she was still alive'. Cognition: attention and concentration poor. Memory not formally tested. Insight: accepts she might be ill, consents to admission; her views on treatment are unclear.

Special investigations: Haemoglobin, electrolytes, TSH, n.a.d.

Treatment and progress: Initially on close observations. Venlafaxine increased to 225 mg/day, augmented by olanzapine, 10 mg nocte. However, condition deteriorated, and given course of six right unilateral ECTs (with consent). Mood improved after several treatments, suicidal ideation reduced, and no longer delusional.

Condition on discharge: Moderate residual depressive symptoms. No suicidal thoughts and realizes her son's epilepsy was not her fault. Hopeful but worried about future of marriage. Childcare—no concerns, husband and patient's sister (lives nearby) are supportive.

Diagnosis: (ICD-10, on admission) F33.3 Recurrent depressive disorder, current episode severe with psychotic symptoms. Now resolving.

Prognosis: Short-term prognosis is good, but at risk of further depressive episodes. Prognosis will be improved by compliance with treatment, and by resolving marital problems

Further management

- Under CPA. Key worker is Jo Smith, community psychiatric nurse, who will visit on 17.8.17.
- Continue venlafaxine 225 mg daily and olanzapine 10 mg nocte. GP to prescribe, and to monitor for metabolic syndrome (due in 1 month). Plan to remain on antidepressant for at least 9 months; olanzapine to be reviewed after 3 months.
- On waiting list for CBT—expected to start in a few weeks.
- Patient and husband will arrange marriage counselling.
- Patient has a copy of her care plan, and she and her husband know who to contact in an emergency.
- First review with psychiatrist in 2 weeks.

Formulations

A formulation is an exercise in clinical reasoning that helps the writer to think clearly about the diagnosis, aetiology, treatment, and prognosis (see Box 3.11).

Although now uncommon in clinical practice, formulations are extremely useful for developing skills in diagnostic reasoning, for understanding how psychiatric knowledge can be applied to the individual patient, and for learning how to prioritize and focus on the problems

Statement of the problem
Differential diagnosis
Aetiology
Plan of treatment
Prognosis

that require attention. We therefore encourage all psychiatrists in training to use formulations as an integral part of their work. Even for an experienced psychiatrist, a formulation remains a valuable exercise and aid.

A formulation is divided into several sections, as in the example shown in Box 3.12. A short opening statement is followed by the differential diagnosis. This consists of a list of reasonable possibilities in decreasing order of probability, together with a note of the evidence for and against each alternative. To produce a good differential diagnosis, it is necessary to have elicited and interpreted the key symptoms and signs (see Chapter 1) and to know the cardinal features of the major psychiatric disorders and how they are classified (see Chapter 2). Under aetiology, predisposing, precipitating, and perpetuating, causes should be identified. This requires a grounding in the causation of psychiatric disorders (see Chapter 5). There follows a list of outstanding problems and any further information that is needed. Next a concise plan of

Box 3.12 Example of a formulation

(Note: This formulation refers to the case summarized in Box 3.10, at the time of admission. By comparing the two ways of condensing information, the reader can appreciate the difference between the two approaches.)

Opening statement

Mrs AB is a 34-year-old married woman with a 3-month history of worsening depression, now with psychotic features. Admitted following serious suicide attempt.

Differential diagnosis

Recurrent depressive disorder (current episode: psychotic). For: subjective and objective low mood, anhedonia, anergia, poor concentration, early-morning waking, loss of appetite and libido, self-blame. Suicidal. Delusional belief that she caused her son's epilepsy. Past history of depressive episode. *Against:* none, unless current depressive episode is better explained by one of the diagnoses listed below.

Bipolar disorder (current episode: depressive). For: depressive symptoms as listed above; longstanding mood variability, family history of bipolar disorder. *Against:* no evidence of past clinically significant mood elevation, nor current hypomanic or mixed affective symptoms.

Organic mood disorder. For: history of hypothyroidism. *Against:* no current symptoms or signs of hypothyroidism (or other abnormalities on physical exam); TSH normal.

Schizophrenia. For: delusional belief regarding her son's epilepsy; hears and sees her dead grandmother. *Against:* the delusion is mood-congruent given her severe depression. The perceptual abnormalities are not true

hallucinations, and are consistent with her supernatural beliefs. She has no first-rank symptom of schizophrenia.

Conclusions: Psychotic depression. F33.3 Recurrent depressive disorder, current episode severe with psychotic symptoms.

Aetiology

Predisposing: genetic—family history of mood disorder. Death of mother when aged 4. Unhappy childhood and not close to father. Personality traits. Previous depressive episode.

Precipitating: discovery of husband's infidelity.

Perpetuating: ongoing marital arguments, worry about debts.

Treatment

Given her diagnosis, and non-response to an adequate trial of venlafaxine, plan to increase dose and augment with an antipsychotic (olanzapine). ECT may be required if no response. Is on waiting list for CBT. Joint interviews with the patient and her husband may help to reduce the marital problems. Suggest sources of financial advice to reduce this stressor.

Prognosis

Mrs AB has a good chance of a full therapeutic response to the planned treatment plan, especially if the marital problems can be improved. However, given her history and the predisposing factors noted above, she is at increased risk of further depressive episodes, particularly at times of stress.

management is outlined, and finally there is a statement about prognosis.

Problem lists

A problem list is useful in cases where there are multiple issues to be addressed, especially complex social problems. The list identifies the range of problems (or needs), summarizes the solution(s) proposed, states who is responsible for each action, and gives a review date. It is best to draw up the list with the patient, to ensure that they are fully involved in the identification of problems and in how these will be addressed. This is formalized in problem-solving counselling (see page 685).

Table 3.2 shows a problem list that might be drawn up following the initial assessment of a man who had taken a serious overdose and was found to have anxiety symptoms, psoriasis, and social problems, including concerns about how he and his partner were caring for their son. As progress is made in dealing with problems in this list, new ones may be added or existing ones modified or removed.

Letters to the general practitioner

When a letter is written to a general practitioner after an initial assessment, consider what they already know about the patient and what questions were asked when they referred them. If the referral letter outlined the salient features of the case, there is no need to repeat these in the reply. If the patient is less well known to the general practitioner, or if the referral has come from another source, more detailed information should be given. The letter should state clearly the diagnosis (if one has been made) or the range of differential diagnoses that are still being considered.

Treatment and prognosis are dealt with next. When discussing treatment, the dosage, timing, and duration of any drug treatment should be stated. Name any key worker, therapists, and other agencies involved, and the nature of their involvement. State the date of the patient's next appointment, and whether you have advised the patient to see the general practitioner in the interim (e.g. for blood tests). Responsibility for physical health care, and for prescribing, should be made clear. Ideally, all these details should be discussed and agreed with the general practitioner by phone before the letter is written to confirm them. The letter should emphasize a collaborative approach, and encourage the general practitioner to get in touch if they are unclear about the arrangements, or are concerned about the patient.

The same principles apply to subsequent correspondence during psychiatric care. That is, keep letters concise, focusing only on those issues that have changed since the last letter (e.g. symptoms, circumstances, treatments, and what is expected of the general practitioner). It is also helpful to highlight at the top of the letter the diagnosis, current state, current treatments (especially drugs and doses), and date of the next appointment.

As noted earlier, it is now standard practice for patients (and their carers, if requested) to be sent copies of all correspondence about them. All letters and other documents should be prepared with this in mind.

Electronic records and new technologies

A switch from paper to electronic health records is occurring in many settings and poses significant challenges, even though the same principles apply with regard to the records' content and nature, whether digital or not (Ennis *et al.*, 2014). For example, it may raise

Table 3.2 A problem list

Problem	Action	Agent	Review
1 Concern over son's care	Initially, discuss with GP	Key worker and GP	2 weeks
2 Relationship problems	Seek counselling	Patient and girlfriend to arrange	3 months
3 Housing unsatisfactory	Visit housing department	Patient	2 weeks
4 Panic attacks	Assess for CBT	Psychologist (via GP)	2 months
5 Psoriasis	GP to review	Patient	1 month

extra concerns about confidentiality, and about responsibility for backdating, updating, and maintaining the electronic records. Equally, developments in computing and 'digital health' provide many opportunities both for clinical practice and research (e.g. Druss *et al.*, 2014). Potential advantages include having access to patient records from any location and at all times, and the ability to keep in contact with patients remotely via mobile phone or internet (e.g. for monitoring of symptoms using apps, or to send text prompts about clinic appointments). Psychiatrists need to be aware of the policies and procedures regarding electronic records and 'digital health' in their own clinical setting, and to keep up to date with the rapid and significant developments that will undoubtedly occur in the coming years (Glenn and Monteith, 2014).

Standardized assessment methods

In research, and sometimes in clinical practice, it is helpful to use standardized methods to assess symptoms and syndromes, as well as disabilities and other consequences of psychiatric disorders. Such methods improve reliability and facilitate comparison of findings across time and between psychiatrists. For a review of rating scales in psychiatry, see Tyrer and Methuen (2007).

Standardized methods of assessment are of four main types. Three are considered in turn below:

- Those that rate symptoms to make a diagnosis; these have been important in the development of contemporary psychiatric classifications, and were introduced in Chapter 2. The Mini-Mental State Examination is another example of this type.
- Those that rate the severity of a symptom or group of symptoms.
- Those that assess the overall evidence for and effects of psychiatric disorder; these are called global rating scales, and they include quality-of-life measures.

In addition there are schedules for the assessment of need, as discussed earlier (see page 53).

Standardized diagnostic assessments

A range of diagnostic assessment schedules has been developed. The leading ones in current use are mentioned here. An important distinction is between those schedules designed for use by interviewers with training in psychiatry, and those for use by interviewers without such training. Schedules in the latter category (generally used in large-scale epidemiological research) require more precise rules for detecting symptoms and for diagnosing syndromes.

Present State Examination and Schedules for Clinical Assessment in Neuropsychiatry

The Present State Examination (PSE) is the archetypal interview schedule for use by trained psychiatrists. Its development began in the late 1950s, and the ninth edition was the first to be published for use by others (Wing *et al.*, 1974). It became widely used, notably in seminal international studies on the diagnosis of schizophrenia (see Chapter 11). The interviewer identifies abnormal phenomena that have been present during a specified period of time and rates their severity. Each of the 140 items is defined in detail in a glossary. Computer programs generate a symptom score, a diagnosis (CATEGO), and a measure of the severity of non-psychotic symptoms (the Index of Definition).

The tenth edition of the PSE was incorporated into the Schedules for Clinical Assessment in Neuropsychiatry (SCAN), a more extensive schedule that can be used to diagnose a broader range of disorders, including eating, somatoform, substance abuse, and cognitive disorders, using ICD-10 or DSM-IV criteria (World Health Organization, 1992a).

Structured Clinical Interview for Diagnosis

The Structured Clinical Interview for Diagnosis (SCID) is a diagnostic assessment procedure designed to make DSM diagnoses (Spitzer *et al.*, 1987). It can be used by the clinician as part of a normal assessment procedure, or in research or screening as a systematic evaluation of a whole range of medical states. SCID-5 is the version released for use with DSM-5.

Composite International Diagnostic Interview

The Composite International Diagnostic Interview (CIDI) combines aspects of an earlier interview schedule, the Diagnostic Interview Schedule (DIS), with the PSE

(Robins *et al.*, 1988). It was designed for lay interviewers to make diagnoses according to ICD and DSM criteria. It is available in many languages and intended for use in different cultures. The interview includes questions about symptoms and problems experienced at any time in life, as well as questions about current state.

Mini International Neuropsychiatric Interview

The Mini International Neuropsychiatric Interview (MINI) is a short structured interview (15–20 minutes, compared to 90 minutes for CIDI) for lay interviewers to make ICD and DSM diagnoses (Lecrubier *et al.*, 1997). It focuses on current disorders only, and is widely used in surveys and screening for clinical trials.

Instruments for measuring symptoms

In addition to instruments designed to make diagnoses, other scales measure the severity of symptoms or their fluctuation with time. Some such instruments rate one or a few symptoms, while others rate a broad group of symptoms as an overall measure of the severity of a disorder.

Ratings of affective symptoms

Hamilton Rating Scale for Depression

The Hamilton Rating Scale for Depression (HAM-D or HRSD; Hamilton, 1967) is available in 17- and 21-item versions, and is filled in by a trained interviewer who uses an unstructured interview. It measures the severity of the depressive syndrome rather than the symptom of depression.

Beck Depression Inventory

The Beck Depression Inventory (BDI; Beck *et al.*, 1961) is a 21-item inventory that is completed by the patient. Each item has four statements, and the patient chooses the one that applies best to their feelings during the previous week.

Montgomery-Åsberg Depression Rating Scale

The Montgomery-Åsberg Depression Rating Scale (MADRS; Montgomery and Åsberg, 1979) inventory has 10 items rated on a 4-point scale by an interviewer using definitions for each point. Only psychological symptoms of depression are rated. Along with the HAM-D, it is widely used in antidepressant drug trials.

Patient Health Questionnaire 9

This self-report questionnaire (PHQ-9; Kroenke *et al.*, 2001) rates each of the nine DSM-IV criteria for depression on a scale of 0 to 3. It is adapted from an American questionnaire called Prime-MD. A score of ≥10 has a sensitivity and specificity of 88% for major depression. The PHQ-9 has been used as a screening tool for depression in primary care, and in monitoring of outcome. A PHQ-2 is also available, in which the two questions ask about depressed mood and anhedonia.

Quick Inventory of Depressive Symptomatology

The Quick Inventory of Depressive Symptomatology (QIDS; Rush *et al.*, 2003) is an increasingly popular 16-item scale for rating of depressive symptoms. It is usually used in a self-report format (QIDS-SR) and is available in many languages. The QIDS has good psychometric properties, is sensitive to change, and is useful for clinical and research purposes.

Ratings of mania

Severity of manic symptoms can be rated by patient and clinician using the 11-item Young Mania Rating Scale (YMRS; Young *et al.*, 1978) or by patients using the briefer Altman Self-Rating Mania Scale (Altman *et al.*, 1997).

Ratings of anxiety symptoms

Hamilton Anxiety Scale

In the Hamilton Anxiety Scale (HAS; Hamilton, 1959), 13 items are rated by an interviewer on 5-point scales, each on the basis of a brief description. The interviewing method is for the rater to decide. Some depressive symptoms are included so that the scale is in fact a measure of the severity of the anxiety syndrome and not of the symptoms of anxiety.

The State–Trait Anxiety Inventory (STAI; Spielberger et al., 1983)

The State–Trait Anxiety Inventory (STAI; Spielberger *et al.*, 1983) is a self-rating scale with 20 statements, which is completed in two ways—as the person feels when they are completing the scale (state), and how they feel generally (trait).

Hospital Anxiety and Depression Scale

The Hospital Anxiety and Depression Scale (HADS; Zigmond and Snaith, 1983) has seven questions about anxiety and seven about depression, and is used to assess symptom severity and caseness in psychiatric and medical patients, and in the general population.

Ratings of other symptoms

Ratings used in the assessment of cognitive impairment and dementia

The Mini-Mental State Examination (MMSE; Folstein *et al.*, 1975) has already been introduced. Other scales that are used to assess cognitive impairment, and the behavioural symptoms of dementia, are discussed in Chapter 14.

Ratings of symptoms of schizophrenia

These are discussed in Chapter 11. The Positive and Negative Syndrome Scale (PANSS) is widely used in research (Kay *et al.*, 1987).

Ratings of motor symptoms

A range of scales is available, especially related to side-effects of antipsychotic medication. They include the Extrapyramidal Symptoms Rating Scale (ESRS; Chouinard *et al.*, 1980) and the Barnes Akathisia Rating Scale (BARS; Barnes, 1989).

Ratings of personality and its disorders

These are discussed in Chapter 15.

Ratings of broad groups of symptoms

General Health Questionnaire

The General Health Questionnaire (GHQ; Goldberg and Hillier, 1979) is designed for use as a screening instrument in primary care, general medical practice, or community surveys. The original instrument contained 60 items, but shorter versions (e.g. GHQ-12 and GHQ-30) have also been developed. Even the full version can be completed within 10 minutes. The symptom ratings are added to a score that indicates overall severity, which is expressed by whether a psychiatrist would judge the patient to be a 'case' or a 'non-case'.

Brief Psychiatric Rating Scale

This instrument (BPRS; Overall and Gorham, 1962) has 16 items, each scored on a 7-point scale. There are criteria to define the symptom items, but not for the severity ratings. The time period is not defined and must be decided by the rater. The BPRS is used mainly for rating psychotic disorders.

Global rating scales

Clinical Global Impression (CGI; Guy, 1976)

The Clinical Global Impression (CGI; Guy, 1976) rating scale has two items. The main one, *global severity*, requires the clinician to rate the overall severity of the patient's illness at the time of interview, relative to other patients with the same diagnosis. The *global change* item rates change relative to a baseline assessment. The CGI is often used as a measure of efficacy in drug trials.

WHO Disability Assessment Schedule 2.0

WHODAS 2.0 is a generic assessment instrument for assessing level of disability. It covers six domains of functioning (e.g. self-care, life activities, cognition) and can be administered in less than 20 minutes.

Global Assessment of Functioning

The Global Assessment of Functioning (GAF) is a 100-point scale, derived from the earlier Global Assessment Scale, on which the clinician rates the overall functioning of the patient (Phelan *et al.*, 1994). Each decile has a brief description of psychological, social, and occupational performance. The GAF was included in DSM-IV and is widely used, but has been removed from DSM-5.

Health of the Nation Outcome Scale

The HoNOS (Wing *et al.*, 1998) is a 12-item scale that rates clinical problems and social functioning. It was developed as an instrument to measure progress towards a UK NHS target to improve the health and social functioning of mentally ill people, and is now being used routinely for this purpose. It was designed to be applicable to all psychiatric disorders, so what it gains in applicability it loses in specificity. The equal weighting of the different variables has attracted criticism but has not limited its use. The HoNOS has been adapted for use in different countries, and for the elderly, those with learning disability, and other clinical groups.

Quality-of-life scales

There is increasing interest in quality of life as a key measure of outcomes throughout medicine. A large number of scales is available. Many are complex and of limited utility. Quality-of-life scales that are commonly used in psychiatry include the relatively simple EuroQol EQ-5D, the SF-36, SF-6D, and the Lancashire Quality of Life scale. Such scales can be helpful in research (e.g. in health economic evaluations) but are of limited value in clinical practice (Gilbody *et al.*, 2002; Brazier, 2010).

Further reading

Cooper JE and Oates M (2009). The principles of clinical assessment in general psychiatry. In: MG Gelder, NC Andreasen, JJ López-IborJr and JR Geddes (eds) *The New Oxford Textbook of Psychiatry*. 2nd edn. Oxford University Press, Oxford. pp. 62–78.

Maguire P and Pitceathly C (2002). Key communication skills and how to acquire them. *British Medical Journal*, **325**, 697–700.

Poole R and Higgo R (2006). *Psychiatric Interviewing and Assessment*. Cambridge University Press, Cambridge.

CHAPTER 4

Ethics and civil law

Introduction

This chapter is concerned with the ways in which general ethical principles, relating to matters such as confidentiality, consent, and autonomy, are applied in the care of people with mental disorders. We assume that the reader has already studied ethical aspects of general medicine, otherwise they should consult Hope *et al.* (2008) or a comparable textbook of medical ethics (Beauchamp and Childress, 2013).

Ethical considerations are important in all branches of medicine. However, in psychiatry they have additional importance because some patients lack the capacity to make judgements about their own need for care, and because of the power of involuntary treatment. Questions about capacity to consent to treatment of psychiatric illness commonly arise, and psychiatrists are sometimes asked by colleagues in other specialties for advice about capacity to consent to treatment for physical illness.

In this chapter we also consider some aspects of the Mental Health Act and the law relevant to psychiatry. These aspects are necessarily general ones because the specific provisions of the law differ from one country to another. It is important that the reader makes themself familiar with legal provisions in their own country and, if in any doubt, always seek expert advice.

The chapter is divided into four parts:

1. General issues.
2. Ethical problems in psychiatry.
3. The Mental Health Act.
4. Some aspects of civil law that are relevant to the practice of psychiatry.

Ethical problems that relate specifically to issues discussed elsewhere in this book are considered in those chapters (see Box 4.1).

General issues

The conclusion that it is ethically right to act in one way rather than another should be:

- based on agreed ethical approaches and principles;
- logically sound;
- consistent across decisions.

Ethical approaches

In psychiatry, as in ethics generally, two broad approaches to ethical problems are employed—a duty-based approach and a utilitarian approach.

The *duty-based approach* sets out clinicians' obligations in a series of rules—for example, doctors must not have sexual relationships with their patients. These rules may be brought together in a code of practice, leaving clinicians in no doubt about their duties. However, this approach is inflexible and is difficult to apply to complex problems.

The *utilitarian approach* balances judgements about benefit and harm. Instead of applying specific rules, each case is assessed individually on the assumption that the correct action is the one with the best foreseeable *overall* consequences. This approach takes into account clinical complexities, but can result in a contested conclusion, as people may give different weight to the benefits and harms in a particular case.

In practice the two approaches overlap. A duty-based approach may include a duty to do that which will result in the best outcome, and in a utilitarian approach the best outcome may result from the application of a rule.

Ethical principles

Three ethical principles are widely adopted in medical ethics (Beauchamp and Childress, 2013).

1. *Beneficence (and non-malevolence)*: doing what is best for patients (and not doing harm). In practice this usually means doing what the body of professional opinion judges to be best.
2. Respect for autonomy: involving patients in health care decisions, informing them so that they can make the decisions, and respecting their views.
3. *Justice*: acting fairly and balancing the interests of different people.

Ethical principles can, and do, regularly conflict with each other. In psychiatry this most often occurs when beneficence is in conflict with respect for autonomy—for example, when a patient refuses treatment that professional opinion judges to be essential, and the Mental Health Act has to be used (see below). The essay 'Two Concepts of Liberty' by the philosopher Isaiah Berlin outlines this dilemma in distinguishing between 'freedom from' and 'freedom to' (Berlin, 1958). Autonomy is not always served simply by ensuring the absence of coercion if the individual is not in a position to act on their liberty. The Nobel Laureate Amartya Sen argues that our sensitivity to injustice informs our balancing of ethical principles, and not vice versa (Sen, 2007).

Codes of practice

Codes of practice and guidelines are prepared and overseen by professional organizations such as the American Psychiatric Association (2013b) and, in the UK, the General Medical Council (2009a) and the Royal College of Psychiatrists (2010). In some countries ethical codes are enforced not by the professions but by government. Loss of confidence in the professions has led to some demands for this arrangement in the UK.

The other professions involved in psychiatric care, such as nursing and psychology, have their own codes of practice, and these are not identical in every respect to those of the medical profession. Such differences may sometimes complicate decisions in multidisciplinary teams.

Values-based practice has recently been proposed as a complement to *evidence-based practice* (Fulford *et al.*, 2012). Ethical values can be in conflict, and routinely need to be balanced. The relative weight assigned to different values by the members of multidisciplinary teams (as well as the patient) may vary considerably. Values-based practice encourages the exploration of this in arriving at decisions, aiming to ensure that the traditional hierarchy in such teams does not inhibit their expression. For example, the psychiatrist may privilege treatment effect, whereas a nurse may privilege the patient's self-respect and the social worker may privilege the patient's rights. All of the team members acknowledge the relevance of all of these values, but they weight them differently and best practice, and effective teamworking, requires that they are accommodated.

Ethical problems in psychiatric practice

In the following sections of this chapter we shall discuss ethical problems relating to:

- the doctor–patient relationship
- confidentiality
- consent
- compulsory treatment
- research.

As mentioned previously, ethical problems that arise in particular aspects of practice are discussed in other chapters (see Box 4.1).

The doctor–patient relationship

A relationship of trust between doctor and patient is the basis of ethical medical practice. This relationship should be in the patient's interests and based on the principles outlined above of respect for autonomy, beneficence, non-maleficence, and justice.

Abuse of the relationship

The more intense the doctor–patient relationship, and the more vulnerable the patient, the more readily that relationship can be abused. For these reasons, particular care has to be taken not to abuse the relationship during psychotherapy. Therapists abuse the doctor–patient relationship when they:

- *Impose their own values and beliefs* on their patients—for example, when counselling about termination of pregnancy. This influence may be overt—for example, when a doctor refuses termination of pregnancy, stating that it is morally wrong. Alternatively, it may be covert—for example, when the doctor expresses no opinion but nevertheless gives more attention to the arguments against termination than to those for it. Similar problems may arise, for example, in marital therapy when therapists' values may intrude on their approach to the question of whether a couple should separate.
- *Put the interests of third parties before those of patients*—for example, the interests of family or employers. This does not mean the interests of patients should be considered in isolation. When allocating scarce resources or with potentially dangerous patients, the interests of the patient have to be balanced against those of others. These difficult decisions are discussed further on page 798.
- *Exploit patients sexually.* Medical codes of practice contain an absolute prohibition against sexual relationships with a patient. Particular care is needed if sexual problems and intimate relationships are prominent in psychotherapy.
- *Exploit patients for financial gain*—for example, by prolonging treatment in private practice beyond that truly necessary.

Confidentiality

Confidentiality is central to the trust between patients and doctors. It is particularly important in psychiatry because information often concerns private and highly sensitive matters. As a general rule, information should not be disclosed without the patient's explicit consent. As will be discussed later, there are defined exceptions to this rule. The rule is an ancient one, stated in the Hippocratic Oath:

Whatever, in connection with my professional practice or not in connection with it, I see or hear in the life of men, which ought not to be spoken abroad, I will not divulge, reckoning that all such should be kept secret.

The rule was restated in 1948 in the Declaration of Geneva, which added the important point that the obligation of confidentiality continues after a patient's death:

I will respect the secrets which are confided in me, even after the patient has died.

In many countries, national professional organizations publish guidelines that deal with common clinical situations such as protecting records, sharing information with relatives, and disclosing information to third parties (see, for example, General Medical Council, 2009a, and the updated website http://www.gmc-uk.org). Confidentiality is also enforced by law and by employment contract. Although professional guidelines do not have the force of law, they are taken seriously by the courts as evidence of generally accepted standards.

Many countries have laws of privacy, and laws that govern the ways in which written and electronic records can be held and that set out patients' rights to see their personal information. Psychiatrists should be aware of the ethical and legal requirements in the place in which they are working. In the UK, the relevant legislation includes the Data Protection Act (1998).

In English law, it is in the *public* interest, as well as that of the individual, that patients should be able to trust their doctors to maintain confidentiality. Whether it is unlawful for a doctor to breach confidentiality is generally answered by balancing two conflicting public interests rather than a private against a public interest.

Ethical principles relating to confidentiality

Safeguarding information

Personal information must be safeguarded and records kept securely, and consideration must be given to the security of mobile phones or email. Unintentional disclosure should be avoided by carrying out consultations where they cannot be overheard, sometimes difficult on home visits or on a medical ward. Discussions between professional staff should be avoided in places where they might be overheard.

Consent to disclosure of information

Confidentiality is not breached when a patient has given informed consent to disclosure. Informed consent implies consent based on a full understanding of the reasons for disclosure, what will be disclosed, and the likely consequences of disclosure. In principle, confidentiality is not breached when the patient cannot be identified—for example, in a disguised case report. Nevertheless, it is usual for journals and books to require that patients give informed, signed consent to publication, even when their identities have been disguised. This obligation, unlike libel laws, continues after death. Poorly anonymized case reports of deceased patients, from which these individuals have been identified, have led to professional complaints from families.

Confidentiality in the care of children

These and other ethical problems in the care of children are discussed in Chapter 16. Here it is sufficient to note that children over a stated age (usually 16 years) have the same rights of confidentiality as adults. For younger children, clinical information is usually shared with parents, who have a legal duty to act in their children's best interests and therefore need to be properly informed.

Situations in which there may be problems regarding confidentiality

Seeking information from others

As a rule, patients' permission should be obtained before information is sought from other individuals. If the patient is too unwell to give an account of himself, the psychiatrist must decide whether to seek it without the patient's consent. The guiding principles are to act in the patient's best interests, and as far as possible to obtain the information from close relatives.

Disclosing information to others

Information should be disclosed only with the patient's consent, except in the special circumstances discussed below. Disclosure should be limited to the minimum necessary information. Relatives often ask for information, but this should usually be given only with the patient's consent. This is a very contentious issue in the era of community care when the family may be the main carers and run the greatest risk (see below). When the patient is unable to consent to disclosure (e.g. as a result of dementia), information may be shared provided that disclosure is in the patient's best interests.

Assessment on behalf of a third party

Often a patient is assessed on behalf of a third party; for example, an assessment of fitness to work carried out for an employer. It is essential to ensure at the outset that the patient understands the purpose of the assessment and the obligations of the doctor towards the third party. Written consent should be obtained. Otherwise disclosure can be made only in the public interest (see below), usually to prevent death or serious harm.

Care in the community

Patients should know from the start that information will be shared as necessary with other members of the care team, and these team members must follow the principles of confidentiality. Some members of the team (e.g. social workers) may be required to discuss information with their supervisors, or to pass on information to other agencies (e.g. when helping patients with housing). It is important to keep such matters in mind as treatment plans develop, and to discuss them with the patient when this becomes necessary. When visits are made to patients, neighbours may become aware of the visits. Moreover, outreach programmes may need to ask neighbours about high-risk patients who have not kept appointments. These and similar potential problems should be anticipated as far as possible and discussed with the patient so that the necessary permissions are obtained in advance. In an emergency, the right to privacy has to be balanced against the risks to the patient or to others, should the necessary enquiries not be made.

If a patient refuses the disclosure of information despite clear information about the likely consequences of non-disclosure, their wishes must be respected unless this would put others at serious risk.

Group therapy

Group therapy presents special problems of confidentiality because patients reveal personal information not only to the therapist but also to other members of the group. Before treatment begins, the therapist should explain the requirement to treat as confidential the revelations of the other group members from everyone in the group.

Therapy with couples

Often couples' therapy is preceded by an interview with each partner separately. Information obtained in this way should not be revealed without an agreement. It is much better if all relevant information is revealed by the partner concerned during the joint sessions. If, during therapy, an individual interview is needed (e.g. to assess symptoms of depression), it may be better to ask a colleague. Similar problems may arise in family therapy.

Exceptions to the rule of confidentiality

Exceptions in the patient's interest

In exceptional circumstances, doctors may disclose information to a third party without the patient's consent, when this disclosure is in the patient's best interest. An example is when information is requested urgently by another doctor who is dealing with the patient in an emergency, or when a patient is incapable of giving informed consent because of severe mental or physical illness, and the disclosure is essential for their care.

Exceptions in the public interest

Although there is a general legal obligation for doctors to keep confidential what patients tell them, there are special circumstances in which doctors are obliged to disclose information. There are *statutory obligations* to do so in relation, for example, to communicable disease, the use of certain controlled drugs, unfitness to drive, and suspected child abuse. There is also an obligation to disclose relevant information in response to a Court Order, and when there is evidence of serious crime, usually a crime that will put some person at risk of death or serious harm (e.g. the abuse of a child). *Child protection* has become a particularly sensitive area for professional confidentiality. Society's tolerance of the potential abuse or neglect of dependent children is almost zero now in most countries. The current expectation is that professionals' threshold for breaking confidentiality should be very low in cases where there are any concerns, even without clear evidence. Every effort should be made to persuade the patient to agree to disclosure but, if they refuse, the reasons for the disclosure should be explained and written down.

Exceptions for legal representatives

A patient's legal representative, like the patient, may read their clinical notes and letters, although there may be restrictions in relation to the possibility of harm to others and for information given in confidence by informants.

For further information about problems related to confidentiality, see Hope *et al.* (2008).

Consent to treatment

Consent is relevant to the whole of medical practice, and in the account that follows we assume that the reader is familiar with the relevant concepts and procedures from their general medical training. Any readers who are not should consult the latest General Medical Council guidelines if they are working in the UK (see http://www.gmc-uk.org) or the equivalent document if they are working elsewhere, and read a textbook of ethics such as that by Hope *et al.* (2008).

Obtaining consent

The patient should:

1. Have a *clear and full understanding* of the nature of the condition to be treated, the procedures available, and their probable side effects.
2. *Agree freely* to receive the treatment.
3. Be *competent* to take decisions (i.e. to *have legal capacity*; see below). (Note that, in the USA, the word 'capacity' is generally used in the clinical sense rather than in the legal sense adopted in the UK.)

Maintaining consent

Some patients consent to treatment of chronic illness but later fail to collaborate with it. When this happens, the clinician should seek to re-establish consent and collaboration. To achieve these, offers of additional help are justified, but threats that help will be reduced are not. This is particularly complex in the long-term community care of individuals with severely disabling disorders such as psychoses. The difference between an 'offer of additional help' and a 'threat that help will be reduced' is not always that clear in practice, and certainly not to the patient. Is a case manager's comment 'I can only really recommend you for this tenancy if I can say you are taking treatment' an offer, or is it a threat? Szmukler and Appelbaum (2008) have explored these gradations of treatment pressures in mental health.

When explicit consent is not required

There are special situations in which explicit consent is not needed (their precise nature depends on local law and precedent). These include:

- *Implied consent*—for example, when a patient holds out his arm to have his blood pressure measured.
- *Necessity*—that is, a circumstance in which grave harm or death is likely to occur without intervention, and there is doubt about the patient's competence (see below).
- *Emergency*—to prevent immediate serious harm to the patient or to others, or to prevent a crime.

When consent to medical treatment is refused

In the UK, the law distinguishes between consent to medical treatment and consent to psychiatric treatment. This section is concerned with refusal of *medical* treatment; refusal of psychiatric treatment is discussed on page 660. Competent adults have a right to refuse medical treatment, even if this refusal results in death or permanent disablement.

If a patient refuses medical treatment, the doctor needs to make two judgements before accepting that the patient has the right to refuse.

1. Does the patient lack competence, i.e. the legal capacity (see below) to consent to or refuse treatment, by reason of mental illness?
2. Has the patient been influenced by others to the extent that a refusal has been coerced or is not voluntary?

Refusal by competent patients

Refusal may, of course, be a rational decision, having weighed up the pros and cons (pain, discomfort, separation from family versus improvement in symptoms or increased life expectancy). However, it is often the result of misunderstanding or fear about the illness and its treatment. Clinicians should set aside the time needed to understand the patient's concerns and understanding of their condition before explaining the medical issues once more. With such an approach, agreement can usually be reached on a treatment plan that is both medically appropriate and acceptable to the patient. Nevertheless, some competent adult patients continue to refuse treatment even after a full discussion, and it is their right to do so.

Refusal by incompetent patients

In the UK and most other countries the doctor has the right to act in the patient's best interests and give immediate treatment in *life-threatening emergencies* when the patient lacks capacity to consent, as when they are unconscious or delirious. Whenever possible, other health workers should be consulted and a careful record should be kept of the reasons for the decision. Doctors should know the relevant law in the country in which they are working. For further discussion of this issue, see Hope *et al.* (2008). The 2005 Mental Capacity Act for England and Wales addresses the previously neglected area of the treatment of incompetent patients who are not actively refusing treatment but who cannot be considered to have consented. It also addresses those who may have previously indicated (when competent) what they would have wished.

Refusal by mentally disordered patients

If a patient who refuses medical treatment has an accompanying mental disorder that appears to impair their ability to give informed consent, the mental disorder should be treated, if necessary and appropriate, under compulsory legal powers. In English law, such powers do not allow treatment of the physical illness against the patient's wishes. However, they do allow the treatment of the mental disorder. After successful treatment of the mental disorder, the patient may then give informed consent for the treatment of the physical illness that was previously refused but, if not, their decision must be respected no matter how perverse it may seem.

Legal aspects of consent

The legal concept of *capacity* to consent relates to a patient's ability to comprehend and retain information about the treatment, to believe this information, and to use it to make an informed choice.

Patients may lack the capacity to give informed consent by reason of the following:

1. Young age—parents give consent for children and adolescents below the age at which, in law, they are able to consent (consent to treatment for children and adolescents is considered in Chapter 16).

2. Learning disability.

3. Mental disorder. Psychiatrists may be asked to assess patients who are thought to be in this third group; they should do so by making the enquiries listed in Box 4.2.

Judgements of legal capacity to consent *are specific to the particular decision*. Thus a patient with a severe mental disorder may be incompetent in other respects, but none the less competent to decide whether to consent

to a particular treatment. For example, a patient with schizophrenia and paranoid delusions may be capable of deciding about medical treatment of a heart attack.

Consent in advance

Advance statements, sometimes called 'living wills', are accepted in many countries. They are designed to ensure that those who previously had the capacity to take decisions but then lose it (usually because of dementia) are treated as they would have wished when competent. To make an advance statement, the person must be competent and well informed at the time. Advance statements respect the principle of autonomy and are generally considered by doctors and patients to be helpful.

Since the 2005 Mental Capacity Act (MCA) regularized the situation, advance statements now have some legal authority in England (the Act does not apply to Scotland). The MCA distinguishes between an advance statement and an 'Advance Decision to Refuse Treatment' (ADRT). Advance statements are relatively informal and may be recorded in notes or care plans (e.g. 'Only use second-generation antipsychotics if I am compulsorily treated', 'Do not inform my sister if I am admitted'). They can even be verbal. They are not legally binding, but it is good practice to follow them if possible and also to encourage patients to update them. If they are not followed, the reasons should be recorded. Because of the relapsing nature of many severe mental illnesses, advance directives are often based on the patient's previous experiences. In general medicine they are more often based on how the individual assumes that they would feel about treatment if and when they lost capacity, usually through dementia. The incorporation of advance statements as part of 'joint care plans' has been tested in some services. Although patients seem reluctant to make them, they do appear to improve relationships and may improve treatment even if they have not been shown to reduce relapses (Thornicroft *et al.*, 2013).

However, the ADRT is binding, even if the decision may result in death. To have this force it must be a written and witnessed statement with confirmation that the individual had capacity at that time. The provision also allows for the naming of a 'surrogate decision-maker', who can give consent on behalf of the patient. The ADRT can be overridden if the Mental Health Act is used, apart from the advance decision to refuse ECT, which is absolute. Compulsory treatment overriding an advance decision may be used in acutely unwell patients most often (but not only) when there are risks to others. Psychiatry is the only area of medicine

> ## Box 4.2 Assessment of competence of adult patients
>
> **Step 1** Identify the decision required and the information relevant to it:
> - the decision to be made
> - the alternative reasonable decisions
> - the pros and cons of each reasonable decision.
>
> **Step 2** Assess cognitive ability.
> Assess whether the patient has the cognitive ability to:
> - understand the information
> - retain the information
> - evaluate the information and reach a decision.
>
> **Step 3** Consider the possible causes of impaired cognitive ability:
> - delirium
> - dementia
> - other neurological disorders that may impair cognition
> - learning disability.
>
> **Step 4** Assess other factors that may interfere with capacity.
> Mental illness:
> - delusions
> - hallucinations
> - mood disorder.
>
> Lack of maturity:
> - assess emotional and cognitive maturity.

where this override is possible, and some view this as discriminatory.

Deprivation of liberty and the 'Bournewood Gap'

An adult man with autism was admitted to Bournewood Hospital against the wishes of his informal carers, but did not himself actively object to being in hospital. An individual was then only considered to have their liberty restricted if they were actively objecting to their treatment. The Bournewood case indicated a 'gap' in the legislation, namely the failure to protect an individual who was deprived of his liberty although not resisting it. This was ruled to conflict with European human rights legislation. The distinction between *deprivation of liberty* and *restriction of liberty* can be a fine judgement. To comply with European legislation it must be clearly in the patient's best interests (i.e. not for the protection

of others). A consequence of this legislation is the Deprivation of Liberty Safeguards, which were introduced in the 2007 amendments to the Mental Health Act. These are complex and usually dealt with by a 'Best Interests Assessor', who may call on a psychiatrist to advise on the capacity or diagnosis of such patients. The implication for psychiatrists is to pay attention to any restrictions on incapacitous patients, even if they are not objecting.

Consent by a proxy

In English law, if an adult patient does not have the capacity to consent to treatment, proxy consent on behalf of that patient can only be given if there is a written advance statement. In some other jurisdictions there is provision for a form of proxy consent such as, in Scottish law, the appointment of a guardian. When there is no legal provision for proxy consent and the patient has not made an advance directive, and a decision as to whether to give treatment must be made, this is done on the basis of the patient's best interests. Best interest is judged by the responsible clinician in accordance with general medical opinion. It is wise to consult relatives and to discuss the case with other professional staff. Detailed notes should be kept of the reasons for the decision and of the consultations that took place.

Ethics of research

Psychiatric research is bound by the ethical principles that apply to all medical research. These derive from the first internationally agreed guidelines on research involving people, referred to as 'The Helsinki Declaration'. The main issues that should always be considered are summarized in Box 4.3. These principles followed the revelations of the appalling abuse of medical research in Nazi Germany, and were first published by the World Medical Association in 1964 (see World Medical Association, 2000). Since then there have been several national and international guidelines, generally enforced by national and local research ethics committees. The ethical problems of psychiatric research are the same as those of other medical research as set out, for example, in the UK General Medical Council guidelines (see http://www.gmc-uk.org) or the website of the UK Health Regulatory Authority (http://www.hra.nhs.uk). They pay particular attention to issues related to consent by competent but vulnerable adults who may feel under pressure to consent, and by those who lack capacity.

Box 4.3 Assessment of some ethical issues relating to research

Note: Ethical problems related to recruitment for and conduct of clinical trials are considered on page 123.

Scientific merits

- Will the findings be of value?
- Are the methods and the size of the groups likely to achieve the aims?
- What are the sources of financial and other support, and are there any potential conflicts of interest?
- Are there any potential conflicts of interest for any of the investigators?
- Could the aims be achieved in an ethically better way?

Safety

- Are the procedures safe? If there is a risk, are all of the necessary precautions being taken?
- Is the assessed level of risk acceptable to investigators, subjects, and relatives?

Consent

- Will the subjects be competent to give consent?
- Will the subjects receive clear and sufficient information?
- Will they have adequate time to consider and, should they wish to do so, to withdraw consent?
- Will it be clear that refusal will not affect the quality or quantity of care provided?
- Is the relationship between subject and investigator potentially coercive (e.g. a supervisor and a student)?
- Is any payment to subjects excessive and acts as an overwhelming incentive to consent?
- Is the researcher under any pressure to recruit subjects (e.g. receiving payments from a sponsoring company)?

Confidentiality

- Have subjects consented to the use of confidential information in the research?
- Will the data from the research be kept securely?

Adapted from Hope T, Savelescu J and Hendrick J, Medical Ethics and Law: The Core Curriculum, 2nd Edition, Copyright (2008), with permission from Elsevier.

Informed consent to research

Informed consent is crucial to the ethical conduct of research.

- Patients must be made specifically aware that the research is not being conducted for their individual benefit.
- Patients must be free from any coercion or inducement.
- Patients have the right to withdraw from the study at any time without any kind of penalty or impact on their broader treatment.
- In addition to the investigator, a family member or other suitable person should be encouraged to monitor the patient's condition and report to the investigator if there are concerns.
- In placebo-controlled trials, patients must understand clearly the probability of receiving placebo, the lack of improvement that might result, and the possibility of symptomatic worsening.

Research involving people who cannot give informed consent

Most psychiatric patients can give informed consent, but a few have a disorder that impairs judgement and decision-making. To exclude these patients from all research could deprive future similar patients of the benefits of research. Ethical protocols for involving such patients have received intense scrutiny in the design of treatment trials for unconscious trauma victims. The decision as to whether to include such patients is made after considering the following:

- any potential benefit of the research to the person who is being asked to consent;
- any possible discomfort or risk to this person;
- the potential benefit to others who have a similar problem and incapacity;
- any signs or other indications that suggest unspoken objection.

It is advisable to consult with relatives or others who may be able to take an informed view of the patient's situation. Jurisdictions vary in the extent to which this is a legal requirement, and investigators should take great care to follow local ethical and legal procedures.

The Mental Health Act

Compulsory treatment for mental disorders

Specific legislation exists to ensure that people with severe mental illness can be treated involuntarily. Such treatment is subject to careful scrutiny, and is found in all developed societies. Legal provision for the detention of disturbed individuals, then described as the 'the furiously mad', was introduced early to the asylum movement in the 1820s. How that legislation is drafted and who has the decision-making powers vary across time and jurisdictions. In the 1825 UK Act it was magistrates who made the decisions and doctors had little say, whereas by the time of the 1959 Mental Health Act, decisions were essentially all clinical. Now, in the light of the European Convention on Human Rights, the emphasis is shifting back more towards greater legal involvement in the process. Compulsory treatment has always been a feature of psychiatry and a legitimate and important responsibility for psychiatrists. In most countries outside the UK its imposition of compulsory admission or treatment is by a legal body (judge, magistrate, etc.). However, the reality in most legislations is that the medical recommendation carries considerable weight. Several states distinguish between compulsory detention and compulsory treatment. In the Netherlands, Austria, and parts of Switzerland a patient can be detained but still must agree to treatment. There is evidence that, after some decades of decline, compulsion is increasing across Europe (Priebe *et al.*, 2005).

When using the Mental Health Act it is essential that psychiatrists familiarize themselves with the local provisions and requirements. Not only do these vary from one country to another, but they can vary within countries. For example, the Scottish and Northern Ireland Mental Health Acts differ in important details from that for England and Wales, each state in the USA has its own legislation, and different cantons of Switzerland impose different conditions. Mental health legislation is often long and obscure—the 2007 amendment runs to several hundred dense pages, and the accompanying Code of Practice likewise. Practising clinicians generally only need to know the main provisions and procedures for the practices outlined in Box 4.4. The major provisions of the 1983/2007 Mental Health Act for England and Wales will be used as the reference point for outlining the principles and practices in what follows. Local training with regular updates is essential and is now obligatory.

Criteria for detention

Until recently all compulsory care required admission to a psychiatric hospital, so the expression 'detained under the Mental Health Act' is still widely used to indicate involuntary care, whether in or outside hospital. The UK Mental Health Acts are broadly very similar, and indeed they all adhere relatively closely to the 1959 Mental Health Act in spirit, differing mainly in detail. The UK acts are 'permissive'—that is, they outline what a doctor *may* do but not what they *must* do. The decision to admit or treat a patient against their will is still a clinical decision. The wording of the new Act is deliberately loose in its definitions of both mental disorder and treatment, allowing considerable scope for clinical discretion. The conditions for detention are worded differently for treatment and assessment, but there are essentially four of them.

1. You consider that the patient is likely to be suffering from a mental disorder (detention may sometimes be necessary to establish this).
2. Detention is necessary for the health or safety of the patient or of others.
3. The patient refuses voluntary admission.
4. Appropriate treatment is available (for treatment orders).

Until the 2007 revision there were four classes of mental disorder subject to detention (mental illness, mental impairment, severe mental impairment, and psychopathic disorder), but these were replaced by a single category of mental disorder. This was to remove individual requirements for specific disorders. The UK criteria are quite paternalistic by international standards—they prioritize the potential for patient benefit. Many

> ### Box 4.4 **Key clinical procedures in the Mental Health Act**
>
> - Criteria for detention
> - Assessment orders
> - Treatment orders
> - Transfer from prisons and courts
> - Police powers and powers of entry
> - Community Treatment Orders

countries (especially those with strong libertarian civil rights traditions, such as the USA) emphasize risk rather than patient benefit. In many US and some European states, patients must pose an *immediate risk* to physical safety (their own or that of others). Finally, patients must always be given the opportunity to accept voluntary treatment ('the least restrictive option') before compulsion can be used.

Historically families (or their formal representatives) made applications for detention, but the 1959 Mental Health Act permitted social workers to do this on their behalf. Over time this has become the accepted practice, although families can still appeal to discharge their members. The social worker has a specific role in ensuring that the patient's civil rights are properly protected and that less restrictive alternatives have not been overlooked. Apart from emergencies, two medical opinions are needed, preferably one who knows the patient (often their GP) and one who is a qualified psychiatrist. Note that this is *preferable*. Although it is worth aiming for, it is not essential. Patients or their families should not be put at risk by delays in trying to comply rigidly with it. Reviews of the legality of detention are conducted by Mental Health Tribunals, which follow automatically at set periods and also if requested by patients. The main sections of the Act used by clinicians are summarized in Table 4.1.

Assessment and treatment sections

The Assessment Order, Section 2, is for 4 weeks (in emergencies, Section 4 is for 72 hours). It allows patients who are not already known and diagnosed to be admitted and assessed if their condition is serious and warrants this. It cannot be repeated. Necessary medication to manage the assessment safely is permitted, but if the diagnosis is confirmed and involuntary treatment is to be instituted, the patient should be transferred to Section 3. There is considerable variation in how much intervention is permitted while the patient is on Section 2. Some social services have advocated for the use of Section 2 as a matter of course, even when patients and their disorders are known to the team. This is to 'assess' their response to this admission. There seems to be little logic to this, and generally a Section 3 should be used when the patient is known to those admitting them, or if the clinical picture is clear and a confident diagnosis can be made. Section 3 is for up to 6 months in the first instance, and can be repeated. Patients on Section 3 can be allowed out of hospital 'on leave' while still under compulsion using Section 17. There is no specific time limit for Section 17 beyond that

imposed by the Section 3, which stays in force. The Code of Practice proposes that it should be reviewed every 7 days and the alternative of a Community Treatment Order considered if extended beyond 7 days. Voluntary patients can be detained for assessment if their condition deteriorates and they attempt to discharge themselves under the provision of Section 5.

Restriction orders and transfers

Patients can be transferred from courts on Section 37 (equivalent to a Section 3) for treatment. Their management is the same as for a Section 3, and they can be discharged when well. Similarly, a prisoner who becomes seriously unwell can be transferred on Section 47 for treatment (again following the same principles as Section 3), but has to be returned to prison when they have recovered. The equivalent assessment order (up to 28 days) is Section 35. The Home Office can impose a restriction order (37/41) on a patient. This means that the psychiatrist cannot

Table 4.1 Sections of the England and Wales Mental Health Act commonly used by clinicians

Section number	Purpose	Duration
Section 2	Assessment	28 days
Section 3	Treatment	6 months, repeatable
Section 4	Emergency assessment	72 hours
Section 5	Detention of informal inpatient	72 hours
Section 17	Leave while on Section 3	Section 3 still in force
Section 17a	Treatment in community (Community Treatment Order)	6 months, renewable
Section 35	Transfer for assessment	28 days
Section 37	Transfer for treatment	6 months
Section 37/41	Restriction order	Imposed by Home Office
Section 135	Forced entry	72 hours
Section 136	Police powers to convey	72 hours

discharge them from their section without permission. However, they can be managed on leave in the community with the Home Office's permission.

Police powers and power of entry

The police have the power to detain anyone whom they find in a public place who is manifestly disturbed and whom they consider to need urgent psychiatric assessment. In the UK this is Section 136 of the Act, and it allows the police to bring the patient to a place of safety for assessment by a psychiatrist and an approved mental health professional (AMHP). The person can be held for up to 72 hours, but the Code of Practice recommends assessment within 6 hours. In the past, police stations were the usual place of safety (and they sometimes still are), but it is considered good practice for assessment to take place in an agreed psychiatric assessment suite. Section 136 is predominantly used in metropolitan settings, and there is little reason to believe that it is overused (the police have quite high thresholds for using it). A local study in North London conducted some years ago indicated that a higher proportion of Section 136s were converted to treatment sections than were Section 2 assessment orders.

The right of individuals to be undisturbed in their own homes is a very ancient one, and one that is vigorously protected. Unless there is overwhelming evidence of immediate risk, entry cannot be forced. Where it is believed that a known patient is deteriorating and requires assessment but they are refusing entry to their home, a warrant from a magistrate is needed. This is Section 135, usually obtained within a day by the social worker. The warrant allows admission by the police officer, accompanied by a psychiatrist and an AMHP, who generally assess for Section 2 or 3.

Community Treatment Orders

The most significant change introduced by the 2007 amendment of the 1983 Mental Health Act was the introduction of Community Treatment Orders (CTOs), often referred to as Section 17a, in official documents. These introduced an effective mechanism for ensuring treatment in the community for patients with established severe disorders and poor compliance with treatment ('revolving-door patients'). Forms of compulsory treatment in the community had been in widespread use in the USA, Canada, Australia, and New Zealand for over three decades (Dawson, 2005). They have attracted strong clinician and family support, although the scientific evidence is that they do not improve outcomes. The three randomized controlled trials that have been published found no impact on relapse and readmission. This has not, however, slowed their use (Swartz et al., 1999; Steadman et al.,2001; Burns et al., 2013). The UK provision can only be applied when a patient is already detained on Section 3. They are subject to a legal requirement to attend for monitoring in the community.

The CTO mirrors the inpatient treatment order (i.e. 6 months repeatable in the first instance, with repeat renewals of 12 months subsequently, and regular tribunal assessments). It is strengthened by a requirement for an independent second opinion in all cases. Beyond this statutory condition for a second opinion, other clinically determined conditions can be added. The commonest are to reside at a stated address and to allow regular access by the clinical team. CTOs do not permit any force outside hospital, but allow for patients to be returned to a clinical setting for up to 72 hours for assessment and treatment. About 4000 CTOs per year are initiated in England and Wales.

CTOs in the UK are generally imposed for substantial periods, and during the first years of their introduction very few of them have been revoked. This reflects the UK's 'paternalistic' approach, with CTOs being used to stabilize functioning in patients with frequently relapsing psychoses. In the USA most are imposed for a short period while patients pose an active risk. However, those who remain on them beyond this early phase stay on them for months or even years.

Informal coercion

Traditionally research into coercion in psychiatry has been based on rates of legal detention. Investigations into how patients perceived their care, however, revealed that it is not so clear-cut. Many voluntary inpatients felt that they were not really free to come and go or refuse treatment (Kaltiala-Heino, 1996; atsakou et al., 2011) and some community patients in Assertive Community Treatment Team care have reported that they found the assertive outreach coercive (Watts and Priebe, 2002; Krupa *et al.*, 2005).

The research focus has shifted from simply enumerating the number of patients legally detained to better understanding their experiences of mental health care. Much of this research has used a rating scale developed by a US research group—the MacArthur Perceived Coercion Scale (Gardner *et al.*, 1993). This simple 15-question scale has three components—perceived coercion, negative pressures, and procedural justice. Initially developed to measure the experience of psychiatric admission, the scale has been adapted for community care. A striking finding is that how a compulsory admission is handled (procedural justice—whether the patient feels listened to and understood) makes a big difference in how coercive they rate the admission (Bonsack and Borgeat, 2005).

Hierarchy of pressures and leverage

With the growing awareness that many community patients experienced their care as coercive, attempts have been made to classify the different types of coercion and to measure some of them. Szmukler and Applebaum (2008) have proposed a hierarchy of treatment pressures arranged on five levels (Box 4.5). Not all levels of persuasion are considered coercive but certainly the last two are.

What Szmukler and Applebaum refer to as inducement has been called 'leverage' in later literature. Leverages are when access to benefits (or avoidance of unwanted consequences) are *explicitly* linked to adherence to treatment. Leverage is when the clinician says to the patient 'if you take your treatment regularly I can help you get a flat, or better benefits, or probation rather than prison'. A survey of leverage with 1011 patients in public mental health services in five states in the US found that nearly half of them reported feeling pressurized in this way into cooperate with treatment (Monahan *et al.*, 2005). The leverages were classified as financial, housing, and criminal justice (usually avoiding or reducing a sentence). A similar pattern, albeit at lower levels (around 30–35%) has been reported in the UK (Burns *et al.*, 2011) and Switzerland (Jäger and Rössler, 2010). Access to separated children has also emerged as

> ### Box 4.5 Levels of persuasion
>
> - Persuasion (includes providing information, appreciation of patient's preferences, and discussion and collaboration between clinician and patient).
> - Interpersonal leverage (based on a patient's emotional dependency on clinician; patient agrees to adhere to please clinician.
> - Inducement (clinician offers reward for adherence).
> - Threats (clinician proposes negative or prevents positive consequences of a patient's non-adherence).
> - Compulsion (involuntary).
>
> Reproduced from Journal of Mental Health, 17(3), Szmukler G and Appelbaum P, Treatment pressures, leverage, coercion and compulsion in mental health care, pp. 233–44, Copyright (2008), with permission from Taylor & Francis.

an important leverage, particularly in individuals with substance abuse (Burns *et al.*, 2011).

Contingency management is a special form of leverage where a direct reward is provided for adherence to treatment. The most controversial schemes involve paying patients to cooperate and have been used mainly with socially marginalized individuals such as homeless sufferers from tuberculosis and even to encourage antenatal care for pregnant teenagers. The approach generates very strong feelings, and many clinicians find it quite unacceptable as it seems to devalue the therapeutic relationship. One trial of paying psychosis patients to comply with their depot injections did find an improvement (Priebe *et al.*, 2013), but there is little evidence of any widespread acceptance of the approach.

The recent focus on informal coercion has underlined just how common it is and also that it is a legitimate part of the therapeutic relationship. All human relationships involve some degree of trying to influence each other, either explicitly or implicitly. The recent attention has made clear the absence of any professional consideration of the practice (Dunn *et al.*, 2014; Valenti *et al.*, 2015) and the need for more structured discussion to permit the emergence of some consensus on what is good practice and what may be overstepping the mark.

Some aspects of civil law

Civil law deals with the rights and obligations of individuals to one another, including family law, which is a particular concern of child psychiatrists. In this respect civil law differs from criminal law, which is concerned with offences against the state (although some are directed against an individual, e.g. homicide). As well as the issues discussed earlier in this chapter, civil law is concerned with property, inheritance, and contracts. Proceedings in civil law are undertaken by individuals or groups who believe that they have suffered a breach of the civil law, in contrast to criminal law proceedings, which are undertaken on behalf of the state.

Psychiatrists are sometimes asked to submit written reports on a patient's mental state in relation to a civil case. Such reports should be prepared only after full discussion with the patient, and only with the patient's informed consent, and they should be concise and factual. The structure should follow the plan set out on page 536 (Box 18.10). It is advisable to seek legal advice about the relevant aspects of law relating to the case. The following sections are based on the law in England and Wales, although the principles apply more widely.

Testamentary capacity

This term refers to the capacity to make a valid will. If someone is suffering from mental disorder at the time of making a will, its validity may be in doubt and other people may challenge it. The will may still be legally valid if the testator was of 'sound disposing mind' (see below) at the time of making it. Psychiatrists may be asked to report in relation to two issues:

1. Testamentary capacity.
2. The possibility that the testator was subjected to undue influence.

To decide whether or not a testator is of sound disposing mind, the doctor should decide whether the person making the will:

- Understands what a will is and its consequences.
- Knows the nature and extent of his property (not necessarily in detail).
- Knows the names of close relatives and can assess their claims to his property.
- *Is free from an abnormal state of mind* that might distort feelings or judgements relevant to making the will. A deluded person may legitimately make a will, provided that the delusions are unlikely to influence it.

To decide these matters, the doctor should first interview the testator alone and then interview relatives or friends to check the accuracy of factual statements. Assessment of undue influence is more complex, and requires an assessment of the relationship between testator and beneficiary, the mental state of the testator, and what is known of the person's earlier intentions.

Power of attorney and receivership

If a patient is incapable of managing their possessions by reason of mental disorder, alternative arrangements need to be made, particularly if the incapacity is likely to last for a long time. Such arrangements may be required for patients who are living in the community as well as for those who are in hospital. In English law two methods are available—power of attorney and receivership.

Power of attorney is the simpler method, and requires only that the patient gives written authorization for someone else to act for them during their illness. In signing such authorization, the patient must be able to understand what they are doing. They may revoke it at any time.

Receivership is the more formal procedure, and is more likely to be in the patient's interests. In England and Wales an application is made to the Court of Protection, which may decide to appoint a receiver. The procedure is most commonly required for the elderly. The question of receivership places special responsibility on the psychiatrist. If a patient is capable of managing their affairs on admission to hospital, but later becomes incapable by reason of intellectual deterioration, then it is the doctor's duty to advise the patient's relatives about the risks to property. If the relatives are unwilling to take action, then it is the doctor's duty to make an application to the Court of Protection. The doctor may feel reluctant to act in this way, but any actions taken subsequently are the Court's responsibility and not that of the doctor.

Aspects of family law

A *marriage contract* is not valid if, at the time of the marriage, either party was so mentally disordered as not to understand its nature. If mental disorder of this degree can be proved, a marriage may be decreed null and void by a divorce court. If a marriage partner becomes of 'incurably unsound mind' later in a marriage, this may be grounds for divorce, and a psychiatrist may be asked to give a prognosis. A doctor may also be asked for an opinion about the *capacity of parents or a guardian* to care adequately for a child.

Torts and contracts

Torts are wrongs for which a person is liable in civil law as opposed to criminal law. They include negligence, libel, slander, trespass, and nuisance. If such a wrong is committed by a person of unsound mind, then any damages awarded in a court of law are usually only nominal. In this context the legal definition of unsound mind is restrictive, and it is advisable for a psychiatrist to take advice about it from a lawyer.

If the person makes a contract and subsequently develops a mental disorder, the contract remains binding. If a person is of unsound mind when the contract is made, in English law a distinction is made between the 'necessaries' and 'non-necessaries' of life. A contract made for necessaries is always binding and that for *non-necessaries* is binding unless it can be shown both that the person did not understand what they were doing and that the other person was aware of the incapacity.

Personal injury

Psychiatrists may be asked to write reports in relation to claims for compensation by patients with post-traumatic stress disorder or one of the other psychological sequelae of accidents (see page 667). Such reports should be set out to accord with the relevant local legal procedures and should state clearly the sources of information, the history of the trauma, the psychiatric and social history, and the post-accident course. They should include a detailed assessment of function and of the relationship between the trauma and any subsequent symptoms and disability.

Fitness to drive

Questions of fitness to drive arise in relation to many psychiatric disorders. Dangerous driving may result from suicidal inclinations or manic disinhibition, panicky or aggressive driving may result from persecutory delusions, and indecisive or inaccurate driving may be due to dementia. Concentration on driving may be impaired in severe anxiety or depressive disorders. The question of fitness to drive also arises in relation to the sedative and other side effects of some psychiatric drugs, such as some anxiolytic or antipsychotic drugs in high dosage.

Doctors should be aware of and follow the legal criteria for fitness to drive in the places in which they are working. These criteria may differ somewhat for drivers of cars and drivers of heavy goods vehicles (the latter are stricter). UK holders of driving licences have a duty to inform the Driver and Vehicle Licensing Agency (DVLA) if they have a condition that may affect their safety as a driver. Doctors should inform patients if they have such a condition, and make sure that they understand their duty to report it. When deciding on a patient's fitness to drive, doctors should consider whether the patient's condition or its treatment is liable to cause loss of control, impair perception or comprehension, impair judgement, reduce concentration, or affect motor functions involved in handling the vehicle. If, after full discussion, a patient with such a condition continues to drive, a doctor working in the UK should disclose the relevant medical information to the medical adviser of the DVLA.

Further reading

In many countries, national medical and psychiatric organizations publish guidelines about the ethical and legal aspects of practice.

American Psychiatric Association (2001). *Ethics Primer of the American Psychiatric Association*. American Psychiatric Association, Washington, DC.

Bloch S, Chodoff P and Green S (eds) (1999). *Psychiatric Ethics*. 3rd edn. Oxford University Press, Oxford. (A series of reviews by leading writers covering the principal theoretical issues.)

Hope T, Savelescu J and Hendrick J (2008). *Medical Ethics and Law: the core curriculum*. 2nd edn. Churchill Livingstone, Edinburgh. (A comprehensive introductory text.)

Montgomery J (2002) *Health Care Law*. 2nd edn. Oxford University Press, Oxford. (A useful work of reference.)

CHAPTER 5
Aetiology

Approaches to aetiology in psychiatry

Psychiatrists are concerned with aetiology in two ways. First, in everyday clinical work they try to discover the causes of the mental disorders presented by individual patients. Secondly, in seeking a wider understanding of psychiatry they are interested in aetiological evidence obtained from *clinical studies, community surveys*, or *laboratory investigations*. Correspondingly, the first part of this chapter deals with some general issues relating to aetiology in the assessment of the individual patient, while the second part deals with the various scientific disciplines that have been applied to the study of aetiology.

General issues relating to aetiology

Aetiology and intuitive understanding

When the clinician assesses an individual patient, he draws on a common fund of aetiological knowledge that has been derived from the study of groups of similar patients, but he cannot understand the patient in these terms alone. He also has to use everyday insights into human nature. For example, when assessing a depressed patient, the psychiatrist should certainly know what has been discovered about the psychological and neuro-chemical changes that accompany depressive disorders, and what evidence there is about the aetiological role of stressful events, and about genetic predisposition to depressive disorder. At the same time he will need intuitive understanding to recognize, for example, that this particular patient feels depressed because he has learned that his wife has cancer.

Common-sense ideas of this kind are an important part of aetiological formulation in psychiatry, but they must be used carefully if superficial explanation is to be avoided. Aetiological formulation can be done properly only if certain conceptual problems are clearly understood. These problems can be illustrated by a case history.

For 4 weeks a 38-year-old married woman became increasingly depressed. Her symptoms started soon after her husband left her, saying that he wanted to live by himself. In the past the patient's mother had received psychiatric treatment on two occasions, once for a severe depressive disorder and once for mania; on neither occasion was there any apparent environmental cause for the illness. When the patient was 14 years old, her father went away to live with another woman, leaving his children with their mother. For several years afterwards the patient felt rejected and unhappy, but she eventually settled down. She later married, and she had two children, aged 13 and 10 years, at the time of her illness. Two weeks after leaving home the patient's husband returned, saying that he had made a mistake and really loved his wife. Despite his return the patient's symptoms persisted and worsened. She began to wake early, gave up her usual activities, and spoke at times of suicide.

When thinking about the causes of this woman's symptoms, the clinician would first draw on knowledge of aetiology derived from scientific enquiries. Genetic investigations have shown that, if a parent suffers from mania as well as depressive disorder, a predisposition to mood disorder is particularly likely to be transmitted to the children. Therefore it is possible that this patient received this predisposition from her mother.

Clinical investigation has also provided some information about the effects of separating children from their parents. In the present case, the information is not helpful because it refers to people who were separated from their parents at a younger age than the patient. On scientific grounds, therefore there is no particular reason to focus on the departure of the patient's father, but *intuitively* it seems very likely that this was an important event. From everyday experience it is understandable that a woman should feel very upset if her husband leaves her. It is also understandable that she is likely to feel even more distressed if this event recapitulates a related distressing experience in her own childhood. Therefore the clinician would recognize intuitively that the patient's depression is likely to be a reaction to the husband's departure and having to manage the distress of her children. The same sort of intuition might suggest that the patient would start to feel better when her husband came back, but in the event she did not recover.

This simple case history illustrates some important aetiological issues in psychiatry:

- the complexity of causes
- the classification of causes

- the concept of stress
- the concept of psychological reaction
- the relative roles of intuition and scientific knowledge in aetiological formulations.

The complexity of causes in psychiatry

In psychiatry, the study of causation is complicated by three problems. These problems are encountered in other branches of medicine, but to a lesser degree.

Lack of temporal association

The first problem is that causes are often *remote in time* from the effects that they produce. For example, it is widely believed that childhood experiences partly determine the occurrence of emotional difficulties in adult life. It is difficult to test this idea, because the necessary information can only be gathered either by studying children and tracing them many years later, which is difficult, or by asking adults about their childhood experiences, which is unreliable.

Cause and effect

The second problem is that a single cause may lead to *several effects*. For example, being deprived of parental affection in childhood has been reported to predispose to antisocial behaviour, suicide, depressive disorder, and several other disorders. Conversely, a single effect may arise from several causes. The latter can be illustrated either by different causes in different individuals or by multiple causes in a single individual. For example, learning disability (a single effect) may occur in several children, but the cause may be a different genetic abnormality or environmental stressor in each child. On the other hand, depressive disorder (a single effect) may occur in one individual through a combination of causes, such as genetic factors, adverse childhood experiences, and stressful events in adult life.

Indirect mechanisms

The third problem is that aetiological factors in psychiatry rarely exert their effects directly. For example, the genetic predisposition to depression may be mediated in part through temperamental factors that make it more likely that the individual concerned will experience adverse life events. Thus aetiological effects are usually mediated through complex intervening mechanisms, which also need to be investigated and understood.

The classification of causes

A single psychiatric disorder, as just explained, may result from several causes. For this reason a scheme for *classifying* causes is required. A useful approach is to divide causes chronologically into those that are *predisposing, precipitating*, and *maintaining*.

Predisposing factors

These are factors, many of them operating from early in life, that determine a person's vulnerability to causal factors acting close to the time of the illness. They include *genetic endowment* and the *environment in utero*, as well as *physical, psychological, and social factors in infancy and early childhood*. The term 'constitution' is often used to describe the mental and physical make-up of a person at any point in their life. This make-up changes as life goes on under the influence of further physical, psychological, and social influences. Some writers restrict the term constitution to the make-up at the beginning of life, while others also include characteristics that are acquired later (this second usage is adopted in this book). The concept of constitution includes the idea that a person may have a predisposition to develop a disorder (e.g. schizophrenia) even though the latter never manifests itself. From the standpoint of psychiatric aetiology, one of the important parts of the constitution is the *personality*.

When the aetiology of an individual case is formulated, the personality is always an essential element. For this reason, the clinician should be prepared to spend sufficient time talking to the patient and to people who know them to build up a clear picture of their personality. This assessment often helps to explain why the patient responded to certain stressful events, and why they reacted in a particular way. The obvious importance of personality in the individual patient contrasts with the small amount of relevant scientific information so far available. Therefore, when evaluating personality it is particularly important to acquire sound clinical skills through supervised practice.

Precipitating factors

These are events that occur shortly before the onset of a disorder and which *appear to have induced it*. They may be physical, psychological, or social. Whether they produce a disorder at all, and what kind of disorder, depends partly on constitutional factors in the patient (as mentioned above). Examples of physical precipitants include cerebral tumours and drugs. Psychological and social precipitants include personal misfortunes such as the loss of a job or an important relationship, and changes in the routine of life, such as moving home. Sometimes the same factor can act in more than one way. For example, a head injury can induce psychological disorder either through physical changes in the brain or through its stressful implications for the patient.

Maintaining factors

These factors *prolong the course of a disorder* after it has been provoked. When planning treatment, it is particularly important to pay attention to these factors. The original predisposing and precipitating factors may have ceased to act by the time the patient is seen, but the maintaining factors may well be treatable. For example, in their early stages many psychiatric disorders lead to secondary demoralization and withdrawal from social activities, which in turn help to prolong the original disorder. It is often appropriate to treat these secondary factors, whether or not any other specific measures are carried out. Maintaining factors are also called *perpetuating factors*.

The concept of stress

Discussions about stress are often confusing because the term is used in two ways. First, it is applied to events or situations, such as working for an examination, which may have an adverse effect on someone. Secondly, it is applied to the adverse effects that are induced, which may involve psychological or physiological change. When considering aetiology it is advisable to separate these components.

The first set of factors can usefully be called *stressors*. They include a large number of physical, psychological, and social factors that can produce adverse effects. The term is sometimes extended to include events that are not experienced as adverse at the time, but which may still have adverse long-term effects. For example, intense competition may produce an immediate feeling of pleasant tension, although it may sometimes lead to unfavourable long-term effects.

The effect on the person can usually be called the *stress reaction*, to distinguish it from the provoking events. This reaction includes *autonomic responses* (e.g. a rise in blood pressure), *endocrine changes* (e.g. the secretion of adrenaline and noradrenaline), and *psychological responses* (e.g. a feeling of being keyed up). Much current neurobiology research is involved in studying the effects of stressors on the brain, and in particular how stressors affect the mechanisms involved in the regulation of mood and processing of emotional information (see Chapter 7).

The concept of a psychological reaction

As already mentioned, it is widely recognized that psychological distress can occur as a reaction to unpleasant events. Sometimes the association between event and distress is evident—for example, when a woman becomes depressed after the death of her husband. In other cases it is far from clear whether the psychological disorder is really a reaction to an event, or whether the two have coincided fortuitously—for example, when a person becomes depressed after the death of a distant relative.

Jaspers (1963, page 392) suggested three criteria for deciding whether a psychological state is a reaction to a particular set of events:

- The events must be adequate in severity and closely related in time to the onset of the psychological state.
- There must be a clear connection between the nature of the events and the content of the psychological disorder (in the example just given, the person should be preoccupied with ideas concerning their distant relative).
- The psychological state should begin to disappear when the events have ceased (unless, of course, it can be shown that perpetuating factors are acting to maintain it).

These three criteria are useful in clinical practice, although they can be difficult to apply (particularly the second criterion).

Understanding and explanation

As already mentioned, aetiological statements about individual patients must combine knowledge derived from research on groups of patients with intuitive understanding derived from everyday experience. Jaspers (1963, page 302) has called these two ways of making sense of psychiatric disorders 'Erklären' and 'Verstehen', respectively.

In German, these terms mean 'explanation' and 'understanding', respectively, and they are usually translated as such in English translations of Jaspers' writing. However, Jaspers used them in a special sense.

He used 'Erklären' to refer to the sort of causative statement that is sought in the natural sciences. It is exemplified by the statement that a patient's aggressive behaviour has occurred because he has a brain tumour. He used 'Verstehen' to refer to psychological understanding, or the intuitive grasp of a natural connection between events in a person's life and his psychological state. In colloquial English, this could be called 'putting oneself in another person's shoes'. It is exemplified by the statement 'I can understand why the patient became angry when her children were shouted at by a neighbour.'

These distinctions are reasonably clear when we consider an individual patient, but confusion sometimes arises when attempts are made to generalize from insights obtained in a single case to widely applicable principles. Understanding may then be mistaken for explanation. Jaspers suggested that some psychoanalytical ideas are special kinds of intuitive understanding that are derived from the detailed study of individuals and then applied generally. They are not explanations that can be tested scientifically. They are more akin to insights into human nature that can be gained from reading great works of literature. Such insights are of great value in conducting human affairs. It would be wrong to neglect them in psychiatry, but equally wrong to see them as statements of a scientific kind.

The aetiology of a single case

How to make an aetiological formulation was discussed in Chapter 3. An example was given of a woman in her thirties who had become increasingly depressed. The formulation showed how aetiological factors could be grouped under headings of predisposing, precipitating, and perpetuating factors. It also showed how information from scientific investigations (in this case genetics) could be combined with an intuitive understanding of personality and the likely effects of family problems on the patient. The reader may find it helpful to re-read this formulation before continuing with this chapter.

Aetiological models

Before considering the contribution that different scientific disciplines can make to psychiatric aetiology, attention needs to be given to the kinds of aetiological model that have been employed in psychiatry. A model is a device for ordering information. Like a theory, it seeks to explain certain phenomena, but it does so in a broad and comprehensive way that cannot readily be proved false.

Reductionist and non-reductionist models

Two broad categories of explanatory model can be recognized. *Reductionist models* seek to understand causation by tracing back to increasingly simple early stages. Examples include the 'narrow' medical model, which is described below, and the psychoanalytic model. This type of model can be exemplified by the statement that the cause of schizophrenia lies in disordered neurotransmission in a specific area of the brain.

Non-reductionist models try to relate problems to wider rather than narrower issues. The explanatory models that are used in sociology are generally of this kind. In psychiatry, this type of model can be exemplified by the statement that the cause of a patient's depression lies in her family; the patient is the most conspicuous element in a disordered group of people. In the same way it can be asserted that certain depressive states are associated with indices of social deprivation and isolation, and can be best understood as being caused by these factors.

The neuroscience approach

The technical and conceptual advances in brain sciences have led to what is often called the *neuroscience approach*. Kandel (1998) outlined the key assumptions underlying this approach to aetiology, which can be summarized as follows.

- All mental processes derive from operations of the brain. Thus all behavioural disorders are ultimately disturbances of brain function, even where the original 'cause' is clearly environmental.
- Genes have important effects on brain function and therefore exert significant control over behaviour.
- Social and behavioural factors exert their effects on the brain in part through changes in gene expression. Changes in gene expression leading to altered patterns of synaptic connectivity underlie the ability of experiences to produce learning and psychotherapy to change behaviour.

The latter concept derives from the ability of a wide range of environmental stimuli to modulate gene expression by various mechanisms, including epigenetic modifications (see below). Thus while genes coding for particular proteins are inherited, environmental and developmental influences are involved in determining whether and to what extent a particular gene is expressed. This provides a plausible mechanism by which nature and nurture interact in the production of a behavioural phenotype.

The neuroscience approach therefore seeks to comprehend the role of social, family, and personal factors in behaviour by relating them to changes in brain function. For example, in understanding the effect of childhood neglect on liability to adult depression, it may be important to find out how adverse childhood experiences might alter relevant brain mechanisms (e.g. the endocrine response to stress), and how this abnormality might predispose to depression when the individual is exposed to difficulties in adulthood. Thus, although a neuroscience approach encompasses the importance of social and personal factors, it seeks to understand their consequences in a *reductionist* way.

Medical models

Several models are used in psychiatric aetiology, but the so-called *medical model* is the most prominent one. It represents a general strategy of research that has proved useful in medicine, particularly in studying infectious diseases. A disease entity is identified in terms of a consistent pattern of symptoms, a characteristic clinical course, and specific biochemical and pathological findings (see Chapter 2 regarding models of disease). When an entity has been identified in this way, a set of necessary and sufficient causes is sought. In the case of tuberculosis, for example, the tubercle bacillus is the necessary cause, but it is not by itself sufficient. However, the tubercle bacillus in conjunction with either poor nutrition or low resistance is sufficient cause.

The importance of personal and social factors in the presentation and course of illness is now well recognized in general medicine, and modern medical models are therefore considerably broader than those based on the elucidation of the mechanism of infectious disease. Modern medical models also recognize that much illness is characterized by quantitative rather than qualitative deviations from normal (e.g. high blood pressure). This also applies to certain disorders in psychiatry, particularly anxiety and milder depressive disorders, which can therefore be accommodated in a broad medical model.

Difficulties with the medical model arise, particularly in relation to disorders that are characterized principally by *abnormalities of conduct and social behaviour*, such as antisocial behaviour and substance misuse. As mentioned above, current neuroscience approaches would seek to understand these disorders through changes in relevant brain systems. This is because causal factors in abnormal social behaviour, such as childhood maltreatment and deprivation, must ultimately express their effects on behaviour through changes in brain mechanisms.

Although the latter view appears theoretically valid, the key decision for both clinician and policy-maker is at what level the disorder is best understood and managed. For example, it is possible to understand problems in substance misuse as arising from a defect in brain reward systems which, in a vulnerable individual, results in 'normal' experimentation with illicit substances leading to substance misuse, with adverse personal and social consequences. Equally, one can see excessive drug misuse in society as a 'symptom' of social deprivation and family disruption (see Chapter 20). Both aetiological models may be valid, but each would suggest different forms of research activity and therapeutic intervention.

The behavioural model

As explained above, certain disorders that psychiatrists treat, particularly those defined in terms of *abnormal behaviour*, do not fit readily into the medical model. The latter include deliberate self-harm, the misuse of drugs and alcohol, and repeated acts of delinquency. The behavioural model is an alternative way of comprehending these disorders. In this model the disorders are explained in terms of factors that determine normal behaviour. These include drives, reinforcements, social and cultural influences, and internal psychological processes such as attitudes, beliefs, and expectations. The behavioural model predicts that there will not be a sharp distinction between the normal and the abnormal, but a continuous gradation. This model can therefore be a useful way of considering many of the conditions that are seen by psychiatrists.

Although the behavioural model is mainly concerned with psychological and social causes, it does not exclude genetic, physiological, or biochemical causes. This is because normal patterns of behaviour are partly determined by genetic factors, and because psychological factors such as reinforcement have a basis in physiological and biochemical mechanisms. Also, the behavioural model employs both *reductionist* and *non-reductionist* explanations. For example, abnormalities of behaviour can be explained in terms of abnormal conditioning (a reductionist model) or in terms of a network of social influences.

Developmental models

Medical and behavioural models incorporate the idea of predisposing as well as precipitating causes (i.e. the idea

that past events may determine whether or not a current cause gives rise to a disorder). Some models place even more emphasis on past events in the form of a sequence of experiences leading to the present disorder. This approach has been called the 'life story' approach to aetiology. One example is Freud's psychoanalysis (see Box 5.1) and another is Meyer's psychobiology. These ideas are considered further below.

Political models ('antipsychiatry', 'critical psychiatry')

The models outlined above rely on a scientific approach to psychiatric aetiology. This implies that psychiatric disorders, like other medical conditions, can be studied and understood in an objective and empirical way using the methods of natural sciences. In the history of psychiatry this view has often been regarded as far from self-evident, and other conceptual frameworks have sometimes been advocated. For example, it was customary in the Middle Ages to explain mental illness in terms of demonic possession and witchcraft (see below). Over the past 50 years, however, criticisms of scientific approaches to aetiology have most often taken the view that psychiatric illness is defined by *social and political imperatives*, and represents at best a cultural value judgement and at worst an abusive means of controlling those whom society finds inconvenient or troubling.

Arguments of this nature were put forward strongly by the French philosopher, Michel Foucault (1926–1984), and were further developed by psychiatrists such as RD Laing (1927–1989), who employed a phenomenological approach to argue that schizophrenia is an understandable response of an individual to a culture of exploitation and alienation. Lack of faith in a scientific approach to mental experience was exemplified by the psychiatrist Thomas Szasz (1920–2012), who commented that 'There is no psychology; there is only biography and autobiography.' These ideas are sometimes called 'antipsychiatry' to emphasize their fundamental contrast with the medical models employed by conventional psychiatry.

Most psychiatrists have believed that these formulations do not advance the understanding of mental illness, and in fact provide rather poor explanations of the range of clinical psychopathology. For example, they seem unable to account for the existence of schizophrenia in all human societies (see Chapter 11). However, *political and cultural perceptions* of mental illness are important because they have powerful effects on the stigma associated with mental illness, the way that

Box 5.1 Psychoanalysis

Psychoanalysis is derived from clinical experience rather than from basic sciences, and consists of elaborate theories of both normal and abnormal mental development. Compared with experimental psychology it is more concerned with *irrational* aspects of mental activity.

Psychoanalytic theories are derived from data obtained in the course of psychoanalytic treatment, and relate to the patient's thoughts, dreams, and fantasies, as well as their memories of childhood experiences and relationships with carers and siblings. Therefore psychoanalytic theories are forms of intuitive understanding ('Verstehen') rather than scientific explanation ('Erklären') (see page 3).

Freud developed a number of ideas about the *unconscious mind*, from which he believed all mental processes originated. The unconscious mind has three key features that are important in the genesis of psychological problems.

1. It is divorced from reality.
2. It is dynamic and contains powerful forces.
3. It is in conflict with the conscious mind.

Freud believed that the unconscious mind could be probed by *dream analysis* and *free association*. The manifest content of a dream can be traced back to a latent content, which is an infantile wish. This wish is disguised by *dreamwork*, which, through various psychological mechanisms, transforms the latent content into a manifest form that is more acceptable to consciousness.

The unconscious mind is the seat of powerful instinctual drives (e.g. sexual and aggressive impulses). The forces in the unconscious mind struggle against the conscious mind, which can give rise to anxiety. This anxiety can be reduced by a variety of *defence mechanisms*, which can be discerned in the behaviour of healthy people as well as those with psychological disorders (see Chapter 7).

Sexual impulses are present from the earliest stages of child development, and there is a progression through different stages of organization (oral, anal, and genital) as the child grows. Failure to pass through these stages effectively can lead to sexual energy (*libido*) becoming fixated, which results in the individual exhibiting infantile patterns of behaviour or regressing to them when under stress. The object of libido also changes with development, first focusing on the self and then focusing on the mother. In the course of this maternal attachment, boys experience angry feelings towards their father (the *Oedipus complex*), while girls develop reverse attachments. Difficulties in resolving these conflicted attachments can give rise to problems in interpersonal relationships later in life.

Freud's theories were developed by many others. Melanie Klein's work, which addresses pre-Oedipal aggressive and sexual drives in a theory of *object relations*, has been influential in the UK.

---

mentally ill people are treated, and the services provided (see Chapter 26). Furthermore, there is no doubt that horrifying abuse of psychiatric patients has occurred, as demonstrated by the cooperation of many leading German psychiatrists with the euthanasia programmes of the Nazi regime (Torrey and Yolken, 2010).

While this is an extreme and abhorrent example, political analyses of psychiatric practice highlight the need for the *rights of patients to be respected* and their experiences understood in a personal and social context as outlined above. (For a discussion of the limits of scientific approaches to psychiatric illness, see Bracken *et al.*, 2012.)

The historical development of ideas of aetiology

From the earliest times, theories of the causation of mental disorder have recognized both *somatic* and *psychological* influences. Greek medical literature referred to the causes of mental disorders, mainly in the Hippocratic writings (fourth century bc). Serious mental illness was ascribed mainly to physical causes, which were represented in the theory that health depended on a correct balance of the four *body 'humours'* (blood, phlegm, yellow bile, and black bile). Melancholia was ascribed to an excess of black bile. Most of the less severe psychiatric disorders were thought to have supernatural causes and to require religious healing. An exception was hysteria, which was thought to be physically caused by the displacement of the uterus from its normal position.

Roman physicians generally accepted the causal theories of Greek medicine, and developed them in some respects. Galen accepted that melancholia was caused by an excess of black bile, but suggested that this excess could result either from cooling of the blood or from overheating of yellow bile. Phrenitis, the name given to an acute febrile condition with delirium, was thought to result from an excess of yellow bile.

Throughout the Middle Ages these early ideas about the causes of mental illness were largely neglected, although they were maintained by some scholars, such as Bartholomeus Anglicus. The causes of mental illness were now formulated in theological terms of sin and evil, with the consequence that many mentally ill people were persecuted as witches. It was not until the middle of the sixteenth century that beliefs in the supernatural and witchcraft were strongly rejected as causes of mental disorder, notably by the Flemish writer Johan Weyer (1515–1588) in his book *De Praestigiis Daemonum*, published in 1563. Earlier, the renowned physician Paracelsus (1493–1541) had emphasized the natural causes of mental illness.

In the seventeenth and eighteenth centuries, a more scientific approach to the causation of mental illness developed as physicians became interested in mental disorders, mainly hysteria and melancholia. The English physician Thomas Willis attributed melancholia to 'passions of the heart', but considered that madness (illnesses with thought disorder, delusions, and hallucinations) was due to a 'fault of the brain'. Willis realized that this fault was not a recognizable gross structural lesion, but a functional abnormality. In the terminology of the time, he referred to a disorder of the 'vital spirits' that were thought to account for nervous action. He also pointed out that hysteria could not be caused by a displacement of the womb, because the organ is firmly secured in the pelvis.

Another seventeenth-century English physician, Thomas Sydenham, rejected the alternative theory that hysteria was caused by a functional disorder of the womb ('uterine suffocation'), because he had observed the condition in men. Despite this renewed medical interest in the causes of mental disorder, the most influential seventeenth-century treatise was written by a clergyman, Robert Burton (1577–1640). This work, *The Anatomy of Melancholy,* published in 1621, described in detail the psychological and social causes (such as poverty, fear, and solitude) that were associated with melancholia and seemed to cause it.

Aetiology depends on *nosology*. Unless it is clear how the various types of mental disorder relate to one another, little progress can be made in understanding causation. From his observations of patients with psychiatric disorders, the Italian physician Giovanni Battista Morgagni (1682–1771) became convinced that there was not one single kind of madness, but many different ones; further attempts at classification followed. One of the best known was proposed by William Cullen, who included a category of neurosis for disorders not caused by localized disease of the nervous system.

The idea that individual mental disorders are caused by lesions of particular brain areas can be traced back to the theory of phrenology proposed by Franz Gall (1758–1828) and his pupil Johann Spurzheim (1776–1832). Gall proposed that the brain was the organ of the mind, that the mind was made up of specific faculties, and that these faculties originated in specific brain areas. He also proposed that the size of a brain area determined the strength of the faculty that resided in it, and that the size of brain areas was reflected in the contours of the overlying skull. Thus the shape of the head reflected a person's psychological make-up. Although the last steps in Gall's argument were erroneous, the ideas of cerebral localization were to develop further. An increased interest in brain pathology led to theories that different forms of mental disorder were associated with lesions in different parts of the brain.

It had long been observed that serious mental illness ran in families, but in the nineteenth century this idea took a new form. Benedict Augustin Morel (1809–1873), a French psychiatrist, put forward ideas that became known as the 'theory of degeneration'. He proposed not only that some mental illnesses were inherited, but also that environmental influences (such as poor living conditions and the misuse of alcohol) could lead to physical changes that could be transmitted to the next generation. Morel also proposed that, as a result of the successive effect of environmental agents in each generation, illnesses appeared in increasingly severe forms in successive generations. It was inherent in these ideas that mental disorders did not differ in kind but only in *severity*, with neuroses, psychoses, and mental handicap being increasingly severe manifestations of the same inherited process.

These ideas were consistent with the accepted theories of the inheritance of acquired characteristics, and they were widely accepted. They had the unfortunate effect of encouraging a pessimistic approach to treatment. They also supported the Eugenics Movement, which held that the mentally ill should be removed from society to prevent them from reproducing. These developments are an important reminder that *aetiological theories may give rise to undesirable attitudes to the care of patients.*

Mid-nineteenth-century views of the causation of mental illness can be judged from the widely acclaimed textbooks of Jean-Étienne Esquirol (1772–1840), a French psychiatrist, and of Wilhelm Griesinger (1817–1868), a German psychiatrist. Esquirol focused on the causes of illness in the individual patient, and was less concerned with general theories of aetiology. He recorded psychological and physical factors, which he believed to be significant in individual cases, and he distinguished between predisposing and precipitating causes. He regarded heredity as the most important of the predisposing causes, but he also stressed that predisposition was acted on by psychological causes and by social (at that time called 'moral') causes such as domestic problems, 'disappointed love', and reverses of fortune. Important physical causes of mental disorder included epilepsy, alcohol misuse, excessive masturbation, childbirth and lactation, and suppression of menstruation. Esquirol also observed that age influenced the type of illness. Thus dementia was not observed among the young, but mania was uncommon in old age. He recognized that personality was often a predisposing factor.

In *Pathology and Therapy of Mental Disorders*, Griesinger maintained that mental illness was a *physical disorder of the brain*, and he considered at length the neuropathology of mental illness. He paid equal attention to other causes, including heredity, habitual drunkenness, 'domestic unquiet', disappointed love, and childbirth. He emphasized the multiplicity of causes when he wrote:

A closer examination of the aetiology of insanity soon shows that in the great majority of cases it was not a single specific cause under the influence of which the disease was finally established, but a complication of several, sometimes numerous causes, both predisposing and exciting. Very often the germs of the disease are laid in those early periods of life from which the commencement of the formation of character dates. It grows by education and external influences.

(Griesinger, 1867).

British views on aetiology in the late nineteenth century can be judged from *A Manual of Psychological Medicine* by Bucknill and Tuke, published in 1858, and from *The Pathology of Mind* by Henry Maudsley, published in 1879. Maudsley described the causes of mental disorder in terms similar to those of Griesinger. Thus causes were multiple, while *predisposing causes* (including heredity and early upbringing) were as important

as the more obvious *proximal causes*. Maudsley held that mistakes in determining causes were often due to 'some single prominent event, which was perhaps one in a chain of events, being selected as fitted by itself to explain the catastrophe. The truth is that in the great majority of cases there has been a concurrence of steadily operating conditions within and without, not a single effective cause' (Maudsley, 1879, *The Pathology of Mind,* page 83).

Although these nineteenth-century writers and teachers of psychiatry emphasized the *multiplicity of causes,* many practitioners focused narrowly on the findings of genetic and pathological investigations, and adopted a pessimistic approach to treatment. However, Adolf Meyer (1866–1950), a Swiss psychiatrist who worked mainly in the USA, emphasized the role of psychological and social factors in the aetiology of psychiatric disorder. Meyer applied the term *psychobiology* to this approach, in which a wide range of previous experiences was considered and then common-sense judgements used to decide which experiences might have led to the present disorder. Meyer acknowledged the importance of heredity and brain disorder, but emphasized that these factors were modified by life experiences, which often determined whether or not a particular disorder would be clinically expressed. Meyer's approach remains the basis of the evaluation of aetiology for the individual patient.

The aetiological theories considered so far have been mainly concerned with the major mental illnesses. Less severe disorders, particularly those that came to be called neurosis, hysteria, and hypochondriasis, and milder states of depression, were treated mainly by physicians. Pierre Charcot, a French neurologist, carried out extensive studies of patients with hysteria and of their response to hypnosis. He believed that hysteria resulted from a functional disorder of the brain and could be treated by hypnosis. In the USA, Weir Mitchell proposed that conditions akin to mild chronic depression were due to exhaustion of the nervous system—a condition he called *neurasthenia.*

In Austria, another neurologist, Sigmund Freud, tried to develop a more comprehensive explanation of nervous diseases, first of hysteria and then of other conditions. After an initial interest in physiological causes, Freud proposed that the causes were psychological, but hidden from the patient because they were in the unconscious part of the mind. Freud took a developmental approach to aetiology, believing that the seeds of adult disorder lay in the process of child development (see Box 5.1). In France, Pierre Janet developed an alternative psychological explanation, which was based on variations in the strength of nervous activity and on narrowing of the field of consciousness.

Interest in psychological explanations of the whole range of mental disorders grew as neuropathological and genetic studies failed to yield new insights. Freud and his followers attempted to extend their theory of the neuroses to explain the psychoses. Although the psychological theory was elaborated, no new objective data were obtained about the causes of severe mental illness. Nevertheless, the theories provided explanations that some psychiatrists found more acceptable than an admission of ignorance. Psychoanalysis became increasingly influential, particularly in American psychiatry, where it predominated until the 1970s. Since that time there has been renewed interest in genetic, biochemical, and neuropathological causes of mental disorder—an approach that has become known as *biological psychiatry* (Guze, 1989).

Perhaps the most important lesson to learn from this brief overview of the history of ideas on the causation of mental disorder is that each generation bases its theories of aetiology on the scientific approaches that are most active and plausible at the time. Sometimes psychological ideas prevail, sometimes neuropathological ones, and sometimes genetic ones. Throughout the centuries, however, observant clinicians have been aware of the *complexity of the causes of psychiatric disorders*, and have recognized that neither aetiology nor treatment should focus narrowly on the scientific ideas of the day. Instead, the approach should be broader, encompassing whatever psychological, social, and biological factors seem to be most important in the individual case. Modern psychiatrists are working in an era of rapid development of the neurosciences, but they need to keep the same broad clinical perspective of aetiology while assimilating any real scientific advances.

The contribution of scientific disciplines to psychiatric aetiology

The main groups of disciplines that have contributed to the knowledge of psychiatric aetiology are shown in Box 5.2. In this section each group is discussed in turn, and the following questions are asked:

- What sort of problem in psychiatric aetiology can be answered by each discipline?
- How, in general, does each discipline attempt to answer the questions?
- Are any particular difficulties encountered when applying its methods to psychiatric disorders?

Box 5.2 Scientific disciplines that contribute to psychiatric aetiology

Clinical descriptive studies
Epidemiology
Social sciences
Experimental and clinical psychology
Genetics
Biochemical studies
Pharmacology
Endocrinology
Physiology
Neuropathology

Clinical descriptive studies

Before reviewing more elaborate scientific approaches to aetiology, attention is drawn to the continuing value of simple *clinical investigations*. Psychiatry was built on such studies. For example, the view that schizophrenia and the mood disorders are likely to have separate causes depends ultimately on the careful descriptive studies and follow-up enquiries carried out by earlier generations of psychiatrists.

Anyone who doubts the value of clinical descriptive studies should read the paper by Aubrey Lewis on 'melancholia' (Lewis, 1934). This paper describes a detailed investigation of the symptoms and signs of 61 cases of severe depressive disorder. It provided the most complete account in the English language and it remains unsurpassed. It is an invaluable source of information about the clinical features of depressive disorders untreated by modern methods. Lewis's careful observations drew attention to unsolved problems, including the nature of retardation, the relationship of depersonalization to affective changes, the presence of manic symptoms, and the validity of the classification of depressive disorders into reactive and endogenous groups. None of these problems has yet been solved completely, but the analysis by Lewis was important in focusing attention on them.

Another good example of this approach is the study conducted by Judd and colleagues (2002) who assessed the natural history of bipolar disorder by prospectively following up 146 patients with bipolar I disorder over a mean of 12 years. Their work showed that bipolar disorder is not, as has often been thought, an illness of discrete episodes of mood disturbance followed by clinical remission. Instead, despite treatment, the patients were symptomatic almost half the time. The majority of this morbidity was attributable to depressive symptomatology. This work stimulated the search for better treatments of depression in bipolar disorder (see Chapter 10). Well-conducted clinical enquiries are likely to retain an important place in psychiatric research for many years to come.

Epidemiology

Epidemiology is the study of the distribution of a disease in space and time within a population, and of the factors that influence this distribution. Its concern is with disease in groups of people, not in the individual person.

Concepts and methods of epidemiology

The basic concept of epidemiology is that of *rate*, or the ratio of the number of instances to the numbers of people in a defined population. Instances can be episodes of illness, or people who are or have been ill. Rates may be computed on a particular occasion (*point prevalence*) or over a defined interval (*period prevalence*).

Other concepts include *inception rate*, which is based on the number of people who were healthy at the beginning of a defined period but became ill during it, and *lifetime expectation or risk*, which is based on an estimate of the number of people who could be expected to develop a particular illness in the course of their whole life. In *cohort studies*, a group of people are followed for a defined period of time to determine the onset of, or change in, some characteristic with or without previous exposure to a potentially important agent (e.g. lung cancer and smoking).

Three aspects of method are particularly important in epidemiology:

- defining the population at risk
- defining a case
- finding cases.

It is essential to *define the population at risk* accurately. Such a population can be all the people living in a limited area (e.g. a country, an island, or a catchment area), or a subgroup chosen by age, gender, or some other potentially important defining characteristic.

Defining a case is the central problem of psychiatric epidemiology. It is relatively easy to define a condition such as Down's syndrome, but until recently the reliability of psychiatric diagnosis has not been satisfactory. The development of standardized diagnostic criteria (see Chapter 2) has greatly improved the reliability and validity of epidemiological studies.

Two methods are used for *case finding*. The first is to enumerate all cases known to medical or other agencies (*declared cases*). Hospital admission rates may give a fair indication of rates of major mental illnesses, but not, for example, of most mood or anxiety disorders. Moreover, hospital admission rates are influenced by many variables, such as the geographical accessibility of hospitals, attitudes of doctors, admission policies, and the law relating to compulsory admissions.

The second method is to search for both declared and undeclared cases in the community. In community surveys, the best technique is often to use two stages— preliminary screening to detect potential cases with a self-rated questionnaire such as the General Health Questionnaire (Goldberg, 1972), followed by detailed clinical examination of potential cases with a standardized psychiatric interview.

Aims of epidemiological enquiries

In psychiatry, *epidemiology* attempts to answer three main kinds of question:

- What is the prevalence of psychiatric disorder in a given population at risk?
- What are the clinical and social correlates of psychiatric disorder?
- What factors may be important in aetiology?

Prevalence can be estimated in community samples or among people attending general practitioners or hospital cases. Studies of prevalence in different locations, social groups, or social classes can contribute to aetiology. Studies of associations between a disorder and *clinical and social variables* can do the same, and may be useful for clinical practice. For example, epidemiological studies have shown that the risk of suicide is increased in elderly men with certain characteristics, such as living alone, misusing drugs or alcohol, suffering from physical or mental illness, and having a family history of suicide.

Causes in the environment

Epidemiological studies of aetiology have been concerned with predisposing and precipitating factors, and with the analysis of the personal and social correlates of mental illness. Among *predisposing factors*, the influence of heredity has been examined in studies of families, twins, and adopted people, as described below in the section on genetics. Other examples are the influence of maternal age on the risk of Down's syndrome, and the psychological effects of parental loss during childhood. Studies of *precipitating factors* include life-events research, which is described below in the section on the social sciences.

Epidemiological approaches to aetiology can be illustrated by the results of studies of environmental correlates of mental disorders. For example, it has been apparent for many years that schizophrenia is more common in urban environments, particularly in disadvantaged inner city areas. This finding could be of aetiological importance or it could be a consequence of the experience of schizophrenia, with, for example, people in the early stages of illness isolating themselves. In a study of this question, van Os *et al.* (2003) confirmed that the prevalence of psychosis increased linearly with the degree of urbanicity (overall odds ratio, 1.57; 95% confidence interval [CI], 1.30–1.89). This significant effect remained after adjustment for factors such as age, gender, education level, parental psychiatric history, and country of birth.

As expected, there was, in addition, an independent and highly significant influence of a family history of psychosis on the risk of an individual developing psychosis (odds ratio, 4.59; 95% CI, 2.41–8.74). Further analysis showed that the effect of urbanicity on increasing the risk of psychosis was much greater in individuals with a family history of psychosis than in those without such a history. These findings suggest an important interaction between genes and environment, such that the adverse environmental effects of urbanicity are expressed particularly in individuals with a genetic predisposition to psychosis.

Social sciences

Many of the concepts used by sociologists are relevant to psychiatry (see Table 5.1). Unfortunately, some of these potentially fruitful ideas have been used uncritically—for example, in the suggestion that mental illness is no more than a label for socially deviant people, the so-called 'myth of mental illness'. This development points to the obvious need for sociological theories to be tested in the same way as other theories by collecting appropriate data.

Some of the concepts of sociology overlap with those of social psychology—for example, attribution theory, which deals with the way in which people interpret the causes of events in their lives, and ideas about self-esteem. An important part of research in sociology, namely the study of life events, uses epidemiological methods.

Transcultural studies

Studies conducted in different societies help to make an important causal distinction. Biologically determined features of mental disorder are likely to be similar in different cultures, whereas psychologically and socially determined features are likely to be dissimilar. Thus the 'core' symptoms of schizophrenia have a similar incidence in people from widely different societies, which suggests that a common neurobiological abnormality is likely to be important in aetiology (see Chapter 11).

By contrast, depressive disorders have a wide range of prevalence. The World Health Survey studied the prevalence of depression in 53 countries using the Composite International Diagnostic Interview to generate ICD diagnoses of depressive episode. Prevalence ranged from 0.4% in Vietnam to 15.7% in Morocco. Interestingly, economic variation between countries accounted for relatively little of the contrasting prevalence rates, and individual factors seemed more important. The latter included female gender, being separated, divorced, or widowed as well as having fewer years of education or material assets (Rai *et al.*, 2013).

The study of life events

Epidemiological methods have been used in social studies to examine associations between illness and certain kinds of events in a person's life. Wolff (1962) studied the morbidity of several hundred people over many years, and found that episodes of illness clustered at times of change in the person's life. Holmes and Rahe (1967) attempted to improve on the highly subjective measures used by Wolff. They used a list of 41 kinds of life event (e.g. in the areas of work, residence, finance, and family relationships), and weighted each according to its apparent severity (e.g. 100 for the death of a spouse, and 13 for a spell of leave for a serviceman).

In later developments the study of the psychological impact of life events has been further improved in a number of ways.

- To reduce memory distortion, limits are set to the period over which events are to be recalled.
- Efforts are made to date the onset of the illness accurately.
- Attempts are made to exclude events that are not clearly independent of the illness (e.g. losing a job because of poor performance).

Table 5.1 Some applications of social theory to psychiatry

Concept	Application
Social class and subculture	Epidemiology of substance misuse
Stigma and labelling	Analysis of social exclusion of the seriously mentally ill in the community
Institutionalization	Negative behavioural effects of institutions
Social deviance	Delinquent behaviour
Abnormal illness behaviour	Psychological consequences of physical illness

- Events are characterized in terms of their nature (e.g. losses or threats) as well as their severity.
- Data are collected with a semi-structured interview and rated reliably.

Although they are significant, life events taken in isolation may be less important than first appears to be the case. For example, in one study, events involving the loss or departure of a person from the immediate social field of the respondent ('exit events') were reported in 25% of patients with depressive disorders, but in only 5% of controls. This difference was significant at the 1% level and appears impressive, but Paykel (1978) questioned its real significance on the basis of the following calculation.

The incidence of depressive disorder is not accurately known, but if it is taken to be 2% for new cases over a 6-month period, a hypothetical population of 10,000 people would yield 200 new cases. If exit events occurred for 5% of people who did not become cases of depressive disorder, in the hypothetical population, exit events would occur for 490 of the 9800 people who were not new cases. Among the 200 new cases, exit events would occur for 25% (i.e. 50 people). Thus the total number of people experiencing exit events would be 490 plus 50, or 540, of whom only 50 (less than 1 in 10) would develop depressive disorders. Thus the greater part of the variance in determining depressive disorder must be attributed to something else; that is, life events trigger depression largely in *predisposed individuals*.

This idea leads us on to the consideration of *vulnerability* and *protective factors*. However, at this point it is also worth noting that studies of genetic epidemiology have taken life events research a stage further by showing that the tendency to experience adverse life events is itself partly genetically determined. For example, individuals differ genetically in their liability to 'select' those environments that put them at relatively higher risk of experiencing adverse life events. Presumably this is one way in which the genetic vulnerability to depression may be expressed (see Kendler *et al.*, 2004).

Vulnerability and protective factors

People may differ in their response to life events for three reasons. First, the same event may have different meanings for different people, according to their *previous experience*. For example, a family separation may be more stressful to an adult who has suffered separation in childhood. Thus adverse experiences that are remote in time from the adverse life event itself may predispose to the later development of psychiatric disorder.

The other reasons are that certain contemporary factors may *increase vulnerability* to life events or *protect* against them. Ideas about these last two factors derive largely from the work of Brown and Harris (1978), who found evidence that, among women, vulnerability factors include being responsible for the care of small children and being unemployed, while protection is conferred by having a confidant with whom problems can be shared. The idea of protective factors has been used to explain the observation that some people do not become ill even when they are exposed to severe adversities.

Causes in the family

It has been suggested that some mental disorders are an expression of emotional disorder within a whole family, not just a disorder in the person seeking treatment (the 'identified patient'). This approach is important in *childhood psychiatric disorders*. Although family problems are also common among adults with psychiatric disorder, their general importance in aetiology is almost certainly overstated in this formulation, as emotional difficulties in other family members may be the result of the patient's problems, rather than its cause. In addition, emotional difficulties in close relatives may result from shared genetic inheritance. For example, the parents of children with schizophrenia have an increased risk of schizotypal personality disorder (see Chapter 11). It seems more likely that family difficulties may modify the course of an established disorder. For example, high levels of 'expressed emotion' from family members increase the risk of relapse in patients with schizophrenia (see Chapter 11). However, in terms of aetiology, twin studies show that shared (family) environment is less important than shared genes in explaining familial clustering in most psychiatric phenotypes.

Migration

Moving to another country, or even to an unfamiliar part of the same country, is a life change that has been suggested as a cause of various kinds of mental disorder. A number of possible mechanisms have been identified:

- *Selective migration.* People in the early stages of an illness such as schizophrenia may migrate because of failing relationships in their country of origin.
- *Process of migration.* Events relating to the process of migration itself (e.g. physical and emotional trauma, prolonged waiting periods, exhaustion, and social deprivation and isolation) may cause several different kinds of stress-related disorder.
- *Post-migration factors.* Many factors come into play after migration that could influence the risk of developing mental illness. These include *social adversity* caused, for example, by *racial discrimination* and *acculturation*, in which the breakdown of traditional cultural structures results in loss of self-esteem and social support. *Social exclusion* and *poverty* are also common problems for migrants. Disparities between aspiration and achievement may also cause stress and depression. Finally, immigrants may be exposed to unfamiliar viruses, which could conceivably affect intrauterine development and predispose to psychiatric disorder in the next generation.

It is fairly well established that immigration is associated with higher rates of psychosis in several ethnic groups, but the mechanisms involved are unclear (see Chapter 11). The effects of immigration on other psychiatric disorders are less consistent, and some groups experience a relative improvement in mental health compared with their native populations. Clearly, refugees who have fled persecution are likely to have elevated rates of stress-related symptomatology, and many of them will meet the formal diagnostic criteria for post-traumatic stress disorder. It is important that such symptoms are interpreted sensitively in the context of the relevant cultural ways of dealing with trauma, but this should not prevent appropriate evidence-based treatment being offered.

Experimental and clinical psychology

The psychological approach to psychiatric aetiology has a number of characteristic features:

- The idea of *continuity between the normal and abnormal*. This idea leads to investigations that attempt to explain psychiatric abnormalities in terms of processes that determine normal behaviour.
- Concern with the *interaction between the person and their environment*. The psychological approach differs from the social approach in being concerned less with environmental variables and more with the person's ways of processing information that is coming from the external environment and from their own body.
- An emphasis on *factors that maintain abnormal behaviour*. Psychologists are less likely to regard behavioural disorders as resulting from internal disease processes, and more likely to assume that persisting behavioural problems are maintained by unhelpful coping mechanisms (e.g. by anxiety-reducing avoidance strategies).

Neuropsychology

Neuropsychological approaches share common ground with biological psychiatry in attempting to identify the neurobiological substrates for psychological phenomena. Various methodologies are employed, but the aim is to understand psychopathology in the context of brain science. Investigations may therefore involve animal experimental work or a range of human studies, including neurological patients with defined brain lesions and patients with psychiatric disorders.

For example, animal experimental models have shown that there is a crucial role for the *amygdala* in fear conditioning. Furthermore, because of its connections to the thalamus, the amygdala is activated by threatening stimuli and can produce autonomic fear responses before there is any conscious awareness of threat. LeDoux (1998) has related this circuitry to traumatic anxiety by proposing an imbalance between the *implicit (unconscious) emotional memory system* involving the thalamus and amygdala and the *explicit (conscious) declarative memory system* in the temporal lobe and hippocampus (see below).

In addition to animal experimental studies, neuropsychological investigations also involve different groups of human subjects. Valuable information may be gained from subjects who have suffered *well-defined brain lesions*. For example, patients with bilateral amygdala lesions can recognize the personal identity of faces, but not the facial expression of fear. This supports the notion that the amygdala is important in the processing of fear-related stimuli.

Current neuropsychological approaches also make extensive use of *functional brain imaging techniques*. This allows localization of the brain regions and neural circuitry involved in specific psychological processes, and facilitates comparisons between healthy subjects and patients who experience abnormalities in the processes concerned. For example, in a magnetic resonance imaging investigation it was found that when patients with depression were shown pictures of sad facial expressions, they exhibited greater activation than controls in brain circuitry related to the processing of emotion, including the amygdala. This increased activation was attenuated by treatment with antidepressant medication (Victor *et al.*, 2010). This suggests that increased activity of the amygdala may play a role in the emotional preoccupations characteristic of depression, and that antidepressants may act by decreasing amygdala function.

Information processing

The *information theory approach* to psychology proposes that the brain can be regarded as an information channel, which receives, filters, processes, and stores information from sense organs, and retrieves information from memory stores. This approach, which compares the brain to a computer, suggests useful ways of thinking about some of the abnormalities in psychiatric disorders. There are various mechanisms involved at different stages of information processing and therefore different points at which dysfunctional processing could give rise to psychiatric disorder. Two of these mechanisms are *attention* and *memory*, changes in which have been linked to psychiatric symptomatology.

Attention

Attention is viewed as an active process of selecting, from the mass of sensory input, the elements that are relevant to the processing that is being carried out at the time. There is evidence that attentional processes are disturbed in some psychiatric disorders. For example, anxious patients attend more than non-anxious controls to stimuli that contain elements of threat, and depressed mothers attend less to the cues of their infants. This can be shown experimentally as a disruption of psychological performance where the task involves ignoring threat-related words. One example is the use of a modified Stroop test, where subjects have to name the colour of a background on which a word is written. When the word is a threatening one (e.g. 'kill'), the latency taken to name the background colour is increased, and this increase is exaggerated in anxious subjects.

Subsequent studies have made two additional observations that are clinically important. First, the attentional bias in anxiety disorders is probably due to a failure to disengage attention from threat-related stimuli, rather than to excessive initial orientation towards them. Secondly, anxious subjects still produce greater responses to threat-related stimuli than controls, even when the stimuli are 'masked' so that they are received outside conscious awareness. Masking is achieved by presenting the stimulus for a very short time (less than 40 milliseconds), immediately followed by the longer presentation of another stimulus (the mask). The fact that masked stimuli elicit greater behavioural responses in anxious subjects suggests that the abnormal attentional mechanisms in anxiety involve the non-conscious threat-processing pathways associated with the amygdala (LeDoux, 1998). Although these findings are of interest, it is important to remember that they may in fact be a *consequence* of the anxiety disorder rather than a *causal* mechanism. However, even in the former case they could still play a role in maintaining symptomatology.

Memory

The *information-processing model* has been applied fruitfully to the study of memory. It suggests that there are different kinds of memory store, namely *sensory stores* in which sensory information is held for short periods while awaiting further processing, a *short-term store* in which information is held for only 20 seconds unless it is continually rehearsed, and a *long-term store* in which information is retained for long periods. There is a mechanism for retrieving information from this long-term store when required, and this mechanism could break down while memory traces are intact. This model has led to useful experiments. For example, patients with the amnestic syndrome (see Chapter 14) score better on memory tests that require recognition of previously encountered material than on tasks that require unprompted recall. This finding suggests a breakdown of information retrieval rather than of information storage.

It is well established that low mood facilitates recall of unhappy events. This can be demonstrated in healthy subjects undergoing a negative mood induction as well as in depressed patients. Once again, it is not clear whether in depressed patients this phenomenon is a manifestation of depressed mood, or one of its causes. However, it is possible that it could play a role in maintaining the depressive state. More recent research has focused on the way that patients with mood disorders recall personal memories. For example, when asked to think of a specific event associated with the word 'happy', a depressed patient may give the response 'when I used to go for long walks by myself', which is a rather general reply. In contrast, a non-depressed person is more likely to respond quite specifically—for example, 'when I went for a walk in Leighton Forest last Sunday with my family'. This over-generalized style of memory recall is associated with a history of negative life events, and might also be linked to impaired problem-solving ability (Hermans *et al.*, 2008).

As noted above, there is increasing interest in how *explicit declarative* and *implicit emotional* memories might be involved in the processing of traumatic events. It has been suggested that, during highly traumatic experiences, explicit memory of the event is relatively poor whereas implicit (unconscious emotional memory) is vivid. This could give rise to the automatic intrusions and poor explicit memory that are seen in post-traumatic stress disorder (Amir *et al.*, 2010).

Beliefs and expectations

The information processing model also predicts that responses to information, including emotional responses, are determined by *beliefs* and *expectations*. This idea proposes that behaviour of all individuals is guided by their beliefs, and that psychopathology is associated with altered *content of beliefs* about the self and the world. Cognitive psychology assumes that such beliefs are organized into *schemas*. Schemas have important properties in relation to different kinds of psychopathology.

- They influence information processing, conscious thinking, emotion, and behaviour.
- Although not necessarily accessible to direct introspection, their content can usually be reconstructed in verbal terms (known as *assumptions* or *beliefs*).
- In patients with psychiatric disorders, these beliefs are dysfunctional, resistant to refutation, and play a part in the aetiology and maintenance of the disorder.

These ideas have been used in the development of *cognitive therapy*, where researchers aim to identify the dysfunctional beliefs associated with particular disorders and apply techniques that help the patient to re-evaluate and change them. For example, experimental work has shown that patients with panic disorder (see Chapter 8) have inaccurate expectations that sensory information about rapid heart action predicts an imminent heart attack. This expectation results in anxiety when the information is received, with the result that the heart rate accelerates further and a vicious circle of mounting anxiety is set up. Changing these expectations can help alleviate panic attacks.

Ethology and evolutionary psychology

Many psychological studies involve quantitative observations of behaviour. In some of these investigations, use is made of methods that were originally developed in the related discipline of ethology. Complex behaviour is divided into simpler components and counted systematically. Regular sequences are noted as well as interactions between individuals (e.g. between a mother and her infant). Such methods have been used, for example, to study the effects of separating infant primates from their mothers, and to compare this primate behaviour with that of human infants separated in the same way.

More recent applications of ethology have used insights from the field of *evolutionary psychology* to understand both normal and abnormal behaviour in an evolutionary context. This approach attempts to explain why various behaviours might have arisen in terms of evolutionary *adaptation*.

For example, because depressive states are ubiquitous in human societies, it is reasonable to ask what their adaptive value may be. One suggestion is that depression may reflect a form of subordination in animals who have lost rank in a social hierarchy. Rather than fighting a losing battle, the depressed individual withdraws and conserves their emotional resources for another day.

Such ideas are not readily testable experimentally, but can give rise to hypotheses concerning possible brain mechanisms. One theoretical difficulty is that psychiatric disorders often appear to represent *maladaptive* rather than adaptive behaviours. For example, Wolpert (1999) has drawn an analogy with cancer, in which the consequences of abnormal cell growth are clearly maladaptive and injurious to the individual. As cancer can be regarded as normal cell division 'gone wrong', so depression might be normal emotion (e.g. sadness) 'gone wrong'. From this viewpoint the question is not what is the adaptive value of the abnormal behaviour, but rather what is the adaptive value of the normal behaviour to which the abnormal state is related.

Genetics

Most psychiatric disorders have a genetic contribution, and a significant amount of aetiological research is currently devoted to identifying the genes concerned, and the mechanisms by which they influence the risk of illness or other *phenotypes* (an observable characteristic, such as a personality trait, or a cognitive ability).

The concepts, methods, and terminology of psychiatric genetics are complex, and will only be introduced briefly here. For more detailed coverage, the textbook by Plomin *et al.* (2013) provides a useful starting point, and can be supplemented by reviews such as that by Doherty and Owen (2014).

The genetic contribution to psychiatric disorders

The first clue that a disorder has a genetic component usually comes from studying aggregation in families. In psychiatry, this is often complemented by adoption studies. However, it is twin studies that provide the most compelling evidence. Positive findings then provide the impetus to use techniques of molecular genetics to locate and identify the genes concerned.

Family studies

In family studies, the investigator determines the risk of a psychiatric condition among the relatives of affected individuals and compares it with the expected risk in the general population. The affected individuals are usually referred to as *index cases* or *probands*. Such studies require a sample that has been selected in a strictly defined way. Moreover, it is not sufficient to ascertain the current prevalence of a psychiatric condition among the relatives, because some of the population may go on to develop the condition later in life. For this reason, investigators use corrected figures known as expectancy rates (or morbid risks).

Family risk studies have been used extensively in psychiatry. Since families share environments as well as genes, these studies by themselves cannot clearly reveal the importance of genetic factors. However, by demonstrating that the disorder of interest shows familial clustering, they are a valuable first step, pointing to the need for other kinds of investigation.

Adoption studies

Adoption studies provide another useful means of separating genetic from environmental influences. The basic method is to compare rates of a disorder in biological relatives with those in adoptive relatives. Three main designs are used:

- *Adoptee study*: the rate of disorder in the adopted-away children of an affected parent is compared with that in adopted-away children of healthy parents.
- *Study of the adoptee's family*: the rate of disorder in the biological relatives of affected adoptees is compared with the rate in adopted relatives.

- *Cross-fostering study*: the rate of disorder is measured in adoptees who have affected biological parents but unaffected adoptive parents, and compared with the rate in adoptees who have healthy biological parents but affected adoptive parents.

Adoption studies are affected by a number of biases, such as the reasons why the child was adopted, the consequences of adoption itself, the non-random nature of the placement (i.e. efforts are made to match the characteristics of the child to those of the adoptive parents), and the effects on adoptive parents of raising a difficult child. A more fundamental limitation is that adoption studies do not control for the prenatal environment, which may be important for disorders associated with intrauterine factors or birth complications. The value and limitations of adoption studies are perhaps best illustrated in schizophrenia research (see Chapter 11).

Twin studies

In twin studies the investigator seeks to separate genetic and environmental influences by comparing rates of *concordance* (i.e. where both co-twins have the same disorder) in uniovular (monozygotic, MZ) and binovular (dizygotic, DZ) twins (Kendler, 2001). If concordance for a psychiatric disorder is higher in MZ twins than in DZ twins, a genetic component is presumed; the greater the difference in concordance, the greater the *heritability* (see below). As well as showing the size of the genetic contribution, modern twin studies allow the environmental contribution to be divided into that which is unique to the individual ('*non-shared*') and that which reflects the common ('*shared*') environment experienced by the twins. This is usually done using a statistical approach called structural equation modelling.

Despite their key role in genetic epidemiology, the results of twin studies should not be accepted uncritically, as they make several assumptions, which are outlined in Box 5.3.

Heritability

Heritability is a measure of the extent to which a phenotype is 'genetic'. More precisely, it refers to the proportion of the liability to the phenotype that is accounted for by additive genetic effects (Visscher *et al.*, 2008). Recent estimates for common psychiatric disorders, based on population-based twin studies, are shown in Table 5.2 (see also Box 5.6). The data show that most psychiatric disorders—like most biological and behavioural traits—are heritable to a degree, and many show a substantial heritability.

Box 5.3 Considerations in the interpretation of twin studies in genetic epidemiology

- Has zygosity been accurately determined? Although MZ co-twins are virtually genetically identical, there can be minor differences.
- It is assumed that MZ and DZ twin pairs both experience the same degree of environmental sharing, and this *'equal environments assumption'* appears to hold for most disorders. However, this may not necessarily be true, especially with regard to the prenatal environment; counterintuitively, this is more dissimilar for MZ than for DZ co-twins. It should also be noted that gene and environment effects interact with each other, and so their effects are not simply additive. For example, parents with antisocial personality disorder may pass on genes that increase the risk that their children will inherit a liability to conduct disorder, but may also produce a family environment that itself increases the risk of behavioural disturbance.
- Most twin studies are now population based, rather than being derived from psychiatric case registers. This reduces the biases of the latter, but does mean that relatively few cases are detected even in large samples, resulting in estimates that can have wide confidence intervals. In addition, the reliability of diagnoses may be less certain.
- Being a twin might in itself affect the risk of developing a psychiatric disorder. However, there is little evidence of this.

Given the importance of the concept, some further comments on heritability estimates and their interpretation are relevant here.

- Estimates of heritability may vary in different populations under different environmental conditions.
- Heritability cannot be applied to an individual, only to a population. For example, some cases may not have a genetic predisposition, and are called *phenocopies*.
- Heritability does not give any indication as to the number, nature, or mechanisms of the genes involved.
- Heritability should not be confused with concordance, or with penetrance. A phenotype can show high concordance in MZ twins without being genetic (e.g. religious faith or football team supported). Equally,

Table 5.2 Heritability estimates for selected psychiatric disorders

Disorder	Heritability estimate (%)
Bipolar disorder	85
Schizophrenia	81
Attention deficit hyperactivity disorder	80
Cocaine use disorder	72
Anorexia nervosa	60
Alcohol dependence	56
Panic disorder	43
Major depression	37
Generalized anxiety disorder	28

Reproduced from Psychological Medicine, 41(1), Bienvenu OJ, Davydow DS and Kendler KS, Psychiatric 'diseases' versus behavioral disorders and degree of genetic influence, pp. 33–40, Copyright (2011), with permission from Cambridge University Press, and other sources.

modest concordance rates between MZ twins may still denote high heritability—it is the *difference* in concordance rates between MZ and DZ twins that denotes heritability. *Penetrance* refers to the likelihood that a specific phenotype occurs in people who carry a particular genotype. This does not always happen, probably reflecting protective genetic or environmental factors, or 'stochastic factors' (i.e. chance). Indeed, only a few conditions are fully penetrant.

The mode of inheritance

A useful intermediate step between finding that a disorder or other phentoype clusters in families and is heritable, and applying molecular methods to find the gene(s) responsible, is to determine the mode of inheritance. In essence, the question is whether the disorder has the characteristics of a Mendelian trait (i.e. whether the family history shows a classic Mendelian pattern of dominant, recessive, or X-linked inheritance). If it does, the disorder can be assumed to be caused by a single major gene. Indeed, in the rare instances where this pattern is observed in psychiatry, causative genes have in many cases already been discovered (e.g. for familial Alzheimer's disease and Huntington's disease). However, such examples are very rare. Most psychiatric disorders, like most common medical disorders, do not show classic Mendelian patterns of inheritance. They are called *non-Mendelian* or *complex genetic disorders*. No gene is either necessary or sufficient to cause the disorder; these *susceptibility genes* are best considered as risk factors that set the genetic threshold of vulnerability.

Within the large category of non-Mendelian disorders, the 'genetic architecture' of most psychiatric disorders (i.e. the number of genes and genetic variants, and how they operate to increase risk) is unclear (Frazer *et al.*, 2009). Most of the heritability is thought to come from genetic variants (*polymorphisms*; see below) that are common in the population and which, although they are important epidemiologically, confer only a small increase in risk to the individual (the *common disease–common variant* model). There may also be genetic variants that are rare in the population, but which, when present, put the individual at a more substantial risk. The relative importance of these two forms of genetic variation is unclear, and likely differs between psychiatric disorders (Gratten et al, 2014).

Linkage and association

The distinction between Mendelian and non-Mendelian disorders has implications for how best to find the genes involved. The former are best studied using *genetic linkage*, in which affected and unaffected individuals within large families are compared with genetic markers to identify which region (*locus*) of which chromosome *segregates* with (shows linkage to) the illness. The result is usually expressed as the *logarithm of the odds of detection of linkage (LOD score)*. A LOD score of 3 or more is conventionally regarded as reasonable evidence for linkage. Having identified the locus, the gene itself is then sought using other approaches.

In contrast, linkage does not work well in non-Mendelian disorders (largely because there is no one gene, nor therefore one locus, to be found). Hence, linkage strategies have been largely unsuccessful in psychiatry. In this situation, *genetic association* is a more feasible and powerful approach. The basic design involves comparing cases with unaffected, unrelated control subjects to find out whether the groups differ in the frequency of specific genetic polymorphisms (see below), measured using a chi-squared test or another similar test. If a significant difference is found, that variant is said to be genetically and statistically associated with the disorder concerned; whether the association reflects a true aetiological role of the variant in the disorder requires further study. Genetic association studies, which have become the work-horse of psychiatric genetics, are described further below.

For a discussion of linkage and association, and other methods for finding genes, see Altshuler *et al.* (2008) and Burmeister *et al.* (2008).

Types of genetic variation and their psychiatric relevance

Genetic differences between individuals are of several different types. Each is relevant in the causation of psychiatric disorders.

Chromosomal (cytogenetic) abnormalities

Cytogenetics is concerned with identifying structural abnormalities in chromosomes. The abnormality can be in the number of chromosomes (*aneuploidy*), a *deletion* or *duplication* of part of a chromosome, or *translocation* of part of one chromosome to another. Cytogenetic abnormalities are usually suspected on the basis of a characteristic physical appearance. They are often associated with learning disability, and can be diagnosed relatively easily by clinical geneticists using *karyotyping*, in which the chromosomes are visualized.

A good example in psychiatry is Down's syndrome, which is usually caused by an additional copy of chromosome 21 (trisomy 21, an example of aneuploidy), although some result from translocation of part of chromosome 21 with a portion of another chromosome. Other examples involve the X and Y chromosomes, such as Turner's syndrome (XO) and Klinefelter's syndrome (XXY). Prominent examples of a more subtle cytogenetic disorder are fragile X syndrome, in which part of the X chromosome is abnormal, and velocardiofacial syndrome (VCFS), in which part of one copy of the long arm of chromosome 22 is deleted.

Although cytogenetic abnormalities are extremely rare causes of psychiatric disorders other than those involving learning disability, their occurrence provides important clues as to where susceptibility genes may be located. For example, it was the observation that Alzheimer's disease occurs earlier and more commonly in Down's syndrome, which encouraged investigators to search chromosome 21 for genes that might cause the disease even in non-trisomic subjects. In this way the role of the amyloid precursor protein (APP) gene was identified (see Chapter 14). Similarly, the markedly increased frequency of psychosis in people with VCFS has focused attention on genes located in that region of chromosome 22 as predisposing to psychosis in general (see Chapter 11).

Mutations and polymorphisms

Most genetic variation between individuals, and their vulnerability to disease, is attributable to changes in one or a few nucleotides (bases) of DNA sequence. These are called mutations or polymorphisms. These and related terms are discussed in Box 5.4 gives three examples of polymorphisms that are relevant to psychiatry.

Copy number variation

Between the extremes of a cytogenetic abnormality and a single nucleotide polymorphism (SNP), an intermediate type of genetic variation has become apparent, called *structural variation* or *copy number variation (CNV)*. CNVs are duplications or deletions of stretches of DNA ranging in size from thousands to millions of nucleotides, and they may be thought of as miniature chromosomal abnormalities. Indeed, there is no absolute distinction from the latter; VCFS is a large CNV.

CNVs are a feature of the normal genome, but they are also genetic risk factors for some psychiatric disorders, notably schizophrenia, autism, and learning disability. The pathogenicity of CNVs depends on their size, their co-occurrence with other variants, and their location in the genome. Large CNVs, and those that disrupt key genes, are more likely to be harmful. Such CNVs are very rare (e.g. less than 1 in 5000 people), yet, when present, typically have a significant effect on disease risk (e.g. an odds ratio of 10); these features contrast with SNPs, which (by definition) are common yet have only a very small effect on risk of a disorder (typically odds ratio of less than 1.2). CNVs can either be inherited or occur *de novo* (i.e. are not seen in either parent). For a review, see Kirov (2015).

Genetic association studies

We have already noted that multiple SNPs appear to underlie much of the genetic predisposition to psychiatric disorders, and that their role is investigated using genetic association. Genetic association studies are of two main types.

Candidate gene studies

As noted earlier, an association study measures the frequency of a genetic polymorphism in a group of

---

Box 5.4 The terminology of molecular genetic variation: polymorphisms, alleles, and mutations

- No two people share precisely the same *genome* (the total genetic information contained on our 23 pairs of chromosomes, about 3 billion base pairs of DNA). Each person has a unique DNA sequence (with the exception of MZ twins). DNA sequence variants are called *polymorphisms or allelic variants*. Most polymorphisms involve a change in a single nucleotide, hence the term *single nucleotide polymorphism* (SNP). SNPs occur on average about every 1000 base pairs (around 2 million SNPs in total), both within genes and in the stretches of DNA between genes. A given polymorphism can be rare, or both variants (*alleles*) can occur at equal frequency in the population.

- The term *mutation* can be used to refer to any very rare polymorphism (i.e. one present in less than 1% of people). However, it is often used in a more restricted way to denote a change in DNA sequence which is by definition harmful—that is, it causes a disease. This differs from polymorphisms in general, which, as noted above, often have no consequences at all; if they do, they can be beneficial, neutral, or harmful, and any effects are not deterministic but merely change the probability of a particular phenotype. The term mutation is therefore used largely with reference to Mendelian disorders.

- Most polymorphisms have no functional significance because they do not lead to an amino acid change in the encoded protein (called *synonymous* or *conservative* polymorphisms), either because the SNP is in non-coding parts of the DNA or because of some redundancy in the coding region. However, some SNPs do have functional correlates, or affect disease risk, and it is these that are sought in genetic association studies.

- Because we have two copies of every autosomal gene (*autosomes* are chromosomes other than X or Y), one from each parent, at any point in the genome the two alleles may be identical (*homozygosity*), or they may differ (*heterozygosity*).

- SNPs that are close together tend to be inherited together. They are said to be in *linkage disequilibrium*, and the SNPs together comprise a *haplotype*. These properties and concepts are important for the conduct and interpretation of genetic association studies. For example, linkage disequilibrium means that if one SNP is measured and shown to be genetically associated with a disorder, it cannot be concluded that it is the biologically important variant; it might simply be a marker for another SNP within the haplotype that is in fact the important one. And the haplotype itself might be more significant than any one of its constituent SNPs. For a review of this subject, see Slatkin (2008).

individuals who have the phenotype of interest, and compares it with the frequency in a group of matched healthy controls. Such studies have been widely used in psychiatry, as it is relatively easy to collect samples (DNA can be extracted from blood or a cheek swab), and then to *genotype* using methods based on the polymerase chain reaction (PCR). Until a decade or so ago, for technical and financial reasons, only a very limited number of genes and SNPs were studied at a time. A gene would be selected for study because researchers considered it to be a *candidate gene*—that is, one that they considered to be a plausible candidate for contributing to the phenotype in question (e.g. a dopamine receptor for schizophrenia). Within the gene, the specific polymorphism was chosen because it was common (providing more statistical power), easy to measure, or had been the subject of a previous positive report.

There have been a huge number of candidate gene association studies in psychiatry. Some findings have proved robust, but most have not, reflecting several major limitations.

- The fundamental problem is that there are about 25,000 protein-coding genes in the human genome, and over two million SNPs. The prior probability that any one gene, let alone any one polymorphism, is truly associated with the phenotype that one is measuring is therefore very small, unless there is already compelling evidence implicating the gene (which is rarely the case in psychiatry). There is therefore a high probability of obtaining a false-positive result, especially as these are more likely to be published than is a negative result.

- The groups that are being compared must have closely similar ethnic backgrounds, as the frequency of polymorphisms can vary markedly. For example, the COMT-Met158 allele (see Box 5.4) varies from 1% to 60% in populations across the world. This can lead to artefactual group differences owing to *ethnic stratification*. One method of avoiding this problem is not to use a control group, but to genotype the parents of the cases to see whether affected children inherit alleles more often than would be expected by chance. These family-based association studies often use the *transmission disequilibrium test*.

- Other problems include genotyping errors and inadequate sample sizes.

Genome-wide association studies

Candidate gene association studies have now been supplanted by genome-wide association studies (GWAS), in which hundreds of thousands of SNPs, selected to cover the whole of the genome, can be tested at the same time. This is done using a silicon 'chip', which contains probes for the SNPs, and on to which the person's DNA is added. A scanner then 'reads' the genotype at each SNP. (It was from these readouts that the existence and importance of CNVs became apparent.) The fundamental advantage of GWAS is that the whole genome is surveyed without the need to have prior hypotheses (or biases). The major problem is that of multiple testing. Because so many SNPs are tested, the criterion for statistical significance between groups must be correspondingly lowered, to approximately $P \leq 10^{-8}$. This in turn requires very large samples to provide the necessary power (tens of thousands of cases, and a similar number of controls).

Studies of this size, and meta-analyses of these, are now being reported for several psychiatric disorders, with significant progress being made in psychosis and autism, as well as in some neurodegenerative disorders. However, there is still considerable debate about the value and limitations of GWAS in psychiatry, and how to interpret the results. For example, GWAS are suited to detecting common but not rare variants. Also, many associations are to regions of the genome with no known genes. Furthermore, the need for large samples often means that the clinical evaluation of the subjects is limited. For a review of GWAS concepts and methods, see Craddock (2013).

Exome and genome sequencing

The latest technologies move on from sampling or 'tagging' the genome (using SNPs) to sequencing the DNA (Bras *et al.*, 2012). *Exome sequencing* is the term used to describe sequencing limited to the stretches of DNA that encode expressed genes (i.e. present in messenger RNA). *Whole genome sequencing* is where the genome is sequenced in its entirety. These methods are rapidly being adopted in genetics research and clinical diagnostics, and data are beginning to emerge in autism and some other psychiatric disorders. Their attraction is that the complete genetic information is captured, but there are several reasons why this is not necessarily an advantage, including the huge amounts of data needing to be stored and analysed, and considerable uncertainty as to how to interpret the results. In particular, sequencing is revealing many more genetic differences between individuals than anticipated, and it is usually unclear which of these are of any functional or pathological significance. For review, see Biesecker and Green (2014).

Other aspects of psychiatric genetics

Relationships between genotype and phenotype

Genes do not code for psychiatric disorders—they code for RNA and protein, and it is these gene products which in turn influence the functioning of cells, tissues, organs, and, ultimately, individuals. This simple point has several implications (Kendler, 2005). First, it is not surprising that genes do not map closely on to our current diagnostic categories. For example, one gene can contribute to various phenotypes (*pleiotropy*). Secondly, it may contribute to the difficulty in finding genes for disorders because there are so many intervening steps that may mask the relationship. In response to this problem, researchers often study *endophenotypes* (also called *intermediate phenotypes*), which are features that are thought to be more closely related to a disorder's underlying genetic basis than is the clinical syndrome itself. For example, eye-tracking dysfunction, impaired working memory, and neuroimaging abnormalities are all endophenotypes in schizophrenia. For a review of the concept, see Gottesman and Gould (2003).

In terms of molecular mechanisms, there are two main ways in which genetic variation can affect phenotype and the risk of a disorder. If the variant alters the sequence of the encoded protein, the function of that protein may be impaired. Even a single amino acid change can be significant—for example, the APP mutations that cause familial Alzheimer's disease, or the apoE4 and COMT Val[158]Met SNPs mentioned in Box 5.5. Larger deletions or insertions within proteins caused by CNVs are also likely to impair, inactivate, or change the function of the protein.

However, most SNPs that have been associated with psychiatric disorders to date do not alter the protein sequence, and may not even be located within a protein-coding gene at all (see Box 5.4). Their effects on disease risk probably occur because they alter the way in which the gene is regulated (i.e. the amount, timing, and location of gene expression and the synthesis of the protein; Harrison, 2015), or they impact on the function of the large number of *non-protein coding genes* now recognized (Barry, 2014). For review see Albert and Kruglyak (2015).

Epistasis

Epistasis refers to the non-additive interactions between two or more genes (Phillips, 2008). For example, an SNP in gene A and an SNP in gene B each confer an odds ratio of 1.2 for a disorder. However, individuals who happen to have both of these risk SNPs have an odds ratio of 6. Epistasis has a major role in the genetics of cancer and many other complex traits. It may well be similarly important in the heritability of psychiatric disorders, but the data are limited for various technical and statistical reasons. For an example of epistasis in schizophrenia, see Nicodemus *et al.* (2010).

Gene–environment interactions and correlations

Genes and the environment are sometimes considered separately, but they are inextricably linked in aetiology (Rutter, 2006). That is, genes affect our susceptibility to environmental factors (*gene–environment interaction*; Thomas, 2010). They also affect our exposure to particular environments (*gene–environment correlation*; Jaffee and Price, 2007). Although this importance is clear from epidemiological studies, few interactions between a specific gene variant and a specific environmental factor have yet been demonstrated in psychiatry (see Box 5.5 for one controversial example), probably because they require very large samples and also careful measurements of the environment. Note that heritability estimates such as those in Table 5.2 can be affected by gene–environment interactions and correlations (Visscher *et al.*, 2008).

Clinical and ethical implications of psychiatric genetics

For some inherited neuropsychiatric conditions (e.g. Huntington's disease and Down's syndrome) genetic counselling and testing are regarded as helpful. Until recently, the only information available for major psychiatric disorders such as bipolar disorder and schizophrenia came from findings from genetic epidemiology indicating, for example, that, while a child of a patient with schizophrenia had a tenfold increase in the risk of schizophrenia, the absolute risk was still only around one in ten. Advances in molecular genetics raise the possibility of moving from risk counselling based on family history to more specific genetic testing of individuals (Gershon and Alliey-Rodriguez, 2013).

As noted above, *GWAS* are increasingly successful at detecting SNPs that contribute to the genetic risk of highly heritable disorders such as schizophrenia, bipolar disorder, and autism. However, the increase in risk conferred by any of these variants considered singly is very small; in addition, even adding the various risk genes together explains only a limited amount of the variance in inherited liability. Therefore current GWAS findings are not likely to be useful in genetic counselling. However some *illness-associated CNVs* carry much larger risk for people in the particular families in which they occur. For example, it has been estimated that an individual with a deletion in 3q29 has a one in three chance of developing schizophrenia. Tracking abnormal CNVs through affected families may therefore provide

Box 5.5 Examples of polymorphisms in psychiatry

Apolipoprotein E4 in Alzheimer's disease

The apoE gene on chromosome 19 exists in three common forms (*alleles*): apoE2, apoE3, and apoE4. ApoE3 is the commonest variant in the population. Since 1993, dozens of studies involving thousands of people have shown an unequivocal association between apoE4 and Alzheimer's disease—a higher proportion of patients have the apoE4 variant of the gene than do age-matched subjects without the disease. In some populations, apoE2 is protective. ApoE4 is thus said to be genetically associated with Alzheimer's disease and, as such, is a genetic risk factor for it. Individuals with one copy of apoE4 (*heterozygotes*, with their other chromosome carrying apoE3 or apoE2) are two to three times more likely to develop Alzheimer's disease, and the risk is over fivefold greater in apoE4 *homozygotes* (in whom both copies of the gene are apoE4). In other words, apoE4 accounts for about one-third of all cases of Alzheimer's disease. However, about half of all Alzheimer's disease occurs in people without an apoE4 allele, and some apoE4 homozygotes never develop it.

ApoE4 represents the best established example of a genetic risk factor for a common psychiatric disorder. However, it also emphasizes that apoE4, like most genes involved in psychiatric disorder, acts as a risk factor, not a determinant; it is neither necessary nor sufficient. The apoE genotype also affects the risk of developing certain other neurological conditions, illustrating the fact that genes can have effects across different disorders. For a further discussion of apoE4, see Chapter 14, and for a review, see Verghese *et al.* (2011).

Catechol-O-methyl transferase and dopaminergic function and dysfunction

The enzyme catechol-O-methyl transferase (COMT) metabolizes monoamines, especially dopamine. It occurs as a high-activity form and a low-activity form, which in turn results in lesser or greater availability of dopamine in the synapse. The difference is due to a SNP in the gene (called Val^{158}Met), which leads to a single amino acid being changed in the COMT protein. The high-activity allele encodes valine (Val-COMT) and the low-activity allele encodes methionine (Met-COMT). Egan *et al.* (2001) showed that subjects with Val-COMT had a less efficient prefrontal cortex, and tended to perform less well during working memory tasks compared with Met-COMT subjects. In other situations (e.g. during emotional processing), Val-COMT subjects are more efficient than Met-COMT subjects.

The COMT Val^{158}Met is perhaps the best psychiatric example of a polymorphism that is known to be functional (i.e. it affects the protein that the gene encodes, and since that protein regulates dopamine, it in turn affects dopamine-mediated brain functions). For that reason it has been extensively studied in a range of behaviours, and in many psychiatric disorders. However, the results have generally not been conclusive, and have led to controversies about the data and their interpretation. Possible reasons for the inconclusive results include the occurrence of sex differences in COMT function, and the presence of other SNPs in the gene which interact with Val^{158}Met to determine COMT activity. For a review of this subject, see Tunbridge *et al.* (2006).

5-HT transporter gene, stress, and depression

The 5-HT transporter (5-HTT) regulates synaptic 5-HT availability and is the target of selective serotonin reuptake inhibitors (SSRIs). Its gene contains a polymorphism in its 'upstream' promoter region (which regulates the expression of the gene). The polymorphism is unlike the above examples in two ways. First, it is non-coding (i.e. it does not change the amino acid sequence of the protein). Secondly, it is not an SNP, but is a polymorphism in the length of the DNA, the two alleles being called short (S) and long (L). Lesch *et al.* (1996) showed that the S allele was associated with neuroticism (trait anxiety), and Caspi *et al.* (2004) found that it influenced whether a person who had experienced adverse early-life events developed depression. The polymorphism may also contribute to individual differences in the therapeutic response to, and side-effects of, SSRIs.

The finding of Caspi *et al.* (2004) is a prominent example of a gene–environment interaction (see below). It is also a prime example of the controversies in the field, since there have been multiple subsequent studies, and controversies as to whether the result is robust, with different meta-analyses coming to opposite conclusions. For a review of this subject, see Karg *et al.* (2011).

information of great clinical significance to members of those families.

The growing availability of knowledge of this nature will require much ethical discussion about issues such as parental genetic testing, the rights of family members to genetic information about each other, as well as preimplantation screening and selection of embryos. Fundamental to such debate are questions about the impact (both positive and negative) of psychiatric disorder for affected individuals, their families, and society. Here the role of stigma must be closely examined. It is sobering that 'genetic' explanations of psychiatric disorder do not guarantee that the stigma of illness will be lessened—if anything, the reverse may be the case (Angermeyer *et al.*, 2011). For a review of these issues, see Gershon and Alliey-Rodriguez (2013).

Epigenetics

Epigenetics describes chemical modifications of DNA and of its binding proteins (called *histones*), which regulate gene activity without changing the DNA sequence. Important examples are methylation of cytosine nucleotides in the promoter region of genes, and the acetylation of specific histone amino acids. A range of environmental factors, including drugs, childhood abuse, and stress, have been shown to affect these modifications. As such, epigenetic regulation provides one mechanism, perhaps the most important one, by which genes and environment interact. There is also interest in the possibility that some epigenetic 'marks' may be heritable. For a review of this subject, see Petronis (2010).

Epigenetics, together with epistasis and gene–environment interactions, may help to reconcile the relatively high heritability of psychiatric disorders with the very small odds ratios associated with all of the individual SNPs discovered so far, and the fact that, cumulatively, SNPs only explain a fraction of the heritability (Maher, 2008). They also provide some of the reasons why finding genes for psychiatric disorders has proved so difficult, as discussed in this section and summarized in Box 5.6.

Biochemical studies

Biochemical studies can be directed either to the causes of diseases or to the mechanisms by which disease produces its effects. The methods of biochemical investigation are too numerous to consider here, and it is assumed that the reader has some knowledge of them. The main aim here is to consider some of the problems of using biochemical methods to investigate psychiatric disorder.

> **Box 5.6 Some reasons why finding genes for psychiatric disorders is difficult**
>
> - Starting with the 'wrong' clinical phenotype. Genes are highly unlikely to map on to current diagnostic categories, yet samples are usually collected based upon the latter. Stronger genotype–phenotype relationships may be seen if categories are broadened (e.g. 'psychosis' rather than schizophrenia and bipolar disorder) or decomposed (e.g. schizophrenia into cognitive deficits and psychotic symptoms, etc.).
> - No 'major genes' exist. Each gene on its own contributes only a small fraction of the heritable risk.
> - Different genes may affect risk in different people (*genetic heterogeneity*).
> - Within a given gene, different variants may affect risk in different people (*allelic heterogeneity*).
> - The presence of phenocopies and *de novo* mutations.
> - Gene–gene interactions (epistasis).
> - Gene–environment interactions.

It will be clear from the above account that the scope for molecular genetic studies is greatly enhanced by the presence of a *biochemical abnormality* that reliably distinguishes patients with a particular psychiatric disorder. The value of such an abnormality would be greater still if the biochemical abnormality concerned played a significant role in the cause of the illness or its pathophysiology. However, the nature of the biochemical changes associated with most psychiatric disorders remains unknown. This is due both to our lack of knowledge about the biochemical complexities of the normal brain and to the difficulty of investigating the biochemistry of the living human brain directly. Moreover, because most psychiatric disorders do not lead to death (other than by suicide), post-mortem material is not widely available except among the elderly.

Because of these problems, workers have adopted a variety of *indirect methods* involving sampling of peripheral tissues and fluids, such as cerebrospinal fluid (CSF), blood cells, and urine. These studies, although more feasible to carry out, are not always easy to interpret. For example, concentrations of neurotransmitters and their metabolites in lumbar CSF have an uncertain relationship to the corresponding functionally active neurotransmitter in the brain. Equally, neurotransmitter receptors and their second messengers in blood platelets and lymphocytes often appear to be regulated in a different way to their brain counterparts. Finally, measures in plasma and urine are very susceptible to confounding dietary and behavioural changes (see below).

The reader will find accounts of the results of biochemical research in subsequent chapters, especially those on mood disorders and schizophrenia. At this point a few examples will be given of the different kinds of investigation that are used.

Post-mortem studies

Post-mortem studies of the brain can provide direct evidence of chemical changes within it. Unfortunately, interpretation of the findings is difficult, because it must be established that any changes in the concentrations of neurotransmitters or enzymes did not occur after death. Moreover, because psychiatric disorders do not lead directly to death, the ultimate cause of death is another condition (often bronchopneumonia or the effects of a drug overdose) that could have caused the observed changes in the brain.

Even if this possibility can be ruled out, it is still possible that the biochemical changes are the result of treatment rather than of disease. For example, the increases in density of dopamine receptors in the nucleus accumbens and caudate nucleus in patients with schizophrenia might be interpreted as supporting the hypothesis that schizophrenia is caused by changes in dopamine function in these areas of the brain. On the other hand, the finding could equally be the result of long-term treatment with antipsychotic drugs which block dopamine receptors and might lead to a compensatory increase in the number of receptors.

As mentioned above, *molecular genetic techniques* can be used to complement biochemical investigations in post-mortem brain or to quantify mRNA or other parameters of gene expression. Although these techniques have the benefits of greater sensitivity and molecular specificity, they suffer from the same inherent limitations.

Brain biochemistry and brain imaging

Over the past few years, effective methods of studying biochemical events in the living brain have become available and have been used in some studies of psychiatric disorders. These methods include the following:

- magnetic resonance imaging (MRI)
- single-photon emission tomography (SPET)
- positron emission tomography (PET).

The use of these techniques to measure cerebral structure and blood flow is discussed below under the relevant headings. However, brain imaging can also be employed to measure aspects of brain biochemistry. For example, it is possible to carry out *in-vivo* receptor binding in different groups of psychiatric patients using positron-labelled ligands and PET or SPET imaging.

Receptor binding with PET and SPET

The 5-HT_{1A} receptor plays an important role in the regulation of 5-HT neurotransmission and is an important target for antidepressant medications. Using PET imaging in conjunction with a positron-labelled 5-HT_{1A}-receptor antagonist, a number of groups have found that the binding of 5-HT_{1A} receptors in the brain is decreased in patients with major depression. Moreover, this abnormality appears to persist in patients who have recovered from depression and are no longer taking medication. This suggests that low 5-HT_{1A}-receptor binding might represent a trait marker for vulnerability to depression. Alternatively, the diminished receptor availability could be a consequence of having been depressed (see Meyer 2013).

For reasons of cost, studies employing PET are likely to remain restricted to a small number of specialist research centres. However, SPET imaging is more widely available, and increasing numbers of specific receptor ligands suitable for SPET studies are being developed. For example, there are already several studies using SPET in conjunction with specific dopamine-receptor ligands examining dopamine-receptor binding in mood disorders and schizophrenia.

Neurotransmitter release *in vivo*

Studies using PET and SPET in conjunction with specific dopamine-receptor ligands have enabled estimation of dopamine release *in vivo*. The principle is to scan subjects on two occasions—after administering a drug that modulates endogenous dopamine release (e.g. amphetamine) and after administering placebo. Amphetamine increases dopamine release presynaptically, and the increased levels of endogenous dopamine compete with the tracer ligand for access to postsynaptic receptors. Therefore the specific binding of the tracer is reduced and the difference in tracer signal between the amphetamine and placebo scans provides a measure of how much dopamine was released by the amphetamine.

A similar approach can be used with drugs that lower endogenous dopamine release, such as the tyrosine hydroxylase inhibitor, α-methyl-para-tyrosine (AMPT). Use of these models has led to the conclusion that dopamine release is increased in patients with acute schizophrenia (see Chapter 11). Current studies are investigating how these techniques can be applied to the release of other neurotransmitters.

Magnetic resonance imaging

MRI has the advantage over SPET and PET that subjects are not exposed to radiation. Although MRI has proved to be an excellent tool for structural brain imaging and, more recently, for the examination of cerebral blood flow (see below), its application to the study of brain biochemistry (magnetic resonance spectroscopy; MRS) has been somewhat limited by its lack of sensitivity. However, there are growing numbers of applications of MRS to the study of psychiatric disorders and their treatment (Dager *et al.*, 2008).

- Proton (^{1}H) MRS can be used to detect a number of compounds of neurobiological interest, including the important amino acid neurotransmitters, gamma-aminobutyric acid (GABA) and glutamate (see Table 5.3).
- MRS can also be used to identify the spectrum of phosphorus-containing compounds, and thus can provide information about energy metabolism and intracellular pH.
- A number of psychotropic drugs (e.g. fluoxetine) possess fluorine atoms, which can be imaged by MRS. This provides a means of imaging the distribution of such drugs at their specific receptor sites in the brain.
- MRS has also been used to image lithium in the human brain, where it appears that brain levels of lithium are about half those seen in plasma.

One reasonably consistent finding from proton MRS is that patients with depression have decreased levels of glutamate in anterior brain regions (Cowen, 2015). This has shed some new light on a condition where aetiological hypotheses have been dominated for decades by the monoamine theory (see Chapter 9).

Peripheral measures

There have been longstanding doubts as to whether changes in the composition of neurotransmitters in the CSF reflect functionally significant changes in the brain. However, there are reasonably reproducible links between lowered CSF levels of 5-hydroxyindoleacetic acid (5-HIAA) and impulsive aggressive behaviour across various psychiatric disorders (Moberg *et al.*, 2011). This suggests that CSF 5-HIAA does correlate with certain defined aspects of behaviour. The major limitation of CSF studies is that it is often ethically and practically difficult to obtain CSF samples from psychiatric patients. In addition, it is not feasible to monitor time-dependent

Table 5.3 **Neuronal metabolites and transmitters measured by MRS**

^{1}H-NMR	^{31}P-NMR
N-Acetyl-aspartate (NAA)	ATP
Creatinine	Phosphocreatine
Myoinositol	Inorganic phosphate
GABA	Phosphodiesters
Glutamate	Phosphomonoesters

changes in neurotransmitter metabolism by repeated sampling.

Ingenious attempts have been made to infer biochemical changes in the brain from measurements of substances in the blood. For example, it is known that the rate of synthesis of 5-HT depends on the concentration of the 5-HT precursor tryptophan in the brain. Several studies have shown that *plasma tryptophan levels are decreased in patients with major depression*, a finding that supports the hypothesis that brain 5-HT function may be impaired in depressive disorders. However, it cannot be assumed that a modest reduction in concentrations of plasma tryptophan will necessarily be associated with impaired brain 5-HT neurotransmission. Furthermore, the same reduction in plasma tryptophan levels is found when healthy people lose weight by dieting. Therefore it is quite possible that the decrease in plasma tryptophan levels found in depressed patients is a consequence of concomitant weight loss. Interestingly, recent theories concerning the role of *inflammation* in depression have suggested that low tryptophan levels in depressed patients may be due to induction of the tryptophan-metabolizing enzyme, indoleamine 2,3-dioxygenase (Maes *et al.*, 2011).

Investigations of biochemical abnormalities in blood and urine have so far not proved particularly fruitful in understanding the aetiology of psychiatric disorders. A recent example of the approach is provided by assay of serum levels of brain-derived neurotropic factor (BDNF) in the hope that such measures might correlate with the elaboration of BDNF in the brain, and therefore permit examination of the neurotropic hypothesis of depression (see Chapter 9). Indeed, the majority of published studies suggest that serum BDNF levels are lowered in depressed patients and increased after antidepressant treatment. However, before the serum measures can be taken as a valid index of BDNF changes in relevant brain regions, it will be necessary to clarify the origin of serum BDNF (Groves, 2007).

In contrast, peripheral biochemical measures have proved useful in the field of learning disability, where measurement of metabolites in blood and urine can provide a valid picture of the abnormalities present in the brain, as well as valuable diagnostic tests. A good example is phenylketonuria (Chapter 17).

Peripheral blood cells such as platelets and lymphocytes possess receptors for neurotransmitters that often resemble the analogous receptor-binding sites in the brain. There have been many studies of monoamine receptors in the platelets of depressed patients, but the findings tend to be inconsistent and easily confounded by factors such as drug treatment. In addition, it is far from clear whether abnormalities found in these peripheral binding sites will necessarily also be present in the brain. Indeed, those studies that have looked simultaneously at peripheral receptor binding and *in-vivo* receptor imaging have not found correlations. Similar comments apply to the use of blood cells to investigate neurotransmitter-linked second messengers and ion flux processes such as calcium entry.

Despite these limited successes, peripheral tissue studies of psychiatric disorder are entering a renaissance because of the ability to create *induced pluripotent stem cells (iPSCs)* from accessible cells such as skin fibroblasts or keratinocytes. iPSCs can in turn be 'reprogrammed' into neurons (or other cell types), and are being used both to study cellular mechanisms of disease and treatment, and may also be viewed as potential therapies of the future (see Haggarty and Perlis, 2014; Licinio and Wong, 2016).

Pharmacology

The study of effective treatment of disease can often throw light on aetiology. In psychiatry, because of the great problems of studying the brain directly, research workers have examined the actions of effective psychotropic drugs in the hope that the latter might indicate the biochemical abnormalities in disease. Of course, such an approach must be used cautiously. If an effective drug blocks a particular transmitter system, it cannot be concluded that the disease is caused by an excess of that transmitter. The example of parkinsonism makes this clear—anticholinergic drugs modify the symptoms, but the disease is caused by a deficiency in dopaminergic transmission and not an excess of cholinergic transmission.

It is assumed here that the general methods of neuropharmacology are familiar to the reader, and attention is focused on the particular difficulties involved in using these methods in psychiatry. There are two main problems. First, most psychotropic drugs have more than one action, and it is often difficult to decide which action is relevant to the therapeutic effects. For example, although lithium carbonate has a large number of known pharmacological effects (see Chapter 25), it has so far not been possible to link any of these effects definitively to its remarkable ability to stabilize mood in bipolar illness.

The second difficulty arises because the therapeutic effects of many psychotropic drugs are slow to develop, whereas most pharmacological effects identified in the laboratory are quick to appear. For example, it has been suggested that the beneficial effect of antidepressant drugs depends on alterations in the reuptake of transmitter at presynaptic neurons. However, changes in reuptake occur quickly, whereas obvious therapeutic effects are usually delayed for a number of weeks, suggesting that 'adaptive' responses of the brain to medication are important in clinical antidepressant action. Over the years several different adaptive responses to antidepressant drugs have been identified, but none of them has yet led to new kinds of antidepressant medication.

Current ideas in this area focus on the effects of antidepressants in modifying synaptic growth and plasticity via actions on gene transcription factors and neurotropins such as BDNF (Duric and Duman, 2013). The introduction of new drugs with different pharmacological actions from conventional compounds can often be used to generate hypotheses about the mode of action of beneficial treatments and the pathophysiology of the disorder concerned. For example, with the introduction of *selective serotonin reuptake inhibitors (SSRIs)*, it became clear that only drugs with potent 5-HT reuptake inhibitor properties are effective in the pharmacological treatment of obsessive–compulsive disorder. Conventional tricyclic antidepressants (with the exception of clomipramine) are not useful in this context. This suggests that the pathophysiology of obsessive–compulsive disorder is likely to differ from that of major depression, for which both classes of compounds are equally effective.

Another drug that has stimulated research in this way is *clozapine*, an antipsychotic drug that is effective in a significant proportion of patients who are unresponsive to traditional antipsychotic agents. Most antipsychotic drugs are believed to produce their therapeutic effects through blockade of dopamine D_2 receptors, but clozapine has a weak affinity for this binding site. In fact, clozapine binds potently to certain 5-HT receptor subtypes, particularly 5-HT_{2A} and 5-HT_{2C} receptors.

This has led to the development of numerous 'atypical' antipsychotic agents, which have combined 5-HT_2 and dopamine D_2 receptor-antagonist properties.

Although these agents may have some advantages over conventional antipsychotic drugs in terms of a lower risk of movement disorders, they do not seem to be as effective as clozapine in patients with treatment-resistant illness (see Chapter 11).

Endocrinology

Changes in circulating concentrations of hormones can have profound effects on mood and behaviour, while abnormalities in endocrine function are responsible for a number of well-defined clinical syndromes, some of which have characteristic neuropsychiatric presentations (e.g. depression in Cushing's disease). The onset of puberty is associated with a sharp increase in rates of anxiety and depression.

Despite these intriguing associations, measurement of basal plasma hormone levels in psychiatric disorders has not, in general, shown consistent abnormalities in psychiatric patients or thrown much light on aetiology. The exception is major depression, in which a significant proportion of patients *hypersecrete cortisol*. Elevated cortisol levels in depression have been postulated to play a role in the pathophysiology of depression, perhaps leading to cellular and synaptic neuropathology. It is also possible that persistent elevation in cortisol may be a factor in the medical comorbidities associated with depression, such as diabetes, cardiovascular disease, and cognitive impairment (see Cowen, 2015).

Peptide-releasing factors

Hormones such as thyroid-stimulating hormone (TSH) and adrenocorticotropic hormone (ACTH) are regulated by peptide-releasing factors that have additional signalling roles in other brain regions, often those involved in the regulation of emotion. These peptides often coexist with classical neurotransmitters—for example, thyrotropin-releasing hormone (TRH) is colocalized with 5-HT in 5-HT neurons. There is growing interest in the development of drugs that act on peptide receptors; for example, the use of corticotropic-releasing hormone (CRH) antagonists in depressed patients who hypersecrete cortisol. However, results from trials of neuropeptide drugs in anxiety and depressive disorders have thus far proved disappointing (Griebel and Holsboer, 2012).

Neuroendocrine tests

Another use of plasma hormone measurement is to monitor the functional activity of brain neurotransmitters. The secretion of pituitary hormones is controlled by a variety of neurotransmitters. Under certain circumstances, changes in the concentration of a plasma hormone can be used to assess the function of the neurotransmitters involved in its release. For example, stimulation of brain 5-HT function with a specific drug gives rise to an increase in plasma prolactin levels. Accordingly, the rise in prolactin concentration that accompanies administration of a standard dose of the drug gives a measure of the functional state of brain 5-HT pathways.

These *neuroendocrine challenge tests* provide dynamic functional measures of brain neurotransmitter pathways, and in certain psychiatric disorders they have yielded consistent evidence of impairments in neurotransmitter function. For example, in depressed patients there is good evidence that the prolactin response to 5-HT stimulation is blunted, and that it remains blunted on clinical recovery.

This suggests that depressive disorders are associated with a deficit in brain 5-HT neurotransmission. However, as with other biological measures, great care must be taken to control for possible confounding effects such as weight loss and impaired sleep (for a review of this field, see Cowen, 2015).

Physiology

Physiological methods can be used to investigate the cerebral and peripheral disorders associated with disease states. The following methods have been used:

- Psychophysiological methods, including measurements of pulse rate, blood pressure, blood flow, skin conductance, and muscle activity.
- Studies of cerebral blood flow.
- Electroencephalographic (EEG) studies.

Psychophysiological measures

Psychophysiological measures can be interpreted in at least two ways. The first interpretation is straightforward. The data are used to provide information about the activity of peripheral organs in disease—for example, to determine whether electromyographic (EMG) activity is increased in the scalp muscles of patients who complain of tension headaches. The second interpretation depends on the assumption that peripheral measurements can be used to infer changes in the state of arousal of the central nervous system. Thus increases in skin conductance, pulse rate, and blood pressure are taken to indicate greater arousal.

Measurement of cerebral blood flow, metabolism, and neuronal function

Advances in brain imaging methods have led to increasing sophistication in the measurement of cerebral blood flow in psychiatric disorders. The use of tomographic techniques allows a three-dimensional measurement of regional cerebral blood flow to be achieved both 'at rest' and following various kinds of challenges, usually either neuropsychological or pharmacological. The aim is to detect abnormal cerebral blood flow, which can then be linked to particular psychiatric disorders or symptom clusters.

Functional MRI

An important development is the demonstration that MRI techniques that use the water proton signal are sufficiently sensitive to define regional increases in cerebral blood flow following neuronal activation. This technique is usually referred to as *functional MRI (fMRI)*. The principal method of fMRI is *blood oxygenation-level-dependent (BOLD) imaging*. The use of BOLD depends on the fact that deoxyhaemoglobin is paramagnetic, and therefore aligns with an applied magnetic field, making the local magnetic field stronger. By contrast, oxygenated haemoglobin is only slightly diamagnetic, and creates weak local field disturbances.

Increases in neuronal activity are associated with increases in local cerebral blood flow, which cause *decreases in deoxyhaemoglobin*. This is because under normal conditions of activation there is a relatively greater increase in blood flow than neuronal oxygen consumption. The change in *local* deoxyhaemoglobin levels can be imaged and measured to provide an indirect measure of cerebral blood flow and thereby of local neuronal activity. The advantages of fMRI are that it has greater spatial and temporal resolution than PET and SPET, and does not require the use of radioactivity.

It is also possible to use fMRI to measure cerebral blood flow more directly than the BOLD signal allows. One method, *dynamic susceptibility contrast*, uses intravenous injection of a gadolinium-based contrast agent. Another less invasive approach is provided by *arterial spin labelling (ASL)*, which uses a radiofrequency inversion pulse to label or magnetically 'tag' the blood water in arterial vessels. A second scan in which the blood is not labelled enables cortical blood flow to be estimated by subtraction. This technique allows the rapid generation of a whole brain map of cortical blood flow (Lu *et al.*, 2013).

PET imaging

PET imaging can be used to measure either *cerebral metabolism* or *cerebral blood flow*. Usually the two measures are closely correlated. In the adult brain, functional activity is almost entirely dependent on oxidative metabolism, which requires glucose and oxygen as substrates. Therefore rates of cerebral metabolism can be determined by measuring the utilization of oxygen or the accumulation of *deoxyglucose*. Measurements of regional cerebral blood flow can be made by assessing the accumulation of radioactivity in the brain during inhalation of suitably labelled CO_2 or H_2O.

SPET

Measurement of blood flow with SPET employs lipophilic radiotracers such as technetium-labelled hexamethylpropyleneamine oxime (^{99m}Tc-HMPAO). Following intravenous administration, these compounds are retained in the brain in a stable form for several hours. This enables high-resolution images to be obtained with the use of a conventional detector such as a rotating gamma camera. The uptake of ^{99m}Tc-HMPAO is linearly related to cerebral blood flow. However, unlike PET, SPET cannot provide an absolute measure of regional cerebral blood flow. Therefore the results of SPET studies are often expressed by comparing the radioactive counts in each brain region of interest with a reference area, usually either whole brain or cerebellum.

Cerebral blood flow in psychiatric disorders

'Resting studies': there have been many studies of 'resting' blood flow in various psychiatric disorders, but the results of different investigations have often been contradictory. To a large extent the conflicting data may result from the considerable methodological difficulties in standardizing the imaging conditions and the patient population. Despite these difficulties, more recent carefully controlled investigations in rigorously assessed drug-free patients are reaching a greater level of consensus. For example, PET studies of patients with depression have revealed decreased metabolic activity and blood flow in brain regions associated with the regulation of emotion (the dorsomedial and dorsolateral prefrontal cortex) and increased blood flow in areas concerned with the perception and experience of emotion (the ventrolateral prefrontal cortex, anterior cingulate cortex, and amygdala) (see Price and Drevets, 2012). In addition, further information can be obtained by correlating basal regional cerebral blood flow with the psychopathology of the patient at the time of scanning. This approach has been successful in mapping symptom clusters in patients with schizophrenia to specific brain regions (see Table 11.1).

More recent work using fMRI has investigated the *functional connectivity* of different brain regions when subjects rest quietly in the camera. Appropriate mathematical modelling can then be used to delineate various *resting state networks* which show synchronized fluctuations in the BOLD signal and presumptively, therefore, in neural activity. These networks often subsume well-characterized functions of brain activity (e.g. the motor and visual networks). Of particular interest to psychiatry is the *default mode network*, consisting of the precuneus, medial frontal, inferior parietal, and temporal regions. This network is more active when subjects are at rest, and has been linked to cognitive activities such as mind wandering and the integration of cognitive and emotional processing (see Lu *et al.*, 2013).

Activation paradigms

Psychological activation paradigms have been widely used in PET and fMRI studies of healthy volunteers to map the brain regions and distributed neuronal circuits involved in fundamental processes such as memory and language. Within-subject activation paradigms can also be applied to patients with psychiatric disorders, with perhaps more consistent results emerging than are usually obtained with 'resting state' blood flow studies. This is because, where patients act as their own controls, potential confounders such as effects of motion, changing mental state, and psychotropic drug treatment are less likely to produce systematic bias (Weinberger and Radulescu, 2016).

For example, when normal control subjects undertake the Wisconsin Card Sorting Test, there is an increase in blood flow in the prefrontal cortex. On this test, patients with schizophrenia perform less well than controls, and produce a different pattern of blood flow in the corresponding cortical area. This suggests that some patients with schizophrenia may have a dysfunction of the *prefrontal cortex*, which is associated with poor performance on tasks that depend on increased neuronal activity in this brain region. More recent studies have linked this altered performance and change in neural activity with polymorphisms of the gene for catechol-O-methyltransferase (COMT), an enzyme involved in the metabolism of dopamine and a candidate gene for schizophrenia (see Box 5.5). Investigations that integrate genetic polymorphisms with variance in cognitive performance and changes in regional cerebral blood flow have been a popular research area but, as often in biological psychiatry, the problem of replication remains substantial (see Murphy *et al.*, 2013).

Electroencephalography

Methods

The electroencephalograph (EEG) provides a measure of *cortical neuronal activity* through detection of potential differences across the scalp. The following techniques are relevant to studies of aetiology in psychiatry:

- standard (analogue) EEG
- quantified (digital) EEG
- sleep EEG (polysomnogram)
- magnetoencephalography (MEG)
- evoked potentials.

Standard EEG

The standard clinical EEG is a *qualitative* assessment of a paper trace by a trained observer using visual inspection. These kinds of recordings have been most helpful when studying the relationships between epilepsy and psychiatric disorders, but otherwise have not been particularly informative about aetiology. About 30% of psychiatric patients who are referred for an EEG are reported to have an abnormal recording, but the relevance of this has proved elusive. Artefacts from drug treatment are probably common. The standard EEG has good temporal but relatively poor spatial resolution.

Quantified EEG

The EEG signal can also be examined *quantitatively* using a number of different mathematical approaches. The most commonly used method employs power spectral analysis with Fourier transformation. Characteristic spectral patterns have been reported for certain disorders, although relating these to underlying brain mechanisms is not straightforward. Statistical removal of EEG artefact is also problematic. So far the main clinical research application has been in the analysis and detection of the effects of different drugs, with the hope of developing an objective method of screening for novel psychotropic compounds.

Sleep EEG (polysomnogram)

During sleep the EEG shows a characteristic recurrent pattern of waves, which can be divided into stages. The fundamental distinction is between *rapid eye movement (REM or dream sleep)* and *non-REM (or quiet)* sleep. The sleep EEG or polysomnogram shows fairly consistent abnormalities in depressed patients, notably a decrease in the *latency to the onset of REM sleep*. Some of these abnormalities may persist into clinical remission and may indicate vulnerability to mood disorder.

The main disadvantage of polysomnography has been the need for a specialized facility (a 'sleep laboratory'). However, the development of home-based monitoring with ambulatory equipment has been helpful in this respect. The polysomnogram has also been useful for measuring the effects of drugs on sleep quality and architecture, and can be helpful in the diagnosis and management of sleep disorders.

Magnetoencephalography

MEG is able to measure changes in extracranial magnetic fields to detect ion fluxes in cortical neurons. Like EEG, MEG has the ability to detect changes in physiological signals over time intervals of the order of milliseconds. It can provide better localization of signals than EEG, but the most useful information may come from using the techniques in combination, or by combining MEG with other imaging modalities. In this way superior temporal and spatial resolution of cortical processing can be obtained. Neither MEG nor EEG is generally helpful in identifying changes in subcortical neuronal activity. MEG can be used to measure cortical oscillations, and particular frequencies have been linked to the activity of the large-scale neuronal networks identified in resting state fMRI studies.

Evoked potentials

EEG techniques can also be used to detect changes in brain electrical activity in response to environmental stimuli. These evoked (or event-related) potentials can be detected by computerized averaging methods, and can be identified as waveforms occurring at particular times after the stimulus. For example, the P300 response is a positive deflection that occurs 300 milliseconds after a subject has identified a target stimulus embedded in a series of irrelevant stimuli.

The P300 wave probably corresponds to the cognitive processes required for the recognition, retrieval from memory, and evaluation of a specific stimulus. In patients with schizophrenia, the amplitude of the P300 wave is reduced. It is notable that the same abnormality can be found in first-degree relatives of schizophrenic patients and those with schizotypal personalities (Bramon *et al.*, 2005).

In these subjects, the change in the P300 response is likely to stem from an abnormality in information processing, and may represent a vulnerability trait marker factor for the development of schizophrenia. However, these changes are not specific in that they can also be found in patients with other disorders, such as bipolar disorder and alcohol misuse. In addition, interpretation of evoked potentials in terms of brain mechanism is not easy, because the potential recorded from the scalp is far from its generational source and is likely to reflect the activity of many different neural systems operating in parallel.

Neuropathology

Neuropathological studies attempt to answer the question of whether a *structural change* in the brain accompanies a particular kind of mental disorder. Brain structure can now be studied in life, usually with MRI scans, as well as by the traditional direct post-mortem examination of the brain. MRI structural imaging continues to develop, and *diffusion tensor imaging (DTI)* can be used to obtain detailed images of white matter tracts *in vivo* by measuring the diffusion of water in neural tissue. A review of studies in mood disorders indicated consistently reduced *anisotropy* of white matter in the frontal and temporal lobes, which suggests a loss of the integrity of white matter, although the precise pathological cause has yet to be established (Sexton *et al.*, 2009).

Neuropathology has been central to the understanding of dementia and a few other psychiatric disorders in which lesions can readily and reliably be found and, if necessary, quantified. It has not shown equivalent diagnostic kinds of lesion in other psychiatric disorders, a factor that contributed to the conventional view that most psychiatric conditions were functional as opposed to organic disorders. However, the advent of MRI and improved neuropathological methods has shown that there are structural correlates of many psychiatric disorders. For example, the brain is smaller and lighter in schizophrenia, associated with changes in its cellular and synaptic composition (see Chapter 11). Similarly, alterations in volume of parts of the limbic system and its cytoarchitecture have been reported in depression (see Chapter 9). Although none of these changes can yet be used for diagnostic purposes (because of overlap in each parameter with comparison subjects, and across diagnostic boundaries), they do argue strongly against the functional versus organic dichotomy.

These research advances are also a useful reminder that the methods of investigation that are available at a particular time may fail to detect relevant biological abnormalities even when the latter are present. For example, Alois Alzheimer (1864–1915) spent a decade searching for the neuropathology of schizophrenia before he came across the case of presenile dementia and identified the lesions which now define the disease that is named after him. In addition, as neuropathological investigations embrace the molecular level, drawing distinctions between 'functional' and 'structural' disorders becomes somewhat arbitrary. Finally, it is worth noting that progress in determining aetiology is most likely to be made through the combination of genetic, pathological, and biochemical investigations, and combining these with epidemiological ascertainment and careful clinical, psychological, and social characterization of subjects. In this way the various approaches can be used to inform and guide each other, and a more integrated view of psychiatric aetiology can ultimately emerge.

Relationship of this chapter to those on psychiatric syndromes

This chapter has reviewed several diverse approaches to aetiology. It may be easier for the reader to put these approaches into perspective when reading the sections on aetiology in the chapters on the different psychiatric syndromes, especially those on mood disorders (see Chapters 9 and 10) and schizophrenia (see Chapter 11).

Further reading

Charney DS *et al.* (2013). *Neurobiology of Mental Illness*. 4th edn. Oxford University Press, Oxford. (A comprehensive overview of the developing methods and concepts in biological psychiatry.)

Jaspers K (1963). *General Psychopathology* (translated by J Hoenig and MW Hamilton). Manchester University Press, Manchester.

pp. 301–11, 355–64, 383–99. (The classical text: these selected pages explain the concepts of meaningful connections and psychological reactions.)

Plomin R *et al.* (2013) *Behavioural Genetics*. 6th edn. Worth Publishers, New York.

CHAPTER 6
Evidence-based approaches to psychiatry

What is evidence-based medicine?

Evidence-based medicine (EBM) is a systematic way of obtaining clinically important information about aetiology, diagnosis, prognosis, and treatment. The evidence-based approach is a *process* in which the following steps are applied:

- formulation of an answerable clinical question;
- identification of the best evidence;
- critical appraisal of the evidence for validity and utility;
- implementation of the findings;
- evaluation of performance.

The principles of EBM can be applied to a variety of medical procedures. For psychiatry, the main use of EBM at present is to assess the value of *therapeutic interventions*. For this reason, in the following sections the application of EBM will be linked to studies of treatment. Applications to other areas, such as diagnosis and prognosis, are discussed later.

History of evidence-based approaches

Examples of what we now might call 'evidence-based approaches' to the investigation of treatments have a long, if sporadic, history in medicine. For example, in 1747 a naval surgeon, James Lind, studied six pairs of sailors 'as similar as I could have them' who were suffering from scurvy. The sailors who received oranges and lemons recovered within a few weeks, in contrast to those who simply received the same housing and general diet. Lind's study was not carried out 'blind', but in 1784 Benjamin Franklin applied blindfolds to the participants in a mesmerism study, who were therefore unaware whether or not the treatment was being applied. The 'blinding' abolished the treatment effect of mesmerism, providing strong evidence that its effects were mediated by suggestion (Devereaux *et al.*, 2002).

The application of modern randomized trial methodology to medicine is attributed to Sir Austin Bradford Hill (1897–1991), who designed the Medical Research Council (MRC) trial of streptomycin treatment of tuberculosis in 1948. Subsequently, Bradford Hill lent his influence to the application of randomized trials in the evaluation of psychiatric treatments, often in the face of vociferous opposition from the profession. The first psychiatric trial to use this methodology was carried out at the Maudsley Hospital in 1955 by David Davies and Michael Shepherd, who demonstrated that, relative to placebo, reserpine had beneficial effects in anxiety and depression. A few years later, Ackner and Oldham (1962) used double-blind randomized methods to debunk insulin coma therapy (see Chapter 25). Subsequently, in 1965, an MRC group reported the first large-scale, multicentre, randomized controlled trial in psychiatry, in which imipramine and electroconvulsive therapy (ECT) were shown to be therapeutically superior to placebo in the treatment of hospitalized depressed patients (see Tansella, 2002).

More recent developments in evidence-based approaches owe much to Archibald Cochrane (1909–1988), an epidemiologist and author of an influential book, *Effectiveness and Efficiency: Random reflections on health services*, which was published in 1972. Cochrane emphasized the need, when planning treatment provision, to use evidence from randomized controlled trials because it is more reliable than any other kind. In a frequently cited quotation (Cochrane, 1979), he wrote: 'It is surely a great criticism of our profession that we have not organized a critical summary, by specialty or subspecialty, adapted periodically, of all relevant randomized controlled trials.'

Cochrane's views were widely accepted, and two further developments enabled his vision to be realized. First, the availability of electronic databases and computerized searching made it feasible to find all (or nearly all) of the relevant randomized trials when gathering evidence on particular therapeutic questions. Secondly, the statistical techniques of meta-analysis enabled randomized trials to be combined, providing greater power and allowing a reliable quantification of treatment effects. Results from studies using these methodologies are called 'systematic reviews' to distinguish them from the more traditional, less reliable, 'narrative reviews' in which the judgement of the authors plays a major role in deciding what evidence to include and what weight to give it. The *Cochrane Collaboration*, which was formed in 1993, is now the largest organization in the world engaged in the production and maintenance of systematic reviews (http://www.cochrane.org). In the UK, the Centre for Reviews and Dissemination, based at the University of York, maintains an up-to-date database of systematic reviews of healthcare interventions (http://www.york.ac.uk/inst/crd/index.htm). Similarly, the *Campbell Collaboration* provides systematic reviews of evidence-based social interventions in the field of education, the criminal justice system, social welfare, and international development (http://www.campbellcollaboration.org/).

Why do we need evidence-based medicine?

There are two main related problems in clinical practice that can be helped by the application of EBM:

- The difficulty in keeping up to date with clinical and scientific advances.
- The tendency of practitioners to work in idiosyncratic ways that are not justified by the available evidence.

With the burgeoning number of clinical and scientific journals, the most assiduous clinician is unable to keep up to date with all of the relevant articles even in their own field. In fact, it has been estimated that to accomplish this task would require scrutiny of at least 20 publications a day! Clinicians therefore have to rely on information gathered from other sources, which might include, for example, unsystematic expert reviews, opinions of colleagues, information from pharmaceutical companies, and their own clinical experiences and beliefs. This can lead to wide variations in practice—for example, those described for the use of ECT (see UK ECT Review Group, 2003).

Kinds of evidence

The fundamental assumption of EBM is that some kinds of evidence are *better* (i.e. more valid and of greater clinical applicability) than others. This view is most easily elaborated for questions about therapy. A commonly used 'hierarchy' is shown in Box 6.1.

In this hierarchy, evidence from randomized trials is regarded as more valid than evidence from non-randomized trials, while *systematic reviews of randomized trials* are seen as the gold standard for answering clinical questions. This assumption has itself yet to be

---

Box 6.1 Hierarchy of the quality of research about treatment

Ia Evidence from a systematic review of randomized controlled trials

Ib Evidence from at least one randomized controlled trial

IIa Evidence from at least one controlled study without randomization

IIb Evidence from at least one other type of quasi-experimental study

III Evidence from non-experimental descriptive studies, such as comparative studies, correlation studies, and case–control studies

IV Evidence from expert committee reports or opinions and/or clinical experience of respected authorities

tested systematically, and some argue that large trials with simple clinically relevant endpoints may be more valid than meta-analyses (see Furukawa, 2004). It is certainly important that clinicians are trained in critical evaluation of systematic reviews before they apply their results to clinical practice (see Geddes, 1999).

Individual treatment studies

Validity

The key criterion for validity in treatment studies is *randomization*. In addition, clinicians entering patients into a therapeutic trial should be unaware of the treatment group to which their patients are being allocated. This is usually referred to as *concealment of the randomization list*. This means that clinicians must not be aware of the likely treatment allocation of the next patient. Such awareness could influence their decision as to whether or not to enter a patient into the trial. Without concealed randomization, the validity of a study is questionable and its results may be misleading.

Other important points to consider when assessing the validity of a study include the following:

- Were all of the patients who entered the trial accounted for at its conclusion?
- Were patients analysed in the groups to which they were allocated (so-called 'intention-to-treat' analysis)?
- Were patients and clinicians blind to the treatment received (a different question to that of *concealed randomization*)?
- Apart from the experimental treatment, were the groups treated equally?
- Did the randomization process result in the groups being similar at baseline?

Presentation of results

Odds ratios and relative risk

When the outcome of a clinical trial is an event (e.g. admission to hospital), a commonly used measure of effectiveness is the *odds ratio*. The odds ratio is the odds of an event occurring in the experimental group divided by the odds of it occurring in the control group. The odds ratio is given with 95% confidence intervals (which indicate the range of values within which we have a 95% certainty that the *true* value falls). The narrower the confidence intervals are, the greater is the precision of the study.

If the odds ratio of an event such as admission to hospital is 1.0, this means the rates of admission do not differ between the control and experimental groups. Therefore if the confidence interval of the odds ratio of an individual study includes the value of 1.0, the study has failed to show that the experimental and control treatments differ from each other.

Relative risk also measures the relative likelihood of an event occurring in two distinct groups. It is regarded as a more intuitive measure of effectiveness than the odds ratio. For example, if action A carries a risk of 99.9% and action B carries a risk of 99.0%, the relative risk is just over 1, which seems intuitively correct for two such similar outcomes. However, the calculated odds ratio is almost 10! With relatively infrequent events, the odds ratio and relative risk become more similar. Measures of relative risk cannot be used in case–control designs and are hard to adjust by covariance for confounding variables.

Effect sizes

In many studies the outcome measure of interest is a continuous variable, such as a mean score on the Hamilton Rating Scale for Depression. It is possible to use the original measure in the meta-analysis, although more often an estimate of *effect size* is made because it is more statistically robust.

Effect sizes are obtained by dividing the difference in effect between the experimental group and the control group by the standard deviation of their difference. The clinical interpretation of the effect size is discussed below.

Clinical utility of interventions

Risk reduction and number needed to treat

An important part of EBM involves using the results of randomized trials of groups of patients to derive the impact of an intervention at the level of the individual patient. A useful concept when assessing the value of a treatment is that of *absolute risk reduction (ARR)*. This compares the proportion of patients receiving the experimental treatment who experienced a clinically significant adverse outcome (e.g. clinical relapse) with the rate in patients receiving the comparison treatment. These rates are known as the *experimental event rate (EER)* and *control event rate (CER)*, respectively, and are calculated as percentages. The difference between these two outcome rates is the ARR.

The ARR can be converted into a more clinically useful number, known as the *number needed to treat (NNT)*. The NNT is the reciprocal of the ARR, and it tells us how many patients would need to be treated to experience one more positive outcome event compared with a comparator treatment (or no treatment) (see Box 6.2). Like odds ratios, NNTs are usually given with 95% confidence intervals.

Example

Paykel *et al.* (1999) randomized 158 patients with residual depressive symptoms following an episode of major depression to either clinical management or clinical management with 18 sessions of cognitive behaviour therapy (CBT). Over the following 68 weeks the relapse rate in the CBT-treated group (29%) was significantly less than that in the clinical management group (47%; *P* = 0.02).

> **Box 6.2 Indices for translating research results into clinical practice**
>
> | | Experimental treatment, X | Control treatment, Y |
> |---|---|---|
> | Positive outcome | a | b |
> | Negative outcome | c | d |
>
> Control event rate (CER) = b/(b + d)
>
> Experimental event rate (EER) = a/(a + c)
>
> Absolute risk reduction (ARR)
>
> The difference in the proportions with a positive outcome on treatments X and Y = (CER − EER)
>
> Relative risk = EER/CER
>
> **Odds ratio (OR)**
>
> The ratio of the odds of a positive outcome on treatments X and Y = (a/c)/(b/d) = ad/bc
>
> **Number needed to treat (NNT)**—the number of patients that need to be treated with treatment X to obtain one more positive outcome than would be expected on treatment Y (= 1/AAR)

The ARR in relapse with CBT is 47 − 29 = 18%. The NNT is the reciprocal of this number, which is approximately six (usually the NNT is rounded up to the next highest integer). This means that six patients with residual depressive symptoms have to be treated with CBT to avoid one relapse. In general, an NNT of less than 10 denotes a useful treatment effect. However, interpretation of the NNT will also depend on the nature of the treatment, together with the extent of its therapeutic and adverse effects. The NNTs for some common psychiatric treatments are shown in Table 6.1. Overall NNTs of psychiatric interventions are comparable to those employed in general medicine (Leucht *et al.*, 2012).

If the outcome measure of an intervention is a beneficial event (e.g. recovery) rather than avoidance of an adverse event, the effect of the intervention is calculated as the *absolute benefit increase (ABI)* in the same way as the ARR (see above), with the NNT being similarly computed. A concept related to NNT is the *number needed to harm (NNH)*, which describes the adverse risks of particular therapies (e.g. extrapyramidal symptoms with antipsychotic drugs).

Computing the NNT from odds ratios

If a study or meta-analysis provides an odds ratio, it is possible to compute an NNT that may be more relevant to the clinical circumstances of the practitioner and their patient. For example, in the example given above (Paykel *et al.*, 1999), relapses occurred in 35 of 78 subjects in the clinical management group, compared with 23 of 80 subjects in the CBT group. This gives an odds ratio of the risk of relapse between the two treatments of 0.49. To obtain an NNT from the odds ratio it is necessary to know, or to estimate, the expected relapse rate in the control group. This is known as the *patient expected event rate (PEER)*. The PEER is combined with the odds ratio (OR) in the following formula:

$$NNT = \frac{1 - PEER(1 - OR)}{(1 - PEER)\,PEER(1 - OR)}$$

If we take the relapse rate in the patients who were in the clinical management group in the above study (45%), we have:

$$NNT = \frac{1 - 0.45 \times (1 - 0.49)}{(1 - 0.45) \times 0.45 \times (1 - 0.49)}$$

This gives an NNT of about 6, which we also derived from the other method of calculation involving the

Table 6.1 Examples of number needed to treat for interventions in psychiatry

Intervention	Outcome	NNT
Maintenance antidepressant treatment	Prevention of relapse	4
Lithium augmentation in resistant depression	Clinical response (50% decrease in symptom score)	4
Antipsychotic drugs in schizophrenia	Relapse prevention	3
Family therapy in schizophrenia	Relapse at 1 year	7
Atypical antipsychotic augmentation of SSRI-resistant depression	Clinical response (50% decrease in symptom score)	9
SSRIs compared with TCAs in acute depression	Remain in treatment at 6 weeks	33

SSRI, Selective serotonin reuptake inhibitor; TCA, tricyclic antidepressant.

ARR. However, if from a local audit we know that in our own service the relapse rate of patients with residual depressive symptoms is about 20% (rather than the figure of 45% reported by Paykel *et al.*), using the above formula the NNT becomes about 11. This means in our own service we would need to treat 11 patients with CBT to obtain one less relapse. Thus odds ratios can be used to adjust NNTs to local clinical conditions, thereby aiding decisions about the applicability of interventions.

Clinical relevance of effect size

Like the odds ratio, the effect size is not easy to interpret clinically. A useful approach is to use the effect size to estimate the degree of overlap between the control and experimental populations. In this way we obtain the proportion of control group scores that are lower than those in the experimental group. (A negative effect size simply means that scores in the control group are *higher* than those in the experimental group.)

For example, in a review of the effects of benzodiazepines and zolpidem on total sleep time relative to placebo, Nowell *et al.* (1997) found an overall effect size of 0.71. From normal distribution tables this means that 76% of controls had less total sleep time than the average sleep time in the hypnotic-treated patients. Effect sizes have been classified in the following way:

- 0.2 = small
- 0.5 = moderate
- ≥0.8 = large.

The effect size of antidepressant medication relative to placebo is about 0.4–0.5. At the kind of response levels seen in antidepressant-treated patients (response rate of around 30% in the placebo group and 60% in the experimental group), an effect size of 0.2 is equivalent

to an NNT of about 10. With an effect size of 0.5, the NNT falls to 5.

Ethical aspects of therapeutic trials

Randomization

As we have seen, randomization is a key process in the conduct of an evidence-based clinical trial, because it is the best way of avoiding bias owing to chance and random error. However, a clinician may feel uncomfortable about randomization if, for example, he has a strong belief in the efficacy of one of the treatments that is being assessed. Randomization is ethical where there is genuine *uncertainty* about the best treatment for the individual concerned. In fact, EBM suggests that this situation is more common than clinicians may realize, in that many strongly held beliefs about the efficacy of therapeutic interventions are based on anecdotal experience rather than systematic evidence.

Use of placebo

The use of drug placebo in trials of psychotropic agents is controversial. However, such studies are required by many drug-licensing authorities before, for example, a new antidepressant drug is licensed. The arguments for the use of placebo in antidepressant drug trials have been summarized as follows (see Kader and Pantelis, 2009):

- The placebo response in major depression is variable and unpredictable, and is not infrequently equivalent in therapeutic effect to active treatment.
- Placebo is required to establish the efficacy of new antidepressants. Comparison against an active treatment is not methodologically sufficient because, while a finding of 'no difference' in antidepressant activity

might mean that the new and established treatments have equivalent efficacy, it might also mean that neither treatment was actually effective under the particular trial conditions employed.

- The lack of placebo-controlled design in antidepressant drug development might lead to the marketing of a drug that is ineffective, thereby harming public health.

These arguments have to be weighed against the knowledge that antidepressants are generally somewhat more effective than placebo in the treatment of depression. Therefore a patient who is treated with placebo in a randomized trial is not receiving the best available therapy. One way of trying to deal with this is to ensure that patients in such trials receive particularly close clinical monitoring, which will result in their being withdrawn from the study if they are not doing well.

An unintended consequence of this problem is that patients in placebo-controlled trials may not be representative of the patients who will receive the treatment concerned in real-world conditions. For example, in placebo-controlled studies of depression, patients are recruited by advertisement, and there can be inflation of depression scores by raters prior to treatment so that individuals will meet the cut-off score for recruitment into the trial. Such patients tend to do well, whether they are receiving placebo or active treatment, making it difficult to show convincing clinical differences between drug and placebo. In addition, the clinical characteristics of such patients differ significantly from those treated routinely (Wisniewski *et al.*, 2009).

Informed consent

The role of informed consent is crucial to the ethical conduct of randomized and placebo-controlled trials. This raises difficulties with some psychiatric disorders in which the judgement and decision-making abilities of patients may be impaired. Kader and Pantelis (2009) have outlined a number of important factors.

- Patients must be made specifically aware that the trial is not being conducted for their individual benefit.
- With placebo treatment there must be clear specification of the probability of receiving placebo, the lack of improvement that might result, and the possibility of symptomatic worsening.
- Patients must be free from any coercion or inducement.
- Patients have the right to withdraw from the study at any time without any kind of penalty.
- In addition to the investigator, a family member or other suitable person should be encouraged to monitor the patient's condition and report to the investigator if there are any concerns.

The key issues therefore are *open and explicit information sharing* with the patient and their family, and all necessary measures to *avoid placebo treatment leading to harm to the subject*. However, the issue remains controversial.

Systematic reviews

Validity

The most common aim of a systematic review is to obtain all of the available *valid* evidence about a specific procedure or intervention, and from this to provide a more precise quantitative assessment of its efficacy. Other uses of systematic reviews (e.g. to examine prognosis) are discussed later in this chapter under the heading, 'Other applications of evidence-based medicine' (page 131). Two advances have greatly increased the feasibility of systematic reviews—first, the availability of electronic databases such as Medline and Scopus and, secondly, new statistical techniques through which results from different studies can be combined in a quantitative manner. Because a meta-analysis uses all of the available valid data, its *statistical power* is greater than that of an individual study. It may therefore demonstrate moderate but clinically important effects of treatment that were not apparent in individual randomized studies.

A problem with systematic review is that, particularly in areas such as psychiatry, where clinical trials are difficult, it can lead to much randomized evidence being excluded from consideration because of perceived lack of quality. For example, a systematic review of the effects of methylphenidate treatment on attention deficit/hyperactivity disorder (ADHD), considered 185 trials of over 12,000 participants, but only six trials, with 183 participants, were regarded as adequate. Such reduction of evidence can lead to much uncertainty about the benefits and harms of widely used interventions. In addition, systematic reviews are rarely able to provide endpoints that are meaningful to clinicians, patients, and their families. This indicates the need, when assessing the value of interventions, to integrate perspectives from multiple research designs, including observational and qualitative studies. This approach may be more helpful in capturing the treatment effects that are most relevant to patients and those caring for them (Fazel, 2015).

Systematic reviews of treatment, like single therapeutic studies, have to be tested for *validity* and *quality*. The following questions should be posed.

- *Is it a systematic review of relevant and randomized studies?* We have already seen that the first task in the EBM process is to ask a clearly formulated question. It is therefore necessary to determine whether the subject of the systematic review is truly relevant to the therapeutic question that needs to be answered. The next step is to make sure that only randomized studies have been included. Systematic reviews that contain a mixture of randomized and non-randomized studies may give misleading results.

- *Do the authors describe the methods by which relevant trials were located?* Although electronic searching greatly facilitates the identification of clinical trials, up to half of the relevant studies may be missed because of miscoding. It is therefore important for authors to make clear whether they supplemented electronic searching with hand-searching of appropriate journals. They may also, for example, have contacted authors of trials, as well as relevant groups in the pharmaceutical industry. In general, negative studies are less likely to be published than positive ones, which can lead to falsely optimistic conclusions about the efficacy and tolerability of particular treatments. For example, analysis of all completed studies of new antidepressants in adolescents indicated that some selective serotonin reuptake inhibitors (SSRIs) and venlafaxine might increase the risk of suicidal behaviour. This potentially important finding was not apparent from analyses of the published data alone (Whittington *et al.*, 2004).

- *How did the authors decide which studies should be included in the systematic review?* In a systematic review, authors have to decide which of the various studies that they identify should be included in the overall analysis. This means defining explicit measures of quality, which will be based on the factors outlined above. Because these judgements are in part subjective, it is desirable for them to be made independently by at least two of the investigators.

- *Were the results of the therapeutic intervention consistent from one study to another?* It is common to see differences in the size of the effect of a therapeutic intervention from one study to another. However, if the effects are mixed, with some studies showing a large clinical effect while others find none at all, the trials are said to show heterogeneity. Sometimes heterogeneity can be accounted for by factors such as lower doses of a drug treatment or differences in patient characteristics. As noted above, systematic reviews should carry a measure of *quality,* and sometimes effects are found only in the high- or low-quality studies. If there is no likely explanation for heterogeneity, the results of the review must be considered tentative.

- *Did the review follow Preferred Reporting Items for Systematic Reviews and Meta-Analyses (PRISMA) guidelines?* The PRISMA guidelines are aimed at standardizing the information provided in publications about how a particular systematic review and meta-analysis was conducted, analysed, and presented (see Moher *et al.*, 2009).

Presentation of results

Combining odds ratios

The results of meta-analyses are often presented as a 'forest plot', in which the findings of the various studies are shown in diagrammatic form (see Figure 6.1). As noted above, studies in which the outcome is an event are presented as odds ratios with 95% confidence intervals.

The aim of meta-analysis is to obtain a *pooled estimate* of the treatment effect by combining the odds ratios or effect sizes of all the studies. This is not simply an average of all the odds ratios, but is *weighted* so that studies with more statistical information and greater precision (with narrower confidence intervals) contribute relatively more to the final result. The pooled odds ratio also has a 95% confidence interval. Once again, if this interval includes the value of 1.0, the experimental intervention does not differ from the control.

In Figure 6.1 some of the studies show a significant effect of assertive community treatment (ACT) in decreasing readmission, while others do not. The two pooled analyses are difficult to interpret because the confidence intervals of one of them (the *fixed effects model*) do not overlap with 1.0, making ACT significantly different from the control, whereas the other (the *random effects model*) just overlaps with 1.0 and is therefore of marginal statistical significance.

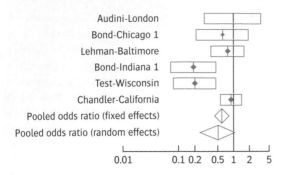

Figure 6.1 Effect of active community treatment on the odds of admission to hospital.

Reproduced from Evidence Based Mental Health, 1(4), Freemantle N, Geddes J, Understanding and interpreting systematic reviews and meta-analyses. Part 2: meta-analyses, pp. 102–4, Copyright (1998), with permission from BMJ Publishing Group Ltd.

We have already seen that the studies in a meta-analysis may indicate *heterogeneity*. This can be tested statistically with a modification of the chi-squared test. If significant heterogeneity is present, the most appropriate meta-analytic technique is a *pooled random effects model*. This model assumes that different treatment effects will occur in different studies, and takes this into account in the pooled estimate. This usually results in wider confidence intervals, as in the pooled random effect odds ratio in the ACT studies (Figure 6.1). If the studies suggest a single underlying population treatment effect (i.e. lack of heterogeneity), the pooled treatment analysis should use a *fixed effects model*. This estimate has narrower confidence intervals that may, however, be misleading in the presence of significant heterogeneity.

In Figure 6.1 there is statistically significant heterogeneity between the studies, and inspection of the data shows that the majority of the benefit is contributed by two of the studies, which are not the largest. The random and fixed effects models find a similar mean benefit of ACT in preventing readmission, but the random effects model has a wider confidence interval and, as noted above, just overlaps with 1.0. Because of the heterogeneity of the studies, the random effects model is the more appropriate way of analysing the data. Overall, therefore, we would be cautious about accepting the efficacy of ACT in lowering readmission rates, unless we were able to find a convincing reason for the variation in the study results. Indeed, heterogeneity can prompt a search for reasons that might explain it. In the ACT example, this might include differences in patient characteristics and the 'control' treatment to which the intervention was compared (Burns *et al.*, 2007c).

Effect sizes

As noted above, where the outcome measure is a continuous variable, the usual method of calculating results is to use effect sizes. As with odds ratios, the effect sizes can be combined to give a pooled estimate of greater precision.

Clinical utility

The clinical utility of meta-analyses is assessed as described for individual studies above. Meta-analyses will often provide figures for the NNT. However, as shown above, it is also possible to calculate NNT values from meta-analysis data using ARR or odds ratios.

Network meta-analysis

Network meta-analysis (NMA), or multiple treatments meta-analysis, is a development in meta-analysis that allows indirect comparisons between multiple treatments even when particular treatments have not been compared directly themselves. This approach provides a useful means of assessing competing interventions and ranking them for efficacy and acceptability. NMA therefore extends the usual pair-wise comparison of two interventions by producing a connected network of interventions in which information flows both directly and indirectly. This provides the important possibility of 'indirect comparison'. As an example we can consider two treatments, A and B, that have both been compared with a common comparator, C. In this case the effectiveness of A versus B can be estimated indirectly through the common comparator C (Mavridis *et al.*, 2015). An example of a network plot of different treatments for acute mania is given in Figure 6.2, and the efficacy and acceptability results of this particular analysis are given in the section on the pharmacological treatment of acute mania (see Chapter 10, Figure 10.1). A problem for NMA is the fact that indirect comparisons cannot control for possible differences between informative studies in trial methodology and patient population. The assumption made is that differing trial characteristics are evenly distributed across studies or do not affect trial outcome. This assumption is known as *transitivity* (Mavridis *et al.*, 2015).

Patient level meta-analysis

Traditional meta-analysis combines data from different investigations by aggregating overall findings from each study, as in Figure 6.1. An increasingly popular approach is to use *individual patient data*, where the original data

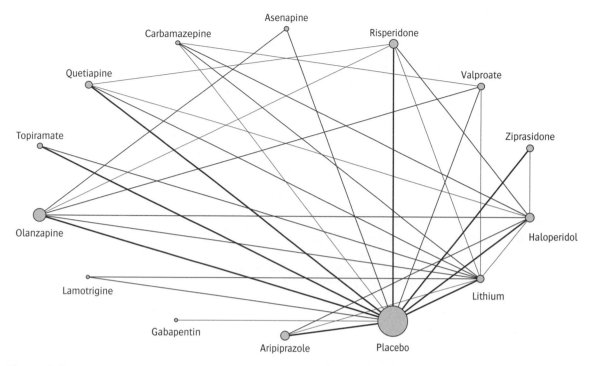

Figure 6.2 Network of eligible comparisons for a multiple-treatments meta-analysis of efficacy and acceptability of different treatments for acute mania. The width of the lines is proportional to the number of trials comparing every pair of treatments, and the size of every node is proportional to the number of randomized participants (sample size).

Reproduced from The Lancet, 378(9799), Cipriani et al, Comparative efficacy and acceptability of antimanic drugs in acute mania: a multiple-treatments meta-analysis, pp. 1306-15, Copyright (2011), with permission from Elsevier.

for each participant is obtained and used in the meta-analysis (Riley *et al.*, 2010). In ideal situations, results from patient level and aggregate meta-analyses should be very similar. However, patient level meta-analyses have the ability to apply consistent inclusion and exclusion criteria across different studies and to harmonize and allow for important patient characteristics, including baseline prognostic factors. This form of analysis also facilitates the inclusion of unpublished data, and the identification of duplicate reporting. Finally, consistent statistical analysis can be applied to the individual studies. The main disadvantage of the approach is the time and practical difficulty involved in obtaining individual data from each investigator, as well as ethical concerns regarding the maintenance of confidentiality (Riley *et al.*, 2010).

Problems with meta-analysis

Biased conclusions

Apart from a systematic location of evidence, the aim of meta-analysis is to combine data from multiple studies into a single estimate of treatment effect. There are a number of ways in which the results of such an exercise can be misleading.

- *Publication bias.* Evidence indicates that studies that show positive treatment effects are more likely to be published than negative studies. If negative studies are not included in the meta-analysis, the effect of treatment will be inflated.

- *Duplication of publication.* Just as negative treatment studies may go unpublished, positive studies may be published several times in different forms, sometimes with different authors! This again will falsely elevate treatment effects if the same study is included more than once.

- *Heterogeneity of studies.* As noted above, individual studies may vary widely in the results obtained, because of quite subtle differences in study design, quality, and patient population. If such heterogeneity is not recognized and accounted for in the meta-analysis, misleading conclusions will be drawn.

How accurate is meta-analysis?

There are some well-known examples where the results of meta-analyses have been contradicted subsequently by single large randomized trials. For example, a meta-analysis that showed that intravenous magnesium improved outcome in patients with myocardial infarction was later decisively refuted by a single large randomized trial of 58,000 patients. The misleading result of the meta-analysis was later explained on the basis of publication bias, poor methodological quality in the smaller trials, and clinical heterogeneity (Baigent et al., 2010).

Reviews of this area have generally found that about 80% of meta-analyses agree with single large trials in terms of direction of effect of treatment, but the size and statistical significance of the effect often differ between the two methods. Furthermore, separate meta-analyses of the same therapeutic intervention may reach rather different conclusions. For example, using the network meta-analysis approach, Cipriani et al. (2009) found clinically significant differences in the efficacy and acceptability of a range of newer antidepressants, whereas Gartlehner et al. (2008), using essentially the same data and approach, found no important differences between the various medications.

Funnel plots

One way of improving the reliability of meta-analyses is by the use of funnel plots. The funnel plot is based on the assumption that the precision (confidence interval) of the estimated treatment effect will be greater in studies with a larger sample size. Therefore the effect sizes of larger studies should cluster around the overall mean difference between experimental and control groups. By contrast, the results from smaller studies should be more dispersed around the mean. Therefore, when the precision of individual studies is plotted against their odds ratios or effect sizes, the resulting graphical plot should resemble a symmetrical inverted funnel (the funnel plot). Statistically significant deviations from this plot suggest the presence of publication bias (for example, that negative studies of treatment are not fully represented). In this case, the findings of the meta-analysis should be treated with caution.

Large-scale randomized trials

As noted above, the advantage of meta-analysis is that by combining individual studies it can assemble sufficient patient numbers to allow detection of moderate-sized but clinically important therapeutic effects. Another way of detecting moderate-sized treatment effects is to randomize very large numbers of patients to a single study. These large-scale randomized (simple) trials (or *mega-trials*) have advantages over meta-analysis in that all of the patients can be allocated to a single study design. Such studies need numerous collaborators and therefore require a *simple study design* and a *clear endpoint*.

This methodology has been most successfully applied to areas of medicine, such as cardiovascular disorders, where interventions can sometimes be simple (e.g. one dose of aspirin daily) and endpoints (e.g. cardiac infarction, or death) clearly identified (Baigent et al., 2010). The challenge for psychiatric trials is to adapt such methodology to conditions for which interventions are more complex and endpoints more subtle.

Applicability

A general problem when applying evidence from randomized trials and meta-analysis to routine clinical work is that clinical trials are often conducted in rather 'ideal' conditions, which in a number of respects may not match routine clinical work:

- *Patient population.* Patients in controlled trials may differ systematically from those in routine clinical care in being less severely ill and having fewer comorbid difficulties. Thus trials may be conducted on patients who are in fact rather unrepresentative of a usual patient population.
- *Level of supervision.* In drug trials, concordance is regularly monitored by frequent review and supervision. Thus patients are less likely to drop out of treatment even when drugs are not particularly well tolerated.
- *Therapist variables.* Particularly in psychotherapy trials, treatment may be administered by skilled and experienced therapists. In routine practice, treatments may be given by people with less experience. Furthermore, in trials the performance of therapists is often monitored closely to ensure that it conforms to the treatment protocol. Everyday practice may match the protocol less well.

Pragmatic trials

To overcome these limitations, it has been suggested that *pragmatic trials* might be a more appropriate way to study the effect of certain psychiatric interventions. Such studies aim to conduct randomized trials in 'real-life' situations. Methodologically they have much in common with the mega-trials described earlier, in that they are designed to answer simple and important clinical questions. As far as possible, pragmatic trials are conducted in a *routine clinical setting*. Other important features include the following:

- Randomization of very large numbers of subjects is necessary to take account of the fact that most advances in treatment will yield only moderate effect sizes. Blinding is seen as less important than randomization, particularly where active treatments are compared.

- The process of recruitment is simplified by avoiding restrictive entry criteria. The principle criterion is that both doctor and patient should feel substantial uncertainty as to which of the trial treatments is best.

- Assessments are streamlined so that they fit in with routine clinical practice: 'Many trials would be of much greater scientific value if they collected 10 times less data ... on 10 times more patients' (Baigent *et al.*, 2010).

- Clinically relevant outcome measures are used. For example, in a trial of a therapeutic intervention in schizophrenia, a rating by a patient and family member on a simple scale of wellbeing may carry more clinical relevance than a score on a standardized rating scale.

Implementation of evidence-based medicine

Implementing evidence-based medicine for the individual patient

Having obtained the best evidence on a therapeutic intervention and decided that it is valid and therapeutically useful, it is necessary to decide how applicable it is to the individual patient you are considering. In large measure this depends on the answers to the questions on 'applicability' listed above. The key issues are as follows:

- How similar is the patient to those in the randomized trials? (This might be particularly relevant to psychiatry, where patients with more severe illness may be underrepresented in randomized trials.)

- Can the local service deliver the intervention successfully? (For example, it is no use recommending applied relaxation for generalized anxiety disorder if there are no trained therapists available to carry it out.)

When making the decision about implementation, it may be useful to adjust the NNT for local clinical conditions if the relevant information is available (see above). A further way of taking more information into account in clinical decision-making is provided by the concept of 'likelihood of being helped or harmed (LHH)'. For example, a meta-analysis of the addition of atypical antipsychotic medication to ineffective SSRI treatment found that the NNT to produce remission was 9, while the NNH to discontinue medication owing to side-effects was 17. The LHH is calculated as the ratio of (1/NNT) to (1/NNH) or (1/9):(1/17), which is about 2 to 1 in favour of the addition

of atypicals in these circumstances. It is also possible to weight the NNT and NNH with factors that incorporate the patient's attitude to the value of improving depression relative to that of experiencing adverse effects. Whether such efforts at quantification add significantly to a careful clinical assessment and discussion with the patient is questionable. The important point is that results from randomized trials need to be adapted to the differing needs of individuals.

Implementing evidence-based medicine at a service level

Haynes (1999) suggested that the following stages are important in the implementation of a new treatment:

- *Efficacy.* Does the intervention work under carefully controlled ('ideal') conditions?

- *Effectiveness.* Does the intervention work when provided under the usual circumstances of health care practice?

- *Efficiency.* What is the effectiveness of the intervention in relation to the resources that it consumes (i.e. its cost-effectiveness or cost–benefit)?

Ideally, the full implementation of EBM would involve successful negotiation of all these stages, and only interventions that have satisfied the three criteria of efficacy, effectiveness, and efficiency would be used. In practice, many therapeutic interventions in psychiatry (particularly drug treatment and cognitive behaviour therapy) are of proven *efficacy*, but there is often uncertainty about their *effectiveness* and *efficiency*. For example, lithium treatment is *efficacious* in the prophylaxis of bipolar disorder, but appears to have disappointing *effectiveness*, mainly because under standard clinical conditions many patients do not take lithium reliably.

Clinical practice guidelines

In some medical fields there is a substantial amount of evidence of different kinds, but still considerable clinical uncertainty about the best therapeutic management. In this situation it may be worth developing *clinical practice guidelines*, which are explicitly evidence-based.

Such guidelines are best developed in the following way.

- A guideline development group, composed of a multidisciplinary group and patient representatives, decides on the precise clinical questions to be answered.
- The available evidence is systematically reviewed and classified according to the hierarchy shown in Box 6.1.
- The guideline development group makes recommendations, explicitly demonstrating how their recommendations are linked to the available evidence.

Clinical guidelines are best developed at a national level by appropriate professional organizations, but usually require modification to take local clinical conditions into account. Guidelines will only be effective if they are actively disseminated and implemented.

In the UK, the National Institute for Health and Care Excellence (NICE) has taken a prominent role in analysing and promulgating evidence about therapeutic interventions in the form of national guidelines (http://www.nice.org.uk/). We cite many of these guidelines in this book. The success of this process in changing clinical practice is not certain, and may depend on other factors such as the strength and stability of evidence, and cost issues (Freemantle, 2004). A further problem is that sometimes the evidence used in guideline development

> ### Box 6.3 Evaluation of utility of therapeutic guidelines
>
> - Did preparation and publication avoid significant conflict of interest?
> - Is the guideline concerned with an appropriate topic and patient group?
> - Did the guideline panel include multidisciplinary, relevant expertise?
> - Have subjective judgements been made explicit and justified?
> - Have all relevant data been obtained and evaluated?
> - Has the evidence been properly synthesised and are results obtained in keeping with the guideline conclusion?
> - Are variations in medical practice addressed?
> - Is the guideline clinically relevant, comprehensive and flexible
> - Does the guideline take into account the acceptability, affordability and practicality of its recommendations?
> - Does the guideline describe how it should be disseminated, implemented and reviewed?
>
> Reproduced from Greenhalgh T, How to Read a Paper, Copyright (2010), with permission from John Wiley & Sons.

is based on a few trials whose relevance to the real world may be questionable. Nevertheless, workable guidelines need relatively definitive advice; this can lead to the issuing of rather arbitrary guidance together with a diminished probability that more informative studies will be carried out subsequently. Clinicians need to be aware of the key guidelines relating to the conditions that they treat, and should be able to justify pursuing different approaches where they have judged this to be necessary in individual cases (Box 6.3).

Evaluation of evidence-based medicine

EBM itself needs to be evaluated through randomized trials of effectiveness. Individual practitioners can also evaluate their EBM performance by:

- auditing what proportion of their clinical decisions are evidence-based;
- recognizing gaps in practice that require a search for and appraisal of relevant evidence;
- auditing the effectiveness of evidence-based practice changes.

In this way the process of EBM can become an integral part of continuing professional development and the audit cycle.

Other applications of evidence-based medicine

The foregoing account has focused on the use of EBM in the assessment of therapeutic interventions in psychiatry. Other applications of EBM include the assessment of evidence relating to diagnosis, prognosis, and aetiology. These applications require rather different methodologies from the randomized trials considered above, and diagnosis and prognosis will be discussed in the remainder of the chapter. Approaches to aetiology have been discussed in Chapter 5. All of these applications start with a focused question, which, as with treatment-related questions, must:

- be directly relevant to the identified problem;
- be constructed in a way that facilitates searching for a precise answer (Geddes, 1999; see Table 6.2).

Diagnosis

If a practitioner is trying to assess the value of a particular study assessing a diagnostic test, they need to consider a number of questions.

- Was there an independent, blind comparison of the test with a diagnostic gold standard?
- Did the sample include the range of patients to whom the test is likely to be applied in clinical practice?

- What is the sensitivity and specificity of the test?
- Will it aid the management of my patients?

Example

Question: How useful is the CAGE questionnaire in detecting problem drinking in medical and surgical inpatients?

The CAGE questionnaire is a simple four-item questionnaire designed to detect patients with alcohol misuse (see Chapter 20). Sackett (1996) describes a study in a community-based teaching hospital in Boston where the CAGE questionnaire was administered to 518 patients. The gold standard to which the CAGE questionnaire was compared was an extensive social history and clinical examination supplemented by liver biopsy where indicated. We can therefore be reasonably confident that cases of alcohol misuse were reliably identified.

On clinical (gold standard) grounds, 117 patients met the criteria for alcohol misuse or dependence. Of the 61 patients who scored positively on the CAGE questionnaire (scores of 3 or 4), 60 were found to have gold standard evidence of alcohol misuse. The CAGE is therefore highly specific (see Figure 6.3). However, the remaining 57 patients with alcohol misuse were not identified by the CAGE. The CAGE therefore has only a modest sensitivity (see Figure 6.3).

Table 6.2 **Common types of clinical question**

Form of the question	Most reliable study architecture
How likely is a patient who has a particular symptom, sign, or diagnostic result to have a specific disorder?	A *cross-sectional study* of patients suspected of having the disorder comparing the proportion of the patients who *really have the disorder and have a positive test result with the proportion of patients who do not have the disorder and have a positive test result*
Is the treatment of interest more effective in producing a desired outcome than an alternative treatment (including no treatment)?	Randomized evidence in which the patients are randomly allocated to receive either the treatment of interest or the alternative (see Box 6.1)
What is the probability of a specific outcome in this patient?	A study in which an *inception cohort* of patients at a common stage in the development of the illness (especially first onset) are followed up for an adequate length of time
What has caused the disorder (or how likely is a particular intervention to cause a specific adverse effect)?	A study comparing the frequency of an exposure in a group of people with the disease of interest (*cases*) with a group of people without the disease (*controls*); this may be a randomized controlled trial, a case–control study, or a cohort study

Number of positive answers to the four CAGE questions		Alcohol abuse or dependency: Yes	Alcohol abuse or dependency: No	
	3 or 4	60 (true +) a	1 (false +) b	61 a+b
	2, 1, or none	57 (false +) c	400 (true +) d	457 c+d
		a+c 117	b+d 401	a+b+c+d 518

$$\text{Sensitivity} = \frac{a}{(a+c)} = \frac{60}{117} = 0.51 \text{ or } 51\%.$$

$$\text{Specificity} = \frac{d}{(b+d)} = \frac{400}{401} = 0.998 \text{ or } 99.8\%.$$

Figure 6.3 The CAGE questions for screening for alcohol abuse/dependency.

Reproduced from Sackett DL, Evaluation of clinical method. In DJ Weatherall, JGG Ledingham and DA Warrell, eds, Oxford Textbook of Medicine, 3rd edn, pp. 15–21, Copyright (1996), with permission from Oxford University Press.

These results show that the CAGE is a useful screening instrument for problem drinking in a general hospital setting, in that a positive response is highly predictive of alcohol problems. However, the test would have to be applied in the knowledge that a negative CAGE response does not rule out alcohol misuse, particularly if there is other evidence of problem drinking.

Prognosis

Studies relating to prognosis should be assessed by considering the following questions.

- Was a defined, representative sample of patients identified at a common point, early in the course of the disorder?
- Was the follow-up sufficiently long and was it complete?
- Were objective outcome criteria applied in a blind fashion?
- Are these follow-up data likely to apply to my own patients?

A common problem with prognostic studies is lack of complete follow-up. As a rule of thumb, less than 5% dropout is ideal, and more than 20% makes the study of questionable validity. As with treatment trials, the applicability of the study will depend critically on the extent to which the patients in it resemble those whom the practitioner is considering.

Example

Question: How much of the time during long-term follow-up do patients with bipolar disorder experience affective symptomatology, and what is the pattern of symptoms?

Judd *et al.* (2002) recruited 146 patients with a diagnosis of bipolar disorder and a current episode of major mood disturbance from five tertiary care centres in the USA. They were followed up with interviews every 6 months for the first 5 years, and annually thereafter. At interview, affective symptoms were elicited using Psychiatric Status Rating Scales, which were linked to the Research Diagnostic Criteria (RDC). Affective symptoms that did not meet the criteria for RDC diagnosis were assigned to subsyndromal categories of depression or mania.

The mean follow-up period was 14.2 years, and 93% of the subjects were followed up for more than 2 years. Patients were symptomatically ill for about half of the time. Overall, about 90% of the patients spent 1 or more weeks during follow-up with depressive symptoms, and almost the same number (86%) experienced at least 1 week of manic or hypomanic symptoms. However, depressive symptoms during follow-up (32% of follow-up weeks) were about three times as common as manic or hypomanic symptoms (9.3%). Most of these depressive states were classified as subsyndromal depression or minor mood disorder rather than major depression. At least 1 week of mood cycling or mixed affective states was noted in about 48% of patients.

This study suggests that patients with bipolar disorder who are referred to a tertiary centre with an episode of major mood disturbance will have some symptoms of mood disturbance for about half of the time over the next few years. Overall, depressive symptoms predominate, particularly minor and subsyndromal depressive states. However, over time patients can experience considerable fluctuation in symptoms (both manic and depressive, or mixed). This study also has some aetiological implications, because it suggests that bipolar disorder and other milder depressive and hypomanic states are different expressions of the same underlying disorder. In terms of applicability, we would note that the patients in the study are tertiary referrals, so the findings might not apply, for example, to patients in primary care.

Qualitative research methods

Qualitative research methods are used to collect and analyse data that cannot be easily represented by numbers (see Brown and Lloyd, 2001). Although current evidence-based approaches in psychiatry have focused on the use of randomized controlled trials with quantitative endpoints, the use of qualitative approaches has a long history and encompasses, for example, the classificatory work of Kraepelin and the case studies of Freud. More modern case series, such as that of Russell (1979) describing bulimia nervosa, also rely on a qualitative approach.

The key differences between qualitative and quantitative research are summarized in Table 6.3.

When should qualitative methods be used?

There are a number of circumstances in which the application of qualitative methods is appropriate in psychiatric research and service development:

- In the initial stages of research, to conceptualize and clarify the relevant questions and to generate hypotheses.
- To gather and collate the attitudes, beliefs, and experiences of service users, carers, and professionals.
- In the development of assessment tools and rating scales.
- To examine the use of evidence-based interventions in practice and to understand problems with their implementation.

From this it can be seen that qualitative and quantitative approaches are not conflicting, but have particular uses in defined situations. For example, Rogers *et al.* (2003) combined a qualitative methodology with a quantitative randomized trial, which aimed to improve the management of antipsychotic medication in patients with schizophrenia. The qualitative study indicated that the trial participants did not readily recall the details of the interventions to which they had been exposed. On the other hand, they valued the opportunity provided by the trial for greater communication and contact with professionals. This was associated with greater feelings of self-efficacy and clinical improvement.

Evaluation of qualitative research

Like quantitative research, qualitative research needs to be relevant and valid. Similar general principles apply to the processes of participant selection, which should be clear and justified. It is important to be explicit about the reasons for choosing a qualitative approach, and to give a clear description of the methods of data collection and analysis. The *concept of permeability,* or the extent to which observations have influenced understanding, is important in qualitative research. The following factors influence study permeability:

- *The degree of engagement with the material.* How far were theories generated by direct contact (e.g. through interviews, naturalistic observation, and familiarity with textual sources)?
- *Iteration.* Did the investigators continually reformulate and re-examine their interpretations in the light of continuing observations?
- *Grounding.* Were the procedures for linking interpretations with observations clearly presented, and were illustrative examples given?

Table 6.3 **Key differences between quantitative and qualitative research**

	Quantitative research	Qualitative research
Fundamental aim	Objectivity, reliability, scientific truth	Understanding through personal encounter and observation; 'permeability'
Sampling	Random selection; designed to represent general population of subjects and avoid bias	'Purposive;' subjects chosen deliberately to possess characteristics relevant to study question
Data collection	Standardized, 'objective'; validated rating scales, biochemical endpoints, etc.	Observation and interview, often interactive and open-ended; systematic study of written material
Analysis of data	Quantitative, statistical, hypothesis testing	Narrative, generation of categories and themes; analysis occurs iteratively with data collection

● *Context.* Were the values and expectations of the investigator disclosed? Was the cultural context of the research and its meaning to the participants made explicit?

Validity

The concept of validity in qualitative research refers to the soundness and reasoning of interpretation, rather than comparison with an objective external criterion. Validity also differs according to role. For example, readers of a study will look for coherence and internal consistency of material, whereas participants must feel that their experiences are accurately described by the interpretations. Finally, the authors of the research need to take into account the effect that the research process itself might have on the data that they have collected ('*reflexivity*').

Assessment of qualitative research is not always straightforward, and the specialist terminology may defeat general readers. Brown and Lloyd (2001) have pointed out the lack of utility of evaluative checklists whose terminology is not readily understood by health service researchers. For a further discussion of the evaluation of qualitative research, see Greenhalgh (2010).

Evidence-based medicine in psychiatry

Practising according to evidence-based principles is an important aspect of modern psychiatry, and is followed as far as possible in this textbook. EBM is probably best viewed as an 'approach' whereby the key tasks for the practitioner are to formulate a relevant clinical question and then identify the best evidence with which to answer it. In addition, EBM provides an important means by which psychiatrists can work in a way that improves both consistency and quality of treatment. However, clinicians work with individual patients with particular needs in specific settings. Therefore EBM needs be tempered with the clinical skills that an expert practitioner brings to each clinical encounter.

Further reading

Greenhalgh T (2014). *How to Read a Paper*. Wiley Blackwell, Oxford. (A concise handbook that provides a clear exposition of the principles of EBM and their implementation.)

CHAPTER 7
Reactions to stressful experiences

Introduction

Stressful events frequently provoke psychiatric disorders. Such events can also provoke emotional reactions that are distressing, but not of the nature or severity required for the diagnosis of an anxiety disorder or a mood disorder. These less severe reactions are discussed in this chapter, together with post-traumatic stress disorder (PTSD), which is an intense and prolonged reaction to a severe stressor. With the exception of normal grief reactions, the conditions described in this chapter are listed as disorders in ICD-10 and DSM-5.

The chapter begins with a description of the various components of the response to stressful events, including coping strategies and mechanisms of defence. The classification of reactions to stressful experience is discussed next. The various syndromes are then described, including acute stress reactions, PTSD, special forms of response to severe stress, and adjustment disorders. The chapter ends with an account of special forms of adjustment reaction, including adjustment to bereavement (grief) and to terminal illness, and the problems of adults who have experienced sexual abuse in childhood.

The response to stressful events

The response to stressful events has three components:

1. An emotional response, with somatic accompaniments.
2. A coping strategy.
3. A defence mechanism.

Coping strategies and *defence mechanisms* are overlapping concepts, but they originated from different schools of thought, and for this reason they are described separately in the following account. Individuals have to adapt to stresses, whether they are trying to make sense of specific one-off events, or facing ongoing difficulties that require a change of expectations. The process of coming to terms with stresses is often referred to as 'working through' them. This term originated in psychoanalysis to designate the subconscious processing or 'work' that was necessary for change. It is now used to mean any coming to terms with emotional difficulties that involves reflection and re-evaluation.

Emotional and somatic responses

These responses are of two kinds:

1. *Anxiety* responses, with autonomic arousal leading to apprehension, irritability, tachycardia, increased muscle tension, and dry mouth.
2. *Depressive* responses, with pessimistic thinking and reduced physical activity.

Anxiety responses are generally associated with events that pose a *threat*, whereas depressive responses are usually associated with events that involve separation or *loss*. These features of these responses are similar to, but less intense than, the symptoms of anxiety and depressive disorders (described in Chapters 8 and 9, respectively).

Coping strategies

Coping strategies serve to reduce the impact of stressful events, thus attenuating the emotional and somatic responses and making it more possible to maintain normal performance at the time (although not always in the longer term; see below). The term *coping strategy* is derived from research in social psychology; it is applied to activities of which the person is aware—for example, deliberately avoiding further stressors. (Responses of which the person is unaware are called *defence mechanisms*; see below.)

Coping strategies are of two kinds: *problem-solving strategies*, which can be used to make adverse circumstances less stressful; and *emotion-reducing strategies*, which alleviate the emotional response to the stressors.

Problem-solving strategies include:

- *Obtaining information or advice* that would help to solve the problem.
- *Solving problems*—making and implementing plans to deal with the problem.
- *Confrontation*—defending one's rights, and persuading other people to change their behaviour.

Emotion-reducing strategies include:

- *Ventilation of emotion*—talking to another person and expressing emotion.
- *Evaluation of the problem*—to assess what can be changed and try to change it (by problem-solving), and what cannot be changed and try to accept it.

- *Positive reappraisal of the problem*—recognizing that it has led to some good (e.g. that the loss of a job is an opportunity to find a more satisfying occupation).
- *Avoidance of the problem*—by refusing to think about it, avoiding people who are causing it, or avoiding reminders of it.

Coping strategies are generally useful for reducing the problem or lessening the emotional reaction to it. However, they are not always adaptive. For example, avoidance may not be adaptive in the early stages of physical illness, because it can lead to delay in seeking appropriate treatment. Therefore a person needs not only the ability to use coping strategies, but also the ability to judge which strategy should be used in particular circumstances.

Maladaptive coping strategies

These strategies reduce the emotional response to stressful circumstances in the short term, but lead to greater difficulties in the long term. Maladaptive coping strategies include the following:

- *Use of alcohol or unprescribed drugs* to reduce the emotional response or to reduce awareness of stressful circumstances.
- *Deliberate self-harm*, either by drug overdose or by self-injury. Some people gain relief from tension by cutting their skin with a sharp instrument to induce pain and draw blood. Others take overdoses to withdraw from the situation or to show their need for help.
- *Unrestrained display of feelings* can reduce tension, and in some societies such behaviour is sanctioned in particular circumstances (e.g. grieving). In other circumstances, such behaviour can damage relationships with people who would otherwise have been supportive.
- *Aggressive behaviour*—aggression provides immediate release of feelings of anger. In the longer term, it may increase the person's difficulties by damaging relationships.

Coping styles

When particular coping mechanisms are used repeatedly by the same person in different situations, they are said to constitute a coping style. Some people change their coping strategies according to the circumstances—for example, they may use problem-solving strategies at work but employ avoidance when unwell. Some people habitually use maladaptive strategies—for example, they repeatedly abuse alcohol or take overdoses of drugs when under stress. More recent research has distinguished between *coping style*, which is seen as a relatively enduring behavioural trait, and *coping response*, which is much more specific to particular stressful environments.

Defence mechanisms

Defence mechanisms (see Box 7.1) are unconscious responses to external stressors as well as to anxiety arising from internal conflict. They were originally described by Sigmund Freud and later elaborated by his

---

Box 7.1 Defence mechanisms

Repression

This is the exclusion from consciousness of impulses, emotions, or memories that would otherwise cause distress. For example, especially painful aspects of the memory of distressing events such as sexual abuse in childhood may be kept out of full awareness for many years.

Denial

This is a related concept, which is inferred when a person behaves as if they are unaware of something that they may reasonably be expected to know. For example, on learning that they are dying of cancer, a patient may continue to live normally as if they are unaware of the diagnosis. In this example, denial is adaptive, as it can help to reduce depression. However, in the early stage of illness, denial may delay help-seeking or lead to refusal of necessary investigations and treatment. In this second example, denial is maladaptive.

Displacement

This is the transfer of emotion from a person, object, or situation with which it is properly associated, to another source. For example, after the recent death of his wife, a man may blame the doctor for failure to provide adequate care, and may thus avoid blaming himself for putting his work before his wife's needs during the last months of her life.

Projection

This is the attribution to another person of thoughts or feelings similar to one's own, thereby rendering one's own thoughts or feelings more acceptable. For example, a person who dislikes a colleague may attribute reciprocal feelings of dislike to him; it is then easier to justify his own feelings of dislike for the colleague.

Regression

This is the adoption of behaviour appropriate to an earlier stage of development—for example, dependence

on others. Regression often occurs among physically ill people. In the acute stages of illness it can be adaptive, enabling the person to acquiesce passively to intensive medical and nursing care. If regression persists into the stage of recovery and rehabilitation, it can be maladaptive because it reduces the patient's ability to make efforts to help themself.

Reaction formation

This is the unconscious adoption of behaviour that is the opposite to that which would reflect the person's true feelings and intentions. For example, excessively prudish attitudes to sex are sometimes (but not always) a reaction to the person's own sexual urges that they cannot accept.

Rationalization

This is the unconscious provision of a false but acceptable explanation for behaviour that has a less acceptable origin. For example, a husband may leave his wife at home because he does not enjoy her company, but he may reassure himself falsely that she is shy and would not enjoy going out.

Sublimation

This is the unconscious diversion of unacceptable impulses into more acceptable outlets—for example, turning the need to dominate others into the organization of good works for charity. (There are, of course, many other motives for charitable work.)

Identification

This is the unconscious adoption of the characteristics or activities of another person, often to reduce the pain of separation or loss. For example, a widow may undertake the same voluntary work that her husband used to do.

daughter, Anna Freud (1895–1982). Defence mechanisms are *unconscious processes* (i.e. people do not use them deliberately and are unaware of their own real motives, although they may become aware of these later through introspection or through another person's comments). Freud identified defence mechanisms in his study of the 'psychopathology of everyday life', a term that he applied to slips of the tongue and lapses of memory. The concept of defence mechanisms has proved useful in understanding many aspects of the day-to-day behaviour of people under stress, notably those with physical or psychiatric illness. Freud also used the concept of mechanisms of defence to explain the aetiology of mental disorders, but this extension of his original observations has not proved useful.

The main mechanisms of defence are described in Box 7.1

Present circumstances, previous experience, and response to stressful events

Brown and Harris (1978) showed that the response to a stressful life event is modified by present circumstances and by past experience. Some current circumstances make a person more vulnerable to stressful life events—for example, the lack of a confidant with whom to share problems. Such circumstances are called *vulnerability factors*. Previous experience can also increase vulnerability. For example, the experience of losing a parent in childhood may make a person more vulnerable in adult life to stressful events involving loss. It is difficult to examine these more remote associations scientifically.

Classification of reactions to stressful events

Although they are included within the classifications of diseases, not all reactions to stressful events are abnormal. Grief is a normal reaction to the stressful experience of bereavement, and only a minority of people have a very severe or abnormally prolonged reaction. There is also a normal pattern of reaction to a dangerous or traumatic event such as a car accident. Most people have an immediate feeling of great anxiety, are dazed and restless for a few hours afterwards, and then recover; a few people have more severe and prolonged symptoms—an abnormal reaction. It is difficult to decide where to draw the separation between normal and abnormal reactions to stressful events in terms of severity or duration, and in practice the division is arbitrary. Similarly, among patients who are in hospital for medical or surgical treatment, most are anxious but a few are severely anxious and show extreme denial or other defence mechanisms that impair cooperation with treatment.

ICD-10 and DSM-5 reactions to stressful experiences are classified into three groups (see Table 7.1).

Acute reactions to stress

This category is for immediate and brief responses to sudden intense stressors in a person who does not have another psychiatric disorder at the time. The ICD-10 definition of *acute stress reaction* requires that the response should start within 1 hour of exposure to the stressor,

and that it begins to diminish after not more than 48 hours, disappearing after a few days.

The DSM-5 definition of *acute stress disorder* states that the onset should occur while or after experiencing the distressing event, and requires that the condition lasts for at least 2 days and for no more than 4 weeks. It is important to recognize that the two definitions capture different phases of the anxiety response as the different terms, *reaction* and *disorder*, suggest. ICD-10 refers to the short-lived normal response, whereas DSM-5 refers to the more prolonged response, which is less common. Both diagnostic systems require that the stressor must be of an 'exceptional' nature and, in the case of DSM-5, that actual or threatened serious injury to self or others or sexual violation has occurred. DSM-5 also requires the presence of clinically significant distress, impairment in social or occupational spheres.

The order of the subgroups has been changed to show the similarities and differences between the two systems.

Post-traumatic stress disorder

This is a prolonged and abnormal response to exceptionally intense stressful circumstances such as a natural disaster or a sexual or other physical assault. It is described further below.

Table 7.1 Classification of reactions to stressful experience

ICD-10	DSM-5
Acute stress reaction	Acute stress disorder
Post-traumatic stress disorder	Post-traumatic stress disorder
Adjustment disorder	Adjustment disorder
• Brief depressive reaction	• With depressed mood
• Mixed anxiety and depressive reaction	• With mixed anxiety and depressed mood
• Predominant disturbance of other emotions	• With anxiety
• Predominant disturbance of conduct	• With disturbance of conduct
• Mixed disturbance of emotions and conduct	• With mixed disturbance of emotions and conduct
• Other specified symptoms	• Unspecified

Source: data from The ICD-10 classification of mental and behavioural disorders: clinical descriptions and diagnostic guidelines, Copyright (1992), World Health Organization; Diagnostic and Statistical Manual of Mental Disorders, Fifth Edition, Copyright (2013), American Psychiatric Association.

Adjustment disorder

This is a more gradual and prolonged response to stressful changes in a person's life. In both ICD-10 and DSM-5, adjustment disorders are subdivided, according to the predominant symptoms, into depressive, mixed anxiety, and depressive, with disturbance of conduct, and with mixed disturbance of emotions and conduct. DSM-5 has an additional category of 'adjustment disorder with anxiety'. ICD-10 has an additional category of 'predominant disturbance of other emotion', which includes not only adjustment disorder with anxiety, but also adjustment disorder with anger.

In ICD-10 the three types of reaction to stressful experience are classified together under 'reactions to stress and adjustment disorders', which is a subdivision of section F4, 'neurotic, stress-related and somatoform disorders'. The defining characteristics of this group of reactions to stress and of adjustment disorders are as follows:

• They arise as a *direct consequence* of either acute stress or continued unpleasant circumstances.

• It is judged that the disorder would not have arisen without these factors.

A similar organizing principle is used in DSM-5.
Adjustment disorder is described later in this chapter.

Additional codes in ICD-10

If any of these reactions is accompanied by an act of deliberate self-harm, another code can be added to record this fact (codes X60–X82 list 23 methods of self-harm). It is also possible to specify certain kinds of stressful event by adding a code from Chapter Z. For example, Z58 denotes problems related to employment and unemployment, and Z63 denotes problems related to family circumstances.

Coding grief reactions

In ICD-10, abnormal grief reactions are coded as adjustment disorders. Reactions to bereavement that are appropriate to the person's culture are not included. If it is appropriate to code them as part of the description of the patient's condition, code Z63.4 (death of a family member) can be used. DSM-5 also codes abnormal grief reactions under adjustment disorder. A more specific set of bereavement-related symptoms is called *persistent complex bereavement disorder*, which is coded under 'Other specified trauma and stressor-related disorder'. Persistent complex bereavement disorder is also listed under 'Conditions for further study'.

Acute stress reaction and acute stress disorder

Clinical picture

The *core symptoms* of an acute psychological response to stress are anxiety or depression. Anxiety is the response to threatening experiences, and depression is the response to loss. Anxiety and depression often occur together, because stressful events often combine danger and loss—an extreme example is a road accident in which a companion is killed. Other symptoms include feelings of being numb or dazed, difficulty in remembering the whole sequence of the traumatic event, insomnia, restlessness, poor concentration, and physical symptoms of autonomic arousal, especially sweating, palpitations, and tremor. Anger or histrionic behaviour may be part of the response. Occasionally there is a flight reaction—for example, when a driver runs away from the scene of a road accident.

Coping strategies and defence mechanisms are also part of the acute response to stressful events. Avoidance is the most frequent coping strategy, where the person avoids talking or thinking about the stressful events, and avoids reminders of them. The most frequent defence mechanism is denial.

Usually avoidance and denial recede as anxiety diminishes; memories of the events can be more readily accessed and the person is able to think or talk about them with less distress. This sequence allows the person to work through and come to terms with the stressful experience, although there may be continuing difficulty in recalling the details of highly stressful events.

Variations in the clinical picture

Not all responses to acute stress follow this orderly sequence, in which coping strategies and defences are maintained for long enough to allow the person to function until anxiety and depression subside, and are then abandoned so that working through can occur. Not all coping strategies are adaptive—an example is the excessive use of alcohol or drugs to reduce distress. Defence mechanisms may also be of a less adaptive type, such as regression or displacement. Sometimes defence mechanisms persist for longer than is adaptive—for example, denial may persist for so long that 'working through' is delayed. Sometimes vivid memories of the stressful events intrude into awareness as *images* and *flashbacks or disturbing dreams. Disassociation* with depersonalization and derealization can also occur.

Diagnostic conventions

As noted above, 'acute stress reaction' in ICD-10 and 'acute stress disorder' in DSM-5 capture different phases of the psychological response to stress. The DSM-5 definition refers to cases of more clinical importance, and it is widely used. The symptomatology of acute stress disorder emphasizes *disassociation and re-experiencing*. People who develop acute stress disorder are more likely to experience subsequent PTSD (indeed, the symptomatology of PTSD is similar to that of acute stress disorder, the main difference being in the timing and duration of symptoms). However, around 50% of those who

eventually develop PTSD after a trauma do not meet the criteria for acute stress disorder soon after it.

Both systems of classification describe typical symptoms of the disorder. In DSM-5 the diagnosis of acute stress disorder requires marked symptoms of anxiety or increased arousal, re-experiencing of the event, and three of the following five 'dissociative' symptoms:

- a sense of numbing or detachment
- reduced awareness of the surroundings ('being in a daze')
- derealization
- depersonalization
- dissociative amnesia.

There must also be avoidance of stimuli that arouse recollections of the trauma, and significant distress or impaired social functioning.

In ICD-10, dissociative and other symptoms are not required to diagnose the disorder in its mild form (F43.00), but two are required for the moderate form (F43.01) and four for the severe form (F43.02), from the following list of seven:

- withdrawal from expected social interaction
- narrowing of attention
- apparent disorientation
- anger and verbal aggression
- despair and hopelessness
- inappropriate or purposeless activity
- uncontrollable and excessive grief.

The terms *acute stress reaction* and *acute stress disorder* are used only when the person was free from these symptoms immediately before the impact of the stressful event. Otherwise the response is classified as an exacerbation of pre-existing psychiatric disorder.

Epidemiology

Rates in the general population are unclear. The rate of acute stress disorder has ranged from around 15% in motor accident survivors to over 50% in women victims of sexual assault. After the Wenchuan earthquake in China, about 30% of the survivors met criteria for acute stress disorder (Zhao *et al.*, 2008).

Aetiology

Many kinds of event can provoke an acute response to stress—for example, involvement in a significant but brief event (e.g. a motor accident or a fire), an event that involves actual or threatened injury (e.g. a physical assault or rape), or the sudden discovery of serious illness. Some of these stressful events involve life changes to which further adjustment is required (e.g. the serious injury of a close friend involved in the same accident). Not all people who are exposed to the same stressful situation develop the same degree of response. This variation suggests that differences in constitution, previous experience, and coping styles may play a part in aetiology. A history of psychiatric disorder and particularly of depression and disassociation prior to the trauma are predisposing factors. *Biological* and *psychological* investigations of the aetiology of acute stress disorder have suggested that similar mechanisms operate as those thought to be important in PTSD (see Ehlers *et al.*, 2009; see page 144).

Treatment

Planning for disaster

Planning is needed to ensure an immediate and appropriate response to the psychological effects of a major disaster. Such a response can be achieved by enrolling and training helpers who can support victims and are willing to be called on at short notice, and by agreeing procedures for contacting these helpers promptly. At the time of the disaster, priorities have to be decided between the needs of the victims of the disaster, those of relatives (including children), and those of members of the emergency services, who may be severely affected by their experiences. The essential elements of psychological assistance for victims of disaster have been described by Alexander (2005) (see Box 7.2).

Box 7.2 The principal components of psychological first aid

- Comfort and consolation
- Protection from further threat and distress
- Immediate physical care
- Helping reunion with loved ones
- Sharing the experience (but not forced)
- Linking survivors with sources of support
- Facilitating a sense of being in control
- Identifying those who need further help (triage)

Debriefing

After a major incident, counselling has often taken the form known as debriefing, or critical incident stress debriefing (CISD), provided either individually or in a group. In debriefing the victim goes through the following stages, after the counsellor has first explained the procedure:

- facts—the victim relates what happened
- thoughts—they describe their thoughts immediately after the incident
- feelings—they recall the emotions associated with the incident
- assessment—they take stock of their responses
- education—the counsellor offers information about stress responses and how to manage them.

Debriefing has been widely used, but current evidence suggests that single-session 'stand-alone' debriefing is not helpful in lowering subsequent psychological distress, and might even be harmful for some (Forneris *et al.*, 2013).

Management

After a traumatic event, many people talk informally to a sympathetic relative or friend, or to a member of the professional staff dealing with any physical injuries that originated during the incident. If anxiety is severe, an anxiolytic drug may be prescribed for a day or two, and if sleep is severely disrupted a hypnotic drug may be given for one or two nights. Since in most cases stress reactions will resolve with time, a policy of watchful waiting is appropriate, although it is good practice to offer a follow-up appointment around two weeks after the trauma to identify people whose symptoms are not settling and who are therefore at increased risk of developing the more long-term and disabling *PTSD*.

If patients show persistent and troublesome symptoms of acute stress disorder at this point, consideration should be given to treatments that may help prevent the onset of PTSD. Approaches of demonstrable efficacy involve verbal exposure to the original event and include *prolonged exposure therapy* (which aims to minimize continuing avoidance) and *trauma-focused cognitive behaviour therapy* (Howlett and Stein, 2016). These treatments are superior to less specific psychological approaches such as supportive counselling. Effective pharmacological treatments would have the advantage of easy implementation, but none are currently established and the use of SSRIs in acute stress disorder to prevent the development of PTSD has not generally proved helpful. On the other hand, research studies indicate that there may in future be a role for treatments that increase corticosteroid levels (Howlett and Stein, 2016).

Post-traumatic stress disorder

This term denotes an intense, prolonged, and sometimes delayed reaction to an intensely stressful event. The essential features of a post-traumatic stress reaction are as follows:

1. Re-experiencing of aspects of the stressful event.
2. Hyperarousal.
3. Avoidance of reminders.

Examples of extreme stressors that may cause this disorder are natural disasters such as floods and earthquakes, man-made calamities such as major fires and serious transport accidents, or the circumstances of war, and rape or serious physical assault on the person. The original concept of PTSD was of a reaction to such an extreme stressor that any person would be affected by it. Epidemiological studies have shown that not everyone who is exposed to the same extreme stressor develops PTSD; thus personal predisposition plays a part. In many disasters the victims suffer not only psychological distress but also physical injury, which may increase the likelihood of PTSD. Other predisposing factors are reviewed below in the section on aetiology.

The condition now known as PTSD has been recognized for many years, although under other names. The term PTSD originated during the study of American servicemen returning from the Vietnam War. The diagnosis meant that affected servicemen could be given medical and social help without being diagnosed as suffering from another psychiatric disorder. Similar psychological effects have been reported (under other names) among servicemen in both world wars, and among survivors of peacetime disasters such as the serious fire at the Coconut Grove nightclub in America in 1942. For a historical review of the concept of PTSD, see Jones and Wessely (2014).

Other reactions to severe stress

PTSD occurs only after exceptionally stressful events, but not every response to such events is PTSD. Six months after a serious accident, major depression may actually be more frequent than PTSD. ICD-10 has a category of 'Enduring personality changes after catastrophic experience' (see Box 7.3). This and other conditions may occur

instead of, but also as well as, PTSD. Also, PTSD is commonly comorbid with other psychiatric disorders, most notably depression, alcohol dependence, substance misuse, and anxiety disorders (Sareen, 2014).

Clinical picture of post-traumatic stress disorder

The clinical features of PTSD can be divided into three groups (see Box 7.4). The most characteristic and diagnostically important symptoms are related to *re-experiencing* (also called *intrusion*) and include flashbacks, recurrent nightmares, and intrusive images or other sensory impressions from the event. The second group of symptoms is concerned with *avoidance*, and includes difficulty in recalling stressful events at will, avoidance of reminders of the events, a feeling of detachment, and inability to feel emotion ('numbing'). The third group of symptoms is related to *hyperarousal*, and includes persistent anxiety, irritability, insomnia, and poor concentration.

Maladaptive coping responses may occur, including persistent aggressive behaviour, the excessive use of alcohol or drugs, and deliberate self-harm and suicide.

Other features

Depressive symptoms are common, and guilt and shame are often experienced by the survivors of a disaster. There can be diminished interest in activities and an inability to experience positive emotions. After some traumatic events, survivors feel forced into a painful reconsideration of their beliefs about the meaning and purpose of life. Some develop exaggeratedly negative views of the world as well as of themselves and others. Dissociative symptoms such as depersonalization are also prominent in some patients.

Onset and course

Symptoms of PTSD may begin very soon after the stressful event, or after an interval, usually of days, but usually within 3 months. It is now accepted, however, that a minority of cases of PTSD can have a delayed onset or, more accurately, that subthreshold symptoms may not develop to fulfil diagnostic criteria for PTSD for

> ## Box 7.3 ICD-10 criteria for 'Enduring personality changes after catastrophic experience'
>
> (A) At least two of the following:
> - a permanent hostile or distrustful attitude towards the world
> - social withdrawal
> - a constant feeling of emptiness or hopelessness
> - an enduring feeling of being on edge or being threatened without external cause
> - a permanent feeling of being changed or being different from others.
> (B) The change causes significant interference with personal or social functioning or significant distress.
> (C) The personality change developed after the catastrophic event, and the person did not have a personality disorder prior to the event that explains the current traits.
> (D) The personality change must have been present for at least 2 years, and is not related to episodes of any other mental disorder (other than PTSD) or to brain damage or disease.
>
> Source: data from The ICD-10 classification of mental and behavioural disorders: clinical descriptions and diagnostic guidelines, Copyright (1992), World Health Organization.

> ## Box 7.4 The principal symptoms of post-traumatic stress disorder
>
> **Hyperarousal**
> Persistent anxiety
> Irritability
> Insomnia
> Poor concentration
>
> **Re-experiencing**
> Intense intrusive imagery
> 'Flashbacks'
> Recurrent distressing dreams
>
> **Avoidance**
> Difficulty in recalling stressful events at will
> Avoidance of reminders of the events
> Detachment
> Inability to feel emotion ('numbness')
> Diminished interest in activities

many months or even years. In DSM-5, PTSD cannot be diagnosed until at least 1 month of symptomatology has elapsed; until then the condition is regarded as an acute stress disorder. However, in these circumstances it is doubtful whether the diagnosis of stress-related disorder and PTSD represents two separate conditions. About one-third of cases of PTSD remit within 3 months, but about 40% of patients have a chronic course (Santiago *et al.*, 2013).

Diagnosis

The diagnostic criteria in ICD-10 and DSM-5 are similar, although the latter are more prescriptive, with ICD-10 requiring only symptoms of *re-experiencing*, while numbing and avoidance, although often present, are not essential to make the diagnosis. In DSM-5, as well as *intrusive symptoms*, patients must also experience symptoms indicating *avoidance, arousal*, and *altered cognitions and mood*. By convention, PTSD can be diagnosed in people who have a history of psychiatric disorder before the stressful events.

Differential diagnoses include the following:

- Stress-induced exacerbations of previous anxiety or mood disorders.
- Acute stress disorder (distinguished by the time course).
- Adjustment disorders (distinguished by the different pattern of symptoms).
- Enduring personality changes after catastrophic experience.

PTSD may present as deliberate self-harm or substance misuse which have developed as maladaptive coping strategies (see page 136).

Prevalence

Estimates of PTSD in the general population have mainly been obtained from the USA, where lifetime rates (using older diagnostic criteria) have been between 6% and 9%. Rates in high-risk groups (for example, soldiers exposed to combat) can be much higher, up to 40% (Sareen, 2014).

Aetiology

The stressor

The necessary cause of PTSD is an exceptionally stressful event. It is not necessary that the person should have been harmed physically or threatened personally; those involved in other ways may develop the disorder—for example, the driver of a train in whose path someone has thrown himself for suicide, and the bystanders at a major accident. DSM-5 describes such events as involving actual or threatened death or serious injury or a threat to the physical integrity of the person or others. In a study of people affected by a volcanic eruption, the highest rate of PTSD was found among those who experienced the greatest exposure to the stressful events (Shore *et al.*, 1989). Even so, not all of those most affected by the stressor developed PTSD, a finding that indicates that some form of personal vulnerability plays a part. Such vulnerability might be genetic or acquired. Epidemiological research has revealed the following findings (Ehlers, 2009):

- The majority of people will experience at least one traumatic event in their lifetime.
- Intentional acts of interpersonal violence, in particular combat and sexual assault, are more likely to lead to PTSD than accidents or disasters.
- Men tend to experience more traumatic events in general than women, but women experience more events that are likely to lead to PTSD (e.g. childhood sexual abuse, rape, and domestic violence).
- Women are also more likely to develop PTSD in response to a traumatic event than men. This enhanced risk is not explained fully by differences in the type of traumatic event.

Genetic factors

Studies of twins suggest that differences in susceptibility to PTSD are in part genetic. True *et al.* (1993) studied 2224 monozygotic and 1818 dizygotic male twin pairs who had served in the US armed forces during the Vietnam War. After allowance had been made for the amount of exposure to combat, genetic variation accounted for about one-third of the variance in susceptibility to self-reported PTSD. Self-reported childhood and adolescent environment did not contribute substantially to this variance. The genetic liability to PTSD is partly explained by a genetic effect on *personality*, which modifies the propensity of individuals to engage in risky behaviours. However, even when allowing for genetic effects on personality, there is an additional genetic influence on the liability to experience PTSD after a given trauma. Several genome-wide association studies (GWAS) of PTSD have been carried out with the aim of identifying causative genes, but reliable findings have not yet emerged (Logue *et al.*, 2015).

Other predisposing factors

The individual factors that increase vulnerability to the development of PTSD have been summarized by Ahmed (2007). They include the following:

- personal history of mood and anxiety disorder
- previous history of trauma
- female gender
- neuroticism
- lower intelligence
- lack of social support.

Neurobiological correlates

Research to date on the neurobiology of PTSD has focused on monoamine neurotransmitters and the hypothalamic–pituitary–adrenal (HPA) axis, both of which are involved in mediating defensive responses to stressful events. In addition, brain imaging studies have implicated changes in the *hippocampus*, a brain region that is important in memory formation, and the *amygdala*, which plays a role in non-conscious emotional processing (see Box 7.5). These findings suggest that hippocampal dysfunction prevents adequate memory processing, while increased activity in noradrenergic innervation of the amygdala increases arousal and facilitates the automatic encoding and partial recall of traumatic memories. Functional imaging studies in PTSD suggest overactivity of the amygdala in the context of decreased regulatory control of the amygdala and other limbic regions by the ventromedial prefrontal cortex.

Psychological factors

Fear conditioning

Some patients with PTSD experience vivid memories of the traumatic events in response to sensory cues, such as smells and sounds related to the stressful situation. This finding suggests that classical conditioning may be involved, as well as failure to *extinguish* conditioned responses.

Cognitive theories

These suggest that PTSD arises when the normal processing of emotionally charged information is overwhelmed, so that memories persist in an unprocessed form in which they can intrude into conscious awareness. In

Box 7.5 Neurobiological abnormalities in PTSD

Hypothalamic–pituitary–adrenal axis

Evidence, albeit somewhat contradictory, for low plasma cortisol levels and increased sensitivity to dexamethasone suppression. Increased levels of corticotropin-releasing hormone in cerebrospinal fluid (CSF).

Noradrenaline

Increased sympathetic tone. Increased startle response. Increased levels of 3-methoxy-4-hydroxy-phenylglycol (MHPG) in CSF. Increased anxiety response to noradrenaline challenge. Decreased levels of neuropeptide Y at baseline and in response to noradrenaline challenge.

Brain imaging

Smaller volume of the hippocampus (which may be a vulnerability factor), overactivity of the amygdala in response to traumatic psychological stimuli, as well as decreased activity in anterior cingulate cortex and prefrontal cortex.

Source: data from Murray KE, Keifer OP, Ressler KJ, Norrholm SD, Jovanovic T, Neurobiology and treatment of PTSD, In: Charney DS, Buxbaum JD, Sklar P, Nestler EJ (Eds), Neurobiology of Mental Illness (4th edition), Copyright (2013), Oxford University Press.

support of this idea, patients with PTSD tend to have incomplete and disorganized recall of the traumatic events. Individual differences in response to the same traumatic events are explained as being because of differences in the appraisal of the trauma and of its effects. Similarly, differences in the appraisal of the early symptoms may explain why these symptoms persist for longer in some individuals. Negative interpretations of intrusive thoughts (e.g. 'I am going mad') after road accidents predict the continuing presence of PTSD after 1 year. The cognitive model of PTSD has been reviewed by Ehlers *et al.* (2012).

Psychodynamic theories

These emphasize the role of emotional development in determining individual variations in the response to severely stressful events. The general approach is plausible, and is supported by the fact that factors such as positive self-esteem, trust, and secure attachment increase resilience and decrease the risk of experiencing PTSD following trauma (see Ahmed, 2007).

Maintaining factors

As noted above, symptoms of PTSD may be maintained in part by negative appraisals of the early symptoms. Other suggested maintaining factors include avoidance of reminders of the traumatic situation (which prevents deconditioning and cognitive reappraisal), suppression of intrusive memories (which is known to make them more likely to recur), and rumination (Ehlers *et al.*, 2012).

Assessment

This should include enquiries about the nature and duration of symptoms, previous personality, and psychiatric history. When the traumatic events have included head injury (e.g. in an assault or transport accident), a neurological examination should be performed. Feelings of anger and thoughts of self-harm are common in PTSD, and an appropriate risk assessment needs to be carried out. Secondary complications such as substance misuse may require treatment in their own right (see Chapter 20).

Treatment

By the time patients with PTSD are assessed for treatment, the disorder may have been present for many months or even years, and comorbidity with depression and substance misuse often complicate management. Psychological treatments are generally preferred in the treatment of PTSD, although pharmacotherapy has a role in patients presenting with significant comorbid depression or where psychological approaches are not beneficial. Where alcohol or substance use disorders coexist with PTSD, it may be advisable to treat the substance misuse prior to offering psychological treatment for PTSD (National Institute for Health and Care Excellence, 2013). Psychological treatments such as *trauma-focused cognitive behaviour therapy* and *eye movement desensitization and reprocessing* are more effective than less specific treatments such as stress management, supportive therapy, and hypnotherapy (Ehlers, 2009). It should be noted that the majority of studies for treating PTSD have been conducted following 'single-episode' events and that those exposed to multiple traumatic events, such as those fleeing humanitarian disasters, conflict, and prolonged sexual abuse might need different treatments.

Cognitive behavioural treatment

Cognitive behaviour therapy is the most appropriate treatment. This treatment has several components:

- Information about the normal response to severe stress, and the importance of confronting situations and memories related to the traumatic events.
- Self-monitoring of symptoms.
- Exposure in imagination and then *in vivo* to situations that are being avoided.
- Recall of images of the traumatic events, to integrate these with the rest of the patient's experience. When first recalled these images are often fragmentary and are not clearly related in time to the other contents of memory.
- Cognitive restructuring through the discussion of evidence for and against the appraisals and assumptions.
- Anger management for people who still feel angry about the traumatic events and their causes.

A meta-analysis of psychotherapy studies of PTSD suggests that cognitive behavioural treatments have a therapeutic effect size of around 1.6 when compared with waitlist control, and around 1.0 when compared with relaxation and supportive therapies. An effect size of 1.0 corresponds to an improvement of one standard deviation on the relevant symptomatic measure, and effect sizes of this nature indicate a large treatment effect (see Chapter 6). At the end of psychological treatment, around 50% of patients no longer meet the criteria for PTSD, although many are still symptomatic to some degree. Although these results are encouraging, further work is required to show that similar benefit can be obtained in everyday clinical settings (Gerger *et al.*, 2014).

Eye movement desensitization and reprocessing was designed for the treatment of PTSD (see Chapter 24). Treatment trials using this technique in subjects with PTSD have shown similar effect sizes to those obtained with cognitive behaviour therapy, but the evidence base is not as large. Some have questioned whether the eye movements associated with this treatment add any specific therapeutic value to the element of exposure.

Narrative exposure therapy (NET) is a more recently developed treatment that aims to enhance autobiographical memory processing of the trauma by embedding it in a chronological life narrative developed collaboratively by patient and therapist. NET was developed originally for those suffering from PTSD following multiple traumatic events and was first trialled in refugee camps in low-income settings. It is a treatment that has been successfully delivered by lay therapists and it has been adapted for use in children (KIDNET). It is being increasingly used in high-income settings as well as low- and middle-income countries, and has a growing evidence-base. For a review see Robjant and Fazel, (2010).

Medication

Anxiolytic drugs such as benzodiazepines should be avoided in patients with established PTSD, because prolonged use may lead to dependence. A number of antidepressant drugs have shown efficacy in clinical trials, including selective serotonin reuptake inhibitors (SSRIs), serotonin and noradrenaline reuptake inhibitors (SNRIs), tricyclic antidepressants (TCAs), and monoamine oxidase inhibitors (MAOIs). There are also more preliminary data supporting the efficacy of mirtazapine, and augmentation with atypical antipsychotic drugs such as olanzapine may have a place in treatment-resistant patients, particularly those with marked sleep disturbance. The anticonvulsant drug topiramate also appears effective but on the basis of a fewer number of studies (National Institute for Health and Care Excellence, 2013).

Meta-analyses reviewed by the National Institute for Health and Care Excellence (2013) indicate that, in patients with PTSD, structured psychotherapies generally have higher effect sizes than drug treatment, and medication should not therefore be a first-line approach unless the patient expresses a preference for it or psychotherapy is not available or is ineffective (Box 7.6).

Response to special kinds of severe stress

Rape and physical assault

Victims of rape or other sexual or physical assault experience acute reactions to stress, PTSD, anxiety and depressive disorders, and psychosexual dysfunction. In one survey of 4000 women in Australia, just over a quarter reported exposure to one or more events of 'gender-based violence' (rape and sexual assault, intimate partner violence, or stalking). Following the trauma around 25% experienced PTSD, but rates for mood and anxiety disorders were even higher (34% and 38%, respectively). Substance use disorder was also common (29%) (Rees *et al.*, 2014).

As well as experiencing symptoms of PTSD, victims of rape and assault often feel humiliated, ashamed, and remain vulnerable to further attack. They lose confidence and self-esteem, question why they were chosen as victims, and blame themselves for putting themselves in unnecessary danger. To these problems are added issues of betrayal and secrecy when the assault is carried out by a family member or a friend. The victim may experience problems in trusting, persistent anger and irritability, and excessive dependence. These problems were first described among women victims of rape, but similar difficulties have been described among male victims of sexual assault (Peterson *et al.*, 2011).

Problems are more likely to persist when there has been an actual or perceived threat to life, previous psychological and social problems, past victimization, particularly abuse in childhood, past psychiatric illness or substance abuse, or a lack of social support (Adshead and Ferris, 2007).

Treatment

Social support is important in providing opportunities for the victim to talk over the problem and to regain self-esteem. Specific treatment for trauma-related symptoms is similar to that for other kinds of PTSD, including prolonged exposure by reliving the events in imagination, with additional emphasis on overcoming feelings of vulnerability and self-blame (Vickerman and Margolin, 2009).

Combatants

'Shell shock', 'battle fatigue', and 'war neurosis' were terms used during the First World War to describe psychological reactions to battle among British and American servicemen. Most of the reactions appear to resemble cases now diagnosed as PTSD; others seem to have resembled panic disorder or depressive disorders. Cases with panic attacks and concerns about the heart, now diagnosed as panic disorder, were known then as Da Costa's syndrome or disorderly action of the heart. Army psychiatrists were few in number, and were unable to deal with the many cases. Moreover, their experience of mental hospital work with severely ill patients did not equip them to treat these reactions to battle. Therefore patients with shell shock were treated mainly by neurologists or psychologists. W. H. Rivers, William Brown, and William McDougall were British psychologists who treated shell shock during the First World War, and used this experience to write influential books on medical psychology in the years after the war.

Treatment

At first, shell shock was treated with the methods in use at the time for neurasthenia, namely evacuation from the combat zone, rest, isolation, massage, and diet, but these methods had a low success rate. Hypnosis achieved some dramatic cures, but was not generally effective. Medical psychologists tried psychotherapeutic methods advocated by Freud, including the recall of stressful events to remove repression and the expression of associated emotion. Later, there was an increasing emphasis on early treatment, keeping the soldier with his colleagues at the front with the explicit aim of rapid return to action ('the soldier's interest and the army's interest are the same'). This approach has been termed *'forward psychiatry'* (Jones and Wessely, 2003). Psychotherapy was combined with military drill to maintain general fitness and morale. This combined treatment led to improved results. It became apparent that chronicity increased dramatically if soldiers were evacuated from the theatre of war.

These general principles of early treatment and maintenance of fitness and morale were widely adopted in the Second World War and in subsequent conflicts. Abreaction with anxiolytic drugs was used extensively in the Second World War. 'Forward psychiatry', with its emphasis on treatment in the combat zone together with an expectation of an early return to frontline duty, is now the approach adopted by most armies in the acute management of 'battle shock', although drug-induced abreaction is no longer employed. It has been claimed that, with this approach, about 70% of soldiers can be returned to duty. However, Jones and Wessely (2003) have cautioned that the proportion of soldiers treated in this way who are able to return to active combat may be much lower, and whether 'forward treatment' decreases the risk of subsequent trauma-related disorders is questionable.

Problems of refugees and victims of torture

Refugees and other forced migrants may have experienced a wide range of traumatic events, either in their countries of origin, in their journey to a place of potential refuge, and then in settling in a new location. The potential exposure to traumatic events can including the following:

- The impact of armed conflict directly on them and on their families and communities, usually through violence.
- Loss by death or separation of relatives and friends.
- Loss of home and possessions.

- Physical injury (including brain injury) either from the actions of war or from assault, rape, or torture, and the witnessing of violence to others.
- Experience of refugee camps or immigration detention facilities and threats by immigration authorities of being returned to their countries of origin.

Those involved may develop any of the reactions to stressful events, especially PTSD, depressive and anxiety disorders, and substance misuse. These conditions have been identified in refugees from many cultures, although the presenting complaints may differ somewhat in people from different cultures, with more emphasis on physical than on psychological symptoms among people from non-western countries. However, it is important to remember that stressors related to a refugee's current situation can be just as difficult to deal with as those that led to flight in the first place (see Box 7.7). In a systematic review, Fazel *et al.* (2005) estimated that, of refugees re-settled in western countries, about 10% met the diagnostic criteria for PTSD, 5% had major depression, and 4% had generalized anxiety disorder. In many individuals these disorders coexisted.

Treatment

Treatment should combine physical and psychiatric care. The latter should be introduced carefully, since it may be resisted as stigmatizing, not only by the refugee but also by humanitarian workers. Special care is needed to establish a trusting relationship. Practical help is often an essential preliminary to engagement. Many refugees have problems related to separation, bereavement, loss of material possessions, and immigration status, so it is important not to focus narrowly on PTSD.

Generally psychological treatments based on cognitive behaviour therapy approaches seem most beneficial for the treatment of PTSD and associated anxiety and depression in refugees (Nickerson *et al.*, 2011). In victims of torture it is helpful, if the patient agrees, to document the episodes of torture that they have experienced. As well as providing valuable information for purposes of advocacy and legal proceedings, the documentation can be developed into *testimonial therapy*, in which patients form a narrative of their experience which can be delivered to others, including their household (Duffy and Kelly, 2015).

Health beliefs and understanding of the 'normal' psychological response to stress may well differ between a health worker from one culture and a forced migrant

Box 7.7 Some stressful issues faced by refugees

Causes

War

Human rights abuses

Persecution on grounds of politics, religion, gender, or ethnicity

Refugee camps and immigration detention centres

Illegal methods of transportation and border crossings, often in the hands of people traffickers

Resultant losses

Country

Culture

Family

Profession

Language

Friends

Possessions

Plans for the future

Issues in country of asylum

Psychological and practical adjustment

Uncertain future

Traumatic life events

Social exclusion and poverty

Racism and bullying

Stereotyping by host country

Immigration policies

Immigration detention centres

Unknown cultural traditions

Reproduced from Advances in Psychiatric Treatment, 8(4), Tribe R, Mental Health of Refugees and Asylum Seekers, pp. 240–7, Copyright (2002), with permission from Royal College of Psychiatrists.

from another. Prior to psychological treatment, or where its use does not seem suitable, provision of language classes, informal support, and acquisition of computer skills can be very beneficial (Duffy and Kelly, 2015). In refugee children and adolescents, psychological interventions have been delivered in community, school, and camp settings with variable effects. The stongest positive effects are for group or individual exposure-based therapies, including trauma-focused cognitive behaviour therapy and narrative exposure therapy (Tyrer and Fazel, 2014).

Care is needed when working through interpreters, especially if these interpreters come from the same cultural group and occasionally from the group representing the 'other side' of the conflict. There are advantages and disadvantages in using family members as interpreters, but it is important to ensure that some therapeutic time is made available with a non-family, non-acquaintance performing the interpretation as the refugee is unlikely to speak of what they regard as shameful experiences in front of family members, community elders, or others they might perceive as likely to speak to people they know.

This point is especially important in situations in which women may have experienced sexual assaults, for these may bring shame on the whole family. Ideally, such problems should be dealt with by a female mental health professional who understands the patient's language and culture, but this may be difficult to arrange. If conducting exposure-based therapy, it is best to try and arrange for all the sessions to be conducted with the same interpreter, who might themselves need emotional support (especially if they have also come from an area of armed conflict).

For further information about the psychiatric problems of refugees and victims of torture, see Duffy and Kelly (2015).

Adjustment disorders

This term refers to the psychological reactions that arise in relation to adapting to new circumstances. Such circumstances include divorce and separation, a major change of work and abode (e.g. transition from school to university, or migration), and the birth of a handicapped child. Bereavement, the onset of a terminal illness, and sexual abuse are associated with special kinds of adjustment, which are discussed below.

Clinical features

The symptoms of an adjustment disorder include anxiety, worry, poor concentration, depression, and irritability, together with physical symptoms caused by autonomic arousal, such as palpitations and tremor. There may be outbursts of dramatic or aggressive behaviour, single or repeated episodes of deliberate self-harm, or the misuse of alcohol or drugs. The onset is more gradual than that of an acute reaction to stress, and the course is more prolonged. Social or occupational function is impaired. The *impairment in social or occupational function*, as well as the *intensity of distress*, is what distinguishes adjustment disorder from normal adaptive reactions.

Stressful life events may precipitate depression, anxiety, schizophrenia, and other psychiatric disorders. For this reason, the diagnosis of adjustment disorder is not made when diagnostic criteria for another psychiatric disorder are met. In practice, therefore, the diagnosis is usually made by excluding an anxiety or depressive disorder. A further requirement for diagnosis is that the disorder starts soon after the change of circumstances. Both ICD-10 and DSM-5 require that the disorder starts *within 3 months*, and ICD-10 indicates that it usually starts within 1 month. An essential point is that the reaction is understandably related to, and in proportion to, the stressful experience when account is taken of the patient's previous experiences and personality. Once the stressor or its consequences are removed, the symptoms resolve within 6 months.

Diagnostic conventions

As explained previously under 'Classification of reactions to stressful events', in ICD-10 adjustment disorders are divided into depressive reactions, mixed anxiety and depressive reactions, reactions with disturbance of other emotions, and reactions with disturbed conduct with or without emotional disturbance. DSM-5 lists six types of adjustment disorder (see Table 7.1).

Epidemiology

The prevalence of adjustment disorder in the community has been little studied. A community study in older people found that the prevalence of adjustment disorders was about 2% (Maercker *et al.*, 2008). It is presumed that in certain settings, such as the general hospital and primary care, prevalence rates are increased. For example, in studies of general hospital inpatients referred for psychiatric consultation, rates of adjustment disorder ranged from 11.5% to 21.5% (Strain *et al.*, 2009). High rates are also seen in people who make suicide attempts (see page 623).

Aetiology

Stressful circumstances are the necessary cause of an adjustment disorder, but individual vulnerability is also important, because not all people who are exposed to the same stressful circumstances develop an adjustment disorder. The nature of this vulnerability is unknown; it seems to vary from one person to another, and may relate in part to previous life experiences.

Prognosis

Clinical experience suggests that most adjustment disorders last for several months, and a few persist for years if the stressor or its consequences cannot be removed. In a review of the literature, Strain *et al.* (2009) concluded that, while the prognosis for adjustment disorder in adults is usually good, the majority of adolescents with adjustment disorder develop psychiatric disorders in adult life. Persistence of adjustment disorder should lead to a review of diagnosis in case symptomatology for a formal anxiety or depressive disorder has developed. As noted above, adjustment disorders can be associated with suicidal ideation and behaviour. Therefore clinical assessments should include careful questioning about risk.

Treatment

Treatment is designed to help the patient to resolve the stressful problems if this is possible, and to aid the natural processes of adjustment. The latter is done by reducing denial and avoidance of the stressful events, encouraging problem-solving, and discouraging maladaptive coping responses. Anxiety can usually be reduced by encouraging the patient to talk about the problems and to express their feelings. Occasionally, an anxiolytic or hypnotic drug is needed for a few days.

Problem-solving counselling (see Chapter 24) encourages the patient to seek solutions to stressful problems, and to consider the advantages and disadvantages of various kinds of action. The patient is then helped to select and implement a course of action to solve the problem. If this action succeeds, another problem is considered. If the first attempt fails, another approach to the original problem is tried. If problems cannot be resolved, the patient is encouraged to come to terms with them. Maina *et al.* (2005) reported that, in patients with adjustment disorder, both brief dynamic and supportive psychotherapy were more effective than a waiting-list control. For a review of adjustment disorder, see Casey (2009).

Special kinds of adjustment

Adjustment to physical illness and handicap

Appraisal of illness

Adjustment to illness cannot be understood simply in terms of the facts about the disease and its objective consequences. Adjustment depends on the patient's beliefs about their disorder and its effects on their life—in other words, on their appraisal of their illness. This appraisal may be similar to that of the professionals who are treating them, or it may be very different because it is based on false information or on emotions rather than on facts, or influenced by cultural beliefs. The appraisal may be reinforced by members of the family who share the patient's views, or it may be contradicted by them, thus adding to the patient's distress. Two terms are much used in the discussions of adjustment to illness and handicap—*illness behaviour* and the *sick role*. These terms will be considered next.

Illness behaviour

Mechanic (1978) suggested the term *illness behaviour* to describe behaviour associated with adjustment to physical or mental disorder, whether adaptive or not. Illness behaviour includes consulting doctors, taking medicines, seeking help from relatives and friends, and giving up inappropriate activities. These behaviours are adaptive in the early stages of illness, but may become maladaptive if they persist into the stage of convalescence when the patient should be becoming independent. Illness behaviour results from the person's conviction that he is ill rather than from the objective presence of disease, and it may develop when no disease is present. Illness behaviour without disease is an important problem in general practice and, once firmly established, it is difficult to treat. The concept of illness behaviour overlaps with that of the sick role (described below), but the two are described separately because they have different origins.

The sick role

Society bestows a special role on people who are ill. The sociologist Talcott Parsons (1951) called this the *sick role*, which is made up of two privileges and two duties:

- exemption from certain social responsibilities
- the right to expect help and care from others

- the obligation to seek and cooperate with treatment
- the expectation of a desire to recover.

While the person is ill, the sick role is adaptive. If they continue in the sick role after the illness is over, recovery is delayed as they continue to avoid responsibilities and depend on others instead of becoming independent.

Adjustment to the onset of physical illness

When a person becomes physically ill, they may feel anxious, depressed, or angry. Usually this emotional reaction is transient, subsiding as the patient comes to terms with the new situation. As in other adjustment reactions, denial or minimization can protect the patient against overwhelming anxiety when the diagnosis is first known. Although helpful in this way, denial can be maladaptive—in the early stage of illness it may lead to delay in seeking help, and at a later stage it may lead to poor compliance with treatment. Other coping strategies can be divided into emotion-reducing and problem-solving groups. Coping strategies that reduce emotion are often appropriate in the early stages of illness, but should give way to problem-solving coping. Coping may fail when demands are very great or when coping resources are limited either in the long term, or as a temporary result of disease of, or trauma to, the brain.

Physical illness as a direct cause of psychiatric symptoms

As well as acting as a stressor, physical illness may induce psychiatric symptoms directly. Anxiety, depression, fatigue, weakness, weight loss, or abnormal behaviour may all be caused directly by physical disorders; common examples are listed in Chapter 22 Box 22.3). Similarly, sexual function may be impaired by physical illness or its treatment (Chapter 13). Any of these symptoms may be the reason for referral, and psychiatrists should always be alert for the possibility of undetected physical illness in their patients.

Psychiatric symptoms due to treatments for physical illness

Some drugs that are used in the treatment of physical illness may affect mood, behaviour, and consciousness. The drugs most likely to have these effects are listed in Chapter 22, Table 22.3).

Help for people who are adjusting to physical illness

Most people adjust well to physical illness, but when adjustment is slow and incomplete, psychological treatment may be needed. This treatment need not be complicated, and can usually be provided effectively by the general practitioner or the hospital doctors or nurses who are managing the physical illness. Generally, the psychiatrist has a role in treating only the more severe problems or in supporting the medical and nursing staff.

The first step is to identify patients who are adjusting badly (i.e. failing to cope). This is generally done by the professional staff who are managing the physical illness. They can do this most easily by looking out for patients who are progressing less well than would be expected on the basis of the severity of the disease. Mood disorders are a common cause of slow progress, but may be dismissed as normal responses to the problems of the illness. Screening questionnaires can be used to detect mood disorders among these patients, but the results should be checked at least by a brief interview, which should be conducted, if possible, in surroundings in which their replies will not be overheard. Generally, one or more members of the family should be interviewed to obtain information about the patient's previous adjustment to problems and illness, and to discover how the family views the illness.

Some patients require medication, but for many counselling (see Chapter 24) is more appropriate. Counselling requires a trusting relationship with the patient, and this in turn requires adequate time for the interviews. Counselling begins with an explanation of the nature of the illness and its treatment. The patient is then helped to accept the implication of the diagnosis, to adjust to the illness, and to give up any maladaptive behaviours, such as excessive dependence on others or denial of the need for treatment. Graded activities, motivational interviewing, and anger management may be useful in some cases. More structured psychological treatment in the form of cognitive behaviour therapy may also be useful (Halford and Brown, 2009).

If the reaction to physical illness is an anxiety or depressive condition, treatment appropriate to that disorder should be given (see Chapters 8 and 9). A large randomized trial of cancer patients with depression showed that, compared to treatment as usual, a collaborative intervention by cancer nurses, psychiatrists, and primary care physicians substantially improved depressive symptomatology as well as diminishing pain and fatigue over the following 6 months (Sharpe *et al.*, 2014).

Adjustment to terminal illness

Among patients referred to palliative care services symptoms of anxiety and depression are common. Particularly in the final days of life, cognitive impairment and delirium can complicate management. Determinants of emotional reactions include the patient's personality, and the amount and quality of support from family, friends, and carers. Understandably, emotional reactions are more common among young dying patients than among the elderly. Surveys indicate that loss of independence and dignity and the management of pain are major concerns (Clarke and Seymour, 2010).

Anxiety

Anxiety may be provoked by the prospect of severe pain, disfigurement, or incontinence, by fear of death, and by concerns about the future of the patient's family. Families and carers sometimes try to spare the patient anxiety by concealing the truth about the condition. Since most patients become aware of the diagnosis, attempts at concealment only serve to increase their fear of possible consequences of the disease, such as pain or incontinence.

Depression

Depression may be provoked by the prospect of separation from family and friends and the loss of valued activities. Changes in physical appearance caused by the illness, the effects of surgery, and the debilitating effects of radiotherapy are other causes of low mood.

Guilt and anger

Some patients experience guilt because they believe that they are making excessive demands on relatives or friends. Patients with religious beliefs may believe that illness is a punishment for previous wrongdoing; conversely, anger may be felt about the unjustness of impending death; this anger may be displaced on to doctors, nurses, and relatives, making care more difficult (see below).

Symptoms induced directly by illness or its treatment

Psychological symptoms may also be induced by the disease or by its treatment, and these may add to the patient's distress. There is a particularly strong association between dyspnoea and anxiety, and drugs may cause or add to delirium. The more frequent associations between disease and psychological symptoms are summarized in Box 22.3. The associations between drug treatment and psychological symptoms are summarized in Table 22.3.

Treatment

In the UK about 60% of deaths occur in hospitals and care homes, and less than 10% in specialist hospice care (Galappathie and Khan, 2016). Dying patients are usually helped to adjust by the staff who are managing the physical illness. Psychiatrists are called upon only when there are special problems (see below) or to assist with staff support and training.

The aims of treatment

Surveys have shown that patients believe the following factors are important in achieving a 'good death':

- managing symptoms
- avoiding prolongation of dying
- achieving a sense of control
- relieving burdens placed on the family
- the strengthening of relationships.

Advance directives can help achieve these aims by preparing for the end of life and communicating future wishes; this might be particularly helpful if there is subsequent loss of capacity (Detering *et al.*, 2010).

Kubler-Ross (1969) formulated an influential model which described five phases of psychological adjustment to death. The phases do not necessarily occur in the same sequence, and some of them may not occur at all, but they are a useful guide for professionals who are helping dying patients. They can be summarized as follows:

- denial and isolation
- anger
- partial acceptance ('bargaining for time')
- depression
- acceptance.

This model has been criticized as being rather mechanistic and failing to capture the complex and unique life experience that each patient and their family bring to the imminent prospect of death. A qualitative study of Danish hospice patients found that patients faced imminent death with sorrow for the separation to come from family and close friends, and concern for how loved ones would fare without them. However, they did not suffer undue anxiety and continued to take significant interest in the daily life of the hospice (Moestrup and Hansen, 2015).

Reducing symptoms

Adequate control of pain and breathlessness and the reduction of confusion due to delirium are particularly important. Anxiety and depression may diminish as pain and breathlessness are controlled. The causes of delirium are listed in Box 14.1. Among dying patients, important remediable causes are dehydration, the side effects of drugs, secondary infection, cardiac or respiratory failure, and hypercalcaemia.

Helping the patient to adjust

It is essential to establish a good relationship with the patient so that they can talk about their problems and ask questions. The nature of the illness should be explained honestly and in simple language. Sometimes doctors are apprehensive that such an explanation will increase the patient's distress. Although excessive detail given unsympathetically can have this effect, it is seldom difficult to decide how much to say about diagnosis and prognosis, provided that patients are allowed to lead the discussion, express their worries, and say what they want to know. If patients ask about the prognosis, they should be told the truth; evasive answers undermine trust in the carers. If a patient does not seem to wish to know the full extent of their problems, it is usually better to save this information until later. At an appropriate stage the patient should be told what can be done to make their remaining time as comfortable as possible.

While the whole account should be truthful, the amount that is disclosed on a single occasion should be judged by the patient's reactions and by their questions. If necessary, the doctor should be prepared to return for further discussion when the patient is ready to continue. It is important to bear in mind that most dying patients become aware of their prognosis whether or not they are told directly, because they infer the truth from the behaviour of those who are caring for them. They notice when answers to questions are evasive and when people avoid talking to them. Patients who are anxious, angry, or despairing need to be able to express these feelings and to discuss the ideas that induce them.

Informing the staff

All of the staff should be made aware of the information that has been given to the patient, otherwise conflicting advice and opinions may be offered. If all those involved know what has been said, they will feel more at ease when talking to the patient. Otherwise they will draw back from the patient, isolating them, and thereby increasing their difficulty in adjusting.

Informing and supporting the relatives

Relatives need to know what has been said to the patient so that they will feel less ill at ease when talking to them. They may need as much help as the patient. They may become anxious and depressed, and they may respond with guilt, anger, or denial. Such reactions make it difficult for them to communicate helpfully with the patient or the staff. Relatives need information, and opportunities to talk about their feelings and to prepare for the impending bereavement, otherwise the patient and their family may become increasingly distant and alienated. Patients might also need specific advice as to how to explain their illness to their children, as sensitively informing children of parental illness is usually to be encouraged.

Special services

In many hospitals, *specialist nurses* work with the family doctor and with the hospital staff who are caring for dying patients. These nurses are trained in the psychological as well as physical care of the dying. Such care is increasingly provided in *hospices*, where it is possible to provide close attention to the details of care that improve quality of life for the dying person. These hospices care for patients when home care is impractical, and provide periods of respite care to relieve those who are caring for the patient at home.

Referral to a psychiatrist

Referral to a psychiatrist is appropriate when psychiatric symptoms or behaviour disturbance are severe. The referrals are concerned with the assessment and management of:

- *Depressed patients*, to determine the cause and whether the patient requires medication or more structured psychotherapy.
- *Uncommunicative patients* who will not talk about the illness.
- *Uncooperative patients* who do not accept the social restrictions imposed by the illness, will not make appropriate plans, or will not take the necessary decisions.
- *Longstanding problems that are made worse by the illness* and that are related to personality or family conflicts.
- *Other symptoms:* although anxiety and delirium are common, these problems are more often dealt with appropriately by medical staff than referred to a psychiatrist; the exception is delirium with paranoid symptoms.

Management of depressive disorders

Depressive disorders may be caused by symptoms such as pain or breathlessness, and all such symptoms should be treated appropriately. Any drugs that can cause depression (see Table 22.3) should be reviewed and, if possible, given at a lower dose or replaced. Some symptoms of depressive disorder are difficult to evaluate in patients with advanced cancer, as weight loss, anorexia, insomnia, loss of interest, and fatigue may be caused by the physical illness. Early-morning wakening, extreme hopelessness, and self-blame are more reliable guides to diagnosis. Suicidal ideation should be assessed carefully. If counselling and improved medical management do not improve the low mood, antidepressant drugs should be prescribed with careful supervision. The starting dose should be small, and medication should be changed if necessary to find a compound that is well tolerated.

Liaison with medical and nursing staff

Liaison with medical and nursing staff is important. Often these staff can provide treatment when the psychiatrist has formulated a plan. For further information about end-of-life care, see Galappathie and Khan (2016) and Box 7.8.

Grief and adjustment to bereavement

Terminology

Although the words 'bereavement', 'mourning', and 'grief' are sometimes used interchangeably, they have separate meanings which incorporate distinctions that are useful in psychiatry.

- *Bereavement* is the loss through death of a loved person.
- *Grief* is the involuntary emotional and behavioural response to bereavement.
- *Mourning* is the voluntary expression of behaviours and rituals that are socially sanctioned responses to bereavement. These behaviours and rituals differ between societies and between religious groups both in their form and in their duration.

The systems of classification do not make these distinctions in consistent ways. In ICD-10, bereavement is coded appropriately as Z63.4—that is, as one of the 'factors influencing health status and contact with health services'. In DSM-5, however, while bereavement itself is not coded, '*persistent complex bereavement*' (a severe grief reaction that has persisted for at least 12 months) is listed

---

Box 7.8 Priorities for care of the dying person

1. The possibility that a person may die within the next few days or hours is recognized and communicated clearly, decisions made and actions taken in accordance with the person's needs and wishes, and these are regularly reviewed and decisions revised accordingly.

2. Sensitive communication takes place between staff and the dying person, and those identified as important to them.

3. The dying person, and those identified as important to them, are involved in decisions about treatment and care to the extent that the dying person wants.

4. The needs of families and others identified as important to dying person are actively explored, respected, and met as far as possible.

5. An individual plan of care, which includes food and drink, symptom control, and psychological, social, and spiritual support, is agreed, coordinated and delivered with compassion.

Source: data from Leadership Alliance for the Care of Dying People, Copyright (2014).

Box 7.9 Normal grief reaction

Stage 1: hours to days

Denial, disbelief
'Numbness'

Stage 2: weeks to 6 months

Sadness, weeping, waves of grief
Somatic symptoms of anxiety
Restlessness
Poor sleep
Diminished appetite
Guilt, blame of others
Experience of a presence
Illusions, vivid imagery
Hallucinations of the dead person's voice
Preoccupation with memories of the deceased
Social withdrawal

Stage 3: weeks to months

Experiences of grief diminish
Social activities resumed
Memories of good times

Symptoms may recur at anniversaries.

---

under 'Conditions for further study'—thus the term is used to denote the response to bereavement, rather than the event itself. ICD-10 codes grief under adjustment disorders, but uses the term 'grief reaction'. Mourning, which is a form of social behaviour, is not a disorder and, appropriately, is not listed in the index to either classification. In this chapter, the term *bereavement reaction* is used to denote all responses to bereavement, both normal and abnormal. Normal reactions are referred to as grief, while abnormal reactions include abnormal grief (also referred to as pathological or complex grief), depressive disorders, and adjustment disorders.

Grief

Grief is a continuous process, but for clarity can be described as having three stages (see Box 7.9).

The *first stage* lasts from a few hours to several days. There is denial, which is manifested as a lack of emotional response ('numbness'), often with a feeling of unreality, and incomplete acceptance that the death has taken place. The bereaved person may be restless, as if searching for the dead person.

The *second stage* usually lasts from a few weeks to about 6 months, but may be much longer. There may be extreme sadness, weeping, loneliness, and often overwhelming waves of yearning for the dead person. Anxiety is common; the bereaved person is anxious and restless, sleeps poorly, lacks appetite, and may experience panic attacks. Many bereaved people feel guilt that they failed to do enough for the deceased. Some feel anger and project their feelings of guilt, blaming doctors or others for failing to provide optimal care for the person who has died. Many bereaved individuals have a vivid experience of being in the presence of the dead person, and about one in ten experience brief hallucinations. The bereaved individual is preoccupied with memories of the dead person, sometimes in the form of intrusive images. Withdrawal from social relationships is frequent, and complaints of physical symptoms are common.

In the *third stage*, these symptoms subside and everyday activities are resumed. The bereaved person gradually comes to terms with the loss and recalls the good times shared with the deceased in the past. Often there is a temporary return of symptoms on the anniversary of the death.

Although these stages are a useful guideline, individual responses vary, and no one feature is universal.

Abnormal grief

Grief is considered to be abnormal if it is delayed or inhibited, or unusually intense and prolonged, when it is referred to as *complicated* or *pathological*. The usual criterion for delay is that the first stage of grief has not occurred by 2 weeks after the death. The criterion for abnormal duration is that the response lasts for more than 6 months. However, many people grieve for longer than this and judgement needs to be used as to whether feelings of grief are continuing to resolve albeit at a slow rate. In all forms of abnormal grief, persistent avoidance of situations and of other reminders of death are common.

Depression in the course of a grief reaction. Depressive symptoms are a frequent component of normal grief, and around 30% of bereaved people meet the criteria for a depressive disorder at some time during their grieving. Most of these depressive disorders resolve within 6 months, but about 20% persist for longer. It might be argued that, if about one-third of bereaved people meet the criteria for depressive disorder at some time, the threshold has been set too low. However, people who meet the criteria for a depressive disorder are more likely to have poor social adjustment, to visit doctors frequently, and to use alcohol. Also, they can respond to medications and psychotherapies employed in depression (Shear *et al.*, 2011). Therefore it is of practical value to use the criterion and to record the additional diagnosis of a depressive disorder in these cases.

If there is doubt whether depressive disorder should be recorded, particular attention should be paid to symptoms of retardation, global loss of self-esteem, and guilt (the latter clearly of greater intensity than the common regrets about omissions of care during the terminal illness), because these features are seldom present in uncomplicated grief. It is also important to assess whether *suicidal feelings* are present. In complicated grief, suicidal thinking usually concerns a wish to be united with the person who has died, whereas in depression the wish to be dead is associated with a pervasive sense of hopelessness (Shear *et al.*, 2011).

Complicated grief. Complicated grief occurs in about 7% of those bereaved (Simon, 2013). People with complicated grief have an intense and prolonged reaction to bereavement. This can include strong yearnings for the person who has died, together with the thought that life now lacks all purpose and meaning. There

is disbelief and anger about the death, and reminders of the loss are avoided or, conversely, persistently sought out to the detriment of other activities and relationships. Complicated grief is also associated with sleep disturbance, increased substance use, and impairment in work and social functioning (Shear *et al.*, 2011). Many of these features are captured in the DSM-5 category of *persistent complex bereavement,* although here the necessary duration of grief since the bereavement is 12 rather than 6 months.

Causes of abnormal grief

Abnormal grief is generally thought to be more likely to occur when:

- The death was sudden and unexpected.
- The bereaved person had a very close, or dependent, or ambivalent relationship with the deceased.
- The survivor is insecure, or has difficulty in expressing their feelings, or has suffered a previous psychiatric disorder.
- The survivor has to care for dependent children and so cannot show their grief easily.

Morbidity after bereavement

Several studies (reviewed by Stroebe *et al.*, 2007) have shown an increased rate of mortality among bereaved spouses and other close relatives, with the greatest increase being in the first 6 months after bereavement. Most studies report increased rates of death from heart disease, and some have reported increased rates of death from cancer, liver cirrhosis, suicide, and accidents. The reasons for these associations are uncertain, and are likely to be different for different conditions.

Management of grief

Grief is a normal response, and most people pass through it with the help of family, friends, spiritual advisers, and the rituals of mourning. In some western societies, many people may not have links with a religion, the rituals of mourning may be attenuated, and family may not be close at hand. For these and other reasons, family doctors have an important part to play in helping the bereaved. Psychiatrists may be asked to help people with abnormal grief.

Although bereaved people have some problems in common, they also have problems that are individual. For example, a young widow with small children will have many difficulties that are not shared by an elderly widow whose adult children can support her. A mother who is grieving for a stillborn child will have special problems (see page 157). When planning management it is important to take into account the individual circumstances of the patient, as well as the general guidelines outlined below.

Counselling

When counselling is appropriate, it is similar to counselling for other kinds of adjustment reaction. The bereaved person needs to talk about the loss, to express feelings of sadness, guilt, or anger, and to understand the normal course of grieving. It is helpful to forewarn a bereaved person about unusual experiences such as feeling as if the dead person is present, illusions, and hallucinations, otherwise these experiences may be alarming. Help may be needed to:

- accept that the loss is real
- work through the stages of grief
- adjust to life without the deceased.

The bereaved person may need help to progress from the first stage of denial of loss to the acceptance of reality. Viewing the dead body and putting away the dead person's belongings help this transition, and a bereaved person should be encouraged to perform these actions. Practical problems may need to be discussed, including funeral arrangements and financial difficulties. A young widow may need help with caring for young children, and in supporting them without inhibiting her own grief excessively. As time passes, the bereaved person should be encouraged to resume social contacts, to talk to other people about the loss, to remember happy and fulfilling experiences that were shared with the deceased, and to consider positive activities that the latter would have wanted survivors to undertake. For further information about grief counselling, see Clark (2004).

Parents who are grieving for a stillborn child need special help. Previous practice has been to advise physical contact with the stillborn baby, and this is something that many parents understandably desire. However, there is growing evidence that holding the body of the baby is associated with greater risk of adverse psychological outcomes, so current advice is that parents should not view or hold the body unless they particularly wish to do so (Turton *et al.*, 2009). Stillbirth increases the risk of subsequent relationship breakdown; lack of support by the partner at the time of the stillbirth and having held the stillborn infant increase this risk.

Medication

Drug treatment cannot remove the distress of normal grief, but it may be needed in specific circumstances. In the first stage of grief, a hypnotic or anxiolytic drug may be needed for a few days to restore sleep or to relieve any severe anxiety. In the second stage, antidepressant drugs may be beneficial if the criteria for depressive disorder are met, although such usage has not been widely evaluated in this special group. Antidepressant medication may also sometimes be helpful in the treatment of complicated grief but is best used in conjunction with a structured psychotherapy (see below; Simon, 2013).

Support groups

Support groups have been developed to help recently bereaved people, particularly young widows and widowers. One such organization in the UK is known as Cruse. By sharing their experience with others who have dealt successfully with bereavement, recently bereaved people can share their grief, obtain practical advice, and discuss ways of coping (Clark, 2004).

Psychotherapy

It is not practicable, nor is there evidence that it is helpful, to provide structured psychotherapies for most bereaved individuals. For abnormal grief, dynamic psychotherapy has a clear rationale and approach, but its effectiveness has not been formally evaluated. However, *complicated grief treatment (CGT)*, which combines aspects of cognitive behavioural therapy and interpersonal therapy, has been reported to be effective in the management of abnormal grief (Simon, 2013).

CGT emphasizes the development of a narrative about the loss, which includes the bereavement itself as well as the positive and negative aspects of life with the deceased. Psychoeducation about grief and its complications is supplemented with exposure to aspects of the bereavement that are being avoided. Cognitive restructuring to re-evaluate maladaptive thinking, for example, that grieving is the only way of honouring the deceased is also employed. Some of the techniques of CGT can be applied by non-specialists; for example, discussion of the bereavement and the previous relationship with the deceased as well as advice for the bereaved person not to avoid events such as family reunions which will bring about reminders of the person and the loss (Simon, 2013).

Long-term adjustment to sexual abuse in childhood

When sexually abused, children may experience anxiety, depression, and PTSD. These effects usually subside during childhood, but people who have been abused in childhood are more vulnerable than others to psychiatric disorder in adult life. Furthermore, sexual abuse in childhood may be followed by persistent low self-esteem and psychosexual difficulties, whether or not a psychiatric disorder develops.

Very occasionally, adults who were previously unaware that they had been sexually abused in childhood suddenly recall the abuse in a vivid and disturbing way. Sometimes this recall occurs spontaneously, often when the person has encountered a reminder of the events. It may also occur during counselling or psychotherapy, at a time when childhood experiences are being discussed. Some of these recollections may be confirmed by other evidence, but many are vigorously denied by the alleged abuser, who is often one of the parents. It has been suggested that many of these unconfirmed reports of abuse are not accurate memories, and that some have been induced by questions, suggestions, or interpretations from the therapists. This phenomenon has been termed false memory syndrome (Brewin, 2009).

Recovered memory and false memory

Many victims of sexual abuse, and of other severe stressful events, have partial amnesia for the most stressful parts of the experience, even though they have suffered no head injury that could lead to post-traumatic amnesia. Indeed, partial amnesia is part of the clinical picture of PTSD. However, complete amnesia is less frequent and, in the view of many psychiatrists, complete amnesia for repeated stressful events followed by their recall is improbable, especially when there is no supporting evidence for the events from another source. This doubt is increased by evidence that 'memories' of single non-abusive childhood events can be implanted by suggestion in about 25% of subjects (Wright *et al.*, 2006).

Evidence for the proposition that true memories can be inaccessible for many years and then be recovered comes mainly from clinical reports. These reports suggest that around 25–50% of people who report childhood sexual abuse describe long periods during which they did not remember the abuse. Furthermore, clinical studies have shown that around 20–60% of people who report childhood sexual abuse state that there were periods during their life when they could not remember that the abuse had taken place. In addition, some people have recovered memories of abuse prior to engaging in therapy, so the effect of suggestion could not have been an influence in these cases.

In the absence of conclusive evidence about the status of memories that are recovered during counselling or psychotherapy, the clinician carrying out these procedures should:

- take special care not to suggest memories of sexual abuse

- consider most carefully apparent recovered memories that arise for the first time in therapy before concluding that they are true memories of actual events.

The state of the current scientific evidence indicates that practitioners should keep an open mind about the possibility and likely frequency of recovered memories of sexual abuse and, of course, of other kinds of traumatic experience. For a review see Brewin (2009).

Epidemiology

Adults who report having experienced sexual abuse in childhood have higher rates of psychiatric disorder in adult life. It is not clear what proportion of children who were sexually abused in childhood go on to develop these disorders in adult life, but some appear to make a good adjustment. An important factor in this kind of resilience is the experience of at least some good quality relationships through childhood and adolescence (Collishaw *et al.*, 2007).

In a prospective study in Australia of over 2750 sexually abused children (80% female) followed for up to 40 years, Cutajar *et al.* (2010) found that 24% of the abused group subsequently had contact with mental health services, compared with 8% of controls. Relative to controls, victims of abuse had higher rates of several adult psychiatric disorders, notably PTSD, substance use disorders, and personality disorders; however, they were also at increased risk of mood and anxiety disorders, and psychosis. More severe sexual abuse and an older age of occurrence were significant predictors of adult psychiatric disorder.

Chen *et al.* (2014) studied over 6000 Han Chinese women with recurrent major depression and a similar number of unaffected controls. They found that any form of reported childhood sexual abuse produced a fourfold risk in the likelihood of experiencing recurrent depression, and the risk increased with the severity of the abuse. Abuse was also associated with suicidality, as well as feelings of guilt and worthlessness.

Aetiology

Childhood sexual abuse may be a direct cause of vulnerability to adult psychiatric disorder or it may be a marker of some other factor, such as disturbed relationships within the family, which is the real cause of the excess psychiatric disorder in adult life. It has become apparent, for example, that sexual abuse frequently coexists and is therefore highly correlated with other kinds of *childhood adversity*, such as other forms of *maltreatment* (physical abuse, emotional abuse, and neglect), *parental loss* (death and other kinds separation such as divorce), and *parental maladjustment* (violence, criminality, substance abuse, and parental mental illness) (Green *et al.*, 2010). Thus studies assessing a single form of childhood adversity on the risk of adult psychiatric disorder may overestimate the impact of that particular kind of adversity. More recent studies have employed measures of a range of childhood adversities followed by multivariate modelling to estimate the relative importance of different kinds of adversity and how far their effects on the risk of developing subsequent psychiatric disorders are additive rather than shared.

McLaughlin *et al.* (2012) studied a population of over 6000 adolescents in the United States and found that over half (58%) had experienced at least one kind of childhood adversity. Over half of these subjects (59%) experienced multiple forms of adversity. The most common childhood adversities were parental divorce (28%), criminality (26%), economic adversity (16%), and mental illness (15%). The reported rate of sexual abuse was 4%. Childhood adversity strongly increased the risk of developing childhood and adolescent psychiatric disorder, and the greatest effects were seen for the combination of *childhood maltreatment* and *parental maladjustment*. The effects of the various individual adversities on the risk of psychiatric disorders were not additive. However, childhood sexual abuse was one of the strongest individual risk factors for future mental illness. A similar finding was observed in a population survey of over 9000 adults (Green *et al.*, 2010).

In these studies different kinds of childhood adversity increase the risk of psychiatric disorder rather generally; that is, particular forms of adversity do not seem to predispose to specific psychiatric disorders. Also, it is still possible that childhood adversity is not strictly causal in the development of subsequent psychiatric illness, perhaps being a risk marker of another causal mechanism; for example, genetic influences on both the risk of parental maladjustment and psychiatric illness in offspring (McLaughlin *et al.*, 2012).

Treatment

The late effects of childhood sexual abuse have been treated with counselling, dynamic psychotherapy, cognitive therapy, and group treatments. The various methods have several common features.

- The general aim is to help the patient to understand the earlier experiences and the effects of these on their life to improve present adjustment.
- The therapeutic relationship is used to help the patient to feel trusted, understood, and respected, and to increase their self-esteem.
- The patient is allowed to set the pace at which they talk about the experience of being abused, otherwise they may be overwhelmed by an extreme emotional response to the memories of abuse, and withdraw from treatment.
- Present problems of adjustment are identified, especially any avoidance of problems and difficulties in expressing anger. Help is given to overcome these difficulties.
- Some patients need help with psychosexual problems.

The main difference between the dynamic and cognitive behavioural approaches is the greater emphasis given in the former to understanding the effects of the trauma on self-esteem and emotional expression, and the greater emphasis given in the latter to more precise specification of the ways in which current patterns of thinking affect present behaviour. In a meta-analysis of 44 studies, Taylor and Harvey (2010) found that many different psychological treatments, ranging from group analytic therapy to individual cognitive behaviour therapy, produced moderate benefits on a range of symptomatology in adults who had suffered sexual abuse in childhood. Generally the largest effect size was seen with cognitive behaviour therapy treatment, particularly for symptoms related to PTSD.

Further reading

Beck JG, Sloan DM (2012) *The Oxford Handbook of Traumatic Stress Disorders*. OUP, Oxford. (A comprehensive overview of traumatic stress disorders, ranging from diagnosis and aetiology to assessment and management.)

National Institute for Health and Clinical Excellence (2005). *Post-Traumatic Stress Disorder (PTSD): the management of PTSD in adults and children in primary and secondary care*. Clinical Guideline 26. National Institute for Health and Clinical Excellence, London. (A periodically updated comprehensive review, available at http://www.nice.org.uk.)

Parkes CM (2010). *Bereavement*. Penguin Books, London. (A comprehensive account of grief, written for the layman, but containing useful information for the professional.)

CHAPTER 8

Anxiety and obsessive–compulsive disorders

Terminology and classification

The symptom of anxiety is found in many disorders. In the anxiety disorders, it is the most severe and prominent symptom, and it is also prominent in the obsessional disorders, although these are characterized by their striking obsessional symptoms. In both ICD-10 and DSM-5 (unlike in DSM-IV), obsessive-compulsive disorder (OCD) is classified separately from anxiety disorder. However, for convenience, both types of disorder are covered in this chapter.

Anxiety disorders

Anxiety disorders are abnormal states in which the most striking features are mental and physical symptoms of anxiety, occurring in the absence of organic brain disease or another psychiatric disorder. The symptoms of anxiety are described in Chapter 1, and are listed for convenience in Box 8.1. Although all of the symptoms can occur in any of the anxiety disorders, there is a characteristic pattern in each disorder, which will be described later. The disorders share many features of their clinical picture and aetiology, but there are also differences:

- In generalized anxiety disorders, anxiety is continuous, although it may fluctuate in intensity.

- In phobic anxiety disorders, anxiety is intermittent, arising in particular circumstances.

- In panic disorder, anxiety is intermittent, but its occurrence is unrelated to any particular circumstances.

These differences (and some exceptions to these initial generalizations) will be explained further when the various types of anxiety disorders are described.

The development of ideas about anxiety disorders

Anxiety has long been recognized as a prominent symptom of many psychiatric disorders. Anxiety and

Box 8.1 Symptoms of anxiety

Psychological arousal

Fearful anticipation
Irritability
Sensitivity to noise
Restlessness
Poor concentration
Worrying thoughts

Autonomic arousal

Gastrointestinal
- Dry mouth
- Difficulty in swallowing
- Epigastric discomfort
- Excessive wind
- Frequent or loose motions

Respiratory
- Constriction in the chest
- Difficulty inhaling

Cardiovascular
- Palpitations
- Discomfort in the chest
- Awareness of missed beats

Genitourinary
- Frequent or urgent micturition
- Failure of erection
- Menstrual discomfort

Muscle tension

Tremor
Headache
Aching muscles

Hyperventilation

Dizziness
Tingling in the extremities
Feeling of breathlessness

Sleep disturbance

Insomnia
Night terror

depression often occur together and, until the last part of the nineteenth century, anxiety disorders were not classified separately from other mood disorders. It was Freud, in 1895, who first suggested that cases with mainly anxiety symptoms should be recognized as a separate entity under the name 'anxiety neurosis'.

Freud's original anxiety neurosis included patients with phobias and panic attacks, but subsequently he divided it into two groups. The first group, which retained the name *anxiety neurosis*, included cases with mainly psychological symptoms of anxiety. The second group, which Freud called *anxiety hysteria*, included cases with mainly physical symptoms of anxiety and with phobias. Thus anxiety hysteria included the cases we now diagnose as agoraphobia. Freud originally proposed that the causes of anxiety neurosis and anxiety hysteria were related to sexual conflicts, although he later accepted a rather wider range of causes. By the 1930s, most psychiatrists considered that a very wide range of stressful problems could cause anxiety neurosis.

Phobic disorders have been recognized since antiquity, but the first systematic medical study of these conditions was probably that of Le Camus in the eighteenth century. The early nineteenth-century classifications assigned phobias to the group of monomanias, which were disorders of thinking rather than of emotion. However, when Westphal first described agoraphobia in 1872, he emphasized the importance of anxiety in the condition. Later, in 1895, Freud divided phobias into two groups—common phobias, in which there was an exaggerated fear of something that is commonly feared (e.g. darkness or high places), and specific phobias, in which there was fear of situations not feared by healthy people (e.g. open spaces). As will be explained later, the term *specific phobia* now has a rather different meaning.

In the 1960s, the different responses of certain phobias to behavioural methods suggested a grouping into simple phobias, social phobia, and agoraphobia, and these groups were also found to differ in their age of onset. (Simple phobias generally begin in childhood, social phobia in adolescence, and agoraphobia in early adult life.) At about the same time, it was observed that, when phobias were accompanied by marked panic attacks, they responded poorly to behaviour therapy and better to imipramine (Klein, 1964). These cases were subsequently classified separately as panic disorder. This advance led to the present scheme of classification into generalized anxiety disorder (GAD), phobic anxiety disorder (simple, social, and agoraphobic), and panic disorder.

The relationship between OCDs and anxiety disorders has been and remains uncertain. Freud initially thought that phobias and obsessions were closely related. He later proposed that anxiety is the central problem in both conditions and that their characteristic symptoms (phobias and obsessions) resulted from different kinds of defence mechanisms against anxiety. Others considered that obsessional disorders were a separate group of neuroses of uncertain aetiology.

As explained above, the two major diagnostic systems no longer classify OCD with anxiety disorders—in DSM-5, OCDs are classified together with other 'obsessive–compulsive-related disorders', which include 'body dysmorphic disorder', 'hoarding disorder', 'trichotillomania', and 'excoriation (skin picking) disorder'. In ICD-10, OCDs have a separate place in the classification and are not grouped with any other conditions.

The classification of anxiety disorders

The classification of anxiety disorders in ICD-10 and DSM-5 is shown in Table 8.1. Although the two are broadly similar, there are two important differences:

- In ICD-10, anxiety disorders are divided into two named subgroups: (a) phobic anxiety disorder (F40); and (b) other anxiety disorder (F41), which includes panic disorder and GAD.
- ICD-10 contains a category of mixed anxiety–depressive disorder, but DSM-5 does not.

The epidemiology of the various anxiety disorders is considered under each condition. The 12-month prevalence rates from a meta-analysis of 85 European studies are shown in Table 8.2 to illustrate the relative frequency of the different disorders in population studies.

Table 8.1 Classification of anxiety disorders

ICD-10	DSM-5
Anxiety disorders	Anxiety disorders*
Phobic anxiety disorder	
Agoraphobia	Agoraphobia
Without panic disorder	
With panic disorder	
Social phobia	Social phobia
Specific phobia	Specific phobia
Other anxiety disorders	
Panic disorder	Panic disorder
Generalized anxiety disorder	Generalized anxiety disorder
Mixed anxiety and depressive disorder	–

* The order of presentation has been altered to facilitate comparison of the schemes.

Source: data from The ICD-10 classification of mental and behavioural disorders: clinical descriptions and diagnostic guidelines, Copyright (1992), World Health Organization; Diagnostic and Statistical Manual of Mental Disorders, Fifth Edition, Copyright (2013), American Psychiatric Association.

Table 8.2 Twelve-month prevalence rates of anxiety disorders and obsessive–compulsive disorder in population studies in the European Union

Diagnosis (DSM-IV)	12-month prevalence range (%)	Median (%)
Specific phobia	3.1–11.1	4.9
Social phobia	0.6–7.9	2.0
Panic disorder*	0.6–3.1	1.2
Generalized anxiety disorder	0.2–4.3	2.0
Agoraphobia†	0.1–3.1	1.2
Obsessive–compulsive disorder	0.1–2.3	0.7

Reproduced from Eur Neuropsychopharmacol., 21(9), Wittchen H U, Jacobi F, Rehm J, Gustavsson A, Svensson M, Jönsson B, Olesen J et al, The size and burden of mental disorders and other disorders of the brain in Europe 2010, pp. 655–679, Copyright (2011), with permission from Elsevier.

* With and without agoraphobia.
† Without panic disorder.

Generalized anxiety disorder

Clinical picture

The symptoms of GAD (see Box 8.2) are persistent and are not restricted to, or markedly increased in, any particular set of circumstances (in contrast to phobic anxiety disorders). All of the symptoms of anxiety (see Box 8.1) can occur in GAD, but there is a characteristic pattern, which consists of the following features:

- *Worry and apprehension* that are more prolonged than in healthy people. The worries are widespread and are not focused on a specific issue as they are in panic disorder (i.e. on having a panic attack), social phobia (i.e. on being embarrassed), or OCD (i.e. on contamination). The person feels that these widespread worries are difficult to control.

- *Psychological arousal*, which may be manifested as irritability, poor concentration, and/or sensitivity to noise. Some patients complain of poor memory, but this is because of poor concentration. If true memory impairment is found, a careful search should be made for a cause other than anxiety.

- *Autonomic overactivity*, which is most often experienced as sweating, palpitations, dry mouth, epigastric discomfort, and dizziness. However, patients may complain of any of the symptoms listed in Box 8.1. Some patients ask for help with any of these symptoms without mentioning spontaneously the psychological symptoms of anxiety.

- *Muscle tension*, which may be experienced as restlessness, trembling, inability to relax, headache (usually bilateral and frontal or occipital), and aching of the shoulders and back.

- *Hyperventilation*, which may lead to dizziness, tingling in the extremities and, paradoxically, a feeling of shortness of breath.

- *Sleep disturbances*, which include difficulty in falling asleep and persistent worrying thoughts. Sleep is often intermittent, unrefreshing, and accompanied by unpleasant dreams. Some patients have night terrors and wake suddenly feeling extremely anxious. Early-morning waking is not a feature of GAD, and its presence strongly suggests a depressive disorder.

- *Other features*, which include tiredness, depressive symptoms, obsessional symptoms, and depersonalization. These symptoms are never the most prominent feature of GAD. If they are prominent, another diagnosis should be considered (see the section on Differential diagnosis below).

Clinical signs

The face appears strained, the brow is furrowed, and the posture is tense. The person is restless and may tremble. The skin is pale, and sweating is common, especially from the hands, feet, and axillae. Being close to tears, which may at first suggest depression, reflects the generally apprehensive state.

> ### Box 8.2 **Symptoms of generalized anxiety disorder**
>
> Worry and apprehension
> Muscle tension[*]
> Autonomic overactivity[*]
> Psychological arousal[*]
> Sleep disturbance[*]
> Other features
> - Depression
> - Obsessions
> - Depersonalization
>
> [*] See Box 8.1.

Diagnostic conventions

There is no clear dividing line between GAD and normal anxiety. They differ both in the extent of the symptoms and in their duration. The diagnostic criteria for both extent and duration are arbitrary, and they differ in several ways between DSM-5 and ICD-10. With regard to *extent*, both DSM-5 and the research version of ICD-10 require the presence of a minimum number of symptoms from a list. However, the ICD-10 list contains 22 physical symptoms of anxiety, whereas there are only six such symptoms in the DSM-5 list. Furthermore, in DSM-5 but not in ICD-10, worry is a key symptom. DSM-5 requires that the symptoms cause clinically significant distress or problems in functioning in daily life.

With regard to *duration*, in DSM-5 and the research version of ICD-10, symptoms must have been present for 6 months. However, the ICD-10 criteria for clinical practice are more flexible—symptoms should have been present on 'most days for at least several weeks at a time, and usually several months'.

Comorbidity of anxiety symptoms

Anxiety and depression

The two classifications differ in their approach to cases that present with significant symptoms of both depressive disorder and generalized anxiety without meeting the full criteria for either condition considered separately. ICD-10 has a separate category for these cases, namely *mixed anxiety and depressive disorder*. These conditions are discussed further below (see page 183) and in Chapter 9. It is also important to note that depressive symptoms are commonly also present in diagnosed anxiety disorders, and that some patients with GAD also suffer from comorbid major depression (Baldwin *et al.*, 2014).

Generalized anxiety disorder and other anxiety disorders

ICD-10 and DSM-5 differ in the guidance that they give about the circumstances in which two diagnoses should be made.

- In ICD-10, GAD is not diagnosed if the symptoms fulfil the diagnostic criteria for phobic anxiety disorder, panic disorder, or OCD.
- In DSM-5, the emphasis that is placed on the worrying ideas in GAD makes it possible to diagnose GAD when those ideas are present even in the presence of symptoms of one of the other three anxiety diagnoses. When this convention is followed, comorbidity between GAD and other anxiety disorders is frequent (social phobia in 23% of cases of GAD, simple phobia in 21%, and panic disorder in 11%) (Tyrer and Baldwin, 2006).

Differential diagnosis

GAD has to be distinguished not only from other psychiatric disorders but also from certain physical conditions. Anxiety symptoms can occur in nearly all psychiatric disorders, but there are some in which particular diagnostic difficulties arise.

Depressive disorder

Anxiety is a common symptom in depressive disorder, and GAD often includes some depressive symptoms. The usual convention is that the diagnosis is decided on the basis of the severity of two kinds of symptom and the order in which they appeared. Information on these two points should be obtained, if possible, from a relative or other informant as well as from the patient. Whichever type of symptoms appeared first and is more severe is considered primary. An important diagnostic error is to misdiagnose the agitated type of severe depressive disorder as GAD. This mistake will seldom be made if anxious patients are asked routinely about symptoms of a depressive disorder, including depressive thinking and, when appropriate, suicidal ideas. Depressive disorders are often worst in the morning, and anxiety that is worst at this time suggests a depressive disorder. As noted above, in some patients a depressive disorder and GAD coexist and both diagnoses can be made.

Schizophrenia

People with schizophrenia sometimes complain of anxiety before the other symptoms are recognized. The chance of misdiagnosis can be reduced by asking anxious patients routinely what they think caused their symptoms. Schizophrenic patients may give an unusual reply, which leads to the discovery of previously unexpressed delusional ideas.

Dementia

Anxiety may be the first abnormality to be complained of by a person developing dementia. When this happens, the clinician may not detect an associated impairment of memory, or may dismiss it as the result of poor concentration. Therefore memory should be assessed in middle-aged or older patients who present with anxiety.

Substance misuse

Some people take drugs or alcohol to relieve anxiety. Patients who are dependent on drugs or alcohol sometimes believe that the symptoms of drug withdrawal are those of anxiety, and take anxiolytic or other drugs to control them. The clinician should be alert to this possibility, particularly when anxiety is severe on waking in the morning, which is the time when alcohol and drug withdrawal symptoms tend to occur. (Anxiety that is worst in the morning also suggests depressive disorder; see above.)

Physical illness

Some physical illnesses have symptoms that can be mistaken for those of an anxiety disorder. This possibility should be considered in all cases, but especially when there is no obvious psychological cause of anxiety, or there is no history of past anxiety. The following conditions are particularly important:

- In *thyrotoxicosis*, the patient may be irritable and restless, with tremor and tachycardia. Physical examination may reveal characteristic signs of thyrotoxicosis, such as an enlarged thyroid, atrial fibrillation, and exophthalmos. If there is any doubt, thyroid function tests should be arranged.
- *Phaeochromocytoma and hypoglycaemia* usually cause episodic symptoms, and are therefore more likely to mimic a phobic disorder or panic disorder. However, they should also be considered as a differential diagnosis of GAD. If there is any doubt, appropriate physical examination and laboratory tests should be carried out.

Anxiety secondary to the symptoms of physical illness

Sometimes the first complaint of a physically ill person is anxiety caused by worry that certain physical symptoms portend a serious illness. If the physical symptoms are non-specific, they may be mistakenly attributed to anxiety. Furthermore, some patients do not mention all of the physical symptoms unless questioned. This is particularly likely when the patient has a special reason to fear serious illness—for example, if a relative or friend died of cancer after developing similar symptoms. It is good practice to ask anxious patients with physical symptoms whether they know anyone who has had similar symptoms.

Generalized anxiety disorder that is mistaken for physical illness

When this happens, extensive investigations may be carried out, which increase the patient's anxiety. Although physical illness should be considered in every case, it is also important to remember the diversity of the anxiety symptoms. Palpitations, headache, frequency of micturition, and abdominal discomfort can all be the primary complaint of an anxious patient. Correct diagnosis requires systematic enquiries about other symptoms of GAD, and about the order in which the various symptoms appeared.

Epidemiology

Estimates of incidence and prevalence vary according to the diagnostic criteria used in the survey, and whether a clinical significance criterion is used. The Adult Psychiatric Morbidity Survey found a 12-month prevalence of 4.4% for GAD in England (McManus *et al.*, 2009), and a similar figure has been reported in US surveys, with rather lower prevalence figures in European countries (around 2%; Wittchen *et al.*, 2011). Rates in women are about twice as high as those in men. GAD is associated with several indices of social disadvantage, including lower household income and unemployment, as well as divorce and separation (McManus *et al.*, 2009). Rates of anxiety, as well as expressions of anxiety, vary across development, and the anxiety disorders *are the most common child mental disorders*, as discussed in Chapter 16.

Aetiology

In general terms, GAD appears to be caused by stressors acting on a personality that is predisposed to anxiety by a combination of genetic factors and environmental influences in childhood. However, evidence for the nature and importance of these causes is incomplete.

Stressful events

Clinical observations indicate that GADs often begin in relation to *stressful events*, and some become chronic when stressful problems persist. A study by Kendler *et al.*

(2003) showed that stressful life events characterized by loss increased the risk of both depression and GAD. However, life events characterized by 'danger' (where the full import of the event was yet to be realized) were more common in those who subsequently developed GAD.

Genetic causes

Early twin studies, such as that by Slater and Shields (1969), showed a higher concordance for anxiety disorder between monozygotic than dizygotic pairs, which suggests that the familial association has a genetic cause. However, the genes involved in the transmission of GAD appear to increase susceptibility to other anxiety conditions, such as panic disorder and agoraphobia, as well as to major depression. Overall, the findings suggest that genes play a significant although moderate role in the aetiology of GAD, but that the genes involved predispose to a range of anxiety and depressive disorders, rather than GAD specifically (Shimada-Sugimoto *et al.*, 2015).

Early experiences

Accounts given by anxious patients of their experience in childhood suggest that *early adverse experience* is a cause of GAD. These accounts have given rise to objective studies and to psychoanalytic theories.

Sociological studies. Brown and Harris (1993) studied the relationship between adverse experience in childhood and anxiety disorder in adult life in 404 working-class women living in an inner city. Adverse early experience was assessed from patients' accounts of parental indifference and of physical or sexual abuse. Women who reported early adversity had increased rates of GAD (and also of agoraphobia and depressive disorder, but not of simple phobia). Parenting styles characterized by *overprotection and lack of emotional warmth* may also be a risk factor for GAD, as well as for other anxiety and depressive disorders in offspring.

Psychoanalytic theories. Psychoanalytical theory proposes that anxiety arises from intrapsychic conflict when the ego is overwhelmed by excitation from any of the following three sources:

- the outside world (realistic anxiety);
- the instinctual levels of the id, including love, anger, and sex (neurotic anxiety);
- the superego (moral anxiety).

According to this theory, in GAD, anxiety is experienced directly unmodified by the defence mechanisms that are thought to be the basis of phobias or obsessions. The theory proposes that in GADs the ego is readily overwhelmed because it has been weakened by a development failure in childhood. Normally, children overcome this anxiety through secure relationships with loving parents. However, if they do not achieve this security, as adults they will be vulnerable to anxiety when experiencing separation or potentially threatening events. Thus both psychoanalytic ideas and objective studies suggest that good parenting can protect against anxiety by giving the child a secure emotional base from which to explore an uncertain world.

Cognitive behavioural theories

Conditioning theories propose that GAD arises when there is an inherited predisposition to excessive responsiveness of the autonomic nervous system, together with generalization of the responses through conditioning of anxiety to previously neutral stimuli. This theory has not been supported by a body of objective data.

Cognitive theory. Particular coping and cognitive styles may also predispose individuals to the development of GAD, although it is not always easy to distinguish predisposition from the abnormal cognitions that are seen in the illness itself. As noted above, it seems likely that people who lack a sense of control of events and of personal effectiveness, perhaps because of early life experiences, are more prone to anxiety disorders. Such individuals may also demonstrate trait-like cognitive biases in the form of increased attention to potentially threatening stimuli, overestimation of environmental threat, and enhanced memory of threatening material. This has been referred to as the *looming cognitive style*, which appears to be a general psychological vulnerability factor for a number of anxiety disorders (Reardon and Nathan, 2007).

More recent cognitive formulations have focused on the process of worry itself. It has been proposed that people who are predisposed to GAD use worry as a positive coping strategy for dealing with potential threats, whereby the individual cannot relax until they have examined all of the possible dangers and identified ways of dealing with them. However, this can lead to 'worry about worry', when a person comes to believe, for example, that worrying in this way, although necessary for them, is also uncontrollable and harmful. This 'meta-cognitive belief' may form a transition between excessive but normal worrying, and GAD (Wells, 2013).

Personality

Personality traits. Anxiety symptoms are associated with *neuroticism,* and twin studies have shown an overlap between the genetic factors related to neuroticism and those related to GAD (Hettema *et al.*, 2004).

Personality disorder. GAD occurs in people with anxious–avoidant personality disorders, but also in individuals with other personality disorders.

Neurobiological mechanisms

The neurobiological mechanisms involved in GAD are presumably those that mediate normal anxiety. The mechanisms are complex, involving several brain systems and several neurotransmitters. Studies in animals have indicated a key role for the *amygdala*, which receives sensory information both directly from the *thalamus* and from a longer pathway involving the *somatosensory cortex* and *anterior cingulate cortex. Cortical involvement* in anxiety is important because it indicates a role for cognitive processes in its expression. The *hippocampus* is also believed to have an important role in the regulation of anxiety, because it relates fearful memories to relevant present contexts. Breakdown of this mechanism could lead to an overgeneralization of fear in response to non-threatening stimuli (Cain *et al.*, 2013).

Animal experimental studies have led to an understanding of the regulation of anxiety in the brain by neurotransmitters and neuromodulators. *Noradrenergic neurons* that originate in the locus coeruleus increase arousal and anxiety, whereas *5-HT neurons* that arise in the raphe nuclei appear to have complex effects, and serve both to signal the presence of anxiety-producing stimuli in the environment and also to restrain the associated behavioural responses. *Gamma-aminobutyric acid (GABA) receptors*, which are widely distributed in the brain, are inhibitory and reduce anxiety, as do the associated benzodiazepine-binding sites. There is probably also an important role for *corticotropin-releasing hormone*, which increases anxiety-related behaviours and is found in high concentration in the amygdala. However, although pharmacological manipulation of 5-HT and GABA mechanisms can be helpful in the treatment of generalized anxiety, there is no firm evidence that changes in these neurotransmitters are fundamentally involved in the pathophysiology of the disorder (Garner *et al.*, 2009).

Functional imaging of the brain during the presentation of aversive stimuli (e.g. fearful faces) has shown inconsistent changes in amygdala reactivity in patients with GAD. There is more reliable evidence of altered activity in cortical regulatory regions such as the *ventrolateral prefrontal cortex* and altered connectivity between this region and the amygdala. This picture is probably best explained by attempts to regulate excessive emotional responses, and perhaps represents the neural expression of the tendency of patients with GAD to use *worry* as an emotional coping strategy (Goodkind *et al.*, 2013).

Prognosis

One of the DSM-5 criteria for GAD is that the symptoms should have been present for 6 months. One of the reasons for this cut-off is that anxiety disorders that last for longer than 6 months have a poor prognosis. Thus most clinical studies suggest that GAD is typically a *chronic condition* with low rates of remission over the short and medium term. Evaluation of the prognosis is complicated by the frequent comorbidity with other anxiety disorders and depression, which worsen the long-term outcome and accompanying burden of disability. In the Harvard–Brown Anxiety Research Program, which recruited patients from Boston hospitals, the mean age of onset of GAD was 21 years, although many patients had been unwell since their teenage years. The average duration of illness in this group was about 20 years and, despite treatment, the outcome over the next 3 years was relatively poor, with only one in four patients showing symptomatic remission from GAD (Yonkers *et al.*, 1996).

However, the participants in the above study were recruited from hospital services, and may not be representative of GAD in community settings. In a naturalistic study in the UK, Tyrer and colleagues (2004a) followed up patients with anxiety and depression identified in primary care and found that, 12 years later, 40% of those initially diagnosed with GAD had recovered, in the sense that they no longer met the criteria for any DSM-III psychiatric disorder. The remaining participants continued to be symptomatic, but in only 3% was GAD still the principal diagnosis. In the vast majority of patients, conditions such as dysthymia, major depression, and agoraphobia were now more prominent. This study confirms the chronic and fluctuating symptomatic course of GAD in many clinically identified patients.

Treatment

Self-help and psychoeducation

A variety of forms of *self-help* have been studied in patients with anxiety disorders, including GAD. Such approaches typically include written and electronic materials with information about the disorder, and practical exercises to carry out based on the principles of cognitive behaviour therapy. Typically self-help has minimal therapist input, but it is also possible for self-help for anxiety disorders to be guided by a trained practitioner *(guided self-help)*. Another form of educational treatment takes place in group form, so-called *group psychoeducation*, where one therapist works with up to a dozen clients in about six weekly sessions of interactive learning and shared experience. The evidence for the benefit of these forms of treatment is limited and the

effects, although superior to no treatment, appear to be modest. However, these approaches are useful as part of an initial stepped-care approach (National Institute for Health and Clinical Excellence, 2010).

Relaxation training

If practised regularly, *relaxation* appears to be able to reduce anxiety in less severe cases. However, many patients with such disorders do not practise the relaxation exercises regularly. Motivation may be improved if the training takes place in a group, and some people engage more with treatment when relaxation is taught as part of a programme of yoga exercises. A structured therapy, known as *applied relaxation*, does appear to be effective in lowering anxiety over 12–15 sessions guided by a trained therapist (Hoyer *et al.*, 2009). A critical element of this treatment is the application of learned relaxation skills to anxiety-provoking situations.

Cognitive behaviour therapy

This treatment combines relaxation with cognitive procedures designed to help patients to control worrying thoughts. The method is described In Chapter 24. Compared with treatment as usual, cognitive behaviour therapy produces quite substantial benefits in terms of symptom resolution, with relatively few dropouts. However, the outcome obtained with cognitive therapy does not appear to differ from that obtained with other kinds of psychological interventions, such as applied relaxation and non-directive counselling, and there are few data on longer-term outcomes (Cuijpers *et al.*, 2014a).

Medication

Anxiolytic drugs are described in Chapter 25. Here we are concerned with some specific points about their use in GADs. Medication can be used to bring symptoms under control quickly while the effects of psychological treatment are awaited. It can also be used when psychological treatment has failed. However, medication is often prescribed too readily and for too long. Before prescribing, it is appropriate to recall that, even though GAD is said to have a poor prognosis, in short-term studies of medication, pill placebo treatment in the context of the clinical care provided by a controlled trial is beneficial for a significant proportion of patients. For example, in a 12-week, placebo-controlled trial of escitalopram and paroxetine, just over 40% of patients responded to placebo, and around 30% reached remission (Baldwin *et al.*, 2006).

Short-term treatment. One of the *longer-acting ben- zodiazepines*, such as diazepam, is appropriate for the short-term treatment of GADs—for example, diazepam in a dose ranging from 5 mg twice-daily in mild cases to 10 mg three times daily in the most severe cases. Anxiolytic drugs should seldom be prescribed for more than 3 weeks, because of the risk of dependence when they are given for longer. *Buspirone* is similarly effective for short-term management of GAD and is less likely to cause dependency, but has a slower onset of action. *Beta- adrenergic antagonists* are sometimes used to control anx- iety associated with sympathetic stimulation. However, they are more often used for performance anxiety than for GAD. If one of these drugs is used, care should be taken to observe the contraindications to treatment, and the advice given in Chapter 25 and in the manufactur- er's literature.

Long-term treatment. Because GAD often requires lengthy treatment, for which benzodiazepines are unsuitable (see above), and is often *comorbid* with depres- sion and other anxiety disorders, treatment guidelines usually recommend *selective serotonin reuptake inhibitors (SSRIs)* as the initial choice (National Institute for Health and Clinical Excellence, 2010). *Serotonin and noradrena- line reuptake inhibitors (SNRIs)* such as duloxetine and venlafaxine are also effective, but are somewhat less well tolerated than SSRIs. The anticonvulsant *pregabalin* is also licensed for the treatment of GAD in the UK. It has a different side effect profile to SSRIs and SNRIs, and might therefore be useful in patients who cannot toler- ate the latter agents. Where patients with GAD respond to medication, the risk of relapse is substantially reduced if treatment is maintained for at least 6 months, and probably longer. For a review of the pharmacological treatment of GAD, see Baldwin *et al.* (2014).

Management

In primary care, many patients are seen in the early stage of an anxiety disorder before a formal diagnosis of GAD can be made. In these circumstances, simple steps such as education and self-help can be tried first. If anxiety is severe, a short course of a benzodiazepine can bring rapid relief. Psychiatrists are more likely to encounter established cases. The steps in the management of such patients can be summarized as follows:

- *What patients need to know.* It can be explained to patients that GAD is a common mental health problem where worries become excessive and out of control. This can make it hard to carry out usual

occupational and social activities. People with gen- eralized anxiety can also experience symptoms of tension and exhaustion and can feel physically very unwell. There are many effective psychological and drug treatments available and discussion with a health care practitioner will assist in finding the best approach for them. It might be helpful for a partner or member of the family to be given an explanation of the symptoms the patient is experiencing and how they can best help.

- *Check the diagnosis and comorbidity*, especially *depres- sive disorder, substance abuse*, or a *physical cause* such as thyrotoxicosis. If any of these are present, treat them appropriately.

- *Evaluate psychosocial maintaining factors* such as persis- tent social problems, relationship conflict, and con- cerns that physical symptoms of anxiety are evidence of serious physical disease.

- *Explain the evaluation and proposed treatment*, especially the origins of any physical symptoms of anxiety. Discuss the way in which the patient might describe the condition to employers, friends, and family. Self- help books reinforce the explanation and describe simple cognitive behavioural techniques that people can use on their own or as part of a wider plan of treatment.

Box 8.3 Stepped-care approach* for generalized anxiety disorder

1. Identification and assessment: education about GAD and treatment options; active monitoring.
2. Low-intensity psychological interventions: pure self- help and guided self-help, group psychoeducation.
3. Choice of a high-intensity psychological interven- tion (cognitive behaviour therapy or applied relaxa- tion) or a drug treatment.
4. Specialist treatment (complex drug and psycho- logical regimens): input from multiagency teams, crisis services, or day hospitals.

* Initiate treatment at Step 3 if the patient presents with more severe symptomatology and/or significant functional impairment.

Source: data from the National Institute for Health and Care Excellence, Generalised anxiety disorder and panic disorder in adults, Copyright (2010), National Institute for Health and Care Excellence.

- *Offer structured psychological treatments, such as cognitive behaviour therapy or applied relaxation.* For patients who do not respond to these initial approaches or who have significant functional disability, benefit can be obtained by using a structured treatment such as cognitive behaviour therapy administered by a trained therapist.
- *Consider the use of medication.* A short course of benzodiazepines may be prescribed to reduce high levels of anxiety initially, but should seldom be given for more than about 3 weeks. Where psychological treatment is not available or has failed, medication—usually with an SSRI initially—is appropriate. The main uses and side effects of medication should be discussed, as when using the same drugs in the treatment of depression (see Chapter 25).
- *Discuss the plan with the patient, the general practitioner, and the community team* and allocate tasks and responsibility appropriately. Plans should recognize that GAD is often a long-term problem.

A guideline from the National Institute for Health and Clinical Excellence (2010) describes a stepped-care approach to the treatment of GAD (see Box 8.3).

Phobic anxiety disorders

Phobic anxiety disorders have the same core symptoms as GAD, but these symptoms occur only in specific circumstances. In some phobic disorders these circumstances are few and the patient is free from anxiety for most of the time. In other phobic disorders many circumstances provoke anxiety, and consequently anxiety is more frequent, but even so there are some situations in which no anxiety is experienced. Two other features characterize phobic disorders. First, the person *avoids* circumstances that provoke anxiety and, secondly, they experience *anticipatory anxiety* when there is the prospect of encountering these circumstances. The circumstances that provoke anxiety can be grouped into *situations* (e.g. crowded places), '*objects*' (a term that includes living things such as spiders), and *natural phenomena* (e.g. thunder). For clinical purposes, three principal phobic syndromes are recognized—specific phobia, social phobia, and agoraphobia. These syndromes will be described next.

Classification of phobic disorders

In ICD-10 and DSM-5, phobic disorders are divided into specific phobia, social phobia, and agoraphobia. In ICD-10, agoraphobia can be diagnosed either as 'with panic disorder' or 'without panic disorder' under 'phobic anxiety disorders' while 'panic disorder' is listed separately under 'other anxiety disorders'. In DSM-5 panic disorder and agoraphobia are coded as two separate diagnoses. A patient who meets criteria for both panic disorder and agoraphobia has both diagnoses assigned.

Specific phobia

Clinical picture

A person with a specific phobia is inappropriately anxious in the presence of a particular object or situation. In the presence of that object or situation, the person experiences the symptoms of anxiety listed in Box 8.1. Anticipatory anxiety is common, and the person usually seeks to escape from and avoid the feared situation. Specific phobias can be characterized further by adding the name of the stimulus (e.g. spider phobia). In the past it was common to use terms such as arachnophobia (instead of spider phobia) or acrophobia (instead of phobia of heights), but this practice adds nothing of value to the use of the simpler names.

In DSM-5, five general types of specific phobia are recognized, which are concerned with:

- animals
- aspects of the natural environment
- blood, injection, medical care, and injury
- situations (for example, aeroplanes, lifts, enclosed spaces).
- other provoking agents (for example, fears of choking or vomiting).

The following specific phobias merit brief separate consideration.

Phobia of dental treatment

Around 5% of adults have a fear of dental treatment. These fears can become so severe that all dental treatment is avoided and serious caries develops. A meta-analysis of 38 studies of behavioural treatment found a significant reduction in fear, with, on average, 77% of treated individuals attending for dental treatment 4 years after the treatment (Kvale *et al.*, 2004).

Phobia of flying

Anxiety during aeroplane travel is common. A few people experience such intense anxiety that they are unable to travel in an aeroplane, and some seek treatment. This fear also occurs occasionally among pilots who have had an accident while flying. Desensitization treatment (see Chapter 24) is provided by some airlines, and self-help books are available. Virtual reality programmes have been used to replace actual and imagined exposure. Good results have been reported, but it is unclear whether the treatment needs to be supplemented with other psychological measures, such as psychoeducation (Da Costa *et al.*, 2008).

Phobia of blood and injury

In this phobia, the sight of blood or of an injury results in anxiety. However, the accompanying autonomic response differs from that in other phobic disorders. The initial tachycardia is followed by a vasovagal response, with bradycardia, pallor, dizziness, nausea, and sometimes fainting. It has been reported that individuals who have this kind of phobia are prone to develop neurally mediated syncope even without the specific blood injury stimulus. Treatment consists of exposure *in vivo* together with the use of muscular tension to help to prevent syncope (Ayala *et al.*, 2009).

Phobia of choking

People with this kind of phobia are intensely concerned that they will choke when attempting to swallow. They have an exaggerated gag reflex and feel intensely anxious when they attempt to swallow. The onset is either in childhood, or after choking on food in adulthood. Some of these individuals also fear dental treatment, while others avoid eating in public. Treatment consists of desensitization.

Phobia of illness

People with this phobia experience repeated fearful thoughts that they might have cancer, venereal disease, or some other serious illness. Unlike people with delusions, people with phobias of illness recognize that these thoughts are irrational, at least when the thoughts are not present. Moreover, they do not resist the thoughts in the way that obsessional thoughts are resisted. Such individuals may avoid hospitals, but the thoughts are not otherwise specific to situations. If the person is convinced that they have the disease, the condition is classified as hypochondriasis (see Chapter 22). If the thoughts

are recognized as irrational and are resisted, the condition is classified as OCD.

Epidemiology

Among adults, the lifetime prevalence of specific phobias has been estimated, using DSM-IV criteria, to be around 7% in men and 17% in women (Kessler *et al.*, 2005a). The age of onset of most specific phobias is in childhood. The onset of phobias of animals occurs at an average age of 7 years, blood phobia at around 8 years, and most situational phobias develop in the early twenties (Öst *et al.*, 2001).

Aetiology

Persistence of childhood fears

Most specific phobias in adulthood are a continuation of childhood phobias. Specific phobias are common in childhood (see Chapter 16). By the early teenage years most of these childhood fears will have been lost, but a few persist into adult life. Why they persist is not certain, except that the most severe phobias are likely to last the longest.

Genetic factors

In one study, 31% of first-degree relatives of people with specific phobia also had the condition (Fyer *et al.*, 1995). Genetic vulnerability may involve differences in the strength of fear conditioning, which has a heritability of around 40% (Hettema *et al.*, 2003). A study of over 1400 female twins indicated that phobias (specific phobias, social phobia, and agoraphobia) were highly comorbid, with heritabilities ranging from 40% to 60%. The study suggested two main genetic liability factors, one of which underpinned the risk of developing specific phobias while the other increased the risk of social phobia and agoraphobia but also weakly increased the risk of specific phobias (Czajkowski *et al.*, 2011).

Psychoanalytical theories

These theories suggest that phobias are not related to the obvious external stimulus, but to an internal source of anxiety. The internal source is excluded from consciousness by repression and attached to the external object by displacement. This theory is not supported by objective evidence.

Conditioning and cognitive theories

Conditioning theory suggests that specific phobias arise through association learning. A minority of specific phobias appear to begin in this way in adulthood, in relation to a highly stressful experience. For example, a phobia of horses may begin after a dangerous encounter with a bolting horse. Some specific phobias may be acquired by observational learning, as the child observes another person's fear responses and learns to fear the same stimuli. Cognitive factors are also involved in the maintenance of the fear, especially fearful anticipation of and selective attention to the phobic stimuli.

Prepared learning

This term refers to an innate predisposition to develop persistent fear responses to certain stimuli. Some young primates seem to be prepared to develop fears of snakes, but it is not certain whether the same process accounts for some of the specific phobias of human children.

Neural mechanisms

Functional imaging studies have revealed hyperactivity of the amygdala upon *presentation* of the feared stimulus, which appears to diminish with successful treatment. *Anticipation* of a phobic stimulus activates the anterior cingulate cortex and the insular cortex. Generally, imaging studies indicate that specific phobias are characterized by increased activation in the regions linked to emotional appraisal and fear (amygdala, insula, anterior cingulate), with a concomitant failure to recruit prefrontal regions such as ventromedial prefrontal cortex, that regulate limbic brain regions (Goodkind *et al.*, 2013).

Differential diagnosis

Diagnosis is seldom difficult. The possibility of an underlying depressive disorder should always be kept in mind, since some patients seek help for longstanding specific phobias when a depressive disorder makes them less able to tolerate their phobic symptoms. Obsessional disorders sometimes present with fear and avoidance of certain objects (e.g. knives). In such cases a systematic history and mental state examination will reveal the associated obsessional thoughts (e.g. thoughts of harming a person with a knife).

Prognosis

The prognosis of specific phobia in adulthood has not been studied systematically. Clinical experience suggests that specific phobias that originate in childhood continue for many years, whereas those that start after stressful events in adulthood have a better prognosis.

Treatment

The main treatment is the *exposure form of behaviour therapy* (see Chapter 24). With this treatment, the phobia is usually reduced considerably in intensity and so is the

social disability. However, it is unusual for the phobia to be lost altogether. The outcome depends importantly on repeated and prolonged exposure, and up to 25% of phobic patients decline exposure-based therapies. Some patients seek help soon before an important engagement that will be made difficult by the phobia. When this happens, a few doses of a benzodiazepine may be prescribed to relieve phobic anxiety until a treatment can be arranged.

Exposure usually takes place over several 1-hour sessions, but it can be carried out in a single very long and intensive session lasting for several hours. Virtual-reality exposure may also be of benefit (Da Costa *et al.*, 2008). In a meta-analysis of 33 studies, Wolitzky-Taylor *et al.* (2008) found that exposure-based treatments were superior to other kinds of therapy; for example, relaxation therapy. Exposure treatment *in vivo* outperformed other kinds of exposure therapy in the short term but not at follow-up. Exposure therapy seemed equally effective across the range of different specific phobias. A significant weakness of most studies was a failure to include dropouts from therapy in the analysis of results.

Although pharmacotherapy has not been regarded as useful in the treatment of specific phobias, there is some evidence that *D-cycloserine*, a partial agonist at the glutamate N-methyl-D-aspartate (NMDA) receptor, may be helpful in augmenting the effectiveness of exposure treatment of phobias (Rodrigues *et al.*, 2014). In animals, D-cycloserine facilitates fear extinction, and it is possible that a similar mechanism may be involved when D-cycloserine is combined with behaviour therapy in humans.

Social phobia

Clinical picture

In this disorder, inappropriate anxiety is experienced in social situations, in which the person feels observed by others and could be criticized by them. Socially phobic people attempt to avoid such situations. If they cannot avoid them, they try not to engage in them fully—for example, they avoid making conversation, or they sit in the place where they are least conspicuous. Even the prospect of encountering the situation may cause considerable anxiety, which is often misconstrued as shyness. Social phobia can be distinguished from shyness by the levels of personal distress and associated social and occupational impairment (Stein and Stein, 2008).

The *situations* in which social phobia occurs include restaurants, canteens, dinner parties, seminars, board meetings, and other places where the person feels observed by other people. Some patients become anxious in a wide range of social situations (*generalized social phobia*), whereas others are anxious only in specific situations, such as public speaking, writing in front of others, or playing a musical instrument in public. In DSM-5 'performance only' social phobia, anxiety is restricted to speaking or performing in public. (In DSM-5 the term 'social anxiety disorder' is preferred to 'social phobia'.)

People with social phobia may experience any of the anxiety *symptoms* listed in Box 8.2, but complaints of blushing and trembling are particularly frequent. Socially phobic people are often preoccupied with the idea of being observed critically, although they are aware that this idea is groundless.

The *cognitions* centre around a fear of being evaluated critically by others. These cognitions are described in more detail in the section on aetiology below.

Other problems. Some patients take alcohol to relieve the symptoms of anxiety, and alcohol misuse is more common in social phobia than in other phobias. Social phobia is also a predictor of alcohol misuse. Comorbid depressive disorders as well as other anxiety disorders are also common (Kessler *et al.*, 2005b).

Onset and development. The condition usually begins in the early teenage years. The first episode occurs in a public place, usually without an apparent reason. Subsequently, anxiety is felt in similar places, and the episodes become progressively more severe with increasing avoidance.

Diagnostic conventions

Table 8.3 shows, in summary form, the criteria for the diagnosis of social phobia in ICD-10 and DSM-5. The requirements are similar (although the original wordings differ more than the paraphrased versions in the table). In ICD-10 there is greater emphasis on symptoms of anxiety—two general symptoms of anxiety, and one of three symptoms associated with social phobia. DSM-5 has an additional criterion that symptoms must have been persistent, lasting for at least 6 months.

Differential diagnosis

Agoraphobia and panic disorder

The symptom of social phobia can occur in either of these disorders, in which case both diagnoses can be made, although it is generally more useful for the clinician to decide which syndrome should be given priority.

Generalized anxiety disorder and depressive disorder

Social phobia has to be distinguished from the former by establishing the situations in which anxiety occurs, and from the latter from the history and mental state examination.

Table 8.3 Abbreviated diagnostic criteria for social phobia in ICD-10 and DSM-5*

ICD-10	DSM-5
Marked fear or avoidance of being the focus of attention or of behaving in an embarrassing or humiliating way—manifested in social situation	Marked fear or avoidance of situations in which the person is exposed to unfamiliar people or to scrutiny, with fear of behaving in an embarrassing or humiliating way
Two symptoms of anxiety in the feared situations, plus at least one from blushing/shaking, fear of vomiting, and fear or urgency of micturition or defecation	Social situations almost always provoke anxiety or are avoided
Significant emotional distress, recognized as excessive or unreasonable	The fear is out of proportion to any actual threat posed by the social circumstances Interferes with functioning, or causes marked distress
Symptoms restricted to or predominate in feared situations or their contemplation	—
Not secondary to another disorder	Not secondary to another disorder Duration at least 6 months

* To facilitate comparison between the two sets of criteria, the wording has been paraphrased and the order of some items has been changed.
Source: data from The ICD-10 classification of mental and behavioural disorders: clinical descriptions and diagnostic guidelines, Copyright (1992), World Health Organization; Diagnostic and Statistical Manual of Mental Disorders, Fifth Edition, Copyright (2013), American Psychiatric Association.

Schizophrenia

Some patients with schizophrenia avoid social situations because they have persecutory delusions. However, when they are in the feared situation, people with social phobia may feel convinced by their ideas that they are being observed, when they are away from the situation they know that these ideas are false.

Body dysmorphic disorder

People with this disorder may avoid social situations, but the diagnosis is usually clear from the patient's account of the problem.

Avoidant personality disorder

Social phobia has to be distinguished from a personality characterized by lifelong shyness and lack of self-confidence. In principle, social phobia has a recognizable onset and a shorter history, but in practice the distinction may be difficult to make, as social phobia usually begins in adolescence and the exact onset may be difficult to recall. Many people have disorders that meet the criteria for both diagnoses (Blackmore *et al.*, 2009).

Inadequate social skills

This is a primary lack of social skills, with secondary anxiety. It is not a phobic disorder, but a type of behaviour that occurs in personality disorders, in schizophrenia, and among people of low intelligence. Its features include hesitant, dull, and inaudible diction, inappropriate use of facial expression and gesture, and failure to look at other people during conversation.

Normal shyness

Some people who have none of the above disorders are shy and feel ill at ease in company. As noted above, the diagnostic criteria for social phobia set a level of severity that is intended to exclude these individuals (Stein and Stein, 2008).

Epidemiology

The National Comorbidity Survey Replication reported a lifetime prevalence rate of social phobia in the community of around 12%. The rate is therefore not much lower than that of specific phobia. Social phobias are about equally frequent among the men and women who seek treatment, but in community surveys they are reported rather more frequently by women (Kessler *et al.*, 2005a, b). As noted above, social phobia is associated with depression and alcoholism.

Aetiology

Genetic factors

Genetic factors are suggested by the finding that social phobia is more common among the relatives of people with social phobia than in the general population, and the risk is greatest in first-degree relatives (about a four-fold increase in incidence), decreasing as the degree of relatedness diminishes. The concordance rate of social phobia in monozygotic twins (around 24%) is higher than that seen in dizygotic twins (around 15%) and *heritability* has been estimated to be around 55%, with shared (familial) environment making relatively little contribution. Avoidant personality disorder also appears more common in families of people affected by social phobia, suggesting that the two conditions may well have a shared genetic aetiology (Isomura *et al.*, 2015).

Conditioning

Most social phobias begin with a sudden episode of anxiety in circumstances similar to those which become the stimulus for the phobia, and it is possible that the subsequent development of phobic symptoms occurs partly through conditioning.

Cognitive factors

The principal *cognitive factor* in the aetiology of social phobia is an undue concern that other people will be critical of the person in social situations (often referred to as a *fear of negative evaluation*). This concern is accompanied by several other ways of thinking, including:

- excessively high standards for social performance
- negative beliefs about the self (e.g. 'I'm boring')
- excessive monitoring of one's own performance in social situations
- intrusive negative images of the self as supposedly seen by others.

People with social phobia often adopt *safety behaviours* (see Chapter 14), such as avoiding eye contact, which make it harder for them to interact normally. For a review of the cognitive model of social phobia, see Moscovitch (2009).

Neural mechanisms

Functional neuroimaging studies have found that patients with social phobia have increased *amygdala* responses to presentation of faces with expressions of negative affect. The *anticipation* of public speaking in individuals with social phobia produced activation in limbic and associated regions, including the *amygdala, hippocampus*, and *insula*, while activation of cortical regulatory areas such as the *prefrontal cortex* was diminished. The insula is thought to represent interoceptive cues, and increased insula activity in patients with social phobia may underpin the preoccupation of patients with bodily autonomic changes; for example, flushing and sweating (Goodkind *et al.*, 2013). Apart from the increased activation in the insula, the pattern of changes in social phobia is similar to that seen in simple phobias.

Course and prognosis

Social phobia has an early onset, usually in childhood or adolescence, and can persist over many years, sometimes even into old age. Only about 50% of people with the disorder seek treatment, usually after many years of symptoms (Pilling *et al.*, 2013).

Treatment

Psychological treatment

Cognitive behaviour therapy is the psychological treatment of choice for social phobia (for a description of this treatment, see Chapter 24). The original cognitive procedures were based on those used successfully to treat agoraphobia and panic disorder and, when added to exposure, did not greatly increase the benefit. A modified form of cognitive behaviour therapy appears to be more effective. This modified treatment is based on the particular cognitive abnormalities that are found in social phobia (see the section on Aetiology above), coupled with measures to reduce safety behaviours, and using video or audio feedback. Cognitive behaviour therapy can be given in a group format, but this may not be as effective as individual treatment (Pilling *et al.*, 2013).

Dynamic psychotherapy. There is limited evidence that dynamic psychotherapy given weekly over 6 months can improve symptoms of social phobia relative to a waitlist control (Pilling *et al.*, 2013). Clinical experience suggests that this treatment may help patients whose social phobia is associated with pre-existing problems in personal relationships. However, there have been no controlled trials to test this possibility.

Drug treatment

SSRIs. Treatment guidelines generally recommend SSRIs as the first choice of pharmacological treatment in the management of social phobia. All of the SSRIs, as well as venlafaxine (an SNRI), have been shown to be effective, although the data for fluoxetine are slightly less consistent. With any of these drugs, the onset of action may take up to 6 weeks. Medication is usually continued for at least 6 months, and often for longer, because the risk of relapse is high if medication is discontinued after an acute response (Baldwin *et al.*, 2014). When medication is reduced, this should be done slowly.

Other drugs. The monoamine oxidase inhibitor, *phenelzine*, is more effective in the treatment of social phobia than placebo. *Moclobemide*, the reversible inhibitor of monoamine oxidase, can also be prescribed, but reported response rates vary, and in some studies the drug was not more beneficial than placebo. Benzodiazepines are effective and can be used for short-term relief of symptoms, but should not be prescribed for long because of the risk of dependency (see Chapter 25). The main use of benzodiazepines is to help patients to cope with essential social commitments while waiting for another treatment to take effect. *Beta-adrenergic blockers* such as propranolol may achieve short-term control of tremor and palpitations, which can be the most handicapping symptoms of specific social phobias, such as performance anxiety among musicians. It is doubtful whether beta-adrenergic blockers are more generally effective in social phobia (Baldwin *et al.*, 2014). There are also positive controlled trials of the antidepressant *mirtazapine* and the anticonvulsants *pregabalin* and *gabapentin*. For a review of the pharmacological treatment of social phobia, see Baldwin *et al.* (2014).

Management

What patients need to know

Patients need to understand that, although constitutional factors may play a part, the extent and severity of their social anxiety are a result of adopting *maladaptive ways of thinking and behaving* when they are socially anxious. These patterns of thinking and behaviour can be reversed either with psychological treatment or with medication. Self-help books can inform patients and help them to use simple cognitive behavioural approaches while awaiting further help. It is important not to misuse alcohol or other substances to deal with the anxiety produced by social situations

The choice of treatment

Guidelines from the National Institute for Health and Care Excellence recommend *individual cognitive behaviour therapy* specifically developed for the treatment of social phobia as first-line treatment. If cognitive behaviour therapy is declined, a further psychological treatment should be offered; for example, an approach based on cognitive behaviour therapy principles applied using supported self-help. Psychodynamic psychotherapy treatment may be used as a third-line psychological option.

Medication

Medication should be reserved for patients who decline psychological treatment or where psychological treatment is ineffective or only partly effective. If medication is to be used, SSRI treatment with either escitalopram or sertraline is recommended, with venlafaxine being offered if SSRIs are not effective. Phenelzine or moclobemide can be employed as third-line drug choices (see Pilling *et al.*, 2013).

Agoraphobia

Clinical features

Agoraphobic patients are anxious when they are away from home, in crowds, or in situations that they cannot leave easily. They avoid these situations, feel anxious when anticipating them, and experience other symptoms. Each of these features will now be considered in turn.

Anxiety

The anxiety symptoms that are experienced by agoraphobic patients in the phobic situations are similar to those of other anxiety disorders (see Box 8.1), although two features are particularly important:

- panic attacks, whether in response to environmental stimuli or arising spontaneously
- anxious cognitions about fainting and loss of control.

Situations

Many situations provoke anxiety and avoidance. They seem at first to have little in common, but there are three common themes, namely *distance from home*, *crowding*, and *confinement*. The situations include buses and trains, shops and supermarkets, and places that cannot be left suddenly without attracting attention, such as the hairdresser's chair or a seat in the middle row of a theatre or cinema. As the condition progresses, the individual increasingly avoids these situations until in severe cases they may be more or less confined to their home. Apparent variations in this pattern are usually due to factors that reduce symptoms for a while. For example, most patients are less anxious when accompanied by a trusted companion, and some are helped by the presence of a child or pet dog. Such variability in anxiety may suggest erroneously that when symptoms are severe they are being exaggerated.

Anticipatory anxiety

This is common. In severe cases anticipatory anxiety appears hours before the person enters the feared situation, adding to their distress and sometimes suggesting that the anxiety is generalized rather than phobic.

Other symptoms

Depressive symptoms are common. Sometimes these are a consequence of the limitations to normal life caused by anxiety and avoidance, while in other cases they seem to be part of the disorder, as in other anxiety disorders. *Depersonalization* can also be severe.

Onset and course

The onset and course of agoraphobia differ in several ways from those of other phobic disorders.

Age of onset. In most cases the onset occurs in the early or mid-twenties, with a further period of high onset in the mid-thirties. In both cases this is later than the average ages of onset of simple phobias (childhood) and social phobias (mostly the teenage years).

Circumstances of onset. Typically the first episode occurs while the person is waiting for public transport or shopping in a crowded store. Suddenly they become extremely anxious without knowing why, feel faint, and experience palpitations. They rush away from the place and go home or to hospital, where they recover rapidly. When they enter the same or similar surroundings, they become anxious again and make another hurried escape. However, not all patients describe such an onset starting from an unexplained panic attack. It is unusual to discover any serious immediate stress that could account for the first panic attack, although some patients describe a background of serious problems (e.g. worry about a sick child), and in a few cases the symptoms begin soon after a physical illness or childbirth.

Subsequent course. The sequence of anxiety and avoidance recurs during the subsequent weeks and months, with panic attacks experienced in a growing number of places, and an increasing habit of avoidance develops. However, sometimes avoidance can occur without the development of panic attacks.

Effect on the family. As the condition progresses, agoraphobic patients become increasingly dependent on their partner and relatives for help with activities, such as shopping, that provoke anxiety. The consequent demands on the partner often lead to relationship difficulties. Alternatively, the partner may become over-involved in supporting the patient, and difficulties in relinquishing this role may complicate efforts at treatment.

Diagnostic conventions

Most, but not all, patients with agoraphobia have panic attacks, which may be situational or spontaneous, and many of these individuals meet the criteria for panic disorder as well as for agoraphobia. In ICD-10, conditions that meet both sets of criteria are diagnosed as agoraphobia (which is coded as with or without panic disorder. In this situation in DSM-5 both diagnoses of agoraphobia and panic disorder are given. Another difference is that the ICD-10 criteria require definitive anxiety symptoms (see Table 8.4). Whether agoraphobia should be seen as an independent disorder, separate from panic disorder, is disputed (Wittchen *et al.*, 2010). The criteria for the diagnosis of panic disorder in DSM-5 are discussed later in the chapter (see page 180).

Differential diagnosis

Social phobia

Some patients with agoraphobia feel anxious in social situations, and some people with social phobia avoid crowded buses and shops, where they feel under scrutiny. Detailed enquiry into the current pattern of avoidance and also the order in which the two sets of symptoms developed will usually decide the diagnosis.

Generalized anxiety disorder

When the agoraphobia is severe, anxiety may develop in so many situations that the condition resembles GAD.

In these cases, the history of development of the disorder will usually point to the correct diagnosis.

Panic disorder

Agoraphobia often includes panic attacks and patients may meet criteria for both disorders, as discussed above.

Depressive disorder

Agoraphobic symptoms can occur in a depressive disorder, and many agoraphobic patients have depressive symptoms. Enquiry about the order in which the symptoms developed will usually point to the correct diagnosis. Sometimes a depressive disorder develops in a person with longstanding agoraphobia, and it is important to identify such cases and treat the depressive disorder (see below).

Paranoid disorders

Occasionally a patient with paranoid delusions (arising in the early stages of schizophrenia or in a delusional disorder) avoids going out and meeting people in shops and other places. The true diagnosis is usually revealed by a thorough mental state examination, which generally uncovers delusions of persecution or of reference.

Epidemiology

A recent community investigation in Europe, using strict DSM-IV criteria, estimated a lifetime prevalence of agoraphobia without panic of 0.6%. However, minor

Table 8.4 Abbreviated diagnostic criteria for agoraphobia in ICD-10 and agoraphobia without panic in DSM-5*

ICD-10	DSM-5
Marked, consistent fear in or avoidance in at least two of the following situations—crowds, public places, travelling alone, and travel away from home	Marked fear or anxiety about two or more of five specific situations, namely: public transport; open spaces; enclosed places; in a crowd; away from home, by oneself
Significant distress caused by the avoidance, or the anxiety, recognized as excessive or unreasonable	These situations are avoided, or endured with distress because of thoughts that escape might be impossible, or that help would not be available in the event of incapacitating or embarrassing symptoms Being in the situations nearly always provokes anxiety
At least one symptom of autonomic arousal plus one other anxiety symptom in the feared situations	The anxiety is disproportionate to any actual danger the situation may pose
Symptoms restricted to, or predominate in, the feared situations or contemplation thereof	The fear, anxiety or avoidance is persistent, typically lasting six months or more. The fear, anxiety or avoidance causes clinically significant distress or functional impairment
Not the result of another disorder, or of cultural beliefs	Not accounted for by another disorder

* The criteria have been abbreviated and paraphrased, and the order has been changed to facilitate comparison of the two systems.
Source: data from The ICD-10 classification of mental and behavioural disorders: clinical descriptions and diagnostic guidelines, Copyright (1992), World Health Organization; Diagnostic and Statistical Manual of Mental Disorders, Fifth Edition, Copyright (2013), American Psychiatric Association.

variations in the diagnostic criteria increased the incidence to 3.4% (Wittchen *et al.*, 2010). In the United States a population study of over 9000 participants using DSM-IV criteria estimated the lifetime risk of agoraphobia to be 2.6% while the risk for panic disorder (with and without agoraphobia) was 5.2% (Kessler *et al.*, 2012). The risk in women for both disorders was two to three times higher than that in men. In clinical samples, agoraphobia without panic appears to be rare, but in the community it may well be more frequent.

Aetiology

Theories of the aetiology of agoraphobia have to explain both the initial anxiety attack and its spread and recurrence. These two problems will now be considered in turn.

Theories of onset

Agoraphobia begins with anxiety in a public place—generally, but not always, as a panic attack. There are three explanations for the initial anxiety.

- The *cognitive hypothesis* proposes that the anxiety attack develops because the person is unreasonably afraid of some aspect of the situation or of certain physical symptoms that are experienced in the situation (see the section on Panic disorder, below). Although such fears are expressed by people with established agoraphobia, it is not known whether they were present before the onset.

- *The biological theory* proposes that the initial anxiety attack results from chance environmental stimuli acting on an individual who is constitutionally predisposed to over-respond with anxiety. There is some evidence for a genetic component to this predisposition, in that relatives of probands with agoraphobia are at increased risk of experiencing an anxiety disorder themselves. There has been disagreement as to whether the liability to agoraphobia and panic might be transmitted separately. For example, a large family study found that parental agoraphobia without panic did not increase the risk of panic attacks or panic disorder in offspring. On the other hand, offspring of parents with panic disorder experienced an increased risk of panic disorder and panic with agoraphobia but not agoraphobia alone. This suggests that, while agoraphobia can occur as a *consequence* of panic disorder, agoraphobia without panic may be genetically transmitted as a separate condition (Knappe *et al.*, 2012).

- *The psychoanalytic theory* essentially proposes that the initial anxiety is caused by unconscious mental conflicts related to unacceptable sexual or aggressive impulses, which are triggered indirectly by the original situation. Although this theory has been widely held in the past, it has not been supported by independent evidence.

Theories of spread and maintenance

Learning theories. Conditioning could account for the association of anxiety with increasing numbers of situations, and avoidance learning could account for the subsequent avoidance of these situations. Although this explanation is plausible and is consistent with observations of learning in animals, there is no direct evidence to support it.

Personality. Agoraphobic patients are often described as dependent, and prone to avoiding rather than confronting problems. This dependency could have arisen from overprotection in childhood, which is reported more often by agoraphobic individuals than by controls. However, despite such retrospective reports, it is not certain that the dependency was present before the onset of the agoraphobia.

Family influences. Agoraphobia could be maintained by family problems, and clinical observation suggests that symptoms are sometimes prolonged by overprotective attitudes of other family members, but this feature is not found in all cases.

Prognosis

Although short-lived cases may be seen in general practice, agoraphobia that has lasted for 1 year generally remains for the next 5 years, and usually the illness runs a chronic course. Episodes of depression are common in the course of chronic agoraphobia, and clinical experience suggests that people are more likely to seek help during these episodes (Wittchen *et al.*, 2010).

Treatment

Much of the available treatment has been developed for panic disorder and for panic disorder with agoraphobia probably because, as noted above, patients with agoraphobia without panic are not common in clinical samples. There has been little systematic investigation of treatment for agoraphobia without panic (Baldwin *et al.*, 2014).

Psychological treatment

Exposure treatment was the first of the behavioural treatments for agoraphobia. It was shown to be effective, but more so when combined with anxiety management (see Chapter 24).

Cognitive behaviour therapy for panic and agoraphobia is described in Chapter 24. Clinical trials (reviewed under panic disorder) indicate that, in the short term, cognitive therapy is about as effective as medication, and that in the long term it is probably more effective.

Medication

The drug treatment of agoraphobia resembles that for panic, except that medication is usually combined with repeated practice in re-entering situations that are feared and avoided. This exposure may account for some of the observed change. Most studies of drug treatment include both agoraphobic and panic disorder patients, and it is difficult to separate the treatment response of the two disorders. The following account should be read in conjunction with the subsequent discussion of medication for panic disorder.

Anxiolytic drugs. Benzodiazepines may be used for a specific, short-term purpose such as helping a patient to undertake an important engagement before other treatment has taken effect. Anxiolytic drugs should not be prescribed for more than a few weeks because of the risk of dependence. Indeed, guidelines issued by the National Institute for Health and Clinical Excellence (2010) for panic disorder and agoraphobia suggest that benzodiazepines should not be used at all, because they may worsen the long-term outcome of the condition. However, in some countries, although seldom in the UK, the high-potency benzodiazepine, *alprazolam*, is used to treat agoraphobia with frequent panic attacks. Some authorities believe that short-term benzodiazepine treatment does have a role in panic disorder—for example, while the patient is being established on more suitable drug treatment. However, it is possible that benzodiazepines could impair the response to psychological treatments (National Institute for Health and Clinical Excellence, 2010).

Antidepressant drugs. As well as the obvious use to treat a concurrent depressive disorder, antidepressant drugs have a therapeutic effect in agoraphobic patients who are not depressed but who have frequent panic attacks. *Imipramine* was one of the first agents to be used in this way, but similar effects have been reported with *clomipramine*. The treatment regime is the same as that described for panic disorder. In addition, several *SSRIs* and *venlafaxine* have been shown to be effective in panic disorder with and without agoraphobia (Baldwin *et al.*, 2014). SSRIs are generally recommended as the most suitable first-line treatment because of their safety and tolerability relative to tricyclic antidepressants (National Institute for Health and Clinical Excellence, 2010). As with other drug treatments for anxiety, maintaining the medication for several months after a clinical response has been obtained significantly lowers relapse rates.

Management

What patients need to know

Patients with agoraphobia and those around them usually have difficulty in understanding the nature of agoraphobia, and may think of it as the result of lack of determination to overcome normal anxiety. A two-stage explanation, starting with the panic attacks, is generally helpful. *Panic attacks* can be likened to *false alarms* occurring in an oversensitive intruder-alarm system. They can occur in most people under stressful circumstances. The excessive sensitivity can be explained in terms of constitution or chronic stress, whichever fits the patient's history. *Avoidance* can be explained in terms of conditioning, with examples such as anxiety after falling from a bicycle or following a car accident. Partners, friends, and relatives can usually understand the principles of behaviour therapy, but may be unsympathetic to drug treatment and puzzled when antidepressants are prescribed for anxiety. In response the patient can say that the medication is to reduce the sensitivity of the 'alarm system', and explain that some antidepressant drugs can do this.

Patients also need to know that medication is only likely to be effective if accompanied by determined and persistent efforts to overcome avoidance. The therapist should explain how to do this, but must emphasize that the result will depend on the patient's own efforts. Self-help books are a useful source of information about the disorder and about the ways in which people with agoraphobia can help themselves.

Behavioural management

In early cases, the patient should be strongly encouraged to return to the situations that they are avoiding. The treatment of choice for established cases is probably a combination of exposure to phobic situations with cognitive therapy for panic attacks. If there is a waiting list for cognitive therapy, the referring clinicians should supervise exposure treatment. Several self-help manuals have been published which reduce the time that therapists need to spend in doing this.

Medication

Medication can be offered as a first treatment, especially when panic attacks are frequent and/or severe. However, it needs to be accompanied by repeated exposure to previously feared and avoided situations. In the UK, the medication is usually an antidepressant, generally an SSRI. Any medication that has proved beneficial should be discontinued only gradually.

Patients who have relapsed after drug treatment can be offered behaviour therapy, although no controlled trials have been carried out specifically with such individuals. Most patients improve, but few of them lose the symptoms completely following treatment. Relapse is common, and patients should be encouraged to seek further help at an early stage should relapse occur.

Panic disorder

Although the diagnosis of panic disorder did not appear in the nomenclature until 1980, similar cases have been described under a variety of names for more than a century. The central feature is the occurrence of *panic attacks*. These are sudden attacks of anxiety in which physical symptoms predominate, and they are accompanied by fear of a serious medical consequence such as a heart attack.

In the past, these symptoms have been variously referred to as irritable heart, Da Costa's syndrome, neurocirculatory asthenia, disorderly action of the heart, and effort syndrome. These early terms assumed that patients were correct in fearing a disorder of cardiac function. Some later authors suggested psychological causes, but it was not until the Second World War (when interest in the condition revived) that the cardiologist, Paul Wood (1907–1962) showed convincingly that the condition was a form of anxiety disorder. From then until 1980, patients with panic attacks were classified as having either generalized or phobic anxiety disorders.

In 1980, the authors of DSM-III introduced the new diagnostic category, *panic disorder*, which included patients whose panic attacks occurred with or without generalized anxiety, but excluded those whose panic attacks appeared in the course of agoraphobia. In DSM-IV, all patients with frequent panic attacks were classified as having panic disorder, whether or not they had agoraphobia. In DSM-5 agoraphobia and panic disorder are diagnosed separately and patients who have both conditions receive both diagnoses. Panic disorder is included in ICD-10, but when patients have concomitant agoraphobia they are diagnosed as suffering from agoraphobia with panic disorder.

Clinical features

The symptoms of a panic attack are listed in Box 8.4. Not every patient has all of these symptoms during the panic attack and, for a diagnosis of panic disorder, DSM-5 requires the presence of only four or more symptoms. The important features of panic attacks are that:

- anxiety builds up quickly
- the symptoms are severe
- the person fears a catastrophic outcome.

Some people with panic disorder hyperventilate, and this adds to their symptoms.

Hyperventilation is breathing in a rapid and shallow way that leads to a fall in the concentration of carbon dioxide in the blood. The resulting hypocapnia may cause the symptoms listed in Box 8.5. The last symptom in the list, the feeling of breathlessness, is paradoxical, as the person is breathing excessively. It is important because it leads to a further increase in breathing, which worsens the condition. Hyperventilation should always be borne in mind as a cause of unexplained bodily symptoms. The diagnosis can usually be made by watching the pattern of breathing when the symptoms are present.

Diagnostic criteria

In DSM-5 the diagnosis of panic disorder is made when: (1) panic attacks occur recurrently (at least twice) and unexpectedly (i.e. not in response to an identified phobic stimulus); and (2) at least one attack has been followed by 4 weeks or more of persistent fear of another attack and worry about its implications (e.g. having a heart attack), *and/or* a significant maladaptive change in behaviour (for example, avoiding exercise or public transport). The research criteria in ICD-10 are similar, except that those concerned with course are rather less

---

Box 8.4 Symptoms of a panic attack

Sudden onset of:
Palpitations
Choking sensations
Chest pain
Dizziness and faintness
Depersonalization
Derealization
Fear of dying, losing control, or going mad

Source: data from The ICD-10 classification of mental and behavioural disorders: clinical descriptions and diagnostic guidelines, Copyright (1992), World Health Organization.

Box 8.5 Symptoms caused by hyperventilation

Dizziness
Tinnitus
Headache
Feeling of weakness
Faintness
Numbness
Tingling in the hands, feet, and face
Carpopedal spasms
Precordial discomfort
Feeling of breathlessness

precise; the attacks must have been recurrent and not consistently associated with a phobic situation or object, or with marked exertion or exposure to dangerous or life-threatening situations.

Differential diagnosis

Panic attacks occur in GADs, phobic anxiety disorders (most often agoraphobia), depressive disorders, and acute organic disorder. Two of the DSM-5 diagnostic criteria help to distinguish these secondary attacks from panic disorder—first, the presence in panic disorder of a persistent marked concern about having further attacks, and secondly, worry about the potentially catastrophic consequences of the attacks.

Epidemiology

The National Comorbidity Survey Replication found a 12-month prevalence rate of DSM-IV panic disorder of 2.7% and a lifetime risk of 4.7% (Kessler *et al.*, 2005a, b). These figures include panic disorder with agoraphobia, which accounts for about 50% of the cases in the general population. In Europe the 12-month prevalence of panic disorder was somewhat less, around 1.2%. In most studies, the prevalence in women is about twice that in men. Patients with panic disorder have increased rates of other anxiety disorders, major depression, and alcohol misuse.

Aetiology

Genetics

Panic disorder is familial, with about a fivefold increase in risk in first-degree relatives (Perez *et al.*, 2013). Rates in monozygotic twins are higher than those in dizygotic twins, indicating that the family aggregation is likely to be at least partly owing to genetic factors, with a heritability of about 40% (Bienvenu *et al.*, 2011). As noted above, *offspring* of patients with panic disorder have an increased risk of panic disorders themselves, both with and without agoraphobia. However, their risk of agoraphobia without panic is not increased (Knappe *et al.*, 2012). Numerous linkage and candidate gene studies have been conducted in panic disorder, and some tentative loci have been identified. One that has been replicated involves the gene for catechol-*O*-methyltransferase (COMT; see Box 5.5), but its effects may depend on ethnicity. It is likely that genes involved in panic disorder affect multiple biological pathways, with differences between populations (Howe *et al.*, 2016).

Biochemistry

Chemical agents, notably sodium lactate and the noradrenaline α_2-adrenoceptor antagonist, yohimbine, but also flumazenil (a benzodiazepine-receptor antagonist), and a 5-HT receptor agonist, m-chlorophenylpiperazine, can induce panic attacks more readily in patients with panic disorder than in healthy individuals (Ballenger *et al.*, 2009). The multitude of chemical agents that provoke panic attacks in panic disorder patients make it difficult to identify a single causal mechanism, and the abnormal responses could reflect altered *psychological attribution*, as described below. However, changes in 5-HT, noradrenaline, and GABA-ergic mechanisms have been suggested. There is most evidence for changes in GABA, with lowered cortical GABA levels measured by magnetic resonance spectroscopy, as well as diminished benzodiazepine-receptor binding in the parietotemporal regions in unmedicated patients with panic disorder (Hasler *et al.*, 2008). Positron emission tomography (PET) studies also suggest a lowering of cortical 5-HT_{1A} receptor binding in patients with panic disorder, similar to that found in depression (Nash *et al.*, 2008). However, this could be attributable to the high comorbidity between panic disorder and depression.

Neural mechanisms

Animal experimental studies suggest that the neural circuitry of fear and particularly escape behaviour (which panic attacks resemble to some extent) involves the amygdala, periaqueductal grey, hippocampus, hypothalamus, and brainstem nuclei, including the locus coeruleus, the origin of noradrenaline cell bodies. The ventromedial prefrontal cortex plays a regulatory inhibitory role. Structural imaging studies in panic disorder have reported altered volumes of amygdala and cingulate cortex, but the findings are not consistent.

Functional imaging studies have described abnormalities both in baseline perfusion and during panic provocation in various elements of this fear-related neural circuitry, but the findings have been variable. The best evidence for changes is in the insula, underlining the important role for interoceptive processes in the pathophysiology of panic disorder (Goodkind et al., 2013).

Cognitive theories

The cognitive hypothesis is based on the observation that fears about serious physical or mental illness are more frequent among patients who experience panic attacks than among anxious patients who do not have panic attacks. It is proposed that there is a spiral of anxiety in panic disorder, as the physical symptoms of anxiety activate fears of illness and thereby generate more anxiety. 'Safety behaviours' prevent disconfirmation of these fears (Helbig-Lang et al., 2014). These observations have led to an effective cognitive treatment for panic disorder.

Hyperventilation as a cause

A subsidiary hypothesis proposes that hyperventilation is a cause of panic disorder. Although there is no doubt that voluntary overbreathing can produce a panic attack, it has not been shown that panic disorder is caused by involuntary hyperventilation.

Course and prognosis

Follow-up studies have generally included patients with panic attacks and agoraphobia as well as patients with panic disorder alone. Earlier studies that used categories such as 'effort syndrome' found that most patients still had symptoms 20 years later, although most had a good social outcome. More recent studies of patients diagnosed with panic disorder also reveal a lengthy course, with fluctuating anxiety and depression. About 30% of patients remit without subsequent relapse, and a similar proportion show useful improvement, although with persistent symptomatology (Ballenger et al., 2009). The prognosis of panic disorder without agoraphobia is somewhat better, and results from controlled trials suggests effective treatment can improve the prognosis of both panic disorder and panic disorder with agoraphobia. Mortality rates from unnatural causes and, among men, from cardiovascular disorders are higher than average, and may be linked to changes in the regulation of the sympathetic nervous system (Davies et al., 2010).

Treatment

Apart from supportive measures and help with any causative life problems, treatment is with medication or cognitive therapy. A number of different kinds of medication can be used.

Benzodiazepines

When given in high doses, benzodiazepines control panic attacks. In these doses, most benzodiazepines cause sedation, but alprazolam, a high-potency compound, is an exception. For this reason it has been used to treat panic disorder, and its effectiveness over placebo has been demonstrated in many controlled trials (see Ballenger, 2009). At the end of treatment, alprazolam should be reduced very gradually to avoid withdrawal symptoms, because even when it is reduced over 30 days, about one-third of patients report significant withdrawal symptoms. This treatment was developed in the USA and has not been widely adopted in the UK, where benzodiazepines are not recommended for the treatment of panic disorder (National Institute for Health and Clinical Excellence, 2010).

Antidepressants

Imipramine was the first antidepressant to be shown to be effective for the treatment of panic disorder, and other tricyclic antidepressants, including clomipramine and lofepramine, are superior to placebo in controlled trials. SSRIs are also beneficial in the treatment of panic disorder, as is the SNRI, venlafaxine, and the selective noradrenaline re-uptake inhibitor, reboxetine (Baldwin et al., 2014). The initial effect of antidepressants in patients with panic disorder is often to produce an unpleasant feeling of apprehension, sleeplessness, and palpitations. For this reason the initial dose should be small (e.g. 5 mg of citalopram), increasing gradually each week until an effective dose is reached. Where patients respond to medication, maintaining treatment for at least 6 months helps to prevent relapse (Baldwin et al., 2014).

Cognitive therapy

Cognitive therapy reduces the fears of the physical effects of anxiety, which are thought to provoke and maintain the panic attacks. Common fears of this kind are that palpitations indicate an impending heart attack, or that dizziness indicates impending loss of consciousness. In treatment, the physical symptoms that the patient fears are induced by hyperventilation or exercise. The therapist points out the sequence of physical symptoms that leads to fear, and explains that a similar sequence occurs in the early stages of a panic attack. The therapist goes on to question the patient's belief in the feared outcome. The procedure is described further in Chapter 24.

Controlled studies have shown that cognitive therapy is as effective as antidepressant medication in the treatment of panic disorder (Cuijpers *et al.*, 2013). Combined treatment with medication and psychotherapy may result in a better response in the acute phase than either treatment modality given alone, but whether this persists in the longer term is uncertain (Cuijpers *et al.*, 2014b).

Management

What patients need to know

Patients need to be able to explain the disorder to relatives and friends, and the explanation outlined in relation to agoraphobia (see above) is usually appropriate. Patients also need to understand how particular ways of thinking and behaviours increase and prolong the disorder (see the section on cognitive therapy, above). Self-help books based on cognitive behaviour principles are available and can be helpful.

Choice of treatment

As cognitive therapy and medication have similar effects on symptoms, the choice of treatment depends on the patient's preference, the availability of cognitive therapy, and considerations of cost and long-term benefit (cognitive therapy is more costly, but probably has more lasting effects). If medication is chosen, one of the SSRIs are preferred to tricyclics because they have fewer side effects. Alprazolam has been used in some countries, but is not recommended in the UK (see above). Information about the main effects and side effects should be the same as that given when the same medication is given for other reasons, including the delayed onset of action, and the need to withdraw medication gradually (see Chapter 25). If there is no improvement after about 12 weeks, the treatment can be changed to an antidepressant of a different class, or cognitive therapy can be started. If cognitive therapy has not been effective, medication can be tried.

If, as often happens, panic disorder is accompanied by some degree of agoraphobic avoidance, exposure treatment should be added to the medication.

Mixed anxiety and depressive disorder

As explained at the beginning of this chapter, anxiety and depressive symptoms often occur together. The overlap is greatest when the symptoms are mild, and least when they are severe enough for a diagnosis of psychiatric disorder. The Adult Psychiatric Morbidity Survey in England found that *mixed anxiety and depression* was the most common psychiatric syndrome in the community, with about 9% of adults fulfilling the symptomatic criteria in the week before interview (McManus *et al.*, 2009). Rates were higher in women, and in households with low disposable income.

Diagnostic conventions

When the anxiety and depressive symptoms are not severe enough to meet the diagnostic criteria for a specific depressive or anxiety disorder, the condition is sometimes referred to as a *minor affective disorder* (see Chapter 9) or as *cothymia*. Other diagnostic terms include the following:

- *Mixed anxiety and depressive disorder*—this category is included in ICD-10 but not in the classification of DSM-5.

- *Adjustment disorder*—this is diagnosed when minor anxiety and depressive symptoms are related to a change in life circumstances.

Aetiology

There are a number of reasons why anxiety and depression may occur together.

- They may have the *same predisposing causes*. Brown and Harris (1993) found that childhood adversity is associated with both anxiety and depressive disorders in adulthood. There is evidence that depression and GAD may have common genetic mechanisms (Hettema, 2008).

- Some *stressful events combine elements of loss and danger*. The former tend to be associated with depression and the latter with anxiety.

- Persistent *anxiety leading to secondary depression*. Follow-up studies have shown that onset of depression among people with persistent anxiety is more common than onset of anxiety among people with persistent depression.

The *prognosis* of mixed anxiety and depressive disorders appears to be worse than that of a specific anxiety disorder (Tyrer *et al.*, 2004a).

Treatment

In community settings, only a minority of individuals with mixed anxiety and depression receives formal treatment. Antidepressant medication is most commonly used, but controlled trials for this indication are lacking. Counselling and brief forms of cognitive behaviour therapy are also employed. A meta-analysis has suggested that both of these forms of psychotherapy have modest beneficial effects, but that the degree of improvement resulting from cognitive behaviour therapy in mixed anxiety and depression is substantially less than in pure anxiety disorders (Cape *et al.*, 2010).

Transcultural variations in anxiety disorder

Anxiety disorders are universal but their prevalence and presentation show important cultural differences (Agorastos *et al.*, 2012). In several cultures the presenting symptoms of anxiety disorder are more often somatic than psychological. Sometimes this difference parallels the different words used to describe anxiety in the corresponding languages. Thus there is no word for anxiety in some African, Oriental, and Native American languages, and instead a phrase denoting bodily function is used. For example, in Yoruba, an African language, the phrase is 'the heart is not at rest'. In addition, several conditions have been described that may be transcultural variants of anxiety disorders, although their exact relationship to these disorders is uncertain. It does appear that in non-western cultures anxiety is experienced more somatically.

Koro: this can occur among men from India, South China, and Japan, and has similarities to panic disorder. Cantonese people call it *suk-yeong*, which means 'shrinking of the penis'. There are episodes of acute anxiety, lasting from 30 minutes to 1 or 2 days, during which the person complains of palpitations, sweating, pericardial discomfort, and trembling. At the same time he is convinced that the penis will retract into the abdomen, and that when this process is complete he will die. Most episodes occur at night, sometimes after sexual activity. To prevent the feared outcome, the patient may tie the penis to an object, or ask another person to hold the organ. This belief parallels the conviction held by patients during a panic attack that the heart is damaged and that they will die. Epidemics of koro have been described among people who are experiencing anxiety because of social stressors (Tseng, 2006).

Variants of social phobia have been described in the east, originally among people in Japan, where it is known as *taijin-kyofu-sho* or 'phobia of interpersonal relations'. There is intense anxiety in social situations and an intense conviction, bordering on the delusional, that the person is being thought of unfavourably by others. Other symptoms include fears of producing body odours, dysmorphophobia, and aversion to eye contact (Agorastos *et al.*, 2012). Tseng (2006) pointed out that, although earlier research in this area tended to focus on 'exotic' presentations of disorder in unfamiliar cultures, all psychiatric syndromes are *culturally influenced*. Therefore a knowledge of how social context alters the presentation of psychological distress is relevant to *all cultures*, particularly in a historical period when cultures in many countries are becoming increasingly diverse.

Obsessive–compulsive disorder

The concise description of OCD, contained in ICD-9, is still valuable:

The outstanding symptom is a feeling of subjective compulsion—which must be resisted—to carry out some action, to dwell on an idea, to recall an experience, or ruminate on an abstract topic. Unwanted thoughts, which include the insistency of words or ideas, ruminations or trains of thought, are perceived by the patient to be inappropriate or nonsensical. The obsessional urge or idea is recognized as alien to the personality but as coming from within the self. Obsessional actions may be quasi ritual performances designed to relieve anxiety, e.g. washing the hands to deal with contamination. Attempts to dispel the unwelcome thoughts or urges may lead to a severe inner struggle, with intense anxiety.

Clinical picture

OCD is characterized by obsessional thinking, compulsive behaviour, and varying degrees of anxiety, depression, and depersonalization. Obsessional and compulsive symptoms are listed in Box 8.6. They were described in Chapter 1, but the reader may find it helpful to be reminded of the main features.

Obsessional thoughts are words, ideas, and beliefs that are recognized by patients as their own, and that intrude forcibly into the mind. They are usually unpleasant, and attempts are made to exclude them. It is the combination of an *inner sense of* compulsion and of *efforts at resistance* that characterizes obsessional symptoms, but the effort at resistance is the more variable of the two. Obsessional thoughts may take the form of single words, phrases, or rhymes, are usually unpleasant or shocking to the person, and may be obscene or blasphemous. Obsessional images are vividly imagined scenes, often of a violent or disgusting kind (e.g. involving sexual practices that the person finds abhorrent).

Obsessional ruminations are internal debates in which arguments for and against even the simplest everyday actions are reviewed endlessly. Some obsessional doubts concern actions that may not have been completed adequately (e.g. turning off a gas tap or securing a door), while other doubts concern actions that might have harmed other people (e.g. that driving a car past a cyclist might have caused him to fall off his bicycle). Sometimes doubts are related to religious convictions or observances ('scruples')—a phenomenon well known to those who hear confession.

Obsessional impulses are urges to perform acts, usually of a violent or embarrassing kind (e.g. leaping in front of a car, injuring a child, or shouting blasphemies at a religious ceremony).

Obsessional rituals include both mental activities (e.g. counting repeatedly in a special way, or repeating a certain form of words) and repeated but senseless behaviours (e.g. washing the hands 20 or more times a day). Some rituals have an understandable connection with the obsessional thoughts that precede them (e.g. repeated hand washing following thoughts about contamination). Other rituals have no such connection (e.g. arranging objects in a particular way). The person may feel compelled to repeat such actions a certain number of times, and if this sequence is interrupted it has to be repeated from the beginning. People who use rituals are usually aware that these are illogical, and usually try to hide them. Some people fear that their symptoms are

> ### Box 8.6 Principal features of obsessive–compulsive disorder
>
> Obsessional symptoms
> Thoughts
> Ruminations
> Impulses
> 'Phobias'
> Compulsive rituals
> Abnormal slowness
> Anxiety
> Depression
> Depersonalization

a sign of incipient madness, and are greatly helped by reassurance that this is not so.

Obsessional slowness. Although obsessional thoughts and rituals lead to slow performance, a few obsessional patients are afflicted by extreme slowness that is out of proportion to other symptoms.

Obsessional phobias. Obsessional thoughts and compulsive rituals may worsen in certain situations—for example, obsessional thoughts about harming other people may increase in a kitchen or other place where knives are kept. The person may avoid such situations because they cause distress, just as people with phobic disorders avoid specific situations. Because of this resemblance, the condition is called an obsessional phobia.

Anxiety. This is a prominent component of OCDs. Some rituals are followed by a lessening of anxiety, while others are followed by increased anxiety.

Depression. Obsessional patients are often depressed. In some patients, depression is an understandable reaction to the obsessional symptoms; in others, depression appears to vary independently.

Depersonalization. Some obsessional patients complain of depersonalization. The relationship between this distressing symptom and the other features of the disorder is unclear.

Relationship to obsessional personality. Obsessional personality (obsessive compulsive personality disorder in DSM-5) is described in Chapter 15. There is no simple, one-to-one relationship between OCD and this kind of personality. Although obsessional personality is over-represented among people who develop OCD, about one-third of obsessional patients have other types of personality (as noted in a classic paper by Lewis, 1936).

Furthermore, people with obsessional personality are more likely to develop depressive disorders than OCDs.

Diagnostic criteria

In DSM-5 the diagnosis of *OCD* requires the presence of *either* obsessions *or* compulsions *or* both. In addition, the obsessions and/or compulsions are required to be *time-consuming* (e.g. taking more than 1 hour daily) and/or to cause *clinically significant distress* and/or *impairment in social or occupational function*. It is also necessary that the obsessive—compulsive symptoms are not attributable to the effects of a substance or another medical condition, and that the disturbance is not better explained by the symptoms of another mental disorder. In DSM-5, it also possible to specify the degree of insight that a patient possesses, ranging from 'good or fair' to 'absent' or 'delusional'. Under these diagnostic criteria, therefore, it is not necessary for the patient with OCD to believe that their obsessions and compulsions are unfounded or nonsensical.

ICD-10 also recognizes that OCD can present with obsessions or compulsions or both. For a definite diagnosis, the obsessional symptoms or compulsive acts must be present on *most days for at least 2 successive weeks* and be a *source of distress and/or interference with usual activities*. As well as the thoughts or impulses being recognized as the person's own, there must be at least one thought or act that is *resisted unsuccessfully*. ICD-10 notes that compulsive acts, while they may relieve tension, are not in themselves *intrinsically pleasurable*. This distinguishes compulsions from acts that are associated with immediate gratification such as those associated with addictions.

ICD-10 also classifies OCD as predominantly taking the form of obsessional thoughts and ruminations, *or* predominantly compulsive acts *or* mixed obsessional thoughts and acts when both are equally prominent. This distinction may be useful because behaviour therapy, for example, is more effective for the treatment of compulsions than it is for disorders characterized chiefly by obsessional thoughts.

Differential diagnosis

OCD must be distinguished from other disorders in which obsessional symptoms occur.

Anxiety disorders

The distinction from GAD, panic disorder, or phobic disorder is seldom difficult provided that a careful history is taken and the mental state is examined thoroughly.

Depressive disorder

The course of OCD is often punctuated by periods of depression in which the obsessional symptoms increase. When this happens the depressive disorder may be overlooked. Furthermore, obsessional symptoms sometimes occur in the course of a primary depressive disorder and may disappear when the depression is successfully treated.

Schizophrenia

Occasionally, the symptoms of OCD may resemble delusions because the content of the obsessional thoughts is peculiar, or the rituals are exceptionally odd, and resistance is weak. The disorder can then be mistaken for a delusional disorder or schizophrenia. In such cases, the correct diagnosis can be made following thorough history-taking and a careful search for other symptoms of psychosis. Obsessive—compulsive symptoms are not uncommon in schizophrenia, and may require separate treatment (Zohar *et al.*, 2009).

Organic disorders

Obsessional symptoms are occasionally found in organic cerebral disorders. They were observed most strikingly in chronic cases of encephalitis lethargica following the epidemic in the 1920s (see page 388).

Childhood-onset disorders

In children, obsessive—compulsive symptoms are frequently comorbid with developmental disorders such as *Gilles de la Tourette syndrome* and *autism* (see page 462).

Epidemiology

In the USA, Narrow *et al.* (2002) found a total 1-year prevalence of OCD of 2.1%, and the 1-year prevalence of OCD not comorbid with another anxiety disorder was 1.2%. In the more recent National Comorbidity Survey Replication, Ruscio *et al.* (2010) found a lifetime risk of 2.1%, and noted high rates of comorbidity, not only with other anxiety disorders but also with mood disorders, impulse control disorders, and substance misuse. Obsessive—compulsive symptomatology that did not meet the full criteria for DSM-IV was reported by 25% of those surveyed, with checking and hoarding being the most common behaviours. Estimates of the female-to-male ratio of lifetime prevalence in the population range from 1.2 (in Puerto Rico) to 3.8 (in New Zealand). However, in clinic populations the ratio is closer to 1 (Zohar *et al.*, 2009).

Aetiology

Healthy individuals experience occasional intrusive thoughts, some of which are concerned with sexual, aggressive, and other themes similar to those of obsessional patients. It is the frequency, intensity, and, above all, the persistence of obsessional phenomena that have to be explained.

Genetics

In the small number of twin studies that have been conducted, the concordance rate was greater in monozygotic than in dizygotic pairs, indicating that at least part of the familial loading is genetic. Familial studies have reached a similar conclusion, and indicate that the risk of OCD in first-degree relatives is increased approximately fourfold compared with control rates (Perez *et al.*, 2013). Molecular genetic studies have found a number of associations between OCD and various genes, including those coding for the glutamate and serotonin transporters, the 5-HT$_{2A}$ receptor, and the gene for brain-derived neurotropic factor. Apart from the glutamate transporter gene (*SLC1A1*), most of these have not been consistently replicated and current genome-wide association studies have not reported findings of genome-wide significance, perhaps owing to sample size limitations (Mattheisen *et al.*, 2015).

Evidence of a brain disorder

Two kinds of evidence suggest a disorder of brain function in OCD—first, associations with conditions that have known effects on brain function, and secondly, evidence from brain imaging.

Associations with other brain disorders. As noted above, obsessional symptoms were recorded frequently among patients affected by encephalitis lethargica after the Spanish 'flu pandemic of 1918–1919. Also, Gilles de la Tourette included obsessional symptoms in his original description of the disorder that now bears his name (de la Tourette, 1885), and more recent studies have confirmed this observation (Zohar *et al.*, 2009). In childhood, 70% of cases of Sydenham's chorea, which affects the caudate nucleus, are reported to have obsessive–compulsive symptoms. The condition, which is referred to as PANDAS (paediatric autoimmune neuropsychiatric disorder associated with streptococcal infection), is considered further in Chapter 16. In addition, the development of OCD in some children has been linked to group A streptococcal infections, although the findings are inconsistent and other infections as well as metabolic disturbances in children can produce neuropsychiatric symptoms, including obsessions and compulsions (Singer *et al.*, 2012).

Brain imaging studies. Structural imaging in patients with OCD has revealed rather variable changes, but the most consistent are an *increase in grey matter volume in the striatum and decrease in orbitofrontal, dorsomedial, and anterior cingulate cortex*. Functional imaging studies also reveal abnormalities in these brain regions both at rest and during psychological challenge paradigms that activate obsessive–compulsive symptomatology. In this situation, patients demonstrate increased activity in orbitofrontal cortex, caudate, anterior cingulate cortex, and thalamus (Ahmari and Simpson, 2013). These findings have led to suggestions that the symptoms of OCD are related to dysfunction in the well-described *cortico-striatal-thalamic loops*, which together support key neuropsychological domains such as affective and reward processing, working memory and executive function, and motor and response inhibition (Milad and Rauch, 2012). In this respect, compulsive behaviour has been linked more specifically to projections from orbitofrontal cortex (OFC) to the medial striatum (caudate nucleus) (Fineberg *et al.*, 2014).

Abnormal serotonergic function

The finding that obsessive–compulsive symptoms respond to drugs that increase 5-HT function suggests that *5-HT mechanisms* might be abnormal in OCD. The full effect of 5-HT uptake inhibitors on obsessive–compulsive symptoms takes several weeks, so the late effects are likely to be most relevant. However, these late effects are complex, and it is not known which of them are important. In any case, the response of obsessive–compulsive symptoms to drugs that affect 5-HT function does not prove that 5-HT function is abnormal in OCD. The situation might resemble that of parkinsonism, in which anticholinergic drugs control symptoms by acting on the normal cholinergic systems of patients whose disorder is caused by abnormal dopaminergic function.

Attempts to assess 5-HT function in OCD have used both neuroendocrine tests and measures of serotonin transporters and serotonin receptors using PET and single photon emission tomography (SPET). The results of these studies have not been consistent. Other studies have examined the effect on obsessive–compulsive symptoms of challenges with agents that have effects specific to particular kinds of 5-HT receptors. Some studies have implicated 5-HT$_{1D}$ and 5-HT$_{2C}$ subtypes, but again the results are contradictory (Ahmari and Simpson, 2013).

Psychoanalytical theories

Although not supported by evidence, these theories are summarized here because of their historical importance.

Freud originally suggested that obsessional symptoms result from unconscious impulses of an aggressive or sexual nature. These impulses could potentially cause extreme anxiety, but anxiety is reduced by the action of the defence mechanisms of repression and reaction formation. This idea reflects the aggressive and sexual fantasies of many obsessional patients, and their restraints on their own aggressive and sexual impulses. Freud also proposed that obsessional symptoms occur when there is a regression to the anal stage of development as a way of avoiding impulses related to the subsequent genital and Oedipal stages. This idea reflects obsessional patients' frequent concerns with excretory functions and contamination.

Neuropsychological function

In psychological terms *'compulsivity'* describes a tendency to perform repetitive acts in a habitual or stereotyped manner to prevent perceived negative consequences. Compulsivity has been contrasted with *impulsivity*, which is seen as a failure to inhibit inappropriate behaviours that are driven by reward and gratification. A tendency to compulsive responding can be detected by neuropsychological tasks that require an altered response once a 'habit' has been established by previous learning. Consistent with this, patients with OCD perform less well on tasks of 'set-shifting' and 'reversal learning' than controls, and a similar abnormality has been detected in first-degree relatives of OCD patients. This suggests that, in people with OCD and those at risk of OCD, actions may be mediated by a relative preponderance of *habit learning* over *goal-directed learning*. This might underpin the development of compulsive behaviours.

It is also worth noting that although *compulsivity* and *impulsivity* are often regarded as opposite behaviours, they can coexist. An anatomical basis for this is that, like compulsivity, impulsivity is thought to arise from dysfunction in *cortico-striatal-thalamic loops,* in the case of impulsivity in pathways involving the ventral striatum, anterior cingulate cortex, and ventrolateral prefrontal cortex. There is therefore significant scope for interaction between the circuits regulating impulsive and compulsive behaviour. Indeed, neuropsychological tasks suggest that patients with OCD and their first-degree relatives manifest significant difficulties in impulse control; for example, by failing to inhibit incorrect responses in tasks assessing motor performance. Thus part of the symptomatology of OCD may arise from failure to inhibit inappropriate responses as well as a compulsion to carry them out. For a review, see Fineberg *et al.* (2014).

Cognitive theory

This theory starts with the premise that it is not the occurrence of intrusive thoughts that has to be explained (as these are experienced at times even by healthy people; see above), but rather the obsessional patient's *inability to control them* and see them in perspective. For example, people with obsessional disorder often respond to such thoughts as if they were personally responsible for their possible consequences (e.g. for harm to another person). It is suggested that this feeling of responsibility leads to excessive attempts to ward off the thoughts and their supposed consequences by adopting compulsive behaviours and avoidance, and seeking repeated reassurance. Although the theory is unproven, it directs attention to aspects of the disorder other than the obvious obsessions and compulsions (see Box 8.7). For a review of the cognitive approach to OCD, see Veale (2007).

Prognosis

About two-thirds of cases improve to some extent by the end of 1 year. Of the cases that last for more than a year, some run a fluctuating course, but others are

---

> ### Box 8.7 **Some key cognitive processes in obsessive–compulsive disorder**
>
> 1. *Thought–action fusion.* Magical thinking—for example, the belief that if one thinks of harming others one is likely to act on the thought or might have done so in the past.
> 2. *Responsibility.* An inflated sense of responsibility for preventing harm to others; the belief that one has power that is pivotal to bringing about or preventing crucial negative outcomes.
> 3. *Compulsions and safety-seeking behaviours.* Compulsions—whether behavioural or mental—are reinforcing because they reduce anxiety temporarily. They strengthen the belief that, had the compulsion not been carried out, discomfort would have increased and harm might have occurred.
> 4. *Overestimation of the likelihood that harm will occur.*
> 5. *Intolerance of uncertainty and ambiguity.*
> 6. *The need for control.*
>
> Source: data from Advances in Psychiatric Treatment, 13(6), Veale D, Cognitive behavioural therapy for obsessive compulsive disorder, pp. 438–46, Copyright (2007), The Royal College of Psychiatrists.

chronic. The prognosis is better when there has been a precipitating event, social and occupational adjustment is good, and the symptoms are episodic. The prognosis is worse when there is a personality disorder, and onset is in childhood. Male gender, tic-related forms of OCD, and overvalued ideas about the obsessions also predict a poor prognosis (Zohar *et al.*, 2009). Marcks *et al.* (2011) studied over 100 patients with OCD, who were recruited to a research programme and followed up for 15 years. Most received treatment with medication and psychotherapy at some point in their course and all had at least one comorbid anxiety disorder. Remission was defined as being essentially free of symptoms for a period of at least 8 weeks. Remission rates in the first year of illness were low (16%), but gradually increased during follow-up to just over 40% at 15 years. The presence of comorbid major depression diminished the chance of recovery.

Treatment

Medication

Clomipramine. The use of clomipramine will be described first because of its historical importance in the development of pharmacological treatment for OCD. However, it is not now used as a first-line agent. Clomipramine is a tricyclic antidepressant with potent 5-HT-uptake-blocking effects. It is more effective than placebo in reducing the obsessional symptoms of patients with OCD (Clomipramine Collaborative Study Group, 1991). Most patients tolerate the treatment, but typical tricyclic side effects are common. and at high doses a few patients develop seizures. A clinically useful effect may not be reached until after about 6 weeks of treatment, and further improvement may take another 6–12 weeks. Many patients relapse during the first few weeks after the drug is stopped, but the relapse rate is reduced if clomipramine is combined with exposure, and if drug treatment is maintained. Other tricyclic antidepressants that are less potent 5-HT-uptake blockers do not have this therapeutic effect in OCD (National Institute for Health and Clinical Excellence, 2005a).

Selective serotonin uptake inhibitors. SSRIs are effective in reducing obsessional symptoms, and it seems unlikely that there are clinically important differences between them, although individual patients may respond better to one SSRI than another. There is some evidence that higher doses are somewhat more efficacious (Bloch *et al.*, 2010). Overall, SSRIs appear to have similar efficacy to clomipramine. However, clomipramine treatment is associated with more dropouts from treatment (National Institute for Health and Clinical Excellence, 2005a).

Since only about 50% of the treated patients improve substantially, attempts have been made to improve the response rate by adding a second drug to the SSRI. The only approach with a consistent, though rather limited therapeutic, effect involves the addition of an antipsychotic agent, usually at a low dose. Beneficial effects have been seen with both typical and atypical antipsychotic drugs, but the latter are usually better tolerated. A meta-analysis suggested that significant, albeit modest, benefit was most likely with the addition of low doses of risperidone and aripiprazole (Veale *et al.*, 2014). As with clomipramine, relapse is common during the first few weeks after an SSRI has been stopped, and longer-term maintenance treatment is advisable.

Anxiolytic drugs. These drugs give some short-term symptomatic relief but should not be prescribed continuously for more than 2–4 weeks at a time.

Cognitive behaviour therapy

Exposure and response prevention. Obsessional rituals usually improve with a combination of response prevention and exposure to any environmental cues that increase the symptoms. About two-thirds of patients with moderately severe rituals can be expected to improve substantially, although not completely (Zohar *et al.*, 2009). When rituals respond to this treatment, the accompanying obsessional thoughts usually improve as well. The results seem to be at least comparable with those of treatment with clomipramine and SSRIs (National Institute for Health and Clinical Excellence, 2005a).

Behavioural treatment is less effective for obsessional thoughts that occur without rituals. The technique of thought-stopping has been used for many years, but there is no good evidence that it has a specific effect. Cognitive approaches to obsessions may well be more successful (see below).

Cognitive therapy. This therapy seeks to reduce the patient's attempts to suppress and avoid obsessional thoughts, as such attempts have been shown to increase, rather than decrease, the frequency of these thoughts. The patient is helped to record the frequency of obsessional thoughts to compare the effects of suppression and distraction. As suppression and avoidance appear to be driven by the conviction that to think something is to make it happen, attempts are made to weaken this conviction by reviewing the evidence for and against it. These techniques may be combined with exposure to audio-recorded repetition of the thoughts, and discussion of any other cognitive distortions along the general lines of cognitive therapy (see Chapter 24 and Shafran *et al.*, 2013). Cognitive therapy by itself may not be as effective as behaviour therapy, but incorporating elements of cognitive approaches into behaviour therapy may enhance the effects of the latter treatment (Ponniah *et al.*, 2013). Current treatments generally incorporate elements of both approaches (National Institute for Health and Clinical Excellence, 2005a).

Dynamic psychotherapy

Exploratory and interpretative psychotherapy seldom helps obsessional patients. Indeed, some are made worse because these procedures encourage painful and unproductive rumination about the subjects discussed during treatment.

Neurosurgery and deep brain stimulation

The immediate result of neurosurgery for severe OCD is often a striking reduction in tension and distress. However, the long-term effects are uncertain, as no prospective controlled trial has been carried out. Hay *et al.* (1993) reported a 10-year follow-up of 26 obsessive–compulsive patients treated with orbitomedial or cingulate lesions, or both. Of the 18 patients who were interviewed, eight had a second operation, two died as a result of suicide, and about one-third of the survivors improved. A similar rate of improvement was found in a survey by Dougherty *et al.* (2002). The frequency of second operations and the modest improvement rates indicate the limitations of this treatment. For a review, see Christmas *et al.* (2004).

Deep brain stimulation (DBS) has also been employed to treat intractable OCD. However, current worldwide experience is still limited. For an account of the use of DBS in intractable OCD, see Chapter 25.

Management

In treatment, it is important to remember that some cases of OCD run a fluctuating course, with long periods of remission. Also, depressive disorder frequently accompanies OCD, and in such cases effective treatment of the depressive disorder often leads to improvement in the obsessional symptoms. For this reason, a thorough search for depressive disorder should be made in every patient who presents with OCD.

What patients need to know

Treatment should begin with an explanation of the symptoms, and, if necessary, with reassurance that these symptoms are not an early sign of insanity (a common concern of obsessional patients). If the patient agrees, their partner or another close relative can be involved in educational sessions about the nature and treatment of the disorder. Patients and family members are often helped by reading a book on OCD.

Obsessional patients may attempt to involve other family members in their rituals. If this happens, the relatives should be helped to find ways of resisting such requests in a way that is firm and appropriately sympathetic. In particular, they need to understand that repeated reassurances about obsessional ruminations do not help.

Choice of treatment

As noted above, medication controls the symptoms of OCD in many cases, but when it is stopped many patients relapse. Exposure with response prevention seems to produce better long-term results, but it is difficult to achieve response prevention when symptoms are severe, and a significant number of patients are unable to tolerate the technique (Veal and Roberts, 2014). For this reason, medication and response prevention should often be combined if the patient finds this acceptable. If there is a waiting list for behaviour therapy, medication can be started first.

First-line medication should generally be an SSRI, and, if this is not effective, a switch to a second SSRI may be considered. If this is unsuccessful, a trial of clomipramine or augmentation with an antipsychotic drug may be considered. Cognitive behaviour therapy should be tried if not used previously. Because patients with OCD may fare better on higher doses of antidepressant medication, it is worth exploring the full recommended dose range if tolerance permits this. If patients respond to medication, long-term maintenance treatment may be needed.

For an account of the management OCD, see Veale and Roberts (2014).

Obsessive–compulsive-related disorders

We have already seen that in DSM-5 a number of disorders are grouped with OCD, including *body dysmorphic disorder*, *hoarding disorder*, and *trichotillomania*. These conditions are listed with OCD principally because all display prominent compulsive features. Here we briefly outline the clinical features, diagnosis, epidemiology, and management of hoarding disorder and trichotillomania. Body dysmorphic disorder is discussed in Chapter 22.

Hoarding disorder

Clinical features

Historically, *pathological hoarding* has been recognized for well over a century, when it became associated with the psychoanalytical concept of 'anal personality'. Subsequently, hoarding behaviour was seen as characteristic of *obsessive–compulsive personality disorder* and, more recently, in DSM-IV, as a symptom of *OCD*. However, in DSM-5, hoarding is now recognized as a disorder in its own right.

Hoarding is a persistent phenomenon typically arising in a middle-aged or elderly person, which is driven by emotional difficulties in parting with or discarding possessions, no matter what their actual value. While normal individuals may collect items in an assiduous way, this collection is systematic and purposeful and does not interfere with the conduct of the individual's life. In hoarding disorder the clutter of material fills up and congests living areas to the extent that their intended use, for example as a kitchen or bedroom, becomes impossible. The most commonly hoarded items are newspapers, magazines, clothing, and paperwork. Some patients also hoard animals in insanitary and unsuitable ways. A form of hoarding in older people that is associated with extreme self-neglect and domestic squalor has been called *Diogenes syndrome or senile squalor syndrome* (see page 555). It is important to note that the latter may be associated with dementia (Pertusa *et al.*, 2010).

Despite the interference of the hoarding behaviour with everyday life and the attendant distress this can cause, affected individuals do not resist the urge to hoard, but feel anxious, upset, or angry if an attempt is made to reduce the accumulated clutter. Unlike OCD, thoughts about hoarding are not experienced as intrusive or repetitive or distressing, and the hoarding behaviour is not seen as senseless or inappropriate. Hoarding remains one of the criteria for *obsessive compulsive personality disorder* in DSM-5; however, hoarding has a low correlation with the other symptoms of obsessive–compulsive personality, and many patients who hoard do not have other features of personality disorder (Mataix-Cols *et al.*, 2010).

Diagnosis

In DSM-5 the diagnosis of 'hoarding disorder' requires that patients show a longstanding problem with getting rid of worthless items and marked distress at the prospect of parting with them. The result is an accumulation of clutter that takes over living areas and makes them impossible to use for their intended purposes, and which eventually can render the home unhygienic and unsafe. When a person meets the diagnosis for both hoarding disorder and obsessive–compulsive personality, both diagnoses should be recorded.

Epidemiology

A moderate degree of hoarding appears common in the general population, so estimates of the population frequency of pathological hoarding vary according to the diagnostic criteria used. A lifetime prevalence between 2% and 4% is probable, and pathological hoarding appears to be familial with a strong genetic component (Pertusa *et al.*, 2010). From a survey of over 700 participants in a personality disorder survey, Samuels *et al.* (2008) estimated that hoarding increased with age, correlated inversely with household income, and was twice as great in men than in women. There was an association with alcohol dependence but not OCD.

Management

Management of patients with hoarding disorder is usually difficult because, in the view of most patients, their hoarding is a not problem. However, improvements in hoarding behaviour compared to waitlist control have been shown with cognitive behaviour therapy given along the same lines as that for OCD. Forms of cognitive behaviour therapy have been developed specifically for hoarding disorder, but whether they confer additional benefit is unresolved (Williams and Viscusi, 2016). There have also been investigations of pharmacotherapy in pathological hoarding, with SSRIs and venlafaxine showing benefit. However, most of the published studies were open label, and randomized controlled trials are needed (Brakoulias *et al.*, 2015).

Trichotillomania

Clinical features

The key feature of trichotillomania is recurrent hair pulling, which results in hair loss. The hair loss is usually visible but in some patients is less apparent because single hairs are pulled from widely distributed sites, or because make-up or a wig is employed. Trichotillomania can involve any site on the body where hair grows, but most often affects the scalp, eyebrows, or eyelashes. Hair pulling can occur in brief episodes throughout the day or in more sustained periods of several hours. Prior to hair pulling, often during a time when the impulse to pull is being resisted, there are increasing feelings of tension, while the act of hair pulling itself is associated with a sense of pleasure or relief. Extracted hair can be chewed and swallowed, thereby causing hair balls in the stomach (trichobezoars) with a risk of bowel obstruction.

Trichotillomania can have an onset in childhood, where there is often less evidence of tension prior to hair pulling. However, it can also begin in adolescence and adulthood. The disorder is more common in women and the course may be episodic or chronic. In clinical samples, trichotillomania is often comorbid with mood and anxiety disorders, as well as impulse control disorders such as substance misuse. Individuals with trichotillomania frequently exhibit other repetitive behaviours involving the body, such as lip chewing or skin picking.

Diagnosis

The DSM-5 diagnosis for trichotillomania requires that the patient repeatedly pulls their hair, despite repeated attempts to stop doing so, and that this hair loss causes distress and/or significant impairment in occupational or social functioning. It is also necessary that the hair loss not caused by another medical condition or mental disorder.

Diagnosis in ICD-10 is similar, although in this classification, trichotillomania is grouped with impulse control disorders such as pathological gambling and pyromania. ICD-10 describes trichotillomania as noticeable hair loss owing to a recurrent failure to resist impulses to pull out hairs. ICD-10 also notes that hair pulling is generally preceded by increasing tension and accompanied by relief or gratification.

Epidemiology

The prevalence of trichotillomania defined by current diagnostic criteria remains to be clarified, but around 1–2% of college students report problematic hair pulling. Family studies indicate that trichotillomania is associated with increased rates of obsessive–compulsive and grooming disorders (trichotillomania, nail biting and skin picking) amongst first-degree relatives. Conversely, first-degree relatives of patients with OCD have higher rates of grooming disorders. These findings suggest some shared genetic diathesis between OCD and trichotillomania (McElroy and Keck, 2009).

Management

Psychological therapies are currently the best validated management for trichotillomania. There are positive studies with behavioural treatment employing habit reversal, and in one study cognitive behaviour therapy proved more effective than clomipramine and placebo. However, when behaviour therapy has been compared to a psychological control procedure such as progressive muscular relaxation it has not been clearly superior. Fluoxetine has not proved reliably beneficial, but good responses to treatment have been reported with clomipramine and the glutathione precursor, N-acetylcysteine (Slikboer *et al.*, 2016).

Further reading

Baldwin DS *et al.* (2014) Evidence-based pharmacological treatment of anxiety disorders, traumatic stress disorder and obsessive-compulsive disorder: A revision of the 2005 guidelines from the British Association for Psychopharmacology. *Journal of Psychopharmacology*, **28**, 403–39. (A comprehensive updated review of the pharmacological treatment of anxiety disorders and obsessive–compulsive disorder.)

Gelder MG *et al.* (eds) (2009). Section 4.7: Anxiety disorders (generalized anxiety disorders; social and specific phobias; and panic disorder and agoraphobia), and Section 4.8: Obsessional disorders. *The New Oxford Textbook of Psychiatry*. Oxford University Press, Oxford.

National Institute for Health and Clinical Excellence (2005a). *Obsessive–Compulsive Disorder: Core interventions in the treatment of obsessive–compulsive disorder and body dysmorphic disorder*. Clinical Guideline 31. National Institute for Health and Clinical Excellence, London. (A periodically updated comprehensive review, available at http://www.nice.org .uk.)

National Institute for Health and Clinical Excellence (2010). *Anxiety: Management of anxiety (panic disorder, with and without agoraphobia, and generalized anxiety disorder) in adults in primary, secondary and community care*. Clinical Guideline 22. National Institute for Health and Clinical Excellence, London. (A periodically updated comprehensive review, available at http://www.nice.org.uk.)

CHAPTER 9

Depression

Introduction

The next two chapters describe depressive disorders and bipolar disorder. These conditions are also called *mood disorders* because one of their main features is abnormality of mood. Nowadays the term is usually restricted to disorders in which this mood is depression or elation, but in the past some authors have included states of anxiety as well. In this book, anxiety disorders are described in Chapter 8. Mood disorders have in the past been referred to as 'affective disorders', a term that is still used fairly widely.

Depressive disorders

It is part of normal experience to feel unhappy during times of adversity. The symptom of depressed mood is a component of many psychiatric syndromes, and is also commonly found in certain physical diseases (e.g. in infections such as viral hepatitis, and some neurological disorders). In this chapter we are concerned neither with normal feelings of unhappiness nor with depressed mood as a symptom of other disorders, but with the syndromes known as *depressive disorders*.

The central features of these syndromes are:

- depressed mood
- negative thinking
- lack of enjoyment
- reduced energy
- slowness.

Of these, depressed mood is usually, but not invariably, the most prominent symptom.

Clinical features

Depressive syndromes

The clinical presentations of depressive states are varied, and they can be subdivided in a number of different ways. In the following account, disorders are grouped by their *severity*. The account begins with a description of the clinical features of an episode of *severe depression*, together with certain important clinical variants that can influence the presentation of depressive disorders. Finally, the special features of the *less severe* depressive disorders are outlined. What constitutes an 'episode' of clinical depression is inevitably a somewhat arbitrary concept. The symptoms listed for the diagnosis of 'depressive episode' in the ICD-10 classification and the various levels of severity are shown in Box 9.1. Similar symptoms (five or more) are required for the diagnosis of 'major depressive episode' in DSM-5 except that the symptomatology in DSM-5 includes psychomotor agitation or retardation. DSM-5 also specifically requires that the symptoms cause clinically significant distress or impairment in social, occupational, or other important areas of functioning.

Severe depressive episode

In a severe episode of depression, the central features are *low mood, lack of enjoyment (anhedonia), negative thinking,* and *reduced energy*, all of which lead to *decreased social and occupational functioning.*

Appearance

The patient's appearance is characteristic. Dress and grooming may be neglected. The facial features are characterized by a turning downward of the corners of the mouth, and by vertical furrowing of the centre of the brow. The rate of blinking may be reduced. The shoulders are bent and the head is inclined forward so that the direction of gaze is downward. Gestures and movements are reduced. It is important to note that some patients maintain a smiling exterior despite deep feelings of depression.

Mood

The mood of the patient is one of *misery*. This mood does not improve substantially in circumstances where ordinary feelings of sadness would be alleviated—for example, in pleasant company or after hearing good news. The low mood is, in this sense, *pervasive*. Moreover, the mood is often experienced as different from *ordinary sadness*. Patients sometimes speak of a black cloud pervading all mental activities. Some patients can conceal this mood change from other people, at least for short periods. Some try to hide their low mood during clinical interviews, which makes it more difficult for the doctor to detect. The mood is often worse first thing in the morning when the patient wakes, improving as the day wears on. This is called *diurnal variation of mood*.

Depressive cognitions

Negative thoughts ('depressive cognitions') are important symptoms that can be divided into three groups:

- worthlessness
- pessimism
- guilt.

In feeling *worthless*, patients think that they are failing in what they do and that other people see them as a failure; they no longer feel confident, and discount any success as a chance happening for which they can take no credit. *Pessimistic thoughts* concern future prospects. Patients expect the worst. They foresee failure in work, the ruin of finances, misfortune for family, and an inevitable deterioration in health. These ideas of *hopelessness* are often accompanied by the thought that life is no longer worth living and that death would come as a welcome release. These gloomy preoccupations may progress to thoughts of, and plans for, *suicide*. It is important to ask about these ideas in every case (the assessment of suicidal risk is considered further in Chapter 21).

> ### Box 9.1 Symptoms needed to meet the criteria for 'depressive episode' in ICD-10
>
> **A**
> - Depressed mood
> - Loss of interest and enjoyment
> - Reduced energy and decreased activity
>
> **B**
> - Reduced concentration
> - Reduced self-esteem and confidence
> - Ideas of guilt and unworthiness
> - Pessimistic thoughts
> - Ideas of self-harm
> - Disturbed sleep
> - Diminished appetite
>
> Mild depressive episode: at least two of A and at least two of B
>
> Moderate depressive episode: at least two of A and at least three of B
>
> Severe depressive episode: all three of A and at least four of B
>
> Severity of symptoms and degree of functional impairment also guide classification
>
> Source: data from The ICD-10 classification of mental and behavioural disorders: clinical descriptions and diagnostic guidelines, Copyright (1992), World Health Organization.

Feelings of *guilt* often take the form of unreasonable self-blame about minor matters—for example, patients may feel guilty about past trivial acts of dishonesty or letting someone down. Usually these events have not been in patients' thoughts for years, but when they become depressed they flood back into their memory, accompanied by intense feelings. Preoccupations of this kind strongly suggest depressive disorder. Some patients have similar feelings of guilt but do not attach them to any particular event. Other memories are focused on unhappy events; patients remember occasions when they were sad, when they failed, or when their fortunes were at a low ebb. These gloomy memories become increasingly frequent as the depression deepens. Patients blame themselves for their misery and incapacity, and attribute it to personal failing and moral weakness (a view not uncommonly held by the wider public).

Goal-directed behaviour

Lack of interest and enjoyment (also known as *anhedonia*) is frequent, although it is not always complained of spontaneously. Patients show no enthusiasm for activities and hobbies that they would normally enjoy. They feel no zest for living and no pleasure in everyday things. They often withdraw from social encounters. Reduced energy is characteristic (although depression is sometimes associated with a degree of physical restlessness that can mislead the observer). Patients feel lethargic, find everything an effort, and leave tasks unfinished. For example, a normally house-proud person may leave the beds unmade and dirty plates on the table. Work outside the home becomes increasingly difficult and academic achievement declines. Understandably, many patients attribute this lack of energy to physical illness. *Anhedonia* is an important symptom because it is an important way of distinguishing depression of at least moderate severity from milder disorders. It is also a key symptom of *melancholic* depression (see 'Classification by symptomatic picture' below).

Psychomotor changes

Psychomotor retardation is frequent (although, as described later, some patients are agitated rather than slowed down). The retarded patient walks and acts slowly. Slowing of thought is reflected in their speech; there is a significant delay before questions are answered, and pauses in conversation may be unusually prolonged. *Agitation* is a state of restlessness that is experienced by the patient as inability to relax, and is seen by an observer as restless activity. When it is mild, patients are seen to be plucking at their fingers and making restless movements of their legs; when it is severe, they cannot sit for long, and instead pace up and down.

Anxiety is frequent, although not invariably present, in severe depression. (As described later, it is common in less severe depressive disorders.) Another common symptom is *irritability*, which is the tendency to respond with undue annoyance to minor demands and frustrations, and can be a core presenting feature in adolescents in particular.

Biological symptoms

There is an important group of symptoms that is often described as 'biological' (also referred to as 'melancholic', 'somatic', or 'vegetative'). These symptoms include *sleep disturbance, diurnal variation in mood, loss of appetite, loss of weight, constipation, loss of libido*, and, among women, *amenorrhoea*. They are very common in depressive disorders of more severe degree (but less usual in mild depressive disorders). Some of these symptoms require further comment.

Sleep disturbance in depressive disorders is of several kinds. The most characteristic type is *early-morning waking*, but delay in falling asleep and waking during the night also occur. Early-morning waking occurs 2 or 3 hours before the patient's usual time of waking. He does not fall asleep again, but lies awake feeling unrefreshed and often restless and agitated. He thinks about the coming day with pessimism, broods about past failures, and ponders gloomily about the future. It is this combination of *early waking and depressive thinking* that is important in diagnosis. It should be noted that some depressed patients sleep excessively rather than waking early, but they still report waking unrefreshed.

Weight loss in depressive disorders often seems to be greater than can be accounted for merely by the patient's reported lack of appetite. In some patients the disturbances of eating and weight are towards excess—that is, they eat more than usual and gain weight. Usually eating brings temporary relief of their distressing feelings.

Complaints about *physical symptoms* are common in depressive disorders. They take many forms, but complaints of constipation, fatigue, and aching discomfort anywhere in the body are particularly common. Complaints about any pre-existing physical disorder usually increase, and *hypochondriacal preoccupations* are common.

Other features

Several other psychiatric symptoms may occur as part of a depressive disorder, and occasionally one of them dominates the clinical picture. They include *depersonalization, obsessional symptoms, panic attacks*, and, more rarely, *dissociative symptoms* such as fugue or loss of function of a limb. Complaints of *poor memory* are also common; depressed patients commonly show deficits on a wide range of neuropsychological tasks, but impairments in the retrieval and recognition of recently learned material are particularly prominent. Sometimes the impairment of memory in a depressed patient is so severe that the clinical presentation resembles that of dementia. This presentation, which is particularly common in the elderly, is sometimes called depressive *pseudodementia* (Chapter 14).

Psychotic depression

As depressive disorders become increasingly severe, all of the features described above occur with greater intensity. There is complete loss of function in social and occupational spheres. Inattention to basic hygiene and nutrition may give rise to concern about the patient's wellbeing. Psychomotor retardation may make interviewing difficult or impossible. In addition, there may be delusions and hallucinations, in which case the disorder is referred to as *psychotic depression* (depressive psychosis is a synonym). As with other psychotic states, insight is impaired and patients (usually of blameless character) regard themselves as wicked and being justly punished for their misdeeds.

The delusions of severe depressive disorders are concerned with the same themes as the non-delusional thinking of moderate depressive disorders. Therefore they are termed *mood-congruent*. These themes are worthlessness, guilt, ill health, and, more rarely, poverty. Such delusions have been described in Chapter 1, but a few examples may be helpful at this point. Patients with a *delusion of guilt* may believe that some dishonest act, such as a minor concealment when filling in a tax return, will be discovered and that they will be punished severely and humiliated. They are likely to believe that such punishment is deserved. Patients with *hypochondriacal delusions* may be convinced that they have cancer or venereal disease, while patients with a *delusion of impoverishment* may wrongly believe that they have lost all of their money in a business venture.

Persecutory delusions also occur. Patients may believe that other people are discussing them in a derogatory way or are about to take revenge on them. When persecutory delusions are part of a depressive syndrome, typically patients accept the supposed persecution as something that they have brought upon themselves. In their view, they are ultimately to blame. This can be a useful diagnostic feature for distinguishing severe depression from non-affective psychosis (see Chapter 11). Some depressed patients experience delusions and hallucinations that are not clearly related to themes of depression (i.e. they are 'mood-incongruent'). Their presence appears to worsen the prognosis of the illness.

Particularly severe depressive delusions are found in *Cotard's syndrome*, which was described by the French psychiatrist, Jules Cotard, in 1882. The characteristic feature is an extreme kind of nihilistic delusion. For example, some patients may complain that their bowels have been destroyed, so they will never be able to pass faeces again. Others may assert that they are penniless and have no prospect of ever having any money again. Still others may be convinced that their whole family has ceased to exist and that they themselves are dead. Although the extreme nature of these symptoms is striking, such cases do not appear to differ in important ways from other severe depressive disorders.

Other clinical variants of depressive disorders

Agitated depression

This term is applied to depressive disorders in which *agitation* is prominent. As already noted, agitation occurs in many severe depressive disorders, but in agitated depression it is particularly severe. Agitated depression is seen more commonly among middle-aged and elderly patients than among younger individuals.

Retarded depression

This name is sometimes applied to depressive disorders in which *psychomotor retardation* is especially prominent. There is no evidence that they represent a separate syndrome, although the presence of prominent retardation is said to predict a good response to electroconvulsive therapy (ECT). If the term is used, it should be in a purely descriptive sense. In its most severe form, retarded depression merges with *depressive stupor*.

Depressive stupor

In severe depressive disorder, slowing of movement and poverty of speech may become so extreme that the patient is motionless and mute. Such depressive stupor is rarely seen now that active treatment is available. Therefore the description by Kraepelin (1921, p. 80) is of particular interest:

The patients lie mute in bed, give no answer of any sort, at most withdraw themselves timidly from approaches, but often do not defend themselves from pinprick. …. They sit helpless before their food; perhaps, however, they let themselves be spoon-fed without making any difficulty.

Kraepelin commented that recall of the events that took place during stupor was sometimes impaired when the patient recovered. Nowadays, the general view is that, on recovery, patients are able to recall nearly all of the events that took place during the period of stupor. It is possible that in some of Kraepelin's cases there was clouding of consciousness (possibly related to inadequate fluid intake, which is common in these patients). Patients in states of depressive stupor may exhibit catatonic motor disturbances (see Chapter 1).

Atypical depression

The term *atypical depression* is generally applied to disorders of moderate clinical severity. The precise meaning of the term has varied over the years, but currently it is applied to disorders characterized by:

- variably depressed mood with *mood reactivity* to positive events
- *overeating and oversleeping*
- *extreme fatigue* and heaviness in the limbs (*leaden paralysis*)
- pronounced *anxiety.*

Many patients with these clinical symptoms have a lifelong tendency to react in an exaggerated way to perceived or real rejection (*rejection sensitivity*), although this character trait can be exacerbated by the presence of a depressive disorder. Patients with atypical depression also have an earlier onset of illness and a more chronic course. The importance of recognizing atypical depression is that, because of their interpersonal sensitivity, patients with this disorder can be hard to manage and may be regarded as having 'difficult' personalities rather than depressive disorder. Traditionally, atypical depression was associated with a poor response to tricyclic antidepressant treatment but had a better outcome with monoamine oxidase inhibitors (MAOIs). However, there is little evidence that the diagnosis of atypical depression predicts response to modern antidepressant drug treatment (see Arnow *et al.*, 2015).

Mixed depression

Mixed affective states have long been recognized in bipolar patients (see Chapter 10), where depressive symptoms are not infrequently detected in patients in whom the main presentation is mania. However, it is possible for patients with major depression to exhibit symptoms that might be seen in mania but do not reach the threshold for diagnosis of bipolar disorder. DSM-5 has a specifier for major depressive episode 'with mixed features'. The most common symptoms in mixed depression are irritable mood, mood lability, distractibility, agitation, and impulsivity (Perugi *et al.*, 2015). Not surprisingly, such symptoms are more common in depressed patients

with a family history of bipolar disorder, and depressed patients with mixed features are more likely themselves to develop bipolar disorder in the future.

Mild depressive states

It might be expected that *mild depressive disorders* would present with symptoms similar to those of the depressive disorders described above, but with less intensity. To some extent this is the case, but in mild depressive disorders there are frequently *additional symptoms* that are less prominent in severe disorders. These symptoms have been characterized in the past as 'neurotic', and they include *anxiety, phobias, obsessional symptoms*, and, less often, *dissociative symptoms*. In terms of classification, both DSM-5 and ICD-10 have categories of *mild depression* where criteria for a depressive episode are met but the depressive symptoms are fewer and less severe (see Box 9.1).

Apart from the 'neurotic' symptoms that are found in some cases, mild depressive disorders are characterized by the expected symptoms of *low mood, lack of energy and interest*, and *irritability*. There is *sleep disturbance*, but not the early-morning waking that is so characteristic of more severe depressive disorders. Instead, there is more often difficulty in falling asleep, and periods of waking during the night, usually followed by a period of sleep at the end of the night. *'Biological' features* (poor appetite, weight loss, and low libido) are not usually found. Although mood may vary during the day, it is usually worse in the evening than in the morning. The patient may not appear obviously dejected, or slowed in their movement. Delusions and hallucinations are not present.

In their mildest forms, these cases merge into the minor mood disorders considered below. As described later, they pose considerable problems of classification. Many of these mild depressive disorders are brief, starting at a time of personal misfortune and subsiding when fortunes have changed or a new level of adjustment has been achieved. However, some cases persist for months or years, causing considerable suffering, even though the symptoms do not increase. These chronic depressive states have been termed *dysthymia*, which is characterized in ICD-10 as the persistence over a number of years of depressive symptoms that are not severe enough to meet criteria for a depressive episode. However, it is not uncommon in such patients for periods of more severe depression to supervene, in which case the diagnosis of depressive episode is made. DSM-5 has a similar category, called 'Persistent Depressive Disorder (Dysthymia)', which requires fewer symptoms than those needed to diagnose 'Major Depressive Disorder' but stipulates that the symptoms must have persisted for at least 2 years. In DSM-5, this category also includes patients who meet full criteria for 'Major Depression' that has persisted for more than 2 years.

Minor anxiety–depressive disorders

We have already seen that anxiety and depressive symptoms often occur together. Indeed, earlier writers considered that anxiety and depressive disorders could not be separated clearly even in patients who had been admitted to hospital with severe disorders. Although most psychiatrists now accept that the distinction can usually be made among the more severe forms that present in psychiatric practice, the distinction is less easy to make in the milder forms that present in primary care.

Classification

As psychiatrists have worked increasingly with general practitioners, the importance of minor anxiety–depressive disorders has been recognized, but without any agreement about classification.

ICD-10 includes a category of 'mixed anxiety and depressive disorder', which can be applied when neither anxiety symptoms nor depressive symptoms are severe enough to meet the criteria for an anxiety disorder or a depressive disorder, and when the symptoms do not have the close association with stressful events or significant life changes that is required for a diagnosis of acute stress reaction or adjustment disorder.

According to ICD-10, patients with this presentation are seen frequently in primary care, and there are many others in the general population who are not seen by doctors. In ICD-10 this diagnosis appears among the anxiety disorders, although some psychiatrists consider that the condition is more closely related to the mood disorders, a view that is reflected in the alternative term, *minor affective disorder*.

In DSM-5, no comparable diagnosis appears in the classification, although there is a category, 'Unspecified Depressive Disorder', for depressive symptoms that cause distress or impairment in social and occupational functioning without meeting criteria for any specific depressive disorder. Although little is known about these conditions or about their relationship to other disorders, patients commonly present to primary care doctors with this group of symptoms. A suitable category is needed even if it is not possible to write strict criteria for diagnosis.

Clinical picture

One of the best descriptions of minor anxiety–depressive disorder is that given by Goldberg *et al.* (1976), who studied 88 patients from a general practice in Philadelphia. The most frequent symptoms were:

- fatigue
- anxiety
- depression
- irritability
- poor concentration
- insomnia
- somatic symptoms and bodily preoccupation.

A similar range of symptoms was found in the Adult Psychiatric Morbidity in England survey (McManus *et al.*, 2009), which surveyed the frequency of 'neurotic' symptomatology in a community sample.

Patients with minor anxiety–depressive disorders commonly present to medical practitioners with *prominent somatic symptoms*. The reason for this is uncertain; some symptoms are autonomic features of anxiety, and it is possible that patients expect somatic complaints to be viewed more sympathetically than emotional problems. Another point of clinical relevance is that minor affective disorders can be prolonged and in some cases may cause quite disabling difficulties in personal and occupational function. Thus the term 'minor' may not capture the serious consequences of the disorder for an individual. In some patients minor affective disorders may represent a residual form of a major mood disturbance (Angst, 2009).

Transcultural factors

There are cultural variations in the clinical presentation of depressive states, but in most countries depression appears to be underdiagnosed, particularly in primary care. In fact, sadness, joylessness, anxiety, and lack of energy are common symptoms of depression in most cultures. While somatic presentations of depression are undoubtedly found in all societies, they are apparently more frequent and prominent in non-western cultures, including in some immigrant groups in western societies. An important factor leading to somatization of depression appears to be the extent to which different cultures stigmatize mental illness (Bagayogo *et al.*, 2013).

It is necessary, however, to distinguish between somatization (see Chapter 22) and somatic metaphors for a painful emotional state. For example, Punjabi women living in London have been found to use expressions such as 'weight on my heart' and 'feelings of heat' to express emotional suffering, the presence of which they were well aware. Particular cultures have their own ways of dealing with painful emotions produced, for example, by loss, and the diagnosis of depression should take this into account by placing suitable emphasis on issues such as degree of distress and level of disability.

Classification of depression

There is no general agreement about the best method of classifying depressive disorders. A number of approaches have been tried, based on the following:

- presumed aetiology
- symptomatic picture
- course.

Classification by presumed aetiology

Historically, depressive disorders were sometimes classified into two kinds—those in which the symptoms were caused by factors within the individual, and were independent of outside factors (*endogenous depression*), and those in which the symptoms were a response to external stressors (*reactive depression*). However, it has been recognized for many years that this distinction is unsatisfactory. For example, Lewis (1934) wrote:

every illness is a product of two factors—of the environment working on the organism—whether the constitutional factor is the determining influence or the environmental one ... is never a question to be dealt with as either/or.

As noted in Chapter 5, when considering the aetiology of individual cases of depression, the relative contributions of a variety of aetiological factors must be considered. Neither ICD-10 nor DSM-5 contains categories of reactive or endogenous depression.

Classification by symptomatic picture

Melancholic depression

It is well recognized that episodes of depression vary in symptomatic profile both within and between subjects. In the section on clinical description it was noted that some depressive conditions are characterized by 'biological' symptoms, such as loss of appetite, psychomotor changes, weight loss, constipation, reduced libido, amenorrhoea, and early-morning waking. These symptoms have sometimes been termed *melancholic*, and they have been used to delineate a specific subgroup of depressive disorders, namely major depression with *melancholia* in DSM-5, or depressive episode with *somatic symptoms* in ICD-10 (see Box 9.2). The difficulty with this classification is that most patients have melancholic symptoms of some kind, although a careful search may be required to reveal them. Therefore the number of symptoms that are needed to fulfil the criterion

> ### Box 9.2 Clinical features of depression with 'somatic' or 'melancholic' features
>
> - Loss of interest or pleasure in usual activities
> - Lack of emotional reactivity to normally pleasurable surroundings and events
> - Early-morning waking (2 hours or more before usual time)
> - Depression worse in the morning
> - Psychomotor agitation or retardation
> - Marked loss of appetite
> - Weight loss (5% or more of body weight in last month)
> - Marked loss of libido (ICD-10 only)
> - Distinct quality of depressed mood (DSM-5 only)
> - Excessive guilt (DSM-5 only)
>
> At least four of these symptoms are required to make a diagnosis of depression 'with somatic features' (ICD-10) or major depression 'with melancholic features' (DSM-5). DSM-5 also specifically requires either 'loss of interest etc' or 'lack of emotional reactivity etc', to be present.

for depression with melancholia is somewhat arbitrary. Despite this caveat, it is generally agreed that clear-cut melancholic depression is associated with the following clinical correlates (see Parker *et al.*, 2015):

- more severe symptomatology
- family history of depression
- poor response to placebo medication
- possibly better response to tricyclic antidepressants than selective serotonin reuptake inhibitors (SSRIs)
- more evidence of neurobiological abnormalities (e.g. decreased latency to rapid eye movement sleep, cortisol hypersecretion).

It is still not clear whether melancholic depression is a distinct subtype or whether it represents a point on a continuum of severity of depression, towards the more severe end. Kendler (1997) attempted to answer this question using a population sample of twins. He found evidence that melancholic depression did represent a valid subtype in that it identified a group of individuals with a particularly high familial risk of depression. However, the diagnosis of melancholia indicated the presence of a *quantitatively* more severe form of depression, rather than a distinct aetiological subtype.

Psychotic depression

As noted above, severe depression can also be manifested with *psychotic features* (although in depressive psychosis the features of melancholia are almost invariably present as well). The presence of psychotic features indicates that treatment with antidepressant medication alone is unlikely to be successful, and that combination with antipsychotic drugs is usually needed (Cowen and Anderson, 2015).

Non-melancholic depression

In this classification by symptom profile, the remaining forms of major depression (*'non-melancholic' depression*) include several different kinds of clinical disorder—for example, mild depressive episodes and atypical depression. These depressions are more likely to have a relative prominence of features, such as *anxiety, hostility, phobias*, and *obsessional symptoms*. In the past, because of these symptoms, non-melancholic depressions were sometimes called 'neurotic depression', but this term does not appear in current diagnostic classifications. As noted above, *atypical depression* has particular clinical characteristics and in DSM-5 atypical depression, like melancholic depression, can be a specifier for a major depressive episode.

Classification by course

Unipolar and bipolar disorders

Mood disorders are characteristically *recurrent*, and Kraepelin was guided by the course of illness when he brought mania and depression together as a single entity. He found that the course was essentially the same whether the original disorder was manic or depressive, and so he put the two together in a single category of *manic–depressive psychosis*.

This view was widely accepted until 1962, when Leonhard and colleagues suggested a division into three groups:

- Patients who had had a depressive disorder only (*unipolar depression*).
- Those who had had mania only (*unipolar mania*).
- Those who had had both depressive disorder and mania (*bipolar*).

Nowadays, it is the usual practice not to use the term 'unipolar mania', but to include all cases of mania in the bipolar group on the grounds that nearly all patients who have mania eventually experience a depressive disorder (see Chapter 10).

Seasonal affective disorder

Some patients repeatedly develop a depressive disorder at the same time of year, usually the autumn or winter. In some cases the timing reflects extra demands placed on the person at a particular season of the year, either in work or in other aspects of their life. In other cases there is no such cause, and it has been suggested that seasonal affective disorder is related in some way to the changes in the seasons (e.g. to the number of hours of daylight). Although these seasonal affective disorders are characterized mainly by the time at which they occur, some symptoms are said to occur more often than in other mood disorders. These symptoms include:

- hypersomnia
- increased appetite, with craving for carbohydrate
- an afternoon slump in energy levels.

The most common pattern is onset in autumn or winter, and recovery in spring or summer. This condition is also called 'winter depression'. Some patients show evidence of hypomania or mania in the summer, which suggests that they have a seasonal bipolar illness. This pattern has led to the suggestion that shortening of daylight hours is important in the pathophysiology of winter depression, and treatment methods include exposure to bright artificial light during hours of darkness. DSM-5 has a specifier of 'seasonal pattern', which can be applied to recurrent major depression with an established seasonal onset. The use of bright light treatment is reviewed in Chapter 25.

Recurrent brief depression

Some individuals experience recurrent depressive episodes of short duration, typically 2–7 days, that are not of sufficient duration to meet the criteria for major depression or depressive episode. These episodes recur with some frequency, about once a month on average. There is no apparent link with the menstrual cycle in female sufferers. Although the depressive episodes are short, they are as severe as the more enduring depressive disorders, and can be associated with suicidal behaviour. Thus recurrent brief depression is associated with much personal distress and social and occupational impairment. Individuals with recurrent brief depression often receive treatment with antidepressant medication, but its value is questionable (see Baldwin and Sinclair, 2015).

Classification in DSM and ICD

The main categories in the sections on depressive disorders in DSM-5 and ICD-10 are shown in Table 9.1 and Box 9.3. Broad similarities are evident, together with some differences. The first similarity is that both systems contain categories for *single episodes* of mood disorder as well as categories for *recurrent episodes*. The second is that both recognize milder but persistent depressive states (*dysthymia*) although, as noted above, in DSM-5 dysthymia has been subsumed into the category of 'Persistent Depressive Disorder', which also includes 'Chronic Major Depression'. In DSM-5, mood disorders that are judged to be secondary to a medical condition are included as a subcategory of mood disorders, whereas in ICD-10 these conditions are classified as mood disorders under 'Organic Mental Disorders'.

Both ICD-10 and DSM-5 classify depressive episodes on the basis of *severity* and whether or not *psychotic features* are present. It is also possible to specify whether the depressive episode has melancholic (DSM-5) or somatic (ICD-10) features. In DSM-5, an episode of major depression with appropriate clinical symptomatology (see above) can be specified as atypical depression. In ICD-10, atypical depression is classified separately under 'Other depressive episodes.' Both ICD-10 and DSM-5 allow the diagnosis of recurrent brief

Table 9.1 **Classification of depressive disorders**

ICD-10	DSM-5
Depressive episode	**Major depressive episode**
Mild	Mild
Moderate	Moderate
Severe	Severe
Severe with psychosis	with psychotic features
Other depressive episodes	
Atypical depression	
Recurrent depressive disorder	**Major depressive disorder**
Currently mild	Recurrent
Currently moderate	
Currently severe	
Currently severe with psychosis	
In remission	
Persistent mood disorders	**Persistent depressive disorder**
Dysthymia	
Other mood disorders	**Other specified depressive disorder**
Recurrent brief	Recurrent brief depression
Depression	

Source: data from The ICD-10 classification of mental and behavioural disorders: clinical descriptions and diagnostic guidelines, Copyright (1992), World Health Organization; Diagnostic and Statistical Manual of Mental Disorders, Fifth Edition, Copyright (2013), American Psychiatric Association.

depression, but under slightly different headings (see Table 9.2). DSM-5 has some additional clinical specifiers which may have implications for treatment and prognosis (Table 9.3).

Classification and description in everyday practice

Although neither DSM-5 nor ICD-10 is entirely satisfactory, it seems unlikely that further rearrangement of descriptive categories would be an improvement. A solution will only be achieved when we have a better understanding of aetiology. Meanwhile, either ICD-10

Box 9.3 Additional specifiers for depressive disorders in DSM-5

- With anxious distress
- With mixed features
- With melancholic features
- With psychotic features
- With catatonia
- With peripartum onset

Source: data from Diagnostic and Statistical Manual of Mental Disorders, Fifth Edition, Copyright (2013), American Psychiatric Association.

Table 9.2 A systematic scheme for the clinical description of depressive episodes

The episode	
Severity	Mild, moderate, or severe
Special features	With melancholic symptoms
	With atypical symptoms
	With prominent anxiety
	With psychotic symptoms
	With agitation
	With retardation or stupor
The course	Single or recurrent episodes
Aetiological factors	Organic
	Family history of mood disorder
	Personal history of mood disorder
	Childhood experiences
	Personality
	Social support
	Life events

Table 9.3 The aetiology of mood disorders

Area of investigation	Relevant studies
Genetic	Genetic epidemiology
	Molecular genetics
Personality	Temperament
	Cognitive style
Early environment	Parental deprivation
	Childhood adversity and abuse
Social environment	Life events
	Chronic difficulties
Psychological	Psychodynamic
	Cognitive
Biological	Monoamines
	Hypothalamic–pituitary–adrenal axis
	Neuropsychology and brain imaging
	Neuropathology
	Neurogenesis, neurotropins, synaptic plasticity

or DSM-5 should be used for statistical recording. For most clinical purposes, it is better to describe disorders systematically than to classify them.

This can be done for every case by referring to the severity, the distinguishing symptomatic features, and the course of the disorder (Table 9.2), together with an evaluation of the relative importance of known aetiological factors (see Table 9.3).

Differential diagnosis of depressive disorders

Depressive disorders have to be distinguished from the following:

- normal sadness
- adjustment disorder
- anxiety disorders
- schizophrenia
- organic brain syndromes.

As already explained, the distinction from *normal sadness* is made on the basis of the presence of other symptoms of the syndrome of depressive disorder. Depressive disorders also have rates of *comorbidity* with a wide range of other disorders—for example, anxiety disorders, eating disorders, substance misuse, and personality disorder. In all of these cases it is important to recognize and treat the depressive disorder. *Adjustment disorders* following a stressor (see page 149) often present with depressed mood, together with tearfulness and feelings of hopelessness. However, the full diagnostic criteria for major depression are not met.

Anxiety disorders

Mild depressive disorders are sometimes difficult to distinguish from anxiety disorders. Accurate diagnosis depends on assessment of the relative severity of anxiety and depressive symptoms, and on the order in which they appeared. Similar problems arise when there are prominent phobic or obsessional symptoms, or when there are *dissociative* symptoms, with or without histrionic behaviour. In all of these cases, the clinician may fail to identify the depressive symptoms and so prescribe the wrong treatment.

Schizophrenia

The distinction from schizophrenia depends on a careful search for the characteristic features of this condition (see Chapter 11). Difficult diagnostic problems may arise when the patient has *depressive psychosis*, but here again the distinction can usually be made on the basis of a careful examination of the mental state, and of the order in which the symptoms appeared. Information about the past psychiatric history may also be useful. Particular difficulties also arise when symptoms characteristic of depressive disorder and of schizophrenia are found in equal measure in the same patient; these so-called *schizoaffective disorders* are discussed in Chapter 11

Dementia and other organic conditions

In middle and late life, depressive disorders are sometimes difficult to distinguish from *dementia*, because some patients with depressive symptoms complain of considerable difficulty in remembering. In fact, patients with severe depression can perform very badly on tests of cognitive function, and distinction between the two conditions purely in terms of the nature of the cognitive impairment may not be possible. Here the presence of depressive symptoms is the key to diagnosis, which should be confirmed with improvement of the memory disorder as normal mood is restored. Numerous other general medical conditions can present with depressive features (see Chapter 22). The key to diagnosis is a careful history and physical examination, supplemented by special investigations where appropriate.

The epidemiology of depressive disorders

It is difficult to determine the prevalence of depressive disorder, partly because different investigators have used different diagnostic definitions. More modern investigations have used structured diagnostic interviews linked to standardized diagnostic criteria, including the Diagnostic Interview Schedule (DIS) and the Composite International Diagnostic Interview (CIDI) (see Chapter 3).

Major depression

Defining the boundaries of depressive episodes in community surveys presents a number of difficulties. However, if the DSM criteria for major depression are applied, recent surveys in industrialized countries suggest that:

- The 12-month prevalence of major depression in the community is around 2–5%.
- The lifetime rates in different studies vary considerably (in the range 4–30%) and the true figure probably lies in the range 10–20%.
- The mean age of onset is about 27 years.
- Rates of major depression are about twice as high in women as in men, across different cultures.
- There may be increased rates of depression in people born since 1945.
- Rates of depression are higher in the unemployed and divorced.
- Major depression has a high comorbidity with other disorders, particularly anxiety disorders and substance misuse.

The reasons for *higher rates of major depression among women* are uncertain. This increase starts to become apparent at puberty, and could be due in part to a greater readiness of women to admit to having depressive symptoms. However, such selective reporting is unlikely to be the whole explanation. It is possible that some depressed men misuse alcohol and are diagnosed as suffering from alcohol-related disorders rather than depression, with the consequence that the true number of major depressive disorders is underestimated (Branney and White, 2008). Again, misdiagnosis of this kind is unlikely to account for the whole of the difference. Furthermore, in many societies women are subject to various kinds of social disadvantage and, for example, are more likely than men to experience sexual abuse and domestic violence. Factors of this sort are also likely to be implicated in their increased risk of depression. It is also important to note that the preponderance of depression in women emerges at puberty and seems more linked to changes in sex hormone levels than chronological age. This suggests a role of certain hormones in sensitizing the brain to the effects of stress (Thapar, 2012).

Although it used to be thought that the risk of depressive disorders increased with age, recent surveys suggest that major depression is most prevalent in the 18–44-year age group. A number of studies have suggested that people born since 1945 in industrialized countries have both a higher lifetime risk of major depression and an earlier age of onset. These studies have mainly been retrospective, and it is possible that the apparent increased rate of major depression in young people is due to the fact that older people forget (or are less willing to reveal) that they have been depressed. For a review of the epidemiology of mood disorders, see Joyce (2009).

Dysthymia and recurrent brief depression

The lifetime risk for *dysthymia* is around 4% (Alonso *et al.*, 2004). Rates of dysthymia are higher in *women* and in the *divorced*. There is less epidemiological information about *recurrent brief depression*, but in the Zurich prospective study the 12-month prevalence for recurrent brief depression was about 2.6%, very similar to the rate found for dysthmia (2.3%) (Pezawas *et al.*, 2003).

Minor anxiety–depressive disorders

Estimates of the frequency *of minor anxiety–depressive disorders* show wide variations because the different studies have not defined cases in the same way. However, these are probably the most prevalent psychiatric disorders in the community. For example, in the Adult Psychiatric Morbidity Survey in England, McManus *et al.* (2009) found that mixed anxiety and depression was the most common mental disorder in the community, with a 1-week prevalence of 9%.

The aetiology of depression

There have been many different approaches to the aetiology of depression. There is substantial knowledge about the *genetic epidemiology* of depression and how certain *childhood experiences* can lay down a predisposition to depressive disorders in adulthood. There is also a good understanding of the role of *current life difficulties and stresses* in provoking depression in predisposed individuals. There is much less knowledge about the mechanisms involved in the translation of these predisposing and provoking factors into clinical symptomatology.

When trying to elucidate these mechanisms (which, of course, have important implications for treatment), investigators have employed two main conceptual approaches, which can be broadly termed *psychological* and *biological*. It is likely, of course, that these approaches represent different levels of enquiry that will eventually inform each other. The aetiology section in the current chapter is structured so as to illustrate to the reader the many ways in which research into the causation of psychiatric disorder can be approached (see Box 9.4). It may therefore be helpful for this section to be read in conjunction with Chapter 5.

Genetic causes

Family and twin studies

It is well recognized that depression tends to run in families, and the risk of depression in a first-degree relative of a proband is increased about threefold. Environmental influences are also important in the aetiology of depression, but the effect of environment is mainly mediated through effects specific to the individual rather than through shared family experiences (Sullivan *et al.*, 2000). Relatives of patients with *unipolar depression* do not have increased rates of bipolar disorder or schizoaffective disorder.

Twin studies confirm that the aggregation of depressive disorders in families is in part due to genetic factors, with the *concordance rate* being higher in monozygotic twins (about 45%) than in dizygotic twins (about 20%). The heritability of major depression has been estimated at 37%, which is considerably less than that of bipolar disorder or schizophrenia (Bienvenu *et al.*, 2011). However, it is possible that certain types of study design (for example, clinical ascertainment of all twin pairs) might yield higher heritability estimates (Cohen-Woods *et al.*, 2013). Twin studies have also suggested that susceptibility to major depression and generalized anxiety disorder involves similar genes but different environmental risk factors (Hettema *et al.*, 2005).

Mode of inheritance

The familial segregation of depression does not fit a simple Mendelian pattern. The *female preponderance of depression* is well established, and it is possible that genetic factors play a somewhat greater aetiological role in women. However, the data are inconsistent, and meta-analyses reveal rather similar heritability estimates for men and women (Lau and Eley, 2010). Overall, it seems likely that the genetic liability to depression results from the combined action of multiple genes of modest, or small, effect—so-called *polygenic inheritance*—in a context of *gene–enviroment interaction*. Although many important environmental

> ### Box 9.4 Multifactorial origin of mood disorders
>
> - An important genetic contribution to mood disorder is made by multiple genes of small individual effect. This genetic contribution may be expressed directly through modification of relevant cortical circuitry, or indirectly through effects on personality and psychological coping mechanisms.
> - Adverse early life experiences also shape personality and limit subsequent attachment behaviour and ability to access social support. In addition, adverse early experience may affect development of the hypothalamic–pituitary–adrenal (HPA) axis and neurobiological responses to stress in adulthood.
> - Depressive disorders are often triggered by current life events, particularly in people who lack social support. The impact of life events is modified by early life experience, personality, and genetic inheritance. The interaction of these factors determines the resilience or vulnerability of an individual to a life event, and the subsequent risk of clinical mood disturbance.
> - The neurobiology of episodes of depression is associated with changes in the activity of monoamine neurons and the HPA axis, which together modify the activity of the neural circuitry involved in emotional regulation. At a cellular level this may involve a loss of synaptic plasticity and dendrite formation. Some structural and functional brain abnormalities in mood disorder suggest persistent biological vulnerability, probably produced by genetic inheritance or early developmental factors.

contributions to depression have been identified (see below), the level at which they interact with genetic predisposition remains unclear.

Molecular genetics

The monoamine theory of depression suggests that allelic variation in genes coding for monoamine synthesis or metabolism or specific receptors may contribute to the risk of mood disorders. There have been numerous association studies of such *candidate genes*, although the results have not been compelling because of the difficulty of replication. The gene coding for the *serotonin transporter* has a number of allelic variants, one of which, in the promotor region, influences the expression of transporter sites. The evidence implicating this polymorphism in major depression in population studies is inconsistent. However, in an influential study, Caspi *et al.* (2003) found evidence which suggested that people carrying a particular allele for the serotonin transporter were more likely to experience a subsequent episode of major depression when exposed to childhood adversity. The robustness of this particular gene–environment interaction has proved controversial (Fergusson *et al.*, 2012).

It is now possible to conduct *genome-wide association studies (GWAS)*, which do not rely on hypothesized candidate genes. Such studies face statistical difficulties with regard to the issue of multiple testing, but results from large investigations are becoming available. In contrast to results from GWAS studies in schizophrenia and bipolar disorder, GWAS studies in depression have not thus far reported any convincingly replicated loci. Cohen-Woods *et al.* (2013) suggest that reasons for this include insufficient sample sizes and the genetic heterogeneity of depression, as well as statistical problems with multiple comparisons. A recent whole genome sequencing study aimed to address the issue of heterogeneity by studying a large sample of Han Chinese women who suffered from severe recurrent depression. Two replicated genetic markers were identified, one of which, near the *SIRT1* gene, may be linked to mitochondrial function (CONVERGE Consortium, 2015).

Personality

Certain kinds of personality could be associated with predisposition to mood disorder. For example, it is a common clinical observation that patients with depression often seem to have high levels of premorbid anxiety. Aspects of personality could be associated with depression in a number of ways.

1. What is recognized as a personality characteristic may in fact represent a milder form of the illness. For example, while dysthymia is now regarded as a mood disorder, previously people with such symptoms might have been classified as having a 'depressive personality'.

2. Some personality features might influence the way in which people respond to adverse circumstances, and thus make depressive disorders more likely. For example, a cognitive style that is characterized by *sociotropy* (a strong need for approval) is associated with increased risk of depression after adverse life events (Mazure and Maciejewski, 2003).

3. Certain kinds of personality development and depressive disorder may share common genes. For example, *neuroticism*, as measured by the Eysenck Personality Questionnaire, predisposes to major depression, but twin studies suggest that neuroticism and major depression have genes in common (Fanous and Kendler, 2004).

Overall, current findings suggest that part of the genetic risk of depression takes the form of inheritance of particular character traits and cognitive styles, which predispose to psychiatric illness in the presence of specific kinds of life stresses (Rihmer *et al.*, 2010).

Early environment

Parental deprivation

Psychoanalysts have suggested that childhood deprivation of maternal affection through separation or loss predisposes to depressive disorders in adult life. Overall, however, epidemiological studies do not suggest that loss of a parent by death in childhood increases the risk of depressive disorder in adulthood. By contrast, there is more support for the proposal that depressive disorder in later life is associated with *parental separation*, particularly divorce. The key factor here appears to be not so much the loss itself as the discord and diminished care that result from it. Indeed, family discord and lack of adequate care predispose to depression even in families where separation does not occur (Brown, 2009).

Relationships with parents

It is clear that gross disruption of parent–child relationships, as occurs, for example, in *physical and sexual abuse*, is a risk factor for several kinds of adult psychiatric disorder, including major depression. It is less certain whether more subtle differences in *parental style* may also predispose to depression. One problem is the difficulty of determining retrospectively what kind of relationship a patient may have had with their parents in childhood. The patient's recollection of the relationship may be distorted by many factors, including the depressive disorder itself. However, it appears that both *non-caring* and *overprotective parenting styles* are associated with non-melancholic depression in adulthood (Parker and Hadzi-Pavlovic, 1992). Mothers with *postnatal depression* may manifest a rearing style that is characterized by neglect and emotional indifference. This could lead to longer-term deleterious effects on self-esteem and attachment style in the child, thus increasing the risk of depression in the subsequent generation (Ramchandani *et al.*, 2009).

Precipitating factors

Recent life events

It is an everyday clinical observation that depressive disorders often follow *stressful events*. However, several other possibilities must be discounted before it can be concluded that stressful events cause the depressive disorders that succeed them. First, the association might be *coincidental*. Secondly, the association might be *non-specific*—there might be as many stressful events in the weeks preceding other kinds of illness. Thirdly, the association might be *spurious*—the patient might have regarded the events as stressful only in retrospect when seeking an explanation for his illness, or he might have experienced them as stressful only because he was already depressed at the time. Finally, the depression itself might have caused the life event.

Research workers have tried to overcome each of these methodological difficulties. The first two problems—whether the events are coincidental, and whether any association is non-specific—require the use of control groups suitably chosen from the general population and from people with other illnesses. The third problem—whether the association is spurious—requires two other approaches. The first approach is to separate events that are undoubtedly independent of illness (e.g. losing a job because a whole factory closes) from events that may have been secondary to the illness (e.g. losing a job when no one else is dismissed). The second approach is to assign a rating to each event according to the consensus view of healthy people about its stressful qualities.

Methodologically reliable research has shown that:

- There is a sixfold excess of adverse life events in the months before the onset of depressive disorder.
- An excess of similar events also precedes suicide attempts, and the onset of anxiety disorders and schizophrenia.
- In general, 'loss' events are associated with depression and 'threat' events are associated with anxiety.
- Life events are important antecedents of all forms of depression, but appear to be relatively less important in established melancholic-type disorders and where there is a strong family history of depression.

Events that lead to feelings of *entrapment and humiliation* may be particularly relevant to the onset of depression, including peer victimization through bullying. In contrast, remission from depression is often associated with 'fresh-start' life events (e.g. establishing a new relationship or starting an educational course; Brown, 2009). It is also important to note that *genetic factors* may be involved in individual liability to experience life events. Thus certain individuals seem to be more prone to select *risky environments*, and genetic factors also play a role in how life events are *perceived* by a particular individual, perhaps through the personality mechanisms discussed above. In general, the importance of life events in the onset of a depressive episode decreases as the number of episodes increases. This suggests that, once a depressive disorder is clearly established, depressive episodes can occur in the absence of major environmental precipitants. This relationship is much less clear where there is a strong family history of depression, raising the possibility that one of the mechanisms by which a family history increases the risk of depression is by diminishing the need for a major environmental stressor during the first few episodes of the illness (Kendler *et al.*, 2001).

Vulnerability factors and life difficulties

It is a common clinical impression that the events immediately preceding a depressive disorder act as the 'last straw' for a person who has been subjected to a long period of adverse circumstances, such as an unhappy marriage, problems at work, or unsatisfactory housing.

In general, there is good evidence that *poor social support*, measured as lack of intimacy or social integration, is associated with an increased risk of depression (Brown, 2009). The mechanism of this association is unclear, and is open to different interpretations. First, it may be that a lack of opportunities to confide makes people more vulnerable. Secondly, it may indicate that depressed people have a distorted perception of the degree of intimacy that they achieved before becoming depressed. Thirdly, some other factor, presumably an abnormality in personality, may result in difficulty in confiding in others, and thus lead to vulnerability to depression.

The effects of physical illness

All medical illnesses and their treatment can act as *non-specific stressors*, which may lead to mood disorders in predisposed individuals. However, sometimes certain medical conditions are believed to play a more direct role in causing the mood disorder (e.g. brain disease, certain infections, including HIV, and endocrine disorders). The resulting mood disorders are known as organic mood disorders (for a further discussion of this subject, see Chapter 14).

Inevitably, the above distinction is arbitrary. For example, major depression occurs in about 50% of patients with *Cushing's disease*. Since not all patients with Cushing's disease suffer from depressive disorder, it follows that variables other than raised plasma cortisol levels are involved. However, organic mood disorders can give clues to aetiology. For example, depressive disorders in patients with Cushing's disease remit after cortisol levels are restored to normal, a finding that led to the proposal that increased cortisol levels may play a pathophysiological role in depression more generally (see hypothalamo-pituitray-adrenal axisbelow). It is also worth noting here that the *puerperium*, although not an illness, is associated with an increased risk of mood disorders (see Chapter 22).

Psychological approaches to aetiology

These theories are concerned with the psychological mechanisms by which recent and remote life experiences can lead to depressive disorders. Much of the literature on this subject fails to distinguish adequately between the symptom of depression and the syndrome of depressive disorder. The main approaches to the problem are derived from the ideas of psychoanalysis (see Box 9.5) and cognitive behavioural theories.

Cognitive theories

Depressed patients characteristically have recurrent and intrusive *negative thoughts* (*'automatic thoughts'*). Beck (1967) proposed that these depressive cognitions reveal negative views of the *self*, the *world*, and the *future* (the depressed patient usually reviews the past in a similar vein). These automatic thoughts appear to persist because of illogical ways of thinking, which Beck called *cognitive distortions*. These include:

- *Arbitrary inference* (drawing a conclusion when there is no evidence for it and even some evidence against it).
- *Selective abstraction* (focusing on a detail and ignoring more important features of a situation).
- *Overgeneralization* (drawing a general conclusion on the basis of a single incident).
- *Personalization* (relating external events to oneself in an unwarranted way).

Although most psychiatrists regarded these cognitions as secondary to a primary disturbance of mood, Beck suggested that another set of cognitions precede depression and predispose to it. These cognitions are *dysfunctional beliefs* or *schemas* such as 'No-one really likes me'. Schemas of this sort are established early in life, usually through childhood adversity, and affect the way in which a person responds to stress and adversity. Such schemas can become activated by 'matching' life experiences. For example, a failure in a relationship is more likely to provoke depression in a person who holds

---

> ### Box 9.5 **Psychoanalytical theory**
>
> - In his seminal paper 'Mourning and melancholia', Freud drew attention to the resemblance between the *phenomena of mourning* and *symptoms of depressive disorders,* and suggested that their causes might be similar (Freud, 1917).
> - Freud suggested that, just as mourning results from loss by death, so melancholia results from *loss of other kinds.* Since it was apparent that not every depressed patient had suffered an actual loss, it was necessary to postulate a loss of 'some abstraction' or internal representation, or, in Freud's terms, the loss of an 'object'.
> - Freud pointed out that depressed patients often appear to be critical of themselves, and he proposed that this self-accusation was really a disguised accusation of someone else for whom the patient 'felt affection'. In other words, depression was thought to occur when feelings of love and hostility were present at the same time (*ambivalence*). When a loved 'object' is lost, the patient feels despair; at the same time, any hostile feelings attached to this 'object' are redirected against the patient himself or herself as self-reproach.
> - Freud's ideas were developed by Melanie Klein (1882–1960), who believed that weaning (loss of the breast) represents a major symbolic loss for the infant, who then feels remorse and guilt about the disappearance of this 'good object'. In normal development this 'depressive anxiety' leads to attempts at reparation and concern for others. Failure to negotiate this process can result in depressive reactions in the face of future losses.
> - John Bowlby (1907–1990) showed that the rearing abilities of the main caregiver play an important role in giving the infant a secure emotional 'attachment', which is of critical importance in the development of satisfactory interpersonal relationships. Insecure attachments can increase the risk of various kinds of adult psychopathology, including depression.
>
> For a review of the psychoanalytical model of depression and its application to treatment, see Taylor (2008).

---

the dysfunctional belief described above (Clark and Beck, 2010) (Figure 9.1).

In fact, more recent investigations suggest that abnormalities in information processing, such as negative

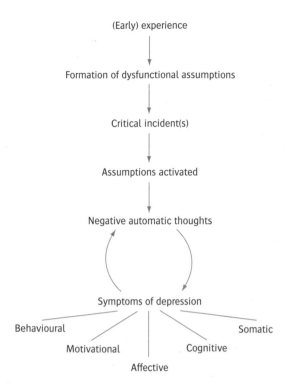

(Early) experience

↓

Formation of dysfunctional assumptions

↓

Critical incident(s)

↓

Assumptions activated

↓

Negative automatic thoughts

↓

Symptoms of depression

Behavioural   Somatic

Motivational   Cognitive

Affective

Figure 9.1 Cognitive model of how latent dysfunctional assumptions (laid down by early experience) are activated by critical incidents, leading to a vicious cycle of negative thinking and depressed mood.

Reproduced from Hawton K, Salkovskis PM, Kirk J, Clark DM, Cognitive Behaviour Therapy for Psychiatric Problems: A Practical Guide, Copyright (1989), with permission from Oxford University Press.

biases in facial expression recognition, can be demonstrated in both recovered depressed patients and those at high risk of depression prior to the development of illness (Victor *et al.*, 2010). Therefore it is possible that longstanding subtle negative biases in information processing may predispose to the development of depression, particularly in the context of psychosocial stress and adverse life events.

Neurobiological approaches to aetiology

Whatever their aetiology, the clinical manifestations of depressive disorders must presumably ultimately be mediated through changes in brain neurochemistry and the circuitry involved in emotional regulation. Biochemical investigations in depressed patients have focused on the *monoamine neurotransmitters* because monoamine pathways appear to play an important role in the actions of effective antidepressant drugs (see

below). Of course, the actions of antidepressant drugs may not reverse the cause of depression, but may merely change the expression of symptoms. However, another reason for studying monoamines is that they play an important role in mediating *adaptive responses to stressful events*, and depressive disorders can be viewed as a failure of these adaptive responses.

Monoamine pathways, particularly those involving noradrenaline and 5-hydroxytryptamine (5-HT), innervate cortical and subcortical brain regions thought to be involved in mood regulation. Recent studies have used structural and functional imaging techniques to elicit changes in the neural circuitry that underpins the expression of clinical affective symptomatology. In hand with this has come the realization that mood disorders, despite their fluctuating and remitting clinical course, are associated with distinct and persistent neuropathological changes in relevant brain regions. Some of these changes are likely to be developmental in origin; this could encompass either genetic inheritance or the consequences of adverse childhood experiences. There is currently much ongoing research effort in both animal and human studies to assess how traumatic experiences in development might affect the subsequent maturation of the hypothalamic–pituitary–adrenal (HPA) axis and thereby influence responses to environmental stress. A final point worth considering is that the prognosis of mood disorders worsens as the number of episodes increases. Although this phenomenon may simply represent an association between severity and poor prognosis, it is also possible that acute episodes of mood disturbance themselves produce neurobiological effects that worsen the subsequent prognosis (a phenomenon that is sometimes known as 'scarring').

The monoamine hypothesis

This hypothesis suggests that depressive disorder is due to an abnormality in a monoamine neurotransmitter system at one or more sites in the brain. In its early form, the hypothesis suggested a changed provision of the monoamine; more recent elaborations postulate alterations in receptors as well as in the concentrations or the turnover of the amines. Three monoamine transmitters have been implicated—*serotonin (5-HT), noradrenaline*, and *dopamine*. The latter two neurotransmitters are called *catecholamines*.

The hypothesis has been tested by observing three kinds of phenomenon:

- The biochemistry of neurotransmitters in patients with mood disorders.

- The effects of selective drugs on measurable indices of the function of monoamine systems—so-called 'challenge tests'.
- The pharmacological properties shared by antidepressant drugs.

The pharmacological effects of antidepressant drugs are considered in Chapter 25. The present chapter will consider the evidence for abnormalities in monoamine neurotransmitters in untreated depressed patients (see Box 9.6).

5-HT function

Plasma trypytophan. The synthesis of 5-HT in the brain depends on the availability of its precursor amino acid, l -tryptophan. *Plasma tryptophan levels* are decreased in untreated depressed patients, particularly in those with melancholic depression. Studies in healthy subjects have shown that weight loss through dieting can lower plasma tryptophan levels, and this factor appears to explain some, but not all, of the reduction in plasma tryptophan concentration that is seen in depression. Decreases in plasma tryptophan levels may contribute to the impairments that are seen in brain 5-HT function in depressed patients, but are probably not an important causal factor (Cowen, 2015).

Studies of cerebrospinal fluid. Indirect evidence about 5-HT function in the brains of depressed patients has been sought by examining cerebrospinal fluid (CSF).

Numerous studies have been carried out, but overall the data do not suggest that drug-free patients with major depression have a consistent reduction in CSF concentrations *of 5-hydroxyindoleacetic acid (5-HIAA)*, the main metabolite of 5-HT formed in the brain. However, there is more consistent evidence that depressed patients who have made impulsive and more dangerous suicide attempts have *low CSF 5-HIAA levels*. This finding is not restricted to patients with depression. It has also been reported in, for example, patients with schizophrenia and personality disorder who have a history of aggressive behaviour directed towards themselves or other people. It has been proposed that low levels of CSF 5-HIAA, although not related specifically to depression, may be associated with a tendency of individuals to respond in an impulsive and hostile way to life difficulties (Moberg *et al.*, 2011).

Studies of post-mortem brain. Measurements of 5-HT and 5-HIAA have been made in the brains of depressed patients who have died, usually by suicide. Although this is a more direct test of the monoamine hypothesis, the results are difficult to interpret for two reasons. First, the observed changes may have taken place after death. Secondly, the changes may have been caused before death, but by factors other than the depressive disorder (e.g. by anoxia, or by drugs used in treatment or taken to commit suicide). Overall there is little consistent evidence that depressed patients dying from natural causes or suicide have lowered brain concentrations of 5-HT or 5-HIAA. Other studies have adopted techniques such as receptor autoradiography and mRNA expression. Such studies have suggested that suicide victims have increased expression of 5-HT$_{2A}$ receptors and decreases in serotonin transporters (5-HT reuptake sites) in the prefrontal cortex. However, the data are not consistent (Stockmeier, 2003).

Neurochemical brain imaging studies. Recent developments in brain imaging with selective labelled ligands have enabled the assessment of certain brain 5-HT receptor subtypes *in vivo*. There is evidence of a widespread modest *decrease in 5-HT$_{1A}$-receptor binding* throughout the cortical and subcortical regions (Meyer, 2013). There also appear to be *reductions in the number of brainstem and limbic region 5-HT reuptake sites* in depressed individuals (Kambeitz and Howes, 2015).

Neuroendocrine tests. The functional activity of 5-HT systems in the brain has been assessed by giving a substance that stimulates 5-HT function, and by measuring an endocrine response that is controlled by 5-HT pathways, usually the release of *prolactin, growth hormone*, or *cortisol*. Neuroendocrine challenge tests have the advantage that they measure an aspect of brain 5-HT

Box 9.6 **Evidence for abnormalities in monoamine activity in depression**

5-HT

- Decreased plasma tryptophan
- Blunted 5-HT neuroendocrine responses
- Decreased brain 5-HT$_{1A}$ receptor binding (PET)
- Decreased brain 5-HT reuptake sites (SPET and PET)
- Clinical relapse after tryptophan depletion

Noradrenaline

- Blunted noradrenaline-mediated growth hormone release
- Clinical relapse after α-methyl-para-tyrosine (AMPT)

Dopamine

- Decreased homovanillic acid (HVA) levels in cerebrospinal fluid
- Clinical relapse after AMPT

function. However, the 5-HT synapses that are involved presumably reside in the *hypothalamus*, which means that important changes in 5-HT pathways in other brain regions could be missed. A number of drugs have been used to increase brain 5-HT function for the purposes of neuroendocrine challenge.

Studies in unmedicated depressed patients have shown consistent evidence that 5-HT-mediated endocrine responses are blunted in depressed patients. A number of these abnormalities persist into clinical recovery, which suggests that there is persistent dysfunction of some aspects of 5-HT neurotransmission in those at risk of depression (Cowen, 2015).

Tryptophan depletion. Although the findings outlined above provide strong evidence that aspects of brain 5-HT neurotransmission are abnormal in depression, they do not reveal whether these changes are central to *pathophysiology* or might instead represent some form of *epiphenomenon*. To assess this, it is necessary to study the psychological consequences of lowering brain 5-HT function in healthy subjects and those at risk of mood disorder.

As mentioned above, the synthesis of brain 5-HT is dependent on the availability in the brain of its amino acid precursor, l-tryptophan. It is possible to produce a transient lowering of plasma tryptophan and brain 5-HT function over a few hours by administering a mixture of amino acids that lacks tryptophan. This procedure is called *tryptophan depletion*. Tryptophan depletion in subjects with no personal or family history of mood disorder has little measurable effect on mood, and does not produce significant clinical depressive symptomatology. By contrast, unmedicated euthymic patients with a personal history of mood disorder undergo a *rapid but temporary depressive relapse* when exposed to tryptophan depletion. People with a strong family history of depression but no previous illness show some lowering of mood after tryptophan depletion, but these changes are relatively mild and not of clinical severity. The following conclusions can be drawn.

- Low brain 5-HT function is *not sufficient* to cause depression, because tryptophan depletion fails to alter mood in those who are not vulnerable to mood disorder.
- Low brain 5-HT function appears to interact with *other vulnerability factors* to cause depressive symptoms.

The nature of these other vulnerability factors remains conjectural. It is possible that the 5-HT pathways of vulnerable individuals react abnormally to precursor deficit. Alternatively, there may be pre-existing deficits in the central mood-regulating circuitry that are 'revealed' in the presence of low brain 5-HT states. For a review of tryptophan depletion studies in depression, see Ruhe *et al.* (2007).

Noradrenaline function

Metabolism and receptors. There is no consistent evidence that *brain or CSF concentrations of noradrenaline* or its major metabolite, *3-methoxy-4-hydroxy-phenylethylene glycol (MHPG)*, are altered in depressed patients (Anand and Charney, 2000). As with 5-HT receptors, noradrenaline receptors in the brain can be divided into a number of subclasses. There is some evidence that depressed patients who die from suicide have increased expression of α_2-*adrenoceptor binding* in some brain regions (Escriba *et al.*, 2004).

Neuroendocrine tests. Increasing brain noradrenaline function elevates plasma concentrations of adrenocorticotropic hormone (ACTH), cortisol, and growth hormone. There is fairly consistent evidence that the *growth hormone* response to both the noradrenaline reuptake inhibitor *desipramine* and the noradrenaline-receptor agonist *clonidine* is blunted in patients with melancholic depression. Clonidine acts directly on *postsynaptic* α_2-*adrenoceptors* in the hypothalamus to increase plasma growth hormone, and therefore the blunted response in depressed patients suggests a decreased responsivity of hypothalamic postsynaptic α_2-adrenoceptors. Clearly this finding appears to be inconsistent with the increased expression of α_2-adrenoceptors in cortical regions noted above.

Catecholamine depletion. It is possible to lower the synthesis of catecholamines by inhibiting the enzyme *tyrosine hydroxylase*, which catalyses the conversion of the amino acid tyrosine to l-DOPA, a precursor of both noradrenaline and dopamine. The drug that is used to achieve this effect is α-*methyl-para-tyrosine (AMPT)*. In healthy subjects, AMPT produces sedation but not significant depressive symptoms. However, as with tryptophan depletion, when administered to recovered depressed patients off drug treatment it causes a *striking clinical relapse in depressive symptomatology* (Ruhe *et al.*, 2007). This could be mediated by diminished function of either dopamine or noradrenaline, or by combined inhibition of both of these neurotransmitters.

These findings suggest that subjects at risk of mood disorder are *vulnerable to decreases in both 5-HT and catecholamine neurotransmission*. This is consistent with the clinical evidence that drugs that act selectively on noradrenaline or 5-HT pathways are effective antidepressant treatments.

Dopamine function

The function of dopamine in depression has been less well studied than that of 5-HT or noradrenaline, but there are a number of reasons for believing that dopamine neurons may be involved in the pathophysiology of the depressed state.

- Dopamine neurons in the mesolimbic system play a key role in incentive behaviour and reward. These processes are disrupted in depression, particularly melancholic states.
- Antidepressant treatments in animals increase the expression of dopamine receptors in the part of the mesolimbic system called the *nucleus accumbens*.

There is some evidence that suggests that dopamine function may be abnormal in depression. For example, CSF levels of the dopamine metabolite *homovanillic acid (HVA)* are consistently low in depressed patients, and some brain imaging studies in depressed patients have found increased binding of dopamine D_2/D_3 receptors in striatal regions. However, this may be restricted to patients with psychomotor retardation. There is also limited evidence for regional reductions in the density of dopamine D_1 receptors (Meyer, 2013). These findings, taken together with the effect of AMPT in causing relapse in recovered depressed patients, suggest that impaired dopamine function may play a role in the manifestation of the depressive syndrome and in the effects of antidepressant drug treatment.

Role of monoamines in depression

There is now good evidence that unmedicated depressed patients have abnormalities in various aspects of monoamine function. However, these abnormalities vary in extent from one case to another, and the changes are not large and are not sufficiently sensitive to be diagnostic. Some abnormalities may also persist into clinical recovery, suggesting that they are related to vulnerability to illness rather than the acute depressive state.

The most convincing studies that show a key role for monoamines in the pathophysiology of depression are the *5-HT and catecholamine depletion paradigms*. This is because lowering of 5-HT and noradrenaline and dopamine function is sufficient to cause clinical depression in those at risk by virtue of a previous illness. It is unclear what neurobiological changes produce this psychological vulnerability to monoamine depletion, but it seems likely that they are at least in part consequences of previous episodes of illness and perhaps their treatment.

Amino acid neurotransmitters

Developments in magnetic resonance spectroscopy (MRS) have facilitated measurement of the amino acid neurotransmitters *gamma-aminobutyric acid (GABA)* and *glutamate* in the brain in patients with mood disorders. Overall, there is evidence for decreased levels of glutamate in the anterior brain regions in depressed patients (Arnone *et al.*, 2015). Brain levels of GABA are also lowered in depression, although for technical reasons much of this work involves measurement in the occipital cortex. GABA concentrations may also be lower in patients with panic disorder, consistent with the known role of GABA in anxiety (Sanacora, 2010).

There is growing interest in the role of glutamate in mood disorders, partly because drugs with glutamatergic properties might be helpful in treatment. For example, the NMDA-receptor antagonist *ketamine* can produce rapid and striking, albeit transient, relief of symptomatology in patients with treatment-refractory depression (McGirr *et al.*, 2015).

Endocrine abnormalities

Abnormalities in endocrine function may be important in aetiology for two reasons.

- Some disorders of endocrine function are followed by mood disorders more often than would be expected by chance, suggesting a causative relationship.
- Endocrine abnormalities found in depressive disorder indicate that there may be a disorder of the hypothalamic centres that control the endocrine system.

Endocrine pathology and depression

About 50% of patients with *Cushing's syndrome* suffer from major depression, which usually remits when the cortisol hypersecretion is corrected. Depression also occurs in *Addison's disease, hypothyroidism*, and *hyperparathyroidism*. Endocrine changes may account for depressive disorders that occur *premenstrually*, during the *menopause*, and after *childbirth*. These clinical associations are discussed further in Chapter 22.

Hypothalamic–pituitary–adrenal axis

Much research effort has been concerned with abnormalities in the control of cortisol in depressive disorders. In about 50% of patients whose depressive disorder is at least moderately severe, *plasma cortisol secretion is increased* throughout the 24-hour cycle. This increase in cortisol secretion is associated with enlargement of the adrenal gland and increased cortisol response to corticotropin (ACTH) challenge.

When studying depressed patients, use has been made of the *dexamethasone suppression test*, which suppresses cortisol levels via inhibition of ACTH release at pituitary level. About 50% of depressed inpatients do not show the normal suppression of cortisol secretion induced by administering 1 mg of the synthetic corticosteroid dexamethasone, an agent which suppresses ACTH via interaction with specific *glucocorticoid receptors*.

Dexamethasone non-suppression is more common in depressed patients with *melancholia*, but it has not been reliably linked with any more specific psychopathological feature. However, abnormalities in the dexamethasone suppression test are not confined to mood disorders; they have also been reported in mania, chronic schizophrenia, and dementia. This lack of diagnostic specificity diminished early hopes that dexamethasone non-suppression could be used as a diagnostic marker of melancholic depression.

The diminished responsivity to dexamethasone that is seen in depressed patients led to the *glucocorticoid-receptor hypothesis* of depression, whereby dysfunction of the HPA axis and the resulting depressive syndrome are linked to genetic or acquired defects of glucocorticoid receptors. This has coincided with findings from animal experimental studies that different classes of antidepressant medication increase expression of glucocorticoid receptors. Therefore one therapeutic mechanism of antidepressant drug action may be to normalize excessive HPA axis activity via increased ability of the glucocorticoid receptors to provide feedback regulation (Gold, 2015).

In general, HPA axis changes in depressed patients have been regarded as *state abnormalities*—that is, they remit when the patient recovers. However, there is some evidence that changes in HPA axis function may persist in recovered depressed subjects. This suggests that some vulnerable individuals may have fairly enduring abnormalities in HPA axis regulation (Cowen, 2015). In experimental animal studies, early adverse experiences produce longstanding changes in HPA axis regulation, indicating a possible neurobiological mechanism whereby childhood trauma could be translated into increased vulnerability to mood disorder. Recent studies have confirmed that adults who were abused as children have altered HPA responses to stress (Juruena *et al.*, 2015)

Corticotropin-releasing hormone (CRH) and depression. In addition to its effects on cortisol secretion, CRH may play a more direct role in the aetiology of depression. It is well established that CRH has a *neurotransmitter role* in limbic regions of the brain, where it is involved in regulating biochemical and behavioural responses to stress. Administration of CRH to animals produces changes in neuroendocrine regulation, sleep, and appetite that parallel those found in depressed patients. Furthermore, CRH levels may be increased in the CSF of depressed patients. Therefore it is possible that *hypersecretion of CRH* could be involved in the pathophysiology of the depressed state, and non-peptide antagonists of CRH receptors may have value as antidepressant agents. For a review of this subject, see Gold (2015).

Thyroid function

Circulating plasma levels of free thyroxine appear to be normal in depressed patients, but levels of *free triiodothyronine* may be decreased. About 25% of depressed patients have a *blunted thyrotropin-stimulating hormone (TSH)* response to intravenous thyrotropin-releasing hormone (TRH). This abnormality is not specific to depression, as it is also found in alcoholism and panic disorder. Like CRH, TRH has a role in brain neurotransmission and is found in brain neurons colocalized with classical monoamine neurotransmitters such as 5-HT. Therefore it is possible that the abnormalities in thyroid function that are found in depressed patients may be associated with changes in central TRH regulation (Bunevicius and Prange, 2010).

Depression and the immune system

There is growing evidence that patients with depression manifest a variety of disturbances of immune function. Earlier studies found decreases in the cellular immune responses of lymphocytes in depressed patients, but more recent research has produced evidence of immune activation, with increases in particular in the release of certain proinflammatory *cytokines* (see Box 9.7). Cytokines are known to provoke HPA axis activity, and therefore changes in immune regulation may play a role in HPA axis dysfunction in depression.

It is also possible that the changes seen in immune activity are secondary to other depressive features (e.g. lowered food intake and diminished self-care). However, the fact that medical administration of some cytokines (e.g. interferon and tumour necrosis factor) can cause significant depressive symptoms suggests that, in some situations, changes in immune function may have a more direct role in provoking mood disorders. Current formulations propose that cytokines can induce expression of the tryptophan-metabolizing enzyme *indoleamine 2, 3-dioxygenase*. This lowers tryptophan levels, which could put vulnerable individuals at risk of depression. Peripheral markers of inflammation have also been linked to treatment resistance in depressed patients (Nanni *et al.*, 2012). For a review of inflammation and depression, see Hodes *et al.* (2015).

- Lowered proliferative responses of lymphocytes to mitogens
- Lowered natural killer cell activity
- Increases in positive acute phase proteins
- Increases in inflammatory cytokine levels (e.g. IL-6 and TNFα)
- Induction of indoleamine 2,3-dioxygenase

Sleep changes in depression

Disturbed sleep is characteristic of depression. Recordings of the sleep EEG (polysomnogram) have shown a number of abnormalities in *sleep architecture* in patients with major depression, including the following:

- impaired sleep continuity and duration
- decreased deep sleep (stages 3 and 4)
- decreased latency to the onset of rapid eye movement (REM) sleep
- an increase in the proportion of REM sleep in the early part of the night.

Decreased REM sleep latency is of interest in relation to aetiology because there is some evidence that it may persist in recovered depressed patients and indicate a vulnerability to relapse. A further link between REM sleep and depression is that many (but not all) effective antidepressant drugs decrease REM sleep time and the latency to its onset. In addition, both *total sleep deprivation* and *selective REM sleep deprivation* can produce a temporary alleviation of mood in depressed patients. For a review, see Steiger and Kimura (2010).

Brain imaging in mood disorder

Structural brain imaging

Changes in brain volume. Computerized tomography (CT) and magnetic resonance imaging (MRI) studies have found a number of abnormalities in patients with depression, particularly in those with more *severe and chronic disorder* (Arnone *et al.*, 2012). The most consistent findings are:

- Enlarged lateral ventricles (predominantly in elderly subjects with late-onset depression).
- Decreased hippocampal volume.
- Decreased volume of basal ganglia structures.

- Decreased grey matter volume in the anterior brain areas, including frontal cortex, orbitofrontal cortex, and cingulate cortex.

The origin of these structural abnormalities is unclear, but might be related to the cellular neuropathological abnormalities that have been described in depression, such as loss of interneurons and glial cells in anterior brain regions (see Falkai and Bogerts, 2009). The *neurotrophic hypothesis* of depression suggests that stress (perhaps aided by cortisol hypersecretion) can lead to atrophy and death of neurons and downregulation of adult neurogenesis, particularly in the hippocampus (Duman, 2009). Conceivably processes of this kind could lead to the kind of structural deficits that are listed above. In elderly subjects with late-onset depression, structural brain changes may be attributable to *cardiovascular disease*.

White matter hyperintensities. Hyperintense MRI signals can be detected in a number of regions in both normal ageing subjects and older patients with major depression. The usual sites are in the deep white matter and periventricular white matter. In major depression, increased deep white matter hyperintensities are associated with the following:

- Late onset of depressive disorder.
- Greater illness severity and poorer treatment response.
- Apathy, psychomotor slowness, and retardation.
- The presence of vascular risk factors.

It has been proposed that major depression with these clinical and radiological features is likely to be caused by vascular disease, which presumably impairs functioning in the pathways involved in mood regulation (Aizenstein *et al.*, 2011).

Cerebral blood flow and metabolism

Cerebral blood flow can be measured in a number of ways—for example, with single-photon emission tomography (SPET), positron emission tomography (PET), or functional magnetic resonance imaging (fMRI). PET can also be used to measure cerebral metabolism. Cerebral blood flow and metabolism are normally highly correlated.

Numerous studies have examined both cerebral metabolism and blood flow in groups of depressed patients. The findings have often been contradictory, and there are many methodological factors, such as patient selection, drug status, and imaging techniques. However, there is a growing consensus that the abnormalities in functional brain imaging in depression support a circuitry model in which mood disorders are associated with *abnormal interactions between several brain regions*, rather than a major abnormality in a single structure. The circuitry that is implicated involves regions of the medial prefrontal cortex, anterior cingulate cortex, amygdala, ventral striatum, thalamus, and hypothalamus (Price and Drevets, 2012). Some tentative correlations between these brain regions and clinical depressive features are listed in Box 9.8.

More recent studies have used 'resting state fMRI' (see Chapter 5) to examine activity in different brain circuits in depression. The *default mode network* becomes active at rest, for example, during 'mind-wandering', and shows decreased activity during specific tasks. Some studies have shown that, in depressed patients, the default mode network remains active even during task-based activity, and this has been proposed to correlate with depressive ruminative thinking and impaired performance on cognitive tasks (Kaiser *et al.*, 2015).

Neuropsychological changes in mood disorder

Patients with acute depression and mania show poor performance on several measures of *neuropsychological*

---

function. Impairment is typically seen over a wide range of neuropsychological domains, including *attention, learning, memory, and executive function*. There is disagreement as to whether these defects are best regarded as global and diffuse, or whether there may be some selectivity with regard to the changes that are seen. However, some authors have suggested that deficits in executive function may be particularly prominent, which would be consistent with the abnormalities seen in prefrontal perfusion in imaging studies.

Most of the cognitive impairments resolve as the mood disorder remits, but a growing literature attests to the persistence of cognitive defects, albeit less striking, in euthymic patients with recurrent depression (Clark *et al.*, 2009). Such deficits are particularly apparent in elderly patients, in whom they have been found to correlate with decreases in hippocampal volume.

As noted above, depression is clinically associated with negative biases in the *processing of emotional information*. Behavioural studies have shown that such biases affect *attention to emotional stimuli* as well as *emotional perception, memory and appraisal*. There is growing understanding of the neural circuitry that underpins emotional processing, in particular the way that limbic brain regions interact with regulatory cortical areas. In patients with depression, functional imaging studies have shown that presentation of negative emotional stimuli (e.g. fearful faces) is associated with overactivity of limbic regions, whereas there is a decrease in activity in the prefrontal regulatory areas. These changes are reversed by antidepressant medication, but are still apparent in recovered patients who have been withdrawn from medication. This suggests that *exaggerated limbic processing of aversive material* may be a trait marker of vulnerability to depression (Victor *et al.*, 2010).

Conclusions

The *predisposition* to develop depressive disorders has an important genetic contribution. The levels at which genetic factors operate are not entirely clear. They could act via effects on the regulation of neural responses to emotion, or through more remote factors such as temperament and the psychological response to stressful life events. Adverse early experiences such as parental conflict, or abuse of various kinds, may play a part in shaping features of personality which in turn determine whether, in adulthood, individuals are able to access emotional support to help to buffer the stressful effects of social adversity. In addition, early life experiences could programme the HPA axis to respond to stress in a

---

> **Box 9.8 Some neuropsychological correlates of altered cerebral perfusion and metabolism in depressed patients**
>
> **Dorsolateral and dorsomedial prefrontal cortex**
> - Cognitive dysfunction (particularly executive dysfunction). Impaired voluntary regulation of emotion
>
> **Medial prefrontal cortex**
> - Abnormal emotional processing
>
> **Anterior cingulate**
> - Impaired attentional processes
> - Altered emotional salience
>
> **Amygdala**
> - Abnormal emotional processing
>
> **Ventral striatum**
> - Impaired incentive behaviour
> - Psychomotor disturbances

way that might predispose to the development of mood disorder.

The *precipitating causes* of mood disorders are stressful life events and certain kinds of physical illness. Some progress has been made in discovering the types of event that provoke depression, and in quantifying their stressful qualities. Such studies show that *loss* can be an important precipitant, but not the only one. The effects of particular events may be modified by a number of background factors that may make a person more vulnerable—for example, being bullied or socially isolated. As noted in the preceding paragraph, the impact of potentially stressful events also depends on early life experience, personality factors, and probably genetic inheritance.

Two kinds of *pathophysiological mechanism* have been proposed to explain how precipitating events lead to the phenomena observed in depressive disorders. The first mechanism is psychological and the second is neurobiological. The two sets of mechanism are not mutually exclusive and, as the neural basis of emotional processing becomes better understood, the two approaches are converging in a way that promises a richer understanding of pathophysiology. In particular it seems that abnormalities in the neural processing of emotion can account for the emotional biases that are characteristic of depression, and can probably account for much of the subjective symptomatology. The relevant brain regions receive a strong innervation from monoamine neurons, and manipulation of 5-HT and noradrenaline neurotransmission is capable of altering emotional processing at both a behavioural level and a neural level (Harmer *et al.*, 2009). This might account for the role of monoamine changes in the pathophysiology of depression, and the ability of monoamine manipulation to produce symptomatic relief in some depressed patients.

Using sophisticated statistical techniques it is possible to derive quantitative estimates of the roles of different *risk factors* in the development of depressive disorders. For example, from a prospective study of 1942 female twin pairs, Kendler *et al.* (2002) calculated that about 50% of the susceptibility to an episode of major depression is attributable to the following factors (in order of relative importance):

- recent stressful life events and difficulties
- adolescent risk factors (neuroticism, early-onset anxiety, and conduct disorder)
- genetic risk
- past history of major depression.

The same study found that adverse childhood experiences also played a significant role in the risk of subsequent depression, but this was expressed indirectly through an increased risk of life events and difficulties and diminished social support. Interestingly, some of the impact of genetic factors was mediated through an increased risk of early adverse experiences. This suggests that part of the genetic risk associated with depression is expressed though greater likelihood of exposure to an adverse family environment. This in turn could be linked to temperamental factors in both parents and children.

Taken together, the findings of recent studies show that major depression is a disorder with important genetic, environmental, and interpersonal determinants. These factors do not interact in a simple additive manner, but modify each other in both direct and indirect ways. Although this formulation precludes the use of simple models to explain the aetiology of major depression, it does correspond more closely with clinical experience. In addition, it suggests that a number of different kinds of intervention could be useful for decreasing the liability of individuals to develop depression.

Course and prognosis of depression

Major depression

When considering course and prognosis of major depression it should be remembered that any sample of patients with unipolar depression will contain a proportion of patients who in fact have a bipolar disorder which has not yet declared itself (since mania or hypomania have not yet occurred). It has been estimated that about 10% of patients who present with a depressive disorder will eventually

have a manic illness. Such patients are more likely to have a family history of mania or to show brief, mild manic mood swings during antidepressant treatment.

- The age of onset of major depression varies widely and can occur at any point in the lifespan. About half of all cases occur before the age of 21. The relative contribution of different aetiological factors probably varies between early- and late-onset cases.

- The average length of a depressive episode is about 6 months, but around 25% of patients have episodes that last for more than 1 year, and around 10–20% develop a chronic unremitting course.

- About 80% of patients with major depression will experience further episodes (i.e. have recurrent major depression).

- Over a 25-year follow-up, patients with recurrent major depression experience on average about four further episodes.

- The interval between episodes becomes progressively shorter.

- About 50% of depressed patients do not achieve complete symptom remission between episodes, and experience continuing subsyndromal depressive symptomatology of fluctuating severity.

- The longer-term prognosis of recurrent major depression is modest. For example, only about 25% of patients with recurrent depression achieve a period of 5 years of clinical stability with good social and occupational performance.

Dysthymia

Dysthymia is by definition a chronic disorder that lasts for many years. Despite this, about 50% of outpatients may be expected to show a clinical recovery over a 5-year follow-up. Over the lifespan, some patients with dysthymia develop major depression (so-called *double depression*), while some patients who originally present with major depression subside into dysthymia. The development of mania is rare.

Minor depressive disorders

Minor depressive conditions are depressive disorders that do not meet threshold criteria for major depression, even of mild severity ('Unspecified Depressive Disorder' in DSM-5). These conditions show a recurrence rate similar to that of major depression. Patients who meet the criteria for minor depression at one point in follow-up may then subsequently be diagnosed as suffering from major depression, and vice versa. Thus, in a similar manner to dysthymia, minor depression is likely to be a *risk factor* for major depression, and may also be a *residual state* following remission of major depression. Overall, the longitudinal data suggest that major and minor depression and dysthymia are not distinct conditions, but represent part of a *spectrum of depressive disorders* (Angst, 2009).

Mortality of depressive disorders

Mortality is significantly increased in patients with depression, largely, although not exclusively, due to *suicide*. The standardized mortality ratio in mood disorders is about twice that found in the general population. Apart from suicide, excess deaths are due to accidents, cardiovascular disease, and comorbid substance misuse. There is now compelling evidence that depressive disorders increase the risk of general medical conditions such as diabetes and cardiovascular disease. Possible common pathophysiological mechanisms include inflammation and increased cortisol secretion (Nemeroff and Goldschmidt-Clermont, 2012). Epidemiological studies suggest that treatment lowers the mortality in patients with depression (Angst *et al.*, 2013).

Rates of suicide in patients with depression are at least 15 times higher than those in the general population, and tend to be higher in unipolar than in bipolar disorder (Angst, 2009). Longer-term follow-up of patients with depression has yielded differing rates of lifetime risk of suicide. In those with severe illnesses who have been treated as inpatients, the risk may be as high as 15%. However, in community samples the risk is lower. The proportion of patients with mood disorders who die by suicide decreases as the period of follow-up increases, presumably because mortality from natural causes becomes more significant. However, it is also possible that the risk of suicide is highest during the early stages of the illness.

Prognostic factors

The best predictor of the future course is the history of *previous episodes*. Not surprisingly, the risk of recurrence is much higher in individuals with a history of *several previous episodes*. Other factors that predict a higher risk of future episodes include the following:

- incomplete symptomatic remission
- early age of onset
- poor social support
- poor physical health
- comorbid substance misuse
- comorbid personality disorder.

The various risk factors, particularly previous pattern of recurrence and the extent of current remission, have important implications for the use of longer-term maintenance treatments (see below). In many patients, depressive disorders are best conceptualized as chronic relapsing conditions that require an integrated long-term treatment approach.

The acute treatment of depression

This section is concerned with the *efficacy of various forms of treatment* in the acute management of depression. Details of treatment with drugs and ECT are provided in Chapter 25, which should be consulted before reading this section. Advice on the selection of treatments and the day-to-day care of patients is given in the section on management (see 'The management of depressive disorders' below).

Antidepressant drugs

Antidepressant drugs are effective in the acute treatment of major depression. The largest effects relative to placebo are seen in patients with major depression whose symptoms are of at least *moderate severity*. Short-term response rates in controlled trials are about 50% for patients on active treatment, and about 30% for those on placebo; the number needed to treat (NNT) is between 5 and 7 (Cleare *et al.*, 2015). In terms of efficacy there is little to choose between the various antidepressants, although some are better than others in certain defined situations.

Similar clinical response rates are seen in *dysthymia*, where again several classes of antidepressant drugs, including tricyclic antidepressants and SSRIs, have shown therapeutic efficacy. A meta-analysis by Levkovitz *et al.* (2011) showed a response rate in patients receiving active treatment of 52%, compared with 29% in those on placebo (NNT = 5). Antidepressants do not appear to be more effective than placebo in the treatment of minor depression (Barbui and Cipriani, 2011).

Tricyclic antidepressants

Tricyclic antidepressants have been extensively compared with placebo in both inpatients and outpatients with major depression. In all but the most severely depressed patients, tricyclic antidepressants are clearly more effective than placebo (Morris and Beck, 1974). There is little evidence that tricyclic antidepressant drugs differ from one another in clinical efficacy, but they do differ in terms of their side effect profile (see Chapter 25). *Lofepramine* is relatively safe in overdose. Among the other classes of antidepressant drug, none is more effective than the tricyclics, although individual patients may show a preferential response to other compounds (see below). Tricyclics are probably not effective treatments for adolescents with depression (for the drug treatment of depression in young people, see Chapter 16).

Selective serotonin reuptake inhibitors and serotonin and noradrenaline reuptake inhibitors

SSRIs have undergone extensive trials both against placebo and against comparator antidepressants. There is good evidence that they are as effective as tricyclic antidepressants in the broad range of depressed patients, although they may be less effective in hospitalized depressed patients. *Venlafaxine,* a serotonin and noradrenaline reuptake inhibitor (SNRI), also appears to be slightly more effective than SSRIs in patients with more severe depressive states. SSRIs are more effective than tricyclic antidepressants (with the exception of clomipramine) where depression occurs in association with *obsessive–compulsive disorder* (Cleare *et al.*, 2015). *Duloxetine* is another SNRI, but current evidence does not suggest that it is more effective than SSRIs. A network meta-analysis suggested that escitalopram and sertraline are the most effective of the SSRIs, but whether these differences are of clinical relevance has been disputed (Gartlehner *et al.*, 2008; Cipriani *et al.*, 2009).

Tolerance of SSRIs relative to tricyclics

In short-term clinical trials, compared with tricyclic antidepressants, SSRIs are associated with *lower dropout rates* due to side effects, but the differences are modest (relative risk of dropout due to side effects = 0.73, NNT = 33). However, the differences in favour of SSRIs increase in routine clinical situations, particularly when the duration of treatment exceeds a few weeks. Clearly, their relative safety in overdose gives SSRIs an advantage in certain clinical situations; however, venlafaxine is less safe in overdose than SSRIs. The relative toxicity of duloxetine in overdose has not been clarified, but fatalities have been reported after consumption of as little as 1000 mg.

Monoamine oxidase inhibitors

The efficacy of MAOIs in the treatment of major depression (particularly with melancholic features) has been a matter of controversy. However, placebo-controlled trials have shown that MAOIs are effective antidepressants and of equal therapeutic activity to tricyclic antidepressants for moderate to severe depressive disorders.

MAOIs are liable to cause dangerous reactions with other drugs and some foods, and for this reason they are not recommended as first-line antidepressant drugs. However, controlled trials have shown that MAOIs can be effective in depressed patients who have not responded to tricyclic antidepressants and SSRIs.

The reversible type-A MAOI *moclobemide* has the advantage of not requiring adherence to a low-tyramine diet. However, it can still produce hazardous interactions with other drugs (see Chapter 25). Controlled trials have shown that moclobemide is more effective than placebo in the treatment of uncomplicated major depression. However, it is doubtful whether moclobemide at standard doses is as effective as conventional MAOIs for patients with resistant depression (Cowen and Anderson, 2015).

Other antidepressants

A variety of other antidepressant drugs are now available (see Chapter 25 and Table 9.4), all of which have established efficacy relative to placebo. The main differences between the various preparations are in side effect profile. Apart from reboxetine, anticholinergic-type side effects are uncommon. Trazodone and mirtazapine are sedating. All of these agents are safer than tricyclic antidepressants in overdose. Agomelatine may have a different mechanism of action, involving the activation of melatonin receptors (Whiting and Cowen, 2013).

Lithium

Lithium as a sole treatment

This section is concerned only with lithium as a treatment for depressive disorders. Placebo-controlled trials suggest that lithium may have some antidepressant efficacy in bipolar depression, but its effects in unipolar depression as a sole treatment are not established (Goodwin *et al.*, 2016).

Lithium in combination with antidepressants

Despite its limited utility as a sole drug treatment for depression, lithium can produce useful therapeutic effects when added to antidepressant medication in treatment-resistant patients (*lithium augmentation*). In a meta-analysis, Nelson *et al.* (2014) found that about 40% of depressed patients responded to lithium augmentation of their antidepressant regimen, compared with about 15% of patients who were given placebo (NNT = 5).

Although some studies have reported a rapid amelioration of the depressed state within as little as 48 hours after the addition of lithium, the more usual pattern of response is a gradual resolution of symptoms over 2–3

Table 9.4 Clinical characteristics of some antidepressant drugs

	Anticholinergic	Sedation	Weight gain	Sexual dysfunction	Toxicity in overdose
Amitriptyline	+++	+++	+++	+	+++
Lofepramine	+	0	0	+	0
SSRIs	0	0	+	+++	0*
Venlafaxine	0	0	+	+++	++
Duloxetine	0	0	+	+++	?
Trazodone	0	+++	+	0	+
Reboxetine	+	0	0	+	0
Mirtazapine	0	+++	+++	0	0
Agomelatine	0	+	0	0	?

0, none; +, mild; ++, moderate; +++, marked.

* Citalopram and escitalopram may be somewhat more toxic than other SSRIs because of an effect to prolong the QTc interval.

weeks. The effects of lithium augmentation in depression do not appear to be restricted to any specific class of antidepressants.

Anticonvulsants

Anticonvulsants such as *carbamazepine, valproate,* and *lamotrigine* are useful in the management of bipolar disorder, and in these circumstances can prevent episodes of major depression. Whether these agents also have acute antidepressant efficacy in unipolar depression is unclear. Lamotrigine has been shown to have antidepressant effects in placebo-controlled trials in *bipolar depressed patients*, particularly those with higher levels of symptomatology, but whether this therapeutic property extends to unipolar depression is currently uncertain (Barbee *et al.*, 2011).

Atypical antipsychotic drugs

Antipsychotic drugs are often combined with antidepressant drugs in the treatment of patients with depressive psychosis, and there is also evidence that atypical antipsychotic agents, used at relatively low dose, can be of benefit when combined with antidepressants in non-psychotically depressed patients who have failed to respond to antidepressant treatment alone. In a meta-analysis of trials involving 3500 patients, Spielmans and colleagues (2013) found that, relative to placebo, the addition of drugs such as aripiprazole, quetiapine, and risperidone to ineffective SSRI treatment was significantly more likely to result in clinical remission (NNT = 9). Olanzapine addition was also of benefit, but the effect was less (NNT = 19).

Electroconvulsive therapy

This treatment is described in Chapter 25, where its unwanted effects are also considered. The present section is concerned with evidence about the therapeutic effects of ECT for patients with depressive disorders.

Comparison with simulated ECT

Six double-blind controlled trials have compared the efficacy of ECT and simulated ECT (anaesthesia with electrode application but no passage of current) in patients with major depression. Five of these studies found ECT to be more effective than the simulation. In the study that did not find the full procedure to be more effective, unilateral low-dose ECT was used, a procedure that is considered on other grounds to be relatively ineffective.

The overall response rate is about 70% for ECT and 40% for simulated treatment (NNT = 3–4) (UK ECT Review Group, 2003; see also Chapter 25).

Comparison with other treatments

Several studies have compared depressed inpatients receiving ECT with those receiving antidepressant drugs. In a total of nine comparisons with tricyclic antidepressants, ECT was therapeutically more effective in six studies and equally effective in the remaining three. In five comparisons with MAOIs, ECT was superior in each trial and worked more quickly. These data suggest that, in severely depressed inpatients, ECT is probably superior to antidepressant drug treatment, at least in the short term (UK ECT Review Group, 2003; see also Box 25.14.

Indications for ECT

Clinicians generally agree that the therapeutic effects of ECT are greatest in severe depressive disorders, especially those in which there is *marked weight loss, early-morning waking, retardation*, and *delusions*. From the trials comparing full ECT with simulated ECT, it appears that delusions and (to a lesser extent) retardation are the features that distinguish patients who respond to full ECT from those who respond to placebo (UK ECT Review Group, 2003).

Other studies have established that patients with *depressive psychosis* respond better to ECT than to tricyclic antidepressants or antipsychotic drugs given alone. However, combined treatment with antidepressants and *antipsychotic drugs* may be about as effective as ECT, although no direct comparisons have been made. Another point of practical importance is that ECT may often prove effective in depressed patients who have not responded to full trials of medication, whether or not psychotic features are present. However, in such patients relapse rates are high (Heijnen *et al.*, 2010).

Psychological treatment

All depressed patients, whatever other treatment they may be receiving, require psychotherapy in a general sense, which provides education, reassurance, and encouragement. These measures ('clinical management') can provide some symptomatic relief, and can also increase the likelihood that pessimistic patients will adhere to specific treatments. Education and reassurance should also be given to the patient's partner, other close family members, and other people involved in their care.

The psychological treatments used for depressive disorders can be divided into the following categories:

- supportive psychotherapy
- cognitive behaviour therapy
- interpersonal psychotherapy
- behavioural activation
- marital therapy
- dynamic psychotherapy.

These psychotherapies can be employed as alternatives to antidepressant medication, or as adjuncts. Psychotherapies have been less well evaluated than antidepressant medication in major depression; the use of 'waitlist' controls or 'treatment as usual' may inflate apparent efficacy of treatment (Cleare *et al.*, 2015). In general, specific psychotherapies are somewhat more effective than treatment as usual in the management of mild to moderate depression, particularly in primary care. In this setting, however, structured treatments such as cognitive behaviour therapy do not appear to be superior to other structured therapies such as interpersonal therapy. This suggests that factors common to all psychological treatments are likely to be important in mediating the therapeutic effect (see Chapter 24). In randomized trials, structured psychotherapies usually perform as well as drug treatment in moderately depressed patients (National Institute for Health and Clinical Excellence, 2009a).

Supportive psychotherapy and problem-solving

Supportive psychotherapy goes beyond clinical management in focusing on the identification and resolution of current life difficulties, and in using the patient's strengths and available coping resources. A development of this approach is *problem-solving*, in which the therapist and the patient identify the main problems of concern and devise feasible step-by-step ways of tackling them. Randomized trials suggest that problem-solving treatment is better than treatment as usual in moderately depressed patients in primary care. Its efficacy relative to drug treatment and other psychotherapies is unclear (National Institute for Health and Clinical Excellence, 2009a).

Cognitive behaviour therapy

For depressive disorder, the essential aim of cognitive behaviour therapy is to help the patient to modify their ways of thinking and acting in relation to life situations and depressive symptoms (for further information, see page 694). There have been numerous studies of cognitive behaviour therapy in acute major depression, which have been reviewed (National Institute for Health and Clinical Excellence, 2009a). Current conclusions can be summarized as follows:

- There is strong evidence that cognitive behaviour therapy is superior to a waiting list control in relieving depressive symptomatology.
- Cognitive behaviour therapy is not generally superior to other structured psychological treatments, such as behavioural activation and interpersonal therapy.
- Cognitive behaviour therapy is as effective as pharmacological treatment in moderately depressed outpatients.
- Combined cognitive behaviour therapy and pharmacological treatment is better than pharmacological treatment alone.

The opinion of many clinicians is that cognitive behaviour therapy is not effective as a sole treatment for patients with severe depression, but this view does not have clear support from trial evidence (Driessen *et al.*, 2010). Issues such as what is meant by 'severity' in different settings, as well as the problem of generalizing from randomized trials to everyday practice, are likely to be implicated in this controversy. In addition, therapist expertise may be a critical factor in the delivery of effective cognitive behaviour therapy.

Behavioural activation

Behavioural activation uses the principles of operant conditioning by tracking the links between actions and emotional outcomes. The goal of therapy is to assist patients, through scheduled activity, to engage in behaviours that will lead to a positive effect on mood (see Chapter 24). Unlike cognitive behaviour therapy, it is claimed that therapist training in behavioural activation techniques is simple and quickly accomplished. A recent meta-analysis of 26 randomized trials of behavioural activation in depression showed that the technique was superior to control procedures (the majority of which were waitlist control). However, follow-up duration was often short (Ekers *et al.*, 2014).

Interpersonal psychotherapy

Interpersonal therapy is a systematic and standardized treatment approach to personal relationships and life problems (see page 687). It has been less studied than cognitive behaviour therapy in depression, but seems to be as effective. The National Institute for Health and

Clinical Excellence (2009a) concluded that, in depressed patients, interpersonal therapy:

- Is more effective than placebo with clinical management and GP treatment as usual.
- Is as effective as antidepressant medication.
- Is more effective when combined with antidepressants than when given alone. However, it is not clear whether the combination of interpersonal therapy and antidepressants is better than antidepressants alone for the treatment of acute depression.

Couple therapy

Couple therapy can be offered to depressed patients for whom *interactions with a partner* appear to have contributed to causing or maintaining the depressive disorder. The aim of the intervention is to understand the nature of these interactions and modify them so that the relationship becomes more mutually supportive. There are few randomized trials available, but the limited evidence suggests that couple therapy is significantly more effective than a waiting list control and as effective as cognitive behaviour therapy. There are insufficient data to indicate how couple therapy compares with antidepressant medication (National Institute for Health and Clinical Excellence, 2009a). In practice, antidepressant treatment and couple therapy are often used together, but the combination has not been well evaluated.

Dynamic psychotherapy

Dynamic psychotherapy has a different aim from the treatments described so far, in that it aims to resolve underlying developmental conflicts and attendant life difficulties that are believed to be causing or maintaining the depressive disorder. While it has been suggested that dynamic psychotherapy may be less effective than cognitive behaviour therapy or antidepressant medication (National Institute for Health and Clinical Excellence, 2009a), more recent meta-analyses have shown equivalent benefit in depressed patients for short-term psychodynamic therapy compared to other psychotherapies (Driessen *et al.*, 2015). Therapist training and patient selection are likely to play an important role in the efficacy of psychodynamic therapy in depression.

Other treatments

Sleep deprivation

Several studies suggest that, in some depressive disorders, rapid short-term changes in mood can be brought about by *keeping patients awake overnight*. The alleviation of depressed mood after total sleep deprivation is nearly always *temporary*; it disappears after the next night's sleep or even during a daytime nap after the night of sleep deprivation. Although the antidepressant effect of sleep deprivation is of great theoretical interest, its brevity makes it unpractical. However, there are reports that sleep deprivation can be used to hasten the onset of effect of antidepressant drugs, and also that some pharmacological manipulations can prolong the effect of sleep deprivation (Hemmeter *et al.*, 2010).

Bright light treatment

Over 50% of patients with recurrent winter depression respond to bright light treatment (about 10,000 lux). Treatment is usually given for an hour or two in the morning, but the timing of light treatment is not always critical, and evening light or even midday exposure can be effective. The duration of exposure usually needs to be 1–2 hours.

Designing placebo-controlled trials of bright light for winter depression presents problems, because most patients are aware before treatment that bright light is believed to be the important therapeutic ingredient. Within this limitation, most studies have found that dim light is less effective than bright light. The usual onset of the antidepressant effect of bright light is within 2–5 days, but longer periods of treatment appear to be needed in some patients. Patients with 'atypical' depressive features such as *overeating* and *oversleeping* appear to respond best. To avoid relapse, light treatment usually needs to be maintained until the usual time of natural remission, in the early spring (see page 769).

Some studies have shown that bright light treatment may also be effective in non-seasonal depression—for example, in elderly people with depression, where circadian rhythm disturbances may be involved in pathophysiology (Lieverse *et al.*, 2011). However, the durability of such an effect has not been established.

The longer-term treatment of depression

Follow-up studies have shown that mood disorders often recur and that, if left untreated, they have a rather poor long-term prognosis. For this reason there is now increasing emphasis on *long-term management*.

Prevention of relapse and recurrence

Strictly speaking, the term *relapse* refers to the worsening of symptoms after an initial improvement during the treatment of a single episode of mood disorder, whereas *recurrence* refers to a new episode after a period of complete recovery. Treatment to prevent relapse should be called *continuation treatment*, and treatment to prevent recurrence should be called *prophylactic or maintenance treatment*. In practice, however, it is not always easy to maintain the distinction between these two kinds of treatment, because a therapy may be given initially to prevent relapse, and may then be used to prevent recurrence.

Drug treatment of unipolar depression

Continuation treatment

It is now well established that stopping antidepressants soon after a treatment response has been obtained is associated with a high risk of *relapse*. About one-third of patients who are withdrawn from medication will relapse during the next year, with the majority of the relapses occurring in the first 6 months. Placebo-controlled studies of the role of continuation therapy have reached the following conclusions (Cleare *et al.*, 2015):

- Continuing antidepressant treatment for 6 months past the point of remission halves the relapse rate.
- Treatment should be at the originally effective dose of medication if possible.
- In patients who are at low risk of further episodes, continuation of antidepressant treatment for longer than 6 months confers little extra benefit except in the elderly, where continuation therapy for 12 months is more appropriate.

Maintenance treatment

Controlled studies involving patients with recurrent depression (usually defined as at least three episodes over the past 5 years) have shown that *maintenance antidepressant treatment* can substantially reduce relapse rates. For example, in a 3-year study of 128 patients, Frank *et al.* (1990) found a relapse rate of 22% in patients taking imipramine, compared with 78% in patients treated with placebo. The effects of longer-term maintenance treatment were confirmed in a systematic review (Geddes *et al.*, 2003) where, over a period of 1–2 years of continued antidepressant treatment, the relapse rate was lowered from 41% on placebo to 18% on active medication (see Figure 9.2). Maintaining the dose of medication at the level that was required to achieve remission appears most effective in prophylaxis if tolerability permits.

Lithium carbonate has also been used in the prevention of recurrent unipolar depression but, while some patients show a clear response, the overall evidence for its efficacy is less robust than for the prevention of bipolar disorder. However, where a therapeutic response to lithium augmentation has been achieved, maintaining lithium together with the antidepressant appears worthwhile (Cleare *et al.*, 2015).

Psychotherapy

Cognitive therapy

As noted above, there is some evidence that cognitive therapy given during an acute phase of depression leads to a more sustained improvement in depressive symptomatology and lessens the risk of subsequent relapse compared to antidepressant drug treatment (National Institute for Health and Clinical Excellence, 2009a). There is also growing interest in the use of continuation and maintenance treatment with cognitive therapy, particularly in patients who have *residual depressive symptomatology* and are therefore at increased risk of relapse. There is good evidence that cognitive behavioural therapy continued (or started) after remission prevents relapse, perhaps to a greater extent than maintenance medication (Bockting *et al.*, 2015).

Mindfulness-based cognitive therapy (MBCT) integrates cognitive behaviour therapy with meditation techniques designed to lower stress by facilitating acceptance and self-compassion. There is evidence that MBCT lowers the risk of relapse in patients with recurrent depression and is as effective as maintenance antidepressant treatment in this respect (Brockting *et al.*, 2015; Kuyken *et al.*, 2015). However, reliable identification of the specific elements of treatment and patient characteristics that may be linked to therapeutic response has proved difficult (Williams *et al.*, 2014).

Interpersonal therapy

Combining interpersonal therapy with medication in the treatment of the acute episode appears to decrease relapse rates over the following 12 months (Bockting *et al.*, 2015). The effect of continuation treatment with combined interpersonal therapy and medication has also been studied in older depressed patients. A benefit of the combined treatment over medication alone was seen with nortriptyline but not with paroxetine (Reynolds *et al.*, 2006). These findings suggest that, in

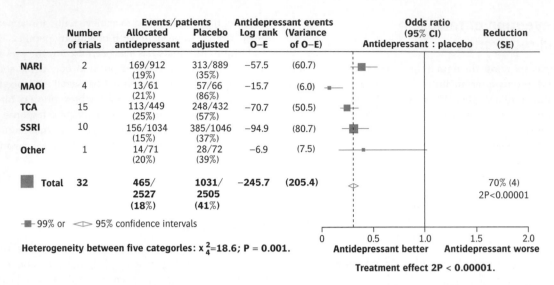

	Number of trials	Events/patients Allocated antidepressant	Placebo adjusted	Antidepressant events Log rank O−E	(Variance of O−E)	Odds ratio (95% CI) Antidepressant : placebo	Reduction (SE)
NARI	2	169/912 (19%)	313/889 (35%)	−57.5	(60.7)		
MAOI	4	13/61 (21%)	57/66 (86%)	−15.7	(6.0)		
TCA	15	113/449 (25%)	248/432 (57%)	−70.7	(50.5)		
SSRI	10	156/1034 (15%)	385/1046 (37%)	−94.9	(80.7)		
Other	1	14/71 (20%)	28/72 (39%)	−6.9	(7.5)		
Total	32	465/ 2527 (18%)	1031/ 2505 (41%)	−245.7	(205.4)		70% (4) 2P<0.00001

■ 99% or ◁▷ 95% confidence intervals

Heterogeneity between five categories: $x^2_4 = 18.6$; P = 0.001.

0   0.5   1.0   1.5   2.0
Antidepressant better   Antidepressant worse

Treatment effect 2P < 0.00001.

Figure 9.2 Meta-analysis of rates of depressive relapse in patients randomly allocated to receive continuation treatment for on average about 1 year with antidepressant medication or placebo.

Reprinted from The Lancet, 361(9358), John R Geddes, Stuart M Carney, Christina Davies, Toshiaki A Furukawa, David J Kupfer, Ellen Frank, and Guy M Goodwin, Relapse prevention with antidepressant drug treatment in depressive disorders: a systematic review, pp. 653-661, Copyright (2003), with permission from Elsevier.

terms of recurrence prevention, the benefit of combined interpersonal therapy treatment over medication alone is equivocal. However, in patients who achieve

remission from depression with interpersonal therapy as a sole treatment, continuation therapy does seem to be helpful in preventing recurrence (Clear *et al.*, 2015).

The assessment of depressive disorders

The aims of the various steps of assessment are as follows:

- To decide whether the diagnosis is depressive disorder.
- To judge the severity of the disorder, including the risk of suicide.
- To form an opinion about the causes.
- To assess the patient's social resources.
- To gauge the effect of the disorder on other people.

Diagnosis depends on thorough *history-taking* and examination of the *physical and mental state*, and has been discussed earlier in this chapter. Particular care should be taken not to overlook a depressive disorder in patients who do not complain spontaneously of being depressed ('masked depression'). It is equally important not to diagnose a depressive disorder simply on the grounds of prominent depressive symptoms, as the latter could be part of another disorder, such as a general medical condition. It should also be remembered

that certain drugs—both legal and illegal—can induce depression (Chapter 20).

The *history of previous mood disturbance* is important in assessment. Some patients will have had recurrent episodes of mood disorder. A history of these episodes often provides clues to the probable course of the current disorder and its response to treatment. It is particularly important to ask about possible previous episodes of *mania and hypomania*, even if these were mild and short-lived. If there is a history of mania, the mood disorder is bipolar. Interviews with relatives and close friends may help to establish whether such episodes have occurred.

The *severity* of the disorder is judged from the symptoms. Considerable severity is indicated by 'biological' symptoms, hallucinations, and delusions, particularly the latter two. It is also important to assess how the depressive disorder has reduced the patient's capacity to work or to engage in family life and social activities. In this assessment, the duration and course of the condition should be taken into account as well as the severity of the present symptoms. Not only does the length of the history affect the prognosis, but it also gives an indication of the patient's capacity to tolerate further distress. A long-continued disorder, even if not severe, can bring the patient to the point of desperation. The *risk of suicide* must be judged in every case (the methods of assessment are described in Chapter 21).

Aetiology is assessed next, with reference to precipitating, predisposing, and maintaining factors. No attempt need be made to allocate the syndrome to an exclusively 'endogenous' or 'reactive' category. Instead, the importance of all relevant risk factors should be evaluated in every case.

Provoking causes may be psychological and social (the 'life events' discussed earlier in this chapter), or they may be physical illness and its treatment. In assessing such cases, it is good practice to enquire routinely about the patient's work, finances, family life, social activities, general living conditions, and physical health. Problems in these areas may be recent and acute, or may take the form of chronic background difficulties such as prolonged marital conflict, problems with children, and financial hardship.

The patient's *social resources* are considered next. Enquiries should cover family, friends, and work. A loving family can help to support patients through a period of depressive disorder by providing company, encouraging them when they have lost confidence, and guiding them into suitable activities. For some patients, work is a valuable social resource, providing distraction and comradeship. For others it is a source of stress. A careful assessment is needed in each case.

The *effects of the disorder on other people* must be considered carefully. The most obvious problems arise when a severely depressed patient is the mother of young children who depend on her. This clinical observation has been confirmed in objective studies, which have demonstrated that depressive disorder in either parent is associated with emotional disorder in the children (Ramchandani *et al.*, 2009). It is important to consider whether the patient could endanger other people by remaining at work (e.g. as a bus driver). If there are *depressive delusions*, it is necessary to consider what would happen if the patient were to act on them. For example, severely depressed parents may harm their children because they believe them to be doomed to suffer if they remain alive.

The management of depressive disorders

This section starts by considering the management of patients with a depressive disorder of moderate or greater severity. The first question concerns the level of care and supervision that may be required. The answer depends on the *severity of the disorder* and the quality of the patient's *social resources*. When judging severity, particular attention should be paid to the *risk of suicide* (or any risk to the life or welfare of family members, particularly dependent children) and to any failure to eat or drink that might endanger the patient's life. Provided that these risks are absent, most patients with a supportive family can be treated at home, even if they are severely depressed. Patients who live alone, or whose families cannot care for them during the day, may need *intensive community treatment or day-patient care*. Inpatient treatment can be considered for patients who are not improving with these measures, or where safety issues raise particular concern. *Involvement of the family* wherever possible is also likely to improve the outcome (see Box 9.9).

The next question is whether the patient should continue to work. If the disorder is of moderate severity, work can provide a valuable distraction from depressive thoughts, and be a source of companionship. If the disorder is more severe, retardation, poor concentration, and lack of drive are likely to impair performance at work, and such failure may add to the patient's feelings of hopelessness. In severe disorders, there may be dangers to other people if patients remain at their jobs.

The need for *antidepressant drug treatment* should be considered next. This treatment is indicated for most patients with a *major depressive syndrome* of at least moderate severity, and particularly those with *melancholic symptoms*. Other indications include a family history or personal history of depression, particularly if there has been a clear response to drug treatment. *Dysthymia* is also an indication for antidepressant medication, but the role of antidepressants in milder depressive conditions is not established. However, where a patient with a clear history of major depression develops symptoms of mild depression, antidepressant medication can be considered. Guidelines for a stepped-care approach to the management of depression have been developed by the National Institute for Health and Clinical Excellence (2009a) (see Box 9.10).

Box 9.9 What patients and families want to know

Particularly for patients with a first episode of moderate to severe depression, questions such as the following are important:

1. What is wrong with me?
2. Can I recover?
3. What treatment do I need?
4. What can I do to improve the situation?
5. Can my family be helped?

The answers to these questions require a good knowledge of patients and their circumstances. Patients will understand and appreciate that a careful practitioner will need to gather information before giving definitive answers to important questions. However, some general advice is given below.

- Depression is as a medical condition and not any fault of the individual concerned. Feelings of guilt are common and are seen as part of the condition.
- The prognosis for individual episodes of depression is good, although people with depression are naturally pessimistic about the future.
- Treatment consists of a comprehensive package with psychological support and medication if indicated. The treatment plan will be developed as a collaborative exercise between the patient and the clinical team, and the patient's rights and choices will be respected.
- Part of the treatment plan will involve a full discussion about the most appropriate level of occupational and social activity for the current circumstances. This will be reviewed frequently to allow adjustment to the patient's changing clinical state.
- It is very useful for the family to be fully involved in discussions about the nature of depression and the treatment plan, as their support can be invaluable. Conversely, critical comments can be demoralizing for depressed people. One of the aims of family involvement is to help to improve mutual communication and support.

Box 9.10 Guidelines for the management of depression

1. Patients with short-lived mild depression who may recover quickly without treatment should be offered an early review ('active monitoring').
2. Antidepressants are not recommended for the treatment of mild depression.
3. Patients with persistent mild depression should be recommended a guided self-help programme based on cognitive behaviour therapy. Group cognitive behaviour therapy is an alternative. An exercise programme and sleep hygiene can also be recommended.
4. For patients with persistent mild depressive symptoms that do not respond to these measures, consider drug treatment with an SSRI or a higher-intensity psychological treatment (cognitive behaviour therapy, behavioural activation, interpersonal therapy, or couple therapy).
5. Patients who present with moderate or severe depression should be treated with a combination of antidepressant medication and a high-intensity psychological intervention.
6. Patients who respond to antidepressant medication should continue treatment for at least 6 months. Patients at high risk of relapse should be advised to continue antidepressant treatment for 2 years.
7. Consider cognitive behaviour therapy for patients who have relapsed despite antidepressant treatment, or mindfulness-based cognitive therapy for patients who are well but who have experienced three or more previous episodes of depression.

Source: data from the National Institute for Health and Clinical Excellence (2009a).

Choice and use of antidepressant drug

Several kinds of antidepressant drug treatment are available, and the choice should be made in collaboration with the patient, with particular consideration of the likely side effects. These are fully described in Chapter 25.

- *SSRIs* are the usual first choice, unless the patient considers that they have done well previously with a different agent. It is also important to be aware of medical contraindications to SSRI drugs, including, for example, concomitant treatment with non-steroidal anti-inflammatory drugs which can increase the risk of bleeding. *Lofepramine*, a tricyclic antidepressant that is relatively safe in overdose, is another non-sedating compound with a different side effect profile (see Table 9.4).

- *Mirtazapine* may be considered if the patient needs concomitant sedation or if there are relative contraindications to the use of SSRIs (for example, concomitant treatment with non-steroidal anti-inflammatory drugs.
- *Tricyclic antidepressants such as amitriptyline* are rarely used now as first choice agents, even for patients with severe depression.

The dosage of these drugs, the precautions to be observed when using them, and the instructions to be given to patients are described in Chapter 25. Here it is necessary only to emphasize again the importance of explaining to the patient that, although side effects will appear quickly, the therapeutic effect is likely to be delayed for 2 weeks, with maximum improvement occurring over 6–12 weeks. During this time the patient should be seen regularly to provide suitable clinical management; those with more severe disorders may need to be seen every few days, and other patients once a week. It is important to make sure that the drugs are taken in the prescribed dose. The patient should be warned about the effects of *taking alcohol*. They should be advised about *driving,* particularly that they should not drive while experiencing sedative side effects or any other effects that might impair their performance in an emergency.

The use of ECT

ECT will very rarely be part of the first-line treatment of depression, and in such circumstances will usually be considered only for patients who have already been admitted to hospital. The only indication for ECT as a first measure is the need to bring about improvement as rapidly as possible. In practice this applies to two main groups of patients:

- Those who refuse to drink enough fluid to maintain an adequate output of urine (including the rare cases of depressive stupor).
- Those who present a highly dangerous suicidal risk.

Occasionally, ECT is indicated for a patient who is suffering such extreme distress that the most rapid form of treatment is deemed justifiable. Such cases are rare. It should be remembered that, with the exception of patients who are unresponsive to antidepressant drugs, the effects of ECT differ from those of antidepressant drugs in terms of greater rapidity of action, rather than the final therapeutic result. In patients with *depressive*

psychosis, ECT is considerably more effective than an antidepressant given alone, but probably about the same therapeutic effect can be achieved, albeit more slowly, if a combination of an antidepressant drug and an antipsychotic drug is used.

Activity

The need for *suitable activity* should be considered for every patient. Depressed patients give up activities and withdraw from other people. As a result they become deprived of social stimulation and rewarding experiences, and their original feelings of depression are increased. It is important to make sure that the patient is occupied adequately, although they should not be pushed into activities in which they are likely to fail because of slowness or poor concentration. Thus there is a fairly narrow range of activity that is appropriate for the individual depressed patient, and the range changes as the illness runs its course. If the patient remains at home, it is important to discuss with the relatives how much they should be encouraged to do each day. For inpatients, this question should be decided by the clinical team.

Psychotherapy

The appropriate kind of psychological treatment should also be decided in each case. As noted earlier, all depressed patients require support, encouragement, and a thorough explanation that they are suffering from illness and not moral failure. Similar counselling of partners and other family members is often useful.

The use of one of the more specific psychological treatments discussed earlier should also be considered. These treatments can be used as the sole therapy for patients with mild to moderate depression without melancholic features, particularly if the patient prefers not to take drug therapy (National Institute for Health and Clinical Excellence, 2009a). The kind of psychological treatment that is used depends largely on the availability of a suitably trained therapist and the preference of the patient, although the more structured therapies (such as interpersonal therapy and cognitive behaviour therapy) have a greater evidence base with regard to the treatment of moderate to severe depression. The therapeutic response to antidepressant drugs is usually faster than that to psychotherapy.

Current recommendations are that in patients with moderate to severe depression it is helpful to add cognitive behaviour therapy to antidepressant medication (National Institute for Health and Clinical Excellence,

2009a). In practical terms, some time is usually needed to arrange cognitive behaviour therapy, and in any event some initial improvement produced by antidepressant medication may enable the patient to make more use of psychological treatment. It is also important to tackle any psychosocial problems that are making an important contribution to the depression. In particular, *couple therapy* can be a helpful addition in depressed patients where problems with a partner are playing a role in maintaining the disorder.

If the depressive disorder is severe, too much discussion of problems at an early stage is likely to increase the patient's feelings of hopelessness. Therapy directed toward self-examination is particularly likely to make the disorder worse. During intervals between acute episodes, such therapy may be offered to patients who have recurrent depressive disorders that are largely caused by their ways of reacting to life events.

Failure to respond to initial treatment

If a depressive disorder does not respond within a reasonable time to a chosen combination of antidepressant drugs, graded activity, and psychological treatment, the plan should be reviewed. The first step is to check again that the patient has been taking medication as prescribed. If not, the reasons for this should be sought. The patient may be convinced that no treatment can help, or may find the side effects unpleasant. The diagnosis should also be reviewed carefully, and a check made that important stressful life events or continuing difficulties have not been overlooked.

If this enquiry is unrevealing, antidepressants should be continued at an increased dose if possible. In general, SSRIs do not have clear dose–response relationships, although some patients respond to higher doses, particularly if a partial response has been observed at a standard dose.

If it becomes clear that the patient is not improving, a number of further steps can be taken (see Box 9.11). There is not a fixed order in which treatments should be offered. Prescribing decisions should be made in collaboration with the individual patient, taking into account factors such as specific symptomatology, how far the condition may have shown a partial response, and the side effect profile of the various treatment options.

Change in antidepressant drug treatment

If a patient does not respond to one antidepressant, the first step is usually to stop the first medication and try

> **Box 9.11 Some pharmacological treatments for resistant depression**
>
> - Increase antidepressant to the maximum dose, if tolerance permits; if the patient has depressive psychosis, add an antipsychotic drug; try a different class of antidepressant drug, including venlafaxine and tricyclic antidepressants
> - Try an antidepressant combination (e.g. an SSRI or venlafaxine with mirtazapine)
> - Add an atypical antipsychotic drug to an SSRI or venlafaxine
> - Add lithium to antidepressant drug treatment
> - MAOIs (can be usefully combined with lithium)
> - ECT

another. Most published studies of this approach have studied patients in an open sequential way; clearly this cannot control for the placebo effect or the possibility of spontaneous remission. Overall, however, there is reasonable evidence that switching to a second antidepressant can produce benefit in about 50% of patients who are unresponsive to an initial medication trial (Cleare *et al.*, 2015).

If a patient has not responded to one kind of antidepressant, it would seem sensible to switch to an antidepressant that has a *different pharmacological profile*. However, it must be acknowledged that open studies have shown equally good response rates when patients who failed to respond to one SSRI were switched to another. A meta-analysis of randomized studies suggested that switching from an SSRI to a different class of drug (mirtazapine, venlafaxine or bupropion) was marginally better in terms of remission rate (SSRI, 23.5% versus non-SSRI, 28%; NNT = 22) than switching to a second SSRI, but this advantage is of doubtful clinical significance (Papakostas *et al.*, 2008). Switching from a drug with serotonergic properties to another serotonergic compound should be carried out cautiously because of the risk of serotonin toxicity. In practice this means that the first compound should be fully withdrawn if at all possible, and the second one started at a half-dose or less. In the case of fluoxetine, because of its long duration of action, at least 1 week should elapse before starting a second serotonergic agent. However, when switching between agents with different pharmacological properties (e.g. from citalopram to mirtazapine or reboxetine), cross-tapering can be employed. Detailed instructions are provided by the Maudsley Prescribing Guidelines (Taylor *et al.*, 2015).

Both amitriptyline and venlafaxine appear to be slightly more effective than SSRIs in patients with severe depression; these drugs are therefore worth trying at some point in the management of patients who are unresponsive to initial medication trials (Cowen and Anderson, 2015). Similar comments apply to the use of conventional MAOIs, which have a clearly beneficial effect in some patients with resistant depression (Nolen *et al.*, 1988). However, the drug and food restrictions associated with MAOIs mean that it is unusual to use them early in drug-resistant depression unless a patient has responded well to them in the past.

Combination treatment with antidepressants

Combination strategies aim to supplement the antidepressant effect of an ineffective or partially effective medication with another antidepressant agent. This approach can therefore be considered an augmentation strategy, although if the patient's condition remits it may be unclear whether the response is due to the combined effect of the two antidepressants or to the second agent acting alone.

The pharmacological rationale of combination treatment is the use of two agents to produce a broader spectrum of activity on monoamine pathways than either agent could produce alone. In practice this means that SSRIs or venlafaxine are usually combined with noradrenergic-promoting agents such as bupropion or mirtazapine (which increases noradrenaline function through blockade of auto-inhibitory α_2-adrenoceptors).

The evidence for any of these strategies is limited, although they are endorsed in case series and expert reviews. Combination of a tricyclic antidepressant with SSRIs must be approached with caution because of the risk of elevation of tricyclic levels (see Chapter 25).

Augmentation of antidepressant drug treatment

When switching antidepressant preparations, one problem is that withdrawal of the first compound may not be straightforward. Patients may have gained some small benefit from the treatment (e.g. improved sleep or reduced tension), and this benefit may be lost. Also, if the first medication is stopped quickly, withdrawal symptoms may result (see Chapter 25). However, if the dose is reduced gradually, the changeover in medication may be protracted and may not be easily tolerated by a depressed and despairing patient.

For this reason, in patients who are unresponsive or partly responsive to first-line medication it may be more appropriate to add a second compound to the antidepressant—so-called *augmentation therapy*. A disadvantage of augmentation therapy is the increased risk of adverse effects due to drug interaction.

Antipsychotic drugs

As noted above, in patients with *psychotic depression* it is usually best to prescribe a combination treatment of antidepressant and antipsychotic medication (Wijkstra *et al.*, 2010). In non-psychotic resistant depression, conventional antipsychotic drugs are of little value except, at low doses, for ameliorating agitation and distress. However, there is good evidence that some *atypical antipsychotic drugs* may have antidepressant effects when used in combination with SSRIs in patients with non-psychotic depression (see above).

The use of atypical antipsychotics to augment SSRIs employs lower doses than would be used to treat schizophrenia, perhaps because the key pharmacological mechanism probably involves 5-HT_2 receptor antagonism rather than dopamine D_2 receptor blockade. Despite this, olanzapine and quetiapine, even at low doses, can cause troublesome sedation and weight gain, while concomitant use of risperidone also produces some degree of weight gain together with hyperprolactinaemia. Aripiprazole is less likely to cause metabolic side effects, but is associated with agitation and restlessness. In randomized studies of SSRI augmentation, the *discontinuation rate* due to adverse effects was significantly greater with atypical antipsychotics than with placebo (odds ratio, 3.9; 95% CI, 2.68–5.72; number needed to harm = 17) (Nelson and Papakostas, 2009). This suggests that, although atypical antipsychotic drug addition can be useful in SSRI-resistant depression, the clinical utility of this approach may be limited by its tolerability.

Lithium augmentation

We have already seen that data from randomized trials indicate that lithium can be effective in the treatment of resistant depression. Provided that there are no contraindications, the addition of lithium to antidepressant drug treatment is usually safe and well tolerated. About 50% of depressed patients will show a useful response over 1–3 weeks. Lithium can be added to any primary antidepressant medication with good effect, although combination with SSRIs and venlafaxine should be undertaken with caution because of the risk of *5-HT neurotoxicity* (see Chapter 25). In the latter case it is appropriate to start lithium at a low dose (200 mg daily) and increase by a maximum of 200 mg weekly. In augmentation treatment, the aim should be to obtain a lithium concentration within the range used for prophylactic purposes

(0.5–0.8 mmol/l); the lower end of the range is appropriate for combination with serotonergic antidepressants. It has been suggested that the combination of lithium with MAOIs or clomipramine (sometimes supplemented with tryptophan) can be effective in depressed patients who are otherwise refractory to treatment (Cowen and Anderson, 2015).

Tri-iodothyronine

Some open and controlled studies have suggested that the addition of tri-iodothyronine (T3) in doses of 20–40 μg daily to ineffective tricyclic antidepressant treatment can bring about a useful clinical response, even where underlying thyroid activity is normal. However, a meta-analysis of four published randomized trials which assessed the efficacy of T3 addition to ineffective tricyclic antidepressant treatment was of borderline significance (Aronson *et al.*, 1996). The evidence for the efficacy of T3 augmentation of newer antidepressant drugs, such as SSRIs, is inconsistent. Despite this, some depressed patients do appear to be helped by the addition of T3, which can start at a dose of 10 μg daily and be increased to 20 μg after 1 week, if tolerance is good (Cowen and Anderson, 2015). At this dose the side effects are mild, but tremor and sweating can occur. It is prudent not to use T3 addition in patients with evidence of cardiovascular disease.

The use of ECT in resistant depression

If severe depression persists, ECT should be considered. ECT is often beneficial to patients who have not responded to antidepressant drugs, and it is probably more effective than drugs in the most severe depressions, particularly when psychotic features are present. Whether medication resistance lowers the response to ECT has been debated. However, a meta-analysis of observational studies suggested that the overall response rate to ECT in patients who failed pharmacotherapy (48%) was significantly lower than the rate in those who did not (65%) (Heijnen *et al.*, 2010).

It is important to note that, among patients who have not responded to full-dose antidepressant medication, the relapse rate in the year after ECT may be as high as 50%. This may be because patients are often continued on the same antidepressant medication to which they previously failed to respond. In these circumstances it seems reasonable to use an antidepressant of a different class, or lithium, for continuation treatment after ECT, but there is currently no unequivocal evidence that this procedure lowers the relapse rate. However, a randomized study of 200 patients found post-ECT prophylaxis with a combination of lithium and nortriptyline to

be as effective as maintenance ECT in sustaining remission in the 6 months following a successful course of treatment. Despite this, just over 50% of the patients in each group relapsed (Kellner *et al.*, 2006).

Other important measures

Continuing support is essential for patients who do not respond to treatment. Lack of improvement increases the pessimism experienced by the depressed patient. Therefore it is important to give reassurance that depressive disorders have a good chance of recovering eventually, whether or not treatment speeds recovery. Meanwhile, if the patient is not too depressed, any problems that have contributed to their depressed state should be discussed further. Particularly in patients who have not received high intensity psychological treatments, the place of structured psychotherapies should be considered. A study of primary care patients who had failed to respond adequately to antidepressant medication found that cognitive behaviour therapy was markedly better than treatment as usual in bringing about a therapeutic response (Wiles *et al.*, 2013).

In patients with prolonged depression, it is particularly important to watch carefully for suicidal intentions. For patients with severe symptoms and particularly long-standing refractory illness, other treatment approaches such as *deep brain stimulation* and *neurosurgery* can be considered. These are discussed in Chapter 25.

Prevention of relapse and recurrence in depression

After recovery, the patient should be followed up for several months by the psychiatric team or general practitioner. If the recovery appears to have been brought about by an antidepressant drug, that drug should usually be continued for about 6 months and then gradually withdrawn over a period of several weeks. If residual symptoms are still present, it is safer not to withdraw medication. At follow-up interviews, a careful watch should be kept for *signs of discontinuation reactions* or *relapse*. It is helpful to discuss with the patient the possible early signs of relapse, and to develop a plan of action should any of these signs appear. If the patient is in agreement, it is helpful to involve the relatives in this plan.

Maintenance treatment

Major depression is often recurrent, and long-term maintenance treatment may need to be considered. The risk factors for recurrence have been noted above. In addition, the clinician will need to take into account the following individual factors:

- the likely impact of a recurrence on the patient's life
- the previous response to drug treatment
- the patient's view of long-term drug treatment.

It is estimated that, among patients who have had three episodes of major depression, the likelihood of another episode is 90%. The usual recommendation is that maintenance drug treatment should be considered if a patient has had two previous episodes of depression within a 5-year period, particularly if there is a family history of recurrent major depression, or personal and social factors predictive of recurrence (Cleare *et al.*, 2015). *Persistent residual symptoms* are also an indication for maintenance treatment.

Choice of medication

For most patients, the choice of antidepressant will be derived from their response in the acute or continuation phase of treatment. In this case, the same medication can be continued, if possible at the same dose. As noted earlier, newer antidepressant drugs are better tolerated in the longer term, and may be preferred for maintenance treatment. If a change needs to be made because of adverse effects (e.g. sexual dysfunction with SSRIs), an alternative choice should be determined on the basis of side effect profile.

Lithium can also be effective for long-term maintenance treatment of recurrent depression in some patients. Its adverse-effect profile and the need for plasma monitoring mean that it will not be a first choice for most patients, but its use should be considered if there is any history of manic episodes, even if these have been mild and transient. In addition, lithium will sometimes be effective in patients with recurrent depression who do not respond to maintenance treatment with antidepressants. Importantly, lithium does seem to lower risk of suicidal behaviour in patients with mood disorders, an action that is not explained completely by its ability to prevent depressive relapse (Cleare *et al.*, 2015).

Other measures

If a depressive disorder was related to self-imposed stressors, such as overwork or complicated social relationships, the patient should be encouraged to change to a lifestyle that is less likely to lead to further illness. These readjustments may be helped by psychotherapy, which may be individual, marital, or group. As noted above, cognitive behaviour therapy appears to be helpful in lowering the risk of relapse, particularly in patients with residual depressive symptomatology. There is also growing interest in the role of MBCT. Community nurses and nurse therapists can play a valuable role in delivering treatment of this kind.

General practitioners play a key and increasing role in the long-term monitoring of patients, and should always be involved in treatment planning. The growing evidence for important comorbidities between depression and general medical conditions such as cardiovascular disease and diabetes gives added importance to the collaboration between mental health services and general practitioners. Annual monitoring of body weight, blood pressure, glucose, and lipids, as is recommended for bipolar patients (see Box 10.4), is advised.

Further reading

Ghaemi N (2013). *On Depression: Drugs diagnosis and despair in the modern world*. The John Hopkins University Press, Maryland. (An intriguing account of the cultural context of modern formulations of depression and the role of psychiatry in identifying and managing depressive conditions.)

Lewis AJ (1934). Melancholia: A clinical survey of depressive states. *Journal of Mental Science*, **80**, 277–378. [Reprinted in Lewis AJ (1967). *Inquiries in Psychiatry*. Routledge and Kegan Paul, London, pp. 30–117]. (This landmark study contains a detailed account of the clinical picture of depressive disorder.)

CHAPTER 10
Bipolar disorder

Introduction

In the previous chapter we considered depressive disorders and we now turn to bipolar disorders, another group of conditions in which depressive episodes are prominent. In bipolar disorder, however, the course is marked by at least one episode of *mania* or *hypomania*. Kraepelin (1921) brought mania and depression together as *manic depressive psychosis,* because he believed that the longer-term clinical course, with its tendency to recurrence of mood disturbance, was similar, whether patients presented with mania or depression. However, Leonhard *et al.* (1962) pointed out that bipolar disorder tends to show a distinct familial clustering. In addition, there are other epidemiological differences between unipolar depression and bipolar disorder (Table 10.1). However, the differences are not great and there must be overlap between the two groups, because a patient who is classified as having unipolar depression at one time may have a manic disorder subsequently. In other words, the unipolar group inevitably contains some bipolar cases that have not yet declared themselves. Despite this limitation, the division into unipolar and bipolar cases is a useful classification because it has implications for treatment, particularly that of bipolar depression.

Clinical features

Mania

The central features of the syndrome of mania are *elevation of mood, increased activity*, and *self-important ideas*.

Mood

When the mood is elevated, the patient appears cheerful and optimistic, and may have a quality described by earlier writers as 'infectious gaiety'. However, other patients are irritable rather than euphoric, and this irritability can easily turn to anger. The mood often varies during the day, although not with the regular 'diurnal' rhythm that is characteristic of many severe depressive disorders. In patients who are elated, it is not uncommon for high spirits to be interrupted by brief episodes of *depression*.

Table 10.1 Epidemiology of bipolar and unipolar (depressive) disorder

	Bipolar disorder	Unipolar disorder
Lifetime risk	About 1%	About 15%
Sex ratio (M:F)	1:1	1:2
First-degree relatives		
Lifetime risk for bipolar disorder	About 10%	About 2%
Lifetime risk for unipolar disorder	20–30%	20–30%
Average age of onset	18 years	27 years
Patients with recurrence	90%	80%
Average number of episodes	10	4

Appearance and behaviour

The appearance of patients often reflects their prevailing mood. Their clothing may be brightly coloured and ill assorted. When the condition is more severe, the patient's appearance is often *untidy and dishevelled*. Manic patients are overactive. Sometimes the persistent overactivity leads to *physical exhaustion*. Manic patients start many activities but leave them unfinished as new ones attract their attention. Appetite is increased, and food may be eaten greedily with little attention to conventional manners. Sexual desires are increased, and sexual behaviour may be uninhibited and quite out of character. Women may neglect precautions against pregnancy, a point that calls for particular attention if the patient is of childbearing age. Sleep is often reduced. Patients wake early, feeling lively and energetic, and often get up and busy themselves noisily, to the surprise (and sometimes annoyance) of other people.

Speech and thought

The speech of manic patients is often *rapid and copious* as thoughts crowd into their minds in quick succession. When the disorder is more severe, there is *flight of ideas* (see Chapter 1), with such rapid changes that it is difficult to follow the train of thought. However, the links are usually understandable if the speech can be recorded and reviewed. This is in contrast to thought disorder in schizophrenia, where changes in the flow of thought may not be comprehensible even on reflection.

Expansive ideas are common. Patients believe that their ideas are original, their opinions important, and their work of outstanding quality. Many patients become *extravagant*, spending more than they can afford (e.g. on expensive cars or jewellery). Others make reckless decisions to give up good jobs, or embark on plans for ill-considered and risky business ventures.

Sometimes these expansive themes are accompanied by *grandiose delusions*. Some patients may believe that they are religious prophets or destined to advise statesmen about major issues. At times there are *delusions of persecution*, when patients believe that people are conspiring against them because of their special importance. Delusions of reference and passivity feelings also occur. Schneiderian first-rank symptoms (see Box 11.3) have been reported in around 10–20% of manic patients. Neither the delusions nor the first-rank symptoms last for long, most of them disappearing or changing in content within a period of days.

Perceptual disturbances

Hallucinations occur. These are usually consistent with the mood, taking the form of voices speaking to the patient about their special powers or, occasionally, of visions with a religious content.

Other features

Insight is invariably impaired in more severe manic states. Patients see no reason why their grandiose plans should be restrained or their extravagant expenditure curtailed. They seldom think of themselves as ill or in need of treatment.

Most patients can exert some control over their symptoms for a short time, and many do so when the question of treatment is being assessed. For this reason it is important to obtain a history from an informant whenever possible. Henry Maudsley (1879, p. 398) expressed the problem well:

Just as it is with a person who is not too far gone in intoxication, so it is with a person who is not too far gone in acute mania; he may on occasion pull his scattered ideas together by an effort of will, stop his irrational doings and for a short time talk with an appearance of calmness and reasonableness that may well raise false hopes in inexperienced people.

Manic stupor

In this unusual disorder, patients are *mute* and *immobile*. Their facial expression suggests elation, and on recovery they describe having experienced a rapid succession of thoughts typical of mania. The condition is rarely seen now that active treatment is available for mania. Therefore an earlier description by Kraepelin (1921, p. 106) is of interest:

The patients are usually quite inaccessible, do not trouble themselves about their surroundings, give no answer, or at most speak in a low voice … smile without recognizable cause, lie perfectly quiet in bed or tidy about at their clothes and bed-clothes, decorate themselves in an extraordinary way, all this without any sign of outward excitement.

On recovery, patients can remember the events that occurred during their period of stupor. The condition may begin from a state of manic excitement, but at times it is a stage in the transition between depressive stupor and mania.

Criteria for manic episode in ICD-10 and DSM-5

The symptoms that are required to make a diagnosis of 'manic episode' in ICD-10 are listed in Box 10.1. The criteria for manic episode in DSM-5 are very similar, although the number of manic symptoms required for diagnosis is specified more precisely. In DSM-5, manic symptoms that occur during treatment with antidepressant medications and persist at a syndromal level despite the antidepressant being stopped are regarded as meeting criteria for a manic episode rather than being coded as a drug-induced manic illness.

ICD-10 notes that some patients with mania present with *psychotic symptoms*, in which case the clinical picture described in Box 10.1 is typically more severe, with inflated self-esteem and grandiose ideas developing into *grandiose delusions*. At the same time irritability and suspiciousness may result in *delusions of persecution*. Sustained physical activity and excitement may result in aggression or violence, and neglect of eating and drinking and personal hygiene can lead to a dangerous state of dehydration and self-neglect.

Criteria for hypomanic episode in ICD-10 and DSM-5

Hypomania refers to a state of elevated mood that is of lesser extent than mania. The criteria in ICD-10 and DSM-5 are similar:

- There is persistent mild elevation of mood for at least several days (in DSM-5, at least 4 days) with increased energy and activity and feelings of wellbeing.
- There is increased sociability, talkativeness and overfamiliarity, increased sexual energy, and decreased need for sleep.
- The mood disturbance, although associated with an unequivocal change in function, which is observable to others, is not sufficiently severe to cause marked

impairment in social or occupational activities, or to necessitate hospital admission.
- Psychotic features are absent.

> ### Box 10.1 Clinical features of a manic episode in ICD-10
>
> - Mood is elevated out of keeping with the individual's circumstances, varying from carefree joviality to almost uncontrollable excitement. In some manic episodes the mood is irritable and suspicious rather than elated
> - Increased energy results in overactivity, pressure of speech, and a decreased need for sleep
> - Social inhibitions are lost, attention cannot be sustained, and there is often marked distractibility
> - Self-esteem is inflated, and grandiose and overoptimistic ideas are freely expressed
> - Perceptual disorders may occur; for example, the appreciation of colours can be especially vivid and beautiful
> - The individual may embark on extravagant and impracticable schemes, spend money recklessly or become aggressive, amorous, or facetious in inappropriate circumstances
> - **For diagnosis**, the episode should last for at least one week and should be severe enough to disrupt ordinary work and social activities more or less completely. The mood change should be accompanied by increased energy and several other symptoms referred to above—particularly *pressure of speech, decreased need for sleep, grandiosity*, and *excessive optimism*.
>
> Source: data from The ICD-10 classification of mental and behavioural disorders: clinical descriptions and diagnostic guidelines, Copyright (1992), World Health Organization.

Other clinical presentations of bipolar disorder

Mixed mood (affective) states

Depressive and manic symptoms sometimes occur at the same time. Patients who are overactive and over-talkative may be having profoundly depressive thoughts. In other patients, mania and depression follow each other in a sequence of rapid changes—for example, a manic patient may become intensely depressed for a few hours and then return quickly to his manic state. These changes were mentioned in early descriptions of mania by psychiatrists such as Wilhelm Griesinger (1817–1868), and have been re-emphasized in recent years because they appear to predict a better response to certain mood stabilizers, such as valproate.

Rapid cycling disorders

Some bipolar disorders recur regularly, with intervals of only days or weeks between episodes. In the nineteenth century these regularly recurring disorders were designated *folie circulaire* (circular insanity) by the French psychiatrist Jean-Pierre Falret (1794–1870). At present, the frequent recurrence of mood disturbance in bipolar patients is usually termed *rapid cycling disorder*. These recurrent episodes may be depressive, manic, or mixed. The main features are that recurrence is frequent (by convention at least four distinct episodes a year), and that episodes are separated by a period of remission or a switch to an episode of opposite polarity. A number of clinical features of rapid cycling disorder are important in management and prevention.

- They occur more frequently in women.
- Concomitant hypothyroidism is common.
- They can be triggered by antidepressant drug treatment.

The lifetime risk of rapid cycling in bipolar populations varies between studies, but is probably in the range 15–30%. Rapid cycling may be a temporary phenomenon, and in most patients it remits within about 2 years. For a review, see Datta and Cleare (2009).

Cyclothymia

The term *cyclothymia* disorder refers to a persistent instability of mood in which there are numerous periods of mild elation or mild depression that do not meet severity criteria for either major depression or hypomania. It is seen as a milder variant of bipolar disorder. It is not unusual, however, for episodes of more severe mood disorder to supervene in the course of the disorder.

Depression

Depressive episodes are common in the course of bipolar disorder and most patients with bipolar disorder present initially with an episode of major depression. The ability to predict which patients first presenting with depression will eventually develop bipolar illness is currently limited, although family history of bipolar disorder can provide a useful clue. The presence of any *hypomanic* or *mixed symptomatology* at initial presentation has some predictive value, but the majority of depressed patients who convert to bipolar illness do not have hypomanic symptoms during the initial episodes of depression. Other clinical features associated with subsequent development of bipolar illness include early age of onset and clinical severity, particularly the presence of *psychosis* (see Fiedorowicz *et al.*, 2011).

There is a high degree of overlap between the clinical symptomatology of unipolar and bipolar depression; however, psychomotor retardation, early morning awakening, morning worsening, and psychotic features are reportedly more common in patients with bipolar disorder (Mitchell *et al.*, 2011).

Transcultural factors

The rates of bipolar disorder are relatively consistent across countries, although there is some evidence for an increased prevalence of bipolar disorder in certain minority groups within a country, such as with black and ethnic minority groups in the United Kingdom. Moreover, patients from these minority groups are more likely to present with a first episode of mania and prominent psychotic features than a comparable white population with bipolar disorder. The reason for this difference is not fully understood, but social exclusion may be a factor, particularly in relation to relatively late access to services (Kennedy *et al.*, 2004).

Classification

Both DSM-5 and ICD-10 delineate hypomania from mania on the basis of duration of symptoms, absence of psychotic features, and lesser degree of social and occupational impairment (see above). A manic episode can be further subdivided according to severity and whether or not psychotic symptoms are present. In DSM-5, the presence of a single episode of mania is sufficient to meet the criteria for bipolar disorder. In ICD-10, however, at least two episodes of mood disturbance (at least one of which must be hypomania or mania) are needed for this diagnosis. DSM-5 also categorizes bipolar disorder as follows (Table 10.2):

- Bipolar I, in which *mania* has occurred on at least one occasion.
- Bipolar II, in which *hypomania* has occurred, but mania has not. However, to make the diagnosis of bipolar II disorder an episode of major depression must also have occurred.

The diagnosis of bipolar II disorder is intended to indicate the importance of detecting mild hypomanic episodes in patients who might otherwise be diagnosed as having recurrent major depression. The presence of such episodes may have implications for treatment response. There is debate about where the line should be drawn between unipolar depression and bipolar disorder, because some patients with definite depressive episodes appear to have features of bipolarity but do not meet the full DSM-5 criteria for mania or hypomania. Such patients may, for example, have elevations of mood that last for less than the required 4 days, or that have little discernible effect on functioning.

In DSM-5, the diagnosis of 'bipolar and related disorder' can be made for such disorders and the reasons why the full criteria fail to be met can be either 'specified' or 'unspecified'. In clinical practice, the term *bipolar spectrum* is also used for these conditions. The pharmacological treatment of bipolar depression differs to some extent from that given to patients with recurrent unipolar depression (see 'Treatment of bipolar depression' below), so making the diagnostic distinction between unipolar and bipolar depression can have important implications for management. However, it is not clear whether depressed patients in the 'bipolar spectrum' do better when treated as having bipolar depression rather than unipolar depression (for a discussion, see Goodwin *et al.*, 2016).

Table 10.2 Classification of bipolar disorder

ICD-10	DSM-5
Manic episode	Hypomanic episode
Hypomania	Manic episode
Mania without psychosis	Mild
Mania with psychosis	Moderate
	Severe
	Severe with psychosis
Bipolar affective disorder	Bipolar I and bipolar II disorders
Currently hypomanic	Current (or most recent episode)
Currently manic	Hypomanic
Currently depressed	Manic*
Currently mixed	Depressed
In remission	Mixed*
Cyclothymia	Cyclothymic disorder

* Excludes bipolar II.
Source: data from The ICD-10 classification of mental and behavioural disorders: clinical descriptions and diagnostic guidelines, Copyright (1992), World Health Organization; Diagnostic and Statistical Manual of Mental Disorders, Fifth Edition, Copyright (2013), American Psychiatric Association.

Differential diagnosis of bipolar disorder

Mania

Manic disorders have to be distinguished from the following:

- schizophrenia;
- organic brain disease involving the frontal lobes (including brain tumour and HIV infection);
- states of brief excitement induced by amphetamines and other illegal drugs.

Schizophrenia

The distinction from schizophrenia can be most difficult. Auditory hallucinations and delusions, including some that are characteristic of schizophrenia, such as delusions of reference, can occur in manic disorders. However, these symptoms usually change quickly in terms of content, and seldom outlast the phase of overactivity. When there is a more or less equal mixture of features of the two syndromes, the term *schizoaffective* is often used. This term is discussed further in Chapter 11. Further clues to diagnosis can often be elicited by a careful personal and family psychiatric history.

Organic brain disorder and drug misuse

An organic brain lesion should always be considered, especially in middle-aged or older patients with expansive behaviour and no past history of affective disorder. In the absence of gross mood disorder, extreme social disinhibition (e.g. urinating in public) strongly suggests *frontal lobe pathology*. In such cases, appropriate neurological investigation is essential. In younger adults, infection with HIV or head injury may lead to the manifestation of mania.

The distinction between mania and excited behaviour caused by *drug misuse* depends on the history and on an examination of the urine for drugs, which is needed before treatment with psychotropic drugs is started. Drug-induced states usually subside quickly once the patient is in hospital. However, it should be remembered that a significant proportion of patients who have bipolar disorder misuse alcohol and other drugs.

Bipolar disorder and recurrent depression

The distinction between bipolar disorder and recurrent unipolar depression depends on the eliciting of symptoms of mania or hypomania in the past history. However, distinguishing recurrent depression from bipolar II disorder can be particularly challenging because brief periods of hypomania can be difficult to identify or may not be remembered clearly by the patient. Moreover, at the time of diagnosis, such symptoms may not yet have declared themselves and it is only subsequently, with the development of mania or hypomania, that the bipolar disorder can be identified. Another point is that patients with bipolar II disorder will almost invariably seek treatment for depressive episodes, tending not to regard spells of hypomania as being illness (Phillips and Kupfer, 2013).

Bipolar disorder and borderline personality disorder

One of the diagnostic features of borderline personality disorder is marked affective instability, which may at times be difficult to distinguish from rapid cycling bipolar disorder. A family history of bipolar disorder may be a useful pointer. Also, shifts in mood in borderline personality disorder can be very rapid over hours and days, which is unusual in bipolar disorder. Classic symptoms of mania, such as increased energy and grandiosity, are not usually present. Finally, mood disturbances in borderline personality are usually triggered by interpersonal issues such as the fear of loss or rejection, while in rapid cycling bipolar disorder such psychosocial triggers are not prominent (Paris and Black, 2015).

Epidemiology

The epidemiology of bipolar disorder depends on the diagnostic criteria used to define it. Including patients in the bipolar spectrum increases rates of bipolar disorder at the expense of recurrent major depression. In addition, as noted above, distinguishing bipolar disorder from recurrent unipolar depression can be challenging.

Community surveys using ICD-10 or DSM-IV criteria for bipolar disorder in industrialized countries have suggested that:

● The lifetime risk for bipolar disorder is in the range 0.3–1.5%.

● The 6-month prevalence of bipolar disorder is not much less than the lifetime prevalence, indicating the chronic nature of the disorder.

● The prevalence in men and women is the same.

● The mean age of onset is about 18 years in community studies.

● Bipolar disorder is highly comorbid with other disorders, particularly anxiety disorders and substance misuse, as well as general medical conditions such as cardiovascular disease.

For a review of the epidemiology of bipolar disorder, see Joyce (2009).

Aetiology

Overview

In earlier studies of aetiology, particularly of depression, the distinction between recurrent unipolar depression and depression in the context of bipolar disorder was not always made. The fact that first-degree relatives of patients with bipolar disorder have an increased risk of recurrent unipolar depression suggests that there is some aetiological overlap between the two conditions. Alternatively, it may be that such relatives make up one particular subtype of the heterogenous disorder which is currently called major depression.

One of the most striking features of bipolar disorder is its high heritability and, accordingly, much recent work has employed molecular genetic techniques in an attempt to implicate genetic loci relevant to pathophysiology. In addition, advances in structural and functional imaging have allowed a clearer description of the brain basis of bipolar disorder and its possible distinction from recurrent unipolar depression. However, none of the brain changes yet identified is sufficiently reliable and distinct to be used as a diagnostic biomarker. In addition, increasing knowledge of possible pathophysiology has not yet led to new treatments, which continue to be developed on an empirical basis.

Genetic causes

Family and twin studies

The risk of both bipolar and unipolar mood disorders is increased in first-degree relatives of bipolar probands. Relatives of bipolar probands also have increased risks of *schizoaffective disorder*. Twin studies have shown that the concordance rate for mood disorder in the monozygotic co-twin of a proband with bipolar disorder is around 60%, but for dizygotic twins the rate is only about 20%. This indicates a high heritability, which has been estimated at around 85% (Bienvenu *et al.*, 2011).

Mode of inheritance

The familial segregation of bipolar disorder does not fit a simple Mendelian pattern. Overall, it seems likely that the genetic liability to the condition results largely from the combined action of multiple genes of modest, or small, effect—so-called *polygenic inheritance*. It is also possible that rare structural chromosomal abnormalities

(copy number variants) and gene–gene interactions (epistasis) contribute to the genetic risk. The fact that the concordance rate of monozygotic twins for bipolar disorder is around 60% indicates that environmental factors are also likely to be important in pathophysiology (Craddock and Sklar, 2013).

Molecular genetics

Molecular linkage studies of mood disorders have so far not been particularly revealing, perhaps because the genes involved are of small effect, or because of genetic heterogeneity. Positive findings have emerged, but have often proved difficult to replicate even in large-scale studies and meta-analyses. Similarly, association studies of 'candidate' genes have not proved fruitful, presumably because lack of understanding of the biology of the disorder inhibits the identification of the most promising candidates (Craddock and Sklar, 2013).

Genome-wide association studies (GWAS) in large numbers of bipolar patients have begun to find risk loci which have some robustness to replication. For example, the Psychiatric Genome-Wide Association Study Consortium Bipolar Disorder Working Group reported on genotype data from over 16,000 bipolar patients and found a replicated genome-wide significant association with *CACNA1C,* which encodes a subunit of the L-type calcium channel. Overall, about 10 replicated loci have thus far been identified (Harrison, 2016).

Overall the data suggest that, as with schizophrenia, the inherited risk of bipolar disorder is conferred by hundreds, or even thousands, of genes of small effect. However, some of the identified genes can be shown to cluster around biologically meaningful processes ('pathway analysis'). For example, a number of genes putatively involved in bipolar disorder impact on the activity of voltage-gated calcium channels, which is of interest in view of the possible mood-stabilizing effects of calcium channel blockers such as verapamil (Craddock and Sklar, 2013). Another point is that many of the genes identified in GWAS studies of bipolar disorder also appear to be risk alleles for the development of schizophrenia. It is striking that molecular genetic studies suggest a greater overlap in risk alleles between bipolar disorder and schizophrenia than for bipolar disorder and unipolar depression (Harrison, 2016). However, this may simply point to the greater heterogeneity of the diagnostic category of major depression.

Environment

The concordance rates for bipolar disorder in monozygotic twins noted above show that environmental factors are likely to be involved in the pathophysiology of bipolar illness. Most of the environmental factors identified thus far do not seem specific for bipolar disorder but rather confer risk of psychiatric disorder more generally. For example, patients with bipolar disorder report higher rates of childhood sexual abuse than healthy controls, but similar or lower rates than other groups of psychiatric patients (Maniglio, 2013). Childhood sexual abuse is known to be linked to the development of psychosis generally in adulthood and in one study in bipolar patients was associated with an increased risk of auditory hallucinations, but not delusions (Upthegrove *et al.*, 2015).

Life events have been shown to precipitate episodes of both depression and mania in bipolar patients, although the effect appears more pronounced in early stages of the illness, suggesting a possible 'kindling' effect (Kemner *et al.*, 2015). Negative life events can trigger episodes of both depression and mania, although mania can also apparently be precipitated by life events associated with goal attainment. One way that life events might lead to illness is through effects on circadian rhythms; for example, decreasing sleep and disrupting regular cycles of sleep and activity (Alloy *et al.*, 2005).

The level of current social support also seems an important factor influencing the course of bipolar disorder. As with schizophrenia, high levels of expressed emotion in a family can worsen affective symptomatology, and the risk of relapse is lessened by treatment addressing this issue (Alloy *et al.*, 2005).

Neurobiological approaches to aetiology

Neurochemistry

An influential hypothesis links *excessive dopamine activity* to the pathophysiology of schizophrenia (see Chapter 11). It has also been proposed that manic states may be attributable to dopamine overactivity because drugs of abuse, particularly those acting to increase central dopamine activity, are associated with many of the symptoms of acute mania, such as elevated mood, decreased need for sleep, talkativeness, and the unguarded pursuit of rewarding behaviours. Also, drugs that block dopamine receptors are commonly employed in the acute treatment of mania.

Studies of dopamine metabolism and function have provided little direct evidence for overactivity of dopamine pathways in patients with manic illness. A study in recovered bipolar patients showed that, while they had a greater psychological response to intravenous amphetamine, there was no greater release of presynaptic dopamine as measured by the technique of raclopride displacement (see Chapter 5). This suggests that there may be a heightened responsivity to changes in dopamine neurotransmission in patients at risk of mania, but this is unlikely to be primarily because of changes in dopamine mechanisms. For a review of the role of dopamine in mania, see Cousins *et al.* (2009).

Many of the drugs used in the longer-term management of bipolar disorder are anticonvulsants, which alter *brain glutamate* levels. Several magnetic resonance spectroscopy (MRS) investigations have been carried out in bipolar patients at various stages of illness. There are suggestions that glutamate levels might be increased in bipolar patients, which makes an interesting point of contrast with findings in major depression (see Chapter 9). The reliability of this finding and its possible utility in diagnosis require further study (Gigante *et al.*, 2012).

Endocrine abnormalities

Cortisol

As in major depression, disturbances of the hypothalamic–pituitary–adrenal (HPA) axis with hypersecretion of cortisol have been reported in patients with bipolar disorder. However, the patients studied have usually been taking medication, making interpretation difficult. There have been suggested links between excessive cortisol secretion in bipolar disorder and the presence of cognitive impairment, with beneficial effects on cognition being reported following treatment with glucocorticoid antagonists (Young, 2014). It is also well recognized that administration of exogenous corticosteroids in the treatment of general medical conditions can give rise to an acute manic illness.

Oestrogen and progesterone

The immediate postpartum period is a time of heightened risk for the development of acute psychotic illness in mothers—usually presenting as a form of bipolar disorder (see Chapter 22). There has therefore been great interest in whether this might be attributable to the abrupt fall in circulating levels of sex steroids that occurs at this time; however, no correlation has been identified and oestrogen treatment does not prevent postpartum psychosis (Hay, 2009).

Brain imaging

Structural brain imaging

Changes in brain volume measured by magnetic resonance imaging (MRI) in bipolar disorder have been inconsistent, and stage of illness and drug treatment, particularly the use of lithium, appear to be important confounding factors. It seems that in bipolar patients not taking lithium, hippocampal volumes are lower, as in recurrent depression. However, this abnormality is reversed in patients taking lithium. There also appears to be a reduction in cerebral volume over the course of bipolar illness, perhaps suggesting a degenerative process in some patients (Hallahan *et al.*, 2011). Studies using diffusor tension imaging (see Chapter 5) in bipolar patients have revealed abnormalities in certain white matter tracts, perhaps representing abnormal myelination or orientation of axons in predominantly frontal and temporal white matter regions (Phillips and Swartz, 2014).

Similarly to patients with major depression (see Chapter 9), there is evidence that neuropathological changes occur in patients with bipolar disorder. For example, studies in the prefrontal cortex have reported reductions in neuronal and glial cell density, the latter consistent with a loss of oligodendroglial cells. Again, as in major depression, there may also be deficits in gamma-aminobutyric acid (GABA) interneurons (Savitz *et al.*, 2014).

Functional imaging

As in patients with unipolar depression, bipolar depressed patients show elevated neural responses in the amygdala and abnormally reduced activity in regulatory lateral and medial prefrontal cortical regions in response to negative emotional cues. Unlike unipolar depressed patients, euthymic bipolar patients show elevated amygdala responses and decreased activity in cortical regions to positive emotional stimuli such as happy faces. Bipolar patients also demonstrate enhanced reactions in ventral striatal and orbitofrontal 'reward' circuitry during tasks that engage reward processing (Phillips and Swartz, 2014). Generally functional imaging studies show a greater range of neural dysregulation in bipolar disorder than in unipolar depression, with abnormalities encompassing not only neural responses to negative emotional stimuli but also positive stimuli, including the experience of reward.

Neuropsychological changes

Cognitive deficits are present in bipolar disorder during both acute illness and periods of euthymia. Deficits are apparent in first-episode patients, suggesting that they may form an integral part of the illness. In comparison to patients with schizophrenia the deficits are relatively modest but cover a wide range of neuropsychological domains, including *executive function, verbal memory, attention,* and *processing speed* (Lee *et al.*, 2015). At the moment there is no clear evidence that cognitive deficits in bipolar disorder increase through the course of the illness. Whether neuropsychological deficits distinguish patients with bipolar I and bipolar II disorder is uncertain.

Conclusions

The *predisposition* to develop bipolar disorder has a major genetic contribution and the relevant genes, which may number many thousands, are starting to be identified. If such genes converge on a number of discrete biological pathways, it will greatly aid elucidation of aetiological mechanisms and may provide clues to new treatments.

In terms of *environmental factors,* adverse early experiences, particularly abuse, may also predispose to bipolar disorder as it does to many other psychiatric conditions. Early episodes of illness are often precipitated by life events but these may become less important as the illness progresses. The psychosocial environment can modify the course of bipolar illness and there may well be an important role for factors that disrupt sleep–wake activity.

Brain imaging studies show functional abnormalities consistent with disordered emotional regulation and reward processes; unlike the abnormalities seen in major depression, these changes also involve exaggerated functional responses to positive emotional stimuli. Modest but widespread neuropsychological deficits can be seen in bipolar disorder and these appear to extend into periods of euthymia.

Course and prognosis

From recent hospital and population-based studies, the following general conclusions can be drawn (Angst, 2009).

Bipolar disorders

- The age of onset of bipolar disorder is typically about 21 years in hospital studies, but earlier (about 18 years) in community surveys. Late-onset bipolar disorder is rare, and may be precipitated by organic brain disease.

- Bipolar disorder usually begins as depression, with the first manic episode manifesting about 5 years later.

- The average length of a manic episode (treated or untreated) is about 6 months.

- At least 90% of patients with mania experience further episodes of major mood disturbance.

- Over a 25-year follow-up, on average bipolar patients experience about 10 further episodes of major mood disturbance.

- The interval between episodes becomes progressively shorter with both age and the number of episodes.

- Over long-term follow-up, patients with bipolar disorder experience mood-related symptomatology of varying severity for about one-third of the time. In both bipolar I and bipolar II disorder this most commonly takes the form of depressive symptoms.

- Nearly all bipolar patients recover from acute episodes, but the long-term prognosis is rather poor. For example, less than 20% of bipolar patients achieve a period of 5 years of clinical stability with good social and occupational performance. Patients with bipolar II disorder have a somewhat better outcome.

Persistent cognitive deficits and mood instability predict a poorer outcome.

Mortality of bipolar disorder

Mortality is significantly increased in patients with bipolar disorders. Over a 40-year follow-up about 8% of men and 5% of women hospitalized for bipolar illness died by suicide (Nordentoft *et al.*, 2011). The high mortality in bipolar disorder is caused not only by suicide but also general medical conditions such as cardiovascular disease and the secondary consequences of comorbid substance misuse, including smoking. A study of 22,00 Danish patients with bipolar disorder found a reduction in life expectancy of about *13 years in men and 9 years in women*. About two-thirds of this reduction was accounted for by natural causes, with the remainder being due to suicide and accidents (Kessing *et al.*, 2015). Cardiovascular disease is an important cause of increased mortality in bipolar patients, which highlights the importance of attending to the medical needs of this population. The metabolic effects of extended treatment with psychotropic medication, particularly antipsychotic drugs, also need careful assessment (Goodwin *et al.*, 2016).

Treatment of mania

General measures

The treatment of mania presents a formidable clinical challenge, which often tests the management skills of the psychiatric team. Drug treatment plays a pivotal role in the management of mania, and has the aim of reducing physical and mental overactivity, improving features of psychosis, and preventing deterioration in health caused by exhaustion, sleep deprivation, and poor fluid intake. It is worth noting that before the advent of modern drug treatment the mortality of mania in the hospital setting was over 20%; nearly 50% of these patients died from exhaustion (Derby, 1933).

Medication

Typical antipsychotic drugs

Several randomized controlled trials have shown the efficacy of *chlorpromazine* and *haloperidol* in treating mania, whether or not patients have clear psychotic features. However, the use of typical antipsychotic drugs

has limitations. Manic patients often receive high doses, and may be particularly susceptible to extrapyramidal side-effects. In addition, conventional antipsychotic drugs do not protect against the depressive downswings that can follow resolution of a manic illness.

Atypical antipsychotic drugs

Because of their improved tolerability profile, atypical antipsychotic agents are being increasingly used in the treatment of mania. Placebo-controlled trials support the efficacy of aripiprazole, asenapine, olanzapine, quetiapine, and risperidone in patients with mania (Cipriani *et al.*, 2011). However, it should be noted that more severely ill patients may not be included in placebo-controlled trials, which could limit the generalizability of these findings.

Lithium

Five placebo-controlled trials have shown that lithium is effective in the acute treatment of mania (Cipriani *et al.*, 2011). In the only study that compared lithium with both placebo and an active comparator, Bowden *et al.* (1994) found a response rate of 49% for lithium, 48% for valproate, and 25% for placebo. In general, lithium is as effective as an antipsychotic medication, but its onset of action is slower. Moreover, in highly active states, antipsychotic medication may be preferable (Goodwin *et al.*, 2016). Prominent depressive symptoms and psychotic features predict a poorer response to lithium alone, as does a rapid cycling disorder.

Carbamazepine

Assessment of the efficacy of carbamazepine in acute mania has been limited by problems with regard to study design. These include small numbers, the use of adjunctive medications, and mixed diagnostic groupings. However, more recent placebo-controlled trials of an extended-release form of carbamazepine found a clinically significantly antimanic effect (Goodwin *et al.*, 2016). Carbamazepine induces drug-metabolizing enzymes in the liver, which can lead to lower plasma levels of concomitantly administered drugs.

Valproate

Several randomized controlled trials have shown that valproate possesses antimanic activity that is greater than that of placebo and equivalent to that of lithium (Cipriani *et al.*, 2011). Valproate may be more effective than lithium in the subgroup of patients with prominent dysphoric symptoms and rapid cycling.

One advantage of valproate is that it has an earlier onset of activity than other mood stabilizers. For example, with 'valproate loading' (20 mg/kg/day) the onset of the antimanic effect can occur as early as within 1–4 days. This is probably because the tolerability of valproate allows rapid dose escalation, whereas lithium and carbamazepine generally need to be introduced more gradually.

Benzodiazepines

Benzodiazepines are useful *adjuncts* in the treatment of mania, because they can rapidly diminish overactivity and restore sleep. They have been used as sole therapy in the treatment of mania, but this carries a risk of disinhibition. Their most useful role is as an adjunct to mood stabilizers, because the latter drugs can take several days to become effective. Benzodiazepines can also be given in combination with antipsychotic drugs, because this lowers the dose of antipsychotic drug required to calm agitated and overactive patients. The benzodiazepines that are usually employed are the high-potency agents, lorazepam and clonazepam. Use should be on an 'as needed' basis and for as short a time as possible, to minimize the risk of tolerance and dependence (Goodwin *et al.*, 2016).

Electroconvulsive therapy

ECT has been widely used to treat mania, although there have been only two prospective controlled trials in the modern era. In one of these trials, bilateral ECT was found to be superior to lithium (Small *et al.*, 1988). In the other study, unilateral and bilateral ECT were compared with a combination of lithium and haloperidol in patients who had not responded to antipsychotic drugs alone. The response rate of these patients to ECT (13 of 22) was greater than that to combined drug treatment (none of five). The efficacy of unilateral and bilateral ECT did not differ (Mukherjee *et al.*, 1988).

Retrospective investigations have shown ECT to be effective in acute mania, with the overall response rate being about 80%. Many of these patients had been unresponsive to medication. ECT is also effective in *mixed affective states* (Valenti *et al.*, 2008). It is often given at shorter intervals in the treatment of mania than in the treatment of depression, but there is no evidence that this regimen is necessary or that it speeds up the treatment response. It is unclear whether bilateral electrode placement is better than unilateral placement in manic patients.

Continuation treatment of mania

It is a common clinical experience that too rapid a reduction in doses of drug treatment can lead to the sudden recrudescence of an apparently treated manic disorder. Since the average length of a manic episode is about 6 months, it seems prudent to continue some form of medication for at least this period. There are several studies involving atypical antipsychotic drugs which show that, compared with placebo, continuation treatment decreases the risk of manic relapse (Goodwin *et al.*, 2016). Patients who have been severely ill may well be taking both a mood stabilizer and an antipsychotic agent. Because of the adverse effects of antipsychotic drugs, it will often be appropriate to withdraw this form of treatment slowly first.

Treatment of bipolar depression

For many years bipolar depression was treated similarly to unipolar depression and, for a number of major issues (for example, clinical assessment and general psychological support), this still holds good. However, in recent years it has become apparent that best pharmacological treatment of depression occurring in the context of bipolar disorder can differ significantly from that employed in unipolar depression.

Medication

Antidepressant drugs

Depression in the context of a bipolar disorder can be problematic because standard antidepressant treatments have a number of disadvantages, which include:

- a possibly lower efficacy than in unipolar depression;
- a risk of inducing mania;
- a risk of inducing rapid cycling.

Whether conventional antidepressant medication is efficacious in bipolar depression has been controversial. However, more recent meta-analyses do indicate some benefit. For example, Vázquez *et al.* (2013) identified 10 placebo-controlled trials involving over 1400 patients with bipolar depression. Response to antidepressants was significantly greater than that to placebo, with a number needed to treat (NNT) of about six. However, compared to studies in unipolar depression the trials are few in number and involve patients with bipolar I and II disorders as well as old and newer antidepressant drugs. It may be that antidepressants are more clinically useful in bipolar II depression than in bipolar I (Malhi, 2015).

It is generally agreed that treatment with tricyclic antidepressants does increase the risk of manic switching in bipolar depressed patients. However, the risk with selective serotonin reuptake inhibitors (SSRIs) seems much less and only slightly greater than that seen with placebo. Venlafaxine is thought more likely than SSRIs to destabilize mood (Vázquez *et al.*, 2014).

Lithium

Lithium may have a role in the *prevention* of depression in bipolar disorder (see page 244), but evidence for its effectiveness in acute bipolar depression is limited and is based on older trials with unsatisfactory designs. A more recent placebo-controlled study in bipolar depression found lithium less efficacious than quetiapine and with few positive differences from placebo (Young *et al.*, 2010).

Atypical antipsychotic drugs

There is growing evidence for the short- and longer-term efficacy of certain *atypical antipsychotic drugs* such as *quetiapine* in the treatment of bipolar depression, and similar effects have been reported for *lurasidone* (Vázquez *et al.*, 2014). The effects of olanzapine as a monotherapy in bipolar depression seem less than those of quetiapine, although in combination with fluoxetine it appears at least as effective (Table 10.3). In contrast, aripiprazole does not appear useful in bipolar depression (Vázquez *et al.*, 2014).

Anticonvulsants

Some *anticonvulsant mood stabilizers* are helpful in the treatment of bipolar depression, with positive evidence from randomized trials for *lamotrigine and valproate*. Both these drugs would be expected to be free from the risk of inducing mania or rapid cycling. A recent large pragmatic trial found benefit at both 12 and 52 weeks for the addition of lamotrigine to ineffective quetiapine therapy. At 12 weeks remission in the lamotrigine group was 31% versus 16% in the placebo group (NNT 6.6) (Geddes *et al.*, 2016). An interesting observation, made possible by the factorial design of the trial, was that

Table 10.3 Meta-analysis of placebo controlled trials of selected pharmacological treatments in bipolar depression

Drug	Drug:placebo response ratio	95% Confidence interval
Valproate	2.08	1.18–3.65
Olanzapine +fluoxetine	1.84	1.44–2.36
Lurasidone	1.72	1.33–2.22
Antidepressants	1.43	1.11–-1.84
Quetiapine	1.36	1.24–1.49
Lamotrigine	1.25	1.07–1.46
Olanzapine	1.25	1.08–1.44
Lithium	1.12	0.92–1.44
Aripiprazole	0.88	0.74–1.04

Reproduced from Advances in Psychiatric Treatment, 20(3), Vázquez GH et al, Pharmacological treatment of bipolar depression, pp. 193–201, Copyright (2014), with permission from Royal College of Psychiatrists.

coadministration of *folic acid* appeared to antagonize the therapeutic effect of lamotrigine.

Electroconvulsive therapy

For resistant depression in bipolar patients, *ECT* can be of benefit. There are few randomized studies of patients specifically diagnosed with bipolar illness. However, in a recent randomized trial of 73 bipolar patients with resistant depression, ECT was more effective than algorithm-based pharmacological treatment in producing an antidepressant response (74% versus 35%). However, remission rates between the two treatments did not differ (Schoeyen *et al.*, 2014). For a review of the treatment of bipolar depression, see Vázquez *et al.* (2014).

Longer-term treatment of bipolar disorder

Medication

Lithium

There is substantial evidence for the efficacy of lithium in the maintenance treatment of recurrent mood disturbances in patients with bipolar disorders. In a systematic review, Geddes *et al.* (2004) found that lithium was significantly more effective than placebo in preventing relapses of all mood disorders (mean relative risk, 0.65; 95% confidence intervals [CI], 0.5–0.84). However, although lithium was clearly effective in preventing manic relapse, its effect in preventing depressive episodes was more equivocal (mean relative risk, 0.72; 95% CI, 0.49–1.07).

In general, about 50% of bipolar patients who are treated with lithium respond well. The following are predictors of a *relatively poorer* response to lithium maintenance treatment:

- rapid-cycling disorders or chronic depression;
- mixed affective states;
- alcohol and drug misuse;
- mood-incongruent psychotic features.

There is also evidence that use of lithium in patients with recurrent mood disorders is associated with a *significant reduction in mortality from suicide*. This effect is most often seen in dedicated lithium clinics, and the mechanism and specificity of the association require further study. Nevertheless, it is clinically important that the carefully supervised use of lithium is associated with a lowered risk of suicidal behaviour. This effect is not necessarily shared by other mood stabilizers (Cipriani *et al.*, 2011).

Valproate

Valproate is increasingly used in the treatment of acute mania, and therefore evidence of its longer-term maintenance effects is needed. Bowden *et al.* (2000) randomized 372 patients to 1 year of maintenance treatment with valproate, lithium, and placebo. There were no significant differences between the three treatment groups on the primary outcome measure of time to recurrence of any mood disorder. However, the number of patients who left the study because of the occurrence of a severe mood episode was significantly less among those taking valproate compared with those on placebo. Patients who were taking valproate experienced more tremor, alopecia, and weight gain than those on placebo. In a pragmatic study in bipolar patients, the relapse rate on lithium (59%) was significantly less than that with valproate (69%) over 24 months. The combination of lithium and valproate was associated with the lowest relapse rate (54%) (BALANCE Study Group, 2010).

Lamotrigine

Two prospective placebo-controlled trials have shown that lamotrigine has prophylactic effects in patients with bipolar illness. Although it may have some modest benefit in the prevention of mania, lamotrigine has a clearer prophylactic effect against depression. Its profile of activity therefore contrasts with those of lithium and valproate, which are more effective in preventing mania (Goodwin *et al.*, 2016). However, lamotrigine is not licensed for the treatment of mood disorder in the UK.

Carbamazepine

Although the number of patients studied in randomized controlled studies is relatively few, carbamazepine appears to have efficacy in the prophylaxis of bipolar disorder. However, it seems to be less effective than lithium in 'classical' bipolar illness (Goodwin *et al.*, 2016). Therefore, carbamazepine can be considered in patients who respond poorly to lithium, particularly those with rapid-cycling disorders. It can be given alone or in combination with lithium. Carbamazepine can induce hepatic metabolizing enzymes, leading to lower levels of coadministered drugs. Therefore it should be used with caution in combination treatments.

Antipsychotic drugs

Patients with bipolar disorder have sometimes been maintained on *typical antipsychotic drugs*, usually given in addition to mood-stabilizing agents. It is usually wise to minimize this form of treatment where possible, because conventional antipsychotic drugs do not protect against depression, and may be more liable to cause tardive dyskinesia in bipolar patients.

Atypical antipsychotic drugs are also being employed in the longer-term maintenance treatment of bipolar disorder, either as a sole treatment or as an adjunct to mood stabilizers. There is evidence from randomized studies for the efficacy of olanzapine and quetiapine in this respect in the prevention of both depression and mania (Goodwin *et al.*, 2016). However, a common design of these studies is to continue antipsychotic treatment in patients who have responded to short-term, open-label treatment, and to compare this with placebo substitution. This sample, enriched for antipsychotic treatment responders, may favour active treatment unduly, and therefore the findings may not be generally applicable to other clinical situations (Cipriani *et al.*, 2010).

Psychotherapy

Studies of structured psychotherapies in bipolar disorder have usually been directed to patients outside acute episodes of mood disturbance. In this situation, therefore, psychotherapy has the aim of improving and sustaining recovery.

Cognitive behaviour therapy

Psychotherapy has been less studied in bipolar patients, but, theoretically, cognitive behavioural techniques may be valuable in helping patients to accept their illness and the need for medical treatment, as well as improving the management of emotionally stressful situations. Some randomized studies have shown that cognitive techniques combined with education about early signs of relapse reduced the rates of relapse in bipolar patients. However, a large pragmatic trial showed no benefit using this approach (Scott *et al.*, 2006). Overall, the benefit of cognitive behaviour therapy in the prevention of relapse in bipolar disorder is uncertain (Geddes and Miklowitz, 2013).

Family focused approaches

The mood swings experienced by bipolar patients, particularly mood elevation, can be very challenging for their families; this may lead to high levels of 'expressed emotion', which in turn worsen the clinical course. Family-based therapy aims to improve relationships and support for the patient within the family by utilizing psychoeducation as well as training in communication skills and problem-solving. In two studies substantial effects of this approach were apparent, with reductions in both hospitalizations and symptomatology by about a third (Geddes and Miklowitz, 2013).

Interestingly, family approaches using the above techniques are also helpful if the patient does not personally attend the sessions. However, the practical utility of this form of therapy will depend much on family structure and the role the patient plays in it, as well as the extent to which the wider culture encourages disclosure of painful feelings within the family (Geddes and Miklowitz, 2013).

Interpersonal and social rhythm therapy

While mood disturbance is almost invariably associated with sleep disruption, the converse is also the case and it is well recognized that sleep deprivation in bipolar patients can trigger episodes of mania. Interpersonal and social rhythm therapy was derived from interpersonal therapy (Chapter 24) and focuses on helping bipolar patients to maintain regular sleep-activity schedules with careful attention to sleep hygiene. Current data suggest that patients who are able to attain stable sleep–wake routines do have a better longer-term outcome (Geddes and Miklowitz, 2013).

Group psychoeducation

Group psychoeducation attempts to deliver psychotherapy in a cost-effective way by educating groups of bipolar patients in a medical understanding of their illness and the best ways of achieving mood stability. As with social rhythm therapy, the importance of regular sleep–wake cycles is stressed, together with the detection of early signs of relapse and how these should be managed. Treatment adherence is also an important treatment goal.

The approach has been pioneered in Barcelona, where a randomized trial of 120 bipolar patients found that psychoeducational group therapy treatment was of benefit in reducing the average number of relapses over a 5-year follow-up period by over 50% (Colom *et al.*, 2009). The best results were shown in people with fewer episodes of illness, which suggests that the intervention should be applied *as early as possible* in the course of the illness.

Practical management of bipolar disorder

Acute mania

Assessment

In the assessment of mania, the important steps can be summarized as follows.

- Decide the diagnosis.
- Assess the severity of the disorder.
- Form an opinion about the causes.
- Assess the patient's social resources.
- Judge the effects on other people.

Diagnosis depends on a careful history and examination. Whenever possible, the history should be taken from relatives as well as from the patient, because the latter may not recognize the extent of their abnormal behaviour. Differential diagnosis has been discussed earlier in this chapter. It is always important to remember that mildly disinhibited behaviour can result from frontal lobe lesions (e.g. tumours) as well as from mania. There should be a urine screen for illegal substances.

Severity is judged next. For this purpose it is essential to interview an informant as well as the patient. Manic patients may exert some self-control during an interview with a doctor, and may then behave in a disinhibited and grandiose way immediately afterwards. At an early stage of mania, the doctor can easily be misled and may lose the opportunity to persuade the patient to enter hospital before causing himself or herself long-term difficulties (e.g. owing to ill-judged decisions or unjustified extravagance). Where possible, it is important to identify any life events that may have provoked the onset of manic illness. Some manic episodes follow physical illness, treatment with drugs (especially steroids or antidepressants), or operations. *Sleep deprivation* may trigger mania in some susceptible individuals.

The patient's resources and the effect of the illness on other people are assessed in the ways described above for depressive disorders. Even the most supportive family will find it extremely difficult to care for a manic patient at home for more than a few days unless the disorder is exceptionally mild. The patient's responsibilities with regard to the care of dependent children, or at work, should always be considered carefully.

Management of mania

Hospital admission

The first decision is whether to *admit the patient to hospital*. In all but the mildest cases, admission is nearly always advisable to protect the patient from the consequences of their own behaviour. If the disorder is not too severe, the patient will usually agree to enter hospital after some persuasion. If the disorder is more severe, compulsory admission is likely to be needed.

General clinical management

Development of a *therapeutic alliance* with the manic patient is an important goal of treatment, although lack of insight into the condition and anger at involuntary detention can make this a testing and time-consuming process. It is best to use an understanding, yet firm, approach that minimizes confrontation. For example, it is often possible to avoid an argument by taking advantage of the manic patient's easy distractibility; instead of refusing demands, it is better to delay until the patient's attention switches to another topic that they can be encouraged to pursue. In hospital, nursing staff play a key role in this kind of management, where they attempt to provide manic patients with a low-stimulus and safe environment that limits confrontations and impulsive behaviour.

Supportive, reality-orientated psychotherapy is an important element of treatment, and may need to be extended to the patient's partner and family, who often will have experienced great strain during the manic episode. *Educational sessions* are important when the patient is more settled. Patients may need much practical help to limit the financial, legal, and occupational repercussions of the illness.

Medication

Medication plays an important role in the acute management of mania. However, all current drug treatments have limitations in terms of their efficacy and tolerability. In the UK, *antipsychotic drugs* are generally used as primary agents in the management of acute mania, with *mood stabilizers* being reserved for longer-term prophylaxis or where the initial response to antipsychotic drugs is unsatisfactory. A network meta-analysis suggested that the most useful acute antimanic drugs in terms of efficacy and tolerability are haloperidol, olanzapine, quetiapine, and risperidone (Cipriani *et al.*, 2011; Figure 10.1).

For patients who are not already taking mood stabilizers, the drug management can be summarized as follows:

- Begin treatment with either olanzapine, quetiapine, or risperidone (a modest dose of haloperidol is an alternative).

- Where necessary, use adjunctive high-potency benzodiazepines (e.g. lorazepam or clonazepam) to avoid the need for high-dose antipsychotic therapy, and to ensure satisfactory sleep.

- Add a mood stabilizer if the response to this treatment is unsatisfactory (use lithium for 'classical' mania, and

valproate for mania with prominent dysphoric or mixed states, or where lithium is contraindicated).

If it is decided to use a mood stabilizer as the initial treatment, the choice lies between lithium and valproate. Valproate is somewhat easier to use and has a faster onset of action. As before, benzodiazepines can be used as an adjunct to reduce overactivity and permit sleep, while antipsychotic agents can be reserved for patients who are unresponsive to these measures. If a patient presents with a manic episode and is already taking a mood stabilizer, the first step is to optimize the mood stabilizer treatment in terms of dosing and adherence. Concomitant treatment with antipsychotic drugs will then probably be needed; addition of a second mood stabilizing drug is an alternative (Goodwin *et al.*, 2016).

Progress of a manic episode can be judged not only by the *mental state* and *general behaviour*, but also by

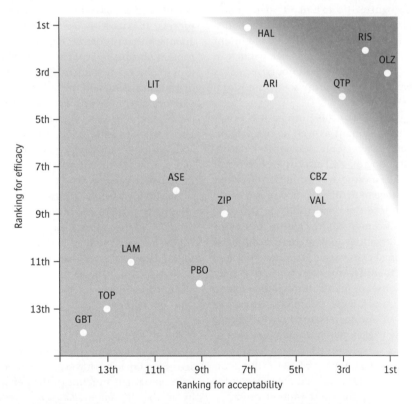

Figure 10.1 Antimanic drugs have been ranked for efficacy (vertical axis) and acceptability (horizontal axis). Treatments in the green section combine the best profile.

ARI=aripiprazole; ASE=asenapine; CBZ=carbamazepine; GBT=gabapentin; HAL=haloperidol; LAM=lamotrigine; LIT=lithium; OLZ=olanzapine; PBO=placebo; QTP=quetiapine; RIS=risperidone; TOP=topiramate; VAL=valproate; ZIP=ziprasidone.

the *pattern of sleep* and the regaining of any weight lost during the illness. As progress continues, antipsychotic drug treatment is reduced gradually. It is important not to discontinue the drug too soon, otherwise there may be a relapse and a return of all the original problems of management.

ECT was used to treat mania before antipsychotic drugs were introduced, but evidence about its effectiveness is still limited (see above). It is appropriate to consider the treatment for the unusual patients who do not respond to drug treatment even when this is given at maximum doses. In such cases, clinical experience suggests that a relatively short course of ECT may often be followed by a significant reduction in symptoms sufficient to allow treatment to be continued with drugs. ECT may also be helpful for *mixed affective states* in which depressive symptoms are prominent.

Whatever treatment is adopted, a careful watch should be kept for symptoms of *depressive disorder*. It should be remembered that transient but profound depressive mood change, accompanied by depressive ideas, is common among manic patients. The clinical picture may also change rapidly to a sustained depressive disorder. If either change happens, the patient may develop suicidal ideas. A sustained change to a depressive syndrome is likely to require additional treatment unless the disorder is mild. For National Institute of Health and Care Excellence (NICE) recommendations on the pharmacological treatment of mania and hypomania see Box 10.2

Continuation treatment

Since the duration of an untreated manic episode can be several months (see above), some form of *continuation treatment,* as in the management of depression, is advisable for at least 6 months. As a guide, treatment should not be withdrawn finally until the patient has been asymptomatic for at least 8 weeks. Withdrawal of lithium should be particularly cautious (e.g. by not lowering the daily dose by more than about 100 mg each week), because sudden discontinuation can lead to 'rebound' mania (Goodwin *et al.*, 2016).

Bipolar depression

Assessment

Depressive episodes are common in bipolar illness and are associated with the majority of the illness burden in both bipolar I and bipolar II disorder (Angst, 2009). Depression may occur as the presenting feature of a new episode of bipolar illness or immediately following

---

> ### Box 10.2 NICE guidance on the pharmacological treatment of mania and hypomania
>
> 1. If a person develops mania or hypomania and is taking an antidepressant; a) consider stopping the antidepressant and b) offer an antipsychotic regardless of whether the antidepressant is stopped.
> 2. If a person develops mania or hypomania and is not taking an antipsychotic or mood stabiliser, offer haloperidol, olanzapine, quetiapine, or risperidone, taking into account any advance statements, the person's preference and clinical context (including physical comorbidity, previous response to treatment, and side effects).
> 3. If the first antipsychotic is poorly tolerated at any dose (including rapid weight gain) or ineffective at the maximum licensed dose, offer an alternative antipsychotic from the drugs listed above taking into account any advance statements, the person's preference and clinical context (including physical comorbidity, previous response to treatment and side effects).
> 4. If an alternative antipsychotic is not sufficiently effective at the maximum licensed dose, consider adding lithium. If adding lithium is ineffective, or if lithium is not suitable (for example, because the person does not agree to routine blood monitoring), consider adding valproate instead.
> 5. If the person is already taking a mood stabiliser such as lithium or valproate consider increasing the dose, up to the maximum therapeutic level if necessary, depending on clinical response. If there is no improvement, consider adding haloperidol, olanzapine, quetiapine or risperidone, depending on the person's preference and previous response to treatment.
>
> Reproduced from the National Institute for Care and Health Excellence, Copyright (2014b).

an episode of mania. The assessment of depression should be carried out as described in Chapter 9, with particular attention to *suicidal thinking*, which may be especially prominent after a sudden switch from mania to depression or during the course of a *mixed affective state.*

Medication

Current guidelines suggest that antidepressant drugs should not be a first line choice for the treatment of bipolar depression. In patients taking mood stabilizers such as lithium and valproate it is important to optimize blood levels as far as tolerance permits. For patients not receiving mood stabilizer treatment, the initial choice lies between treatment with quetiapine or the combination of olanzapine and fluoxetine. Both may cause problems with sedation and weight gain. Lurasidone is an alternative if these side effects prove too problematic (Box 10.3).

Lamotrigine is an alternative as a monotherapy (and can be added to ineffective quetiapine), but the slow dose escalation required to minimize the risk of rash, means that the usual therapeutic dose of around 200 mg daily will not be reached for several weeks. Lamotrigine probably does not induce mania but may not protect against it.

Where bipolar patients with depression are already taking mood stabilizers, the treatments outlined above can be added. However, where lamotrigine is initiated in a patient taking valproate, lamotrigine dosing must be particularly cautious and the *British National Formulary* consulted.

Some patients with bipolar disorder do seem to require conventional antidepressants to achieve a therapeutic response, and short-term treatment can be justified although it is advisable for patients with bipolar I disorder to be on concomitant treatment with a mood stabilizer or an antimanic dose of an atypical antipsychotic. If benefit is obtained consideration should be given to stopping the antidepressant treatment after about 12 weeks to lessen the risk of mood destabilization. Whether the same cautions around antidepressant use should apply to depressed patients with bipolar II disorder is not fully clear (Malhi, 2015). ECT can be considered in patients whose depressive symptoms are severe and require urgent treatment (see Chapter 9) or where sustained attempts at pharmacotherapy have been ineffective.

Psychotherapy

There are very few studies examining the role of structured psychotherapies in acute bipolar depression. In the circumstances, depending on the severity of the depressive disorder and the preferences of the patient, it seems reasonable to offer a structured psychotherapy; for example, cognitive behaviour therapy or interpersonal therapy, that has been shown to be effective in unipolar depression (National Institute for Care and Health Excellence, 2014).

Prevention of relapse and recurrence

Medication

We have already seen that the majority of patients with bipolar disorder will experience recurrence, suffering both depressive and manic episodes, although the pattern in individual patients is variable. For patients who have had two or more episodes of illness in less than 5 years, particularly where the illnesses have proved personally disruptive or hazardous, longer-term maintenance treatment should be considered. This will usually involve long-term treatment with a mood stabilizer or an atypical antipsychotic drug such as quetiapine or perhaps a combination of both. It is worth noting that *valproate* taken during pregnancy is established to be a significant cause of *neurodevelopmental defect*. Therefore valproate should not be prescribed to women of childbearing age unless

---

Box 10.3 NICE guidance on the pharmacological treatment of bipolar depression

1. If a person develops moderate or severe bipolar depression and is not taking a drug to treat their bipolar disorder, offer fluoxetine combined with olanzapine, or quetiapine on its own, depending on the person's preference and previous response to treatment.
2. If the person prefers, consider either olanzapine (without fluoxetine) or lamotrigine on its own.
3. If there is no response to fluoxetine combined with olanzapine, or quetiapine, consider lamotrigine on its own.
4. If a person develops moderate or severe bipolar depression and is taking either lithium or valproate, first (if tolerance permits) increase the mood stabiliser to within the maximum permitted by the therapeutic range. If this is unsuccessful add one of the options above.[1]

[1]Carefully follow the guidance of the British National Formulary when adding lamotrigine to valproate because of the likelihood of elevated lamotrigine levels.

Reproduced from the National Institute for Care and Health Excellence, Copyright (2014a).

all other appropriate treatments have proved ineffective or poorly tolerated.

People with bipolar disorder are often reluctant to consider long-term treatment with medication. There are usually a number of reasons for this, and it is necessary to spend time in discussion with patients so that their point of view can be fully appreciated and understood. An excellent personal account has been provided by Jamison (1997). The reasons for reluctance to consider such treatment may include:

- Difficulties in accepting a diagnosis of a lifelong condition and the need for maintenance treatment with medicines; issues of stigma are usually important.
- A belief that it should be possible to control mood without medication, and that the use of medication for this purpose is a sign of personal weakness.
- A fear that medication will blunt the patient's emotional life, and sometimes specifically that mood stabilizing drugs will decrease feelings of joy and creativity. If the latter feelings are associated with hypomania, it is indeed possible that they will be lessened by medication. For some individuals this can represent a significant loss, which needs to be balanced against the prevention of disabling episodes of depression.

In the UK, lithium is still regarded as the first choice of mood stabilizer, although in the USA valproate is the most popular choice because of its better tolerability. However, the evidence for its long-term prophylactic efficacy is less complete. In addition, there is evidence that the supervised use of lithium is associated with a decreased risk of suicidal behaviour in bipolar illness.

The practical aspects of using lithium to prevent further episodes are discussed in Chapter 25. There are two aspects of maintenance that require emphasis. First, the patient should be seen and their plasma lithium levels and renal and thyroid function assessed at regular intervals. Secondly, some patients stop lithium of their own accord because they fear that the drug may have harmful long-term effects, or because it makes them feel 'flat'. The risk associated with stopping lithium suddenly is that it may well lead to acute relapse. Therefore patients should be advised to discontinue lithium slowly under supervision.

With carefully supervised follow-up, the likelihood of relapse can be substantially reduced by maintenance treatment, although lesser degrees of mood change often continue. These mood changes may require adjunctive antidepressant or antipsychotic drug treatment. For patients who do not show a good response to lithium, alternative mood stabilizing drugs can be used. It is possible to use combinations of mood stabilizers, although the risk of adverse reactions is increased. When using combinations of mood stabilizers it is helpful to bear in mind that lamotrigine appears to be more effective in preventing depression than in preventing mania, while the reverse is true for lithium and valproate. Quetiapine appears to be effective in preventing both depression and mania, although its longer-term use is associated with weight gain and metabolic abnormalities (Vieta et al., 2008).

Current guidelines stress the importance of *regular clinical and biochemical monitoring of the physical health of bipolar patients*, as well as monitoring of their psychological status (Box 10.4)

Psychosocial approaches

Bipolar disorder is often a lifelong, disruptive illness which carries a substantial morbidity. There are several areas of psychosocial function where problems may arise:

- adjustment to the diagnosis, and the need for lifestyle limitations;
- interpersonal and relationship difficulties, and occupational problems;
- misuse of both illegal and legal substances;
- problems relating to concordance with medication.

Box 10.4 Monitoring physical health in bipolar disorder

Ensure that the physical health check for people with bipolar disorder, performed at least annually, includes:
- weight or BMI, diet, nutritional status and level of physical activity
- cardiovascular status, including pulse and blood pressure
- metabolic status, including fasting blood glucose, glycosylated haemoglobin (HbA_{1c}) and blood lipid profile
- liver function
- renal and thyroid function, and calcium levels, for people taking long-term lithium.

Reproduced from the National Institute for Care and Health Excellence, Copyright (2014a).

Psychological treatment approaches designed to help with these important problems employ a number of theoretical approaches (see above). However, they have a number of features in common which centre around education about the illness and enhancing self-management (Goodwin *et al.*, 2016) (Box 10.5).

Although there are some useful drug therapies for bipolar illness, the effectiveness of treatment in clinical practice can be disappointing. The use of the psychosocial measures outlined above should enhance the overall effectiveness of treatment plans and randomized trials of certain approaches, such as psychoeducational programmes and family intervention, are promising in this respect (Geddes and Miklowitz, 2013).

> **Box 10.5 Psychological approaches to bipolar disorder**
>
> - Advice about lifestyle (regular social and sleep routines, avoidance of illegal drugs).
> - Identification and avoidance of triggers for relapse (e.g. sleep deprivation, substance misuse).
> - Identification of early subjective signs of relapse (e.g. feeling driven, sleeping badly), with contingency plans for action.
> - Education about the importance of medication, and discussion of sensitivity to side effects and active measures to reduce these.

Further reading

Jamison KR (1997). *An Unquiet Mind*. Picador, London. (A superb autobiographical account of the experience of bipolar illness and its treatment.)

Kraepelin E (1921). *Manic-Depressive Insanity and Paranoia* (translated by RM Barclay). Churchill Livingstone, Edinburgh [reprinted in 1976 by Arno Press, New York]. pp. 1–164. (The classical account. Of particular interest is the description of untreated mania, which is seldom seen today.)

Miklowitz DJ, Gitlin MJ (2014) *Clinicians Guide to Bipolar Disorder*. Guilford Press, London. (Very readable account of the assessment and practical management of bipolar disorder with excellent coverage of both pharmacological and psychosocial approaches.)

CHAPTER 11
Schizophrenia

Introduction

Of all the major psychiatric syndromes, schizophrenia is perhaps the most difficult to define and describe. This partly reflects the fact that, over the past century or more, widely divergent concepts have been held in different countries and by different people. Although there is now a greater consensus, substantial uncertainties remain. Indeed, schizophrenia remains the best example of the fundamental issues with which psychiatry continues to grapple—concepts of disease, classification, and aetiology. Here, we start with an introduction to the major symptoms and other important clinical features.

Clinical features

In this section, it is assumed that the reader has read the descriptions of symptoms and signs in Chapters 1 and 3, which include definitions of many of the cardinal features of schizophrenia. These have classically been divided into two groupings:

- *Positive symptoms.* These are delusions and hallucinations, the most florid and well-known types of symptom of schizophrenia. Particular types of delusion and hallucination (called *first-rank symptoms*, discussed below) carry greater weight in the diagnosis and help distinguish schizophrenia from other psychotic disorders.
- *Negative symptoms.* These are called 'negative' symptoms because they reflect a loss of normal functioning.

They are often listed as 'four As': *alogia* (decreased spontaneous speech), *avolition* (decreased motivation), *affective flattening* (lack of emotional expressivity, but not depression) and *anhedonia*. (These 'four As' are related to but distinct from Bleuler's 'four As' described in Box 11.5.)

In recent years, other features of schizophrenia have been grouped together in two further categories:

- *Behavioural disorganization.* This includes *formal thought disorder* (abnormalities in the flow and sequence of thoughts; in the past this was often considered as a positive symptom) as well as *inappropriate affect* and *bizarre behaviour*.

- *Cognitive symptoms.* The extent and significance of attentional and memory impairments in schizophrenia, discussed below, has been increasingly recognized, and hence they are now often considered as a separate symptom category.

The predominant symptoms differ between *acute schizophrenia* and *chronic schizophrenia*, and the further description of the clinical syndrome is divided on this basis. Briefly, the acute syndrome is dominated by positive symptoms, with subtypes of acute schizophrenia classically recognized based upon the relative prominence of different positive symptoms. Many patients recover from the acute illness, but progression to the chronic syndrome is also common. Chronic schizophrenia is characterized by negative symptoms; once the chronic syndrome is established, few patients recover completely. Note, however, that the acute versus chronic distinction is an oversimplification; all features of schizophrenia can occur, and co-occur, at any phase of the illness.

For review of the clinical features of schizophrenia, see Arango and Carpenter (2011). For review of negative symptoms, see Marder and Galderisi (2017).

Acute schizophrenia

In acute schizophrenia, positive symptoms predominate, and are often florid. Behavioural disorganization, especially formal thought disorder, is also prominent. Negative symptoms are less common and cognitive deficits less apparent, although this is partly because they are masked by the positive symptoms.

The vignette in Box 11.1 illustrates several common features of acute schizophrenia, including prominent persecutory delusions, with accompanying hallucinations, gradual social withdrawal and impaired performance at work, and the idea that other people can read one's thoughts.

In appearance and behaviour some patients with acute schizophrenia are entirely normal. Others seem changed, although not always in a way that would immediately point to psychosis. They may be preoccupied with their health, their appearance, religion, or other intense interests. Social withdrawal often occurs—for example, spending a long time in their room, perhaps lying immobile on the bed. Some patients smile or laugh without obvious reason. Some appear to be constantly perplexed, while others are restless and noisy, or show sudden and unexpected variability of behaviour.

The speech often reflects an underlying *thought disorder*. In the early stages, there is vagueness in the patient's talk that makes it difficult to grasp the meaning. Some

> ### Box 11.1 A vignette of acute schizophrenia
>
> A previously healthy 20-year-old student had been behaving in an odd way. At times he appeared angry and told his friends that he was being persecuted; at other times he was seen to be laughing to himself for no apparent reason. For several months he had seemed increasingly preoccupied with his own thoughts. His academic work had deteriorated. When interviewed, he was restless, suspicious, and exhibited odd mannerisms. He described hearing voices commenting on his actions and abusing him. He believed that the police had conspired with his university teachers to harm his brain and interfere with his thoughts. He also suspected that they could read his thoughts.

patients have difficulty in dealing with abstract ideas. Other patients become preoccupied with vague pseudo-scientific or mystical ideas. Thought disorder is reflected in the *loosening of association* between expressed ideas, and may be detected in illogical thinking (e.g. *'knight's move' thinking*) or talking past the point (*vorbeireden*). In its severest form, the structure and coherence of thinking are lost, so that utterances are jumbled (*word salad* or *verbigeration*). Some patients use ordinary words or phrases in unusual ways (metonyms or paraphrases), and a few coin new words (*neologisms*). Disorders of the form (or stream) of thought include pressure of thought, poverty of thought, thought blocking, and thought withdrawal; some of these constitute first-rank symptoms (see Boxes 11.2 and 11.3).

Auditory hallucinations are among the most frequent symptoms. They may take the form of noises, music, single words, brief phrases, or whole conversations. They may be unobtrusive, or so severe as to cause great distress. Some voices seem to give commands to the patient. Some patients hear their own thoughts apparently spoken out loud either as they think them (*Gedankenlautwerden*) or immediately afterwards (*echo de la pensée*), and some voices discuss the patient in the third person or comment on his actions; these are first-rank symptoms (see Box 11.3). Visual hallucinations are less frequent, and usually occur together with other kinds of hallucination. Tactile, olfactory, gustatory, and somatic hallucinations are reported by some patients. They are often interpreted in a delusional way—for example, hallucinatory sensations in the lower

Box 11.2 Schneider's symptoms of the first rank

First-rank symptoms (Box 11.3) were described by Kurt Schneider (1887–1967), not to be confused with Carl Schneider, who categorized types of thought disorder. First-rank symptoms were an attempt to make the diagnosis of schizophrenia more reliable by identifying a group of symptoms characteristic of schizophrenia and rarely found in other disorders. It is worth noting that, unlike Bleuler's fundamental symptoms (Box 11.4), Schneider's symptoms were not supposed to have any central psychopathological role, merely that they were valuable in making the diagnosis:

Among the many abnormal modes of experience that occur in schizophrenia, there are some which we put in the first rank of importance, not because we think of them as basic disturbances, but because they have this special value in helping us to determine the diagnosis of schizophrenia. When any one of these modes of experience is undeniably present and no basic somatic illness can be found, we may make the diagnosis of schizophrenia. …. Symptoms of first rank importance do not always have to be present for a diagnosis to be made. (Schneider, 1959)

Studies have shown that first-rank symptoms are probably the most sensitive and specific means of making a diagnosis of schizophrenia. However, they are not always present in schizophrenia, and occur in 10–20% of people with other psychotic disorders. Moreover, in schizophrenia they do not predict outcome. For these and other reasons, first-rank symptoms were removed from the diagnostic criteria in DSM-5, and are expected to be omitted from ICD-11 (Tandon et al., 2013).

abdomen are attributed to unwanted sexual interference by a persecutor.

Delusions are almost invariable in acute schizophrenia, although primary delusions are infrequent and are difficult to identify with certainty. Delusions may originate against a background of so-called primary delusional mood (*Wahnstimmung*). Persecutory delusions are common, but are not specific to schizophrenia, as they also characterize delusional disorders and occur in all psychoses (see Chapter 12). Less common, but of greater diagnostic value, are delusions of reference and of control (passivity), and delusions about the possession of thought. The latter are delusions that thoughts are being inserted into or withdrawn from one's mind, or 'broadcast' to other people. Some of these symptoms are first-rank symptoms (Box 11.3).

Insight is almost always impaired. Most patients do not accept that their experiences result from illness, but usually ascribe them to the malevolent actions of other people.

Orientation is usually normal, although this may be difficult to determine if there is florid thought disorder or if the patient is too preoccupied with their psychotic experience to attend to the interviewer's questions.

Alterations in mood are common and are of three main kinds. First, there may be symptoms of anxiety, depression, irritability, or euphoria. These can be clinically significant, but if such features are sufficiently prominent and sustained, the possibility of schizoaffective disorder or other affective psychosis should be considered. Secondly, there may be blunting (or flattening) of affect—that is, sustained emotional indifference or diminution of emotional response. Thirdly, there may be incongruity of affect, in which the expressed mood is not in keeping with the situation or with the patient's own feelings.

Finally, we emphasize the variability of the clinical picture. Few patients experience all of the symptoms introduced above, while others already have features of the 'chronic' syndrome at first presentation. Moreover, the overall pattern and duration of features are also taken into account before making a diagnosis. These issues, together with some additional clinical features, are discussed later in the chapter.

Box 11.3 First-rank symptoms

Hearing thoughts spoken aloud

Third-person hallucinations

Auditory hallucinations in the form of a 'running commentary'

Somatic (bodily, tactile) hallucinations

Thought withdrawal or insertion

Thought broadcasting

Delusional perception

Feelings or actions experienced as made or influenced by external agents (*passivity*)

Chronic schizophrenia

Although the positive symptoms of the acute syndrome may persist, the chronic syndrome is characterized by the *negative symptoms* of underactivity, lack of drive, social withdrawal, and emotional apathy. The vignette in Box 11.4 illustrates several of the negative features of what is sometimes called a 'defect state' or *deficit syndrome*. The most striking feature is diminished volition—that is, a lack of drive and initiative. Left to himself, the patient may remain inactive for long periods, or may engage in aimless and repeated activity. He withdraws from social encounters, and his social behaviour may deteriorate in ways that embarrass other people. Self-care may be poor, and the style of dress and presentation may be careful but somewhat inappropriate. Some patients collect and hoard objects, so that their surroundings become cluttered and dirty. Others break social conventions by talking intimately to strangers or shouting obscenities in public.

Speech is often abnormal, showing evidence of thought disorder of the kinds found in the acute syndrome described above. Affect is generally blunted and, when emotion is shown, it is incongruous or shallow. Hallucinations and delusions occur, but are by no means universal. They tend to be held with little emotional response. For example, patients may be convinced that they are being persecuted but show neither fear nor anger.

Various disorders of movement occur, including stereotypies, mannerisms and other catatonic symptoms, and dyskinesias (see below). The latter are primarily but not entirely due to antipsychotic medication. Cognitive impairment is common, if not universal, in chronic schizophrenia (see below), and, together with the negative symptoms, contributes to the low level of functioning and poor outcome that still bedevils chronic schizophrenia. However, the cognitive deficits are rarely of sufficient magnitude to be apparent unless detailed cognitive testing is undertaken, and this is rarely the case in clinical practice.

As with acute schizophrenia, the symptoms and signs of the chronic illness are variable. At any stage, positive symptoms may recur or become exacerbated; this may be in response to life events, or to discontinuation of medication.

Subtypes of schizophrenia

Schizophrenia is conventionally divided into several subtypes, based upon the predominant clinical features, especially during the acute phase(s) of the illness.

- *Paranoid schizophrenia* is the commonest form. It is characterized by persecutory delusions, often systematized, and by persecutory auditory hallucinations. Thought disorder and affective, catatonic, and negative symptoms are not prominent. Personality is relatively well preserved.

- In *hebephrenic schizophrenia*, also called *disorganized schizophrenia*, thought disorder and affective symptoms are prominent. The mood is variable, with behaviour often appearing silly and unpredictable. Delusions and hallucinations are fleeting and not systematized. Mannerisms are common. Speech is rambling and incoherent, reflecting the thought disorder. Negative symptoms occur early, and contribute to a poor prognosis.

- In *catatonic schizophrenia*, the most striking features are motor symptoms, as noted in Chapter 1, and changes in activity that vary between excitement and stupor. At times the person may appear to be in a dream-like (*oneiroid*) state. Formerly common, catatonic schizophrenia is now very rare, at least in industrialized countries. Possible reasons for this include a change in the nature of the illness, improvements in treatment, or past misdiagnosis of organic syndromes with catatonic symptoms. It has also been argued that catatonia is a distinct syndrome (Fink *et al.*, 2010) and this is reflected to a degree in DSM-5 (see Box 11.6).

- *Simple schizophrenia* is characterized by the insidious development of odd behaviour, social withdrawal, and declining performance at work. Positive symptoms are not apparent. Given the limited utility of the category and its history of abuse—for example, in the detention of political dissidents in the former Soviet

---

Box 11.4 A vignette of chronic schizophrenia

A middle-aged man lives in a supported hostel and attends a sheltered workshop. He spends most of his time alone. He is usually dishevelled and unshaven, and cares for himself only when encouraged to do so by others. His social behaviour seems odd and stilted. His speech is slow, and its content is vague and incoherent. He shows few signs of emotion. For several years this clinical picture has changed little except for brief periods of acute symptoms, which are usually related to upsets in the ordered life of the hostel.

Union ('sluggish schizophrenia')—its use is now rare, and should be avoided.

- *Undifferentiated schizophrenia* is the term used for cases that do not fit readily into any of the above subtypes, or where there are equally prominent features of more than one of them.

- *Residual schizophrenia* refers to a stage of chronic schizophrenia when, for at least a year, there have been persistent negative symptoms but no recurrence of positive symptoms.

Despite their widespread use, research has shown that these subsyndromes of schizophrenia are not reliable, stable over time, nor associated with clear differences in pathophysiology nor prognosis. For these reasons, they have been removed from DSM-5 (Tandon *et al.*, 2013).

Other subclassifications of schizophrenia have also been proposed, intended to reflect biologically more valid entities. Two examples are given here: Liddle's three subsyndromes, and Crow's type I and type II schizophrenia.

Three clinical subsyndromes

Liddle (1987) studied patients with chronic schizophrenia and, based on clustering of symptoms, described three overlapping clinical syndromes, which he called reality disturbance, disorganization, and psychomotor poverty (see Table 11.1). In many respects, these are comparable to the groupings of positive symptoms, behavioural disorganization, and negative symptoms introduced earlier. Liddle then linked these symptom clusters to distinct patterns of neuropsychological deficit and to regional cerebral blood flow (Liddle *et al.*, 1992). The most reproducible finding is the link between psychomotor poverty, impaired performance on frontal lobe tasks, and decreased frontal blood flow.

Type I and type II schizophrenia

Crow (1985) described two syndromes of schizophrenia, based upon a combination of clinical and neurobiological factors. Type I has an acute onset, mainly positive symptoms, and preserved social functioning during remissions; there is a good response to antipsychotic drugs, associated with dopamine overactivity. By contrast, type II has an insidious onset, mainly negative symptoms, and poor outcome and response to antipsychotic drugs, without evidence of dopamine overactivity but with structural brain changes (especially ventricular enlargement). Subsequent research has not strongly supported the biological subtypes and correlations predicted by the model. However, it was important as an example of the renewed focus on the neurobiological aspects of schizophrenia which occurred around that time.

Other aspects of the clinical syndrome

Cognitive features

Despite Kraepelin's original term *dementia praecox*, cognitive impairment was for many years a neglected component of schizophrenia. However, contemporary studies have emphasized its extent and importance (Schaefer *et al.*, 2013). Deficits are seen across all domains of learning and memory, with disproportionate involvement of semantic memory, working memory, and attention. The deficits average about one standard deviation below expected performance, and are present at the first episode; IQ is also reduced (Mesholam-Gately and Giuliano, 2009). Executive function and attention may be the core deficits, in that they are seen even in patients with otherwise intact cognition. Patients also have deficits in *social cognition*—the perception, storage,

Table 11.1 Cerebral and psychological correlates of three subsyndromes of chronic schizophrenia

Syndrome	Symptoms	Regional cerebral blood flow correlates	Impaired psychological performance
Reality disturbance	Delusions, hallucinations	Left medial temporal lobe, cingulate cortex	Disorders of self-monitoring
Disorganization	Formal thought disorder, inappropriate affect, bizarre behaviour	Anterior cingulate, right ventral frontal cortex, bilateral parietal regions	Tests of selective attention
Psychomotor poverty	Flat affect, poverty of speech, decreased spontaneous movement	Underactivity of frontal cortex ('hypofrontality')	Word generation tasks, planning tests

and utilization of information about other people and ourselves—leading to many difficulties in social interactions and daily life (Green *et al.*, 2015). The social cognitive deficits include marked impairments in *theory of mind* (Bora and Pantelis, 2013).

The time course of neuropsychological involvement in schizophrenia is complex. People who later develop schizophrenia already have reduced IQ scores during childhood (Khandaker *et al.*, 2011). The onset of illness is associated with further cognitive impairments, which may partially improve after resolution of the acute episode. However, most of the cognitive deficits appear to be trait features, largely independent of other symptom domains. Later in the illness, the risk of overt dementia is markedly increased (Ribe *et al.*, 2015), but the dementia is not attributable to Alzheimer's disease or other recognized neurodegenerative disorder. Like many other features of schizophrenia, impaired cognitive performance is also observed in attenuated form in unaffected first-degree relatives.

Cognitive aspects of schizophrenia are currently being emphasized for several reasons (Kahn and Keefe, 2013). First, they are a major determinant of poor functional outcome (Green, 2006; Green *et al.*, 2015). Second, they are now viewed as potential targets for both drugs and psychological therapies (*cognitive remediation*). Third, cognitive features are increasingly conceptualized as being central to the disorder and as underlying the psychotic symptoms (Cannon, 2015); for example, there is a causal and genetically mediated relationship between low IQ and schizophrenia (Kahn and Keefe, 2013).

Methods have been developed to promote and standardize cognitive assessments in schizophrenia (e.g. the MATRICS Battery; Nuechterlein *et al.*, 2008); however, this has yet to become widespread in clinical practice. Failure to achieve this goal, together with uncertainty about the diagnostic specificity of the cognitive deficits, contributed to their omission from DSM-5 diagnostic criteria for schizophrenia, despite their importance in the origins and outcomes of the disorder (Tandon *et al.*, 2013).

Depressive symptoms

Depressive symptoms commonly occur in schizophrenia, in any phase of the illness. They are also prominent features of the prodrome (see below). About 25% of patients exhibit persistent and significant depression, called *postschizophrenic depression*. Comorbid depression in schizophrenia worsens the functional outcome.

There are several reasons why depressive symptoms may be associated with schizophrenia.

- Depression may be an integral part of schizophrenia. This view is supported by the observation that about 50% of patients with acute schizophrenia experience significant depressive symptomatology, which improves as the psychosis remits.
- In the postpsychotic phase, depressive symptoms may be a response to recovery of insight into the nature of the illness and the problems to be faced. Again, this may happen at times, but it does not provide a convincing general explanation.
- Depression may be a side effect of medication. This is not the only explanation, as depressive symptoms can occur in the absence of antipsychotic drug therapy.

Depressive symptoms in schizophrenia should not be confused with negative symptoms nor for the parkinsonian side effects of antipsychotic medication. These distinctions are important, but can be difficult to make. The Calgary Depression Scale for Schizophrenia can be useful in this regard.

For review, see Castle and Bosanac (2012).

Neurological signs

Neurological signs are another neglected clinical feature of schizophrenia (Chan *et al.*, 2010). They are called 'soft signs' because they do not localize pathology to a particular tract or nucleus. They include abnormalities in sensory integration, coordination, and sequencing of complex motor acts; catatonic features and dyskinesias may also be considered under this category (Koning *et al.*, 2010). Neurological signs are seen in unmedicated, first-episode patients (and are therefore at least partially separate from the effects of antipsychotic drugs), but are more common in chronic schizophrenia. The presence of neurological signs correlates with cognitive dysfunction, evidence for developmental anomaly, and diffuse brain pathology, and they are thought to be a manifestation of the neurodevelopmental origins of schizophrenia (Liddle, 2013). A neurological examination that focuses upon the extrapyramidal system should be part of the routine assessment of a patient who presents with schizophrenia.

Olfactory dysfunction

Patients with schizophrenia have deficits in olfactory function, which affect the identification of, sensitivity to, and memory for, odours (Moberg *et al.*, 2014). The deficits are not attributable to medication or smoking, and are associated with cognitive and negative symptoms.

Pain insensitivity

A diminished sensitivity to pain in patients with schizophrenia has long been noted by clinicians, and can on occasion be extreme (Engels *et al.*, 2014). Its cause is unknown. Proposed explanations include thalamic lesions, and the possibility that psychotic symptoms render the patient less concerned by, or distracted from, the pain.

Factors that modify the clinical features

The social and cultural background of the patient affects the content of symptoms. For example, religious delusions are less common now than they were a century ago, and have been replaced by delusions concerned with cloning, HIV, or terrorism. Age also seems to modify the picture. In adolescents and young adults, the clinical features often include thought disorder, mood disturbance, passivity phenomena, thought insertion, and withdrawal. With increasing age, paranoid symptomatology is more common, with more organized delusions.

Intelligence also affects the clinical features, and the psychiatrist's ability to elicit them. Patients with intellectual disability usually present with a simple clinical picture, sometimes referred to as *pfropfschizophrenie*. In contrast, highly intelligent people develop complex delusional systems, and are also better able to articulate, or conceal, their experiences.

The amount of social stimulation has a considerable effect. Understimulation is thought to increase negative symptoms, whereas overstimulation precipitates positive symptoms. Psychosocial approaches to treatment are designed to avoid both extremes.

The prodrome of schizophrenia

In recent years increasing attention has been paid to the prodrome of schizophrenia—that is, the period of time during which psychosis is 'brewing', when there are identifiable symptoms but before diagnosable criteria are met, and before the patient typically presents for help (Yung and McGorry, 1996). The terms 'at-risk state' or 'high-risk state' are also used to describe the prodrome. The focus on the prodrome reflects the fact that in many patients this period may last for several months or years and, the longer the duration of untreated psychosis, the worse the outcome (Penttilä *et al.*, 2014). There are several possible explanations for this association:

- A prolonged, insidious onset is a feature of a severe and treatment-resistant form of schizophrenia.
- Untreated psychosis is 'neurotoxic' and makes the illness less responsive to treatment.
- Illness is more severe by the time treatment is initiated and therefore harder to treat.
- A longer prodrome leads to greater psychosocial impairments and loss of functioning, hampering full recovery.

These considerations have led to a rapid growth in 'early intervention', with services designed to detect and then prevent emerging cases of schizophrenia. These have been driven by the hope that this will improve long-term outcome, although note that this would be unlikely if the first of the four explanations listed above is correct. The therapeutic and service implications are discussed later in this chapter.

The prodrome is characterized by insidious and shifting profiles of largely non-specific symptoms, including mild psychotic-like positive and negative symptoms, and also commonly depressive and anxiety symptoms. Cognitive and social functioning also deteriorates. Various criteria are available to define, assess, and rate the prodrome, including the Comprehensive Assessment of At Risk Mental State (CAARMS). Importantly, many people who are considered to be prodromal do not progress to overt psychosis; typically, less than 25% do so during a 2- to 3-year follow-up. This has important implications for treatment interventions. Studies are attempting to identify the predictors of conversion (Fusar-Poli *et al.*, 2013a).

Diagnosis and classification

This section is concerned mainly with the diagnostic criteria for and classification of schizophrenia as specified in DSM-5 and ICD-10. However, the current approach—and its problems—can be understood better with some knowledge of the historical perspective.

Historical development of ideas about schizophrenia

The development of ideas about schizophrenia is discussed in Box 11.5. To a large extent, they mirror the development of ideas about psychiatric illness in general, reflecting the central position in psychiatry held by schizophrenia during the last century. For a review, see Andreasen (2009).

In the 1960s it was noticed that there were wide divergences in the use of the term schizophrenia, and marked differences in diagnostic practice. This was unsurprising, given the multiple views and traditions summarized in Box 11.5. For example, in the UK and continental Europe, psychiatrists generally employed Schneider's first-rank symptoms (Box 11.2 and 11.3) to identify a narrowly delineated group of cases. In the USA, however, interest in psychodynamic processes led to diagnosis on the basis of mental mechanisms, and to the inclusion of a much wider group of cases. First-admission rates for schizophrenia were also much higher in the USA than in the UK.

These discrepancies prompted two major cross-national studies of diagnostic practice, discussed in Chapter 2 (see page 30), which proved highly influential not just for schizophrenia but also for the development of diagnostic criteria and classificatory systems, namely the US–UK Diagnostic Project (Cooper *et al.*, 1972) and the International Pilot Study of Schizophrenia (IPSS) (World Health Organization, 1973). These findings led to a consensus that agreed diagnostic criteria were required, and the development of standardized methods by which these could be defined and identified, culminating in the current ICD-10 and DSM-5 criteria for schizophrenia.

Box 11.5 Development of schizophrenia concepts and terminologies

In the nineteenth century, one view was that all serious mental disorders were expressions of a single entity, which Griesinger called *Einheitspsychose* (unitary psychosis). The alternative view, put forward by Morel in France, was that mental disorders could be separated and classified. Morel searched for specific entities, and argued for a classification based on cause, symptoms, and outcome. In 1852 he gave the name *démence précoce* to a disorder which he described as starting in adolescence and leading first to withdrawal, odd mannerisms, and self-neglect, and eventually to intellectual deterioration. A few years later, Kahlbaum (1863) described the syndrome of *catatonia*, and Hecker (1871) wrote an account of a condition he called *hebephrenia*.

Emil Kraepelin (1856–1926) derived his ideas from studying the course and outcome of the disorder. His observations led him to argue against the idea of a single psychosis, and to propose a division into *dementia praecox* and *manic–depressive psychosis*. This grouping brought together as subclasses of dementia praecox the previously separate entities of hebephrenia and catatonia. (His adoption of the word *dementia* emphasizes the prominence he attributed to the cognitive impairments of the disorder.) Kraepelin's description of dementia praecox appeared for the first time in 1893, in the fourth edition of his textbook, and the account was expanded in subsequent editions. He described the illness as occurring in clear consciousness, and consisting of 'a series of states, the common characteristic of which is a peculiar destruction of the internal connections of the psychic personality' (Kraepelin, 1919). Kraepelin originally divided dementia praecox into three subtypes (catatonic, hebephrenic, and paranoid), and later added a fourth subtype (simple). He separated the condition that he named *paraphrenia* (Box 12.2) from dementia praecox on the grounds that it started in middle life and seemed to be free from the changes in emotion and volition found in dementia praecox. It is commonly held that Kraepelin regarded dementia praecox as invariably progressing to chronic deterioration. However, he reported that, in his series of cases, 13% recovered completely (although some relapsed later) and 17% were ultimately able to live and work without difficulty.

Eugen Bleuler (1857–1939) based his work on that of Kraepelin, and in his own book wrote 'the whole idea of dementia praecox originates with Kraepelin' (Bleuler, 1911). He also acknowledged the help of his younger colleague, Carl Jung, in trying to apply some of Freud's ideas to dementia praecox. Compared with Kraepelin, Bleuler was concerned less with prognosis and more with the mechanisms of symptom formation. Bleuler proposed the name *schizophrenia* to denote a 'splitting' of psychic functions, which he considered to be of central importance. He believed in a distinction between *fundamental* and *accessory* symptoms. Fundamental symptoms included four features sometimes known as Bleuler's 'four As': *Associations* (thought disorder), *Affect* (blunting, flattening, and incongruity of affect), *Ambivalence* (lack of motivation), and *Autism* (social withdrawal and failure of theory of mind). It is interesting that, in Bleuler's view, some of the most frequent and striking symptoms were accessory (secondary)—for example, hallucinations, delusions, catatonia, and abnormal behaviours. Bleuler was interested in the psychological study of his cases, but did not rule out the possibility of a neuropathological cause of schizophrenia. Since Bleuler was preoccupied more with psychopathological mechanisms than with symptoms themselves, his approach to diagnosis was less precise than that of Kraepelin, but remained influential in many parts of the world even into the 1980s. In addition, Bleuler took a more optimistic view of the outcome, but still held that one should not 'speak of cure but of far-reaching improvement'. He also wrote: 'as yet I have never released a schizophrenic in whom I could not still see distinct signs of the disease, indeed there are very few in whom one would have to search for such signs' (Bleuler, 1911).

Several German psychiatrists tried to define subgroupings within schizophrenia. Kleist, a pupil of the neurologist Wernicke, looked for associations between brain pathology and different subtypes of psychotic illness. He accepted Kraepelin's main diagnostic framework, but used careful clinical observation in an attempt to distinguish various subdivisions within schizophrenia and other atypical disorders. His attempt to match these subtypes to specific kinds of brain pathology was ingenious but unsuccessful.

Leonhard continued this approach of careful clinical observation, and published a complicated classification that distinguishes schizophrenia from the *'cycloid'* *psychoses*—a group of non-affective psychoses of good outcome (Leonhard, 1957). He also divided schizophrenia into two groups. The first group is characterized by a progressive course, and is divided into catatonias, hebephrenias, and paraphrenias. Leonhard gave this group a name, which is often translated as *systematic*. The second group, referred to as *non-systematic*, is divided into *affect-laden paraphrenia*, *schizophasia*, and *periodic catatonia*. Affect-laden paraphrenia is characterized by paranoid delusions and the expression of strong emotion about their content.

In schizophasia, speech is grossly disordered and difficult to understand. Periodic catatonia is a condition with regular remissions. During an episode, akinetic symptoms are sometimes interrupted by hyperkinetic symptoms.

Scandinavian psychiatrists were influenced by Jaspers' distinction between process schizophrenia and reactive psychoses. In the late 1930s, Langfeldt, using follow-up data on patients in Oslo, proposed a distinction between true schizophrenia, which had a poor prognosis, and *schizophreniform states*, which had a good prognosis. True schizophrenia was defined narrowly and was similar to Kraepelin's dementia praecox. Schizophreniform states were described as often precipitated by stress and accompanied by confusional and affective symptoms. Langfeldt's distinction between cases with good and bad prognoses has been influential, but research has not found that his criteria predict prognosis accurately. According to modern diagnostic criteria, most of Langfeldt's schizophreniform states would be classified as mood disorders. (Note also that in DSM-5 the term schizophreniform disorder is used in a different way.)

In Denmark and Norway, cases of psychosis arising after stressful events have received much attention. The terms *reactive psychosis* or *psychogenic psychosis* are commonly applied to conditions that appear to be precipitated by stress, are to some extent understandable in their symptoms, and have a good prognosis. In current diagnostic schemes such disorders would be classified as *brief psychotic disorder* or *schizophreniform disorder*.

Current debates about schizophrenia nomenclature and classification centre on two issues. Firstly, whether the word schizophrenia should be abolished, as has already occurred in Japan and South Korea. This is advocated to reduce stigma, and in order to replace it with a term that better fits current views about its nature and boundaries, such as *psychosis spectrum syndrome* (van Os, 2016). Secondly, whether schizophrenia (and other psychotic disorders) should be a dimensional rather than categorical diagnosis (Linscott and van Os, 2013; see Chapter 2). For review see Lawrie *et al.* (2016a).

In summary, a wide range of views about schizophrenia have been held over the past century since Kraepelin and Bleuler established the concept. With the advent of current classificatory systems, the term now refers to a syndrome that can be diagnosed reliably, which is essential for rational clinical practice. However, as noted in Chapter 3, reliability is not in itself sufficient. Because the cause of schizophrenia is still largely unknown, the syndrome remains of uncertain validity. Until this fundamental question is answered, there will continue to be dispute as to its most important features, diagnostic boundaries, and internal subdivisions.

Table 11.2 Classification of schizophrenia and schizophrenia-like disorders in ICD-10 and DSM-5[*]

ICD-10	DSM-5
Schizophrenia	**Schizophrenia**
• Paranoid	
• Hebephrenic	
• Catatonic	
• Undifferentiated	
• Residual	
• Simple schizophrenia	
• Postschizophrenic depression	
• Other schizophrenia	
• Unspecified schizophrenia	
Schizoaffective disorder	**Schizoaffective disorder**
Persistent delusional disorders	**Delusional disorder**
• Delusional disorder	
• Other persistent delusional disorders	
Acute and transient psychotic disorder	**Brief psychotic disorder**
• Acute schizophrenia-like psychotic disorder	**Schizophreniform disorder**
• Acute polymorphic psychotic disorder	
• Other acute psychotic disorders	
Induced delusional disorder	**Other specified schizophrenia spectrum and other psychotic disorder**
Other non-organic psychotic disorders	
Unspecified non-organic psychosis	**Unspecified schizophrenia spectrum and other psychotic disorder**
Schizotypal disorder	**Substance/medication-induced psychotic disorder**
	Psychotic disorder due to another medical condition

[*] The order of categories in the two systems has been changed to compare their features more clearly.
Source: data from The ICD-10 classification of mental and behavioural disorders: clinical descriptions and diagnostic guidelines, Copyright (1992), World Health Organization; Diagnostic and Statistical Manual of Mental Disorders, Fifth Edition, Copyright (2013), American Psychiatric Association.

Classification of schizophrenia in DSM-5 and ICD-10

The classification of schizophrenia and schizophrenia-like disorders in DSM-5 and ICD-10 is outlined and compared in Table 11.2. The classifications are broadly similar but do have some important differences.

DSM-5

In this classification, schizophrenia is defined in terms of the symptoms, course, and impaired functioning (Box 11.6). The cardinal acute symptoms are given in criterion A, which comprise delusions, hallucinations, disorganized speech, disorganized or catatonic behaviour,

> ### Box 11.6 Simplified description of criteria for schizophrenia in DSM-5
>
> A. Two or more of the following, each present for at least 1 month (or less if successfully treated). At least one of these must be 1, 2 or 3:
>   1. Delusions
>   2. Hallucinations
>   3. Disorganized speech (e.g. frequent derailment or incoherence)
>   4. Grossly disorganized or catatonic behaviour
>   5. Negative symptoms (i.e. diminished emotional expression or avolition).
>
> B. Impaired level of functioning in one or more domain (e.g. work, relationships) for a significant portion of the time since onset. If the onset is in childhood or adolescence, there is a failure to achieve the expected level of functioning.
>
> C. Continuous signs of the disturbance persist for at least 6 months. This 6-month period must include at least 1 month of symptoms that meet Criterion A.
>
> D. The patient does not meet criteria for schizoaffective disorder, or a mood disorder with psychotic features.
>
> E. The disturbance is not attributable to the psychological effects of a substance (e.g. a drug of abuse, a medication) or another medical condition.
>
> F. If there is a history of autism spectrum disorder, the additional diagnosis of schizophrenia is made only if there are prominent delusions or hallucinations present for at least 1 month, in addition to the other required symptoms of schizophrenia.
>
> Source: data from Diagnostic and Statistical Manual of Mental Disorders, Fifth Edition, Copyright (2013), American Psychiatric Association.

and negative symptoms. At least two of these must have been present for at least 1 month (unless treated). In addition, there must be evidence of impaired level of functioning (criterion B), and continuous signs of disturbance for at least 6 months (criterion C). The other criteria address the boundaries of schizophrenia with mood disorders, organic and substance abuse disorders, and autistic spectrum disorders.

Patients who have schizophrenia-like symptoms of less than the 1- and 6-month duration criteria are classified as suffering from schizophreniform disorder or brief psychotic disorder. Other related disorders include delusional disorder (see Chapter 12) and psychotic disorders not otherwise classified (see below).

After at least 1 year has elapsed since the onset of active-phase symptoms, DSM-5 allows the disorder to be classified by the number of acute episodes that have occurred, and whether the patient is currently in an episode, or in partial or full remission. The current severity for each of the category A items can also be rated on a 5-point scale.

Catatonia. As noted earlier, DSM-5 does not divide schizophrenia into the classical subtypes such as paranoid, hebephrenic, or catatonic. However, it does include catatonia as a category that can be diagnosed as being comorbid with a disorder such as schizophrenia.

For review of schizophrenia in DSM-5, see Tandon *et al.* (2013).

ICD-10

The ICD-10 criteria for schizophrenia (see Box 11.7) place more reliance than DSM-5 on specific types of psychotic symptoms, including first-rank symptoms. The diagnosis can be made after a duration of only 1 month, excluding prodromal symptoms, and hence can be applied to recent onset cases which in DSM-5 would be categorized as schizophreniform disorder. Unlike DSM-5, ICD-10 subclassifies schizophrenia into the subtypes described earlier.

Certain aspects of personality are associated with schizophrenia, clinically and genetically. ICD-10 includes *schizotypal disorder* among the spectrum of schizophrenic disorders, whereas in DSM-5 this condition is classified as a personality disorder. Schizotypal disorder is associated with social isolation and restriction of affect; in addition, there are perceptual distortions, with disorders of thinking and speech and striking eccentricity or oddness of behaviour.

Similar to DSM-5, ICD-10 classifies delusional disorders separately from schizophrenia. In addition, ICD-10 includes a group of acute and transient psychotic disorders that have an acute onset and complete recovery within 2–3 months (see below).

Note that schizophrenia-like disorders that occur in recognized organic disorders, or secondary to substance use, are classified separately in ICD-10, but are included in the schizophrenia chapter of DSM-5.

Summary of key differences between DSM-5 and ICD-10

- ICD-10 places weight on Schneider's first-rank symptoms; DSM-5 emphasizes course and functional impairment.
- ICD-10 requires a duration of illness of 1 month; DSM-5 requires a duration of 6 months.
- ICD-10 recognizes traditional subtypes of schizophrenia (e.g. paranoid schizophrenia); DSM-5 does not.
- Schizotypal disorder is included in ICD-10, but is categorized as a personality disorder in DSM-5.

Schizophrenia-like disorders

Whatever definition of schizophrenia is adopted, there will be cases that resemble schizophrenia in some respects and yet do not meet the criteria for diagnosis. In DSM-5 and ICD-10, these disorders can be considered within four groupings:

1. Delusional disorders (paranoid psychoses).
2. Brief psychotic disorders.
3. Psychotic disorders accompanied by prominent affective symptoms.
4. Psychotic disorders without all of the symptoms required for schizophrenia.

Delusional disorders are discussed in Chapter 12. The latter three groups are discussed here.

Brief psychotic disorders

DSM-5 uses the term *brief psychotic disorder* to refer to a syndrome characterized by at least one of the acute-phase positive symptoms shown in Box 11.6. The disorder lasts for at least 1 day but not more than 1 month, by which time recovery has occurred, including full return to premorbid level of functioning. The disorder may or may not follow a stressor, but psychoses induced by the direct physiological effects of drugs or medical illness are excluded.

In DSM-5, *schizophreniform disorder* is a syndrome similar to schizophrenia (meeting criterion A) which has lasted for more than 1 month (and so cannot be classified as brief psychotic disorder), but for less than the 6 months required for a diagnosis of schizophrenia to be made. Social and occupational dysfunction are not required to make the diagnosis.

In ICD-10, the grouping is *acute and transient psychotic disorder*. These disorders are of acute onset, and complete recovery within 2–3 months is the rule. The disorder may or may not be precipitated by a stressful life event. The category is then subdivided into several overlapping and somewhat confusing subtypes. In the first two, *acute polymorphic psychotic disorders, with or without symptoms of schizophrenia,* hallucinations, delusions, and perceptual disturbance are obvious, but change rapidly in nature and extent. There are often accompanying changes in mood and motor behaviour. *Bouffée délirante* and *cycloid psychosis* (see Box 11.5) are given as synonyms for these categories. A third subtype, *acute schizophrenia-like psychotic episode,* is a non-committal term for cases that meet the symptom criteria for schizophrenia but last for less than 1 month. Residual cases that do not fit these subtypes of acute psychosis are called *other acute psychotic episodes.* The term schizophreniform disorder is not used as a discrete category in ICD-10.

For review of brief psychotic disorders and their outcome, see Fusar-Poli et al (2016).

Schizophrenia-like disorders with prominent affective symptoms

Some patients have a more or less equal mixture of schizophrenic and affective symptoms. Such patients are classified under *schizoaffective disorder* in both DSM-5 and ICD-10.

The term schizoaffective disorder has been used in several distinct ways. It was first applied by Kasanin (1994/1933) to a small group of young patients with severe mental disorders characterized by a very sudden onset in a setting of marked emotional turmoil. The psychosis lasted a few weeks and was followed by recovery.

The current definitions differ substantially from this description. DSM-5 requires that there should have been an uninterrupted period of illness during which there is a major depressive or manic episode concurrent with symptoms that meet criterion A for schizophrenia. During this continuous episode of illness, acute psychotic symptoms must have been present for at least 2 weeks in the absence of prominent mood symptoms (or the diagnosis would be a mood disorder with psychotic features). However, the episode of mood disturbance must have been present for a substantial part of the illness.

The definition of schizoaffective disorder in ICD-10 is similar. It also specifies that the diagnosis should only be made when both definite schizophrenic and definite affective symptoms are equally prominent and present simultaneously, or within a few days of each other. (This is an important point. The label 'schizoaffective' should not be applied just because a patient has an isolated symptom or two consistent with both diagnoses, or because the assessment has not been sufficiently detailed to identify the primary diagnosis). ICD-10 classifies schizoaffective disorder according to whether the mood disturbance is depressive, manic, or mixed. In DSM-5 schizoaffective disorder is specified as either depressive type or bipolar.

The reliability and nosological status of schizoaffective disorder is questionable (Kotov *et al.,* 2013), with neither genetic nor neurobiological separation from schizophrenia or bipolar disorder (Cardno and Owen, 2014). The outcome of schizoaffective disorder is generally thought to be better than that for schizophrenia, with negative symptoms rarely developing; however, the data are limited.

As noted above, it is not uncommon for patients with schizophrenia to develop depression as the symptoms of acute psychosis subside. This is recognized in ICD-10 as *postschizophrenic depression,* where prominent depressive symptoms have been present for at least 2 weeks while some symptoms of schizophrenia (either positive or negative) still remain.

Persistent disorders without all of the required symptoms for schizophrenia

A difficult problem is presented by cases that have long-standing schizophrenia-like symptoms but which do not fully meet the diagnostic criteria. There are four groups.

- Patients who have exhibited the full clinical picture of schizophrenia in the past, but who no longer have all of the symptoms required to make the diagnosis. These cases are classified as *residual schizophrenia* in ICD-10.

- People who from an early age have behaved oddly or eccentrically and shown features seen in schizophrenia—for example, ideas of reference, persecutory beliefs, and unusual types of thinking. These disorders can be classified as personality disorders in DSM-5 (*schizotypal personality disorder*), or with schizophrenia in ICD-10 (*schizotypal disorder*). Because of a suggested close relationship to schizophrenia, these disorders have also been called *latent schizophrenia,* or part of the *schizophrenia spectrum.*

- People with social withdrawal, lack of initiative, odd behaviour, and blunting of emotion, in whom positive psychotic symptoms are never known to have occurred. A variety of terms may be applicable, including *simple schizophrenia, schizoid personality disorder,* and *Asperger's syndrome.* (We advise caution in using the terms simple schizophrenia or latent schizophrenia. Both of these lack utility—since treatment is rarely indicated or sought—and represent speculative diagnostic labels for what many would consider simply to be eccentricity.)

- People with stable, persistent delusions but without other features of schizophrenia (see Chapter 12).

Comorbidity

Many patients with schizophrenia also meet the criteria for another psychiatric diagnosis, complicating diagnosis and treatment, and worsening the outcome. The example of depression (which occurs in 50% of cases) has already been mentioned. The estimated lifetime prevalence of any substance abuse is 47%, and of alcohol abuse is 21%. Psychiatric disorders often comorbid with schizophrenia include post-traumatic stress disorder (29%), obsessive–compulsive disorder (23%), and panic disorder (15%). For a review, see Buckley *et al.* (2009).

Differential diagnosis

We have already described how current classifications include schizophrenia-like disorders as well as schizophrenia, but the boundary between them is blurred and to some extent arbitrary. Similarly, there is no clear distinction between disorders that are considered to be variants of schizophrenia, some of which are viewed as being part of its differential diagnosis. For example, delusional disorders and schizotypal disorder are often included in both categories. Such difficulties reflect the unknown validity of the syndrome(s), and are unlikely to be resolved until the classification is based upon aetiology or other empirically validated markers (Lawrie *et al.*, 2016b). In this regard, the distinction between schizophrenia and organic schizophrenia-like disorders is also not only unhelpful (Chapter 2) but becomes increasingly blurred as potential causes of some cases of 'schizophrenia' are discovered, such as copy number variants and antineuronal antibodies (see below).

With these caveats in mind, current diagnostic practice requires schizophrenia to be distinguished from a number of other disorders, summarized in Box 11.8.

Organic syndromes. Acute schizophrenia can be mistaken for *delirium*, especially if there is pronounced thought disorder and a rapidly fluctuating affect and mental state. Careful observation is needed for clouding of consciousness, disorientation, and other features of delirium (see Chapter 14).

> **Box 11.8 Differential diagnosis of schizophrenia**
>
> **Cases meeting some but not all criteria for schizophrenia**
> Brief psychotic disorder
> Delusional disorder
> Schizotypal disorder
>
> **Cases with affective and psychotic symptoms**
> Schizoaffective disorder
> Psychotic depression
> Bipolar disorder
>
> **Schizophrenia-like disorders attributable to a specific cause**
> Schizophrenia-like disorder due to psychoactive substance use
> Organic schizophrenia-like disorder
>
> **Other**
> Autism and related disorders
> Obsessive–compulsive disorder
> Body dysmorphic disorder
> Schizoid personality disorder
> Paranoid personality disorder

Schizophrenia-like disorders can also occur, in clear consciousness, in a range of neurological and medical disorders. These conditions are referred to as a *psychotic disorder due to another medical condition* (DSM-5), *organic delusional disorder* (ICD-10), or simply as *secondary schizophrenia*. Classic examples include temporal lobe epilepsy (complex partial seizures), general paralysis of the insane, and metachromatic leukodystrophy (see Chapter 14, and Hyde and Ron, 2011). Visual, olfactory, and gustatory hallucinations are said to be suggestive of an organic aetiology. The occurrence of organic schizophrenia-like disorders emphasizes the importance of a careful medical history and physical examination (and investigations, if indicated) in all such patients. One study in London found that 10 out of 268 cases (3.7%) of 'first-episode schizophrenia' had an organic cause other than substance misuse (Johnstone *et al.*, 1987).

Drug-induced states (including substance misuse). Certain prescribed drugs, particularly steroids and dopamine agonists, can cause florid psychotic states. Psychoactive substance misuse, particularly with psychostimulants or phencyclidine, and also alcohol, should always be considered in the presentation of schizophrenia-like psychoses. Urine or hair testing can be helpful in diagnosis, as is the temporal association between drug use and symptoms. However, the high prevalence of recreational drug use in young adults means that a clear distinction between a drug-induced psychosis and schizophrenia is not always possible. See also Chapter 20.

Mood disorders with psychotic features. The distinction of schizophrenia (and schizoaffective disorder) from affective psychosis depends on the degree and persistence of the mood disorder, the relationship of any hallucinations or delusions to the prevailing mood, and the nature of the symptoms in any previous episodes. The distinction from mania in young people can be particularly difficult, and sometimes the diagnosis can only be clarified by longer-term follow-up. A family history of mood disorder may be a useful pointer.

Delusional disorders. These disorders (see Chapter 12) are characterized by chronic, systematized paranoid delusions, but lack other symptoms of schizophrenia, and many areas of the mental state are unremarkable.

Personality disorder. Differential diagnosis from personality disorder, especially of the paranoid, schizoid, or schizotypal forms, can be difficult when insidious changes are reported in a young person, or paranoid ideas are present. Prolonged observation may be required to detect genuine symptoms of psychosis, and the additional features indicative of schizophrenia. Some patients with borderline personality disorder also exhibit transient psychotic symptoms, although the presence of affective instability and other features means that there should rarely be diagnostic confusion with schizophrenia.

Epidemiology

Schizophrenia is a disorder with a low incidence and a high prevalence. Estimates of both have varied, reflecting the methodology and diagnostic criteria used, as well as probable differences between populations. Recent reviews and meta-analyses have helped to clarify the estimates and their confidence intervals (McGrath *et al.*, 2008; Jablensky *et al.*, 2011).

Incidence

The annual incidence using current diagnostic criteria is 0.16–1.00 per 1000 population using a broad definition; for more restrictive diagnoses (e.g. DSM-IV criteria), the incidence is about two to three times lower (Jablensky *et al.*, 2011). A meta-analysis reported a mean incidence of 0.24 per 1000 population but a median incidence of 0.15 per 1000 (McGrath *et al.*, 2008). The difference reflects a skew, with many estimates in the upper tail of the distribution, which in turn results from studies that sampled from within populations with a high incidence (e.g. migrant groups, as discussed below). Another meta-analysis found an incidence of schizophrenia in England of 15.2 per 100,000 person years (Kirkbride *et al.*, 2012a).

These recent analyses strongly question the belief, which arose largely from the WHO Ten-Country Study (Jablensky *et al.*, 1992), that schizophrenia has a similar incidence (and prevalence) in all populations. Indeed, data indicate a fivefold global variation in incidence, with rates higher in developed than developing countries (McGrath *et al.*, 2008). There are also variations in incidence related to a number of other environmental factors (see below).

Suggestions made in the latter part of the last century that the incidence of schizophrenia was falling have not been borne out; indeed, the incidence of diagnosed early-onset schizophrenia has, if anything, increased over the past four decades (Okkels *et al.*, 2013).

Prevalence

Systematic reviews indicate a lifetime prevalence of about 5 per 1000 (Simeone *et al.*, 2015), and a lifetime morbid risk of 7.2 per 1000 (McGrath *et al.*, 2008). These are median values because the data are skewed; the means are higher, at 5.5 and 11.9 per 1000, respectively. The latter figure is more consistent with the frequent statement that about 1 in 100 people develop schizophrenia, but the value of 7 in 1000 is statistically more appropriate.

Age at onset

Schizophrenia can begin at any stage of life, from childhood to old age. The usual onset is between 15 and 54 years, most commonly in the mid-twenties; more detailed analyses suggest that there are two peaks, one at 20 years, and a second peak at 33 years. Gender differences in age of onset may explain these observations, as men have a single peak in their early twenties, whereas women have a broader range of age of onset, and a second peak in their fourth decade. However, the gender difference in mean age of onset is smaller and less robust than often stated (Eranti *et al.*, 2013).

For review of schizophrenia in children see Chapter 16 and Hollis (2015); for review of late-onset schizophrenia see Chapter 19 and Cohen CI *et al.* (2015).

Gender

In addition to possible gender differences in age of onset, meta-analyses show that schizophrenia is more common in men than in women, with a male:female ratio of 1.4:1. The difference is more marked for severe cases, and is not due to differences in referral, identification, or age of onset. It has been attributed to the neuroprotective effects of oestrogen, but the evidence for this is poor. Gender differences in genetic and epigenetic risk factors may also be relevant. For a review of gender issues in schizophrenia and its management, see Abel *et al.* (2010).

Fertility

Whether patients with schizophrenia show decreased fertility has been a controversial topic, not least because of its implications for debate about whether schizophrenia is a 'disease', and with regard to its genetic basis. A meta-analysis showed a substantial reduction in fertility in people with schizophrenia (about 40% of that expected), which was greater in men than in women (Bundy *et al.*, 2011). These figures are difficult to interpret as being an intrinsic feature of schizophrenia, since opportunities for patients to have children have historically been limited by institutionalization, as well as by the amenorrhoea and sexual dysfunction caused by antipsychotic drugs. On the other hand, fertility is also decreased before the onset of psychosis (Zimbron *et al.*, 2013) and is slightly reduced in the unaffected siblings of patients (Bundy *et al.*, 2011). There are various theories but no explanation as to why schizophrenia persists in the population despite the apparent reduction in fertility.

Other aspects of schizophrenia epidemiology

Epidemiological aspects relevant to aetiology are considered in the next section. The course and outcome of schizophrenia are discussed later in the chapter.

Aetiology

Overview

Views about the aetiology of schizophrenia have been inextricably linked with the controversies regarding its nature and classification discussed earlier in this chapter. Schizophrenia therefore exemplifies the whole range of biological, psychological, and social factors considered to be important in psychiatric causation and the methods that have been applied to try to identify them. This section summarizes the current knowledge and theories in each domain, and also mentions some outdated but influential views. Table 11.3 lists the main evidence-based contemporary aetiological factors and theories.

Key aspects of the present consensus regarding the aetiology of schizophrenia can be summarized as follows. The most important influence is genetic, with about 80% of the risk being inherited. The mode of inheritance is complex, and the genes—some of which have recently been identified—act as risk factors, not determinants of

illness. A number of environmental factors contribute too, many of which act early in life, and which interact with the genetic predisposition. Together, these and subsequent risk factors lead to a neurodevelopmental disturbance that renders the individual vulnerable to the later emergence of symptoms, and that manifests itself premorbidly in a range of behavioural, cognitive, and biological features. In schizophrenia, there are minor but clear differences in brain structure and function, and their characteristics support the view that the syndrome is a disorder of brain connectivity. Acute psychosis is associated with excessive dopamine neurotransmission in the basal ganglia, which may be secondary to abnormalities of the glutamate system. Various psychosocial factors significantly influence the onset, and course, of illness. Finally, it is emphasized that there are few certainties about the aetiology of schizophrenia, and even where the facts are robust, their interpretation often remains unclear.

Table 11.3 Schizophrenia: aetiological factors and theories

Category	Examples
Genetic	Single nucleotide polymorphisms in many genes (e.g. ZNF804A)
	Copy number variation (e.g. 22q11 deletion)
	Rare variants (e.g. SETD1A)
Early environment	Maternal malnutrition
	Maternal infection
	Birth complications
	Urban birth
Social	Migration
	Ethnic minority status
Other	Early cannabis use
Hypotheses	Neurodevelopmental
	Gene–environment interactions
	Dopamine
	Glutamate
	Dysconnectivity
	Immune/inflammatory

In this section, we discuss the genetic and environmental risk factors for schizophrenia. In the following sections we discuss in turn the key neurobiological, social and psychological elements, and the major explanatory models proposed regarding the nature of the disorder.

For contemporary reviews of the aetiology of schizophrenia, see van Os *et al.* (2010), Howes and Murray (2014), and Owen *et al.* (2016).

Genetics

Family, twin, and adoption studies have all been applied extensively in schizophrenia, and cumulatively provide irrefutable evidence for a major genetic contribution to the syndrome. Such studies set the context for the current wave of genomic and molecular studies designed to identify the individual genes and mechanisms by which the risk for schizophrenia is mediated.

Family studies

The first systematic family study was conducted in Kraepelin's department by Rudin, who showed that the rate of dementia praecox was higher among the siblings of probands than in the general population. Gottesman (1991) reviewed the combined results of many studies and provided estimates for the lifetime risk of schizophrenia in various classes of relatives (Table 11.4). Whilst some of these estimates may be questioned, they do provide clear evidence of a familial aetiology, and the greater concordance rates in monozygotic compared to dizygotic twins indicates that this arises primarily from shared genes. Equally, the higher incidence in dizygotic twins than in siblings supports a role for shared environmental factors.

Family studies can also be used to determine whether the liability to schizophrenia and other disorders (e.g. bipolar disorder) is transmitted independently, which should be the observed pattern if the two disorders are separate syndromes with differing aetiology. Earlier studies gave inconclusive or inconsistent results, but recent large studies indicate clearly that there is no such independent transmission. For example, Lichtenstein *et al.* (2009) show in the Swedish population that schizophrenia and bipolar disorder coexist in families. It is also known that the risk of schizophrenia, schizoaffective disorder, and schizotypal and paranoid personality disorders is increased in first-degree relatives of patients with schizophrenia. These findings support the concept of a *schizophrenia spectrum*, in which the familial

Table 11.4 Lifetime risk of schizophrenia in relatives of a proband with schizophrenia

Relative type	Lifetime risk of schizophrenia
Monozygotic twin	48%
Dizygotic twin	17%
Sibling	9%
Half-sibling	6%
Child with one affected parent	17%
Child with two affected parents	46%
First cousin	2%
Baseline risk	1%

Source: data from Gottesman I, Schizophrenia Genesis: the origins of madness, Copyright (1991), W. H. Freeman.

predisposition is to a range of disorders, not simply schizophrenia itself. This is also consistent with recent findings from genome-wide studies, discussed below.

Twin studies

Twin studies were introduced in Chapter 5. They have been of considerable importance in research on schizophrenia, providing unequivocal evidence of the heritability of this disorder.

The first substantial twin study was conducted in Munich by Luxenberger in the 1920s. He found concordance in 11 of his 19 monozygotic (MZ) pairs and in none of his 13 dizygotic (DZ) pairs. Subsequent investigations all agree that concordance is several-fold higher in MZ than in DZ twins, with representative estimates of 40–50% concordance for MZ twins and about 10% for DZ twins (Box 11.4, and see Cardno and Gottesman, 2000).

Modern twin studies also produce estimates of *heritability* (the proportion of liability to schizophrenia in the population that can be attributed to genes; see page 103), and can separate environmental factors into those that are unique to the individual and those that are shared with others. A meta-analysis of twin studies (Sullivan *et al.*, 2003) confirmed the substantial heritability of schizophrenia (81%; 95% confidence interval [CI], 73–90%). These data unambiguously show that inheritance (i.e. genes) contribute the majority of the risk for schizophrenia. However, there are caveats about the interpretation of heritability figures. For example, the estimates make some assumptions about the 'genetic architecture' (i.e. how the genetic factors operate) and include gene–environment interactions. The meta-analysis also showed that most of the environmental contribution comes from shared rather than individual-specific influences (11%; 95% CI, 3–19%). The identity of these shared environmental factors is unknown. It is also worth noting that estimates for schizophrenia heritability from population studies are somewhat lower (e.g. 64% in the study by Lichtenstein *et al.*, 2009) than those of twin studies, for reasons which are not entirely clear.

Among discordant MZ twins, the risk of schizophrenia is increased equally in children of the unaffected and the affected co-twin. This indicates that the unaffected co-twin indeed had a similar genetic susceptibility to developing schizophrenia as the affected twin, but for some reason did not express the phenotype. This is most probably due to environmental protective factors, or chance ('stochastic processes'), affecting the penetrance or expression of the genetic predisposition. Moreover, as a group, unaffected identical co-twins do exhibit some mild features of schizophrenia (in terms of symptoms and biological findings), which fall short of being diagnostically significant, but which are on average greater than those seen where neither member of a twin pair has schizophrenia. This probably reflects a partial expression of the risk genotype.

Adoption studies

Adoption studies provide another way to try and disambiguate genetic from family environmental factors. Heston (1966) studied 47 adults who had been born to mothers with schizophrenia and separated from them within 3 days of birth. As children they had been brought up in a variety of circumstances, although not by the mother's family. At the time of the study their mean age was 36 years. Heston compared them with controls matched for circumstances of upbringing, but whose mothers had not suffered from schizophrenia. Among the offspring of the affected mothers, five were diagnosed as having schizophrenia, compared with none of the controls. The rate for schizophrenia among the adopted-away children was comparable with that among children with a schizophrenic parent who remained with their biological family.

Further evidence came from a series of Danish studies that started in the 1960s (Petersen and Sorensen, 2011). In one project, two groups of adoptees were identified—a group of 33 adoptees who had schizophrenia, and a matched group who were free from schizophrenia. Rates of disorder were compared in the biological and adoptive families of the two groups of adoptees. The rate for schizophrenia was higher among the biological relatives of the adoptees with schizophrenia than among the relatives of the controls, a finding which supports the genetic hypothesis. Furthermore, the rate for schizophrenia was not increased among couples who adopted the affected children, which suggests that environmental factors were not of substantial importance. Follow-up studies using a national sample of Danish adoptees confirmed that biological first-degree relatives of patients with schizophrenia have an approximately tenfold increased risk of suffering from schizophrenia or a related ('spectrum') disorder (Kety *et al.*, 1994).

The data from adoption studies thus strongly support the view that genetic factors explain the familial clustering of schizophrenia. However, it should be noted that they cannot control for the prenatal environment, which other studies, discussed below, suggest is important. Nor can they rule out an interaction between environmental causes in the adoptive family and genetic predisposition; indeed, Finnish data show that adoptees at high genetic risk of schizophrenia are more sensitive to adverse upbringing (Tienari *et al.*, 2004).

The mode of inheritance

As pointed out in a seminal paper by Gottesman and Shields (1967), the frequency profile of schizophrenia among people with different degrees of genetic proximity to the proband does not fit any simple Mendelian pattern, as would be expected if the disorder was caused by a single major gene. Instead, the pattern indicates that schizophrenia arises from the cumulative effect of many genes, each of small effect, as a so-called *polygenic disorder*, also known as a *complex genetic* or *non-Mendelian* disorder. The liability to schizophrenia lies along a continuum in the population, and is expressed when a certain threshold of genetic susceptibility is exceeded. No genes are either necessary or sufficient, and they act as risk factors, not determinants. Indeed, no families in which schizophrenia is inherited as a single-gene dominant or recessive disorder have been identified. Within a polygenic model, there can be a range of different kinds of genetic variation and genetic mechanisms (sometimes called *genetic architecture*), which ongoing genomic and related approaches are beginning to reveal.

Schizophrenia susceptibility genes

Despite the high heritability, and a considerable research effort, it has proved difficult to identify schizophrenia genes. This difficulty reflects a number of factors (Box 11.9). However, significant progress has been made in the past decade, due mainly to advances in genomics knowledge (e.g. copy number variants [CNVs]) and methods (e.g. genome-wide association studies [GWAS]), coupled with larger sample sizes and more sophisticated analyses. The findings now show that three types of genetic variation contribute to schizophrenia risk:

- Single nucleotide polymorphisms (SNPs).
- Copy number variants (CNVs).
- Rare variants.

Single nucleotide polymorphisms

Much of the genetic risk for schizophrenia comes from SNPs (see Chapter 5), as revealed by GWAS. These SNPs affect many hundreds or thousands of genes, with each one contributing a very small effect (odds ratios typically about 1.05). The largest study to date, in over 35,000 cases and 80,000 controls, identified 108 genomic loci, containing over 600 known protein-coding genes, that were each statistically associated with schizophrenia risk (Schizophrenia Working Group of the Psychiatric Genomics Consortium, 2014). These genes include a number that are consistent with prior hypotheses about

---

Box 11.9 Why finding schizophrenia genes has been difficult

Knowing the right phenotype to study. Most genetic studies have been conducted on subjects who meet diagnostic criteria for schizophrenia, yet there are no grounds for assuming this syndrome has a specific genetic basis. As discussed, there is good evidence that the genetic predisposition is to a broader range of disorders than just schizophrenia. Equally, different genes may contribute to different aspects of schizophrenia (e.g. cognitive deficits, negative symptoms), sometimes called *endophenotypes* or *intermediate phenotypes*.

No single or major gene, but multiple genes of small effect. Many previous studies used genetic linkage to identify regions of the genome that segregated with schizophrenia. Linkage works best when a single gene is causing the phenotype being studied, explaining why it proved of very limited value in schizophrenia. Finding multiple genes of small effect requires very large samples (tens of thousands) of cases and controls.

Genetic heterogeneity. Beyond simply the large number of genes, schizophrenia is genetically heterogeneous in that the genetic risk (as explained below) comes from three kinds of variation—SNPs, CNVs, and rare variants—which likely vary between individuals, as well as between ethnic groups. These factors further confound detection of statistically robust genetic signals.

Gene–gene interactions (epistasis). Epistasis is common for many complex traits and disorders. Existing studies have rarely been designed or powered to investigate epistasis in schizophrenia. Its importance thus remains unknown.

Gene–environment interactions. Many genes may affect schizophrenia risk indirectly, by affecting an individual's response to environmental factors, as discussed in the following section. Since environmental data are rarely collected in genomic studies, most of these interactions will have been missed.

Lack of good candidate genes. Until genome-wide methods became available (in the early 2000s), a 'candidate gene' approach was required, in which researchers studied one or a few genes, believed for whatever reason to be involved in schizophrenia. This led to both false-positive and false-negative findings and means that most of the pre-GWAS era findings are now given little credence.

schizophrenia (e.g. dopamine D2 receptor, several gluta-mate genes) but also many that were not. These results are a major advance in schizophrenia genetics, but they also leave many questions unanswered. For example, these multiple loci still only explain a small amount of the heritability. Neither is it clear which genes, and what mechanisms, explain the statistical association. These issues are discussed below; see also Harrison (2015a).

Copy number variants

CNVs were introduced in Chapter 5. There is now strong evidence that specific CNVs are associated with schizophrenia. The major schizophrenia associated CNVs are shown in Table 11.5; the best known CNV is deletion of chromosome 22q11 (*velocardiofacial syndrome*; Box 11.10). The CNVs can either be deletions or duplications of a length of DNA. In contrast to SNPs, each CNV is extremely rare but, if present, confers a significant effect on risk. For example, as shown in Table 11.5, deletion of 1.35 million nucleotides from chromosome 15q11.2, affecting seven genes, occurs in about 0.14% of cases of schizophrenia compared to 0.02% of controls: an odds ratio of 7. Overall, about 2.5% of patients and 0.9% of controls carry a CNV strongly supported as a schizophrenia risk factor. For review, see Kirov *et al.* (2015).

About half of the CNVs associated with schizophrenia are inherited, the others are *de novo*—that is, they are not seen in either parent of the affected person; in effect, they are sporadic mutations, and the person's illness has not been inherited. However, if the affected person has children, each child has a 50% chance of inheriting the CNV, and their illness would therefore have been inherited.

Most schizophrenia-associated CNVs are also associated with a risk of one or more other neuropsychiatric phenotypes. However, there is not a clear excess of CNVs in bipolar disorder (Green *et al.*, 2016), and this may be one of the points of separation in the aetiology of these disorders.

Rare variants

A further proportion of cases of schizophrenia are due to rare single nucleotide (or dinucleotide) variants in individual genes which, if present, confer a high risk of the disorder. The variants are predicted to cause a loss-of-function of the gene concerned, and are sometimes referred to as mutations. The best example to date concerns a gene called *SETD1A*, of which 10 such variants were seen amongst 5000 cases, but in only two out of 45,000 controls, conferring an odds ratio of 32 (Singh *et al.*, 2016). As with CNVs, some rare variants are inherited, some occur *de novo*. The overall importance of rare variants in schizophrenia will become apparent from ongoing studies are using exome or genome sequencing in large samples.

Table 11.5 Copy number variants associated with schizophrenia risk

Locus	Size (kb)	Genes affected	Frequency in cases	Frequency in controls	Odds ratio	P value	Other phenotypes
1q21.1 del	820	11	0.17%	0.02%	8	10^{-13}	Microcephaly, heart defects
1q21.1 dup	820	11	0.13%	0.04%	3	10^{-4}	
NRXN1 del	Varies	1	0.18%	0.02%	9	10^{-11}	
15q11.2 del	290	4	0.59%	0.28%	2	10^{-10}	Epilepsy
15q13.3 del	1350	7	0.14%	0.02%	7	10^{-10}	Epilepsy
16p13.11 dup	790	8	0.31%	0.13%	2	10^{-5}	ADHD
16p11.2 dup	560	26	0.35%	0.03%	11	10^{-24}	ASD, microcephaly
22q11.2 del	1240	40	0.29%	0.0%	n.a.	10^{-40}	Multiple, including cardiac

Adapted from Advances in Psychiatric Treatment, 21(3), Kirov G et al, What a psychiatrist needs to know about copy number variants, pp. 157–163, Copyright (2015), with permission from The Royal College of Psychiatrists.

Only CNVs with a frequency in schizophrenia greater than 0.1% are included. NRXN1, neurexin 1; del, deletion; dup, duplication; kb, kilobases; ASD, autism spectrum disorder; ADHD, attention deficit hyperactivity disorder.

> ## Box 11.10 Velocardiofacial syndrome: a schizophrenia-associated CNV
>
> Unlike most CNVs associated with schizophrenia, which were discovered by chance from GWAS, *velocardiofacial syndrome* (VCFS, also known as *di George syndrome*) was already well known, being detectable using standard clinical genetic techniques. VCFS is caused by deletion of one copy of chromosome 22q11 (hence its alternative name, *22q11 hemideletion syndrome*). It is a relatively common cytogenetic anomaly, occurring in 1 in 4000 live births, and causes a range of physical abnormalities. Of relevance here, it is also associated with psychosis (either schizophrenia-like or affective) in about 30% of individuals. Even though VCFS is a rare cause of schizophrenia overall, 22q11 is implicated as a locus for schizophrenia genes in general, and several such genes within this region have been identified. 22q11 hemideletion is also associated with other neurodevelopmental and neuropsychiatric syndromes (e.g. intellectual disability, attention deficit hyperactivity disorder [ADHD]), illustrating how one CNV can produce different phenotypes (*pleiotropy*). For review, see Jonas *et al.* (2014).

Disrupted in schizophrenia 1

Disrupted in schizophrenia 1 (*DISC 1*) deserves mention because it has a unique place in schizophrenia genetics. It was identified from extensive studies of a large Scottish family in which a translocation between chromosomes 1 and 11 is linked with a high incidence of schizophrenia and several other disorders. *DISC 1* is the gene thought to be affected ('disrupted') by the translocation, and to be the likely cause of the observed phenotypes. However, it is unclear as to the role of *DISC 1* in schizophrenia outside this one family, and the heated debate illustrates broader controversies about the genetics of schizophrenia (Sullivan, 2013; Porteous *et al.*, 2014).

The 'missing heritability'

Much of the heritability of schizophrenia is still unexplained (or 'missing'), despite the large numbers of SNPs, CNVs, and rare variants already identified. It has been estimated that SNPs collectively will explain about 30% of the genetic risk, and CNVs perhaps another 5–10%. The remainder likely arises from four sources:

- Many additional genetic variants, especially rare variants, which will be identified as sample sizes increase and extensive whole genome sequencing is carried out.
- Epistasis (see Box 11.9).
- Gene–environment interactions (Iyegbe *et al.*, 2014).
- Epigenetic factors, some of which are heritable. See Dempster *et al.* (2013) and Toth (2015).

The relative importance of these four factors in explaining the missing heritability is unknown.

Crow's lateralization hypothesis

A very different view of the aetiology of schizophrenia was proposed by Crow (2002). He argued that schizophrenia is due to a single gene, which is also responsible for cerebral asymmetry and language. For various reasons, the gene is postulated to reside at a particular location on the sex chromosomes. The theory is ingenious but not widely supported.

The biology of schizophrenia genes

The discovery of multiple loci and genes associated with schizophrenia has been followed by attempts to understand the biological implications and the molecular mechanisms. Although these are at an early stage, several broad conclusions can be drawn:

- The genes converge on several functional networks and biochemical pathways. In particular, current data highlight aspects of N-methyl-D-aspartate (NMDA) receptor-mediated signalling and synaptic plasticity, immune function, calcium signalling, and histone modification. See Box 11.11; Hall *et al.* (2015).
- CNVs likely exert their effects through gene dosage. That is, a deletion leads to insufficient levels of gene expression, and duplications to excess. Deletions may also be pathogenic by revealing the effects of a harmful recessive allele on the undeleted chromosome.
- The mechanism by which SNPs alter gene function to affect the risk of schizophrenia is more complicated to determine, for several reasons. Firstly, GWAS does not identify the causal variant, merely one that is 'tagging' the genetic risk. Secondly, even where the causal variant has been inferred, very few are coding substitutions (c.f. ApoE4, see Box 5.5), and so their functional significance is unclear. The mechanism is likely to be that they affect how the gene is regulated—for example, when and where it is transcribed, or spliced—with some data suggesting that this particularly affects prenatal brain development.

Box 11.11 Convergence of schizophrenia genes: the examples of immune function and NMDA receptor signalling

Immune function. The major histocompatibility complex (MHC) locus on chromosome 6 shows the strongest statistical association to schizophrenia (Schizophrenia Working Group of the Psychiatric Genomics Consortium, 2014). There are two main interpretations of this finding. The first is that it supports a role for immune, autoimmune, or inflammatory factors in schizophrenia, consistent with a range of epidemiological and biological evidence discussed later in this chapter. The alternative interpretation is that is also known that many 'immune genes' (such as the classical complement pathway) also play a role in brain development, influencing synaptogenesis and other processes, and this might be the basis for the genetic association. In support, Sekar *et al.* (2016) showed that the genetic signal to the MHC locus arises mainly from the complement component 4 (C4) gene, which is expressed by developing neurons and synapses. They also showed that individuals with the risk forms of C4 express the gene at higher levels, and that (at least in mice) this is associated with more pruning of synapses during brain development.

NMDA receptor signalling. A role for glutamate and NMDA receptor hypofunction has long been postulated in schizophrenia. It is now supported by clear evidence that genes involved in NMDA receptor signalling, and synaptic function more generally, are overrepresented among the genes affected by schizophrenia risk SNPs and CNVs (Hall *et al.,* 2015).

For review, see Harrison (2015a).

Clinical and therapeutic implications of schizophrenia genetics

At present there is no direct clinical role of genetic testing for schizophrenia in clinical practice, since none of the genetic findings are diagnostic and they do not have clearly established prognostic or therapeutic implications. The only possible exception is testing for CNVs, which some authorities argue may now be justified, and which raises several ethical issues (Rees *et al.*, 2014).

Genetic discoveries are also providing new potential drug targets and encouraging investment in the field, but seem unlikely to lead directly to new pharmacotherapies in the near future because of the many complexities involved (Schubert *et al.*, 2014).

Environmental risk factors

Despite the prominent genetic component, the twin studies discussed earlier, along with many epidemiological and other studies, show that environmental factors are also important in the aetiology of schizophrenia. A range of factors, especially prenatal and perinatal ones, have been identified (Table 11.6); for some, the relative risks they confer have been estimated from meta-analyses (Table 11.6, and see text).

For review, see van Os *et al.* (2010) and McGrath and Murray (2011).

Several issues are worth bearing in mind when considering the individual risk factors to be discussed:

- The causality of most environmental risk factors for schizophrenia is often unknown, and differing interpretations of the reported associations are possible.
- Many of the environmental risk factors are not specific to schizophrenia but, like the genetic factors, are shared by one or more other disorders.
- The distinction between genetic and environmental factors is an oversimplification. In fact, as noted earlier, interactions between them are common, and

Table 11.6 Environmental risk factors for schizophrenia, and the relative risk conferred

Factor	Relative risk
Maternal infections	?
Maternal malnutrition	2
Birth complications	2
Winter birth	1.1
Advanced paternal age	1.7
Urban birth and upbringing	1.9
Childhood trauma and adversity	2.8
Being an immigrant	2.9
Cannabis smoking	2
Tobacco smoking	2.2
Life events	3.2

can complicate identification of both types of factor (Iyegbe *et al.*, 2014). Some specific examples are given in the following sections.

Obstetric complications

Rates of schizophrenia are increased in individuals who experienced obstetric complications, compared with their unaffected siblings or normal controls. Meta-analyses suggest an odds ratio of about 2 (Cannon *et al.*, 2002). A range of exposures is associated with increased risk, including antepartum haemorrhage, diabetes, low birth weight, asphyxia, and Rhesus incompatibility. Obstetric complications may be more relevant in individuals who also have a genetic predisposition to schizophrenia (Nicodemus *et al.*, 2008).

The association of obstetric complications with schizophrenia has several possible explanations. They might be directly causal (e.g. via fetal hypoxia), or a reflection of pre-existing fetal abnormality, or even a reflection of maternal characteristics.

Infective and inflammatory factors

Several studies have suggested that fetuses exposed during the second trimester to influenza, especially the 1957 influenza A2 pandemic, have an increased risk of schizophrenia. Some biological support for this association was provided by animal studies, which showed that prenatal influenza affects fetal brain development. Additional support emerged with the demonstration that serological evidence of influenza infection during early pregnancy was associated with an increased risk of schizophrenia in the offspring. However, other studies, and a meta-analysis of the 1957 pandemic, yielded negative results (Selten *et al.*, 2010), and a relationship between influenza and schizophrenia has been hard to establish (Khandaker *et al.*, 2013). Several other maternal (and childhood) infections have also been associated with schizophrenia, including toxoplasmosis, herpes simplex virus 2, and rubella, with varying degrees of support (Khandaker *et al.*, 2013).

A number of studies have measured inflammatory markers (such as interleukins, cytokines, and C-reactive protein) in serum collected during pregnancy and related this to schizophrenia risk in the offspring (Khandaker *et al.*, 2013; Canetta *et al.*, 2014). Although these markers are often taken as supportive of an infective origin, inflammation may occur for various reasons (Cannon *et al.*, 2014).

Genetic factors may well modify the relationship between maternal infection and schizophrenia. For example, a large population study found that the association between maternal infection and schizophrenia risk was only observed in women with a history of psychiatric disorder (Blomstrom *et al.*, 2016).

For review of maternal infection, inflammation, and schizophrenia, see Brown and Derkits (2010).

Maternal malnutrition

Children born to mothers who experienced famine early in their pregnancy have an increased risk of schizophrenia, with an odds ratio of about 2. This was shown initially in children born after the Dutch 'Hunger Winter' of 1944, and subsequently in two large Chinese populations exposed to famines in the 1960s. The mechanism is proposed to be epigenetic—viz. that malnutrition alters DNA methylation and other processes regulating gene expression in the affected offspring (Kirkbride *et al.*, 2012b). It is not known whether the cause is related to general malnutrition or lack of specific micronutrients (e.g. vitamin D), nor is it clear whether less extreme fluctuations in nutritional status during pregnancy affect schizophrenia risk. For review, see Brown and Susser (2008).

Winter birth

Schizophrenia is slightly more frequent among people born in the late winter than among those born in the summer (Davies *et al.*, 2003). This season of birth effect has been shown in both the northern and southern hemispheres, and becomes more prominent at higher latitudes. The explanation is unknown. It has been linked to the prevalence of influenza earlier in the winter, and to sunshine and vitamin D levels around the time of birth; it could also be related to factors related to the time of conception, via seasonal fluctuations in the genetic make-up of gametes.

Paternal age

A replicated finding is that schizophrenia is associated with paternal age, especially in those without a family history of psychosis. A meta-analysis found a relative risk of 1.66 for fathers over 50 years old compared to those aged 25–29 (Miller *et al.*, 2011). The favoured explanation is that the frequency of mutations in sperm increases with age. However, the phenomenon is only observed for a man's first-born child, and not for subsequent ones (Petersen *et al.*, 2011). This suggests that the paternal age effect may instead be related to how personality (or relationship factors) modify the age at which a man first fathers a child.

Child development

Parnas *et al.* (1982) reported a study of 207 children of mothers with schizophrenia who were first assessed when they were 8–12 years of age and then again, as adults, 18 years later, by which time 13 individuals had developed schizophrenia and 29 had 'borderline schizophrenia'. Of the measures that were used on the first occasion, those that predicted schizophrenia were poor rapport at interview, being socially isolated from peers, disciplinary problems mentioned in school reports, and parental reports that the person had been passive as a baby.

In a national birth cohort of more than 16,000 children prospectively studied over a 16-year period, those who developed schizophrenia could be distinguished at the age of 11 years, if not earlier, by greater hostility towards adults, and by speech and reading difficulties (Done *et al.*, 1994). This difference was apparent compared to those who grew up to develop neurotic illness, as well as those who remained well. In another large prospective cohort study, Jones *et al.* (1994) found that children who eventually developed schizophrenia showed delayed milestones and speech problems, together with lower education test scores and less social play. A graded relationship between delayed milestones (e.g. age at walking) and schizophrenia has been confirmed in several subsequent cohorts. The behaviour of children (including motor acts in infants), as recorded in home movies and videotapes, is also associated with later schizophrenia (Schiffman *et al.*, 2004).

These and other studies provide good evidence that individuals who will develop schizophrenia show increased rates of intellectual and motor dysfunction and poor social competence in childhood. However, it is unclear how specific these changes are, or how they are related to the subsequent development of the illness. Most of the children who were destined to develop schizophrenia were not considered clinically abnormal at the time, and many children who perform poorly on these indices do not develop schizophrenia. Nevertheless, the findings support an early neurodevelopmental contribution to schizophrenia.

Substance use

The high prevalence of drug and alcohol use in patients with schizophrenia is well established, but whether substance misuse plays a causal role in schizophrenia is more controversial. If substance use is considered to have directly caused or precipitated the psychosis, it is diagnosed as such, and not as schizophrenia. However, there is evidence that prior use of some drugs, particularly cannabis, is associated with an increased risk of later developing schizophrenia. Andreasson *et al.* (1987) followed up over 45,000 Swedish conscripts for 15 years, and found that the relative risk of developing schizophrenia was 2.5 times higher in subjects who used cannabis, with a sixfold increase in risk for heavy users. Subsequent longitudinal studies show a consistent association between cannabis use and psychosis (with an odds ratio of about 2), which may be modified by interaction with genetic and other factors, such as the strain of cannabis (Gage *et al.*, 2015). Cannabis use is also associated with an earlier age of onset of psychosis (Large *et al.*, 2011). However, the causality and specificity of the relationship between cannabis use and psychosis, and hence the implications for public health policy, remain controversial (Hall and Degenhardt, 2011) (see also Chapter 20).

Tobacco smoking is also a risk factor for development of psychosis, and is associated with an earlier onset of symptoms (Gunillo *et al.*, 2015). As with cannabis use, it is not certain whether this is causal; for example, given the strong effects of nicotine on the dopamine system, the relationship could reflect an attempt at self-medication (Kumari and Postma, 2005).

Social and psychosocial factors

Although neglected in recent years compared to biological risk factors, social and psychosocial factors are also important in schizophrenia. For review, see van Os *et al.* (2010) and Bebbington and Kuipers (2011).

Occupation and social class

Schizophrenia is overrepresented among people of lower social class. In Chicago, Hollingshead and Redlich (1958) found both the incidence and the prevalence of schizophrenia to be highest in the lowest socioeconomic groups. At first, these findings were thought to be of aetiological significance, but they could be a consequence of schizophrenia. For instance, Goldberg and Morrison (1963) found that people with schizophrenia were of lower social status than their fathers, and that this was usually because they had changed status after the onset of the illness. However, Castle *et al.* (1993) found that, compared with controls, patients with schizophrenia were more likely to have been born into socially deprived households. Those authors proposed that some environmental factor of aetiological importance was more likely to affect individuals of lower socioeconomic status.

Place of birth and residence

Faris and Dunham (1939) studied the place of residence of mentally ill people in Chicago, and found that individuals with schizophrenia were overrepresented in the disadvantaged inner-city areas. This distribution has been confirmed in other cities, and it has been suggested that unsatisfactory living conditions can cause schizophrenia. These findings have often been ascribed to the occupational and social decline ('*social drift*') described above, or to a search for social isolation by people who are about to develop schizophrenia.

However, recent data suggest that schizophrenia is associated with place of birth and early upbringing, findings that cannot be explained as a consequence of illness. Specifically, population-based studies in several countries show that urban birth is associated with an increased risk of schizophrenia. Larger cities carry a higher odds ratio than small towns or suburban areas (Pedersen and Mortensen, 2001). The cause of the association remains unclear, and may relate to social deprivation, migration, infections, stress, or interactions between genetic vulnerability and urban environments (Peen and Dekker, 2004). Recent data support the view that genetic liability to schizophrenia plays a significant part in the social drift (Sariaslan *et al.*, 2016).

Migration and ethnicity

In a study of Norwegians who had migrated to Minnesota, Ødegaard (1932) found that the inception rate for schizophrenia was twice that of Norwegians living in Norway. Many subsequent studies have confirmed high rates of schizophrenia among migrants. Meta-analyses confirm that schizophrenia is more common in migrants, and in their children, and show that this cannot be explained solely by selection (Bourque *et al.*, 2011). The relative risk ranges from about 2 to 4.5, and tends to be higher in migrants from lower- and middle-income countries.

A particularly controversial aspect of migration and schizophrenia concerns the Afro-Caribbean population in the UK. This group has a strikingly increased incidence of schizophrenia, particularly in the 'second generation', who were born in the UK. The relative risk for all psychosis ascertained in the multicentre first-onset AESOP study was 6.7 for the Afro-Caribbean population and 1.5 for the Asian population, compared with the white population in the UK (Fearon *et al.*, 2006). Overall, rates in Caribbean-born migrants and their descendants in England are increased 4.7-fold (Tortelli *et al.*, 2015). There has been concern that the high rates in the UK represent misdiagnosis because of poor diagnostic practice, and even 'institutional racism' (Singh and Burns,

2006). However, several studies have compared the diagnoses in Afro-Caribbean and white patients using structured research instruments, and found them to be equivalent (Singh and Burns, 2006). The most rigorous test was the AESOP study mentioned, which, despite the raised rates, found that symptom profiles were broadly the same across the ethnic groups, and the association with known risk factors was also similar. Thus, there is now strong evidence that the raised incidence is a real phenomenon, but its explanation is unclear (Morgan *et al.*, 2010). The increased rate of schizophrenia has sometimes been attributed to a disproportionate migration of people who are unsettled because they are becoming mentally ill. Alternatively, the effect of migration could be due to exposure to environmental factors in the host country, especially in those who are genetically or otherwise predisposed. Thus both 'social selection' and 'social causation' may contribute to an excess of schizophrenia among migrants. Amongst the latter category, evidence indicates that experiential factors likely play a significant part. Studies show that the high incidence in ethnic-minority patients varies according to where they grew up in the host country. Controlling for known risk factors (e.g. cannabis use and deprivation), the rates are still more than doubled when these individuals grow up in areas where they are members of a small minority as opposed to areas where they are a relatively large minority. The mechanism by which this differential 'ethnic density' impacts upon rates of schizophrenia is unclear. For review, see Shaw *et al.* (2012).

Life events and difficulties

Life events and difficulties have often been proposed as precipitants of schizophrenia. In one of the most convincing studies, Brown and Birley (1968) used a standardized procedure to collect information from 50 patients newly admitted with a precisely datable first onset or relapse of schizophrenia. By comparison with a control group, the rate of 'independent' events in those with schizophrenia was increased during the 3 weeks before the onset of the acute symptoms. Paykel (1978) calculated that experiencing a life event doubles the risk of developing schizophrenia during the subsequent 6 months. A recent meta-analysis yielded an odds ratio of 3.2 for life events and psychosis (Beards *et al.*, 2013).

For review, see Bebbington and Kuipers (2011).

Childhood trauma

There is an increased prevalence of childhood trauma and abuse, including bullying, in individuals who

---

Box 11.12 Psychodynamic and family theories of aetiology

Psychodynamic theories

Freud elaborated his theory of schizophrenia in his 1911 analysis of the Judge Schreber case. He proposed that libido was withdrawn from external objects and attached to the ego, resulting in exaggerated self-reference. The withdrawal of libido deprived the external world of salience so meaning was derived from abnormal beliefs. The libidinal withdrawal meant the patient could not form a transference and therefore could not be treated by psychoanalysis. Although Freud developed his general ideas later and elaborated his theory he did not replace it.

Melanie Klein (1952) believed that schizophrenia originated in infancy. In the *'paranoid schizoid position'*, the infant neutralized innate aggressive impulses by splitting his ego and his experience of his mother into two parts, one wholly bad and the other wholly good. Only later did the child realize that the same person could be good at one time and bad at another. Failure to pass through this stage adequately was the basis for the later development of schizophrenia and the sense of persecution common in it.

The family as a cause of schizophrenia

The family has been proposed as a cause of schizophrenia, either through *deviant role relationships* (associated with Fromm-Reichmann and Lidz) or *disordered communication* (associated with Bateson and Wynne). The role of the family in influencing the *course* of schizophrenia is discussed later.

The *'schizophrenogenic'* mother, a cold and distant figure unable to foster emotional growth, was suggested by the analyst Fromm-Reichmann in 1948, whilst Lidz and his colleagues used intensive psychoanalytical methods to study the families of 17 wealthy patients with schizophrenia, and suggested two abnormal family patterns:

- *Marital skew,* in which one parent yielded to the other's (usually the mother's) eccentricities, which dominated the family.
- *Marital schism,* in which the parents maintained contrary views, and consequently the child had divided loyalties.

The *double bind* (Bateson *et al.*, 1956) is said to occur when an instruction is given overtly, but is contradicted by a second more covert instruction. For example, a mother may overtly tell her child to come to her, while conveying by her manner and tone of voice that she rejects him. Double binds are only pathogenic within families that implicitly prohibit the acknowledgement of this contradiction. They are (after all) far from uncommon. Double binds trap the child in ambiguous responses and inhibit the development of logical thinking.

An association between abnormal social communication in parents and schizophrenic illness in children may in fact be a consequence of a shared genetic inheritance or, indeed, as a response to the stresses of relating to the child. These and other speculations about the causative role of family relationships have had the unfortunate consequence of inducing unjustified guilt in parents.

---

develop schizophrenia, with an odds ratio of about 3. The risk is greater for multiple and severe adversities. The relationship is not explained fully by genetic factors or other potential confounders, and may therefore be at least partly causal. For review, see Morgan and Gayer-Anderson (2016).

Psychological factors

Personality

Several early writers, including Bleuler, commented on the frequency of abnormalities of personality preceding the onset of schizophrenia. In the 1930s, Kretschmer proposed that both personality and schizophrenia were related to the asthenic type of body build.

He suggested a continuous variation between normal personality, schizoid personality, and schizophrenia. He regarded schizoid personality as a partial expression of the psychological abnormalities that are manifested in their full form in schizophrenia. Such ideas must be treated with caution, as it is difficult to distinguish between premorbid personality and the prodromal phase of emerging illness. However, Kretschmer's ideas are similar to the current concept of the schizophrenia spectrum, in which schizophrenia represents the most severe end of a continuum. Taken together, the findings suggest that abnormal personality features are not uncommon among people who later develop schizophrenia, and among their first-degree relatives. However, many people with schizophrenia have no obvious disorder of personality before the onset of the illness, and only a minority of people with schizotypal or schizoid personalities develop schizophrenia. For review of personality and psychosis, see Ohi *et al.* (2012).

Psychological theories

In the past, psychological theories of schizophrenia were based on psychodynamic concepts and often centred on a pathogenic role of family (see Box 11.12). Such theories are now largely of historical interest, since they lack empirical evidence. However, it is important to know about them because they help focus attention on interpersonal and developmental aspects, and because they remain influential with some families and health professionals.

Current psychological models of schizophrenia are more grounded within neuroscience, and reflect the increasing focus on cognitive aspects of schizophrenia introduced earlier. For review, see Palmer *et al.* (2009).

An early neuropsychological model of schizophrenia proposed that positive symptoms arise from a failure to integrate stored memories with current stimuli (Gray *et al.*, 1991). The *aberrant salience* model of Kapur (2003), mentioned later, shares some features with Gray's model and links neuropsychology to the dopamine hypothesis of schizophrenia.

Frith (1996) argued that in schizophrenia there is a breakdown in the internal representation of mental events. For example, a failure to monitor and identify one's own willed intentions might give rise to the idea that thoughts and actions arise from external sources, resulting in delusions of control. This theory has a counterpart in models of aberrant connectivity and brain networks, to be discussed below (Menon, 2011).

Neurobiology

Schizophrenia is at the forefront of attempts to understand psychiatric disorders in terms of alterations in brain structure and function, utilizing the whole range of contemporary neuroscientific concepts and techniques. For general reviews, see Kahn *et al.* (2015) and Owen *et al.* (2016). See Kahn and Sommer (2015) for review of the neurobiology of onset and first-episode psychosis, and Remington *et al.* (2014) for the neurobiology of relapse.

Structural brain changes

Whether there is a neuropathology associated with schizophrenia has been a matter of debate for over a century. The search began with Alzheimer, who spent a decade studying the brains of patients with dementia praecox (Box 11.5) before he reported the case of presenile dementia with which his name is associated. The failure of Alzheimer and others to identify a neuropathology was central to the view of schizophrenia as a functional disorder rather than an organic one. However, evidence has accrued over the past 40 years which disproves the null hypothesis that there are no structural differences in the brain in schizophrenia, albeit their details and interpretation remain poorly understood, and the findings are not clinically useful in the diagnosis of individual patients. The main findings are summarized in Box 11.13.

Structural brain imaging

In a landmark study, Johnstone *et al.* (1976) used the novel technique of computerized tomography, and found significantly larger ventricles and cerebral

---

Box 11.13 Summary of structural brain changes in schizophrenia

Brain imaging

- Decreased brain volume
- Decreased intracranial volume
- Enlarged lateral and third ventricles
- Smaller hippocampus and thalamus
- Thinner cortical grey matter
- Altered white matter pathways

Neuropathology

- Decreased brain weight
- Absence of neurodegenerative changes or gliosis
- Reductions in synaptic and dendritic markers
- Decreased markers of some interneurons
- Smaller pyramidal neurons in some areas
- Fewer thalamic neurons

atrophy in 17 elderly hospitalized patients with schizophrenia than in eight healthy controls. Lateral ventricular enlargement in schizophrenia had been reported decades previously using pneumoencephalography, but it was the study by Johnstone and colleagues that stimulated renewed interest. A large number of subsequent imaging studies, mostly using MRI, have confirmed and extended those findings. A meta-analysis of brain volumes in over 18,000 subjects (Hajima *et al.*, 2013) concluded that, in schizophrenia, ventricular volumes are increased by about 30%, brain volume decreased by 2.6%, and intracranial volume reduced by 2%. The latter finding suggests strongly that much of the structural brain changes occur early in childhood. Effect sizes were largest in hippocampus and thalamus, and greater for grey matter than white matter. The results were broadly similar in antipsychotic-naïve as in medicated patients.

Longitudinal studies have attempted to identify the course of structural brain changes. The results are complex. Some of the volume reductions are present before the onset of symptoms, and likely relate to the genetic predisposition to the disorder, while others emerge at the first episode. Thereafter, there is some further loss of grey and white matter, but the timing, magnitude, and explanation, remain unclear (Weinberger and Radulescu, 2016). For example, the extent to which progressive volume reductions are attributable to the disease process versus antipsychotic medication or other confounders, and whether typical and atypical antipsychotics differ in this regard (Fusar-Poli *et al.*, 2013b).

Other notable aspects of structural brain imaging in schizophrenia include:

- There is no evidence for an 'organic' subtype. Rather, there is a unimodal shift in ventricular and brain volumes in the disorder.
- There are few clear clinicopathological associations, although particular structural alterations have been associated with specific symptoms; for example, thought disorder with smaller superior temporal gyri.
- Despite their robustness, the changes are small, with significant overlap between patients and controls. Furthermore, the findings are not diagnostically specific—for example, some of the findings are also seen in bipolar disorder (Ellison-Wright and Bullmore, 2010).

As well as volume changes, MRI methods such as diffusion tensor imaging have shown alterations in white matter connectivity. A range of differences has been reported in schizophrenia, generally indicative of decreased or otherwise aberrant white matter pathways, especially involving the frontal cortex (Samartzis *et al.*, 2014).

Neuropathology

Post-mortem neuropathological studies have sought to explain the cellular and molecular basis for the neuroimaging findings (see Box 11.13). For review, see Harrison (1999) and Dorph-Petersen and Lewis (2011). A few findings deserve mention here.

- Brain weight is decreased by 2–3%.
- There is no evidence of any neurodegenerative processes. This supports a neurodevelopmental origin of the pathology, and also argues that any progression of pathology during the illness, as inferred from some MRI studies, is not neurotoxic or degenerative in nature (Zipursky *et al.*, 2013).
- The main positive findings are reductions in some markers of synapses and dendrites, and in specific neuronal populations (e.g. the parvalbumin subclass of interneurons, and layer III pyramidal neurons).
- An abnormal position or clustering of some neurons, notably in the entorhinal cortex and in the subcortical white matter, has been reported in several studies.
- Studies of gene expression are consistent with the involvement of neurons and oligodendroglia in schizophrenia.

The nature of the neuropathological changes is strongly suggestive of an origin early in life, and has contributed to the neurodevelopmental hypothesis of schizophrenia. However, virtually all of the patients whose brains are studied post mortem had been ill, and medicated, for many years. It is therefore difficult to determine the extent to which the findings in schizophrenia are confounded by the consequences of illness, antipsychotic medication, and other factors (e.g. smoking).

Functional brain imaging

As described in Chapter 5, a number of imaging techniques, particularly positron emission tomography (PET), single-photon emission tomography (SPET), and functional magnetic resonance imaging (fMRI), have been used to assess patterns of brain activity in schizophrenia. Study designs usually compare groups of patients with groups of controls, either at rest, or during performance of different kinds of cognitive task. For a review, see Meyer-Lindenberg (2010).

Cerebral blood flow

The first study was conducted by Ingvar and Franzen (1974), who used injections of radioactive xenon, and found decreased perfusion of the frontal cortex compared with the posterior regions in chronic, medicated patients with schizophrenia. This 'hypofrontality' has sometimes been considered to be a feature of schizophrenia and, although many studies have given negative results, was confirmed in a meta-analysis (Hill *et al.*, 2004). However, stronger relationships with hypofrontality are seen if the phase of illness and symptom profile are taken into account (e.g. the association with psychomotor poverty) (see Table 11.1).

BOLD signal on fMRI

Altered frontal activity is also apparent in fMRI studies of schizophrenia, particularly in the prefrontal cortex during performance of working memory tasks, such as the Wisconsin Card Sorting Test and the N-back task. The profile of changes is complex (Minzenberg *et al.*, 2009). When patients are matched with controls for performance, patients require more frontal cortex activation to achieve the same level of performance as controls, which suggests that there is a reduced 'efficiency' of cortical processing (Callicott *et al.*, 2003). Other fMRI studies have looked at the cerebral correlates of specific symptoms—for example, the cortical regions that are activated during auditory hallucinations (Jardri *et al.*, 2011)—whilst there is also emerging interest in alterations in 'resting state' brain activity (Kuhn and Gallinat, 2013).

Aberrant connectivity

Bleuler conceptualized the fundamental symptoms of schizophrenia as 'psychic splitting' or a failure of integration of mental functions, and Wernicke and other neuroanatomists of the late nineteenth century took a 'connectionist' view (Collin *et al.*, 2016). A similar view is currently framed in terms of 'dysconnectivity', whereby the activity of different brain circuits or networks is aberrant in schizophrenia (Stephan *et al.*, 2009). Some variants of this model also involve a structural component (changes in the 'wiring' of the brain), consistent with the structural imaging and neuropathology findings mentioned earlier. Recent studies focus on brain oscillations and network activity, the coordinated firing of ensembles of neurons between brain areas underlying cognition, and other brain operations (Gonzalez-Burgos *et al.*, 2015).

Neurophysiological findings

Neurophysiological function in schizophrenia has been examined using a range of methods. For a review, see Winterer and McCarley (2011).

Electroencephalography

The electroencephalogram (EEG) in schizophrenia generally shows increased amounts of theta activity, fast activity, and paroxysmal activity. The significance of these findings is not known. More sophisticated combinations of EEG and event-related potential analyses show a decreased synchronization or coherence of electrical activity in the prefrontal cortex in schizophrenia, suggestive of 'noisy' or inefficient cortical processing (Winterer and Weinberger, 2004).

Sensory evoked potentials: P300 and P50

The P300 response is an auditory evoked potential that occurs 300 milliseconds after a subject has identified a target stimulus embedded in a series of irrelevant stimuli. The response provides a measure of auditory information processing. In patients with schizophrenia, and a proportion of their first-degree relatives, the amplitude of the P300 wave is reduced.

Abnormalities in another evoked potential, the P50 wave, have also been reported in patients with schizophrenia and their relatives. Moreover, molecular genetic studies in families with schizophrenia have shown that P50 deficits are linked to the gene coding for a subunit of the nicotinic cholinergic receptor. This suggests that alterations in cholinergic neurotransmission could underlie abnormalities in information processing in schizophrenia.

A meta-analysis confirmed the presence of P300 and P50 deficits in schizophrenia (Bramon *et al.*, 2004).

Biochemical findings

Dopamine

Two early lines of research converged and implicated dopamine as having a key role in schizophrenia. The first concerned the effects of amphetamine which, among other actions, releases dopamine at central synapses. Repeated use of amphetamine at high doses can induce a disorder similar to acute schizophrenia, and acute amphetamine administration worsens psychotic symptoms in people with schizophrenia. The second approach starts from the finding that all antipsychotic drugs are dopamine-receptor antagonists, and that their affinity at dopamine D$_2$ receptors is the property that correlates best with their clinical potency. These observations led to the well-known 'dopamine hypothesis' of schizophrenia, which emerged during the early 1970s and has persisted.

Despite the prominence and longevity of the theory, evidence that dopamine neurotransmission is excessive or otherwise abnormal in schizophrenia was hard to obtain, in part because of the difficulty in distinguishing drug effects from disease effects in medicated patients. However, the use of PET and SPET techniques to image dopamine receptors and dopamine synthesis has now provided good evidence to support the presumed 'hyperdopaminergia' in acute schizophrenia. There is a slight increase in dopamine D$_2$ receptors, and an increased occupancy of D$_2$ receptors, but the main finding is that the synthesis and release of striatal dopamine are markedly increased (Howes *et al.*, 2012). Moreover, the extent of this increase predicts the response to antipsychotic medication. The abnormality develops during the prodrome and is not seen in patients during remission. Contrary to expectations, the excess dopamine function occurs primarily in the associative and not the ventral striatum (i.e. in the mesocortical rather than the mesolimbic dopamine pathway). For review, see Howes *et al.* (2015).

Other phases and aspects of schizophrenia may be associated with different abnormalities in dopamine function. In particular, various lines of evidence suggested that there is deficient dopaminergic activation of the prefrontal cortex, relevant to the enduring cognitive deficits of the illness. The first direct evidence to support the presence of dopamine deficits in the cortex in schizophrenia came from Slifstein *et al.* (2015), using a new PET ligand. There are plausible pathways and mechanisms to link these opposing dopaminergic abnormalities in striatum and frontal cortex.

The cause of dopaminergic involvement in schizophrenia is unclear. There may be a genetic component, but current theories emphasize dysregulation secondary to glutamatergic and developmental abnormalities, as outlined below. A phenomenological account has been proposed by Kapur (2003). He argues that the known roles of dopamine in cognition and behaviour suggest that it mediates the 'salience' of external events and internal representations, and that in schizophrenia the dopamine abnormalities lead the patient to misattribute stimuli and their meaning. Delusions and hallucinations are viewed as the consequence of these experiences and the patient's attempt to make sense of them.

Glutamate

The excitatory neurotransmitter amino acid glutamate is second only to dopamine in neurochemical theories of schizophrenia. The key finding that triggered this interest was that antagonists of the NMDA type of glutamate receptor (e.g. phencyclidine and ketamine) can induce a schizophrenia-like psychosis (Javitt and Zukin, 1991). This finding is now complemented by several other lines of evidence (see Box 11.14). For review, see Howes *et al.* (2015).

The origins of glutamatergic involvement in schizophrenia are not known. The 'NMDA receptor hypofunction' model postulates a developmental abnormality in the receptor (Olney and Farber, 1995). As mentioned earlier, there is a genetic component, and a small percentage of cases may be attributable to anti-NMDA receptor antibodies (Lennox *et al.*, 2012, 2017).

The glutamate and dopamine systems are intricately linked, and their dysfunction in schizophrenia is also thought to reflect shared factors. Glutamate is generally considered to be the more primary or 'trait' abnormality, with the dopamine abnormality downstream and 'state'-related. Alternatively, there may be differential involvement of glutamate and dopamine in different patients (Howes *et al.*, 2015).

Gamma-aminobutyric acid

Gamma-aminobutyric acid (GABA) is the major inhibitory transmitter in the brain, and it is implicated in

---

Box 11.14 Evidence for glutamatergic involvement in schizophrenia

NMDA-receptor antagonists induce or exacerbate schizophrenia symptoms

NMDA-receptor co-agonists (e.g. D-serine) reduce some symptoms

Alterations in glutamate markers and receptors in schizophrenia brain

Altered levels of glutamate and its metabolites in schizophrenia brain shown using spectroscopy (Merritt *et al.*, 2016)

Schizophrenia risk genes affect glutamate signalling

Anti-NMDA receptor antibodies in some cases of schizophrenia

schizophrenia for several reasons. There is a decrease in its synthetic enzyme, glutamic acid decarboxylase (GAD), in the cerebral cortex, and reductions in the connections made by a type of GABA neuron (parvalbumin-containing interneurons). There are also alterations in the expression of $GABA_A$ receptors, and reduced GABA levels as measured by spectroscopy. The relationship between GABA and glutamate alterations in schizophrenia is unclear; one point of convergence is that NMDA receptors on GABA neurons may be especially vulnerable in the disorder. For review see Gonzalez-Burgos et al. (2015).

Serotonin (5-hydroxytryptamine; 5-HT)

A role for serotonin (5-HT) in schizophrenia has long been considered, because the hallucinogen, lysergic acid diethylamide (LSD), is an agonist at $5\text{-}HT_2$ receptors. Other evidence that suggests such a role is that $5\text{-}HT_2$-receptor antagonism may contribute to the atypical profile of some antipsychotics, and alterations in 5-HT receptor densities in schizophrenia, notably a reduction in the number of frontal cortex $5\text{-}HT_{2A}$ receptors and an increase in $5\text{-}HT_{1A}$ receptors.

Inflammatory markers

The possible involvement of inflammation in the causation of schizophrenia has been mentioned with regard to risk genes and prenatal factors. There are also many studies showing alterations in various inflammatory markers in the blood in patients with the disorder, suggestive of a proinflammatory state. Such activation can in turn influence the dopamine, glutamate, and 5-HT systems (Muller et al., 2015). Evidence of inflammation in the brain was provided by Bloomfield et al. (2016), who used PET to show activation of microglia (resident inflammatory cells of the brain) in patients with schizophrenia and during the prodrome. However, the finding awaits replication, and overall the significance of inflammation in schizophrenia remains unclear (Manu et al., 2014; van Kesteren et al., 2017).

Neurodevelopmental model

The notion that schizophrenia is a disorder of neurodevelopment was proposed by Clouston in 1892 and by others, including Kraepelin, at the turn of the last century. The current interest can be traced to Murray and Lewis (1987), and especially to Weinberger (1987). Specific forms of the neurodevelopmental model implicate the second trimester in utero, adolescence, or an interaction between the two. Evidence in favour of the model has accrued from several sources and is summarized in Box 11.15. Many of the factors have already been discussed in this chapter.

There are no serious challenges to the neurodevelopmental model as a hypothesis of schizophrenia pathogenesis. This partly reflects its vagueness, which allows most findings to be interpreted as being consistent with it. Its weaknesses include a failure to readily explain the variable course of the disorder or provide a convincing explanation for late-onset schizophrenia.

For review, see Weinberger and Levitt (2011) and Howes and Murray (2014).

Box 11.15 Findings that support the neurodevelopmental hypothesis of schizophrenia

Structural brain changes present at or before illness onset

Limited progression of brain changes after onset

Motor, cognitive, and social impairments in children who later develop schizophrenia

Neuropathological changes without gliosis implies a prenatal timing

Most environmental risk factors relate to prenatal and perinatal period

'Soft' neurological signs at presentation

Minor physical anomalies and aberrant dermatoglyphics

Increased frequency of large cavum septum pellucidum

Schizophrenia risk genes affect brain development

Findings from animal models

Course and prognosis

The course and long-term outcome of schizophrenia has been a fiercely debated issue, in part due to differing ways in which diagnosis was made, patients followed up, and recovery defined.

Kraepelin initially believed that dementia praecox had an invariably poor outcome, although later reported that 17% of his patients eventually were socially well-adjusted. Manfred Bleuler (1974), son of Eugen Bleuler, personally followed up 208 patients who had been admitted to his hospital in Switzerland between 1942 and 1943. He concluded that the outcome was not so gloomy: 20 years after admission, 20% exhibited complete remission, 35% had good social adjustment, and 24% remained severely disturbed. When full recovery had occurred, this was usually within the first 2 years. In recurrent illnesses subsequent episodes usually resembled the first one in clinical features. Bleuler's conclusions were broadly supported by Ciompi (1980). Using well-kept records of 1642 schizophrenia patients followed up for an average of 37 years, he found one-third had a good or fair social outcome, with symptoms becoming less severe in the later years. However, Ciompi reported his percentages of followed-up subjects rather than recruited subjects, many of whom had died, so his outcomes are probably overoptimistic.

A more recent 15- and 25-year follow-up study of patient cohorts in 15 countries found that one-sixth of the patients had achieved full recovery (Harrison et al., 2001); importantly, late recovery was seen in a significant minority, challenging the therapeutic pessimism that such improvements are very rare. A 10-year follow-up of first-episode psychosis in the UK AESOP study found that 23% had had an unremitting illness, and 45% had been free of psychotic symptoms for at least 2 years; this study also highlighted that social outcomes are often worse than symptomatic ones (Morgan et al., 2014). A recent meta-analysis, defining recovery as requiring improvement in both symptoms and social/functional roles, persisting for at least 2 years, reported that about 14% of patients met this criterion (Jaaskelainen et al., 2013).

Whether the outcome of schizophrenia has improved since Kraepelin's era remains unclear. A meta-analysis found a 'recovery rate' of 35% prior to 1955, and 49% for the period 1956–1985, a difference that may reflect the introduction of antipsychotic drugs. However, the rate fell back to 36% between 1986 and 1992 (Hegarty et al., 1994). Any apparent time trends must be interpreted very cautiously because of changes in diagnostic practice and outcome measures during the twentieth century.

For a review of the course and clinical outcome of schizophrenia, see an der Heiden and Häfner (2011). Kooyman and Walsh (2011) have reviewed the societal outcomes.

Physical health, mortality, and suicide in schizophrenia

Originally reported by Ødegaard in Norway in 1951, there is an increased mortality in patients with schizophrenia. In an early meta-analysis, Harris and Barraclough (1998) found that the risk of death from all causes was increased 1.6-fold. Subsequent studies have found a higher figure, typically around threefold, and suggest that the 'mortality gap' is increasing (Saha et al., 2007). Expressed another way, men with schizophrenia die approximately 20 years prematurely, and women 15 years prematurely. All-cause mortality rates are increased several-fold further in patients with schizophrenia who have comorbid alcohol and substance misuse (Hjorthoj et al., 2015).

About 60% of the excess early mortality in schizophrenia is accounted for by unnatural causes (suicide and accidents), and the rest from natural causes. The latter are especially cardiovascular disease, partly reflecting the high rates of smoking, as well as poor diet, sedentary lifestyle, and higher rates of obesity, type 2 diabetes, and other physical illnesses. Lower rates of diagnosis and less active treatment of these disorders may also contribute (Shiers et al., 2015). Medication, especially atypical antipsychotics, has been postulated to contribute significantly to this excess mortality, from metabolic syndrome. However, moderate levels of antipsychotic use are associated with the lowest mortality in patients with schizophrenia, and even high doses are associated with lower mortality than no treatment (Torniainen et al., 2015). As an aside, the incidence of, and mortality from, some cancers and autoimmune disorders is lower than expected in individuals with schizophrenia and in their relatives (Catts et al., 2008). The mechanisms involved are not known.

The lifetime risk of suicide in schizophrenia is often quoted as 10% or more, but recent meta-analyses suggest a figure of about 5%. The risk is greatest early in the illness, and in those with affective symptoms, a history of suicide attempts, recent discharge from hospital, and number of psychiatric admissions (Popovic et al., 2014).

For review of early mortality in schizophrenia, see Laursen *et al.* (2014).

Predictors of outcome

The outcome of schizophrenia is, as noted earlier, heterogeneous and still largely unpredictable (an der Heiden and Häfner, 2011). However, epidemiological data, and some characteristics of the first presentation, have identified a number of poor prognostic factors, including younger age of onset, male sex, poor premorbid functioning, a prolonged duration of untreated psychosis, and early negative symptoms and cognitive impairment. See Box 11.16 for a list of factors influencing outcome in schizophrenia. However, their modest predictive value is emphasized, and caution should always be exercised when asked to predict the outcome of individual cases.

International studies suggest that the course and outcome of schizophrenia may differ between countries. The International Pilot Study of Schizophrenia (World Health Organization, 1973) found the 2-year outcome was better in India, Colombia, and Nigeria than in western countries, particularly for the proportion achieving complete remission. A 15- and 25-year follow-up study confirmed the stability of geographical differences in course, and suggested that a difference in the severity and type of illness at first presentation is an important contributory factor (Harrison *et al.*, 2001). Nevertheless, the better outcome of schizophrenia in developing countries, and its explanation, remains controversial.

Social stimulation

In the 1940s and 1950s, clinicians recognized that among people with schizophrenia living in institutions, many clinical features were associated with an unstimulating environment. Wing and Brown (1970) investigated patients at three mental hospitals. One was a traditional institution, another had an active rehabilitation programme, and the third had a reputation for progressive policies and short admissions. The research team devised a measure of 'poverty of the social milieu', which took into account little contact with the outside world, few personal possessions, lack of constructive occupation, and pessimistic expectations on the part of ward staff. Poverty of social milieu was found to be closely related to three aspects of the patients' clinical condition, namely social withdrawal, blunting of affect, and poverty of speech. The causal significance of these

> ### Box 11.16 Factors predicting a poor outcome in schizophrenia
>
> **Demographic factors**
>
> Male
> Single
> Younger age at onset
> Family history of schizophrenia
> Comorbid substance abuse
>
> **Clinical features**
>
> Poor premorbid adjustment
> Insidious onset
> Long duration of untreated psychosis
> Hebephrenic (disorganized) subtype
> Negative symptoms
> Cognitive impairment
> Absence of affective symptoms
> Poor insight
>
> **Other factors**
>
> High expressed emotion in family
> Poor adherence with treatment

social conditions was strongly supported by a further survey 4 years later; improvements had taken place in the environment of the hospitals, and these changes were accompanied by corresponding improvements in the three aspects of the patients' clinical state. It is possible that similar factors also apply to patients living in the community, where environments can also be impoverished or understimulating in various ways.

Family life and expressed emotion

Overstimulation also appears to be associated with poorer outcomes. Brown and colleagues found that patients with schizophrenia returning to their families generally did worse than those entering hostels. Relapse rates were greater in families with *high expressed emotion* ('*high EE*') (Brown *et al.*, 1962). This consisted of making critical comments, expressing hostility, and showing signs of emotional overinvolvement. In such families the risk of relapse was greater if there were high levels of contact (measured as more or less than 35 hours a week). The association with expressed emotion appeared to be mediated by antipsychotic medication, with the highest rates of relapse (92%) occurring in those with high EE, intense contact, and no medication (Vaughn and Leff, 1976).

Further studies (Leff *et al.*, 1985) demonstrated that relapse rates could be reduced in high EE families by a behavioural programme involving family sessions. Training in this intervention became an integral part of the Thorn Course for psychiatric nurses. Despite the strong evidence base and its inclusion in clinical guidelines (see below), it has struggled to be adopted in routine practice (Couldwell and Stickley, 2007).

Effects of schizophrenia on the family

Relatives caring for patients with schizophrenia describe two main kinds of problems: social withdrawal and episodes of disturbed behaviour. Patients tend not to interact with other family members; they seem slow, lack conversation, have few interests, and neglect themselves and stay in bed. Qualitative studies with families indicate that this self-neglect is experienced as a greater burden than the problems of more obviously disturbed or socially inappropriate behaviour, and occasional threats of violence.

Relatives of patients with schizophrenia may feel anxious, depressed, guilty, or bewildered. They may be understandably uncertain about how to deal with difficult and odd behaviour. It is this 'anticipatory anxiety' and sense of stigma rather than the practical burden of caring that families find wearing and demoralizing. Further difficulties can arise from differences in opinion between family members, and from a lack of understanding and sympathy among neighbours and friends. Although few mental health professionals still harbour discredited theories of family causation of schizophrenia (Box 11.12), there is still considerable popular support for such ideas. While this is less than it was a generation ago, families do often feel blamed and blame themselves. Community services and support for patients with schizophrenia and their relatives are often less than adequate, but improving help, advice, and services to carers of patients is a priority in many countries. In the UK all carers are now entitled to an annual assessment of their needs.

Treatment

Antipsychotic drugs are the mainstay of treatment for schizophrenia, but are used with increasing caution, and complemented by specific psychological and psychosocial interventions. This section is concerned with the evidence regarding individual treatments. The following section, on Management, deals with how these treatments are used together and delivered in clinical practice.

Clinical guidelines for schizophrenia

Several recent consensus guidelines are available for the treatment and management of schizophrenia. There is broad agreement on most key issues, but also some differences:

- NICE have produced updated UK guidelines for the management of schizophrenia in adults (National Institute for Health and Clinical Excellence, 2014a) and in children and adolescents (National Institute for Health and Clinical Excellence, 2013b). Compared to the two guidelines mentioned below, the NICE guidelines are relatively short on details, and the adult guideline has been criticized for overemphasizing psychological and psychosocial interventions (Taylor and Perera, 2015).

- Scottish guidelines (Scottish Intercollegiate Guidelines Network, 2013) give a greater focus upon the use of antipsychotic medication, on treatment-resistant schizophrenia, and on perinatal issues.

- Australasian guidelines (Galletly *et al.*, 2016) are the most detailed. They provide specific recommendations for a wide range of situations (such as comorbid substance abuse, acute behavioural disturbance, older patients, etc.), and include an algorithm for the pharmacological treatment of first-episode psychosis.

Pharmacological treatment

There is a strong evidence base supporting the use of antipsychotic drugs in the treatment of schizophrenia for prevention of relapse. However, there are important limits to their effectiveness, and significant side effects and other potential harms. Some of the key issues are listed in Box 11.17, and in the evidence summarized below, together with data regarding other physical treatments used in schizophrenia. As noted, discussion of how medication is used in practice and integrated with other aspects of treatment is deferred to the following section.

The pharmacology of antipsychotic drugs is covered in Chapter 25.

Effectiveness and side effects of antipsychotic drugs

The effectiveness of antipsychotic medication in the treatment of acute schizophrenia is well established by multiple placebo-controlled and active comparator studies (Leucht *et al.*, 2009; 2013). The median effect size compared to placebo is 0.44 (Leucht *et al.*, 2013). About two-thirds of patients show a significant therapeutic response, but at present there are no clinically useful ways of predicting whether an individual patient will respond. Importantly, antipsychotic drugs only treat the positive symptoms of schizophrenia. They have little or no clinically significant effect on negative (Fusar-Poli *et al.*, 2015) or cognitive (Nielsen *et al.*, 2015) symptoms, although a recent clinical trial reports efficacy of the new atypical antipsychotic cariprazine against negative symptoms (Nemeth *et al.*, 2017).

There are no substantial differences in efficacy between one antipsychotic and another (with the exception of clozapine), nor between typical and atypical antipsychotics. However, this does not mean that all antipsychotics are the same. There are considerable differences in their side effect profile (discussed in Chapter 25). These were confirmed in a recent multiple-treatments meta-analysis, which also showed slight but robust differences in efficacy and overall tolerability for individual drugs (Leucht *et al.*, 2013; see Table 11.7). These factors should be taken into account when discussing the choice of antipsychotic drug with a patient, as discussed in the section on Management.

Onset of action

Antipsychotics do not have a delayed onset of action, as is sometimes believed (Agid *et al.*, 2003). Improvement in psychotic symptoms, as well as sedation, can often be detected within 24 hours (Kapur *et al.*, 2005). Moreover, if there has not been a 20% improvement in symptom score after 2 weeks, the chances of a later response to that drug and dose are small (Samara *et al.*, 2016).

Dosage

Studies using PET and SPET to measure dopamine D_2 receptor occupancy, discussed in Chapter 25, provide a rationale for the dosing of antipsychotic drugs. This evidence complements clinical guidelines, which

---

> **Box 11.17 Key points in the pharmacological treatment of schizophrenia**
>
> **Acute episode**
> - Initiate antipsychotic medication at lower end of the licensed dose range.
> - Do not use loading doses ('rapid neuroleptization'). If sedation is needed, use adjunctive benzodiazepines.
> - The choice of drug should be based on patient preference, effects of previous treatments, and relative liability of the drug to cause serious side effects (especially extrapyramidal and metabolic syndromes).
> - Titrate dose within licensed range, monitoring for effects and side effects.
> - Aim to achieve optimum dose with good adherence for 2 weeks. If no response at that time, consider changing drug.
> - Record the indications for medication, the anticipated benefits and time course, and discussions with patient and carers.
> - Consider psychological interventions whenever medication is being introduced or changed.
>
> **Maintenance and relapse prevention**
> - Continue medication for a year, or longer, using the same principles as for the acute episode.
> - Ensure that dose, duration, and adherence are adequate before switching drug.
> - Drug withdrawal should be gradual, and the mental state should be monitored.
> - Continuous treatment is more effective than intermittent treatment.
> - Monitor adherence regularly.
> - Monitor for side effects, including metabolic syndrome, regularly.
> - Consider depot formulations, especially if adherence is a problem.
> - Always consider psychological interventions together with pharmacological options.

Table 11.7 Antipsychotic drugs ranked by effect sizes for efficacy, side effects, and tolerability (excluding clozapine)

	Greatest effect/ Most likely to	Smallest effect/ Least likely to
Efficacy	Amisulpride	Lurasidone
	Olanzapine	Asenapine
	Risperidone	Chlorpromazine
Continue on the drug	Amisulpride	Haloperidol
	Olanzapine	Lurasidone
	Paliperidone	Asenapine
Weight gain	Olanzapine	Haloperidol
	Chlorpromazine	Lurasidone
	Quetiapine	Aripiprazole
Extrapyramidal side effects	Haloperidol	Olanzapine
	Chlorpromazine	Quetiapine
	Lurasidone	Aripiprazole
Increased prolactin	Paliperidone	Aripiprazole
	Risperidone	Quetiapine
	Haloperidol	Asenapine
QTc prolongation	Amisulpride	Lurasidone
	Risperidone	Aripiprazole
	Asenapine	Paliperidone
Sedation	Chlorpromazine	Amisulpride
	Quetiapine	Paliperidone
	Olanzapine	Aripiprazole

Three drugs are highlighted in each category, but note that in many instances there are other drugs that have very similar properties. Clozapine, and antipsychotics not currently licensed in the UK, have been omitted from the table.

Adapted from Lancet, 382(9896), Leucht S et al, Comparative efficacy and tolerability of 15 antipsychotic drugs in schizophrenia: a multiple-treatments meta-analysis, pp. 951–962, Copyright (2013), with permission from Elsevier.

emphasize that antipsychotic drugs should be used at the lowest effective dose. The latter is lower in the first episode than subsequently (Kahn and Sommer, 2015), and applies particularly to adolescents requiring antipsychotic medication (National Institute for Health and Clinical Excellence, 2013).

Clozapine is the only antipsychotic for which it is often worth measuring plasma levels (see page 295).

Maintenance treatment and prevention of relapse

Since the original demonstration by Pasmanick *et al.* (1964), many controlled trials have confirmed the effectiveness of continued antipsychotic medication in preventing relapse. A meta-analysis reported a 1-year relapse rate of 65% in those who discontinued medication, compared to 27% in those who had continued it, with an NNT of 3 (Leucht *et al.*, 2012). Antipsychotic continuation was also associated with a better quality of life. An even more striking effect was seen in a systematic review, which looked selectively at recurrence after a first episode of psychosis. It reported a 1-year recurrence rate of 77% in those who discontinued medication, but only 3% in those who remained on medication (Zipursky *et al.*, 2014). Continuous medication is more effective than intermittent treatment strategies (De Hert *et al.*, 2015).

These meta-analyses emphasize the effectiveness of maintenance antipsychotic treatment in schizophrenia, as noted in all clinical guidelines, and notwithstanding some concerns about their long-term use (Moncrieff, 2015). However, there is less evidence as to how long maintenance treatment should last after an acute episode, reflected in differences between guidelines: National Institute for Health and Clinical Excellence (2014a) suggests 1–2 years, whereas Galletly *et al.* (2016) recommends 2–5 years.

Treatment adherence

Partial or non-adherence to treatment with antipsychotic drugs is common, and is associated with worse outcomes. A recent meta-analysis reported non-adherence rates of up to 52%, with non-adherence being related to poor insight and negative attitudes to medication; other variables, such as severity of illness and side effects showed inconsistent effects (Sendt *et al.*, 2015). Frequency of administration is an important factor, with adherence greatest for once-daily dosing, declining successively with twice and three times daily dosing (Medic *et al.*, 2013).

Depot antipsychotics (long-acting injectables)

Long-acting depot injections of antipsychotics (more recently called *long-acting injectables*) were introduced to deal with the problem of non- (or uncertain) adherence to treatment. Depot injections are more successful than oral medication in preventing relapse, presumably due to improved compliance, with a meta-analysis showing a relative risk reduction of about 30% (Leucht *et al.*,

2012). Long-acting injectables are prescribed to about 30% of patients with schizophrenia in the UK (Barnes *et al.*, 2009).

Clozapine

At least 30% of patients do not respond to antipsychotics, or are intolerant of them. The only proven drug intervention for this group is clozapine, which is effective in about one-third of such patients, as shown by the key trial by Kane *et al.* (1988), and confirmed in subsequent studies and meta-analyses (Leucht *et al.*, 2009). There is no evidence that any other atypical antipsychotic shares this greater efficacy. Clozapine may also have benefits with regard to suicide risk, aggression, and substance misuse, although earlier suggestions that it might improve persistent negative symptoms have not been borne out. Nevertheless, its beneficial properties give clozapine a unique place in the treatment of schizophrenia, despite its risks and side effects (see Chapter 25, and below).

A recent network meta-analysis challenges the widely accepted superiority of clozapine over other antipsychotics in treatment-resistant schizophrenia (Samara *et al.*, 2016). Limiting their analysis to the small number of double-blind randomized studies, it found few significant differences between drugs; clozapine was superior to haloperidol and chlorpromazine but was not more effective than olanzapine or risperidone. Interpretation of this study is unclear, not least since it contrasts with the finding of another methodologically similar meta-analysis (Leucht *et al.*, 2013). Issues include generalization from the blinded trials to clinical practice, shifting definitions of treatment resistance, and clozapine dosage (Kane and Correll, 2016).

There is little evidence-based guidance on the appropriate treatment of patients who are unresponsive to, or unable to take, clozapine. There are two common augmentation strategies. The first is to add an antipsychotic such as amisulpride that has a high affinity for the dopamine D_2 receptor; there is also a vogue for using aripiprazole. This is the only situation that justifies prescribing two antipsychotics at once. The other strategy is to add a mood stabilizer, especially lamotrigine. Occasionally, ECT is used to augment clozapine, and a recent systematic review suggest that it merits greater consideration in this situation (Lally *et al.*, 2016). However, overall there is limited evidence for any clinically or statistically significant clozapine augmentation strategy, nor for how to deal with treatment resistance if clozapine cannot be used (Miyamoto *et al.*, 2015).

Other drug classes used in schizophrenia

Antidepressants. Despite the prevalence of depression in schizophrenia, and the frequent use of antidepressant drugs, there is limited evidence regarding their efficacy in this situation, and recommendations for their use vary between clinical guidelines. A recent meta-analysis does show clear but modest beneficial effects against depressive and negative symptoms, especially for SSRIs, and a good safety profile (Helfer *et al.*, 2016).

Mood stabilizers. The value of mood stabilizers in treating schizophrenia is unproven. There is no evidence that they have an antipsychotic effect, and the beneficial effects reported in some trials could be due to treatment of affective symptoms. A systematic review confirmed that the benefits of lithium in schizophrenia occur in patients with affective symptoms (or with schizoaffective disorder) (Leucht *et al.*, 2004). The use of mood stabilizers in enhancing clozapine response was mentioned earlier.

Benzodiazepines. There is no role for benzodiazepines in augmenting antipsychotic drugs (Dold *et al.*, 2013), but they are useful acutely as part of rapid tranquillization (see below).

Future drug treatments. A diverse group of medications are under investigation, especially for negative and cognitive symptoms (Vreeker *et al.*, 2015). These include minocycline, non-steroidal anti-inflammatories, and polyunsaturated fatty acids. Some have clinical trial data suggesting efficacy but none is ready for routine clinical use.

Electroconvulsive therapy

The traditional indications for electroconvulsive therapy (ECT) in schizophrenia are catatonic stupor, severe comorbid depressive symptoms, and severe behavioural disturbance. In each situation the clinical impression is that the effects of ECT can be dramatic, but data are limited (Pompili *et al.*, 2013). ECT is used infrequently in the treatment of schizophrenia in the UK. However, it remains more widely used in some other countries and, as noted above, it may have value in clozapine augmentation.

Psychosocial approaches

The development of community-based services, and concerns about the limitations of medication, has led to an increasing emphasis on psychosocial interventions in the treatment of schizophrenia. These interventions

> ### Box 11.18 Psychosocial interventions for schizophrenia
>
> Family therapy (psychoeducation)
> Cognitive behaviour therapy
> Cognitive remediation
> Art therapy
> Social skills training
> Illness management skills
> Supported employment
> Integrated treatment for comorbid substance misuse

are of several different kinds (Box 11.18), but share the following aims:

- Enhancement of interpersonal and social functioning, including promotion of independent living in the community.
- Attenuation of symptom severity and associated comorbidity.

Family therapy

Family therapy, both formal and informal, is often employed at various stages of treatment. The most systematically evaluated intervention is that designed to decrease expressed emotion in family members. The procedure is usually combined with education about the illness and its consequences, together with practical advice on management (see Box 11.19). A meta-analysis confirmed that such interventions lower rates of relapse (NNT = 7) and improve medication compliance (NNT = 6). However, the studies showed a wide range of outcomes and may overestimate the treatment effect (Pharoah *et al.*, 2010). Psychoeducation alone is effective

> ### Box 11.19 Elements of family intervention in schizophrenia
>
> Education about schizophrenia
> Improving communication
> Lowering expressed emotion
> Expanding social networks
> Adjusting expectations
> Reducing number of hours of daily contact

in improving family members' knowledge and coping, but is of less effectiveness in reducing expressed emotion (Sin and Norman, 2013).

Cognitive behavioural therapy

The use of cognitive behavioural therapy (CBT) in schizophrenia is based on the rationale that positive psychotic symptoms are amenable to structured reasoning and behavioural modification. Several trials, and meta-analyses, have found CBT to be effective in schizophrenia, following Tarrier et al. (1998), who reported that it was more effective than supportive counselling in decreasing positive symptoms (see Turner *et al.*, 2014). In patients with delusional beliefs, for example, individual ideas are traced back to their origin and alternative explanations are explored. Similarly, it may be possible to modify a patient's beliefs about the omnipotence and origin of auditory hallucinations, with a resulting decrease in the distress that accompanies the experience and, perhaps, in the intensity of the hallucinations. Although normally used as an adjunct to medication, a recent study found CBT to be effective in patients who had chosen not to take an antipsychotic (Morrison *et al.*, 2014).

All current guidelines recommend CBT as part of an integrated treatment package for schizophrenia. However, there have also been studies with negative findings, and other reviews that have come to more cautious conclusions, especially regarding its use in routine clinical settings. Indeed, a recent systematic review concluded that CBT for schizophrenia has only a very small effect (Jauhar *et al.*, 2014) and the NICE guideline (National Institute for Health and Clinical Excellence, 2014a) has been criticized for overemphasizing the evidence for, and role of, CBT (Taylor and Perera, 2015).

Cognitive remediation

As noted above, cognitive impairments are important determinants of poor outcome in schizophrenia, and current pharmacological strategies have little, if any, effect. At present, the evidence is stronger for psychological approaches. Most of these rely on mental exercises and training to improve performance through practice. One of the most extensively tested is *cognitive remediation therapy*, and there is now good evidence that it has some effect both on cognitive performance and on functional outcomes, especially if there is real world practice of the learned cognitive skills (Medalia and Saperstein, 2013).

Other psychosocial interventions

Social skills training uses a range of approaches to teach the patient complex interpersonal skills, including behavioural reversal, feedback, and training. It is not recommended in current UK guidelines (National Institute for Health and Clinical Excellence, 2014a). However, a recent meta-analysis does indicate some efficacy against negative symptoms (Turner *et al.*, 2014).

Arts therapies are included in NICE guidelines amongst psychosocial interventions that should be considered (National Institute for Health and Clinical Excellence, 2014a). However, there is little evidence for their effectiveness (Scottish Intercollegiate Guidelines Network, 2013), and a recent multicentre randomized clinical trial was negative (Crawford *et al.*, 2012).

In the past, *dynamic psychotherapy* was commonly used in the treatment of schizophrenia (more so in the USA and France than in the UK). Evidence from clinical trials is sparse, but does not support the use of this kind of psychological treatment. In addition to the lack of convincing evidence for efficacy, there are concerns that dynamic psychotherapy may cause overstimulation and relapse.

Exercise is effective in improving a range of symptoms, quality of life, and global functioning in schizophrenia (Dauwan *et al.*, 2016). It is also valuable more generally for physical health, and for counteracting the weight gain propensity of many antipsychotic drugs.

Adherence therapy (previously referred to as *compliance therapy*) is a brief intervention using motivational interviewing, which aims to improve outcome by enhancing adherence to treatment use. UK guidelines state that it should not be offered (Scottish Intercollegiate Guidelines Network, 2013; National Institute for Health and Clinical Excellence, 2014a). However, a recent meta-analysis found that adherence therapy had a significant effect on reducing symptoms, even though it did not improve adherence or alter attitudes to medication adherence (Gray *et al.*, 2016).

Management

Successful management of schizophrenia depends on first establishing a good relationship with the patient. This can be difficult because of the nature of the illness but, with skill and patience, progress can usually be made. All plans that are made should be realistic, and acceptable to the patient and their carers. The importance of medication needs to be carefully explained, as well as its limitations and its side effects. The same principle applies to all other interventions. Such discussions should be informed by an up-to-date knowledge of the evidence, as outlined in the preceding section on Treatment. Novel modes of service delivery are likely to impact on the management of schizophrenia over the next few years, and it is important to keep up to date with these developments too.

Box 11.20 summarizes the key elements of the management of schizophrenia. When reading the following sections, the reader is also referred to the various current clinical guidelines available to inform and guide management decisions (Scottish Intercollegiate Guidelines Network, 2013; National Institute for Health and Clinical Excellence, 2013b; 2014a; Galletly *et al.*, 2016).

The acute illness

Admission to hospital for assessment and treatment is usually needed for the first episode of schizophrenia and for severe relapses, and not infrequently requires use of the Mental Health Act. Hospital admission allows a thorough assessment, provides a safe environment, and gives a period of relief to the family, who will often have experienced considerable distress during the emergence of the illness. However, for less severe episodes, and with adequate resources, home treatment is possible and has some advantages, including patient preference (Killaspy *et al.*, 2006). This is reflected in the development of crisis teams, who aim to treat and support acutely ill patients at home, although the evidence that such teams reduce admissions is relatively weak (Jacobs and Barrenho, 2011).

A drug-free observation period is a counsel of perfection, and is rarely attempted now, in part because of the pressure on inpatient beds. The main difficulty in establishing the diagnosis is often to elicit all of the symptoms from a withdrawn or suspicious patient. This procedure may require several interviews, as well as information

> **Box 11.20 Components and principles of the management of schizophrenia**
>
> Therapeutic partnership with patient and carers
> Early intervention for the first episode, and prompt intervention for later episodes
> Integrated, multidisciplinary working, involving primary and secondary care
> Antipsychotic drugs for treatment and maintenance, with attention to side effects and adherence
> Trial of clozapine for all patients who meet the criteria
> Cognitive behavioural therapy
> Family interventions
> Cognitive remediation
> Assertive outreach for vulnerable patients
> Regular assessment of needs
> Crisis resolution and home treatment teams as alternatives to admission
> Maintain realistic therapeutic optimism

from relatives or close friends and careful observations by nursing staff.

A physical examination and routine investigations should be carried out as soon as the mental state permits, for two reasons. The first is to exclude the possibility of an 'organic' or drug-induced psychosis; the second is to ensure that medical comorbidities are detected and to provide baseline data for metabolic syndrome monitoring (see below).

While the diagnosis is being established, a social assessment should be carried out. This includes a history of the patient's personality, level of functioning, work record, accommodation, and leisure pursuits, and the attitudes to the patient of relatives and any close friends. The current social functioning and capabilities can be assessed by other members of the multidisciplinary team, notably occupational therapists, social workers, and nurses. Discussions about the appropriate use and choice of psychosocial interventions (such as CBT) can also be carried out, although the patient is unlikely to be able to engage fruitfully in specific psychological therapies at this stage.

Drug treatment of the acute episode

Antipsychotic medication is the mainstay of the treatment of schizophrenia and other psychoses. It will usually be initiated soon after the diagnosis is made—or even while this remains uncertain—and will often continue for several years. Therefore the use of medication, and appropriate involvement of the patient and their carer in decision-making, are key aspects of management.

If the patient is acutely disturbed, *rapid tranquillization* may be required (Chapter 25). However, in other situations, treatment with *low to moderate doses* of an oral antipsychotic drug should be started. In general, in patients presenting with a first episode of psychosis, antipsychotic drug doses should be towards the lower end, certainly at the initiation of treatment; for example, risperidone (1–4 mg/day), amisulpride (100–400 mg/day), or aripiprazole (5–20 mg/day). It has been suggested that olanzapine should be avoided as a first-line treatment in first episode psychosis because of its greater propensity to cause metabolic syndrome (Dixon and Stroup, 2015); however, it is widely used, and its sedative properties can be valuable in the acute situation. As discussed earlier, the choice of drug should be based on an understanding of their differences in likely side effect profile, drug interactions, presence of any contraindications, and other clinical considerations (see Chapter 25).

Metabolic syndrome is prevalent even in unmedicated first-episode psychosis, being present in about 10% of patients (Mitchell *et al.*, 2013). The rate rises significantly later in the illness, presumably as a result of antipsychotic medication and lifestyle factors (Vancampfort *et al.*, 2013). Hence baseline examination and investigations for metabolic syndrome (Chapter 25) should be carried out before initiating antipsychotic medication and at recommended intervals thereafter (Cooper *et al.*, 2016).

As soon as the patient's mental state permits—and ideally before initiating antipsychotic medication—it is essential to explain the need for drug treatment and to obtain full consent, especially in view of the risk of serious and long-term side effects. If the patient is judged to be unable to make decisions of this nature, the appropriate legal safeguards under the Mental Health Act and its code of practice should be employed. The patient's family should be involved as far as possible in all decisions about treatment as a matter of principle, and because they will have a role in encouraging compliance. The use of patient advocates is also helpful.

In the early stages of treatment, the choice and timing of doses should be adjusted if necessary from one day to the next, until the most acute symptoms have been brought under control. Thereafter, regular once- or twice-daily doses are usually appropriate. It is important to be alert for acute dystonic reactions in the early days of treatment. A careful watch should also be kept for parkinsonian side effects as treatment progresses. For the elderly or physically ill, observations of temperature and blood pressure should be made to detect hypothermia or postural hypotension.

Although patients usually become rapidly more settled after starting antipsychotic drugs, improvement in psychotic symptoms is usually gradual, with full resolution taking a number of weeks. Current trends are to maintain the dose of antipsychotic drugs at a modest steady level and not to escalate the dose in the hope of speeding up the rate of improvement. For patients in whom agitation and distress continue to cause concern, (re)introduction of short-term intermittent treatment with a benzodiazepine is a better option than increasing the dose of antipsychotic.

If there are doubts about whether the patient is swallowing tablets, the drug can be given as syrup or as an orally dispersible tablet. Short-acting depot preparations (of zuclopenthixol acetate or olanzapine) are available, but are not recommended in patients whose tolerance of antipsychotics has not been determined. Anticholinergic drugs should be prescribed if extrapyramidal side effects are troublesome, but should not be given routinely or for sustained periods. As noted earlier, the acute symptoms of excitement, restlessness, irritability, and insomnia can be expected to improve rapidly after instituting treatment. Delusions, hallucinations, and other psychotic symptoms also begin to respond during this time, with improvement developing further over a period of several weeks.

By the time that meaningful symptomatic improvement has occurred, and prior to discharge, the team should have formulated a provisional plan for continuing care, based upon the social assessment that has been carried out. In the UK, this will occur within the framework of the Care Programme Approach (CPA).

Care plans and the Care Programme Approach

Care plans are important because of the need for coordinated multidisciplinary working, risk management, and clear documentation of responsibilities for their delivery. In the UK this responsibility has been formalized in the CPA (see Chapter 26). CPA is particularly appropriate for those with schizophrenia, who often require complex and long-term support. The essential elements of a care plan are to identify and record:

- A systematic assessment of health and social needs.
- A treatment plan agreed by the relevant staff, the patient, and relatives.
- The allocation of a key worker whose task is to maintain contact with patients, monitor their progress, and ensure that the treatment programme is being delivered.
- Regular review of patients' progress and needs.

Management after the acute episode

Once the acute episode has settled, the priorities for management are to maximize and maintain recovery. This will usually require maintenance medication which, as noted earlier, should normally continue for at least 1–2 years, and for longer after a second or subsequent episode. For many patients, depot injections are a helpful way to ensure adherence with medication (Box 11.21).

The emphasis on medication in no way diminishes the importance of multidisciplinary care in the long-term management of schizophrenia. It is important to use medication as part of an integrated package of care. This can involve supporting realistic structured activity, whether it be attending a day centre, pursuing education, or seeking a job. Advice should be given about avoiding obviously stressful events. CBT and other psychological interventions should continue, or be reconsidered if they have not previously been implemented. The patient should be seen regularly as an outpatient or at home by a member of the community mental health team (often a psychiatric nurse).

The extent and duration of ongoing care after an acute episode of schizophrenia depend on the severity and nature of the residual symptoms and impairments. At one extreme, following a single episode with excellent recovery, medication and other interventions can gradually be tailed off, and the patient returned to the care of the GP with a cautiously good prognosis. At the other end of the spectrum, the patient whose schizophrenia proves refractory to treatment requires long-term and intensive support.

Between these extremes lie the majority of patients, whose illness is relapsing and remitting, who never return to their premorbid level of functioning, and who have persistent difficulties or problems that need to be

> **Box 11.21 Use of antipsychotic depot preparations**
>
> For a number of reasons, some patients do not take their drugs reliably, and in these circumstances one of the intramuscular depot preparations may be useful. At the start of treatment a small test dose is given to find out whether serious side effects are likely to occur with the full dose, although this is not considered necessary with atypical antipsychotic preparations (Taylor *et al.*, 2015). The appropriate maintenance dose is then established by observation and careful follow-up. Since depot preparations have long half-lives, it may take several weeks for maximum plasma concentrations to be reached (see Table 25.4). This has implications for the rate at which dose increases and decreases should be made, and also for the tapering of doses of oral antipsychotic medication once depot treatment has started. It should be noted that treatment with olanzapine pamoate has been associated acutely with excessive sedation, confusion, and sometimes coma. Although these reactions are not common (they affect about 2% of patients) and full recovery occurs within 24–72 hours, all patients receiving this preparation require medical observation for at least 3 hours post injection.

identified and managed. This group includes patients with prominent negative symptoms, poor social adjustment, and cognitive and behavioural deficits characteristic of chronic schizophrenia. In patients who fail to return to their premorbid level of functioning and activities, despite resolution of their positive symptoms, it is important to consider the cause. For example, it may be due to negative symptoms, depressive symptoms, cognitive impairments, or the side effects of medication. If a cause is identified, appropriate action should be taken; this may include interventions for depression, a change in medication, or referral for psychological treatment.

Despite the above steps, the reality is that many patients progress to an illness state in which few specific new treatment options remain. Once a clinical picture of chronic schizophrenia has become established, the main emphasis is on a programme of support, tailored to the needs of the individual patient. An occupational therapist and clinical psychologist can make valuable contributions. The following specific issues require attention.

- Living accommodation and circumstances. Will the patient be able to live alone or will they return to live with their parents or other relatives? Will accommodation need to be arranged?
- Occupational activities. Will the patient be able to undertake some form of paid employment or voluntary work?
- Activities of everyday living. Patients often need help to re-learn and implement basic living skills such as cooking, budgeting, shopping, housework, and personal hygiene.
- If available, cognitive remediation, social skills training, or related therapies mentioned earlier that are aimed at improving cognition and social functioning.
- Monitoring and management of any comorbid condition or substance misuse.
- Monitoring and management of physical health problems.
- Optimization of the efficacy and tolerability of medication, while recognizing that any further response beyond that achieved earlier in the illness is unlikely.
- The family, and any other carers, must be fully supported, to help them to understand the patient's illness, to have realistic expectations of what the patient can accomplish, and to decrease their emotional involvement where appropriate. Work of this nature can be undertaken by community psychiatric nurses, social workers, psychiatrists, and GPs working together. Support groups for families and carers are also valuable. Specific interventions to help such carers have been trialled, and the evidence suggests that both support and psychoeducation reduce distress (Yesufu-Udechuku *et al.*, 2015).

Some patients with chronic schizophrenia understandably tend to withdraw from treatment and follow-up. For those who are judged to be at continuing risk of relapse, more assertive outreach (see Chapter 26) has a useful role to play (Burns and Firn, 2016).

Treatment-resistant schizophrenia

About one in three patients with schizophrenia come into this category, also known as *refractory schizophrenia*. For review, see Howes *et al.*, (2017). Management is particularly challenging because of the nature of the illness and the lack of evidence-based treatment options other than clozapine. The use of clozapine is hampered by the need for regular blood monitoring and the risks of agranulocytosis, as well as by other serious side effects, notably weight gain, sedation, and hypersalivation (Chapter 25). Nevertheless, because of its efficacy, clozapine should be recommended to all patients who do not respond to or cannot tolerate at least two other antipsychotics. In practice, only a minority of suitable patients have a trial of the drug, and often this does not occur until many years into the illness.

Assessment involves a detailed review of the history and establishment of the current symptom profile (Box 11.22). It is also worth trying to establish that the patient is refractory to treatment and not simply non-adherent; a recent study found that half of patients considered treatment-resistant had low or undetectable antipsychotic plasma levels (McCutcheon *et al.*, 2015).

The use of clozapine in clinical practice requires skill and experience to optimize adherence and efficacy, and to minimize and manage the common side effects and the rare but serious adverse events (Mortimer, 2011). Plasma levels are worth measuring if there are concerns about non-response or non-compliance. A minimum trough level of 200 µg/l should be attained; higher levels, up to 500 µg/l or more, may increase response, but at the cost of more side effects. For practical advice on clozapine use and monitoring, see Chapter 25 and Taylor *et al.* (2015).

Despite the focus on clozapine, management of refractory schizophrenia should also pay due attention to optimizing all other aspects of care, including physical health and psychosocial functioning, as described above for other patients with chronic schizophrenia.

For review of management of refractory schizophrenia, see Beck *et al.* (2014).

Other aspects of management

Early intervention

As noted earlier in the chapter, there is now a consensus that early treatment of schizophrenia may improve the long-term prognosis, based on a number of lines of evidence (Penttilä *et al.*, 2014).

- In conventional practice, patients have often been psychotic for many months before the diagnosis is made and treatment is initiated. Patients with a longer duration of untreated psychosis have a poorer longer-term prognosis.
- The treatment response becomes slower and less frequent during subsequent psychotic episodes.
- Much of the deterioration in social function takes place during the first 2 years after diagnosis.

These observations imply that it may be worth attempting to identify patients with psychosis as early as possible, so that effective treatment can be instituted. Specific 'Early Intervention in Psychosis Service' (EIS) teams were mandated in the UK in the 2000 NHS Plan, and are endorsed in the current NICE guidelines (National Institute for Health and Clinical Excellence, 2014a). These teams are described in Chapter 26.

Despite the widespread introduction of EIS teams, the evidence that they are effective remains limited and actively debated. There is no convincing evidence that early intervention reduces the duration of untreated psychosis (Lloyd-Evans et al., 2011), and the effectiveness, desirability, and cost-effectiveness of such interventions remain controversial (Castle, 2012; McGorry, 2015).

The EIS approach has also been extended to trials of treatment in individuals thought to be in the prodrome of illness but who do not have overt psychotic symptoms, and even to those considered to be at 'ultra-high risk' of developing schizophrenia. There is some evidence that low-dose medication and cognitive behavioural approaches may decrease the conversion to psychosis, and in one study, omega-3 polyunsaturated fatty acids significantly reduced the risk of onset of psychosis over the subsequent 6 years (Amminger *et al.*, 2015). For review, see Thompson *et al.*, 2016).

Box 11.22 Assessment of treatment-resistant schizophrenia

Review diagnosis (e.g. possibility of organic psychosis)

Review comorbidities (e.g. substance misuse, physical health)

Review treatment history (e.g. drugs, doses, psychological therapies)

Rate current symptoms and severity using established scales (e.g. BPRS, PANSS, CGI)

Physical examination (e.g. for metabolic syndrome)

Discuss patient's views regarding treatment

Check for treatment adherence (e.g. drug levels)

Consider routine blood tests and further investigations (e.g. imaging)

Substance misuse

Schizophrenia patients who misuse drugs and alcohol are now more the rule than the exception. They tend to have a worse symptomatic course and to be more difficult to engage in treatment. In addition, substance misuse is associated with increased risks of homelessness, violent behaviour, poor general health, and a substantial excess early mortality (Hjorthoj *et al.*, 2015). Comprehensive outpatient and assertive community programmes that address both substance misuse and psychotic illness in an integrated way have been proposed for this group, although evidence for their efficacy is limited. Antipsychotic drugs, especially clozapine, show some efficacy in reducing cannabis use (Wilson and Bhattacharyya, 2016).

The violent patient

Overactivity and disturbances of behaviour are common in schizophrenia, and although major violence towards others is not common, it does occur. Using data linkage for the entire Swedish population, Fazel *et al.* (2014a) found that 10.7% of male and 2.7% of female schizophrenia patients were convicted of a violent offence within 5 years of diagnosis. Comorbid substance misuse is probably the main factor implicated in the increased risk of violence (Fazel *et al.*, 2009a), but Fazel *et al.* (2014a), showed that this risk is reduced by medication. However, patients with schizophrenia are much more at risk of being victims of violence than of being perpetrators (Dean *et al.*, 2007). Careful follow-up and close community supervision may reduce the likelihood of victimization.

General management for the potentially violent patient is the same as that for any other patient with schizophrenia, although compulsory treatment is more likely to be required. Much can be done by providing a calm, reassuring, and consistent environment in which provocation is avoided. Threats of violence should be taken seriously, especially if there is a history of such behaviour, whether or not the patient was ill at the time. The danger usually resolves as acute symptoms are brought under control, but a few patients pose a continuing threat. In patients with persistent hostility and violence, clozapine and paliperidone extended release were highlighted as beneficial by a recent systematic review (Victoroff *et al.*, 2014).

The management of violence is considered further in Chapter 18.

Suicide risk

We have already seen that the rate of suicide is markedly increased in schizophrenia. As in other psychiatric disorders, demographic risk factors apply, such as male gender, social isolation, unemployment, and a previous episode of suicidal behaviour (Popovic *et al.*, 2014). Other risk factors include:

- comorbid depression and hopelessness
- frequent exacerbations of psychosis
- being in the early stage of the disorder
- during hospitalization or shortly after discharge.

Patients with pronounced negative symptoms are less likely to make suicide attempts. Although suicide may be associated with active positive symptoms such as delusions of control or auditory hallucinations, more often it occurs in those with previously high levels of educational attainment who are relatively well at the time. Such patients often have depressive symptoms in the context of high premorbid expectations of themselves and dismay at how their illness has damaged their future prospects.

Lowering the risk of suicide in schizophrenia involves being aware of and managing the relevant risk factors, and treating depressive symptoms vigorously. Clozapine (Meltzer *et al.*, 2003) and antidepressants (Tiihonen *et al.*, 2012) have been associated with reduced suicide rates in schizophrenia.

Management of schizophrenia in children and adolescents

There is relatively little evidence to guide management in this population. Guidelines agree that the same principles apply as to adults with schizophrenia, but greater caution is advised concerning the use and dosage of antipsychotic medication, with a correspondingly more prominent role for psychological interventions (Stafford *et al.*, 2015). For review, see National Institute for Health and Clinical Excellence (2013b), and also Chapter 16.

Management of schizophrenia in older patients

See Chapter 19 and Cohen CI *et al.* (2015).

Discussing schizophrenia with patients and carers

There is probably more stigma and misunderstanding associated with schizophrenia than with any other psychiatric diagnosis. It is therefore particularly important that the term is used carefully and sensitively, and all patients and their carers should have regular opportunities to ask questions, express their views, and raise any concerns that they may have. The involvement of the family in all decisions about treatment and management has already been mentioned.

There should be discussion about the nature of the illness, identification of any misapprehensions, and an explanation of the current meaning of the term schizophrenia. It is worth discussing what is known about the aetiology, in part to ensure that misconceptions do not lead to unnecessary guilt. For example, some parents worry, incorrectly, that their behaviour may have caused the illness. Mention of its heritability may lead to questions about the risks of schizophrenia in other relatives or future generations. These can be answered using the figures in Table 11.4, acknowledging the increased risk while emphasizing the probability that offspring and unaffected relatives will remain well. If, after discussion, the family continue to have very different concepts of schizophrenia from those of the clinical team, such views should be respected.

The prospects for recovery should be portrayed realistically but optimistically, given that some people wrongly believe schizophrenia is untreatable and inevitably follows an unremitting or deteriorating course. The key role of medication, together with psychosocial factors (e.g. family environment, substance misuse), in influencing outcome should be emphasized. Note that the family may have very different views about the meaning of recovery. The 'Recovery Approach' (sometimes referred to as the 'Recovery Movement') has achieved considerable prominence and influence in UK policy (Slade *et al.*, 2014). Originating in the USA and well established in New Zealand, it is a relatively loose collection of ideas and principles that emphasize the priority of the patient's aspirations and the goal of living life as fully as possible with the illness. Recovery advocates often criticize psychiatrists for having too pessimistic a view of the prognosis in schizophrenia, and insist on the need for optimism.

A further area in which there may be a difference in emphasis between psychiatrist and carer or patient is the focus upon the content rather than the nature of the patient's beliefs. That is, the psychiatrist is usually more concerned as to whether a thought is or is not delusional, or whether a perception is or is not a hallucination, whereas patients wish to discuss the thought or percept itself and its meaning for them. The psychiatrist should give the patient or carer adequate time to voice these concerns, while also explaining why it is necessary to ask detailed questions about the nature of the experiences.

Other than noting these broad themes, the psychiatrist must be prepared to adapt to the circumstances of each case. As noted, the full involvement of the patient and their carers should be an integral part of the management of schizophrenia. It is reasonable to assume that establishing and maintaining a genuine therapeutic alliance in this way will increase the likelihood that the patient maintains contact with psychiatric services, is adherent with treatment, and thereby has an improved prognosis.

Further reading

Bleuler E (1911). *Dementia Praecox or the Group of Schizophrenias* (English edition 1950). International University Press, New York.

Kraepelin E (1919). *Dementia Praecox and Paraphrenia*. Churchill Livingstone, Edinburgh.

Weinberger DR, Harrison PJ (2011). *Schizophrenia*, 3rd edn. Wiley-Blackwell, Oxford.

CHAPTER 12

Paranoid symptoms and syndromes

Introduction

The term *paranoid* can be applied to symptoms, syndromes, or personality types. Paranoid symptoms are overvalued ideas or delusions that are most commonly persecutory, but not always so (see Box 1.4, page 12). Paranoid syndromes are those in which paranoid delusions form a prominent part of a characteristic constellation of symptoms, such as pathological jealousy or erotomania. In paranoid personality disorder, there is excessive self-reference and undue sensitiveness to real or imaginary humiliations and rebuffs, often combined with self-importance and combativeness. Thus the term paranoid is descriptive; if we recognize a symptom or syndrome as paranoid, this does not constitute making a diagnosis, but it is a preliminary to doing so. In this respect it is like recognizing stupor or depersonalization.

Paranoid syndromes present considerable problems of classification and diagnosis. The difficulties can be reduced by dividing them into two distinct groups:

- Paranoid symptoms occurring as part of another psychiatric disorder, such as schizophrenia, mood disorder, or an organic mental disorder.

- Paranoid symptoms occurring without evidence for any underlying disorder. This group of disorders has gone by a variety of names, commonly *paranoid states* or *paranoid psychosis*, but the ICD-10 and DSM-5 category is *delusional disorder*. It is this second group that has caused persistent difficulties in several respects—for example, regarding their terminology, their relationship to schizophrenia, and their forensic implications.

This chapter begins with definitions of the common paranoid symptoms, expanding upon their descriptions in Chapter 1, and then reviews the causes of such symptoms. Next there is a short account of paranoid personality. This is followed by a discussion of primary psychiatric disorders with which paranoid symptoms are frequently associated, and the differentiation of these disorders from delusional disorders. The general features of delusional disorder and its major subtypes are then reviewed. A historical perspective is also given, with particular reference to paranoia and paraphrenia. The chapter ends with a summary of the assessment and treatment of patients with paranoid symptoms.

Paranoid symptoms

Although the vast majority of paranoid delusions are persecutory, the term is also applied to the less common delusions of grandeur and jealousy, and sometimes to delusions concerning love, litigation, or religion. It may seem puzzling that such varied delusions should be grouped together. The reason is that the central abnormality implied by the term paranoid is a morbid distortion of beliefs or attitudes concerning relationships between oneself and other people. If someone believes falsely or on inadequate grounds that he is being victimized, or exalted, or deceived, or loved by a famous person, then in each case he is construing the relationship between himself and other people in a morbidly distorted way.

The varieties of paranoid symptom were discussed in Chapter 1, but important ones are also outlined in Box 12.1 for convenience. The definitions are derived from the glossary to the Present State Examination (see page 66; Wing *et al.*, 1974).

Causes of paranoid symptoms

When paranoid symptoms occur as part of another psychiatric disorder, the main aetiological factors are those that determine the primary illness. However, the question still arises as to why some people develop paranoid symptoms, while others do not. This has usually been answered in terms of premorbid personality and social isolation.

Premorbid personality

Many writers, including Kraepelin, have held that paranoid symptoms are most likely to occur in patients with premorbid personalities of a paranoid type (see next section). Kretschmer (1927) also believed this, and thought that such people developed sensitive delusions of reference ('*sensitive Beziehungswahn*') as an understandable psychological reaction to a precipitating event. Subsequent studies of so-called late-onset paraphrenia have supported

---

Box 12.1 **Some paranoid symptoms**

Ideas of reference

Ideas of reference are held by people who are unduly self-conscious. The subject cannot help feeling that people take notice of him in buses, restaurants, or other public places, and that they observe things about him that he would prefer not to be seen. He realizes that this feeling originates within himself and that he is no more noticed than other people, but all the same he cannot help the feeling, which is quite out of proportion to any possible cause.

Delusions of reference

Delusions of reference consist of an elaboration of ideas of reference, to the point that the beliefs become delusional. The whole neighbourhood may seem to be gossiping about the subject, far beyond the bounds of possibility, or he may see references to himself in the media. He may hear someone on the radio say something connected with a topic he has just been thinking about, or he may seem to be followed, his movements observed, and what he says recorded. The importance of distinguishing a delusion of reference from an idea of reference is that the former is a symptom of psychosis.

Delusions of persecution

When a person has delusions of persecution he believes that a person, organization, or power is trying to kill him, harm him in some way, or damage his reputation. The symptom may take many forms, ranging from the direct belief that he is being hunted down by specific people, to complex, bizarre, and impossible plots.

Delusions of grandeur

These may be divided into delusions of grandiose ability and delusions of grandiose identity. The subject with delusions of grandiose ability thinks that he is chosen by some power, or by destiny, for a special purpose because of his unusual talents. He may think that he is able to read people's thoughts, is much cleverer than anyone else, or has invented machines or solved mathematical problems beyond most people's comprehension.

The subject with delusions of grandiose identity believes that he is famous, rich, titled, or related to prominent people. He may believe that he is a changeling and that his real parents are royalty.

these views (see Box 12.2). Thus Kay and Roth (1961) found paranoid or hypersensitive personalities in over half of a group of 99 subjects with late-onset paraphrenia.

Freud proposed that, in predisposed individuals, paranoid symptoms could arise through a convoluted process involving the defence mechanisms of denial and projection, based upon his study of Daniel Schreber, the presiding judge of the Dresden Appeal Court. Freud never met Schreber, but read the latter's autobiographical account of his paranoid illness (now generally accepted as being paranoid schizophrenia), together with a report by Weber, the physician in charge. Freud speculated that Schreber could not consciously admit his homosexuality, and projected his unacceptable desires ('I do not love him, he loves me') and then inverted this with another denial ('he does not love me, he hates me'). This configuration was abandoned fairly early on, and never had much clinical support.

Social isolation and deafness

Social isolation may also predispose to the emergence of paranoid symptoms. Prisoners (especially those in solitary confinement) and migrants have been considered to be prone to paranoid symptoms and syndromes, with social isolation being the common factor. However, there are no data that unambiguously support this view, and there are some which suggest other explanations. For example, the association between migration and psychosis is better explained in terms of broader psychosocial factors or marginalization, rather than just isolation (Singh and Burns, 2006; see also Chapter 11).

There is better evidence that the social isolation produced by deafness increases the risk of paranoid symptoms, as originally noted by Kraepelin. For example, Kay and Roth (1961) found hearing impairment in 40% of patients with late-onset paraphrenia. Subsequent studies have confirmed that hearing impairment is a risk factor for disorders in which paranoid symptoms occur, especially in the elderly (David *et al.*, 1995). However, it should be remembered that the great majority of deaf people do not become paranoid, and that many deaf people are not socially isolated.

Paranoid personality disorder

The concept of personality disorder is discussed in Chapter 15, and paranoid personality disorder is also briefly described there. It is characterized by the following:

- extreme sensitivity to setbacks and rebuffs
- suspiciousness
- a tendency to misconstrue the actions of others as hostile or contemptuous
- a combative and inappropriate sense of personal rights.

This definition embraces a wide range of types. At one extreme is the excessively sensitive young person who shrinks from social encounters and thinks that everyone disapproves of him. At the other is the assertive and challenging woman who flares up at the least provocation. An American study found a 4.4% prevalence of paranoid personality disorder, which is higher than previous estimates; the study also showed that the disorder had a significant impact on social and role functioning (Grant *et al.*, 2004).

Because of the implications for treatment, it is important to distinguish paranoid personality disorder from the delusional disorders to be described later. The distinction can be very difficult to make, and is based on the fact that in paranoid personality disorder there are no delusions (only overvalued ideas), and no hallucinations. Considerable skill is needed to separate paranoid ideas from delusions. The criteria for doing so were given in Chapter 1, and exemplified by the comparison between ideas of reference and delusions of reference (Box 12.1). In reality, the conditions probably lie along a continuum. Thus family studies indicate a genetic relationship between paranoid personality disorder and delusional disorder, and individuals with paranoid personality traits are at increased risk of developing delusional disorder.

For review of paranoid personality disorder and its management, see Carroll (2009) and Triebwasser *et al.* (2013).

Paranoid symptoms in psychiatric disorders

Paranoid symptoms are often secondary to a primary psychiatric disorder. Thus when paranoid symptoms, especially persecutory delusions, are elicited it is important to assess for the other features of these disorders. The diagnosis of delusional disorder, to be considered below, is in many respects a 'residual' category, used for patients whose delusions cannot be attributed to one of these other conditions. As the primary disorders are described at length in other chapters, they will be mentioned only briefly here.

Paranoid symptoms in organic disorders

It is important to consider an organic aetiology for paranoid symptoms, especially in the elderly or in cases where there is other evidence for a medical illness. In such situations, paranoid symptoms are likely to be a feature of *delirium*. Impaired grasp of what is going on around the patient may give rise to apprehension and misinterpretation, and so to suspicion. Delusions may then emerge, which are usually transient and disorganized; these may lead to disturbed behaviour, such as querulousness or aggression. Similarly, persecutory delusions commonly occur at some stage in *dementia*, and are occasionally the presenting feature. Paranoid symptoms and delusional disorders may occur with *focal brain lesions* of various causes, including tumour, stroke, and trauma. Some examples are given later in this chapter when the specific delusional disorders are considered. Finally, paranoid symptoms can occur in learning disability and other neurodevelopmental disorders.

Paranoid symptoms in substance misuse disorders

Paranoid symptoms occur in many substance misuse disorders, especially those associated with amphetamines, cocaine, and alcohol. An important example is the association between alcohol misuse and morbid jealousy, described below. Some therapeutic drugs can also precipitate paranoid symptoms, such as l-DOPA.

Paranoid symptoms in mood disorders

Paranoid symptoms are not uncommon in patients with severe depressive disorders, and paranoid delusions are a feature of psychotic depression. Conversely, depressive symptoms often occur in delusional disorders, although the diagnostic criteria for the latter require that their total duration is relatively brief (see Box 12.3). In practice, it is sometimes difficult to determine whether the paranoid symptoms are secondary to depressive disorder, or vice versa, as both scenarios are common. The distinction is of some importance, as the two disorders differ with regard to treatment and prognosis. A depressive disorder is likely if the mood changes have occurred earlier and are of greater intensity than the paranoid features. Previous psychiatric history and family history may also be useful pointers. Finally, in depressive disorder the patient typically accepts the persecution as justified by their own guilt or wickedness. This is a useful point clinically, as it contrasts with non-affective psychoses, in which such persecutions are bitterly resented.

Paranoid symptoms also occur in mania, and are typically mood-congruent and thus grandiose rather than persecutory.

Paranoid symptoms and paranoid schizophrenia

Paranoid schizophrenia was described in Chapter 11. Its distinction from delusional disorders has been problematic, both conceptually and practically (see Box 12.2; Opjordsmoen, 2014). A relatively large recent study

---

Box 12.2 Historical background: paranoia and paraphrenia

The terms *paranoia* and *paraphrenia* have played a prominent part in psychiatric thought. Although the classic studies are now several decades old, much can still be learned from reviewing the issues and the conceptual difficulties involved.

The term *paranoia*, from which the adjective *paranoid* is derived, has a long and chequered history. It has probably given rise to more controversy and confusion of thought than any other term used in psychiatry. A comprehensive review of the large body of literature, which is mostly German and from the period before the 1970s, has been provided by Lewis (1970) (see also Box 1.4). The word is derived from the Greek *para* (beside) and *nous* (mind). It was used in ancient Greek literature to mean 'out of mind' (i.e. of unsound mind or insane). This broad usage was revived in the eighteenth century, but when it came into prominence in the second half of the nineteenth century, in German psychiatry, it became particularly associated with conditions characterized by delusions of persecution and grandeur. The German term *Verrucktheit* was often applied to these conditions, but was eventually superseded by *paranoia*. There were many different conceptions of these disorders. The main issues, most of which remain today, can be summarized as follows.

● Did these conditions constitute a primary disorder, or were they secondary to another disorder?

● Did they persist unchanged for many years, or were they a stage in an illness which later manifested deterioration of intellect and personality?

● Did they sometimes occur in the absence of hallucinations?

● Were there forms with a good prognosis?

Kahlbaum raised these issues as early as 1863, when he classified paranoia as an independent primary condition which would remain unchanged over the years. Kraepelin had a strong influence on the conceptual history of paranoia, although he was never comfortable with the term, and his views changed strikingly over the years. In 1896 he used the term only for incurable, chronic, and systematized delusions without severe personality disorder. In the sixth edition of his textbook he wrote:

The delusions in dementia praecox [schizophrenia] are extremely fantastic, changing beyond all reason, with an absence of system and a failure to harmonize them with events of their past life; while in paranoia the delusions are largely confined to morbid interpretations of real events, are woven together into a coherent whole, gradually becoming extended to include even events of recent date, and contradictions and objects are apprehended and explained.

(Kraepelin, 1904, p. 199)

In later descriptions, Kraepelin (1919) used the distinction made by Jaspers (1913) between personality development and disease process. He proposed paranoia as an example of the former, in contrast to the disease process of dementia praecox. In his final account, Kraepelin (1919) developed these ideas by distinguishing between dementia praecox, paranoia, and a third paranoid psychosis, namely paraphrenia. He made the following suggestions:

● Dementia praecox had an early onset and a poor outcome, ending in mental deterioration, and was fundamentally a disturbance of affect and volition.

● Paranoia was restricted to patients with late onset of completely systematized delusions and a prolonged course, usually without recovery, but not inevitably deteriorating. An important point was that the patient did not have hallucinations.

● Paraphrenia was somewhat intermediary, in that the patient had unremitting systematized delusions but did not progress to dementia. The main difference from paranoia was that the patient with paraphrenia had hallucinations.

Bleuler's concept of the paranoid form of dementia praecox (which he later called paranoid schizophrenia) was broader than that of Kraepelin (Bleuler, 1906, 1911). Bleuler did not regard paraphrenia as a separate condition, but as part of dementia praecox. However, he accepted Kraepelin's view of paranoia as a separate entity, although he differed from Kraepelin in maintaining that hallucinations could occur in many cases. Bleuler was particularly interested in the psychological development of paranoia; at the same time he left open the question of whether paranoia had a somatic pathology.

From this time, two views of paranoia predominated. The first was that paranoia was distinct from schizophrenia and psychogenic in origin. The second view was that paranoia was part of schizophrenia. Some celebrated studies of individual cases appeared to support the first theme. For example, Gaupp (1974) made an intensive study of the diaries and mental state of the mass murderer Ernst Wagner, who murdered his wife, four children, and eight other people as part of a careful plan to revenge himself on his supposed enemies. Gaupp concluded that Wagner suffered from paranoia in the sense described by Kraepelin. At the same time, he believed that Wagner's first recognizable delusions developed as a psychogenic reaction. The most detailed argument for psychogenesis was put forward by Kretschmer (1927) in his monograph *Der Sensitive Beziehungswahn*. Kretschmer believed that paranoia should not be regarded as a disease, but as a psychogenic reaction occurring in people with particularly sensitive personalities. However, many of Kretschmer's cases would nowadays be classified as schizophrenia. In 1931, Kolle put forward evidence for the second view, that paranoia is part of schizophrenia. He analysed a series of 66 patients with so-called paranoia, including those diagnosed by Kraepelin in his Munich clinic. For several reasons, both symptomatic and genetic, Kolle came to the conclusion that paranoia was really a mild form of schizophrenia.

Considerably less has been written about paraphrenia. However, it is interesting that 50 of Kraepelin's series of 78 paraphrenic patients later developed schizophrenia. Indeed, paraphrenia has increasingly been regarded as late-onset schizophrenia or schizophrenia-like disorder of good prognosis. Kay and Roth (1961) used the term 'late paraphrenia' to denote paranoid conditions in the elderly that were not due to primary organic or affective illnesses. These authors found that a large majority of their 99 patients had the characteristic features of schizophrenia.

In current classifications, the term paranoia has, in effect, been replaced by delusional disorder. Paraphrenia does not feature either, but it continues to be used clinically to describe chronic, atypical, paranoid psychoses of middle and late life.

emphasized a number of ways in which delusional disorder differed from paranoid schizophrenia, including a later age of onset and better premorbid adjustment and overall functioning, but more severe delusions, and poorer response to antipsychotic medication (Peralta and Cuesta, 2016). When diagnosing an individual case, it is useful also to focus on the differences in the core features of delusional disordere compared to paranoid schizophrenia:

- The diagnosis of paranoid schizophrenia is suggested if the delusions are particularly odd in content (often referred to by psychiatrists as *bizarre delusions*), whereas the delusional themes are more 'plausible' in delusional disorder. Criterion A of the DSM-IV diagnostic criteria for delusional disorder specified that the delusions were non-bizarre. However, because of the poor reliability of this distinction, the specifier was removed in DSM-5 (Cermolacce *et al.*, 2010). Neither is it included in ICD-10.

- In schizophrenia, delusions tend to be fragmented and multiple, whereas in delusional disorder they are *systematized* and based around a single, internally consistent theme. In delusional disorder, the delusional system is also characteristically encapsulated, such that the rest of the mental state can appear remarkably normal, in contrast to schizophrenia.

- Patients with paranoid schizophrenia often have auditory hallucinations, and the content of these appears to be unrelated to their delusions. In delusional disorder, hallucinations are very rare, and when they do occur they are fleeting and clearly related to the delusions.

Paranoid symptoms in schizophrenia-like syndromes

Paranoid symptoms are features of several schizophrenia-like syndromes, which were discussed in Chapter 11. These include the DSM-5 categories of brief psychotic disorders and schizophreniform disorder, and the ICD-10 categories grouped under the heading 'Acute and transient psychotic disorders'.

Delusional disorders (paranoid psychoses)

As mentioned in the introduction, the terminology and classification of psychoses which are neither affective, organic, nor schizophrenia have been disputed for many years. Box 12.2 summarizes the main historical terms and themes, and provides the backdrop to the way in which the disorders are currently categorized. In this section, the core features of delusional disorders—the current terminology for these conditions—are described. The specific types of delusional disorder are covered in the following section.

Classification of delusional disorder

DSM-5 uses the term *delusional disorder* to describe a disorder with one or more persistent delusions that is not due to any other disorder. It is synonymous with the widely used term *paranoid psychosis*, and includes the non-specific term *paranoid states*. ICD-10 has a similar category of *persistent delusional disorders*. The essence of the modern concept of delusional disorder is that of a stable delusional system that develops insidiously in a person in middle or late life. The delusional system is encapsulated, and there is no impairment of other mental functions. The patient can often continue working, and his social life may be maintained fairly well.

The criteria for delusional disorder in DSM-5 are summarized in Box 12.3, with the subsequent description of five specific subtypes of delusional disorder and two other categories:

- persecutory
- jealous
- erotomanic
- somatic
- grandiose
- mixed
- unspecified.

Of these, persecutory is much the commonest subtype.

ICD-10 gives a similar definition for the principal category (F22.0) of persistent delusional disorders. Unlike DSM-5, the symptoms must have been present for at least 3 months. ICD-10 also includes litigious and self-referential subtypes, and has a separate subcategory (F22.8) of 'other persistent delusional disorders'. The latter includes delusional dysmorphophobia, whereas DSM-5 groups all types of body dysmorphic

> **Box 12.3 DSM-5 criteria for delusional disorder**
>
> A. One or more delusions, of at least 1 month's duration.
> B. Criterion A for schizophrenia has never been met. Hallucinations, if present, are not prominent, and are related to the delusional theme.
> C. Apart from the impact of the delusion(s) or its ramifications, functioning is not markedly impaired and behaviour is not obviously odd or bizarre.
> D. The total duration of any mood episodes has been brief relative to the duration of the delusional periods.
> E. The disturbance is not due to the direct physiological effects of a substance (e.g. a drug of abuse, a medication) or a general medical condition.
>
> Source: data from Diagnostic and Statistical Manual of Mental Disorders, Fifth Edition, Copyright (2013), American Psychiatric Association.

disorder together within the category of obsessive–compulsive disorders (Phillips *et al.*, 2006).

For review of delusional disorder, see Munro (2009).

Epidemiology of delusional disorder

Delusional disorder is regarded as being an uncommon illness, although there are relatively few data. Kendler (1982) reviewed the literature and reported an incidence of 1–3 per 100,000 per year, with delusional disorder constituting 1–4% of all psychiatric admissions. In a large population survey, delusional disorder had a lifetime prevalence of 0.18% (Peraala *et al.*, 2007).

In a large case series, the mean age of onset of delusional disorder was 46 years, and the diagnosis remained stable over a 10-year period, with only 21% being rediagnosed with schizophrenia (Marneros *et al.*, 2012).

Significant depressive symptoms are common in delusional disorder (note category D in Box 12.3; Peralta and Cuesta 2016)

Aetiology of delusional disorder

What little is known about the aetiology of delusional disorder is based upon its relationship to, and comparison with, schizophrenia, paranoid personality disorder,

and depressive disorder (Kendler, 1982). This question has been addressed by family and neurobiological studies. However, the relatively small sample sizes and varying diagnostic definitions mean that few conclusions can be drawn. Psychological explanations for delusional disorder centre upon the delusions themselves (see Garety and Freeman, 2013).

Family studies of delusional disorder

First-degree relatives of patients with delusional disorder have an increased incidence of paranoid personality disorder (Kendler *et al.*, 1985). The familial relationship of delusional disorder to schizophrenia is less clear. Although the risk of delusional disorder is increased in first-degree relatives of patients with schizophrenia, relatives of patients with delusional disorder do not have an increased risk of schizophrenia or schizotypal personality (Kendler *et al.*, 1995; Kendler and Walsh, 1995; Tienari *et al.*, 2003). This familial association pattern has been called asymmetric coaggregation, and may be because of a number of factors:

- Differences in the incidence rates of the two disorders in the general population.
- Differences in the diagnostic error rate between probands and relatives (probands are usually subject to more intensive assessment).
- A higher genetic loading for severe illness in those who come to medical attention (and are therefore assessed as probands).

Overall, there appears to be a weak genetic link between delusional disorder and, on the one hand, schizophrenia, and on the other, paranoid personality disorder. However, the extent of this overlap is unclear, and no individual loci or genes associated with delusional disorder have been identified.

There is also a familial clustering of delusional disorder and alcoholism (Kendler and Walsh, 1995), which could contribute to the association between morbid jealousy and alcohol misuse (see page 306).

Neurobiological studies

Very little is known regarding biological correlates of delusional disorder, nor the extent to which they overlap with or differ from schizophrenia. One MRI study reported that elderly patients with delusional disorder have enlarged cerebral ventricles (Howard *et al.*, 1995). A recent study of younger patients with delusional disorder found alterations in brain activation and cortical thickness, especially in the insula and cingulate cortex (Vicens *et al.*, 2016).

Specific delusional disorders

As noted above, specific subtypes of delusional disorder are recognized, on the basis of the content of the predominant delusion(s) (see Box 12.4). Historically, these symptoms have been of particular interest to French psychiatrists. Classification in this area is confusing for two reasons.

- Some of the disorders are often referred to by older, eponymous, terms, or by categories that are not included in ICD-10 or DSM-5 but which remain in common usage.
- Some of the syndromes can be viewed as symptoms (e.g. delusional misidentification), or can occur secondary to other psychiatric disorders.

In this section we also consider stalking and persistent litigants, as both behaviours may be secondary to delusional disorder.

Pathological jealousy

Pathological or *morbid jealousy* (other synonyms are listed in Box 12.4) will be described first and in most detail as it is the archetypal delusional disorder; it is also the commonest (other than 'persecutory delusional disorder', not otherwise specified) and, importantly, appears to carry the greatest risk of dangerousness.

The essential feature is an abnormal belief that the patient's partner is being unfaithful. The condition is termed pathological because the belief, which may be a delusion or an overvalued idea, is held on inadequate grounds and is unaffected by rational argument. The belief is often accompanied by strong emotions and characteristic behaviour, but these do not in themselves constitute pathological jealousy. A man who finds his wife in bed with a lover may experience extreme jealousy and may behave in an uncontrolled way, but this should not be called pathological jealousy. The term should be used only when the jealousy is based on unsound evidence and reasoning.

The main sources of information about pathological jealousy come from the classic paper by Shepherd (1961), and from surveys by Langfeldt (1961), Vauhkonen (1968), and Mullen and Maack (1985). Shepherd examined the hospital case notes of 81 patients in London, and Langfeldt did the same for 66 patients in Norway. Vauhkonen conducted an interview study of 55 patients in Finland, and Mullen and Maack examined the hospital case notes of 138 patients.

Pathological jealousy is more common in men, with the surveys mentioned above finding that about two men were affected for every woman. The frequency of the condition in the general population is unknown, but it is not uncommon in psychiatric practice. Each case merits careful attention, not only because of the great distress that the condition causes within relationships, but also because these individuals may be highly dangerous.

Clinical features of pathological jealousy

As indicated above, the main feature is an abnormal belief in the partner's infidelity. This may be accompanied by other abnormal beliefs—for example, that the partner is plotting against the patient, trying to poison him, taking away his sexual capacities, or infecting him with venereal disease. The mood of the pathologically jealous patient may vary with the underlying disorder, but often it is a mixture of misery, apprehension, irritability, and anger.

Typically, the behaviour involves an intensive search for evidence of the partner's infidelity—for example, by

---

Box 12.4 Types of delusional disorder

Type	Synonymous with, or includes
Jealous	Morbid jealousy, pathological jealousy, erotic jealousy, sexual jealousy, Othello syndrome
Erotic	Erotomania, De Clèrambault's syndrome
Somatic	Monosymptomatic hypochondriacal psychosis, delusional body dysmorphic disorder
Querulous	Persecutory
Shared	Induced delusional disorder, folie à deux, communicated insanity
Other	Delusional misidentification syndrome, Capgras syndrome, Fregoli delusion, intermetamorphosis, syndrome of subjective doubles

looking through diaries and by examining bed linen and underwear. The patient may follow the partner about, or engage a private detective. The jealous person often cross-questions the partner incessantly. This may lead to violent quarrelling and paroxysms of rage in the patient. Sometimes the partner becomes exasperated and worn out, and is finally goaded into making a false confession. If this happens, the jealousy is inflamed rather than assuaged. An interesting feature is that the jealous person often has no idea who the supposed lover may be, or what kind of person they may be. Moreover, he may avoid taking steps that could produce unequivocal proof one way or the other.

Behaviour may be strikingly abnormal. A successful city businessman carried a briefcase that contained not only his financial documents but also a machete for use against any lover who might be detected. A carpenter installed an elaborate system of mirrors in his house so that he could watch his wife from another room. A third patient avoided waiting alongside another car at traffic lights, in case his wife, who was sitting in the passenger seat, might surreptitiously make an assignation with the other driver.

Aetiology of pathological jealousy

Pathological jealousy, like other paranoid symptoms and syndromes, can occur in a range of primary disorders (see Box 12.5). In the surveys mentioned, the frequencies of disorders varied, probably reflecting the population studied and the diagnostic scheme used. For example, paranoid schizophrenia was reported in 17–44% of patients, depressive disorder in 3–16%, neurosis and personality disorder in 38–57%, alcoholism in 5–7%, and organic disorders in 6–20%.

The role of personality in the genesis of pathological jealousy should be emphasized. It is often found that the patient has a pervasive sense of inadequacy, together with low self-esteem. There is a discrepancy between his ambitions and his attainments. Such a personality is particularly vulnerable to anything that may threaten this sense of inadequacy, such as loss of status or development of sexual dysfunction. In the face of such threats the person may project the blame on to others, and this may take the form of jealous accusations of infidelity. As mentioned earlier, Freud believed that unconscious homosexual urges played a part in all jealousy, but clinical studies do not support an association between homosexuality and pathological jealousy. Similarly, although pathological jealousy has sometimes been attributed to the onset of sexual difficulties, there is no good evidence of such an association.

Prognosis of pathological jealousy

Little is known about the prognosis of pathological jealousy. It probably depends on a number of factors, including the nature of any underlying psychiatric disorder and the patient's premorbid personality. When Langfeldt (1961) followed up 27 of his patients after 17 years, he found that over 50% of them still had persistent or recurrent jealousy. This confirms a general clinical impression that the prognosis is often poor.

Risk of violence

Although there are no reliable estimates of the risks of violence, there is no doubt that people with pathological jealousy can be dangerous (Silva et al., 1998). In addition to homicide, the risk of physical injury inflicted by jealous patients is considerable. In one series, around 25% had threatened to kill or injure their partner, and 56% of men and 43% of women had been violent towards or threatened the supposed rival (Mullen and Maack, 1985). Schanda et al. (2004), studying convicted murderers in Austria, found that delusional disorder (subtype not specified) is associated with homicide, with an odds ratio of 6. There is also a risk of suicide, particularly when an accused partner finally decides to end the relationship.

Assessment of pathological jealousy

The assessment of a patient with pathological jealousy should be particularly thorough, and should always include the partner, who should be interviewed separately whenever possible.

The partner may give a much more detailed account of the patient's morbid beliefs and actions than can be elicited from the patient. The doctor should try to find out tactfully how firmly the patient believes in the

---

> ### Box 12.5 Disorders associated with pathological jealousy
>
> Schizophrenia
> Mood disorder
> Organic disorder
> Substance misuse (especially alcohol)
> Paranoid personality disorder

partner's infidelity, how much resentment he feels, and whether he has contemplated any vengeful action. What factors provoke outbursts of accusations and questioning? How does the partner respond to such outbursts? How does the patient respond in turn to the partner's behaviour? Has there been any violence so far? Has there been any serious injury?

In addition to these enquiries, the doctor should take a detailed relationship and sexual history from both partners, and assess for underlying psychiatric disorder, as this will have implications for treatment.

Treatment of pathological jealousy

The treatment of pathological jealousy, as with other delusional disorders, is in principle fairly straightforward, the mainstay being antipsychotic drugs, but in practice can be very difficult because of the patient's lack of insight and their reluctance to collaborate with the treatment plan. Furthermore, there is a lack of randomized evidence.

Adequate treatment of any associated disorder, such as schizophrenia or a mood disorder, is a first requisite. If alcohol or other substance misuse is present, specific treatment will be needed. In other cases the pathological jealousy may be the symptom of a delusional disorder, or an overvalued idea in a patient with low self-esteem and personality difficulties.

If the jealousy appears to be delusional in nature, a careful trial of an antipsychotic drug is worthwhile, although the results are often disappointing. As noted above, even when depressive disorder is not the primary diagnosis, it frequently complicates pathological jealousy and may worsen it. Treatment with an antidepressant may help in these circumstances, and also when the jealousy appears to be an overvalued idea rather than a delusion.

Psychotherapy may be attempted in cases where the jealousy appears to arise from personality problems. One aim is to reduce tensions by allowing the patient (and their partner) to ventilate their feelings. Behavioural methods include encouraging the partner to produce behaviour that reduces jealousy; for example, by refusal to argue, depending on the individual case. A study of the use of cognitive therapy, in which patients were encouraged to identify faulty assumptions and were taught strategies of emotional control, gave superior results compared with a waiting list control group (Dolan and Bishay, 1996).

If there is no response to outpatient treatment, or if the risk of violence is high, inpatient care may be necessary. Not uncommonly, however, the patient appears to improve as an inpatient, only to relapse on discharge.

If there appears to be a risk of violence, the doctor should warn the partner, even if this involves a breach of confidentiality. In some cases the safest procedure is to advise separation. It is not uncommon for feelings of pathological jealousy to wane once a relationship has ended. Sometimes, however, the problem re-emerges if the patient enters a new relationship.

Erotomania and erotic delusions

Erotic delusions can occur in any psychotic disorder, especially paranoid schizophrenia, but they are the predominant and persistent symptom in a form of delusional disorder called *erotomania*. It was a French psychiatrist, De Clérambault, who in 1921 proposed that a distinction should be made between paranoid delusions and delusions of passion. The latter differed in their pathogenesis and in being accompanied by excitement. This distinction is of historical interest only, but the syndrome is still sometimes known as *De Clérambault's syndrome*.

Erotomania is rare and occurs almost entirely in women, though Taylor *et al.* (1983) reported four cases in a series of 112 men charged with violent offences. The woman, who is usually single, believes that an exalted person is in love with her. The supposed lover is usually inaccessible, as he is already married, or is a famous person. According to De Clérambault, the infatuated woman believes that it is the supposed lover who first fell in love with her, and that he is more in love with her than she is with him. She derives satisfaction and pride from this belief. She is convinced that the supposed lover cannot be a happy or complete person without her. The patient often believes that the supposed lover is unable to reveal his love for various unexplained reasons, and that he has difficulties in approaching her, has indirect conversations with her, and has to behave in a paradoxical and contradictory way. The woman may cause considerable nuisance to the supposed lover. She may be extremely tenacious and impervious to reality. Other patients turn from a delusion of love to a delusion of persecution, become abusive, and make public complaints about the supposed lover. This was described by De Clérambault as two phases—hope followed by resentment.

There are few data regarding the treatment and outcome of erotomania. For review see Seeman (2016). For a review of the concept of erotomania, see Berrios and Kennedy (2002).

Stalking

A proportion of 'stalkers' appear to suffer from delusional disorders, including erotomania, which is why the topic is mentioned here.

There is no clear consensus about the definition of stalking. Most formulations contain the following elements:

- a pattern of intrusive behaviour
- the intrusive behaviour is associated with implicit or explicit threats
- the person being stalked experiences fear and distress.

Stalkers typically follow their victims around and loiter outside their house or place of work. Unwanted communications by telephone, letter, or graffiti, and, in more recent times, by email or social media, are very common. Behaviour can then become more threatening, with hoax advertisements or orders for services, scandalous rumour mongering, damage to the victim's property, threats of violence, and actual assault.

Stalkers are a heterogeneous group with differing underlying psychopathologies (Dressing et al., 2006). Some, usually women, have erotomania or erotic delusions secondary to other psychotic disorders. More commonly, stalkers suffer from a personality disorder, predominantly with borderline, narcissistic, and sociopathic traits. They have often had a relationship with their victim that may have been quite superficial; in other cases, however, a serious relationship has cooled. A previous history of domestic violence in the relationship puts the victim at particularly high risk of assault and injury. Whether or not the victim suffers actual assault, they invariably experience severe psychological stress, which can lead to anxiety and mood disorders and post-traumatic stress disorder. Risk assessment is important (Mullen et al., 2006).

For a review of stalking, see Mullen et al. (2009).

Somatic delusional disorder

People with somatic delusional disorder believe that they suffer from a physical illness, deformity, or infestation (e.g. delusional parasitosis, also called Morgellons disease). The term encompasses monosymptomatic hypochondriacal psychosis, as there is often a single, intense delusional belief of this kind. Somatic delusional disorder needs to be distinguished from the hypochondriacal delusions (and somatic hallucinations) that can occur in other disorders (e.g. schizophrenia, psychotic depression, cocaine abuse), and from genuine somatic symptoms that occur secondary to organic disorders

(e.g. the pruritus of hepatic failure). It must also be distinguished from the common occurrence of obsessional thoughts or overvalued ideas about similar bodily issues. A specific example of the latter is body dysmorphic disorder (also called dysmorphophobia). In fact there is much overlap clinically, and perhaps therapeutically, between delusional and non-delusional forms of body dysmorphic disorder (Phillips et al., 2006). The difference between how ICD-10 and DSM-5 classify these disorders was noted earlier.

Because of the content of the belief, somatic delusional disorders often present to the relevant medical specialism—for example, body dysmorphic disorder to plastic surgeons, or delusional parasitosis to dermatologists (e.g. Lepping et al., 2010). To ensure correct identification and appropriate treatment, it is necessary that the physician recognizes the nature of the disorder, and is able either to treat it or to involve a psychiatrist in its management. However, this does not always occur, and in any event patients are often reluctant to accept the diagnosis.

Querulant delusions and reformist delusions

Querulant delusions were the subject of a special study by Krafft-Ebing in 1888. Patients with this kind of delusion indulge in a series of complaints and claims lodged against the authorities. Closely related to querulant patients are paranoid litigants, who undertake a succession of lawsuits, and become involved in numerous court hearings, in which they may become passionately angry and may make threats against the magistrates. The characteristics of persistent litigants have been reviewed by Lester et al. (2004).

Baruk (1959) described 'reformist delusions', which are based on religious, philosophical, or political themes. People with these delusions constantly criticize society and sometimes embark on elaborate courses of action. Their behaviour may be violent, particularly when the delusions are political. Some political assassins fall within this group. It is extremely important that this diagnosis is made on clear psychiatric grounds rather than on political grounds, as occurred in the former Soviet Union (see Chapter 2).

Delusional misidentification syndrome

Another group of delusions involves different aspects of misidentification, either of the self or of others. Like all delusions, they often occur in other psychotic disorders, especially schizophrenia and organic disorders, but they can also occur in isolation, and have been given the collective label of delusional misidentification syndrome (Christodoulou, 1991). The category is not named in ICD-10 or DSM-5, but constitutes an example of 'other persistent delusional disorders' coded in the former. One argument for bringing them together is that they all appear to be 'face-processing disorders', and associated with abnormalities in the posterior part of the right hemisphere, where the systems responsible for face recognition are located. Note also the seemingly close relationship of these disorders to the neurological category of *prosopagnosia* (the inability to recognize familiar faces). Interestingly, the delusions are specific to a few, usually familiar, people, and recognition of other faces (and objects) is not impaired. Although the beliefs are delusional, the patient is aware that something is wrong with the 'replacement' person. The patient may be extremely distressed, and may occasionally act against individuals whom they believe to be impostors.

Four main variants of delusional misidentification are recognized. In each case there is debate as to whether they constitute a symptom or a syndrome.

Capgras syndrome

In this rare condition—which is really a delusion rather than a syndrome, hence its alternative name, *Capgras delusion*—the patient, usually a woman, believes that a person closely related to her (often her partner) has been replaced by a double. She accepts that the misidentified person has a strong resemblance to the familiar person, but still believes that they are different people. Some patients with Capgras syndrome may behave dangerously by attacking the presumed double. A history of depersonalization, derealization, or déjà vu is not unusual. Schizophrenia is said to be the most frequent diagnosis (Berson, 1983), although in older subjects, Lewy body disease or other neurodegenerative disorders are common (Josephs, 2007). The syndrome is an example of a reduplicative paramnesia.

The name derives from the classic description by Capgras and Reboul-Lachaux in 1923, who called it *l'illusion des sosies (illusion of doubles)*. However, as noted above, it is a delusion, not an illusion. For review, see Edelstyn and Oyebode (1999).

Fregoli syndrome

In this condition, also called the *Fregoli delusion*, the patient believes that one or more individuals have changed their appearance to resemble familiar people, usually in order to persecute the patient in some way. The symptom is usually associated with schizophrenia or with organic brain disease. Its name derives from an actor called Fregoli who had remarkable skill in changing his facial appearance. Originally described by Courbon and Fail in 1927, the condition is even rarer than the Capgras delusion. For review, see Langdon *et al.* (2014).

Intermetamorphosis

In this syndrome, the patient believes that one or more individuals have been transformed, both physically and psychologically, into another person or people, or that people have exchanged identities with each other. As with the other forms of delusional misidentification, note that intermetamorphosis is not a hallucination—the abnormality is one of interpretation, not misperception.

The syndrome of subjective doubles

In the syndrome of subjective doubles, the patient has the delusion that another person has been physically transformed into his own self, like a doppelganger.

Shared (induced) delusional disorder

Sometimes a person who is in a close relationship with someone who already has an established delusional system develops similar ideas. The commonest term is a *folie à deux*, although the ICD-10 category is *shared delusional disorder*. The condition has also been called *communicated insanity*. The frequency of induced psychosis is not known, but it is low. Sometimes more than two people are involved (*folie à plusieurs*), but this is exceedingly rare. It has also been speculated that some apocalyptic cults involve phenomena of this kind.

Over 90% of reported cases are members of the same family. Usually there is a dominant partner with fixed delusions who appears to induce similar beliefs in a dependent or suggestible partner, sometimes after initial resistance. The beliefs in the recipient may or may not be truly delusional. Generally the two people have lived together for a long time in close intimacy, often in isolation from the outside world. Once established, the condition runs a chronic course.

It is usually necessary to advise separation of the affected individuals. This may lead to resolution of the quasi-delusional state in the recipient; the original patient should be treated in the usual fashion for delusional disorder. For a review of shared delusional disorder, see Silveira and Seeman (1995).

Assessment of paranoid symptoms

The assessment of paranoid symptoms involves two stages—first, the recognition of the symptoms themselves, and, secondly, the diagnosis of the underlying condition.

Sometimes it is obvious that the patient has persecutory ideas or delusions. At other times recognition of paranoid symptoms may be exceedingly difficult, and considerable skill is required by the interviewer. The patient may be suspicious or angry. They may be very defensive, say little, or speak fluently about other topics while steering away from persecutory beliefs or denying them completely. The psychiatrist should be tolerant and impartial, acting as a detached but interested listener who wants to understand the patient's point of view. The interviewer should show compassion, but not collude in the delusions or give promises that cannot be fulfilled. When an apparently false belief is disclosed, considerable time and effort may then be needed to determine whether or not it meets the criteria for a delusion rather than an overvalued idea or other form of belief. This is of crucial diagnostic significance, as the presence of a delusion is likely to be the symptom upon which a diagnosis of psychotic disorder is based, whereas non-delusional thoughts which may be similar in content are consistent with a range of other diagnostic categories.

If delusions are detected, the next step is to diagnose the type of psychosis, based upon the diagnostic features of the disorders noted earlier in this chapter. It is also important to determine whether the patient is likely to try to harm the alleged persecutor. A full risk assessment is needed. This calls for close study of the patient's personality, history of violence, and the characteristics of their delusions and any associated hallucinations. Hints or threats of homicide should be taken seriously. The doctor should be prepared to ask tactfully about possible homicidal plans and preparations to enact them. In many ways the method of enquiry resembles the assessment of suicide risk: 'Have you ever thought of doing anything about it?', 'Have you made any plans?', and 'What might prompt you to do it?'

The assessment of dangerousness is discussed further in Chapter 18.

Treatment of paranoid symptoms and delusional disorder

General principles

Management of paranoid symptoms and delusional disorder is frequently difficult. Patients will typically regard their delusional beliefs as justified, and therefore see no need for treatment. Or, they may be suspicious and distrustful, believing that psychiatric treatment is intended to harm them. Considerable tact and skill are needed when dealing with such patients, not only to encourage them to describe their symptoms fully, as discussed above, but also to persuade them to accept treatment and then to adhere to it. Sometimes treatment can be made acceptable by offering to help non-specific symptoms such as anxiety or insomnia, or by pointing out the harmful consequences of the beliefs. Thus a patient who believes that he is surrounded by persecutors may agree that his nerves are being strained as a result, and that this needs treatment.

A decision must be made as to whether to admit the patient for inpatient care. This may be indicated if there is a significant or immediate risk of violence to others, or of suicide. When assessing such factors, it is important to consult other informants and obtain a history of the patient's behaviour. If voluntary admission is refused, compulsory admission may be justified to protect the patient or other people, although this is likely to add to the patient's resentment.

Drug treatment

Paranoid symptoms in delusional disorder are treated with antipsychotic drugs just as in other psychoses, although there are few randomized trial data to guide decision-making (Manschreck and Khan, 2006; Lepping *et al.*, 2007). Pimozide was advocated as the antipsychotic of choice for monosymptomatic hypochondriacal psychosis (delusional disorder, somatic type) and pathological jealousy (Munro, 2009). However, the assertion is not supported by good evidence, and the cardiotoxicity of pimozide should also be taken into account. In general, any high-potency, non-sedating antipsychotic is suitable (e.g. risperidone), always starting with a low dose. Signs of improvement, notably a decrease in preoccupation with the delusion(s) and a reduction in agitation, may be seen within a few days. The importance of establishing a good therapeutic relationship to improve collaboration with treatment has already been emphasized.

With regard to the delusional form of body dysmorphic disorder, some data suggest that selective serotonin reuptake inhibitors (SSRIs) rather than antipsychotics should be used as first-line treatment, with antipsychotic augmentation for those patients who do not respond (Phillips *et al.*, 2006). The role of antidepressants in other delusional disorders remains unclear, although they are often used at some stage in treatment, reflecting the frequency of comorbid depressive symptoms, and their emergence during treatment. The risk of suicide should be monitored regularly.

Psychological treatment

Patients with paranoid symptoms require support, encouragement, and reassurance. This form of nonspecific psychological treatment is an integral part of management, and essential if the patient is to be persuaded of the benefits of more targeted interventions. Of the latter, drugs are the mainstay of treatment, but specific psychological therapies may have a role, too. In particular, cognitive therapy, as used for the treatment of delusions in schizophrenia, may be worth trying if a sufficiently good therapeutic rapport exists. Interpretative psychotherapy and group psychotherapy are unsuitable, because suspiciousness and hypersensitivity may easily lead the patient to misinterpret what is being said.

Prognosis of delusional disorder

There are no reliable data on long-term outcomes. Clinical impression suggests that the prognosis in delusional disorder is poor, although Munro (2009) claims that in patients who are compliant with medication, recovery occurs in 50% of cases, with substantial improvement in a further 30%. Certainly, compared to schizophrenia, long-term outcome and overall functioning are relatively good (Marneros *et al.*, 2012). In some patients, medication can be reduced or stopped without ill effects, while in others (probably the majority) delusions recur rapidly on discontinuation, and treatment must be maintained for prolonged periods. This issue can be judged only by a careful clinical trial with regular monitoring of the patient's mental state, and it requires discussion with the patient of the risks and benefits of long-term medication.

Further reading

Enoch MD and Ball HN (2001). *Uncommon Psychiatric Syndromes*, 4th edn. Edward Arnold, London. (Fascinating descriptions of many delusional disorders and eponymous psychiatric syndromes.)

Hirsch SR and Shepherd M (eds) (1974). *Themes and Variations in European Psychiatry*. John Wright, Bristol. (See the following sections: E Strömgren, *Psychogenic psychoses*; R Gaupp, *The scientific significance of the case of Ernst Wagner* and *The illness and death of the paranoid mass murderer schoolmaster Wagner: a case history*; E Kretschmer, *The sensitive delusion of reference*; H Baruk, *Delusions of passion*.)

Lewis A (1970). Paranoia and paranoid: A historical perspective. *Psychological Medicine*, **1**, 2–12. (A scholarly review of the origin and development of the term paranoid and related concepts.)

Munro A (1999). *Delusional Disorders*. Cambridge University Press, Cambridge.

CHAPTER 13
Eating, sleep, and sexual disorders

The drives to eat, sleep, and have sex can all become impaired or dysfunctional in many psychiatric and medical disorders. They can also all be primary disorders, and it is the latter which are the focus of this chapter.

Eating disorders

Eating disorders are characterized by abnormalities in the pattern of eating and the amount and nature of food eaten. These behaviours are determined primarily by the patients' attitudes to their weight and shape. The disorders share a distinctive core psychopathology, which is best described as an overevaluation of weight and shape, such that patients judge their self-worth in terms of their shape and weight and their ability to control these. The disorders covered in this are anorexia nervosa and bulimia nervosa, as well as a number of related conditions. Obesity is not covered, as it is not a psychiatric disorder (Marcus and Wildes, 2009), although it is associated with an increased risk of various psychiatric disorders, and there may be shared mechanisms (Lopresti and Drummond, 2013).

Until the late 1970s, eating disorders were believed to be uncommon. Following the description of bulimia nervosa, they have increasingly been seen as conspicuous and disabling. It remains uncertain whether the rapid rise in presentation and diagnosis reflects a true increase in incidence or an increase in detection and diagnosis. Many eating disorders go clinically unrecognized, and it is estimated that only about 50% of the cases of anorexia nervosa in the general population are detected in primary care; for bulimia nervosa the figure is substantially less, and the majority of individuals with bulimia are untreated. Within secondary care, eating disorders are seen and managed by general psychiatrists as well as by specialist eating disorder services. For introductory reviews, see Jones *et al.* (2012) and Nicholls and Barrett (2015).

Classification

Although anorexia nervosa and bulimia nervosa are the two best known eating disorders, many cases show significant features of one or both disorders but do not meet the specified diagnostic criteria of either. ICD-10 and DSM-5 differ in how they classify eating disorders and deal with this complexity (Table 13.1). For example, DSM-5 includes the diagnoses 'binge eating disorder' and 'other specified eating or feeding disorder', whereas ICD-10 uses the prefix 'atypical' and the category of 'eating disorder, unspecified' (sometimes abbreviated as EDNOS). ICD-11 is likely to move closer to the DSM-5 approach (Uher and Rutter, 2012).

Adding to the uncertainties about the most appropriate classification, even patients who do meet criteria for anorexia nervosa or bulimia nervosa 'migrate' between

Table 13.1 **Diagnostic classification of eating disorders**

DSM-5 Feeding and eating disorders	ICD-10 Eating disorders
Anorexia nervosa	Anorexia nervosa
Bulimia nervosa	Bulimia nervosa
Avoidant/restrictive food intake disorder	Atypical anorexia nervosa
Binge eating disorder	Atypical bulimia nervosa
Other specified feeding or eating disorder	Other eating disorders (e.g. pica)
Unspecified feeding or eating disorder	Eating disorder, unspecified
Pica	

Source: data from The ICD-10 classification of mental and behavioural disorders: clinical descriptions and diagnostic guidelines, Copyright (1992), World Health Organization; Diagnostic and Statistical Manual of Mental Disorders, Fifth Edition, Copyright (2013), American Psychiatric Association.

categories over time (Figure 13.1), suggesting that they share a common pathophysiology, and that the boundaries between them are largely arbitrary (Fairburn and Harrison, 2003). These issues should be borne in mind when reading the following sections.

The order of categories has been modified to facilitate comparison. ICD-10 also has categories of overeating and vomiting associated with other psychological disturbances; DSM-5 also has a category of rumination disorder.

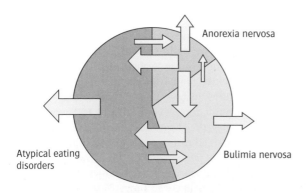

Figure 13.1 Schematic representation of temporal movement between the eating disorders. The size of the arrow indicates the likelihood of movement in the direction shown. Arrows that point outside of the circle indicate recovery.

Reproduced from The Lancet, 361(9355), Fairburn CG, Harrison PJ, Eating disorders, pp. 407–16, Copyright (2003) with permission from Elsevier.

Anorexia nervosa

Although there were many previous case histories, anorexia nervosa was first named in 1868 by the English physician William Gull, who emphasized the psychological causes of the condition, the need to restore weight, and the role of the family. The other key description at this time was by Charles Lasegue in Paris.

The main features of anorexia nervosa are:

- Very low body weight (defined as being 15% below the standard weight, or body mass index (BMI) of less than 17.5 kg/m²), which is maintained by restriction of energy intake.

- Extreme concern about weight and shape, characterized by an intense fear of gaining weight and becoming fat and a strong desire to be thin.

- An undue influence of body weight or shape on self-evaluation.

- Lack of recognition of the seriousness of low body weight.

- ICD-10, but not DSM-5, includes amenorrhoea as a criterion in women.

Most patients are young women (see the section on Epidemiology, below). The condition usually begins in adolescence, although childhood-onset and older-onset cases are encountered. It generally begins with ordinary efforts at dieting, which then get out of control. The central psychological features are the characteristic overvalued ideas about body shape and weight (Fairburn *et al.*, 1999).

The *pursuit of thinness* may take several forms. Patients generally eat little and set themselves very low daily calorie limits (often between 600 and 1000 kcal). Some try to achieve weight loss by inducing vomiting, exercising excessively, and misusing laxatives (*purging*). Patients are often preoccupied with thoughts of food, and sometimes enjoy cooking elaborate meals for other people. Some patients with anorexia nervosa admit to stealing food, either by shoplifting or in other ways.

Binge eating. A subgroup of patients have repeated episodes of binge eating. (A binge is an episode of eating when a large amount of food is consumed in a short period of time, and during which there is a sense of loss of control.) This behaviour becomes more frequent with chronicity and increasing age. During binges, the patient typically eats foods that are usually avoided. After overeating they feel bloated and may induce vomiting. Binges are followed by remorse and intensified efforts to lose weight. If other people encourage them to eat, the patient is often resentful; they may hide food or vomit in private as soon as the meal is over. In DSM-5, anorexia nervosa with binge eating and purging (self-induced vomiting or the misuse of laxatives or diuretics) is recognized as a distinct type, which differs from the restricting subtype. This distinction is supported by evidence that they have different trajectories and cognitive features (Treasure *et al.*, 2015).

Amenorrhoea is one of several physical abnormalities that have traditionally been incorporated in diagnostic criteria (but not, as noted, in DSM-5). It occurs early in the development of the condition, and in about 20% of cases it precedes obvious weight loss, although careful history-taking generally reveals that these patients had already started dieting. Some cases first come to medical attention with amenorrhoea rather than disordered eating.

Other symptoms. Depressive, anxiety, and obsessional symptoms, lability of mood, and social withdrawal are all common. Three-quarters of patients report a lifetime history of major depressive disorder. Lack of sexual interest is usual.

For a review of anorexia nervosa, see Zipfel *et al.* (2015).

Physical consequences

A number of important symptoms and signs of anorexia nervosa are secondary to starvation. Several body systems can be affected, with increasing involvement as BMI falls (see Box 13.1). Some cases first come to medical attention because of one of these complications rather than because of disordered eating itself. For a review of the physical consequences, see Mitchell and Crow (2006).

Epidemiology

The incidence of anorexia nervosa based upon primary care and mental health surveys is about 5 per 100,000. Rates in the community are considerably higher. Incidence is greatest among young women, with 40% of all incident cases occurring in 15–19-year-old females. Reported incidence rates increased from the beginning of the twentieth century up to the 1970s, but have remained fairly stable since then. It is rare in children under 13 years of age, and in this age group the sex ratio is closer to one.

Prevalence estimates vary depending on the method of ascertainment, country, and age range studied, and whether atypical anorexia nervosa is included. If so, population studies find a lifetime prevalence of between 0.9% and 4% in women; rates in men are always lower, but the sex ratio is less than the 10:1 figure often stated. The condition is thought to be more common in the upper than the lower social classes, and is reported to be rare in non-western countries and in the non-white population of western countries.

For review of anorexia nervosa epidemiology, see Smink *et al.*, (2012).

Onset, course, and prognosis

In its early stages, anorexia nervosa often runs a fluctuating course, with exacerbations and periods of partial remission. The long-term prognosis is difficult to judge owing to incomplete follow-up, or because there may be normalization in weight or menstrual function but persistent abnormalities of eating habits and attitudes to weight and shape. A review of 119 studies reported that weight and menstrual function recover in about 60% of patients, and eating behaviour becomes normalized in almost 50% (Steinhausen, 2002). A more recent population study found that about two-thirds of women with anorexia nervosa had largely or fully recovered at 5 years (Smink *et al.*, 2012). Poor prognostic factors include onset before puberty or in adulthood, long history (>3 years), premorbid personality problems, comorbid substance misuse, and childhood obesity. Recognition and management of the group of patients with severe and enduring anorexia nervosa poses particular challenges (Robinson, 2014). In addition to their chronic psychopathology and physical health problems, they have significant impairments in social functioning and employment, and impose a major burden on carers (Schmidt *et al.*, 2016).

Anorexia nervosa has the highest mortality rate of any major psychiatric disorder, with a fourfold to fivefold increase in mortality (Arcelus *et al.*, 2011; Franko *et al.*, 2013). One in five deaths is from suicide; the others reflect the many adverse health consequences of the disorder, notably cardiac events and sepsis. There is evidence that the excess mortality rate has fallen in recent years.

Aetiology

Genetics

Anorexia nervosa is strongly familial, with a reported heritability of 28–74%, suggesting that much of the familiality reflects genetic predisposition (Yilmaz *et al.*, 2015). A proportion of the genetic risk is shared with other psychiatric disorders, including obsessive–compulsive disorder and, perhaps more surprisingly, schizophrenia (Bulik-Sullivan *et al.*, 2015). However, no individual risk genes for anorexia nervosa have yet been identified by genome-wide association studies, in part because of their insufficient sample size. The genetic risk

> ### Box 13.1 Main physical features of anorexia nervosa
>
> #### Physical symptoms
>
> Heightened sensitivity to cold
> Gastrointestinal symptoms—constipation, fullness after eating, bloating
> Dizziness and syncope
> Amenorrhoea
> Lack of sexual interest
> Poor sleep, with early-morning wakening
>
> #### Physical signs
>
> Emaciation
> Stunted growth and failure of breast development (if onset is prepubertal)
> Dry skin, with orange discoloration of the palms and soles
> Fine downy hair (*lanugo*) on the back, forearms, and sides of face
> Salivary gland swelling
> Erosion of the inner surface of the front teeth (perimylolysis) in those who vomit frequently
> Cold hands and feet; hypothermia
> Bradycardia; hypotension; cardiac arrhythmias (especially in those with electrolyte abnormalities)
> Peripheral oedema
> Weak proximal muscles (e.g. difficulty in rising from a squatting position)
>
> #### Abnormalities on physical investigation
>
> ##### Endocrine abnormalities
>
> Low luteinizing hormone, follicle-stimulating hormone, and oestradiol levels
>
> Low T_3, with T_4 in low normal range and normal concentrations of thyroid-stimulating hormone (low T_3 syndrome)
> Increase in cortisol and dexamethasone non-suppression
> Raised growth hormone concentration
> Hypoglycaemia
>
> ##### Cardiovascular abnormalities
>
> Conduction defects, especially prolongation of the QT interval
>
> ##### Gastrointestinal abnormalities
>
> Delayed gastric emptying
> Decreased colonic motility (if chronic laxative misuse)
> Acute gastric dilatation (rare, secondary to binge eating or excessive re-feeding)
>
> ##### Haematological abnormalities
>
> Normocytic normochromic anaemia
> Mild leucopenia with relative lymphocytosis
> Thrombocytopenia
>
> ##### Other metabolic abnormalities
>
> Hypercholesterolaemia
> Raised serum carotene
> Hypophosphataemia (exaggerated during re-feeding)
> Dehydration
> Electrolyte disturbances, especially hypokalaemia (in those who vomit frequently or misuse laxatives or diuretics)
>
> ##### Other abnormalities
>
> Osteopenia and osteoporosis
>
> Adapted from The Lancet, 361(9355), Fairburn CG, Harrison PJ, Eating disorders, pp. 407–16, Copyright (2003) with permission from Elsevier.

may also vary with age of onset, with a lesser heritability of eating disorder symptoms in preadolescent and early adolescent cases.

Neurobiology

There have been many brain imaging and other neurobiological studies of anorexia nervosa, and a range of structural, functional, and biochemical abnormalities reported. These include reductions in brain volume, and alterations in the 5-HT (serotonin) system. However, it is often difficult to determine whether

abnormalities are causal, or are the result of starvation and weight loss. Nevertheless, some findings are of interest:

- Cognitively, there are difficulties in switching between tasks, and relative impairment of strategic planning compared to detailed focusing on tasks.
- Structurally, grey matter volume is increased in the orbitofrontal cortex and insula, regions known to be involved in assessing reward and in introspection, respectively.

• Functional neuroimaging also indicates involvement of brain regions involved in responses to food rewards.

Linking neuroimaging with neurochemistry, one theory is that the restrictive eating of anorexia nervosa is a maladaptive attempt to reduce the negative affect caused by an imbalance between the aversive (serotonergic) and reward (dopaminergic) systems of the brain (Kaye *et al.*, 2013).

Sociocultural factors

The fact that anorexia nervosa is more common in certain societies suggests that cultural factors play a part in its development. Important among such factors is likely to be the notion that thinness is desirable and attractive. Surveys in affluent societies show that most schoolgirls and female college students diet at one time or another. However, when other risk factors are taken into account, people who develop anorexia nervosa have no greater exposure to factors that increase the risk of dieting. This suggests that the problem is more due to how an individual reacts to dieting than to dieting itself. Emerging evidence supports the importance of media and peer groups in influencing weight and shape concerns in adolescents (Keel and Forney, 2013).

Individual psychological causes

Bruch (1974) was one of the first writers to discuss the psychological antecedents of anorexia nervosa. She suggested that these patients are engaged in 'a struggle for control, for a sense of identity and effectiveness, with the relentless pursuit of thinness as a final step in this effort'. These clinical observations are supported by epidemiological studies, which implicate low self-esteem and perfectionism in the development of the disorder (Fairburn, 1999). It has been suggested that these premorbid personality traits can make it particularly difficult for an individual to negotiate the demands of adolescence.

Causes within the family

Disturbed relationships are often found in the families of patients with anorexia nervosa, and some authors have suggested that they have an important causal role. Minuchin *et al.* (1978) held that a specific pattern of relationships could be identified, consisting of 'enmeshment, overprotectiveness, rigidity and lack of conflict resolution'. They also suggested that the development of anorexia nervosa in the patient served to prevent dissent within the family.

Epidemiological studies suggest that people who develop anorexia nervosa are more likely than healthy controls to be exposed to a range of childhood adversities, including poor relationships with parents and parental psychiatric disorder, particularly depression. However, these risk factors are not specific to anorexia nervosa, but are found with equal frequency among people who subsequently develop other psychiatric disorders (Fairburn, 1999). It seems likely that these general risk factors interact with specific factors within the individual, such as perfectionism and low self-esteem, to increase the risk of developing anorexia nervosa. For review, see Keel and Forney (2013).

Assessment

Most patients with anorexia nervosa are reluctant to change their behaviour, let alone see a psychiatrist, so it is important to try to establish a good relationship. This means listening to the patient's views, explaining the treatment alternatives, and being willing to consider compromises. A thorough history should be taken of the development of the disorder, the present pattern of eating and weight control, and the patient's ideas about body weight (see Boxes 13.2 and 13.3). In the mental state examination, particular attention should be given to depressive symptoms, as well as to the characteristic psychopathology of anorexia nervosa itself. More than one interview may be needed to obtain this information and gain the patient's confidence.

In children and adolescents, gathering information on early feeding and parental weight and shape concerns are important; and parents and teachers should be interviewed.

It is essential to perform a full physical examination. Particular attention should be paid to the degree of emaciation (including measurement of weight and BMI), cardiovascular status (blood pressure, heart rate), and temperature. Routine investigations include full blood count, urea and electrolytes, blood glucose, liver function tests, and ECG. The results may also reveal that the patient is at high risk of medical complications and may require further urgent investigations or inpatient treatment (Box 13.4).

A range of medical and psychiatric disorders may present with weight loss or loss of appetite, and lead to the possibility of anorexia nervosa being raised (Box 13.5). However, there should rarely be significant diagnostic uncertainty once the presence or absence of the cardinal psychopathology of anorexia nervosa has been determined.

Box 13.2 Assessment of eating

What is a typical day's eating? What are the mealtime arrangements at home and at school/work?

To what degree is the patient attempting restraint?

Is there a pattern? Does it vary? Is eating ritualized?

Does the patient avoid particular foods? If so, why?

Does she restrict fluids?

What is the patient's experience of hunger or of any urge to eat?

Does she binge? Are these objectively large binges? Does she feel out of control?

How do binges begin? How do they end? How often do they occur?

Does she make herself vomit? If so, how?

Does she take laxatives, diuretics, emetics, or appetite suppressants? If so, with what effects?

Does she fast for a day or longer?

Can she eat in front of others?

Does she exercise? Is this to 'burn off calories'?

Reproduced from Palmer B, Helping People with Eating Disorders: A clinical guide to assessment and treatment, Copyright (2000), with permission from John Wiley and Sons.

Box 13.3 Assessment of psychological issues

What does the patient feel about her body and her weight?

If she is restraining her eating, what is her motivation?

Does she feel fat? Does she dislike her body? If so, in what way?

Does she have a distorted body image? If so, in what way?

What does she feel would happen if she did not control her weight or her eating?

Does she fear loss of control? Is she able to say what she means by this?

Does she feel guilt or self-disgust? If so, what leads her to feel this?

Does anything about her disorder lead her to feel good?

If she binges, what are her feelings before, during, and afterwards?

What has she told others about her eating disorder—if anything?

How does she think about her disorder? What does she make of it?

Reproduced from Palmer B, Helping People with Eating Disorders: A clinical guide to assessment and treatment, Copyright (2000), with permission from John Wiley and Sons.

Treatment of anorexia nervosa

There has been a lack of good evidence about treatment and management of anorexia nervosa, meaning that clinical experience and expert opinion are prominent in guidelines. However, since the National Institute of Health and Clinical Excellence (NICE) guidelines were published in 2004 (National Institute for Health and Clinical Excellence, 2004a; see Box 13.6), the evidence base for specific psychotherapeutic and pharmacotherapeutic interventions has increased considerably. For recent reviews and guidelines, see Watson and Bulik (2013) and Hay *et al.* (2014). In addition, there is current interest in the possibility that deep brain stimulation may be of benefit in severe, intractable cases, but the evidence is very preliminary and there are significant ethical issues (Park *et al.*, 2017).

Psychotherapy

Psychotherapies are the mainstay of treatment for anorexia nervosa. In the past, these were based on

psychodynamic concepts, but these have largely been superseded by cognitive behavioural therapy (CBT) and related therapies. Both family and individual interventions have been used.

Family therapy has been widely advocated, reflecting the belief that family factors are important in the origins of anorexia nervosa. Various kinds of family therapy have been used. Evidence suggests that, for children and adolescents, family-based treatments that focus on the eating disorder and related issues are more effective than those addressing broader family processes, and more so than individual psychotherapy (Lock, 2015).

In adults, individual treatments predominate. Generic CBT has only modest benefits, but a specifically tailored form ('CBT-E') has efficacy in weight restoration and in weight maintenance (Fairburn *et al.*, 2009a, 2013). As discussed below, CBT-E is also highly effective for bulimia nervosa, and is the first evidence-based

Box 13.4 **Abnormalities requiring urgent follow-up or intervention in anorexia nervosa**

General

BMI <14 kg/m^2

Temperature <35.5°C

Cardiovascular

Bradycardia (<50 beats/minute)

Blood pressure <80/50 mmHg

Postural hypotension >20 mmHg

Postural tachycardia (increase >20 beats/minute)

Arrythymia

QTc >50 msec

Blood tests

Hypokalaemia (<3.0 mmol/l)

Hypophosphataemia (<0.5 mmol/l)

Hypoglycaemia

Neutropenia

Adapted from Australian and New Zealand Journal of Psychiatry, 48(11), Hay P et al., Royal Australian and New Zealand College of Psychiatrists clinical practice guidelines for the treatment of eating disorders, pp. 977-1008, Copyright (2014), with permission from SAGE Publications; Lancet Psychiatry, 2(12), Zipfel S et al., Anorexia nervosa: aetiology, assessment, and treatment, pp. 1099-1111, Copyright (2015), with permission from Elsevier.

Box 13.5 **Differential diagnosis of anorexia nervosa**

Medical disorders

Neoplasia (e.g. gastrointestinal, hypothalamic, lymphoma, cachexia)

Inflammatory bowel disease

Malabsoprtion syndromes (e.g. coeliac disease, chronic pancreatitis)

Hyperthyroidism

Chronic infection

Diabetes mellitus

Pituitary failure

Cystic fibrosis

Psychiatric disorders

Other eating disorders

Depression

Somatoform disorders

Obsessive–compulsive disorder

'trans-diagnostic' eating disorder therapy. Other psychological interventions with some support include *focal psychodynamic psychotherapy* and a form of cognitive–interpersonal therapy (Zipfel *et al.*, 2015). Nevertheless, anorexia nervosa remains difficult to treat, with many patients reluctant to engage in treatment or proving refractory to it.

For review of psychological treatments in anorexia nervosa, see Hay (2013).

Medication

Both antidepressants and antipsychotics are used in anorexia nervosa, with antidepressants sometimes prescribed in high dosage. However, systematic reviews show no clear effect of antidepressants on weight gain, maintenance, or psychological symptoms during re-feeding

(de Vos *et al.*, 2014). Small trials have suggested possible benefit from olanzapine (Kishi *et al.*, 2012), but overall the evidence is similarly negative for the use of antipsychotics and they are not recommended.

Antidepressants are also used to treat depression in anorexia nervosa. The evidence for their effectiveness in this situation is weak, and guidelines suggest that antidepressants should not be used until it is apparent that the symptoms are not merely due to starvation, and that they persist during restoration of weight (Hay *et al.*, 2014). Particular care in prescribing is required in patients under 18 years old, and because of the high risks of medical complications and side effects in underweight patients.

Management

Starting treatment

Success largely depends on establishing a good relationship with the patient. It should be made clear that achieving an adequate weight is essential to reverse the physical and psychological effects of starvation. It is important to agree a specific dietary plan, while emphasizing that weight control is only one aspect

Box 13.6 NICE (2004) guidelines for anorexia nervosa

- Most people with anorexia nervosa should be managed on an outpatient basis, with psychological treatment and monitoring of their physical condition.

- Psychological therapies for anorexia nervosa include cognitive analytic therapy (CAT), cognitive behaviour therapy (CBT), interpersonal psychotherapy (IPT), focal psychodynamic therapy, and family interventions focused explicitly on eating disorders.

- Outpatient psychological treatment for anorexia nervosa should normally be of at least 6 months' duration. Failure to improve or deterioration should lead to more intensive forms of treatment (e.g. a move from individual therapy to combined individual and family work, or day care, or inpatient care). Dietary counselling should not be provided as the sole treatment for anorexia nervosa.

- For inpatients with anorexia nervosa it is important to monitor the patient's physical status during re-feeding. Psychological treatment should be provided that has a focus both on eating behaviour and attitudes to body weight and shape, and on wider psychosocial issues with the expectation of weight gain. Rigid inpatient behaviour modification programmes should not be used in the management of anorexia nervosa.

- Following inpatient weight restoration, people with anorexia nervosa should be offered outpatient psychological treatment that focuses both on eating behaviour and attitudes to body weight and shape, and on wider psychosocial issues, with regular monitoring of both physical and psychological risk.

Adapted from National Institute for Clinical Excellence, Eating Disorders: core interventions in the treatment and management of anorexia nervosa, bulimia nervosa and eating disorders, Clinical Guideline 9, Copyright (2004a), with permission from National Institute for Clinical Excellence.

of the problem, and help should be offered with the accompanying psychological problems, as well as dealing with any medical complications. Educating patients and their families about the disorder and its treatment is important. There is good evidence that early intervention (within 3 years of onset) is associated with better outcomes, and so every effort should be made to engage with the patient as promptly as possible. Conversely, in longstanding cases of anorexia nervosa, treatment goals may be more modest, and include helping patient and carers cope with a serious and chronic illness (Hay et al., 2012).

Setting of treatment

Most cases may be treated on an outpatient or day-patient basis, ideally within a specialist eating disorder service. There is no good evidence that inpatient care is more effective, and admission to hospital is now unusual. However, it may be indicated in two situations: to a medical ward, if there are serious and imminent physical health risks (Box 13.5), or to psychiatric inpatient care if there is acute suicidal ideation or if sustained attempts at out-patient or day-patient treatment have failed.

Compulsory treatment for anorexia nervosa is controversial both legally and ethically (see Chapter 4). It is rarely used, although re-feeding is accepted as a treatment for eating disorders under the Mental Health Act. For children and adolescents unable or unwilling to give informed consent, either the Mental Health Act or Children Act (1989) may be utilized. The views of the parents as well as the patient are critical in decisions of this kind (Nicholls and Barrett, 2015).

Restoring weight

A reasonable aim is an increase of 0.5 kg a week, which will usually require an extra 500–1000 calories a day. More rapid re-feeding is potentially dangerous. The target weight should be above a minimum healthy level (a BMI above 18.5); it is not a good idea to agree a compromise target lower than this except in severe and refractory cases. It is good practice to monitor the patient's physical state regularly, and to prescribe vitamin supplements if indicated. It is also important to assess and modify other weight-reducing strategies that the patient may employ, such as overexercising and laxative misuse.

Previously, for those receiving inpatient treatment, the patient would usually stay in hospital until her agreed target weight was reached and maintained, and strict behavioural regimes were often used. Currently, much shorter admissions, with a more collaborative therapeutic approach, are the norm, followed by outpatient or day-patient care. Whilst in hospital, eating should be supervised by a nurse, who has three roles—to reassure the patient that she will not lose control over her weight, to be clear about the agreed targets, and to ensure that the patient does not induce vomiting or take laxatives.

Bulimia nervosa

The term *bulimia* refers to binge eating, defined earlier. As mentioned, binge eating occurs in some cases of anorexia nervosa, and is also the hallmark of binge eating disorder (see below). The syndrome of bulimia nervosa was first described by Russell (1979) in an influential paper in which he named the condition and described the key clinical features in 30 patients who were seen between 1972 and 1978. The prevalence of bulimic behaviours and the associated harms soon became apparent, and the syndrome was first included in DSM-III.

The central features of bulimia nervosa are as follows:

- A preoccupation with eating, with an irresistible and recurrent urge to overeat, manifesting in repeated 'binges' when large amounts of food are consumed in a short time, accompanied by a sense of loss of control.
- The use of extreme measures to control body weight, especially self-induced vomiting and use of laxatives, as well as periods of starvation or excessive exercise.
- Overvalued ideas concerning shape and weight, of the type seen in anorexia nervosa.

DSM-5 specifies that these behaviours have occurred at least once a week for 3 months, and that they do not occur solely during times when the person met criteria for anorexia nervosa. (As an aside, many of the cases in Russell's original series also suffered from concomitant anorexia nervosa and would thus not currently be diagnosed with bulimia nervosa.) Bulimia nervosa also needs to be distinguished from binge eating disorder, described below. DSM-5 classifies the severity of bulimia nervosa according to the frequency of 'inappropriate compensatory behaviours', ranging from mild (1–3 per week) to extreme (14 or more per week). ICD-10 does not have these elements.

Patients with bulimia nervosa are usually of normal weight (BMI 18.5–25), not least since patients who are substantially underweight usually qualify for a diagnosis of anorexia nervosa, which takes precedence.

There is a profound loss of control over eating. Episodes of binge eating may be precipitated by stress, or by the breaking of self-imposed dietary rules, or may occasionally be planned. During the episodes, large amounts of food are rapidly consumed, on average over 2000 kcal (e.g. a loaf of bread, pot of jam, cake, and biscuits). This voracious eating usually takes place when the patient is alone. At first it brings relief from tension, but this is soon followed by guilt and disgust, and the patient induces vomiting or engages in another compensatory behaviour.

Depressive symptoms are very common, and usually secondary to the eating disorder. A high proportion of patients meet the criteria for major depression. The depressive symptoms usually remit as the eating disorder improves.

For review of bulimia nervosa, see Fairburn *et al.* (2009b).

Physical consequences

Bulimia nervosa can impact on physical health, mostly due to repeated vomiting or use of laxatives or other drugs. With vomiting, reflux symptoms are common, and teeth become pitted by the acidic gastric contents. *Russell's sign* describes callouses on the knuckles caused by repeatedly putting fingers down the throat to induce vomiting. More serious physical health problems can occur, but all are very rare (Box 13.7).

The physical complications are best treated by cessation of the causative behaviour, but symptomatic treatments are also available for some; for example, proton pump inhibitors for oesophageal reflux, or spironolactone for peripheral oedema. However, medication for these purposes should be used with caution, and only in severe cases.

For review, see Sachs and Mehler (2016).

Epidemiology

As with anorexia nervosa, the prevalence and incidence of bulimia nervosa are uncertain. In the community, the prevalence is around 1% among women aged between 16 and 40 years in western societies (Kessler *et al.*, 2013). It is at least 10 times less common in men. The dramatic increase in presentation and diagnosis seen in the UK in the early 1990s has been followed by stability or a modest decline.

For review, see Smink *et al.* (2012).

Onset, course, and prognosis

Bulimia nervosa usually has an onset in late adolescence or early adulthood (i.e. several years later than anorexia nervosa). It often follows a period of concern about body shape and weight, and 25% of patients have a history of anorexia nervosa (see Figure 13.1). There is commonly an initial period of dietary restriction which, after a variable length of time, but usually within 3 years, breaks down, with increasingly frequent episodes of overeating. As the overeating becomes more frequent, the body weight returns to a more normal level. At some stage, self-induced vomiting or laxative abuse are adopted to compensate for the overeating. However, this may result in even less control of eating.

Box 13.7 Physical complications of bulimia nervosa

General

Menstrual irregularities
Non-specific gastrointestinal symptoms

Related to vomiting

Cardiac arrhythmias
Oesophageal reflux
Oesophageal tears
Gastric rupture
Epistaxis and subconjunctival haemorrhage
Damage to teeth (perimyolysis)
Parotid gland enlargement (sialadenosis) and raised salivary amylase
Metabolic alkalosis
Peripheral oedema
Myopathy and cardiomyopathy[*]

Related to stimulant laxatives

Metabolic abnormalities as described for vomiting
Hyponatraemia
Chronic constipation
Melanosis coli

[*]When syrup of ipecac is used to induce vomiting.

Despite the original assertion by Russell (1979) that bulimia nervosa was an 'ominous variant', its outcome is clearly better than anorexia. Nevertheless, even 5–10 years later between one-third and a half of individuals still have a clinical eating disorder, although in many of these cases it will take an atypical form (Fairburn *et al.*, 2000). No convincing predictors of course or outcome have been identified, although childhood obesity and low self-esteem may be associated with a worse prognosis (Fairburn *et al.*, 2000).

The mortality rate is approximately doubled, but the excess is significantly less than that for anorexia nervosa (Franko *et al.*, 2013).

Aetiology

Like anorexia nervosa, bulimia nervosa appears to be the result of exposure to general risk factors for psychiatric disorder, including a family history (in part, reflecting a genetic predisposition), especially depression and substance misuse, and a range of adverse childhood experiences. No risk genes have been identified. It was thought that childhood sexual abuse was especially common, but the evidence suggests that the rate is no higher than among those who develop other types of psychiatric disorder (Fairburn, 1999). Epidemiological studies also suggest that, unlike those with anorexia nervosa, patients with bulimia nervosa have increased exposure to factors that specifically promote dieting, such as childhood obesity, parental obesity, and early menarche. Perfectionism appears to be less of a risk factor than in anorexia nervosa (Fairburn, 1999).

The neurobiological mechanisms appear to be broadly similar to those described above for anorexia nervosa (Kaye *et al.*, 2013). There are also recent models of bingeing, which conceptualize it as 'food addiction' (Smith and Robbins, 2013), or note its similarities to impulsive/compulsive behaviours (Pearson *et al.*, 2015), but these remain speculative.

Treatment of bulimia nervosa

There has been much more research into the treatment of bulimia nervosa than into that of anorexia nervosa, at least amongst adults, and more evidence for effective psychological and pharmacological treatments. For a few people, guided self-help according to CBT may be sufficient, but in most cases formal treatment is indicated. For review, see Fairburn *et al.* (2009b).

Psychotherapy

Both CBT and interpersonal therapy are effective in bulimia nervosa. Of those who complete treatment (about 20% drop out), 60% will have stopped binge eating, and there is an 80% reduction overall. Psychological aspects improve in parallel. Early response is a strong predictor of outcome. The effect is maintained, with low relapse rates seen over 12 months.

The most striking evidence comes from a specifically tailored CBT-based approach ('CBT-E'), mentioned above in the description of anorexia nervosa treatment. In a relatively large study, CBT-E reduced or abolished core behavioural and psychological symptoms of eating disorders, and showed sustained efficacy (Fairburn *et al.*, 2009a). The treatment was delivered in two forms—a 'simple' intervention which focused solely on the eating disorder, and a 'complex' intervention in which personality, mood, and interpersonal issues were also addressed. The authors suggested that the simple treatment is the default version and widely applicable to bulimia nervosa (and other eating disorders), whereas the latter could be limited to individuals with additional psychopathology. Subsequent studies have confirmed the efficacy of CBT-E and showed its superiority over psychoanalytic psychotherapy (Poulsen *et al.*, 2014) and interpersonal psychotherapy (Fairburn *et al.*, 2015).

As with anorexia nervosa, family-based treatments may have some advantages over individual therapy in adolescents with bulimia nervosa (Le Grange *et al.*, 2015).

Medication

Antidepressants are effective, producing a reduction of about 50% in the frequency of binge eating, and cessation in 20% of cases. The onset is more rapid than in depression, but a higher dose may be needed (e.g. fluoxetine 60 mg daily). However, long-term data are less encouraging and show poor compliance. Antidepressants should be used rarely, and viewed as second-line treatment and only if an effective psychological treatment is unavailable or unsuccessful. Topiramate is effective in suppressing binge eating, but side effects limit its usefulness and its use in bulimia nervosa is not advocated.

For review of the drug treatment of bulimia nervosa, see McElroy *et al.* (2012).

Management

The management of bulimia nervosa is easier than that of anorexia nervosa because the patient is more likely to wish to recover, and a good working relationship can often be established. Furthermore, there is no need to manage the complications of starvation nor restore weight. However, it is necessary to assess the patient's physical state and to measure electrolyte status in those who are vomiting frequently or misusing laxatives (Box 13.7).

As with many common disorders, a 'stepped-care' approach appears to be the best way of providing appropriate care for large numbers of people with varying degrees of severity of disorder (National Institute for Clinical Excellence, 2004a).

Step 1. Identify the small minority (less than 5%) of individuals who need urgent specialist care because of severe depression, physical complications, or substance abuse that requires treatment in its own right.

Step 2. Offer guided cognitive behavioural self-help, using a self-help book and with the guidance of a non-specialist facilitator. Treatment usually takes about 4 months and requires eight to ten meetings with the facilitator. Guided self-help is appropriate for primary care, and appears to lead to good progress in about one-third of patients.

Step 3. Patients who do not show benefit within 4–6 weeks of commencing Step 2 require CBT-E. In a minority of cases, where concomitant depressive symptoms are severe or persistent, it is worthwhile adding an antidepressant drug such as fluoxetine in doses of up to 60 mg daily.

Step 4. Patients who do not improve with CBT require comprehensive specialist reassessment. In some cases, measures to provide more intensive cognitive therapy or an antidepressant drug may be useful. It is important to review the initial treatment with the patient, with the aim of agreeing a treatment approach that the patient finds acceptable.

Binge eating disorder

This is a new diagnostic category in DSM-5. It is characterized by recurrent bingeing episodes in the absence of the other diagnostic features of bulimia nervosa; in particular, there are no compensatory behaviours such as vomiting or purging. In ICD-10, such patients would be classified as eating disorder, unspecified. Patients may have depressive symptoms and some dissatisfaction with their body weight and shape; however, this is usually less severe than in bulimia nervosa. Nevertheless, binge eating disorder is of comparable severity to bulimia nervosa in terms of personal and public health (Kessler *et al.*, 2013) and increased mortality, likely related to the comorbid obesity (Smink *et al.*, 2012; Franko *et al.*, 2013).

The risk factors for, and mechanisms underlying, binge eating disorder are thought to be similar to those for bulimia nervosa (Balodis *et al.*, 2014). About 25% of patients who present for treatment for obesity have features of binge eating disorder. The condition generally affects an older age group than bulimia nervosa, and up to 25% of those who present for treatment are men.

Binge eating disorder has a relatively high spontaneous remission rate and larger effect sizes for response to CBT, interpersonal therapy, and antidepressants. Recently, lisdexamfetamine was licensed for binge eating disorder in the USA.

For review of treatment of binge eating disorder, see McElroy *et al.* (2015).

Other eating disorders

Other specified feeding or eating disorder

As noted earlier, many patients with eating disorders do not meet criteria for anorexia nervosa or bulimia nervosa. Whilst some are now accounted for in the DSM-5 category of binge eating disorder, others are not. In DSM-5, most of the remainder are diagnosed as 'Other specified feeding or eating disorder', which largely comprises atypical or mixed forms of the three aforementioned disorders. The ICD-10 equivalent is 'Eating disorder, unspecified'. These states share much of the core psychopathology of anorexia nervosa and bulimia nervosa, and respond well to CBT-E.

Psychogenic vomiting

Psychogenic vomiting is chronic and episodic vomiting without an organic cause, which usually occurs after meals and in the absence of nausea. It differs from bulimia nervosa, in which self-induced vomiting follows episodes of binge eating. It must also be distinguished from diabetic gastroparesis and other causes of vomiting. Psychogenic vomiting appears to be more common in women than in men, and usually presents in early or middle adult life. It is reported that both psychotherapeutic and behavioural treatments can be helpful.

For a review of idiopathic vomiting disorders, see Olden and Chepyala (2008).

Pica

Pica is the repeated eating of non-nutritional, 'non-food' substances. A wide range of substances may be ingested, such as hair, paper, or stones. In some cases, the ingested substance may be correcting a mineral deficiency. Pica is particularly common in people with intellectual disability, and is also seen in several other psychiatric disorders, including autism and schizophrenia. It is also associated with pregnancy and iron deficiency. In each of these situations, a diagnosis of pica should only be made if the behaviour is sufficiently persistent or severe to require clinical attention.

Pica can lead to medical or surgical emergencies due to poisoning, obstruction, nutritional deficiencies, or parasitosis. The differential diagnosis includes anorexia nervosa, factitious disorder, and personality disorder. Behavioural approaches are usually used; SSRIs or atypical antipsychotics are sometimes tried in refractory cases.

Avoidant/restrictive food intake disorder

DSM-5 introduced this category, which occurs in children who have insufficient dietary intake to the point where there is nutritional deficiency, failure to thrive, and impaired psychosocial functioning. The child may lack interest in food, or be worried about its sensory characteristics, or its adverse consequences. However, there is no disturbance of body image or preoccupation with weight. It replaces a previous category of 'Feeding disorder of infancy and early childhood'.

Sleep disorders

There has been increasing recognition in recent years of the prevalence and clinical significance of sleep problems for mental and physical health, and a resulting growth of the specialty of sleep medicine. However, psychiatrists are often still asked to see patients whose main problem is either difficulty in sleeping (*dyssomnia*, which includes insomnia and hypersomnia) or behaviours associated with sleep (*parasomnias*). Many other patients seen by psychiatrists also complain about sleep problems as one of their symptoms.

Sleep problems are important for several reasons.

- They may represent primary sleep disorders (which are the focus of this section).
- They may be symptoms of psychiatric disorder, especially mood disorders, or occur in a range of medical disorders. In these situations they may be called *secondary sleep disorders*.
- They may be causes of psychological symptoms and contribute to the onset of psychiatric disorders.

- Persistent sleep difficulties are significantly associated with a range of adverse physical health outcomes.

For a review of the biology of sleep and its disorders, see Siegel (2009), and for its impact on psychiatric disorders and physical health, see Wulff *et al.* (2010).

Classification

DSM-5 recognizes 10 categories of sleep disorders, which it calls *sleep–wake disorders* (Box 13.8). Classification in ICD-10 is rather different, with sleep disorders occurring in different parts of the classification (Box 13.9). Unlike DSM-5, ICD-10 distinguishes sleep disorders based on their presumed aetiology. Only the category of 'Non-organic sleep disorders' (defined as those 'in which emotional causes are considered to be a primary factor') is located within Chapter V. Other sleep disorders are considered either to be organic (such as Kleine–Levin syndrome) or non-psychogenic (e.g. narcolepsy).

Box 13.8 Classification of sleep–wake disorders in DSM-5

Insomnia disorder
Hypersomnolence disorder
Narcolepsy
Breathing-related sleep disorders
Circadian rhythm sleep–wake disorders
Non-rapid eye movement (REM) sleep arousal disorders
Nightmare disorders
REM sleep behaviour disorder
Restless legs syndrome
Substance/medication-induced sleep disorder

Source: data from Diagnostic and Statistical Manual of Mental Disorders, Fifth Edition, Copyright (2013), American Psychiatric Association.

Box 13.9 Classification of sleep disorders in ICD-10

Non-organic sleep disorders (F51)
Non-organic insomnia
Non-organic hypersomnia
Non-organic disorder of the sleep–wake cycle
Sleepwalking (somnambulism)
Sleep terrors (night terrors)
Nightmares
Other non-organic sleep disorders
Non-organic sleep disorder, unspecified

Sleep disorders of organic origin (G47)
Narcolepsy
Kleine–Levin syndrome
Sleep apnoea
Episodic movement disorders

Other (R33)
Primary nocturnal enuresis

Source: data from The ICD-10 classification of mental and behavioural disorders: clinical descriptions and diagnostic guidelines, Copyright (1992), World Health Organization.

A more complex classification of sleep disorders intended for use by specialists in sleep medicine is the third edition of the International Classification of Sleep Disorders (ICSD 3). It has 80 types of sleep disorder.

Epidemiology

Sleep disorders are frequent, but there is a wide range of variation in estimates, depending on the definition and the population studied; for example, 22% of adults meet the DSM-IV criteria for insomnia (DSM-5 data are not available), but only 4% meet the ICD-10 criteria (Roth *et al.*, 2011). Excessive sleepiness occurs in 5% of adults, and about 15% have some form of chronic sleep–wake disorder.

Groups at particular risk of persistent sleep problems include young children and adolescents (Stores, 2015), the elderly, the physically ill, and those with learning disability (Heussler, 2016).

Assessment

Assessment requires a full psychiatric and medical history, together with detailed enquiries about the sleep complaint (see Box 13.10). In some cases specialist investigation, including polysomnography, is necessary.

Insomnia

Insomnia is a condition of unsatisfactory quality and/or quantity of sleep, with difficulty falling asleep, remaining asleep, or waking early and being unable to return to sleep.

Transient insomnia occurs at times of stress or as 'jet lag'. Short-term insomnia is often associated with personal problems—for example, illness, bereavement, relationship difficulties, or stress at work. Sleep-onset insomnia can be a relatively common complaint among adolescents.

Insomnia in clinical practice is usually secondary to other disorders, notably painful physical conditions, depressive disorders, and anxiety disorders; it also occurs with excessive use of alcohol or caffeine, and in dementia. It can also be provoked by prescribed drugs.

In about 15% of cases of insomnia, no cause is found. For diagnosis, ICD-10 requires insomnia to have been present for at least three nights per week for 1 month, and to cause distress or affect daytime functioning; DSM-5 is similar but requires a 3-month duration.

For a review of insomnia, see Winkelman (2015).

Assessment of insomnia

Usually the diagnosis of insomnia is made on the basis of the account given by the patient, or parent/carer in the

Box 13.10 Assessment of sleep disturbance

Screening questions

Do you sleep well enough and long enough?
Are you very sleepy during the day?
Is your sleep disturbed at night?

Sleep history

Detailed history of the sleep complaint and a typical sleep–wake cycle
Factors that improve or worsen sleep
Effect on mood and functioning
Past and present treatment
History from bed partner

Sleep diary

Systematic 2-week or longer record

Possible investigations

Video recording
Actigraphy (wrist-worn)
Polysomnography
HLA typing
Cerebrospinal fluid orexin (hypocretin) levels

Box 13.11 Treatments for insomnia

Cognitive and behavioural interventions

Sleep hygiene
Sleep restriction
Stimulus control
Cognitive therapy
Relaxation therapy

Pharmacological treatments

Short-acting benzodiazepines (e.g. temazepam)
'Z drugs' (zolpidem, zopiclone)
Low-dose sedative antidepressants (e.g. trazodone, mirtazapine)
Melatonin or melatonin agonists

Box 13.12 Principles of sleep education (sleep hygiene)

Sleep environment

Familiar and comfortable
Dark
Quiet

Encourage

Bedtime routines
Consistent time for going to bed and waking up
Going to bed only when tired
Thinking about problems *before* going to bed
Regular exercise

Avoid

Late-evening exercise
Caffeine-containing drinks late in the day
Using mobile devices or watching TV in bed
Excessive alcohol and smoking
Excessive daytime sleep
Large late meals
Too much time in bed lying awake

case of children. Assessment should focus on the nature of the sleep problem and its daytime consequences, as well as screening for psychiatric and medical disorders and use of alcohol and drugs. Sleep studies are rarely undertaken.

Treatment of insomnia

Both non-pharmacological and pharmacological approaches can be used to treat insomnia (Riemann *et al.*, 2015). Hypnotic drugs were widely prescribed in the past, but non-pharmacological approaches are now recommended as first-line treatment. These include a range of cognitive and behavioural components (Box 13.11), including sleep hygiene (Box 13.12). *Sleep hygiene* refers to a series of steps that are useful for all patients with insomnia and can be applied in primary care. For more serious or persistent insomnia, a range of additional specific non-pharmacological treatments have been shown to be effective. For example, *stimulus control* focuses on the principle that one only goes to bed when sleepy, and, if not asleep within 20 minutes, one should get up and engage in a relaxing activity before returning to bed. Adaptations of CBT for insomnia for delivery via the internet are being evaluated and show promise.

Medication has a limited role to play. Although it is sometimes justifiable and useful to give a hypnotic for short-term use (e.g. in the early stages of SSRI treatment), demands for prolonged medication should be resisted. Apart from the risks of tolerance, dependence, and 'hangover' effects, withdrawal of hypnotics can lead to insomnia that is as distressing as the original sleep disturbance. Low doses of sedative antidepressants, such as trazodone or mirtazapine, are an alternative pharmacological treatment for insomnia.

For guidelines on the use of medication to treat insomnia and other sleep disorders, see Wilson *et al.* (2010).

Hypersomnia and excessive daytime sleepiness

Excessive daytime sleepiness is common (with a reported prevalence of 3–5%) and underdiagnosed. Many cases are secondary to loss of night-time sleep. Box 13.13 lists the principal causes. For review, see Zeman *et al.* (2004). For a discussion of the treatment of excessive daytime sleepiness, see Billiard (2009).

Narcolepsy

Narcolepsy is an important cause of chronic sleepiness, affecting about 1 in 2000 people. It usually begins with the sudden onset of persistent daytime sleepiness between the ages of 10 and 20 years, although diagnosis is often delayed by several years. A useful diagnostic clue is that, unlike daytime sleepiness caused by insufficient sleep or that which is often observed in teenagers, people with narcolepsy typically feel refreshed after a full night's sleep. In addition, narcolepsy is characterized by a disturbance in rapid eye movement (REM) sleep, which can occur at any time and lead to unusual states in between sleep and wakefulness (such as hypnopompic and hypnogogic hallucinations). The most striking of these REM-like states is *cataplexy*: sudden episodes of partial or complete paralysis of voluntary muscles,

> **Box 13.13 Causes of excessive daytime sleepiness**
>
> Insufficient sleep
> Narcolepsy
> Depression
> Other medical disorders (e.g. hypothyroidism, Prader–Willi syndrome)
> Shift-work sleep disorder
> Use of sedative medications
> Obstructive sleep apnoea

sometimes causing the person to fall to the ground. Cataplexy does not occur in all patients, being limited to type I narcolepsy (see below). Additional clinical features of narcolepsy include a tendency to obesity (owing to a low metabolic rate), and depression is common.

For review of narcolepsy, see Scammell (2015).

Aetiology and pathology

Considerable progress has been made in understanding narcolepsy in recent years, and has led to the delineation of two types. Type 1 narcolepsy is characterized by cataplexy and by marked reduction of a peptide called orexin-A (also called hypocretin-1) in the cerebrospinal fluid (CSF). This occurs because of a severe and selective loss of the hypothalamic neurons that make this peptide, which is known to be involved in regulation of wakefulness. Type 2 narcolepsy is not associated with cataplexy, and CSF orexin-A levels are normal; its diagnosis is therefore more challenging, and its biological basis less well understood.

The predominant genetic association to narcolepsy is HLA-DQB1*06:02. More than 98% of patients with type 1 narcolepsy (and 50% of those with type 2 narcolepsy, have this genotype, compared to about 15–30% of the general population. HLA-DQB1*06:02 has been estimated to increase the risk of narcolepsy by a factor of 200. Other genes involved in immune function are also implicated in narcolepsy risk. There is increasing evidence that narcolepsy may be an autoimmune disorder, triggered by infections or other stimuli (Mahlios *et al.*, 2013). For example, its onset is most common in late spring, and may follow streptococcal infections. Strikingly, there was a marked increase in cases of narcolepsy in children given a specific brand of influenza vaccine in 2009–2010, but only in those with HLA-DQB1*06:02 genotype. It is thought that these genetic and environmental triggers lead to an immune response that damages the orexin-A producing cells.

Assessment

Narcolepsy usually presents to neurologists. The differential diagnosis is from other causes of excessive daytime sleepiness (Box 13.13). A full history, especially a sleep history, is the main assessment tool. The Epworth Sleepiness Scale is often used. In specialist settings the *multiple sleep latency test* (in which the latency to daytime naps, and the occurrence of REM sleep during them) is carried out. Measurement of HLA status and orexin-A levels in CSF is sometimes undertaken, but is not routine.

A psychiatrist may be involved in the care of a person with narcolepsy for several reasons:

- To assist in the diagnostic assessment.
- If cataplexy is triggered by strong emotions, as is often observed.
- If the patient has comorbid psychiatric disorder, or is distressed by the psychological and social consequences of their symptoms, especially cataplexy.
- To advise regarding the use of psychotropic medication for treatment of narcolepsy.

Treatment of narcolepsy

Patients need considerable help in adjusting to a disabling chronic illness. They should be encouraged to follow a regular routine, with good quality sleep at night and planned naps during the day. If stressful events or other factors (e.g. fatigue) appear to provoke cataplexy, efforts should be made to avoid them or to arrange the patient's lifestyle so as to minimize their impact. Particular caution should be taken with driving and other activities where sudden drowsiness or cataplexy may be dangerous.

Most patients require treatment with stimulant drugs. For mild or moderate cases, modafinil, a non-amfetamine stimulant, reduces daytime sleepiness and increases alertness. Amfetamines are more potent but have more side effects and risk of abuse. Venlafaxine, clomipramine, and other antidepressants can be used to decrease cataplexy. Night-time sleep can be improved by sodium oxybate, with beneficial effects on daytime functioning, but its side effects restrict its use to severe cases.

For guidelines on the treatment of narcolepsy, see Scammell (2015).

Breathing-related sleep disorder

This syndrome consists of daytime drowsiness together with periodic respiration, recurrent apnoeas, and excessive snoring at night. It is usually associated with upper airways obstruction, hence the term *obstructive sleep apnoea syndrome*. The prevalence is about 4% in the male population. The typical patient is a middle-aged overweight man who snores loudly. Treatment consists of relieving the cause of the respiratory obstruction and encouraging weight loss. Continuous positive pressure ventilation using a face mask is often effective. Compliance with advice is often poor. Obstructive sleep apnoea is a risk factor for stroke.

Some children with a history of problems with tonsils, adenoids, and/or ear infections can have frequent arousals during sleep, diminishing the overall quality of sleep from obstructed airways, leading to daytime difficulties with irritability and attentional problems.

Kleine–Levin syndrome

This very rare secondary sleep disorder consists of episodes of somnolence, increased appetite, and hypersexuality, often lasting for days or weeks, with long intervals of normality between them. It usually affects adolescent boys. The symptoms suggest a hypothalamic disorder, but its aetiology is unknown. There is no established treatment, but stimulants, lithium, and other mood stabilizers, are used. For review, see Miglis and Guilleminault (2014).

Circadian-rhythm sleep disorder (sleep–wake schedule disorders)

There are several forms of circadian-rhythm sleep disorder, of which jet lag is the most familiar. Shift-work sleep disorder is a common and increasing problem, the consequences of which are widely underestimated. Fatigue and transient difficulties in sleeping accompany regular changes of shift, or the irregular alternation of night work and days off may lead to chronic problems of poor sleep, fatigue, impaired concentration, and an increased risk of accidents as well as adverse physical and social effects (Wulff *et al.*, 2010).

Puberty triggers a change towards an evening preference in a sizeable proportion of adolescents (up to 40%), exacerbated by a range of social and behavioural factors. The most prevalent sleep complaint therefore tends to be an inability to wake up for school, with significant impairment in a small subset of adolescents.

For a review of the assessment and treatment of circadian-rhythm sleep disorders, see Morgenthaler *et al.* (2007).

Parasomnias

Parasomnias are abnormal behaviours or physiological events occurring in association with sleep, specific sleep stages, or sleep–wake transitions. Some types of parasomnia are especially common in children (Stores, 2015), whereas others occur mostly in older adults and may be associated with neurodegenerative disorders.

For review, see Howell (2012).

Nightmares (dream anxiety disorder)

A nightmare is an awakening from REM sleep to full consciousness with detailed dream recall. Children experience nightmares with a peak frequency around the age of 5 or 6 years. Nightmares may be stimulated by frightening experiences during the day, and frequent nightmares usually occur during a period of anxiety. Other causes include post-traumatic stress disorder, fever, psychotropic drugs, and alcohol detoxification.

Night terror disorder

Night terrors are much less common than nightmares. They are sometimes familial. The condition begins and usually ends in childhood, but occasionally persists into adult life. A few hours after going to sleep, the child, while in stage 3–4 non-REM sleep, sits up and appears terrified. They may scream, and they usually appear confused. There are marked increases in heart rate and respiratory rate.

After a few minutes the child slowly settles and returns to normal calm sleep. There is little or no dream recall. A regular bedtime routine and improved sleep hygiene have been shown to be helpful. Benzodiazepines and imipramine have been shown to be effective in preventing night terrors, but their prolonged use should be avoided.

Sleepwalking disorder

Sleepwalking is an automatism that occurs during deep non-REM sleep, usually in the early part of the night. It is most common between the ages of 5 and 12 years, and 15% of children in this age group walk in their sleep at least once. Occasionally, the disorder persists into adult life. Sleepwalking may be familial. Most children do not actually walk, but sit up and make repetitive movements. Some walk around, usually with their eyes open. They do not respond to questions, and are very difficult to wake. They can usually be led back to bed. Most episodes last for a few seconds or minutes.

As sleepwalkers can occasionally harm themselves, they need to be protected from injury. Doors and windows should be locked and dangerous objects removed. Adults with severe problems should be given advice about safety, avoidance of sleep deprivation, and any other circumstances that might make them excessively sleepy (e.g. drinking alcohol before going to bed).

Other parasomnias

Rapid eye movement (REM) sleep behaviour disorder is a parasomnia that should be considered when behavioural problems, particularly agitation or aggression, occur during the night. It is thought to occur when the normal atonia of REM sleep is lost, so that dreams are acted out. It is more common in the elderly, particularly men. It is associated with, and can precede the onset of, neurodegenerative disorders, particularly Parkinson's disease and Lewy body dementia (Boeve *et al.*, 2013). Clonazepam and donepezil may be effective.

Restless legs syndrome is a distressing and painful condition that can result in severe insomnia and periodic limb movements during sleep. It is common, with 2.5% of the population having significant symptoms. Risk factors include female gender, pregnancy, ageing, low iron status, and parkinsonism. The syndrome can be mistaken for a psychiatric symptom or disorder (e.g. anxiety, akathisia), and it can be comorbid, especially with depression. For review, see Yeh *et al.* (2012).

Sleep paralysis is an inability to perform voluntary movements during the transitions between sleep and wakefulness, either at sleep onset (hypnagogic) or during awakening (hypnopompic). The episodes are often accompanied by extreme fear.

Disorders of sexual function, preference, and gender identity

In the past, as reflected in earlier editions of this book, sexual matters were more prominent in psychiatry than is now the case, for several reasons:

- Sexual factors were considered to be important in psychodynamic theories of causation and, perhaps related to this historical view, more attention was paid to the patient's sexual history, attitudes, and behaviour than is now usual.
- Disorders of sexual function, preference, and gender identity were often attributed to mental illness and therefore in the domain of psychiatry. Notably, homosexuality was a category of psychiatric disorder until the 1970s.
- Sex therapy was more widely practised by psychiatrists (Althof, 2010).

In contemporary psychiatry, there has been a marked shift in the psychiatric relevance of, and involvement in, disorders of sexual function, preference, and gender identity. These are now seen primarily in specialized clinics, where a multidisciplinary approach is taken. Within this setting, the psychiatrist's main role is to identify and manage any comorbid mental illness or distress that has arisen. Much less emphasis is placed on the 'psychiatric' basis of sexual disorder itself.

This chapter reflects these developments, whilst recognizing that current classifications use categories and concepts that retain many elements of the earlier views. Hence, we discuss the main features of the three categories of disorders affecting sex and gender that are recognized in ICD-10 and DSM-5 (see Table 13.2). In ICD-11, substantial changes to terrminology and classification in this area are anticipated (Reed *et al.*, 2016).

- *Sexual dysfunction* denotes impaired or unsatisfying sexual enjoyment or performance. Such conditions are common. They are subdivided, according to the stage of the sexual response that is mainly affected, into disorders of sexual desire, disorders of sexual arousal, and disorders of orgasm. There are also categories for the painful conditions vaginismus and dyspareunia. For a DSM-5 diagnosis, these disorders need to last at least 6 months.
- *Abnormalities of sexual preference (paraphilias)* are uncommon, but they take many forms and have forensic implications.
- Gender identity refers to one's sense of being male or female. When this sense of identity is at variance with an individual's anatomical sex, that person is said to have a *gender dysphoria* (formerly *gender identity disorder*).

Note that a brief sexual history continues to be an integral part of assessment (Chapter 3), and knowledge of how psychiatric disorders and treatments can impair sexual function remains important. The psychiatric aspects of childhood sexual abuse are discussed in Chapter 16, and forensic aspects of sexual offences covered in Chapter 18.

The epidemiology, physiology, and psychology of sexual behaviour are not covered here. Regarding sexual orientation, a 2013 study on 18–44-year-olds in the US showed that 92% of women and 95% of men said they were 'heterosexual or straight'; 1.3% of women and 1.9% of men said they were 'homosexual, gay, or lesbian'; 5.5% of women and 2.0% of men said they were bisexual; and 0.9% of women and 1.0% of men said 'don't know' or declined to answer (Copen *et al.*, 2016). For review of psychiatric aspects of sexual orientation, see Meyer (2013).

Sexual dysfunction

In men, sexual dysfunction refers to repeated impairment of normal sexual performance, and less often to impairment of sexual interest and pleasure. In women it more often refers to a repeated unsatisfactory quality to the experience, or to impaired desire for it. Note also that there is no agreed definition of 'dysfunction' in this context. What is regarded as 'normal' (e.g. in terms of the frequency or duration of sexual activity) depends in part on the expectations of the individuals concerned.

As explained above, problems of sexual dysfunction are classified into those that affect:

- sexual desire and sexual enjoyment
- the genital response (erectile impotence in men, and lack of arousal in women)
- orgasm (premature or delayed ejaculation in men, and orgasmic dysfunction in women).

To this list can be added problems that result in pain during sex (vaginismus and dyspareunia in women, and painful ejaculation in men).

It is important to remember that sexual function may not be disclosed directly, but only revealed during enquiries about another complaint, such as depression or poor sleep, or gynaecological symptoms.

Table 13.2 Classification of sexual and gender identity disorders

DSM-5	ICD-10
Sexual dysfunctions	**Sexual dysfunction not caused by organic disorders**[*]
Sexual desire/arousal disorders	Lack or loss of sexual desire
	Sexual aversion and lack of sexual enjoyment
● Female sexual interest/arousal disorder	Failure of genital response
● Male hypoactive sexual desire disorder	
● Erectile disorder	
Orgasm disorders	**Orgasmic dysfunction**
● Female orgasmic disorder	
● Delayed ejaculation	
Premature ejaculation	Premature ejaculation
Genitopelvic pain/penetration disorder (classified under specific phobia)	
Substance/medication-induced sexual dysfunction	
	Non-organic dyspareunia
	Non-organic vaginismus
	Excessive sexual drive
Paraphilic disorders	**Disorders of sexual preference**[†]
Anomalous sexual preferences	
Exhibitionistic disorder	Exhibitionism
Voyeuristic disorder	Voyeurism
Frotteuristic disorder	
Sexual masochism disorder	Sadomasochism
Sexual sadism disorder	
Anomalous target preferences	
Paedophilic disorder	Paedophilia
Fetishistic disorder	Fetishism
Transvestic disorder	Fetishistic transvestism
Gender dysphoria	**Gender identity disorders**[‡]
In children	
In adolescents and adults	

[*] In ICD-10, sexual dysfunction is part of F5, 'Behavioural syndromes associated with physiological disturbances and physical factors'.
[†] In ICD-10, these disorders are part of F6, 'Disorders of adult personality and behaviour'.
[‡] In ICD-10, gender identity disorders are part of F6.

Source: data from The ICD-10 classification of mental and behavioural disorders: clinical descriptions and diagnostic guidelines, Copyright (1992), World Health Organization; Diagnostic and Statistical Manual of Mental Disorders, Fifth Edition, Copyright (2013), American Psychiatric Association.

For comprehensive review of assessment and treatment of sexual dysfunction see Wincze and Weisberg (2015).

Prevalence of sexual dysfunction

In the UK, a sample of over 11,000 people aged 16–44 years were asked about sexual problems that had lasted for more than 1 month and for more than 6 months (Mercer *et al.*, 2003). The response rate was 65%. It is not known whether the self-reported problems would have met the diagnostic criteria for the corresponding sexual dysfunction. The reported rates are shown in Table 13.3. More women than men reported problems, and among both the majority of problems lasted for less than 6 months. Nazareth *et al.* (2003) surveyed patients from 13 general practices in London, with a 70% response rate to the questionnaire. Around 22% of the men and 40% of the women met the criteria for an ICD-10 diagnosis of a sexual problem. The most frequent problems were inhibited female orgasm (19%), lack or loss of sexual desire (17% of women and 7% of men), male erectile dysfunction (9%), and female sexual arousal dysfunction (3.6%).

A systematic review of 135 studies of female sexual dysfunction showed considerable heterogeneity, with an overall estimate in premenopausal women of 41%

Table 13.3 **Reported frequency of sexual dysfunction among people aged 16–44 years with a sexual partner (respondents could report more than one disorder)***

	Lasting 1 month	Lasting 6 months
Males		
Lack of sexual interest	17%	2%
Erectile difficulty	6%	1%
Premature orgasm	12%	3%
Anxiety about performance	9%	2%
Females		
Lack of sexual interest	40%	10%
Inability to reach orgasm	14%	4%
Pain during coitus	12%	3%
Anxiety about performance	7%	2%

*Adapted from British Medical Journal, 327(7412), Mercer CH et al, Sexual function problems and help seeking behaviour in Britain: national probability sample survey, pp. 426–7, Copyright (2003), with permission from BMJ Publishing Group Ltd.

(95% confidence interval [CI] = 37–44). Prevalence rates of individual sexual disorders ranged from 21% (lubrication difficulties) to 28% (hypoactive sexual desire disorder). Further analyses showed significantly higher rates in studies in Africa (McCool *et al.*, 2016).

Erectile dysfunction is common and increases with age, but overall rates for sexual dysfunction, estimated at 35%, are lower than those for women (Angst *et al.*, 2015; Shamloul and Ghanem, 2013). The more restrictive DSM-5 criteria (requiring a 6-month duration) will produce lower prevalence rates.

Causes of sexual dysfunction

The aetiology of most sexual dysfunction will be multiply determined, as often both physical and psychological factors are present. Causes can be split into three broad categories: biological/medical, psychological, and as a result of sociocultural influences.

For a review of female sexual dysfunction see McCool *et al.* (2016), and for a review of male dysfunction, see Shamloul and Ghanem (2013).

Biological/medical causes

Sexual dysfunction sometimes dates from a period of abstinence associated with the debilitating effects of physical illness (see Box 13.14). Of the diseases that have a direct effect on sexual performance, *diabetes mellitus* is particularly important, due both to autonomic neuropathy and vascular disease. For example, the presence of penile microangiopathy in a middle-aged male diabetic can cause erectile difficulties. Erectile dysfunction can also be an early marker for cardiovascular disease. Similarly, hormonal changes that can accompany menopause in women can produce vaginal dryness and dyspareunia. Other important organic causes of sexual dysfunction include neurological disorders (Rees *et al.*, 2007), as well as a range of general medical conditions (Basson and Schulz, 2007).

Several commonly used classes of drugs—psychiatric, medical, and recreational—have side effects that involve sexual function (see Box 13.15). The psychotropic medications most likely to negatively affect sexual functioning are: serotonergic antidepressants, prolactin-inducing antipsychotic medications, and mood stabilizers or anticonvulsants that lower bioavailable testosterone (Clayton *et al.*, 2016). Intoxication from or the excessive use of alcohol and illicit drugs can also impair sexual performance.

Psychological causes

Psychological contributions to dysfunction include negative body image and performance anxiety (fear of

Box 13.14 Medical conditions and surgical procedures commonly associated with sexual dysfunction

Medical conditions

Endocrine
- Diabetes, hyperthyroidism
- Addison's disease, hyperprolactinaemia

Gynaecological
- Vaginitis, endometriosis, pelvic infections

Cardiovascular
- Hypertension, myocardial infarction, peripheral vascular disease

Respiratory
- Asthma, obstructive airways disease

Other
- Prostate cancer
- Arthritis
- Renal failure
- Pelvic autonomic neuropathy, spinal cord lesions, stroke

Surgical procedures

Mastectomy
Colostomy, ileostomy
Prostate surgery
Prolapse surgery

Box 13.15 Some drugs that may impair sexual function

Therapeutic agents

Diuretics and antihypertensive agents
- β-blockers, calcium channel blockers, spironolactone

Antidepressants and mood stabilizers
- SSRIs, tricyclic antidepressants, monoamine oxidase inhibitors, lithium

Anxiolytics and hypnotics
- Benzodiazepines

Antipsychotics

Antihistamines and histamine H_2-receptor antagonists
- Diphenhydramine
- Ranitidine

Parkinson's disease medications

Misused substances

Alcohol, heroin, amphetamine, MDMA, cocaine, marijuana

negative evaluation, hypervigilance, or rejection). Many psychiatric disorders may impair sexual function, as discussed in other chapters. There is a strong relationship with depression, in which rates of sexual dysfunction are estimated to be up to 50%, compounded by treatment-emergent sexual dysfunction with rates of 37–62% (Reichenpfader *et al.*, 2014).

Sociocultural influences

Causes of sexual dysfunction can also arise from a person's social context. For example communication and relationship inequalities can foster sexual dysfunction, whilst larger sociocultural influences such as sex-role or religious proscriptions may also have an impact on sexual functioning. Furthermore, there are impacts of the environment under which sexual activity occurs, such as a lack of privacy and disparate work schedules, which have been identified as significant contributors to sexual dysfunction.

Assessment of patients with sexual dysfunction

History-taking

The interviewer needs to be particularly sensitive when enquiring about sexual function and dysfunction, and when detecting and dealing with embarrassment experienced by the patient. Whenever possible, the patient and their sexual partner should be interviewed, both separately and together. The major areas of enquiry are listed in Box 13.16. In addition to full characterization of the dysfunction itself, the assessment should search for evidence of any of the medical and psychiatric disorders noted earlier that can lead to sexual dysfunction.

Physical examination and special investigations

If the general practitioner or another specialist has not already done so, a physical examination should be performed, especially in men (see Box 13.17). Laboratory tests or other investigations should be arranged in appropriate cases—for example, fasting blood sugar, testosterone, and other hormones in men with erectile dysfunction.

Box 13.16 Assessment of sexual dysfunction

Define the problem (ask both partners)

Origin and course
Prior (baseline) sexual function
With other partners?
Sexual drive
Knowledge and fears
Social relationships generally
Relationship between the partners
Psychiatric disorder
Substance misuse
Medical illness; medical or surgical treatment
Why seek help now?

Physical examination

Laboratory tests

Box 13.17 Physical examination of male patients presenting with sexual dysfunction

General examination (directed especially to evidence of diabetes mellitus, thyroid disorder, and adrenal disorder)

Hair distribution
Gynaecomastia
Blood pressure
Peripheral pulses
Ocular fundi
Reflexes
Peripheral sensation

Genital examination

Penis: congenital abnormalities, foreskin, pulses, tenderness, plaques, infection, urethral discharge

Testicles: size, symmetry, texture, sensation
Prostate

Treatment of sexual dysfunction

The main treatments for sexual dysfunction are shown in Box 13.18. The first step, after a detailed assessment, is to provide advice and reassurance, since the problem is often longstanding by the time the patient presents, and it may have led to adverse secondary effects—for example, by increasing anxiety or impairing the quality of the relationship generally. Where possible, the underlying causes should be treated.

Specific interventions include a range of psychological and behavioural treatments, including *sex therapy/sensate focus techniques*. Psychological interventions have been shown in a systematic review to be effective treatment options for sexual dysfunction (effect size 0.58) (Frühauf *et al.*, 2013), with the strongest evidence for female hypoactive sexual desire disorder and female orgasmic disorder. There are also physical treatments, of which drug therapy with phosphodiesterase type 5 (PDE-5) inhibitors is by far the most widely used (Shamloul and Ghanem, 2013). The roles of the various treatment modalities and the evidence for their efficacy vary according to the specific type of sexual dysfunction, as discussed below.

Sex therapy

As noted above, many patients benefit from simple advice and reassurance. Other cases resolve with treatment of the cause of the sexual dysfunction, or the use of medication. For some people, a formal type of behavioural therapy, known as *sex therapy*, may be appropriate. In the UK, its availability within the National Health Service is very limited, although it is also provided by the charity Relate.

Sex therapy owes much to the work of Masters and Johnson (1970), and has four characteristic features.

1. The partners are treated together.
2. They are helped to communicate better about their sexual relationship.
3. They receive education about the anatomy and physiology of sexual intercourse.
4. They complete a series of graded tasks, often called *Sensate Focus*, which are a hierarchical series of structured touching opportunities with a focus as much on what must not yet be attempted as what is to be done. This prohibition often significantly reduces 'performance anxiety', resulting in increased confidence and subsequent success through a system of systematic desensitization (Linschoten *et al.*, 2016).

> ### Box 13.18 Treatments for sexual dysfunction
>
> **Advice, information, and reassurance**
>
> **Treatment of underlying cause**
>
> **Psychological methods**
> Sexual skills training
> Sex therapy (including sensate focus exercises)
> CBT
> Marital therapy
> Systematic desensitization
> Educational intervention
>
> **Drug treatments**
> PDE-5 inhibitors
>
> **Other physical treatments**
> Vacuum devices
> Dilators

As with the majority of treatments for sexual dysfunction, there are few adequately controlled studies of sex therapy.

Types of sexual dysfunction

In this section we discuss the features and treatment of the more common categories of sexual dysfunction.

Lack or loss of sexual desire (hypoactive sexual desire disorder)

Complaints of diminished sexual desire are much more common among women than among men. There is controversy about the extent to which lack of sexual desire, especially in women, should be considered a psychiatric disorder (Angel, 2010). Lack of desire can be categorized as either a lack or a loss, and as either global or situational.

Hypoactive sexual desire disorder can be treated effectively with psychological interventions—especially sexual skills training or CBT (Frühauf *et al.*, 2013). Testosterone may be used in men with hypogonadism (Snyder *et al.*, 2016).

Female sexual arousal disorder

This category is now combined with hypoactive sexual desire disorder in DSM-5. Lack of sexual arousal in the female is manifested as reduced vaginal lubrication. This may be due to inadequate foreplay, lack of sexual interest, anxiety, or low oestrogen levels (typically related to the menopause).

Male erectile disorder (erectile dysfunction; impotence)

This condition is the inability to achieve an erection or to sustain it for long enough for satisfactory coitus. It may be present from the first attempt at intercourse (primary male erectile disorder) or develop after a period of normal function (secondary male erectile disorder). It is more common among older than younger men (in contrast with premature ejaculation; see below).

Primary cases may occur because of a combination of low sexual drive and anxiety about sexual performance. Secondary cases may arise from diminishing sexual drive in the middle-aged or elderly, loss of interest in the sexual partner, anxiety, depressive disorder, or organic disease and its treatment. It is thought that abnormalities of the vascular supply to the penile erectile tissue are important factors in erectile failure associated with physical disease, including diabetes and peripheral vascular disease (as above).

The following aspects of the assessment are particularly important.

- Has there been a previous period of normal function?
- Does erection occur during foreplay?
- Does erection occur on waking or in response to masturbation? Erection in these circumstances suggests psychological causes for the failure of erection at other times.
- Is there evidence of alcohol or drug abuse? (Ask the partner as well as the patient.)
- Are there possible effects of any medication?

If the aetiology is uncertain after history-taking, physical examination, and blood tests, several special investigations may be considered, including measurements of tumescence and blood flow using ultrasound.

Any reversible causes should be treated. The first-line specific therapy is now the use of PDE-5 inhibitors—sildenafil (Viagra), vardenafil, and tadalafil—which are effective in about 70% of cases (Tsertsvadze *et al.*, 2009). These inhibit the breakdown of cyclic GMP by a phosphodiesterase located in the vascular smooth muscle of the penis. They do not initiate arousal but enhance the effects of sexual stimulation. Care should be taken to observe the manufacturer's advice about contraindications and interactions. The most common side effects are headache, flushing, dyspepsia, and nasal congestion.

PDE-5 inhibitors have almost entirely supplanted earlier physical treatments for erectile dysfunction (i.e. intra-cavernosal injections, vacuum devices, and surgical methods).

For review of erectile dysfunction, see Shamloul and Ghanem (2013).

Female orgasmic disorder

Many women do not regularly reach orgasm during intercourse, but do so in response to clitoral stimulation. Whether failure to reach orgasm regularly should be regarded as a disorder has been questioned (Heiman, 2002). Nevertheless, some women regard it as a problem and ask for advice and help. The best evidence is for sexual skills training.

Male orgasmic disorder

This term refers to serious delay in, or absence of, ejaculation. It is usually associated with general inhibition about sexual relationships, but it may be caused by drugs, including SSRIs, antipsychotics, and monoamine oxidase inhibitors.

Premature ejaculation

This term refers to habitual ejaculation either before penetration or so soon afterwards that the woman has not experienced pleasure. It is more common among younger men, especially during their first sexual relationships. When it persists, it is often caused by fear of failure.

Psychological causes should be treated initially with advice and reassurance. If the partner is willing, the 'squeeze technique' can be useful. When the man indicates that he will soon have an orgasm, his partner grips the penis for a few seconds and then releases it suddenly. Intercourse is then continued. There are also other methods designed to regulate and reduce the amount of sexual stimulation in order to delay orgasm, which can be implemented as part of sex therapy. Sometimes SSRIs, which delay ejaculation, are used in treatment, but continued use is required.

Genitopelvic pain/penetration disorder

Dyspareunia. This refers to pain on intercourse, and implicitly relates to women, although it can occur in men. Such pain can have many different causes. Pain that is experienced after partial penetration may result from impaired lubrication of the vagina, from scars or other painful lesions, or from the muscle spasm of vaginismus. Pain on deep penetration strongly suggests pelvic pathology such as endometriosis, ovarian cysts or tumours, or pelvic infection, although it can be caused by impaired lubrication associated with low sexual arousal. For a review, see Steege and Zolnoun (2009).

Vaginismus. This refers to spasm of the vaginal muscles, which causes pain when intercourse is attempted, in the absence of a physical cause. The spasm is usually part of a phobic response to penetration, and may be made worse by an inexperienced partner. Spasms often begin as soon as the man attempts to enter the vagina; in severe cases they occur even when the woman attempts to introduce her own finger. Points of special relevance in the sexual history include the circumstances and objects that provoke spasm, the partner's sexual technique, and any history of traumatic sexual experience.

There have been very few trials of treatment for dyspareunia and vaginismus, so therapy has to be based on clinical experience (Frühauf *et al.*, 2013). Treatment employs the general sex therapy techniques described above, with emphasis on an initial ban on attempts at intercourse. Fears are treated by using psychological approaches, and the woman is helped to desensitize herself gradually by inserting first her finger and then dilators of increasing size.

Abnormalities of sexual preference (paraphilias)

The concept of abnormal sexual preference has a social aspect—that is, the behaviour does not conform to some generally accepted view of what is normal. The accepted view is not the same in every society or at every period in history. For centuries, abnormalities of sexual preference were regarded as offences against the laws of religion, rather than conditions that doctors should study and treat. The systematic investigation of these disorders began in the 1870s. Krafft-Ebing, a professor of psychiatry in Vienna, wrote a systematic account of paraphilias in his book *Psychopathia Sexualis*, which was first published in 1886. In England, Havelock Ellis (1859–1939) wrote extensively about these and other sexual disorders, which at the time included masturbation.

In a current psychiatric context, the status of paraphilia remains controversial. The important feature that delineates abnormal sexual preference is *harm* or *mental distress* to the person or to others (McManus *et al.*, 2013).

This distinction is recognized in DSM-5, in which 'a paraphilic disorder is a paraphilia that is currently causing distress or impairment to the individual or … harm, or risk of harm, to others'. The specific paraphilic disorders are classified in Table 13.2. All are much commoner in men than in women. Some carry major legal implications and interactions, and so the more serious disorders are primarily in the domain of forensic psychiatrists. However, any doctor may encounter abnormalities of sexual preference in their clinical work—for example, as a request for help, or an expression of concern by a third party.

For a review of this subject, see Beech *et al.* (2016) and Konrad *et al.* (2015).

Types of abnormality of sexual preference

Abnormalities of sexual preference can be divided into two groups—abnormalities of the *object* of the person's sexual interest, and abnormalities in the preference of the sexual *act*. Abnormalities of the sexual object include paedophilic disorder and fetishistic disorder. Abnormalities of preference of the target for the sexual act include exhibitionistic disorder, voyeuristic disorder, and sexual masochism disorder.

Aetiology of abnormalities of sexual preference

The aetiology of paraphilias remains unknown, although a range of theories have been proposed, none of which are supported by good evidence.

- *Behavioural models.* According to these models, sexual preference is shaped by events and reinforcements during development. For example, in 1877 Alfred Binet proposed that fetishism arises from the chance co-occurrence of sexual excitement with the object that later becomes the fetish object.
- *Psychoanalytical models.* For example, Freud argued that fetishism arises when castration anxiety is not resolved in childhood, with each fetish object representing a phallus.
- *Biological models.* These include reports linking paraphilias with abnormal brain activity or structure, or with genetic predisposition.
- *Disease models.* Paraphilias that begin in middle age or later may be secondary to dementia or other organic disorders, or to their treatment. For example, high-dose dopamine agonists that are used to treat Parkinson's disease are associated with a range of abnormal sexual

behaviours and might elucidate aspects of the pathophysiological process (Solla *et al.*, 2015).

Assessment of abnormalities of sexual preference

Assessment often takes place in the context of possible or actual legal proceedings. It is important therefore to explain the relationship of the interview to any such proceedings, to explain the position with regard to confidentiality and its limits, and to obtain the necessary consent. People who are seen for the assessment of abnormality of sexual preference are often reluctant to disclose the true nature of their desires, or of their sexual behaviour. Whenever possible, consent should be obtained for an interview with any regular sexual partner, and with other informants who may be able to assist with, for example, the assessment of personality.

Assessment includes a psychiatric history, and should incorporate the following steps.

- *Exclude another psychiatric disorder*, especially if the patient first presents with the abnormal sexual preference in middle age or later. Abnormal sexual preference is sometimes secondary to dementia, alcoholism, or mania.
- *Document the sexual behaviour and its effect.* Obtain details of the normal and abnormal sexual behaviour, both currently and in the past. Remember that it is not uncommon for people to have more than one form of abnormal sexual preference. Find out what part the abnormal sexual preference is playing in the patient's life other than as a source of sexual arousal.
- *Assess the patient's motivation.* This will influence decisions about management. Patients' motives for seeking treatment are often mixed. Individuals who have little wish to change their sexual behaviour may consult a doctor because of pressure from a sexual partner, a relative, or the police. Such people may hope to be told that no treatment can help, so as to justify the continuation of their paraphilia. Others seek help when they are depressed and feel guilty about their behaviour. A strong desire for change, expressed during a period of depression, may fade quickly as the patient's normal mood is restored.
- *Psychophysiological assessment.* Some specialists use penile plethysmography or polygraphy to assess sexual interests. These methods are not part of routine assessment.

The management of abnormalities of sexual preference

Some aspects of management apply to all kinds of abnormality of sexual preference. Management specific to particular disorders is described below, along with the other aspects of those disorders. The following outline is suggested:

- Complete the assessment to make a provisional diagnosis.
- Assess the immediate risks—for example, whether the patient should be reported to the authorities, or whether their level of distress requires urgent treatment or admission. Often it is a crisis that first leads the person to present—for example, if they have been accused of a sexual offence or have been caught in a compromising sexual act.
- Decide what treatment is indicated and acceptable to the patient. This includes agreement about the aims of treatment, and the patient's motivation. It may also include incentives or punishments determined by the legal system.
- Treatments for the paraphilias are of three types, although the field is hampered by little available high-quality evidence:
  - psychotherapy—individual, couple, or group based on behavioural or psychodynamic theories
  - pharmacotherapy—SSRIs, synthetic steroidal analogues and gonadotropin-releasing hormone analogues
  - rehabilitation—counselling, education, social skills training.

An algorithm to assist clinicians in determining appropriate biological treatments for individuals with paraphilic disorders has been developed, which provides guidance on treatments depending on severity of impairment and risk of harm (Thibaut *et al.*, 2010).

For an overview of treatments for paraphilias see Bradford (2014) and for a review on biological treatments see Holoyda *et al.* (2016).

Types of abnormality of preference for the sexual object

These abnormalities involve preferences for an 'object' other than another adult for the achievement of sexual excitement. The alternative 'object' may be inanimate, as in fetishistic disorder, or may be a child (paedophilic disorder) or an animal (zoophilia). The more common paraphilias are mentioned below.

Fetishistic disorder

In sexual fetishism, the preferred or only means of achieving sexual excitement are inanimate objects or parts of the human body that do not have direct sexual associations. The objects that evoke sexual arousal are many and varied, the most common being female items of clothing, but for each individual there is usually only a small number of such objects. Contact with the object causes sexual excitement, which may be followed by solitary masturbation or by sexual intercourse that incorporates the fetish. The disorder merges into normal sexual behaviour, but is considered to be abnormal when the behaviour takes precedence over the usual patterns of sexual intercourse. The estimated prevalence is 1–18% in men, and the disorder is very rare in women. There are no good data on natural history or treatment outcome.

Transvestic disorder

Transvestic disorder ranges from the occasional wearing of a few articles of clothing of the opposite sex to complete cross-dressing (Beech *et al.*, 2016). The prevalence of the disorder in men is estimated to be around 1%, although 3% of males report having been sexually aroused by dressing in clothes associated with the opposite gender. Onset usually occurs at around the time of puberty. Most are heterosexual and many have sexual partners, who may or may not know about the behaviour. Transvestic disorder is rare among women. There have been no reliable follow-up studies or evaluated treatments.

Paedophilia

In contrast to the generally benign effects of fetishism on others, paedophilia has serious forensic and clinical implications. Paedophilia is repeated sexual activity (or fantasizing about such activity) with pre-pubertal children as a preferred or exclusive method of deriving sexual excitement. Like most paraphilias, it is most prevalent in the male population, although female cases are recognized (Gannon and Rose, 2008). Paedophilia has to be distinguished from intercourse with young people who have passed puberty but not yet reached the legal age of consent (which differs between legislations).

Paedophiles usually choose a child aged between 6 years and puberty, but some prefer very young children. The child may be of the opposite sex (heterosexual paedophilia) or the same sex (homosexual paedophilia). Some paedophiles approach children within their extended family, or in their professional care, while others befriend unrelated children. Although most paedophiles who are seen by doctors are men of middle age, the condition is usually established early in life. With younger children, fondling or masturbation is more likely to occur than full coitus, but sometimes young children are injured by forcible attempts at penetration. There are rare and tragic cases of paedophilia associated with sexual sadistic disorder.

Estimates of the prevalence of paedophilic disorder range from 1% to 5% in the male population (Konrad *et al.*, 2015; Beech *et al.*, 2016). It occurs in all ethnic and socioeconomic groups. As is evident from the existence of child prostitution in some countries, the ready sale of pornographic material depicting sex with children and the number of internet sites that show such material, interest in sexual relationships with children is not rare.

Treatments are discussed in the Forensic chapter under child sexual abuse (Chapter 18).

Abnormalities in the preference for the sexual act

The second group of abnormalities of sexual preference involves variations in the behaviour that is engaged in to obtain sexual arousal.

Voyeuristic disorder

Voyeurism refers to observing the sexual activity of others repeatedly as a preferred means of sexual arousal. The rates are estimated to be as high as 12% in males and 4% in females for lifetime prevalence of this disorder (Beech *et al.*, 2016), with some co-occurrence with exhibitionistic disorder. The voyeur spies on individuals (occasionally with video cameras) who are undressing or without clothes, but does not attempt to engage in sexual activity with them. Voyeurism is usually accompanied by or followed by masturbation. There is limited treatment efficacy reported with either pharmacological or psychoanalytical approaches.

Exhibitionistic disorder

Exhibitionistic behaviour—broadly defined as the exposing of the genitals to an unsuspecting stranger—is the most commonly reported of all sex offences (McNally and Fremouw, 2014). Exhibitionistic behaviour is estimated to occur at rates as high as 2–4% in the general population. It is almost entirely a male disorder, and adolescents account for approximately 10% of exhibitionistic offences. It is less frequent than voyeuristic disorder but perpetrators often commit multiple offences on multiple occasions (Beech *et al.*, 2016). It is usually done for the purpose of achieving sexual excitement, without any attempts at further sexual activity with

the person. The name *exhibitionism* was suggested by Lasègue in 1877. (This technical use of the term is clearly different from its everyday meaning.)

Over a 5-year follow-up, 5–10% of exhibitionistic perpetrators were found to escalate to contact sexual offending, while approximately 25% recidivated with a subsequent exhibitionistic offence. The strongest risk factor for escalation was a general clustering of antisocial behavior, including a history of sexual and non-sexual convictions (McNally and Fremouw, 2014).

As a generalization, two groups of exhibitionists can be described. The first group includes men of inhibited temperament who struggle against their urges and feel much guilt after the act; they sometimes expose a flaccid penis. The second group includes men who have aggressive traits, sometimes accompanied by features of antisocial personality disorder; they usually expose an erect penis. They gain pleasure from any distress they cause, and often feel little guilt. Few evidence-based treatments exist, but those that are most effective are along the lines of treatment for sex offenders and can include CBT (Beech *et al.*, 2016).

Frotteuristic disorder

In *frotteurism*, the preferred form of sexual excitement is by rubbing the male genitalia against another person, or by fondling the breasts of an unwilling participant, who is usually a stranger, generally in a crowded place. Frotteuristic activity usually starts in adolescence, with most acts occurring between the ages of 15 and 25 years, and prevalence estimates suggest that approximately 30% of the population has committed acts that would qualify as frotteuristic (Beech *et al.*, 2016).

Sexual sadism disorder

Sadism is named after the Marquis de Sade (1740–1814), who inflicted extreme cruelty on women for sexual purposes. Sexual sadism refers to the achievement of sexual arousal habitually, and in preference to heterosexual intercourse, by inflicting pain on another person, by bondage, or by humiliation. The acts may be symbolic, causing little actual harm. However, at times serious injuries are caused, including severe acts of mutilation in a murder. In these rare cases, ejaculation may occur during the sadistic act, or later, during intercourse with the dead body (necrophilia).

Sexual sadism as the predominant sexual practice is uncommon, but sexual sadism as a part of 'normal' sexual activity has an estimated prevalence of 3–20%. No treatment has been shown to be effective. Men who have committed serious injury are dealt with by legal means. The risks must not be underestimated when potentially dangerous behaviour has been planned or has taken place.

Sexual masochism disorder

Sexual masochism disorder involves using the experience of suffering or humiliation as a preferred or exclusive practice for achieving sexual excitement. The condition is named after Leopold von Sacher-Masoch (1836–1895), an Austrian novelist, who described sexual gratification from the experience of pain. The suffering may take the form of being beaten, trodden upon, or bound, or the enactment of various symbolic forms of humiliation. Masochism, unlike most other sexual deviations, occurs relatively commonly in women, although its prevalence in both genders is difficult to gauge. There is little data on treatment efficacy.

Gender dysphoria

Gender dysphoria (formerly *gender identity disorder*) is a term that denotes persistent discomfort with one's biologic sex or assigned gender. It is receiving significant attention, and referrals to gender-confirming clinics (formerly known as *sex reassignment clinics*) are dramatically rising, as is the prominence of the subject in all forms of the media (Zucker *et al.*, 2016). The management of gender dysphoria should be multidisciplinary, as endocrine, surgical, and psychological input are all often needed. There is, however, a growing argument that these dysphorias should not necessarily sit within a psychopathological or psychiatric model (Wylie *et al.*, 2016). Such models are seen as outdated and not able to reflect the multitude of different experiences and terms used to describe individuals whose gender identity or gender role behaviour does not match up with societal expectations or stereotypes associated with the (biological) male–female binary (Drescher *et al.*, 2012; Zucker *et al.*, 2016). Reflecting the changing views, DSM-5 adopted the term *gender dysphoria* to replace '*gender identity disorder*', placing emphasis on the emotional distress that can result when there is a marked incongruence between one's experienced/expressed gender and one's assigned gender. An increasing number of other terms are also being used with regard to gender and gender dysphoria (see Box 13.19, also Winter et al., 2016). Subtypes have been described that include sexual orientation—whether sexually attracted to males, females, both, or neither, as well as age of onset of the gender dysphoria, with early-onset usually denoting the preschool period. The implications of these subtypes are unclear, although they have played a historical role in assessments for sex

---

> ### Box 13.19 Some terms used relevant to gender dysphoria
>
> *Transgender*: an umbrella term for people whose gender (identity, expression, general sense of self) is different from the sex they were assigned at birth
>
> *Transsexual*: someone who has transitioned from one sex to the other through the use of hormones and/or surgical procedures
>
> *Transgender woman/trans woman/MtF*: someone who was assigned male at birth but living as a woman (male to female)
>
> *Transgender man/trans man/ FtM*: someone who was assigned female at birth but living as a man (female to male)
>
> *Sexual orientation*: refers to an individual's enduring physical, romantic, and/or emotional attraction to another person. Transgender people may be straight, bisexual, lesbian, gay, or asexual
>
> *Non-binary*: someone who does not identify with either gender, or has a gender that changes over time, or feels in between genders
>
> *Cisgender*: someone who identifies with the gender they were assigned at birth

---

reassignment surgery. For review of gender dysphoria in adults see Zucker *et al.* (2016) and in adolescents and children see Zucker *et al.* (2015). For review of transgender people and mental health, see Wylie *et al.* (2016) and Winter *et al.* (2016).

Epidemiology

Prevalence rates are difficult to determine. Previous data were drawn from numbers of referrals to specialist centres and also on numbers requesting a change to the gender they had been assigned in their passports. This, however, is unlikely to be a true prevalence rate because of the stigma attached to individuals with gender dysphoria and the limited services available. As public understanding has increased, there has been an increase in the reported prevalence rates; this might reflect a bona-fide increase or, more likely, just an increase in those who would previously not have sought treatment.

Conron *et al.* (2012) conducted telephone interviews on over 28,000 adults (aged 18–64 years) and found that

0.5% considered themselves to be transgender. Studies using stricter caseness criteria, such as Dhejne *et al.* (2014), reported a point prevalence in Sweden of 1:7750 adult males and 1:13,000 females who had applied for a legal name change. Judge *et al.* (2015) reported a prevalence of 1:10,000 adult males and 1:28,000 females referred for hormonal treatment in Ireland. A meta-analytic review of 21 studies concluded that the prevalence of transsexualism in males was 1:15,000 and 1:38,000 in females (Zucker and Lawrence, 2009).

Associated psychopathology

Comorbid psychopathology is significantly more prevalent in adults with gender dysphoria than in the general population. Mood and anxiety disorders are the most common. A study of all persons in Sweden who had undergone sex reassignment surgery, a cohort of over 300 individuals, showed that 19% of males-to-females and 17% of females-to-males had been hospitalized for psychiatric problems other than gender dysphoria prior to undergoing sex reassignment surgery (compared to 3–4% of controls) (Dhejne *et al.*, 2014). Their risk for hospitalization for psychiatric problems remained over double that of controls after surgery, and they were 4.9 times more likely to have made a suicide attempt, and 19 times more likely to have died from suicide.

Another large study of over 300 people with gender dysphoria treated in clinics across Europe showed that 38% had a current Axis I disorder and 69% had a lifetime Axis I disorder—predominantly mood and anxiety disorders (Heylens *et al.*, 2014). This is consistent with many other studies that have shown a high prevalence of comorbid psychopathology (Zucker *et al.*, 2016).

Aetiology

A number of causal mechanisms have been proposed. These are predominantly based on general principles of 'normative' or 'sex typical' psychosexual development—that becomes inverted in the development of gender dysphoria.

Genetic causes: family and twin studies demonstrate that there is some genetic contribution to gender dysphoria, but no genes have been identified. In a study of twins with gender dysphoria, 39% of monozygotic twins were concordant for gender dysphoria, whereas none of the dizygotic twins were concordant (Heylens *et al.*, 2012).

Prenatal sex hormones: it has been hypothesized that feelings of gender incongruence may arise from atypical sexual differentiation of the brain under the influence of prenatal hormones (Swaab, 2009).

Sex-dimorphic brain structure and function: brain structure and function have been studied to determine whether they show atypical sexual differentiation. The studies demonstrate that homosexual male-to-females are dissimilar to their natal sex in grey matter volume (Simon *et al.*, 2013), cortical thickness (Zubiaurre-Elorza *et al.*, 2013), and white matter microstructure (Rametti *et al.*, 2011). For non-homosexual male-to-females the picture is less clear. For natal females, who are more likely to be similar in sexual orientation (homosexual), female-to-males had larger grey matter volumes than female controls, and the majority of studies have shown support for atypical sexual differentiation of their brains (Zucker *et al.*, 2016).

Psychosocial processes: in some children and adults, gender identity can be observed as more fluid and less trait-like. For example, clinical populations of children with gender dysphoria show a diminution of their cross-gender behaviour over time, which may lead to a shift in their underlying gender identity or identification, especially in samples in which a social transition to living as the desired gender has not occurred prior to puberty (Steensma *et al.*, 2013). There were also historical studies exploring the relationship quality and warmth between mothers and fathers with the person with gender dysphoria, but it is difficult to draw conclusions from these studies. For review, see Zucker *et al.* 2016).

Treatment

The treatment of adults with gender dysphoria has been standardized across many high-income countries, reflecting the influence of a number of clinical guidelines. The Standards of Care for the Health of Transsexual, Transgender and Gender-Nonconforming People, Version 7 (SOC-7) is the most influential (Coleman *et al.*, 2012). A key change in these latest guidelines is that the diagnosis can be made by any appropriately trained health professional, not only by a mental health professional. The latter historically played a gatekeeper role to receiving hormone therapy, but this might have inadvertently undermined individual autonomy in a person who might need the treatment and not have a mental illness. Nevertheless, a psychological and psychiatric assessment is important to rule out and treat any significant comorbid mental illness, as well as provide interventions that might help in alleviating the dysphoria.

The guidelines generally follow expert consensus rather than evidence from clinical trials. Current treatment includes the following steps:

Counselling and psychotherapy should deal with the full range of options available. It emphasizes the need to set realistic goals and to consider the full consequences of any contemplated changes, both for the person and for their family. It is now considered unethical to make the focus of therapeutic work a goal for that person's gender identity to be more congruent with the sex they have been assigned at birth, as, although gender dysphoria can remit in some cases, the agreed consensus at present is to make the focus of therapeutic involvement the 'long-term comfort in … gender identity expression, with realistic chances for success in … relationships, education and work' (Coleman *et al.*, 2012).

Real life experience in the preferred gender role. Almost all individuals with gender dysphoria will have to live in their new gender role for a period of 1 year prior to surgery. During this time, appropriate hormone treatment (see below) is prescribed. At the end of the year, an individual who can demonstrate to an assessment panel that they are better adjusted in the new gender role than in the old one may be considered for surgery. Despite the widespread requirement to live in the new gender role for a year, there is little evidence to support it, and it carries psychosocial risks, including loss of employment, impaired relationships, and gender-based discrimination; thus it has been argued that, if a person with gender dysphoria can achieve satisfactory relief with hormone therapy and sex reassignment surgery, it is unclear why they have to undertake the real life experience (Zucker *et al.*, 2016).

Hormonal therapy. Hormone therapy is effective and reasonably safe in adults with gender dysphoria; those undergoing hormone therapy demonstrate significant improvement in quality of life if they undergo concomitant sex reassignment surgery (Murad *et al.*, 2010) than if they do not (Gorin-Lazard *et al.*, 2012). The treatments for males-to-females include testosterone suppression, spironolactone, cyproterone acetate, or gonadotropin-releasing hormone (GnRH) agonists. Androgens may be prescribed to females-to-males, as a result of which the voice deepens, hair increases on the face and body, menstruation ceases, the clitoris enlarges, and sex drive increases.

Gender-confirming (sex reassignment) surgery. Opinions differ about the merits of sex reassignment, and decisions should be taken with the person and members of the multidisciplinary team. For a male-to-female, possible surgical procedures include mammoplasty, penectomy, orchidectomy, and the creation of a vagina-like structure. For a female-to-male, surgical procedures include mastectomy, ovariectomy, and phalloplasty.

Follow-up studies show that outcomes after surgery are generally favourable. In a study of 46 males-to-females and 11 females-to-males, objective psychological measures improved after hormone therapy and became similar to those of the general population, but no further improvement was noted following sex reassignment surgery (Heylens *et al.*, 2014). A meta-analysis showed that 86% of females-to-males and 71% of males-to-females reported improvement in quality of life (Murad *et al.*, 2010); equally, it is important to note that a significant minority do not. Factors predictive of less satisfactory functioning include non-homosexual orientation relative to natal sex, greater dissatisfaction with secondary sex characteristics, and more comorbid psychopathology (Smith *et al.*, 2005).

Gender identity disorders in children

Children with gender dysphoria display behaviours that reflect identification with the other sex. There are early-onset forms (before 12 years, and usually between 2–4 years) and later-onset forms. The early-onset form in both biological males and females is associated with later homosexual orientation, whereas the late-onset form is typically non-homosexual (Lawrence, 2010).

Boys are referred more often than girls. It is not clear whether this is because such behaviour is less frequent or more socially acceptable in girls. Parents should be discouraged from making attempts to force children into stereotyped 'gender-based' behaviours and roles, as this has no demonstrated benefits and can cause discord and distress. There is emerging evidence that, for a proportion of adolescents for whom gender dysphoria is persistent, the negative impacts on social adaptation, general mental health, and peer and family relations might encourage biomedical treatments, including initiating hormonal therapies to delay or suppress somatic puberty.

For further information, see Giordano (2013) and Zucker *et al.* (2015). For a summary of the controversies, see Drescher *et al.* (2016).

Further reading

Fairburn CG (2008). *Cognitive Behavior Therapy and Eating Disorders*. Guilford Press, New York.

Kryger MH *et al.* (2016). *Principles and Practice of Sleep Medicine*. 6th edn. Elsevier, Philadelphia, PA.

Wincze, J. P., and Weisberg, R. B. (2015). *Sexual dysfunction: A guide for assessment and treatment*, Guilford Publications, 3rd edition, New York.

CHAPTER 14

Dementia, delirium, and other neuropsychiatric disorders

Introduction

Neuropsychiatry comprises psychiatric disorders that arise from demonstrable abnormalities of brain structure and function. Cognitive impairments are the most prominent feature, especially in dementia and delirium, but behavioural and emotional disturbances are also common, and may be the sole manifestations.

The term *neuropsychiatry* is sometimes used interchangeably with *organic psychiatry* (see David, 2009a). However, the latter category is broader, including psychiatric disorders that arise from general medical disorders with their basis outside the brain (e.g. endocrine and metabolic disorders). Moreover, the term *organic* has the fundamental problem that it wrongly implies that other psychiatric disorders do not have any such basis (Spitzer *et al.*, 1992; see Chapter 2). Finally, regardless of terminology, there is always the risk that psychological and social factors will be neglected if a disorder is considered to be 'physical', and vice versa.

In this chapter we cover the range of disorders conventionally considered under the heading of neuropsychiatry, which include:

- delirium—acute, generalized impairment of attention and cognition in the setting of altered consciousness

- dementia—chronic, generalized cognitive impairment in clear consciousness. As with delirium, the syndrome of dementia can be caused by many separate disease processes. (This chapter covers the clinical features and aetiology of dementia; its treatment and management are covered in Chapter 19).

- amnesic (or amnestic) syndromes (or disorders)—circumscribed deficits in memory

- cerebrovascular disorders

- movement disorders

- epilepsy

- head injury

- other neuropsychiatric disorders, including focal cerebral syndromes, encephalitis, tumours, and multiple sclerosis
- secondary or symptomatic neuropsychiatric disorders—disorders such as depression and anxiety, which in particular cases can be attributed directly to a neuropsychiatric cause (e.g. psychosis due to cerebral vasculitis). Psychiatric disorders secondary to diseases elsewhere in the body are covered in Chapter 22.

Classification

In ICD-10, organic psychiatric disorders are grouped together in category F00–F09, as *organic, including symptomatic, mental disorders*. In DSM-5, the equivalent chapter is entitled *neurocognitive disorders*; as in DSM-IV, the term 'organic' is not used. The two classifications are compared in Table 14.1 (the order of diagnoses has been modified to facilitate the comparison). Despite many similarities, ICD-10 and DSM-5 differ to a significant extent, and more so than in most other areas of psychiatric diagnosis:

- The most substantial difference is that DSM-5 introduces the new category of *neurocognitive disorder*, and divides it into major and minor forms (Sachdev *et al.*, 2014). *Major neurocognitive disorder* subsumes the conventionally distinct categories of dementia and amnestic disorder. The term dementia is still used descriptively in DSM-5, but amnesic syndrome is not. *Mild neurocognitive disorder* describes cases that show lesser degrees of cognitive and functional impairment (and which would not meet criteria for dementia). Both major and minor neurocognitive disorders are then subcategorized by their presumed aetiology (e.g. due to Alzheimer's disease). Neurocognition in DSM-5 is divided into six domains: complex attention, executive function, learning and memory, language, perceptual–motor, and social cognition. The individual neurocognitive disorders vary as to the relative involvement of these domains. In this chapter, we follow the ICD-10 approach, and retain the terms dementia and amnesic disorder.

- In ICD-10, the category of organic disorder includes subcategories for any mental disorder that is due to brain damage and dysfunction and to physical disease, and for personality and behavioural disorders that are due to brain disease, damage, and dysfunction (e.g. 'organic anxiety disorder, thyrotoxicosis'). In DSM-5, such conditions are classified separately, under the relevant psychiatric disorder, with the addition of a code to indicate that the disorder is secondary to a medical condition.

- Conversely, DSM-5 includes cases of delirium or dementia (major neurocognitive disorder) that are due to use of psychoactive substances, whereas ICD-10 excludes these conditions and records them in a separate section on 'mental and behavioural disorders due to psychoactive substance abuse' (F10–F19). Thus, for example, amnestic syndrome that is due to alcohol dependence is classified as a psychoactive substance abuse disorder.

Symptoms associated with regional brain pathology

Before considering the various syndromes, it is helpful to consider the characteristic features associated with lesions in different regions of the brain, and the neuroanatomical basis of memory. Knowledge of the regional affiliation of neurological and psychopathological findings is relevant when attempting to localize neuropsychiatric conditions. However, the clinical features are not diagnostically specific and the clinicopathological correlations are often modest rather than strong. For a review of this subject, see David (2009a).

Frontal lobe

The frontal lobes, together with their reciprocal connections to other cortical and subcortical regions, have a crucial role in personality and judgement. Patients with a frontal lobe syndrome may present with a variety of clinical syndromes.

- They may be disinhibited, overfamiliar, tactless, and garrulous, make fatuous jokes and puns (*Witzelsucht*),

Table 14.1 Classification of organic mental disorders in ICD-10 and DSM-5

ICD-10 F00–F09. Organic, including symptomatic, mental disorders	DSM-5 Neurocognitive disorders
Delirium (not induced by alcohol and other psychoactive substances)	Delirium Substance intoxication delirium Substance withdrawal delirium Medication-induced delirium Delirium due to another medical condition Delirium due to multiple aetiologies
Dementia Dementia in Alzheimer's disease Vascular dementia Dementia in Pick's disease Dementia in Creutzfeldt–Jakob disease Dementia in Huntington's disease Dementia in Parkinson's disease Dementia in HIV disease Unspecified dementia	Major neurocognitive disorder (dementia) Due to Alzheimer's disease Due to vascular disease Due to frontotemporal lobar degeneration Due to prion disease Due to Huntington's disease Due to Lewy body disease Due to HIV infection Due to traumatic brain injury Due to substance/medication use Due to another medical condition Due to multiple aetiologies Unspecified
Organic amnesic syndrome (not induced by alcohol and other psychoactive substances)	Minor neurocognitive disorder Subcategories as listed for major neurocognitive disorder
Other mental disorders due to brain damage and dysfunction and to physical disease Organic hallucinosis Organic catatonic disorder Organic delusional disorder Organic mood disorders Organic dissociative disorder Mild cognitive disorder	
Personality and behavioural disorders due to brain disease, damage, and dysfunction	
Unspecified organic or symptomatic mental disorder	

Source: data from The ICD-10 classification of mental and behavioural disorders: clinical descriptions and diagnostic guidelines, Copyright (1992), World Health Organization; Diagnostic and Statistical Manual of Mental Disorders, Fifth Edition, Copyright (2013), American Psychiatric Association.

commit errors of judgement and sexual indiscretions, and disregard the feelings of others.

- They may appear inert (abulic) and apathetic, with a paucity of spontaneous speech, movement, and emotional expressions.

- They may engage in obsessive, ritualistic behaviours, with perseveration of thought and gesture.

Measures of formal intelligence are generally unimpaired in frontal lobe disease. However, there may be difficulties in abstract reasoning (e.g. 'How are glass and ice different?') and cognitive estimates are typically inaccurate but precise (e.g. '364 miles from London to New York'). Concentration and attention are reduced, and insight is often markedly impaired. Verbal fluency, assessed using word generation by letter (e.g. number of words beginning with 's' in 1 minute) and category (e.g. number of animals), is reduced, and unusual (low-frequency) examples may be volunteered. The patient has difficulty switching between tasks (perseveration), carrying out sequenced movements, and understanding rules. Utilization behaviour (e.g. donning several pairs of spectacles) may be evident.

Posterior extension of a dominant frontal lobe lesion may involve Broca's area and produce an expressive (non-fluent) dysphasia. Encroachment on the motor cortex or deep projections may result in a contralateral hemiparesis. Other signs may include ipsilateral optic atrophy or anosmia, a grasp or other primitive reflexes and, if the process is bilateral or in the midline, incontinence of urine.

Parietal lobe

Lesions of the parietal lobe may cause various neuropsychological disturbances that are easily mistaken for conversion disorder (see page 648). Involvement of the non-dominant parietal lobe characteristically gives rise to visuospatial difficulties, with neglect of contralateral space, and constructional and dressing apraxias. Lesions of the dominant lobe may be associated with receptive dysphasia, limb apraxia, body image disorders, right–left disorientation, dyscalculia, finger agnosia, and agraphia. Other signs may include contralateral sensory loss, astereognosis, and agraphaesthesia, and (with more extensive lesions) a contralateral hemiparesis or homonymous inferior quadrantanopia.

Persistent unawareness of neurological deficit (anosognosia) is not uncommon, especially with non-dominant parietal lesions. In extreme cases, the patient may deny that a paretic limb belongs to him. This should be distinguished from denial due to a psychological unwillingness to recognize disability and its consequences.

Temporal lobe

The temporolimbic syndromes are characterized by complex and wide-ranging neuropsychiatric clinical pictures. There may be personality change resembling that of frontal lobe lesions, but more often accompanied by specific cognitive deficits and neurological signs. The relatively florid behavioural disturbances that characterize the frontotemporal dementias reflect the combined temporal and frontal involvement, and their interconnections.

Unilateral medial temporal lobe lesions, especially those involving the hippocampus, produce lateralizing memory deficits—left hippocampal damage impairs verbal memory (and semantic impairment and fluent dysphasia), whereas right hippocampal damage affects non-verbal (spatial) aspects of memory. Some evidence also suggests that left medial temporal lobe lesions are more likely to produce psychotic symptoms, and right-sided lesions produce affective ones.

Occipital lobe

Occipital lobe lesions rarely present to psychiatrists, but they may cause disturbances of visual processing that are easily misinterpreted as being of psychological origin. Such phenomena occasionally accompany migraine or occipital lobe seizures. Complex visual hallucinations may occur with lesions involving visual association areas, sometimes referred to a hemianopic field. These include multiple visual images (polyopia), persistent aftertraces of the features of an image (visual perseveration or palinopsia), and distortions of the visual scene (metamorphopsia). Lesions that impinge anteriorly on the parietal or temporal lobes may produce visual disorientation (inability to localize objects in space under visual guidance) with asimultagnosia (difficulty in perceiving the visual scene as a unity), or prosopagnosia (inability to recognize familiar faces). In patients with suspected occipital lobe pathology, the visual fields should be mapped using perimetry, and neuropsychological tests performed to delineate visual agnosias and other higher-order derangements of visual processing. Some patients who are blind due to occipital lobe damage deny that they are blind (*Anton's syndrome*).

Corpus callosum

Corpus callosum lesions (classically, the 'butterfly glioma') typically extend laterally into both hemispheres. They then produce a picture of severe and rapid intellectual deterioration, with localized neurological signs varying with the degree and direction of extension into adjacent structures. Pure callosal lesions (usually iatrogenic, following surgery for intractable epilepsy) can be surprisingly difficult to identify, and require specialized neuropsychological testing to expose a 'disconnection syndrome', reflecting disruption of interhemispheric communication. These unique 'split-brain' patients raise intriguing questions concerning the mechanisms that normally bind the two hemispheres together to generate a consistent, unitary sense of the self (Gazzaniga, 2000). Callosal degeneration is a hallmark of the rare Marchiafava–Bignami syndrome, which is seen in severe alcohol dependence.

Subcortical structures and cortico-subcortical circuits

The regional cortical associations with cognitive, affective, and behavioural features reflect the classic 'locationist' approach to neurology and neuropsychiatry. Increasingly, this has been replaced by a 'connectionist' approach, in which emphasis is placed on distributed neural systems in which cortical regions are linked with subcortical structures, and with the white matter pathways that connect them.

Mesulam (1998) described five networks:

- a right-hemisphere spatial awareness network, including the posterior parietal cortex and frontal eye fields
- a left-hemisphere language network, including Broca's and Wernicke's areas
- a memory–emotion network, including the hippocampus, amygdala, and cingulate cortex
- a working memory–executive function network, including the prefrontal cortex and posterior parietal cortex
- a face and object recognition network in the temporo-parietal and temporo-occipital cortex.

Another influential model is that of Alexander and Crutcher (1990), who proposed four parallel circuits linking different parts of the cerebral cortex with specific basal ganglia and thalamic nuclei. Each circuit mediates different functions. For example, the 'limbic' circuit, which is involved in emotional and motivational processes, links the anterior cingulate cortex and medial prefrontal cortex with the ventral striatum, ventral pallidum, and mediodorsal thalamus.

Thalamus, basal ganglia, and cerebellum

A variety of cognitive and psychiatric consequences have been described following lesions of subcortical nuclei. These structures, which were previously considered to be primarily involved in sensory processing (the thalamus) or in motor control (the basal ganglia and cerebellum) are now all known also to be integrally involved in cognition and behaviour, and lesions therein may present with psychiatric as well as neurological features (DeLong and Wichmann, 2007; Schmahmann and Pandya, 2008), and include disturbances of memory, language, and mood. Reduced initiation of actions is also characteristic of basal ganglia pathology, and impaired consciousness with thalamic lesions.

Rostral brainstem

Behavioural disturbances frequently accompany lesions of the rostral brainstem. The most characteristic features are an amnestic syndrome (see below), hypersomnia, and the syndrome of *akinetic mutism* ('vigilant coma') or stupor.

White matter

As well as the corpus callosum, mentioned earlier, damage to other white matter tracts—both subcortical and periventricular—has important neuropsychiatric and behavioural consequences. The clinical features of white matter pathology depend on the location of the damage and whether it is focal or diffuse. For review, see Schmahmann *et al.* (2008).

Memory systems and their neuroanatomy

Clinical, neuropsychological, and brain imaging studies (both structural and functional) support the existence of multiple memory systems in the human brain. These functions may all be affected more or less selectively by brain lesions. The most basic division lies between implicit (i.e. procedural) and explicit (i.e. declarative) memory. The former includes a range of phenomena that are not usually subject to conscious analysis, such as motor skills, conditioned behaviours, and repetition priming. Explicit memory is subclassified into episodic (memory of autobiographical events) and semantic (knowledge of the world) functions.

The short-term store underpins working memory (e.g. when dialling an unfamiliar telephone number). Distinct anatomical substrates for short-term storage of verbal and visuospatial information, both controlled by a central executive, have been proposed. In neuropsychological terms, 'short-term' refers to immediate recall. By contrast, the concept of 'short-term' memory, as sometimes applied by clinicians to recall over minutes and days, does not correspond to an anatomical substrate.

Specific types of memories, such as faces and topographical information, may engage dedicated subsystems. Episodic memory has both anterograde (new learning) and retrograde (recall of past events) components. It appears to be mediated by a network of cortical and subcortical structures, which include the hippocampus, parahippocampal and entorhinal cortices, amygdala, mammillary bodies, fornix, cingulate, thalamus, and frontobasal cortex, whereas semantic memory may be subserved by a partly independent network overlapping the language areas. Broadly speaking, verbal memories are mediated by the left (dominant) hemisphere and non-verbal memories by the right hemisphere.

For a review of the classification and neuroanatomical basis of memory and its dysfunction, see David and Kopelman (2009) and Ranganath and Ritchey (2012).

Assessment of the 'neuropsychiatric patient'

The assessment of cognitive function was introduced in Chapters 1 and 3 as part of the general psychiatric assessment, and in this chapter the evaluation of amnesia, delirium, and dementia will be discussed. In this section, we introduce key aspects of the initial approach to the patient who has a suspected neuropsychiatric disorder. For a more detailed discussion, see Kipps and Hodges (2005) and David (2009b).

Before embarking upon the assessment, it is worth bearing in mind the range of major diagnostic possibilities. One question to be addressed early on is whether there is clouding of consciousness, as this defines delirium, and the assessment can proceed to determine its cause. If there is no impaired consciousness, the main diagnostic categories to consider are amnesia, dementia, or a 'functional' cause of cognitive impairment. The key feature of an amnestic syndrome is a specific deficit in episodic memory, as outlined above; although rare, amnestic syndrome needs to be considered in patients presenting with memory impairment, especially in those with alcohol dependence. A functional cause should always be considered, as memory impairment may occur secondary to many psychiatric disorders; in particular, depression in the elderly may present as *pseudodementia* (see Chapter 19). Distinction between organic and functional causes requires positive evidence to be sought for both forms of disorder, and is an important distinction to make, as it has a significant impact upon treatment and prognosis. Once these other causes of cognitive impairment (delirium, amnestic syndrome, and functional disorder) have been ruled out, a provisional diagnosis of dementia can be made (assuming that the impairment is of sufficient severity), and attention can then turn to determining the type of dementia from which the patient is suffering, as discussed later.

History and mental state examination

Although physical examination and laboratory investigations play a much larger role than elsewhere in psychiatry, the history remains essential: 'the difference between a good neuropsychiatrist and a mediocre one is a good history' (David, 2009b). An informant is especially important, as the presence of impaired cognition or consciousness will necessarily limit the patient's ability to provide a full and accurate history. Key points in the history include the onset, duration, and progression of the impairment—for example, an acute onset suggests delirium or, if it began after a fall, may indicate a subdural haematoma. The neurological, medical, and family history is important too, as many causes of cognitive impairment are secondary to pre-existing disorders or have a genetic basis.

Physical examination

The physical examination needs to be comprehensive and careful, as signs may not be conspicuous. Particular attention should be paid to the nervous system, as well as to searching for peripheral stigmata of systemic disease and alcohol dependence. Specific signs may provide diagnostic clues (Cooper and Greene, 2005) (e.g. the Argyll–Robertson pupil of neurosyphilis, optic disc pallor in vitamin B_{12} deficiency, or cranial nerve involvement in neurosarcoidosis).

Investigations

The choice and extent of investigations will depend on the findings from the history, mental state examination, and physical examination, but usually include a core set of tests, such as the cognitive tests and blood tests used in evaluation of dementias noted below. In difficult or atypical cases, and in younger patients, investigations may be extensive, and the opinion and assistance of a neurologist, physician, or neurosurgeon may be required.

Some examples of specialized investigations used in neuropsychiatric evaluation are listed here. Many are described later in the chapter with regard to investigation of dementia.

- *Structural brain imaging* with CT or MRI. Neuroimaging can detect focal and diffuse pathologies, and longitudinal scans can map progressive changes that mirror clinical decline. MRI is superior to CT for most purposes, including evaluation of white matter disease, and the ability to perform volumetric measurements. *Functional brain imaging* with fMRI, MRS, SPECT, or PET is a valuable research tool, but is not in widespread clinical use.

- *Neuropsychological testing* is less widely used than previously, in part because of the increasing availability of brain imaging. However, it can still play a valuable part in characterization of the cognitive impairment (e.g. the cognitive domains that are most affected), and measurement of severity and progression (David, 2009b). Rating scales for the assessment of dementia are considered below.

- *Electroencephalogram (EEG) studies* retain a limited but valuable role in several situations where EEG findings are characteristic—for example, in delirium, prion disease, and detection of non-convulsive status epilepticus. They are also useful in the differential diagnosis of stupor, as a normal EEG would suggest a dissociative state.

- *Cerebrospinal fluid (CSF) examination* after lumbar puncture is essential if an inflammatory or infective process is suspected. It may also become more widely used in the evaluation or prediction of dementia, as different proteins are discovered to have diagnostic or prognostic value as biomarkers.

- *Genetic testing* has a key role in the diagnosis (and prediction) of a very limited range of familial disorders in which the mode of inheritance, and the causative gene, are known (e.g. Huntington's chorea).

- *Brain biopsy*, usually of the right frontal lobe, is occasionally indicated as a last resort in the diagnosis of unexplained cognitive impairment or in suspected prion disease. However, the risks of this procedure must always be weighed against the diagnostic and prognostic information that will be obtained from it.

Delirium

Delirium is characterized by global impairment of consciousness (*clouding of consciousness*), resulting in reduced level of alertness, attention, and perception of the environment, and thence cognitive performance. A number of other terms, such as *acute confusional state, acute brain failure*, and *acute organic syndrome*, have also been used, but delirium is the preferred term in both ICD-10 and DSM-5.

For a review of delirium and its management, see Inouye *et al.* (2014a) and O'Connell *et al.* (2014).

Epidemiology

The prevalence of delirium in the elderly is 1–2% in community samples, 8–17% in emergency departments, 18–35% on admission to hospital, with an overall occurrence in inpatients of 29–64% (Inouye *et al.*, 2014a). Rates of about 8% have been reported in residential care homes (Boorsma *et al.*, 2012). Delirium is much more common in the elderly than in younger people, and in individuals with diminished 'cerebral reserve', notably those with pre-existing dementia and other medical factors (Box 14.1). Delirium is thus a common disorder in all medical settings, especially for older people. Moreover, it is associated with several adverse outcomes, discussed below, and so its prompt recognition and treatment are important.

Clinical features

The cardinal feature of delirium is disturbed consciousness. It is manifested as drowsiness, decreased awareness of one's surroundings, disorientation in time and place, and distractibility. At its most severe the patient may be unresponsive (stuporose), but more commonly the impaired consciousness is quite subtle. Indeed, the first clue to the presence of delirium is often one of its other features, which include mental slowness, distractibility, perceptual anomalies, and disorganization of the sleep–wake cycle (see Box 14.2).

Symptoms and signs vary widely between patients, and in the same patient at different times of day, typically being worse at night. For example, some patients are hyperactive, restless, irritable, and have psychotic symptoms, while others are hypoactive, with retardation and perseveration. Repetitive, purposeless movements are common in both forms. Thinking is slow and muddled, but often rich in content ('dream-like'). Ideas of reference and delusions (often persecutory) are common, but are usually transient and poorly elaborated. Visual perception is often distorted, with illusions, misinterpretations, and visual hallucinations, sometimes with fantastic content. Tactile and auditory hallucinations also occur. Anxiety, depression, and emotional lability are common. The patient may be frightened, or

Box 14.1 Delirium: predisposing and precipitating factors

Predisposing factors

Dementia
Previous episode of delirium
Functional impairment
Sensory impairment
History of cerebrovascular disease
Alcohol misuse
Older age

Precipitating factors

Substance-related
    Prescribed medical drugs (e.g. steroids, digoxin, diuretics)
    Psychotropic medication (e.g. sedatives, opiates, hypnotics)
    Alcohol—intoxication, withdrawal, delirium tremens
    Use of more than one drug
Physiological causes
    Septicaemia
    Infection (e.g. urinary tract, respiratory)
    Hypoxia (e.g. postoperative)
    Organ failure (e.g. renal, hepatic, cardiac)
    Abnormal albumin
    Metabolic acidosis
    Hypoglycaemia or hyperglycaemia
    Dehydration
Neurological causes
    Post-ictal
    Head injury
    Space-occupying lesion
    Encephalitis
Use of physical restraints
Bladder catheter
Pain
Sleep deprivation
Constipation

Adapted from Lancet, 383(9920), Inouye SK, Westendorp RGJ and Saczynski JS, Delirium in elderly people, pp. 911-922, Copyright (2014a), with permission from Elsevier.

Box 14.2 Clinical features of delirium

Clouding of consciousness
Impaired attention
Disorientation for time and place
Impaired memory
Psychotic-like symptoms
Perceptual disturbances
Delusions
Perplexity
Thought disorder
Behavioural and other symptoms
Agitation
Irritability
Labile affect
Word-finding difficulties
Temporal course
Rapid onset
Fluctuation over 24-hour period
Reversal of sleep—wake cycle

of delirium screening tools are available (De and Wand, 2015), of which the Confusion Assessment Method is most widely used.

Aetiology

The main causes of delirium are listed in Box 14.1. In practice, most cases are multifactorial, and sometimes idiopathic. In elderly people in medical settings, drugs (especially polypharmacy) and infection are probably the commonest causes; in other settings and populations, delirium has a wide range of causes and hence requires urgent and wideranging investigations (see below).

The pathophysiological basis of delirium is unclear. The severity of clinical disturbance correlates with the degree of slowing of cerebral rhythms on EEG, and the neurotransmitters dopamine and acetylcholine are implicated in a final common pathway. Inflammatory, metabolic, and genetic factors also contribute (Inouye *et al.*, 2014a).

Management of delirium

Prevention

There are more effective interventions to prevent delirium than to treat it. This applies to pharmacological

perplexed. Experiences of depersonalization and derealization are sometimes described. Attention and registration are particularly impaired, and on recovery there is usually amnesia for the period of the delirium. A range

and particularly to non-pharmacological strategies. The latter include a range of validated approaches such as the Hospital Elder Life Program (HELP) and targeting of delirium risk factors (e.g. reorientation, promotion of sleep) (Inouye *et al.*, 2014a). Low doses of antipsychotics, gabapentin, and melatonin also have some efficacy in preventing delirium (Friedman *et al.*, 2014). In practice, however, preventative interventions are often not possible, or resources not available, and it becomes necessary to treat delirium.

Treatment

Delirium is a medical emergency. Although it is a clinical diagnosis, it is essential to identify and treat the underlying cause, and a range of investigations may be required (see Box 14.3). Many are routine (e.g. electrolytes, full blood count, urinalysis), whereas others are carried out depending on the context (e.g. lumbar puncture). Vital signs need regular measurement. As delirium is often caused by drugs (due to side effects or withdrawal effects), these should always be suspected until there is evidence of another cause.

The mainstay of treatment should be non-pharmacological, since there is little evidence that any medication improves outcome, and antipsychotics (which are commonly used) have known adverse effects (Inouye *et al.*, 2014b). General measures should always be used to relieve distress, control agitation, and prevent exhaustion. These include frequent explanation, reorientation, and reassurance. Unnecessary changes in the staff caring for the patient should be avoided. The patient should ideally be nursed in a quiet single room. Relatives should be encouraged to visit regularly. At night, lighting should be sufficient to promote orientation, while not preventing sleep. In many cases, use of these behavioural measures can be sufficient to manage the patient whilst the cause of the delirium is being investigated and treated.

Nevertheless, despite such interventions, in practice many patients with delirium are treated with medication to control agitation and distress, and to allow adequate sleep. Antipsychotics are usually first-line medication. They should be limited to cases with severe agitation (endangering the patient) and for psychotic symptoms causing distress (hallucinations or delusions) (Inouye *et al.*, 2014b). Haloperidol has conventionally been used, starting at a very low dose, and then carefully titrated to

---

Box 14.3 Investigations for delirium

Blood tests

Full blood count
Urea and electrolytes
Renal function tests
Liver function tests
Calcium
Random blood glucose
Blood cultures
Arterial blood gas
Syphilis serology

Other tests

Urinalysis
Chest X-ray
Drug screen
Cardiac enzymes
MRI or CT brain scan
EEG
Lumbar puncture

---

achieve the desired calming effect without excess sedation or side effects. If necessary, the first dose can be given intramuscularly, followed by doses every 6 hours (typically 1–5 mg per day, although elderly patients may require less). Atypical antipsychotics are now often prescribed instead of haloperidol; the same principles of careful administration and monitoring apply. Some causes of delirium require avoidance of antipsychotics, or particular caution when using them. This includes all patients with coexisting dementia, especially dementia with Lewy bodies, (see page 368).

Antipsychotics should be avoided in delirium associated with alcohol withdrawal (delirium tremens; see page 570) or with epilepsy, because of the risk of seizures. In delirium tremens, a benzodiazepine is the standard treatment (either lorazepam or chlordiazepoxide; see page 581). All drugs should be used with caution in liver failure because of the danger of precipitating hepatic coma.

For a practical review of delirium management, see O'Connell *et al.* (2014).

Outcome

Many cases of delirium recover rapidly. The prognosis is related to the underlying cause, and is worse in the elderly and in those with pre-existing dementia or physical illness. Patients with a 'hypoactive' behavioural profile have a worse outcome than those who are 'hyperactive'. There is an elevated mortality rate following delirium, with an estimated 25% mortality at 3 months, although published estimates vary markedly; a recent meta-analysis of elderly patients found that an episode of delirium was associated with a twofold increased risk of death in the next 2 years (Witlox et al., 2010).

The relationship between delirium and dementia is complex and bidirectional (Inouye et al., 2014a). As noted earlier, pre-existing dementia is a major risk factor for delirium, and there is now increasing evidence that delirium has a role in the onset of dementia. The Witlox et al. (2010) meta-analysis reported a fivefold increase in incidence of dementia 2 years after an episode of delirium, and subsequent studies find similar or even greater effects (Davis et al., 2012). A large recent study shows that delirium acts synergistically with underlying dementia neuropathology to accelerate the pace of cognitive decline (Davis et al., 2017).

Amnesia and amnesic disorders

Amnesia is loss of memory, and *amnesic (also called amnestic) disorders or syndromes* are those in which episodic memory is specifically and persistently affected, and with a decline from previous level of functioning. In ICD-10 and in routine clinical practice, these criteria together distinguish amnesic disorders from dementia, delirium, or neurodevelopmental disorders (see Box 14.4). However, as noted earlier, DSM-5 subsumes amnesic disorders within the broader category of major neurocognitive disorder, removing the distinction from dementia.

Amnesic disorders manifest as an inability to learn new information (anterograde amnesia) and to recall past events (retrograde amnesia). To make the diagnosis, there should be a significant impairment in social or occupational functioning, and evidence of a general medical condition which can be aetiologically related to the memory impairment. *Korsakov syndrome* (also called *Korsakoff syndrome*) is sometimes erroneously referred to synonymously with amnesic disorder, but is in fact a specific form of it, as described below.

For a review of amnesia and amnesic disorders, see Markowitsch and Staniloiu (2012).

> ### Box 14.4 Causes of amnesia
>
> **Transient**
> Transient global amnesia
> Transient epileptic amnesia
> Head injury
> Alcoholic blackouts
> Post-electroconvulsive therapy
> Post-traumatic stress disorder
> Psychogenic fugue
> Amnesia for criminal offence
>
> **Persistent** (amnestic syndrome)
> Korsakov syndrome
> Herpes encephalitis
> Posterior cerebral artery and thalamic strokes
> Head injury

Clinical features

The cardinal feature is a profound deficit in episodic memory. The full clinical picture is striking. There is disorientation for time, loss of autobiographical information (often extending back for many years), severe anterograde amnesia for verbal and visual material, and lack of insight into the amnesia. Events are recalled immediately after they occur, but forgotten a few minutes later. Thus the digit span, which tests the short-term memory store, is typically normal. New learning is grossly defective, but retrograde memory is variably preserved and shows a temporal gradient, with older memories being better preserved. Other cognitive functions are relatively intact, although some emotional blunting and inertia are often observed.

The other classic feature, seen particularly in Korsakov syndrome, is *confabulation*, in which gaps in memory are filled by a vivid and detailed but wholly fictitious account of recent activities, which the patient believes to be true. The confabulating patient is often highly suggestible.

Aetiology and pathology

Amnesia results from lesions in the medial thalamus, other midline diencephalic structures, or medial temporal lobes (hippocampus and adjacent temporal cortex) (Markowitsch and Staniloiu, 2012). Cases due to damage in the medial temporal lobe typically produce the 'purest' amnesia, with little in the way of disorientation or confabulation; these features are characteristic of thalamic and diencephalic lesions.

Korsakov syndrome

The commonest cause of amnesic disorder is *Korsakov syndrome*, named after the Russian neuropsychiatrist who described it in 1889. The alternative term, *Wernicke–Korsakov syndrome*, was proposed by Victor *et al.* (1971), because the syndrome often follows an acute neurological syndrome called *Wernicke's encephalopathy*, consisting of delirium, ataxia, pupillary abnormalities, ophthalmoplegia, nystagmus, and a peripheral neuropathy. Korsakov syndrome is usually caused by thiamine deficiency, secondary to alcohol abuse, although it occasionally results from other causes, such as hyperemesis gravidarum and severe malnutrition (Scalzo *et al.*, 2015). The classic neuropathological findings are neuronal loss, gliosis, and microhaemorrhages in the periaqueductal and paraventricular grey matter, the mammillary bodies, and the anterior and mediodorsal thalamus (Kril and Harper, 2012).

Other causes of amnesic syndrome include tumours and infarcts in the medial thalamus (diencephalic amnesia) and encephalitis.

Investigation and management

Alertness to the possibility of amnesic syndrome is essential; the patient may not fit the stereotype of chronic alcohol misuse associated with Korsakov syndrome, and this is a potentially reversible condition. Useful findings from investigations include a reduced red cell transketolase level, which is a marker of thiamine deficiency, and an increased MRI signal in midline structures.

In practice, Korsakov syndrome should be assumed to be the cause of amnesic syndrome until another aetiology (see Box 14.5) can be demonstrated, and should be treated urgently with thiamine without awaiting the results of investigations. Thiamine is given parenterally in an acute presentation, together with rehydration, general nutritional support, and treatment of supervening alcohol withdrawal. Thiamine replacement should always precede administration of intravenous glucose-containing solutions. Close liaison with physicians and neurologists is important. Apart from thiamine, there are no interventions of proven efficacy for amnesic disorders.

In the longer term, amnesic syndrome may require substantial rehabilitation and support, as the condition markedly impairs normal activities and ability to provide self-care.

Course and prognosis

In the series of Victor *et al.* (1971), consisting of 245 patients with Wernicke–Korsakov syndrome, 96% of the patients presented with Wernicke's encephalopathy. Mortality was 17% in the acute stage, and 84% of the survivors developed a typical amnesic syndrome. There was no improvement in 50% of cases, complete recovery in 25%, and partial recovery in the remainder. Favourable prognostic factors were a short history before diagnosis and prompt commencement of thiamine replacement.

The prognosis is poor in cases of amnesic syndrome resulting from viral encephalitis and other causes of irreversible bilateral hippocampal or diencephalic damage. However, amnesic syndrome owing to head injury has a better outlook. Progressive amnesia suggests a slowly expanding structural lesion, such as a midbrain tumour.

Transient global amnesia

The syndrome of *transient global amnesia* is important in the differential diagnosis of paroxysmal neurological and psychiatric disturbance (see Box 14.5). It occurs in middle or late life. The clinical picture is of sudden onset of isolated, often profound, anterograde amnesia in a clear sensorium, generally lasting for between 15 minutes and 24 hours. Functional imaging studies during transient global amnesia have demonstrated localized transient hypoperfusion or hyperperfusion consistent with dysfunction of circuits that mediate episodic memory.

Box 14.5 Differential diagnosis of transient amnesia and other paroxysmal neuropsychiatric symptoms

Organic

Syncope (cardiogenic, vasovagal, reflex)

Transient ischaemic attacks

Migraine

Epileptic seizure (ictal or post-ictal)

Hypoglycaemia

Phaeochromocytoma

Transient global amnesia

Narcolepsy and other parasomnias

Tonic spasms of multiple sclerosis

Treatment-related complications in Parkinson's disease

Drug abuse

Medial temporal lobe tumour

Functional

Panic attacks and hyperventilation

Dissociative disorder

Schizophrenia

Bipolar affective disorder

Aggressive outburst in personality disorder

Temper tantrums (in children)

Breath-holding spells (in children)

The patient appears bewildered, and requires repeated reorientation, only to ask the same questions moments later. However, there is no disturbance of alertness, and (in contrast to psychogenic fugue) personal identity is retained. Procedural memory is spared—for example, the patient may carry on driving competently during the episode. Apart from the memory disturbance, the neurological examination is entirely normal.

Complete recovery, with amnesia for the period of the episode, is usual and recurrence is rare. However, investigation is always indicated, to exclude other causes of amnesia (see above and Box 14.5). Patients with transient global amnesia often present as emergencies, and the syndrome may be misdiagnosed as a dissociative fugue.

For a review see Arena and Rabinstein (2015).

Dementia

Dementia is an acquired global impairment of intellect, memory, and personality, but without impairment of consciousness (Burns and Illiffe, 2009). It is usually but not always progressive. The syndrome of dementia is caused by a wide range of diseases, but the majority of cases are due to Alzheimer's disease, which is the commonest cause, followed by vascular dementia and dementia with Lewy bodies (Box 14.6). Only a small proportion of cases (4% in one large series) are currently potentially reversible (Hejl *et al.*, 2002).

Although dementia is a global or generalized disorder, it often begins with focal cognitive or behavioural disturbances. However, ICD-10 requires impairment in two or more cognitive domains (memory, language, abstract thinking and judgement, praxis, visuoperceptual skills, personality, and social conduct), sufficient to interfere with social or occupational functioning. Deficits may be too mild or circumscribed to fulfil this definition, and are then called *mild cognitive impairment* (see page 360).

In this section, the main features of the dementia syndrome are described, followed by the principles of assessment. We then discuss the clinical, aetiological, and neuropathological features of the major diseases that produce dementia. Note in Box 14.6 that many other neuropsychiatric disorders and some medical disorders can also include cognitive impairment; these conditions are considered later in this chapter and in Chapter 22, respectively. Dementia as a result of substance misuse, especially alcohol misuse, is discussed in Chapter 20. The management of dementia, and the relationships between dementia and ageing, are deferred until Chapter 19.

Box 14.6 Causes of dementia

Primary neurodegenerative disorders

Alzheimer's disease*, dementia with Lewy bodies, frontotemporal dementias*,
Parkinson's disease*, prion diseases*, Huntington's disease*

Vascular causes

Vascular dementia*, strokes, focal thalamic and basal ganglia strokes, subdural haematoma

Inflammatory and autoimmune causes

Systemic lupus erythematosus, other forms of cerebral vasculitis, Behçet's disease, neurosarcoidosis, Hashimoto's encephalopathy, multiple sclerosis

Trauma

Severe head injury, repeated head trauma ('dementia pugilistica')

Infections and related conditions

HIV, iatrogenic and variant CJD (prion disease), neuro-syphilis, postencephalitic

Metabolic and endocrine causes

Renal failure, hepatic failure, hypothyroidism, hyperthyroidism,

hypoglycaemia, Cushing's syndrome, hypopituitarism, adrenal insufficiency

Neoplastic causes

Intracranial space-occupying lesions, carcinomatous or lymphomatous meningitis, paraneoplastic limbic encephalitis

Post-radiation

Acute and subacute radionecrosis, radiation thromboangiopathy

Post-anoxia

Severe anaemia, post-surgical (especially cardiac bypass), carbon monoxide poisoning, cardiac arrest, chronic respiratory failure

Vitamin and other nutritional deficiencies

Vitamin B_{12} deficiency, folate deficiency

Toxins

Alcohol, poisoning with heavy metals, organic solvents, organophosphates

Other

Normal-pressure hydrocephalus
Leucodystrophy*

* Can occur in genetically determined forms.

Clinical features of dementia

The presenting complaint is usually of poor memory. Other features include disturbances of behaviour, language, personality, mood, or perception.

The clinical picture is much determined by the patient's premorbid personality, as well as by the underlying cause. People with good social skills may continue to function adequately despite severe intellectual deterioration. Dementia is often exposed by a change in social circumstances or an intercurrent illness. The elderly, socially isolated, or deaf are less likely to compensate for failing intellectual abilities; however, their difficulties may go unrecognized or be dismissed.

Forgetfulness is usually early and prominent, but may sometimes be difficult to detect in the early stages. Impaired attention and concentration are common and non-specific. Difficulty with new learning is usually the most conspicuous feature. Memory loss is more evident for recent than for more remote material. Disturbed episodic memory is manifested as forgetfulness for recent day-to-day events, with relative preservation of procedural memory (e.g. how to ride a bicycle) and, at least initially, general knowledge about the world at large. By contrast, words and, ultimately, the very objects to which they refer, lose their meaning for patients with semantic memory impairment (as in certain frontotemporal dementias).

Loss of flexibility and adaptability in new situations, with the appearance of rigid and stereotyped routines ('organic orderliness'), and, when taxed beyond restricted abilities, sudden explosions of rage or grief ('catastrophic reaction') may occur. As dementia worsens, patients are less able to care for themselves and they neglect social conventions. Disorientation for time, and later for place and person, is common. Behaviour becomes aimless, and stereotypies and mannerisms may appear. Thinking slows and becomes impoverished in content and perseverative. False ideas, often of a persecutory kind, gain ground easily. In the later stages, thinking becomes grossly fragmented and incoherent. This is reflected in the patient's speech, with syntactical and dysnomic errors. Eventually the patient may become mute. Mortality is increased, with death often following bronchopneumonia and a terminal coma (Mitchell *et al.*, 2009).

Behavioural, affective, and psychotic features often accompany the cognitive deficits. They appear to be part of the underlying biology of the disease process, although in the early stages, while insight is retained, they may also be a psychological response to the realization of cognitive decline. Mood disturbances are particularly common, together with distress, anxiety, irritability, and sometimes aggression. Later, emotional responses become blunted, and sudden, apparently random, mood changes occur. Psychotic symptoms are also a common and fluctuating feature during dementia.

The balance of these core symptoms and signs, together with some additional features, forms the basis for the clinical differentiation between the various causes of dementia, as summarized in Table 14.2 and described in the following sections.

Subcortical and cortical dementia

A distinction is sometimes drawn between subcortical and cortical dementia, based upon their putative neuroanatomical basis. Although the distinction is blurred, clinically and pathologically, the terms have descriptive utility (Turner *et al.*, 2002). The key features are summarized in Table 14.3, and examples of the diseases are listed in Box 14.7. The term *subcortical dementia* is seen to refer to a syndrome of slowness of thought, difficulty with complex, sequential intellectual tasks, and impoverishment of affect and personality, with relative preservation of language, calculation, and learning. It contrasts with the spectrum of dysfunction (including early, prominent impairments of memory, word finding, or visuospatial abilities) that is seen in *cortical dementias*.

Presenile and senile dementia

Another traditional distinction was that made between dementia occurring in those under 65 years of age (presenile or early-onset dementia) and dementia beginning later in life (senile or late-onset dementia). It arose in part because of the belief that the major causes were different—Alzheimer's disease in the former, and

vascular dementia in the latter. With the realization that Alzheimer's disease is the commonest form of dementia in both groups, less attention is now paid to this categorization. However, presenile dementia does differ in certain respects from late-onset dementia (Rossor *et al.*, 2010). Frontotemporal dementia and prion disease are relatively more common, vascular dementia is rarer, and a higher proportion of cases are due to genetic diseases. Patients with presenile dementia are more likely to be referred to and investigated by neurologists before psychiatrists become involved in their care. Investigations are more intensive and extensive to give a definite diagnosis and provide a clear prognosis. The clinical course tends to be more rapid than in late-onset cases.

Assessment of dementia

Assessment of a patient who is presenting with a complaint of cognitive impairment involves several stages. A key question to be addressed initially is whether the impairment is due to dementia. This involves ruling out other causes, notably delirium, amnesia, and depression. Other patients will have mild cognitive impairment.

Having established the probable diagnosis of dementia, its characteristics (including severity, symptom and behaviour profile, and associated risks) are considered, together with assessment of its cause, and identification of potentially reversible causes. In the study mentioned earlier, the latter consisted mostly of hydrocephalus and space-occupying lesions (Hejl *et al.*, 2002).

Assessment of the severity and clinical profile

Screening tests are useful in the assessment of dementia and its severity, and for monitoring progression. Different scales are available to assess cognition, behavioural symptoms, global functioning and activities of daily living, and depression; the latter is useful because depression can coexist with dementia and worsen functioning. Some commonly used screening tests, most of which take 10 minutes or less, are listed in Box 14.8. For review of screening tests for dementia, see Sheehan (2012) and Velayudhan *et al.* (2014).

For cognitive impairment, the benchmark is the Mini-Mental State Examination (MMSE), which has a sensitivity and specificity for dementia of around 80% when a cut-off score of 23 is chosen (Mitchell, 2009). The MoCA and clock test are valuable and brief alternatives. The ADAS-cog is specifically designed for suspected Alzheimer's disease, and is widely used in clinical trials

Table 14.2 Clinical features that help to distinguish between major causes of dementia

	Prominent symptoms and signs	Other clinical features
Alzheimer's disease	Memory loss, especially short-term	Relentlessly progressive
	Dysphasia and dyspraxia	Survival 5–8 years
	Sense of smell impaired early on	
	Behavioural changes (e.g. wandering)	
Vascular dementia	Personality change	Stepwise progression
	Labile mood	Signs of cerebrovascular disease
	Preserved insight	History of hypertension
		Commoner in men, and in smokers
Dementia with Lewy bodies	Fluctuating alertness	Frequent adverse reactions to antipsychotics
	Parkinsonism	
	Visual hallucinations	
	Falls and faints	
Frontotemporal dementia	Prominent behavioural change	Onset usually before the age of 70 years
	Expressive dysphasia	Range of clinical subtypes
	Early loss of insight	
	Early primitive reflexes	
Prion disease	Myoclonic jerks	Often early-onset
	Seizures	Rapid onset and progression
	Cerebellar ataxia	Transmissible
	Psychiatric symptoms (vCJD)	
Normal-pressure hydrocephalus	Mental slowing, apathy, inattention	Commonest in 50–70-year age group
	Urinary incontinence	Commonest reversible dementia
	Problems walking (gait apraxia)	

to monitor treatment response. The CAMCOG is largely a research tool. Note that these tests are validated for use in the diagnosis of dementia, and are not recommended for 'case finding' in the population (Brown, 2015).

Careful evaluation of the behavioural symptoms of dementia is an integral part of the assessment, and needs to be repeated during the illness, since these symptoms are common, fluctuate, and pose many difficulties for carers.

Assessment of the cause of dementia

Definitive diagnosis of the cause of dementia can usually only be made neuropathologically or, in rare cases, by identification of genetic mutations. However, the differing profiles of the various dementias allow 'probable' diagnoses to be made by experienced clinicians with reasonable accuracy. The use of biochemical, radiological, and genetic investigations only modestly

Table 14.3 **Features of cortical and subcortical dementias**

	Subcortical dementia	Cortical dementia
Memory impairment	Moderate	Severe, early
Language	Normal	Dysphasias, early
Mathematical skills	Preserved	Impaired, early
Personality	Apathetic, inert	Indifferent
Mood	Flat, depressed	Normal
Coordination	Impaired	Normal
Cognitive and motor speed	Slowed	Normal
Abnormal movements	Common, e.g. tremor	Rare

increases the diagnostic accuracy for common dementias, but is important for ruling out rarer and reversible causes. Box 14.9 summarizes the investigations for dementia. An MRI or CT scan is recommended as routine in many guidelines but, in practice, brain scanning, like most investigations, is used in some but not all patients. Recent findings have shown the value of PET imaging with ligands to detect β-amyloid, and of CSF measurement of specific proteins in the differential diagnosis of dementia (Skillback *et al.*, 2015; Scheltens *et al.*, 2016). However, these tests are not yet routinely available. The extent to which investigations are carried out, as well as the addition of more specialized tests, depends upon the patient's age and history, the results of the initial tests, and the subsequent differential diagnosis.

Assessment of risk in dementia

Patients with dementia are at risk from self-neglect, poor judgement, wandering, and abuse. Their physical health is often a problem. Risks to others may occur because of aggressive or disinhibited behaviour. Fitness to drive is a specific issue to consider, and may be difficult to determine in the early stages (Wilson and Pinner, 2013); current UK regulations allow those with 'sufficient skills' and whose 'progression [of dementia] is slow' to continue to drive, subject to annual review. Thus risk assessment is part of a full assessment of dementia. A good history from carers and other informants is essential, and an occupational therapist has an important role to play in assessment of functional ability.

Early detection of dementia

Mild cognitive impairment

Increasing attention is being given to the earlier diagnosis of dementia in those with equivocal evidence, or subjective complaints, of worsening memory. This is in part driven by the research focus on developing treatments to delay or prevent progression to dementia. This intermediate category, which was introduced in ICD-10, is called *mild cognitive impairment (MCI)*. In people presenting with features of MCI, it is important to consider

---

Box 14.7 Examples of cortical, subcortical, and mixed causes of dementia

Cortical

Alzheimer's disease
Frontotemporal dementias

Subcortical

Huntington's disease
Parkinson's disease
Focal thalamic and basal ganglia lesions
Multiple sclerosis

Mixed

Vascular dementia
Dementia with Lewy bodies
Corticobasal degeneration

Box 14.8 Screening tests for dementia

Cognitive function

Mini-Mental State Examination (MMSE)
Six-Item Cognitive Impairment Test
Seven-minute screen
Clock drawing test
Hopkins Verbal Learning Test (HVLT)
Mental Test Score (MTS)
Alzheimer's Disease Assessment Scale—cognitive subscale (ADAS-cog)
Montreal Cognitive Assessment (MoCA)
Cambridge Examination for Mental Disorders of the Elderly, cognitive section (CAMCOG)

Behavioural and psychological features

Neuropsychiatric Inventory
MOUSEPAD
BEHAVE-AD
Cohen—Mansfield Aggression Inventory

Activities of daily living

Bristol Scale
Alzheimer's Disease Functional Assessment and Change Scale
Disability Assessment for Dementia

Depression

Cornell Scale
Geriatric Depression Rating Scale

Global assessment

Clinical Dementia Rating (CDR)

Box 14.9 Investigations for establishing the cause of dementia

In primary care

Full blood count
Erythrocyte sedimentation rate
Urea and electrolytes
Liver function tests
Calcium and phosphate
Thyroid function tests
Vitamin B_{12} and folate

In secondary care

MRI or CT brain scan
Urinalysis
Syphilis serology
HIV status
Chest radiograph
Neuropsychological assessment
Genetic testing[*]
EEG[*]
PET: amyloid or fluorodeoxyglucose imaging[*]
CSF: measurement of amyloid Aβ1-42 and tau[*]

[*]Tests not routinely available.

Adapted from The BMJ, 338, Burns A and Illiffe S, Dementia, b75, Copyright (2009), with permission from BMJ Publishing Group Ltd.

and exclude depression and other 'non-dementia' causes of cognitive impairments. *Amnesic MCI* refers to cases in which memory loss is the most prominent feature, and which is thought to be prodromal Alzheimer's disease.

It is important to note that the clinical and prognostic significance of MCI remains unclear. Only 5–20% of patients convert to dementia each year, and 40–70% of MCI patients have not progressed to dementia 10 years later. For review of MCI, see Langa and Levine (2014); for management of MCI see page 560.

Presymptomatic diagnosis and biomarkers

There is increasing evidence that dementia, especially Alzheimer's disease, can be detected premorbidly, long before overt symptoms of any kind (including MCI) are present. The category of *preclinical Alzheimer's disease*, or *at-risk for Alzheimer's disease*, has been introduced to describe people with evidence of Alzheimer's pathology (from biomarker studies, discussed below) but who are cognitively intact.

Features and biomarkers of the preclinical and prodromal phase of Alzheimer's disease are listed in Table 14.4. Longitudinal studies show that there are selective and characteristic neuropsychological impairments detectable up to 20 years before the onset of symptoms. Olfactory deficits are also a simple and valuable marker (Devenand *et al.*, 2015). Imaging and CSF biomarkers are also positive well in advance of clinical disease. The most sensitive and specific biomarkers are provided by the PET imaging and CSF protein markers, but the availability of these in clinical practice is limited. Hippocampal atrophy, either determined visually or quantitatively, using CT or MRI, is a more feasible imaging biomarker. The occurrence of these various biomarkers is consistent with the realization that the neuropathological changes begin, and progress, decades before the onset of Alzheimer's disease dementia (Braak and Del Tredici, 2015).

For review of biomarkers in preclinical and early dementia, see Jack *et al.* (2013) and Scheltens *et al.* (2016). The use of biomarkers in the differential diagnosis of established dementia was considered earlier.

Alzheimer's disease

In 1907, Alois Alzheimer reported the case of Auguste D, a woman with presenile dementia whose brain exhibited unusual neuropathological features. It was Alzheimer's colleague, Emil Kraepelin, who named the disease (Maurer *et al.*, 1997). For many years the disease was thought to be rare and limited to presenile forms of dementia, but classic studies by Roth and colleagues (Blessed *et al.*, 1968) suggested that it is the commonest cause of senile dementia, a conclusion that has been confirmed by many subsequent studies. About 60% of dementia is attributable to Alzheimer's disease (Neuropathology Group of the Medical Research Council Cognitive Function and Ageing Study, 2001), occurring either in isolation or together with features of vascular dementia and other neurodegenerative disorders. The rate of Alzheimer's disease doubles every 5 years in the elderly, with an overall prevalence in those aged 60 or older of 5–7%. See Chapter 19, page 542 for the epidemiology of Alzheimer's disease.

For reviews of Alzheimer's disease, see Lovestone (2009a) and Scheltens *et al.* (2016).

Clinical features

The main features of dementia have been described above, and Box 14.10 summarizes the clinical features of Alzheimer's disease (strictly, 'dementia of the Alzheimer type', since formal diagnosis awaits neuropathology) (see also Lovestone, 2009a).

The first evidence of the condition is often minor forgetfulness, which may be difficult to distinguish from normal ageing. The condition progresses gradually for the first 2–4 years, with increasing memory disturbance

Table 14.4 Possible biomarkers of preclinical Alzheimer's disease

Clinical	Comments
Neuropsychological deficits	E.g. in verbal episodic memory
Olfactory deficits	
Biochemical	
Cerebrospinal fluid	
Amyloid Aβ42	Correlates with cortical amyloid deposition
Total tau	Correlates with intensity of neurodegeneration
Phosphorylated tau	Correlates with neurofibrillary changes
Brain imaging	
Structural	
Hippocampal atrophy	More apparent and progressive than in controls
Functional	
Fluorodeoxyglucose PET	Normal scan has high negative predictive value
Amyloid PET	Normal scan has high negative predictive value
Tau PET	Not yet in clinical use

and lack of spontaneity. Memory is lost for recent events first. Language is usually affected early on, with difficulty in finding words or naming objects, and impairments in the ability to construct fluent and informative sentences. Visuospatial skills may be affected, with difficulties in tasks such as copying pictures or learning the way round unfamiliar environments (e.g. when on holiday or in an unfamiliar house). Disorientation in time gives rise to poorly kept appointments and changes in the diurnal pattern of activity.

Depression

The relationship between Alzheimer's disease and depression is complex. Depression is a probable risk factor for the disease, may be confused with it, or may occur as part of the syndrome. Regarding the latter point, major depression occurs in about 10% of cases, with less marked episodes and symptoms occurring in

> ## Box 14.10 Key clinical features of Alzheimer's disease
>
> ### Core features
>
> Memory impairment (amnesia), with gradual onset and continuing decline
>
> Aphasia
>
> Apraxia
>
> Agnosia
>
> Anosmia
>
> Disturbance in executive functioning (e.g. planning, reasoning)
>
> ### Other features
>
> Depression
>
> Psychosis
>
> Behavioural symptoms (e.g. agitation, wandering)
>
> Personality change

over 50% of cases. Patients who experience depression have greater decreases in serotonin and noradrenergic markers than other patients with Alzheimer's disease.

Psychotic symptoms

Delusions and hallucinations occur in a significant minority of patients at some stage in the illness. Their prevalence is unclear, as many studies did not distinguish Alzheimer's disease from dementia with Lewy bodies (see below). Recent estimates suggest rates of 10–50% for delusions and 10–25% for hallucinations. The commonest delusions are persecutory, concerning theft (however, as this idea often arises from the patient's forgetfulness, it is questionable whether it is helpful to regard this as a true delusion).

Behaviour

Changes in behaviour are common, and are of particular concern to carers. The patient may be restless and wake at night, disorientated, and perplexed. Motor activity may increase in the evening ('*sundowning*'), and eventually the sleep–wake cycle may become completely disorganized. *Aggression* (both verbal and physical) is common, and often takes the form of resistance to help with personal care. Serious physical violence towards others is rare. Both increases and reductions in level of activity are common, involving varying degrees of purposefulness. *Wandering* can refer to a variety of different

behaviours, but patients may place themselves at risk by going into unsafe environments. Patients with dementia may undereat or overeat, with associated changes in weight and nutritional state. Changes in sexual behaviour occur, usually with a reduction in drive, although sexual disinhibition occasionally occurs.

Self-care and social behaviour decline, although some patients maintain a good social facade despite severe cognitive impairment, particularly if carers are able to assist with these functions.

Course

In the early stages of Alzheimer's disease, the clinical features are modified by the patient's premorbid personality, and their traits tend to be exaggerated. In the middle and later stages of the illness, the cognitive impairments increasingly predominate, together with the neurological and behavioural features noted above. Incidental physical illness may cause a superimposed delirium, resulting in a sudden deterioration in cognitive function. Median survival from diagnosis is 5–7 years, and is slightly less in men than in women. Shorter survival is also associated with an older age of onset, and a rapid rate of cognitive decline.

Investigations

The investigation of suspected Alzheimer's disease follows the same principles as the investigation of dementia in general, outlined above. In addition, a comment on genetic testing is warranted. Such testing is indicated in the very rare cases of familial early-onset Alzheimer's disease, for which three causative genes are known (see below). Although the apoE4 allele of the apolipoprotein E gene is a major risk factor in all forms of Alzheimer's disease (see below and Box 5.4), routine testing for this variant in the differential diagnosis of dementia is not recommended, and there is no place for genetic screening of healthy subjects to predict future dementia. The scientific and ethical issues involved have been discussed by Loy *et al.* (2014).

Neuropathology

On gross examination the brain is shrunken, with widened sulci and enlarged ventricles. Brain weight is reduced. On microscopic examination, the cardinal diagnostic features are *neurofibrillary tangles* and *senile plaques* (also called *amyloid plaques*) in the cerebral cortex and many subcortical regions. The diagnostic criteria are based upon the abundance and distribution of plaques and tangles—the Consortium to Establish a Registry for Alzheimer's Disease (CERAD) criteria (Mirra *et al.*, 1991).

However, it should be noted that these features are also seen, to some extent, in some non-demented elderly people, and the relationship between clinical dementia and neuropathology is more complex than is sometimes assumed to be the case.

In addition to the tangles and plaques, there is selective loss of neurons in the hippocampus and entorhinal cortex, proliferation of astrocytes (gliosis), and loss of synapses. The latter is the strongest neuropathological correlate of cognitive impairment. Other histological findings include amyloid deposits in blood vessel walls (so-called *vascular amyloid* or *congophilic angiopathy*), *Hirano bodies* (intracellular crystalline deposits) and *granulovacuolar accumulation* (vacuoles or 'holes' within neurons).

For a review of the neuropathology of Alzheimer's disease, see Duyckaerts *et al.* (2009).

Progression of neuropathology

The disease process starts in the entorhinal cortex, before spreading to the hippocampus, association areas of the parietal lobe, and some subcortical nuclei. Six neuropathological stages based upon β-amyloid deposition are recognized, called *Braak stages*, which correlate with clinical severity (Braak and Braak, 1991), and which complement the evidence noted earlier that the onset of neuropathology long precedes the symptoms of dementia (Braak and Del Tredici, 2015). The spread of pathology along cortico-cortical projections leads to an effective 'disconnection' between affected regions.

Senile (amyloid) plaques

Senile plaques are deposits of insoluble proteins, together with degenerating neurites (neuronal processes) and glia. They occur in the space between neurons (the neuropil). Both neuritic and diffuse plaques are recognized, depending on their appearance using silver stains; neuritic plaques have a dense-staining core, whereas diffuse plaques have been likened to cotton wool. The neuritic plaques are pathologically more significant. The protein at the heart of all senile plaques is β-amyloid (also called amyloid-β, Aβ, or βA4), a 39–42-amino acid peptide. This molecule and its encoding gene are central to the aetiology of the disease (see below).

Neurofibrillary tangles

Neurofibrillary tangles occur within the cell body of neurons, especially pyramidal neurons of the cerebral cortex and hippocampus. They are formed of paired helical filaments, which are comprised of the microtubule-associated protein tau. The normal function of tau is in axonal transport and maintenance of the neuronal cytoskeleton. Tangles are thought to occur because tau becomes hyperphosphorylated, rendering it insoluble. The presence of a tangle causes dysfunction and death of the neuron.

Aetiology and pathogenesis

Genes

In rare families, usually those with an early onset of illness (before the age of 60 years), there is an autosomal dominant mode of inheritance. Causative mutations have been identified in three genes—amyloid precursor protein (*APP*, on chromosome 21), presenilin 1 (*PSEN1*, on chromosome 14), and presenilin 2 (*PSEN2*, on chromosome 1). Discovery of *APP* as the first 'Alzheimer gene' was a seminal event (see Box 14.11). These three genes together account for most familial cases of the disease, but at least one other gene is likely to exist. Different mutations are known in each gene, and the age of onset, features, and progression of disease vary depending on the causative mutation.

Despite the importance of these findings, the vast majority of Alzheimer's disease is not inherited in a Mendelian fashion, and it is often termed 'sporadic'. However, first-degree relatives of patients with late-onset Alzheimer's disease have an elevated risk of developing the disorder, and a genetic predisposition is now confirmed by the unequivocal association between polymorphisms in the apolipoprotein E (*apoE*) gene and all forms of Alzheimer's disease. As discussed in Box 5.4, the *apoE4* variant of this gene accounts for about 50% of the vulnerability to late-onset Alzheimer's disease. Its main effect is to promote an earlier onset of disease, by about a decade. *ApoE4* heterozygotes have a threefold greater risk, and homozygotes have an eightfold greater risk of the disease. Other data suggest that *apoE4*-positive cases may show some differences from *apoE4*-negative cases in terms of pathology, course, and response to medication. In Caucasians, the *apoE2* variant reduces the risk of Alzheimer's disease (compared with the commonest *apoE3* form), but this does not hold in all other ethnic groups. The (lack of a) role of genetic testing for *apoE4* was mentioned above. It is stressed that *apoE4* is not a determinant of disease; at least one-third of patients with Alzheimer's disease are *apoE4*-negative, and many *apoE4* homozygotes never develop the disease. It is not known how *apoE4* elevates the risk of Alzheimer's disease, but it is likely to reflect its interaction with β-amyloid metabolism and clearance from the brain, cholesterol metabolism, and other cellular functions (Liu *et al.*, 2013).

For review of Alzheimer's disease genetics, see Karch and Goate (2015).

Box 14.11 Discovery of *APP* gene mutations in familial Alzheimer's disease

In 1984, the protein that accumulates in senile plaques, cerebral vasculature, and meninges in Alzheimer's disease was discovered to be the β-amyloid peptide. Knowledge of its amino acid sequence allowed the encoding gene, called amyloid precursor protein (*APP*), to be identified and localized to chromosome 21. It was already known that there was a relationship between Alzheimer's disease and Down's syndrome (trisomy 21), suggesting that *APP* was a 'candidate gene' for Alzheimer's disease. Researchers collected DNA from families with autosomal dominant Alzheimer's disease to test this hypothesis. The work culminated in the landmark discovery in 1991 of an *APP* mutation (a point mutation changing valine to isoleucine at position 717), which caused Alzheimer's disease (Goate *et al.,* 1991). Since then, different *APP* mutations have been found in other families. Any doubt that the *APP* mutations are causative for the disease was removed by the demonstration that transgenic mice containing a mutated *APP* gene become cognitively impaired and deposit β-amyloid (Games *et al.,* 1995). *APP* mutations are pathogenic primarily because they affect metabolism of APP, promoting the formation of β-amyloid. The other two genes causing familial Alzheimer's disease are the presenilins (*PSEN1* and *PSEN2*). They provide the catalytic subunit for the enzyme that cleaves APP, called γ-secretase, and hence all three genes share a common influence on APP processing. *APP* and *PSEN* mutations explain most cases of familial Alzheimer's disease, but only a tiny fraction (<0.1%) of all cases of Alzheimer's disease. However, mis-metabolism of APP and β-amyloid, caused by a range of other factors, is involved in all forms of Alzheimer's disease, as described in the text.

There is now statistically convincing evidence for about 20 other susceptibility genes for Alzheimer's disease. Many of these contain common variants with small effects on disease risk (e.g. *CLU, PICALM*), while a few genes (e.g. *TREM2*) have rarer variants with larger effect sizes. All are of much lesser importance, epidemiologically speaking, than *apoE4*. They implicate pathways involved in immune function, inflammatory responses, and lipid recycling.

Environmental factors

Various environmental factors are associated with an altered risk of developing dementia in general, or Alzheimer's disease in particular (see Box 14.12). However, for many of them, it is not clear to what extent they are causal, act independently, or interact with genetic predisposition.

The most powerful studies are those in which people have been followed up since early adulthood or middle age. These have revealed that a number of 'lifestyle' factors, such as diabetes, and physical and mental inactivity, as well as indices of vascular health, present at or before middle age, predict later onset of dementia, especially Alzheimer's disease. This relationship indicates the potential for primary prevention, but this has yet to be fully explored (Norton *et al.,* 2014). The robust finding that higher levels of educational attainment, as well as cognitive activity, are protective against Alzheimer's disease, supports a 'use it or lose it' hypothesis, whereby such attributes are thought to increase cerebral reserve. The relationship between body mass index in middle age and dementia is unclear; several studies report an association with obesity, but a large UK population database found that low body mass index in middle age predicted later dementia (Qizilibash *et al.,* 2015).

With regard to non-steroidal anti-inflammatory drugs (NSAIDs), hormone replacement therapy (HRT), and statins, there is considerable evidence that people who have used these drugs have a decreased rate of dementia and Alzheimer's disease (Wong *et al.,* 2013b). For each class of drug there is also a plausible biological explanation for this effect. On the other hand, randomized trials have failed to find any beneficial effect of these drugs in treating or preventing dementia. The significance of the observational data is therefore unclear. Aluminium exposure has been implicated, but the evidence is weak, and it is not an established risk factor for Alzheimer's disease.

The amyloid cascade hypothesis

The *APP* research summarized in Box 14.11 led to the 'amyloid cascade hypothesis', originated by Hardy and Higgins (1992), which became the dominant molecular model for the disorder. It proposes that the central, pathogenic event is increased formation and deposition of β-amyloid, particularly the 42-amino acid variant. APP is a transmembrane protein, which can be cleaved by one of three enzymes, called secretases. Normally, α-secretase

> ### Box 14.12 Risk factors for non-familial Alzheimer's disease
>
> **Demographic factors**
>
> Increasing age
> Family history
> Down's syndrome
>
> **Genetic factors**
>
> *ApoE4*
> Other genetic polymorphisms
>
> **Environmental and medical risk factors**
>
> Low educational attainment
> Head injury
> Cerebrovascular disease
> History of depression
> History of dementia
> High homocysteine levels
> Diabetes mellitus
> Herpes simplex virus
>
> **Protective factors**
>
> Cognitive and physical activity in mid-life
> Mediterranean diet
> ?Use of non-steroidal anti-inflammatory drugs (NSAIDs)
> ?Use of hormone replacement therapy (HRT)
> ?Use of statins

activity predominates, and this does not give rise to β-amyloid. However, in Alzheimer's disease, more APP is processed via β- and γ-secretase pathways, leading to increased β-amyloid formation. The increased production of β-amyloid leads to disease because it tends to aggregate, becomes insoluble, and is toxic to synapses and neurons. Decreased removal of β-amyloid from the brain also contributes. The other pathological changes of Alzheimer's disease, including neurofibrillary tangles and the involvement of tau, are all seen as downstream in the causal process.

Although the amyloid cascade hypothesis is a convincing explanation of familial Alzheimer's disease, its relevance to sporadic forms of the disease remains controversial (Harrison and Owen, 2016). For example, PET imaging has shown that cortical β-amyloid pathology is common in cognitively healthy elderly individuals,

suggesting that additional factors are required for development of dementia (Jansen *et al.*, 2015). It is currently thought that β-amyloid is only one component of a more complex, non-linear, process, which also involves tau protein, and a range of other molecules and events (Jack *et al.*, 2013; Krstic and Knuesel, 2013). In one formulation, β-amyloid is a necessary, but not sufficient, cause for Alzheimer's disease (Musiek and Holtzman, 2015).

Inflammatory mechanisms

Inflammation, including microglial activation, is a well-known component of the neuropathology of Alzheimer's disease, but until recently was generally considered to be a response to the ongoing neurodegeneration. However, inflammatory, and immune, factors are now thought to be an important part of the disease process itself (Krstic and Knuesel, 2013). The evidence is diverse. It includes interactions with β-amyloid, and the fact that *TREM2*, one of the risk genes for Alzheimer's disease mentioned above, is a microglial receptor involved in β-amyloid clearance. For review, see Heppner *et al.* (2015).

The cholinergic hypothesis

Prior to the amyloid hypothesis, the prevailing view was the *cholinergic hypothesis* of Alzheimer's disease, based on findings in the 1970s that there is a severe and widespread loss of acetylcholine in the cerebral cortex. The loss occurs because of pathology and atrophy in the cells of origin, in the nucleus basalis of Meynert. The findings led to the development of the current cholinergic therapies for the disease. However, although cholinergic deficits may well explain some of the symptoms, they do not appear to have a primary causal role. Cholinergic pathology may in fact be of more relevance in dementia with Lewy bodies, and it is possible that the earlier studies of Alzheimer's disease included patients in this category.

Vascular dementia

The dementia caused by cerebrovascular disease was in the past referred to as 'atherosclerotic psychosis'. Following the separation of distinct syndromes of psychiatric disorder in late life (Roth, 1955), it became apparent that dementia was often associated with multiple infarcts, and Hachinski *et al.* (1974) suggested the term *multi-infarct dementia*. Subsequent research has shown that these patients are in fact a small subgroup of those with cognitive impairment due to cerebrovascular disease, and the umbrella term of *vascular dementia* (or *vascular cognitive impairment*) is now preferred, within which a range of subtypes is recognized (see Box 14.13). Small-vessel disease affecting subcortical regions is now considered the commonest form of vascular dementia. However, the neuropathological findings of vascular dementia are very varied, and include embolus, vasculitis, angiopathy, and haemorrhage, as well as infarcts.

For review, see Series and Esiri (2012) and O'Brien and Thomas (2015).

Vascular dementia is usually said to be the second commonest cause of dementia after Alzheimer's disease, of comparable prevalence to dementia with Lewy bodies. However, there is considerable uncertainty over these figures, because of the pathological heterogeneity of vascular changes, the absence of accepted neuropathological criteria for vascular dementia, and their frequent coexistence with Alzheimer-type pathology, which makes it difficult to know the causal contribution of vascular pathology. Recent estimates suggest that 'pure' cerebrovascular disease is a relatively rare cause of dementia (O'Brien and Thomas, 2015).

Clinical features

Onset is usually in the late sixties or the seventies. With large-vessel disease, onset is often relatively acute and follows a stroke, in which case the term *post-stroke dementia* is sometimes used. Emotional and personality changes may appear first, followed by impairments of memory and intellect that characteristically progress in stages. Depression is frequent, and episodes of emotional lability and confusion are common, especially at night. Transient ischaemic attacks or mild strokes may recur from time to time. Insight is often maintained until a late stage. Apathy, behavioural retardation, and anxiety are more common than in Alzheimer's disease, but cognitive impairment itself is more variable and often of lesser degree. Attention, information processing, and executive function are typically most affected, and tests that focus on these domains (such as the Montreal cognitive assessment scale [MoCA] or vascular dementia assessment scale [VADAS-cog]) are more likely to identify deficits than the MMSE.

The course of vascular dementia is classically a stepwise progression, with periods of deterioration that are sometimes followed by partial recovery for a few months. About 50% of patients die from ischaemic heart disease, and others from cerebral infarction. From the time of diagnosis the lifespan varies widely. However, most studies show somewhat shorter survival than in Alzheimer's disease.

The diagnosis is difficult to make with confidence unless there is a clear history of strokes or localizing neurological signs. Suggestive features are patchy psychological deficits, erratic progression, and relative preservation of the personality. On physical examination there may be signs of hypertension and of arteriosclerosis in peripheral and retinal vessels, and there may be neurological signs such as pseudobulbar palsy, rigidity, akinesia, and brisk reflexes. CT or MRI imaging are valuable to demonstrate the nature and severity of vascular pathology. CT is sufficient to show established infarcts and large areas of white matter damage, but MRI is more sensitive in revealing the full profile of involvement.

Aetiology

It is assumed that vascular dementia results from the neuronal dysfunction and death, and the damage to white matter tracts, that follow from the cumulative focal areas of ischaemia and necrosis (Iadecola, 2013). About 10% of people develop dementia after a first stroke, and more than one-third after recurrent stroke (Pendlebury and Rothwell, 2009). The risk factors for vascular dementia are essentially those of cerebrovascular disease (Box 14.14). Prevention and optimal management of these risk factors is predicted to reduce the incidence of vascular dementia, but this has yet to demonstrated. The overlap of these risk factors with those posing risk for Alzheimer's disease is consistent with the frequent co-occurrence of the two pathologies and the emerging concept of mixed dementia (see below). The main genetic form of vascular dementia is the rare autosomal dominant disorder CADASIL, caused by a mutation in the *Notch* gene on chromosome 19 (Box 14.13). There are no other well-established genetic

---

> ### Box 14.13 Subtypes of vascular dementia
>
> **Multi-infarct dementia** (cortical vascular dementia)
> **Small-vessel dementia** (subcortical vascular dementia; includes Binswanger's disease)
> **Hypoperfusion dementia**
> **Haemorrhagic dementia**
> **Hereditary vascular dementia** (CADASIL: cerebral autosomal dominant arteriopathy with subcortical infarcts and leucoencephalopathy)

Box 14.14 Risk factors for vascular dementia

History of stroke—risk related to number, location, and size

Increasing age—risk doubles every 5 years

Low education

Hypertension

Orthostatic hypotension

Evidence of vascular disease (e.g. carotid bruit, cardiac disease)

Vascular risk factors (e.g. smoking, hyperlipidaemia, obesity)

High blood homocysteine

Late-life depression

Box 14.15 Terminology of dementia involving Lewy bodies

Dementia with Lewy bodies. Dementia occurring before or concurrently with, or within a year of the onset of, parkinsonism. However, not all patients develop parkinsonism

Parkinson's disease dementia. Dementia occurring a year or more after the onset of established Parkinson's disease

Lewy body dementias. Umbrella term that includes both the above categories

Lewy body disease. A pathological diagnosis, based on the presence and distribution of Lewy body-type pathology

Adapted from Lancet, 386(10004), Walker Z *et al.*, Lewy body dementias, pp. 1683- 1697, Copyright (2015), with permission from Elsevier.

---

risk factors for vascular dementia, although *apoE* and *MTHFR* (a gene involved in homocysteine metabolism) have been implicated.

Dementia with Lewy bodies

A hitherto unrecognized type of dementia with a relatively distinct pathology and clinical course was described in the late 1980s using various terms, including cortical Lewy body disease, diffuse Lewy body disease, and Lewy body variant of Alzheimer's disease. *Dementia with Lewy bodies* is now the consensus term. Box 14.15 summarizes some relevant terminology. The disorder accounts for 4–25% of cases of dementia; the wide range of estimates (and the belated 'discovery' of dementia with Lewy bodies) probably reflects sampling bias in some studies (e.g. underrepresentation in patients coming to autopsy) and the fact that cortical Lewy bodies are difficult to see using routine neuropathological stains.

For a review, see Walker *et al.* (2015).

Clinical features

The core clinical features, which form the recognized criteria for diagnosis of dementia with Lewy bodies, are summarized in Box 14.16 (McKeith *et al.*, 2017). The fluctuating level of dementia with recurrent delirium-like phases, together with visual hallucinations and parkinsonism, is characteristic, although the motor features are not always apparent. Use of these criteria allows dementia with Lewy bodies to be diagnosed with good specificity and sensitivity, but it remains underdiagnosed

in routine clinical practice. The average survival is 5–7 years.

Neuropathology

The characteristic histopathological feature of dementia with Lewy bodies is the presence of Lewy bodies in the cerebral cortex. Lewy neurites are also seen. As in Parkinson's disease, these features are also seen in the substantia nigra, and their biochemical composition is the same in both diseases. Lewy bodies are intraneuronal inclusions, composed mainly of abnormal aggregations of a protein called α-synuclein. They also contain other proteins, including ubiquitin, detection of which is widely used in the routine detection of Lewy bodies. There is also a significant neuropathological overlap with Alzheimer's disease, with dementia with Lewy bodies often exhibiting abundant senile plaques and widespread reductions in choline acetyltransferase in the neocortex; however, neurofibrillary tangles are rare. Brain atrophy is less marked than in Alzheimer's disease, especially in the hippocampus. For a review, see Irwin *et al.* (2013).

Aetiology

Dementia with Lewy bodies is closely related to Parkinson's disease, and both are characterized as 'synucleinopathies', reflecting the abnormal aggregation of

> ### Box 14.16 Abbreviated clinical criteria for dementia with Lewy bodies
>
> **Key features**
>
> Progressive cognitive decline, especially in attention and visuospatial ability
> Pronounced fluctuations in cognition and attention
> Recurrent visual hallucinations, usually well formed and detailed
> Motor features of parkinsonism
>
> **Supportive features**
>
> Repeated falls
> Syncope
> Transient loss of consciousness
> Systematized delusions
> Non-visual hallucinations
> Adverse reactions to antipsychotics
>
> **Diagnosis made less likely in the presence of**
>
> Evidence of cerebrovascular disease or stroke
> Evidence of other disorder sufficient to account for the clinical picture

For review of frontotemporal dementia, see Bang *et al.* (2015).

Clinical features and subtypes

Frontotemporal dementia encompasses a range of neurodegenerative diseases affecting the frontal and temporal lobes and which are characterized clinically by progressive deficits in behaviour, language, and memory. Compared to most other dementias, cognitive impairment is a relatively minor feature, with behavioural, psychiatric, and linguistic aspects being more prominent. There is a significant clinical and aetiological overlap with motor neuron disease, and with parkinsonian syndromes (Baizabal-Carvallo and Jankovic, 2016). The diagnostic terminology is complicated because of the clinical, neuropathological, and genetic heterogeneity; Box 14.17 lists some of the older terms, including Pick's disease, which are now subsumed within the category of frontotemporal dementia (but note that ICD-10 still uses 'dementia in Pick's disease').

Based upon the clinical profile, two major subtypes of frontotemporal dementia are now recognized: *behavioural-variant frontotemporal dementia* and *primary progressive aphasia*. The latter is then divided into *semantic-variant* and *non-fluent variant* forms. All forms can exhibit the features shown in Box 14.18, but the clinical features that characterize each subtype are summarized in Box 14.19. About one in eight patients

α-synuclein protein present in Lewy bodies. There is a modest familial aggregation for dementia with Lewy bodies, and there are associations with some of the genes implicated in Parkinson's disease and Alzheimer's disease (Loy *et al.*, 2014). However, neither genetic nor environmental risk factors for dementia with Lewy bodies have been well established.

Frontotemporal dementias

Frontotemporal dementias are the second most common form of presenile dementia, and also underlie about 7% of late-life dementias. The term was proposed in 1994 when the Lund–Manchester criteria were developed to better classify Pick's disease (see below) and related disorders, based upon their shared clinical features and regional neuropathology, as described below. For current diagnostic criteria, see Galimbeti *et al.* (2015). The term *frontotemporal lobar degeneration* is the neuropathological counterpart (Mackenzie *et al.*, 2010).

> ### Box 14.17 Diagnostic categories subsumed within frontotemporal dementia
>
> Pick's disease
> Lobar atrophy
> Frontal lobe degeneration of non-Alzheimer type
> Dementia lacking distinctive histology
> Semantic dementia
> Motor neuron disease with dementia
> Progressive non-fluent aphasia
> Progressive aphasic syndrome
> Frontotemporal dementia with parkinsonism
> Corticobasal degeneration*
> Progressive supranuclear palsy*
> Parkinsonism–dementia complex of Guam*
>
> * Not always included.

Box 14.18 Clinical features of frontotemporal dementias

Behavioural features

Insidious onset, slow progression
Early loss of insight
Early signs of disinhibition and lack of judgement
Mental inflexibility
Stereotyped and imitative behaviour
Hyperorality (e.g. craving for sweet foods)
Distractibility and impulsivity

Language and speech features

Progressive decrease in speech output
Perseveration
Echolalia

Affective features

Depression
Apathy
Emotional blunting
Hypochondriasis

Physical signs

Early primitive reflexes
Early incontinence
Late parkinsonism
Low and labile blood pressure

Box 14.19 Features characteristic of the three clinical subtypes of frontotemporal dementia

Behavioural-variant

Personality change
Disinhibition
Apathy
Selfishness
Self-neglect
Overeating
Behavioural stereotypies
Mental rigidity

Semantic-variant primary progressive aphasia

Anomia (especially for nouns)
Word-finding difficulties
Impaired verbal comprehension
Increased pain responses
Prosopagnosia
Irritability

Non-fluent variant primary progressive aphasia

Slow, laboured speech
Misuse of grammar
Speech sound errors
Anomia (especially for verbs)
Irritability

Adapted from Lancet, 386(10004), Bang J, Spina S and Miller BL, Frontotemporal dementia, pp. 1672-1682, Copyright (2015), with permission from Elsevier.

with frontotemporal dementia develop motor neuron disease, and another 20–30% exhibit features of parkinsonism. As discussed below, the presence of these additional neurological elements is related to the neuropathological features and, in familial cases, to the causal gene.

Frontotemporal dementia is difficult to diagnose, since in the early stages it can easily be mistaken for depression or psychosis, and hard to distinguish from other forms of dementia. The history should concentrate on the past psychiatric history, family history, and premorbid personality and functioning. The assessment should also include a careful evaluation of the behavioural features and language abilities. Physical examination of the motor system, looking for muscular weakness and parkinsonism, is also important.

Structural brain imaging can play a useful role, with MRI or CT showing focal, often asymmetrical, atrophy of the temporal and frontal poles (behavioural and language symptoms being associated with right and left hemisphere involvement, respectively). Functional imaging shows disproportionate hypometabolism and hypoperfusion in these regions.

The average survival of frontotemporal dementia is 6–11 years from symptom onset (and about 2–6 years from diagnosis); patients with concurrent motor neuron disease have the worst prognosis.

Pick's disease

Arnold Pick described the disease that bears his name in 1892. Pick's disease remains the archetypal fronto-temporal dementia, and is sometimes referred to synonymously with it but, if defined properly (including the neuropathological features), it explains only a small proportion of cases. The clinical features that he noted were of aphasia with dementia, such that the case would probably be diagnosed today as a primary progressive aphasia. The pathological findings of Pick's original case were reported by Alzheimer, and were striking, with focal 'knife-blade' atrophy of the frontal and temporal poles, with ballooned neurons (Pick cells) that contained inclusions called Pick bodies. Pick bodies also occur in other areas, notably the hippocampus. They are composed of tau, ubiquitin, and other proteins.

Neuropathology

The classic features of Pick's disease have been summarized above. Other forms of frontotemporal dementia also show gross atrophy of the temporal and frontal lobes, with neuronal loss, gliosis, microvacuolar changes, and often ballooned cells. Different neuropathological subtypes of frontotemporal dementia are now recognized, based primarily upon the identity of the protein which is aberrantly deposited: tau, TDP-43, or FUS. However, there is only a modest correspondence between clinical and pathological subtypes of frontotemporal dementia (Bang *et al.*, 2015).

Aetiology

About 10% of cases are caused by autosomal dominant mutations, with three genes (*C9orf72, MAPT* [which encodes tau], and *GRN*) accounting for the majority of these cases (Loy *et al.*, 2014). In Caucasian populations, *C9orf72* is the commonest cause, particularly for frontotemporal dementia with motor neuron disease (Rohrer *et al.*, 2015). The *C9orf72* mutations are due to hexanucleotide repeats (a repeated sequence of six nucleotides, which occurs up to 20 times in the normal gene, but hundreds of times in those with disease). The *GRN* mutations are null, preventing production of the encoded protein; the *MAPT* mutations disrupt the expression and structure of tau. Each of the three genes is closely associated with a particular neuropathological profile (for example, *C9orf72* cases have TDP-43 neuropathology), but less strongly with the clinical picture

(Bang *et al.*, 2015). The pathogenic mechanisms by which the gene mutations cause neurodegeneration are uncertain, and may be different for each gene. Genetic testing is now available and should be considered for all patients with frontotemporal dementia with a family history suggestive of autosomal dominant inheritance of neurodegenerative disorders. For review, see Loy *et al.* (2014).

The causes of the commoner non-familial forms of frontotemporal dementia are not known.

Prion diseases

Prion diseases are a unique category of neurodegenerative disorders, grouped together because of the central causal role of a specific protein, called prion protein (PrP). They also share neuropathological features, including diffuse spongiosis (hence the older term, '*spongiform encephalopathy*'), neuronal loss, gliosis, and, in many cases, amyloid plaques. They can be inherited, or acquired infectiously or iatrogenically, while other cases are sporadic and idiopathic. Because of these properties, their interest and importance are out of all proportion to their rarity (about 100 cases per year in the UK). In the UK, all cases of suspected prion disease should be referred to the National Surveillance Centre in Edinburgh.

For reviews of prion diseases, see Collinge (2009) and Prusiner (2013).

Creutzfeldt–Jakob disease

Creutzfeldt–Jakob disease (CJD) is the main prion disease, with an approximate annual incidence of one case per million. A small number of cases are inherited as an autosomal dominant disorder due to mutations in the *PrP* gene (see below). Other cases have been transmitted iatrogenically, via pituitary-derived growth hormone, contaminated neurosurgical instruments or graft material, and possibly by blood transfusion. The incubation time in these cases can exceed 20 years. Because of the potential infectivity, no patients with dementia should be organ donors.

Sporadic CJD affects both sexes equally. Onset is typically between 50 and 65 years of age. It is usually heralded by memory impairment, which may be accompanied by prominent behavioural abnormalities or personality change, prompting initial referral to a psychiatrist (Thompson *et al.*, 2014). Visual hallucinations, cerebellar signs, involuntary movements, myoclonic jerks, and other motor features are frequent. Seizures occur later in the course. There is usually a relentless and rapid progression to death, often within 6 months. The EEG classically shows a triphasic 1–2 Hz discharge which, together with the history and rapid course, is diagnostically characteristic. The biochemical profile of the CSF, notably the presence of '14-3-3 proteins', is also suggestive. However, definitive diagnosis in life requires a brain biopsy.

Variant Creutzfeldt–Jakob disease

Intense interest in prion disease followed the description of variant Creutzfeldt–Jakob disease (vCJD), which was first identified in the UK in 1996. This was linked with bovine spongiform encephalopathy (BSE), which was epidemic in British dairy herds at that time. BSE and vCJD are, in effect, the same disease (see below), and it is beyond reasonable doubt that vCJD occurred as a result of eating contaminated bovine products. The incidence of vCJD peaked around the year 2000, with only one new case diagnosed since 2013. A total of 177 cases had been identified by January 2016. It is now considered highly unlikely that a human epidemic will occur; however, abnormal PrP has been found in about 1 in 200 appendixes in a large UK survey, suggesting a vCJD 'carrier state' (Gill *et al.*, 2013). There is a common polymorphism at codon 129 of the *PrP* gene that encodes either methionine or valine; all vCJD patients except one have been homozygous for methionine (compared with 40% in the population), which suggests that this genetic subgroup is more susceptible to development of vCJD.

Compared with other forms of CJD, vCJD has an earlier onset, slower course, and usually presents with psychiatric symptoms, notably depression and personality change (Thompson *et al.*, 2014). EEG abnormalities are less common. The 'pulvinar' sign on MRI (hyperintensity over the posterior thalamus) is a useful and non-invasive diagnostic sign.

Other prion diseases

Kuru, described in the Fore tribe of New Guinea highlanders, was transmitted by ritual cannibalism; the disease has disappeared since this practice was abolished in the 1950s. Transmission of kuru to monkeys in 1970 was the first experimental proof of the infectivity of prion disease.

Other inherited prion diseases are Gerstmann–Sträussler-Scheinker syndrome and fatal familial insomnia. Like familial CJD, both of these are caused by autosomal dominant mutations of the prion protein gene. Both are extremely rare.

Aetiology

The name 'prion' denotes proteinaceous infectious particles. It was coined in 1982 by Prusiner, who received the 1999 Nobel Prize for Medicine. Prion protein (PrP) is encoded by a gene on chromosome 20. The functions of 'normal' PrP (denoted PrP^C) are unknown, but it is expressed by neurons and may serve as a receptor and influence synaptic properties. Prion diseases are caused when PrP^C takes on an abnormal conformation, called PrP^{Sc} (named after scrapie, the prion disease that affects sheep). PrP^{Sc} is both the core molecular marker and presumed causative agent of prion diseases. Compared with PrP^C, PrP^{Sc} is resistant to breakdown by proteases, and tends to self-aggregate and be deposited in the brain. PrP^{Sc} can spread trans-synaptically from neuron to neuron, thereby promoting synaptic and neuronal loss and gliosis, and producing the resulting spongiform appearance of the brain.

In familial cases, the mutated PrP is assumed to be intrinsically more likely to self-aggregate. In forms that are acquired (either iatrogenically or through diet), it is postulated that the normal PrP^C becomes 'corrupted' by the acquired PrP^{Sc}, which changes the conformation of PrP^C into PrP^{Sc}, thus propagating ever more PrP^{Sc}. The molecular details of this remarkable process remain obscure. In the case of peripheral acquisition, PrP^{Sc} may spread via the nerves, lymphatics, and blood to reach the brain. Different PrP conformations and modifications (glycosylation patterns) give rise to various disease 'strains'. The aetiology of 'sporadic' prion disease is not known. It may result from spontaneous mutation or conversion of PrP^C to PrP^{Sc}, or it may arise from occult environmental sources. It is not known why PrP^{Sc} is infectious, when other misfolded, amyloidogenic proteins (such as β-amyloid and α-synuclein) do not appear to be. Prion diseases are not caused by 'slow viruses', as was formerly believed.

For review, see Prusiner (2013).

Dementia due to HIV disease

See Chapter 22.

Dementia due to alcohol misuse

See Chapter 20.

Emerging concepts of dementia

Classification and clinical practice are based on the dementia syndromes described above. However, epidemiological and biological research is increasingly calling current diagnostic concepts into question.

Mixed dementia

The frequency and importance of 'mixed dementia' are becoming apparent, particularly the coexistence of Alzheimer's disease and vascular dementia. This occurs in at least 20% of cases (and in the majority of cases if lower thresholds for cerebrovascular disease are used). Indeed, in the over 80s, mixed dementia 'is the norm not the exception' (O'Brien and Thomas, 2015). The coexistence of Alzheimer's disease with cerebrovascular disease worsens the severity of dementia (Toledo et al., 2013). The clinical overlap is now complemented by the increasing evidence that risk factors and disease mechanisms for Alzheimer's disease overlap with those for vascular dementia (Saito and Ihara, 2016).

Molecular classification of neurodegenerative diseases

There is further blurring of diagnostic boundaries at the molecular level, in that the same core biochemical processes—misfolding and accumulation of specific proteins, and their spread along neuronal pathways in the brain—appears to be central to many neurodegenerative disorders, including β-amyloid in Alzheimer's disease, PrP in prion disease, and α-synuclein in Parkinson's disease (Hardy and Revesz, 2012; Arnold et al., 2013). Equally, it is apparent that there is not a one-to-one correspondence between protein and syndrome, as exemplified by the involvement of tau in both Alzheimer's disease and some forms of frontotemporal dementia (Iqbal et al., 2016). These factors are leading to the molecular reclassification of dementias as 'tauopathies', 'synucleinopathies', etc. These issues are likely to influence diagnostic and clinical practice as their prognostic and treatment implications become clear.

Movement disorders

Parkinson's disease, and other disorders in which movement and coordination are the cardinal features, are usually managed by neurologists. However, they usually also include prominent and clinically significant psychiatric features, including cognitive impairment, psychosis, and mood disorders. It is the psychiatric aspects that will be considered here.

Parkinson's disease

Clinical features

The cardinal triad of idiopathic Parkinson's disease is a rest tremor, cog-wheel rigidity, and bradykinesia. The main psychiatric consequences are cognitive impairment, depression, psychosis, and behavioural problems (Aarsland et al., 2009; Box 14.20). Impaired olfaction is a neglected feature, and can pre-date other symptoms by several years (Doty, 2012); constipation, sleep disturbances, and depression are also common well before the onset of motor symptoms. The differential diagnosis includes other parkinsonian syndromes, and, of particular relevance to psychiatrists, the parkinsonian side effects of antipsychotic drugs. In clinicopathological terms, Parkinson's disease is part of the spectrum of Lewy body disease, discussed earlier.

For review of Parkinson's disease, see Kalia and Lang (2015).

Dementia

The prevalence of cognitive impairment in Parkinson's disease is about 30%, with up to 80% of patients eventually developing dementia. The diagnosis is 'Parkinson's disease dementia' if the dementia begins more than 1 year after the onset of established Parkinson's disease; if dementia occurs less than a year after Parkinson's disease, the diagnosis is dementia with Lewy bodies (see page 368) (Box 14.15). Dementia is more common in later-onset cases and those in whom bradykinesia is more prominent than tremor. The clinical picture is of a subcortical dementia (see page 358), although other profiles of cognitive impairment are seen in Parkinson's disease, notably a 'dysexecutive syndrome' in which planning and working memory are especially affected (Kehagia et al., 2010). For treatment of dementia in Parkinson's disease see Chapter 19.

Depression

The association of Parkinson's disease with depression is well established; clinically significant depressive symptoms (including apathy) are present in 35% of cases, and a major depressive disorder in about

> **Box 14.20 Psychiatric manifestations in Parkinson's disease**
>
> Delirium, stupor (especially due to drugs, or intercurrent infection)
>
> Cognitive decline (subcortical dementia, dysexecutive syndrome)
>
> Depression, apathy, mania
>
> Hallucinations (chiefly visual)
>
> Delusions
>
> Sleep attacks, REM sleep behaviour disorder
>
> Sexual disorders
>
> Impulse control disorders, e.g. gambling (largely medication-related)

20%. Depression is most common in the early and the very advanced stages of the disease. The mechanism is uncertain; depression correlates poorly with degree of disability and disease duration, and may be related to frontal lobe abnormalities and disturbed dopaminergic mechanisms. Antidepressants must be used with care to avoid exacerbation of cognitive impairment or induction of delirium. SSRIs and newer-generation agents, which have less anticholinergic activity, are preferable to tricyclic antidepressants. Pramipexole is also used.

Psychotic symptoms

Psychotic symptoms occur at some stage in around 20% of patients. Visual hallucinations are associated with dopaminergic medication, increasing age, disease duration and severity, depression, cognitive impairment, and reduced visual acuity. Delusions are less frequent and are usually paranoid in content. Anti-parkinsonian drugs have been implicated as causes, and whenever possible these should be reduced. If antipsychotic medication is necessary, clozapine or quetiapine should be used.

Other neuropsychiatric manifestations

Excessive somnolence, a disordered sleep–wake cycle, sleep attacks, and REM sleep behaviour disorder are more common in (and before the onset of) Parkinson's disease. As a result, patients with Parkinson's disease must be counselled about the risks of driving, even in the absence of dementia. Pathological gambling and other impulsive behaviours are also a recognized and

sometimes problematic feature, especially in patients treated with dopamine agonists such as pramipexole.

Aetiology

Idiopathic Parkinson's disease is usually a disorder of later life, occurring in around 1% of the population over the age of 55 years, and rising rapidly with age thereafter. It is more common in men than women, with a ratio of 3:2. The disease results primarily from degeneration of dopaminergic neurons in the zona compacta of the substantia nigra, although the first site of pathology is in the IX/X cranial nerve nuclei, and it later extends to other regions and pathways. The pathological hallmark is Lewy bodies (α-synuclein inclusions within dopaminergic neurons), as described for Lewy body dementia. The dementia of Parkinson's disease involves more widespread pathology, and involves β-amyloid and tau as well as α-synuclein (Irwin *et al.*, 2013).

Risk factors for Parkinson's disease are summarized in Box 14.21. Rarely, cases are inherited as autosomal dominant or autosomal recessive disorders, caused by mutations in several genes, including the *SCNA* gene, which encodes α-synuclein. However, the large majority of cases are sporadic, reflecting a combination of a complex genetic predisposition and a range of environmental factors. Of these risk genes, variation in *GBA* is the most important, conferring an odds ratio of more than 5; *GBA* encodes β-glucocerebrosidase, the lysosomal enzyme that is deficient in Gaucher's disease. The environmental risk factors include a range of toxins and drugs. Tobacco smoking is associated with a decreased risk of Parkinson's disease, but this appears to be due to people who develop the disease being more able to quit smoking, rather than a true protective effect of nicotine. Pathophysiologically, the disease process is thought to be due to impairment of mitochondrial and synaptic functioning, and oxidative stress. Neuroinflammation may also play a role. For review, see Schapiro *et al.* (2014).

Huntington's disease

This autosomal dominant disease, also called *Huntington's chorea*, was described by the New England physician George Huntington in 1872. It has a worldwide distribution, with an estimated prevalence of 4–7 per 100,000. Onset is typically in middle life, although adolescent cases are well recognized.

The clinical features of Huntington's disease are shown in Box 14.22. They comprise a triad of movement abnormalities, cognitive impairment, and psychiatric features. The classical choreiform movement

Box 14.21 Risk factors for Parkinson's disease

Genetic

Autosomal dominant: *SCNA; LRRK2; VIP35; EIF4G1; DNAJC13; CHCHD2*

Autosomal recessive: *Parkin, PINK1, Dj-1*

Risk polymorphisms: *GBA; INPP5F;* and many others

Environmental risk factors

Pesticide exposure

Head injury

Rural living

Drinking well water

Agricultural occupation

Use of beta-blockers

Environmental protective factors

Tobacco smoking

Coffee drinking

Use of NSAIDs

Use of calcium channel blockers

Alcohol

Adapted from Lancet, 386(9996), Kalia LV and Lang AE, Parkinson's disease, pp. 896-912, Copyright (2015), with permission from Elsevier.

Box 14.22 Features of Huntington's disease

Motor abnormalities

Involuntary movements

 Chorea

 Fidgeting

Impairment of voluntary movements

 Incoordination

 Gaze apraxia

 Failure to sustain tongue protrusion ('serpentine tongue')

 Bradykinesia

 Rigidity

Cognitive impairment

Cognitive slowing

Decreased attention

Reduced mental flexibility and planning

Impaired emotional recognition

Poor visuospatial function

Psychiatric and behavioural features

Depression

Irritability

Apathy

Delusions and hallucinations

Early loss of insight

abnormality is required for diagnosis, but significant cognitive impairment and psychiatric symptoms frequently occur in the decade before chorea appears (the 'prodrome' of Huntington's disease), and individuals may therefore present to psychiatrists during this time (Epping *et al.*, 2016). Apathy is commonly the first psychiatric manifestation. Most subjects will be aware of their family history, and many will have had predictive genetic testing (see below), and so the psychiatrist will need to deal with the resulting implications and concerns (MacLeod *et al.*, 2013). After presentation, the motor and cognitive symptoms are invariable and progress inexorably, whereas the psychiatric symptoms are much more variable. Depression is seen in over 50% of cases at some stage, and irritability and apathy are also common. Psychotic symptoms, both schizophrenia-like and affective in nature, occur in about 10% of cases.

For review of Huntington's disease, see Ross *et al.* (2014). For review of treatment of the psychiatric features, see Chapter 19 and Videnovic (2013).

Neuropathology

The pathological changes mainly affect the caudate nucleus and frontal lobes. The basal ganglia, especially the caudate nucleus, is markedly atrophic and gliotic. The shrinkage of the caudate can be seen using MRI; it begins many years before diagnosis and its extent correlates strongly with the motor and cognitive impairments (Ross *et al.*, 2014). There is also some involvement of the frontal cortex, with thinning of the grey matter and pyramidal neuronal loss. Polyglutamine nuclear inclusions are present within some cells, reflecting the causative gene mutation described below. Neurochemically, there are decreased concentrations of the inhibitory transmitter gamma-aminobutyric acid (GABA) in the caudate nucleus.

Aetiology

Huntington's disease is one of the few single gene, autosomal dominant disorders in psychiatry. The gene, on chromosome 4p, is called *huntingtin (HTT)*. The mutation, identified in 1993, is a multiple repeat of the codon CAG, which codes for glutamine. It is therefore known as a '*triplet repeat*', '*trinucleotide repeat*' or '*CAG repeat*' mutation, giving rise to a 'polyglutamine' sequence in the HTT protein. Normal individuals have less than 30 CAG repeats in the gene; disease occurs in those who have more than 36 copies, with full penetrance (i.e. all carriers of the mutation develop the disease) at 40 copies or more. New mutations are very rare; most apparently sporadic cases reflect an incomplete family history, or lack of knowledge of true paternity. The expansion tends to increase in succeeding generations, leading to an earlier age of onset, a feature called *anticipation*, which is characteristic of trinucleotide repeat diseases. The normal function of huntingtin, and the pathogenic mechanism by which the mutation causes disease, remain unclear, but a range of molecular pathways leading to cellular dysfunction and death are implicated (Ross *et al.*, 2014). Diagnostic and predictive genetic testing is widely available. Because of the devastating implications for the sufferer and their descendants, genetic counselling is required (MacLeod *et al.*, 2013).

Dystonias

Dystonias are uncontrolled focal muscle spasms that lead to involuntary movements of the eyelids, face, neck, jaw, shoulders, larynx, hands, and (rarely) other parts of the body. The aetiology is uncertain. In the past, dystonias were regarded as conversion phenomena. However, there is now strong evidence that some cases are caused by gene mutations, whilst others are due to infection, brain injury, neurotoxicity, drugs, and a range of other causes (Albanese *et al.*, 2013), and that psychogenic cases are rare. However, psychiatric factors may exacerbate symptoms and disability. Clinical types include blepharospasm, torticollis, writer's cramp, and laryngeal dystonia. The most effective treatment is the injection of botulinum toxin directly into the affected muscles. Deep brain stimulation is also being used. Psychiatric symptoms secondary to the physical disorder can be treated with antidepressants or behavioural therapy. For review, see Henderson and Mellers (2009).

Occupational dystonia

Muscular problems are common among musicians, and may threaten to end their careers. There are many causes, including overuse injury, pressure on peripheral nerves, and focal dystonias. These problems should be assessed by a physician with experience in the field. Performance anxiety is also frequent, and may impair or prevent performance. Beta-blockers alleviate this symptom and are used by many musicians, sometimes without medical supervision. Anxiety management is effective in some cases. Other occupations also have characteristic dystonias (e.g. golfers' 'yips').

Tics

Tics are purposeless, stereotyped, and repetitive jerking movements that most commonly occur in the face and neck. They are much more common in childhood than in adulthood, although a few cases begin at up to 40 years of age. The peak of onset is about 7 years, and onset often occurs at a time of emotional disturbance. Tics are especially common in boys. Most sufferers have just one kind of abnormal movement, but a few people have more than one (multiple tics). Like almost all involuntary movements, tics are worsened by anxiety. Unlike dystonias, they can be controlled briefly by voluntary effort, but this results in an increasing unpleasant feeling of tension. Many tics that occur in childhood last for only a few weeks, and 80–90% of cases improve within 5 years. Tics in children are associated with a range of psychiatric disorders, notably obsessive–compulsive disorder, attention deficit hyperactivity disorder, and anxiety disorders. For review, see Knight *et al.* (2012). Tics are treated primarily with behavioural interventions, including exposure and response prevention, and habit reversal therapy. Occasionally, atypical antipsychotics such as risperidone, or alpha-2 adrenergic agonists, are used (Roessner *et al.*, 2013).

Tourette syndrome

This condition was first described by Jean Itard in 1825 and subsequently by Georges Gilles de la Tourette in 1885. It is the most common tic disorder. The syndrome is defined by the onset in childhood of both motor and vocal tics (grunting, snarling, and similar ejaculations), lasting for at least a year. Up to a third of affected individuals exhibit *coprolalia* (involuntary uttering of obscenities). Around 10–40% exhibit echolalia or echopraxia. There may be stereotyped movements, such as jumping and dancing. The tics are often preceded by premonitory sensations. Associated features include overactivity, difficulties in learning, emotional disturbances, and social problems. Comorbidity with attention deficit hyperactivity disorder and obsessive–compulsive disorder occurs in over 50% of cases.

The prevalence in children is estimated at 0.5–1%. The disorder is three to four times more common in males than in females. There is a substantial genetic contribution to the syndrome and an overlap with the genetic predisposition to obsessive–compulsive disorder. Prenatal maternal smoking, perinatal hypoxia, and autoimmune abnormalities are also implicated. The neural basis of the syndrome is thought to involve altered dopamine function and aberrant cortico-striatal connectivity. For review see Paschou (2013).

Mild cases may not require specific treatment. The tics are treated as described above (Roessner *et al.*, 2013), together with treatment of any comorbid psychiatric disorders. There are few good outcome data. Clinical experience suggests that two-thirds of patients can expect an improvement or lasting remission by early adulthood, but the outcome is frequently poor.

For a review of Tourette syndrome, see Cohen *et al.* (2013).

Cerebrovascular disorders

Stroke

Cognitive deficits

Strokes may lead to vascular dementia, as described earlier. However, they have other neuropsychiatric implications, too. Overt strokes usually present as a neurological emergency, with hemiparesis, dysphasias, and other focal symptoms and signs. Subsequently, survivors may be left with these and other impairments, in addition to a range of psychiatric symptoms, which depend largely on the site and size of the vascular event. For review, see Fleminger (2009).

Personality change

Irritability, apathy, lability of mood, and occasionally aggressiveness may occur. Inflexibility in coping with problems is common, and may be observed in extreme form as a catastrophic reaction. These behavioural changes are often as disabling, and as distressing to carers, as residual hemiplegia or dysphasia. They are probably due more to associated widespread arteriosclerotic vascular disease than to a single stroke, and they may continue to worsen even when the focal signs of a stroke are improving.

After a stroke, some people become abnormally emotional, with mixtures of spontaneous laughter and crying, and the emotional display is frequently at odds with the patient's apparent mood. Antidepressants are considered to be helpful.

Post-stroke depression

Depressed mood is common after stroke and may contribute to the apparent intellectual impairment or impede rehabilitation. The prevalence of depression is about 30% and remains stable for up to 10 years post-stroke; there is a cumulative incidence of about 45% for depression within 5 years of a stroke (Ayerbe *et al.*, 2012). The main risk factors are the extent of post-stroke impairment in activities of daily living, the degree of cognitive impairment, and a past history of depression (Ayerbe *et al.*, 2012). Suggestions that the risk of depression is related to the location of the stroke (being greater following a left frontal or left basal ganglia stroke) have not been well confirmed. Post-stroke depression is associated with a reduced quality of life, and increased disability and mortality compared to non-depressed stroke survivors.

Treatment of post-stroke depression depends in part on active rehabilitation. Antidepressants, especially SSRIs, are effective, and they may also enhance recovery after stroke independent of their effects on mood. Medication should, however, be used cautiously in this population, as side effects are frequent and patients are at risk of further cerebrovascular events.

For review of post-stroke depression, see Robinson and Jorge (2016).

Subarachnoid haemorrhage

In the survivors of subarachnoid haemorrhage, cognitive impairment, personality change, and anxiety and depression are all common. The long-term outcome is poor, and psychosocial problems are often prominent. There are also anecdotal reports that a subarachnoid haemorrhage can be precipitated by emotionally stressful events. For review, see Fleminger (2009).

Subdural haematoma

Subdural haematoma may follow a fall in elderly patients, especially in those with a history of alcoholism. However, a history of head trauma is commonly lacking. Acute haematomas may cause coma or fluctuating impairment of consciousness, associated with hemiparesis and oculomotor signs. The psychiatrist is more likely to see the chronic syndromes, in which patients present with headache, poor concentration, vague physical complaints, and fluctuating consciousness, but often with few localizing neurological signs. It is particularly important to consider this possibility as a cause of accelerated deterioration in patients with a neurodegenerative dementia. Treatment is by surgical evacuation, which may reverse the symptoms.

Head injury

The psychiatrist is likely to see two main groups of patients who have suffered a head injury:

- a relatively small group with persistent, serious cognitive and behavioural sequelae
- a larger group with emotional symptoms and personality change.

The severity of non-penetrating (closed) head injury is best assessed by the duration of post-traumatic amnesia (PTA)—that is, the interval between the injury and the return of normal day-to-day memory. This measure has the advantage of being reasonably accurate even when assessed retrospectively (i.e. by asking the patient several months later what they remember of the immediate post-injury period). A PTA of less than 1 week is associated with a reasonable outcome (e.g. return to work) in the majority of cases, but a PTA of more than 1 month often results in failure to return to work. Retrograde amnesia (i.e. loss of memory of events prior to the injury) is much less predictive of outcome. An MRI scan is useful for defining the extent of brain injury, but a normal MRI scan does not preclude some degree of brain damage.

The vast majority of closed head injuries are due to acceleration and deceleration forces. When loss of consciousness occurs for a few seconds it is thought to be due to disruption of cholinergic transmission in the brainstem. With more severe injuries, haemorrhagic areas of damage and diffuse axonal injury and shearing in white matter are the two main pathological events (Blennow *et al.*, 2012). Both contribute to coma duration. Other complications include extradural and subdural haemorrhage and anoxia. Deposition of β-amyloid occurs in some cases, which may explain the link between head injury and later development of Alzheimer's disease, and with dementia pugilistica (see below). Apolipoprotein E4 (*apoE4*) genotype may increase the risk of death or cognitive deficits after head injury.

For review of the psychiatric aspects of head injury, see Fleminger (2009) and Bryant *et al.* (2010).

Acute psychological effects

After severe injury, a phase of delirium may follow awakening from coma. Prolonged delirium may be accompanied by a transient confabulatory state. Occasionally, delusional misidentification or reduplicative paramnesia (see page 309) is observed—for example, ward staff may be identified as old friends, or the ward may be identified as a duplicate in a distant town. Agitation and disinhibition (often sexual) are often present, and may take days or weeks to resolve.

Chronic psychological effects

Both primary and secondary (due to the effects of brain swelling and raised intracranial pressure) damage determine the neurological and cognitive deficits. The long-term outcome is also influenced by premorbid personality traits, occupational attainment, availability of social support, and compensation issues. Post-traumatic epilepsy may be a further significant complicating factor in more serious injuries. The risk of suicide is increased threefold after head injury.

Post-concussional syndrome

After mild head injury, 15–30% of patients describe a group of symptoms known as the post-concussional syndrome (Hou *et al.*, 2012). The main features are anxiety, depression, and irritability, accompanied by headache, dizziness, fatigue, poor concentration, and insomnia. The duration and severity of these symptoms are highly variable. Most cases resolve without specific medical intervention.

Lasting cognitive impairment

The particular vulnerability of frontal and temporal lobes to closed head injury hints at the usual pattern of neuropsychological deficits, with memory and executive function being most affected. The patient may show significant impairments in these domains (e.g. organizing and planning activities) without an overall decline in performance in terms of IQ.

Personality change

Personality change is common after severe injuries, particularly if there is frontal lobe damage, when there may be irritability, apathy, loss of spontaneity and drive, disinhibition, and occasionally reduced control of aggressive impulses. ICD-10 has a category of 'organic personality disorder' to describe this group. Management is difficult, demanding considerable social support and, in some cases, prolonged rehabilitation. Such resources are scarce and often unavailable. Head injury has been associated with an increased rate of violence (Fazel *et al.*, 2009b) and of violent crime and suicide (Fazel *et al.*, 2014b).

Depression and emotional disorder

Depression, anxiety, and emotional lability are very common after brain damage, although estimates of prevalence vary widely (Rapoport, 2012). Post-head-injury mania is much less common, and can be mistaken for personality change.

Psychosis

Transient psychotic symptoms are common during the delirium after head injury. However, it is unclear whether there is an increased risk of schizophrenia-like psychosis after this phase has passed. A famous study by Davison and Bagley (1969) reported a twofold to three-fold greater risk of schizophrenia in survivors of war injuries. However, later studies do not support such an association (David and Prince, 2005).

Boxing and head injury

In 1969, Roberts drew attention to the tendency for professional boxers to develop a chronic traumatic encephalopathy, sometimes called *punch-drunk syndrome* or *dementia pugilistica* (Roberts, 1969), related to the cumulative extent of head injuries suffered during their boxing careers. The principal early features are executive dysfunction, bradyphrenia, mild dysarthria, and incoordination. The fully developed syndrome may consist of a range of motor features, cognitive deficits, and a variety of behavioural manifestations. Neuropathologically, there is loss of neurons in the cortex, substantia nigra, and cerebellum, together with neurofibrillary tangles and diffuse amyloid plaques (Fleminger, 2009). Changes to the rules of boxing, and more careful medical assessments, have reduced the risks, but similar concerns are now being raised with other activities involving regular head trauma (Smith *et al.*, 2013).

Treatment of head injury

Early assessment of the extent of neurological signs provides a useful guide to the likely pattern of long-term physical disability. Neuropsychiatric problems should be assessed and their impact anticipated, and a comprehensive social assessment is crucial. The clinical psychologist can sometimes contribute behavioural and cognitive techniques. Practical support is needed for the patient's family and carers. Issues of compensation and litigation should be settled as quickly as possible.

Medication is often used to treat aggression, depression, apathy, psychosis, or concentration problems, but evidence (as for psychological treatments) is lacking. If drugs are considered to be necessary, always start with a low dose and choose agents that have less potential for seizure generation and anticholinergic or extrapyramidal side effects. For review of the management of head injury, see Fleminger (2009).

Most improvement after a head injury occurs within the first year. Late deterioration should raise suspicion of a progressive or second event, such as a subdural haematoma or hydrocephalus, epilepsy, the development of a psychiatric disorder (e.g. depression), or drug toxicity.

Epilepsy

Epilepsy is the tendency to recurrent seizures, where a seizure consists of a paroxysmal electrical discharge in the brain and its clinical sequelae. The tendency to recurrent seizures, which defines epilepsy, must be distinguished from isolated seizures that may be provoked by many factors, including drugs, hypoglycaemia, and intercurrent illnesses. Epilepsy is managed primarily by neurologists, and for a full description the reader is advised to refer to a neurology textbook. However, epilepsy also has several important psychiatric aspects, reflecting its description as the 'bridge' between psychiatry and neurology:

- the differential diagnosis of episodic disturbances of behaviour (particularly 'atypical' attacks, aggressive behaviour, sleep problems, and 'pseudoseizures')
- the treatment of the psychiatric and social complications of epilepsy
- seizures caused by psychotropic medication
- the psychological side effects of anticonvulsant drugs.

Types of seizures

The current classification of seizures was proposed by the International League Against Epilepsy (1989). A simplified outline is shown in Box 14.23. The principal distinction is between seizures which are generalized from the start and those with a focal onset, called partial seizures. Since focal-onset seizures may become generalized, an accurate description of the onset is essential. It is also necessary to distinguish between types of epilepsy and types of seizure. Older terms such as *'petit mal'* and *'grand mal'* are ambiguous, and are best avoided. It should be remembered that an 'aura' is in fact a partial seizure; most so-called 'absences' and 'petit mal' are actually complex partial seizures, implying a focal rather than generalized disturbance, as in true absences.

A brief clinical description of the more common types of seizure follows.

Simple partial seizures

The content depends upon the site of the focus. Simple partial seizures include Jacksonian motor seizures and a variety of sensory seizures in which the phenomena are relatively unformed. Awareness is not impaired. Focal neurological or cognitive dysfunction may persist for a variable period following the seizure.

Complex partial seizures

Complex partial seizures are characterized by altered awareness of self and the environment, and include a wide range of 'psychiatric' features (see Table 14.5), hence the earlier term *'psychomotor epilepsy'*—making them the form of epilepsy of most importance to psychiatrists, and frequently forming part of the differential diagnosis.

Consciousness is not lost, unless secondary generalization occurs. However, during this period subjects appear out of touch with their surroundings, and often have great difficulty in describing their experiences later.

Box 14.23 Simplified classification of seizures

Seizures beginning focally

Simple motor or sensory (without impaired consciousness)
Complex partial (with impaired consciousness)
Partial seizures with secondary generalization

Generalized seizures without focal onset

Tonic–clonic
Myoclonic
Atonic
Absence

Unclassified

Table 14.5 Clinical features of complex partial seizures

Domain	Features
Consciousness	Altered
Autonomic and visceral	'Epigastric aura', dizziness, flushing, tachycardia, and other bodily sensations
Perceptual	Distorted perceptions, *déjà vu*, *jamais vu*, visual, auditory, olfactory, gustatory, somatic hallucinations
Cognitive	Disturbances of speech, thought, and memory, derealization, depersonalization
Affective	Fear and anxiety; occasionally, euphoric or ecstatic states
Psychomotor	Automatisms, grimacing, and other bodily movements; repetitive or more complex stereotyped behaviours

The seizures arise most commonly in the temporal lobe, reflecting the additional former term 'temporal lobe epilepsy'. However, that is not an appropriate term, as complex partial seizures can also begin in the frontal lobes and other sites. Seizures that originate in the latter region are particularly likely to be misdiagnosed as functional, as they are frequently accompanied by bizarre posturing and other semi-purposeful, complex motor behaviours. Complex partial seizures of temporal lobe origin are often heralded by an *aura*, which may take the form of olfactory, gustatory, auditory, visual, or somatic hallucinations. Particularly common is the 'epigastric aura'—a sensation of churning in the stomach that rises towards the neck. The patient may also experience odd disturbances of thought or emotion, including an intense sense of familiarity (*déjà vu*) or unfamiliarity (*jamais vu*), depersonalization, or derealization, or, rarely, vivid hallucinations of past experiences ('experiential phenomena'). The sequence of events during the seizure tends to be stereotyped in the individual patient, which is an important diagnostic aid. The whole ictal phase usually lasts for up to 1–2 minutes. After recovery, only the aura may be recalled. Non-convulsive status epilepticus may take the form of a prolonged single seizure, or a rapid succession of brief seizures. In such cases, a protracted period of automatic behaviour may be mistaken for a dissociative fugue or other psychiatric disorder.

Absences

The key feature of an absence attack is loss of awareness that starts suddenly, without an aura, lasts for seconds, and ends abruptly. Simple automatisms (e.g. eyelid fluttering) often accompany the attack. There are no post-ictal abnormalities. For the purposes of diagnosis and treatment, it is essential to distinguish between absence seizures and complex partial seizures. The latter last longer, automatisms during the episode are more complex, recovery occurs more slowly, and the patient may subsequently recall an aura. Absence attacks in children were previously called 'petit mal', and are classically associated with 3 per second 'spike-and-wave' EEG discharges.

Generalized tonic–clonic seizures

This is the familiar epileptic convulsion with a sudden onset, tonic and clonic phases, and a succeeding period of variable duration (up to many hours) in which the patient may be unrousable, sleepy, or disorientated. Incontinence and tongue-biting or other injuries may occur during the seizure. During the post-ictal phase the patient may present with delirium, which may cause diagnostic uncertainty if the convulsion was not witnessed. Generalized tonic–clonic seizures may be initiated by a partial seizure, implying localized brain disease, which is often overlooked. This is an issue of importance, as primary and secondary generalized seizures differ in significance and management.

Myoclonic, atonic, and other seizure types

There are several types of seizures with predominantly motor symptoms, including myoclonic jerks and drop attacks with loss of postural tone. They are unlikely to present to the psychiatrist.

Epidemiology

In the UK, general practice data indicate that the prevalence of epilepsy in adults is about 7 per 1000. About 1 in 30 people have a seizure at some stage. The inception rate is highest in early childhood, and there are further peaks in adolescence and over the age of 65 years. Epilepsy is usually of short duration, and only becomes a chronic condition in about 20% of subjects. This means that regular attenders at specialist clinics are a minority of all those with epilepsy, and who are especially likely to suffer from its medical and social complications. There is psychiatric comorbidity in 20–40% of people with epilepsy (Agrawal and Govender, 2011), and there are particular psychiatric and cognitive implications for children with epilepsy (Lin *et al.*, 2012).

Aetiology

Age at onset is an important clue to aetiology. For example, in the newborn, birth injury, congenital brain malformations, and metabolic disorders are common causes. Infantile febrile convulsions, especially status epilepticus, are classically associated with later complex partial epilepsy, via damage to the hippocampus (hippocampal sclerosis). About 30% of epilepsy is thought to have a primarily genetic basis. However, although many individual genetic mutations and copy number variants are being identified, to date they account for only a small proportion of cases. In adults, identifiable causes include cerebrovascular disease, brain tumours, head injury, autoimmune disorders, and neurodegenerative disorders.

Patterns of alcohol and other drug use should always be established, particularly in young adults. Seizure threshold may be lowered by drug therapy, including antipsychotics, tricyclic antidepressants, and bupropion. Sudden withdrawal of substantial doses of any drug with anticonvulsant properties, most commonly diazepam or alcohol, can precipitate seizures.

For review, see Moshe *et al.* (2015).

Making the diagnosis

Epilepsy is essentially a clinical diagnosis that depends upon detailed accounts of the attacks provided by witnesses as well as by the patient. The background history, physical examination, and special investigations are directed towards establishing the aetiology. The extent of investigation is guided by the initial findings, the type of attack, and the patient's age. Only an outline can be given here; for a full account the reader is advised to refer to a neurology or epilepsy textbook. An EEG can confirm but cannot exclude the diagnosis. It is more useful for determining the type of epilepsy and site of origin. The standard EEG recording may be supplemented by sleep recording, ambulatory monitoring, and split-screen video (telemetry) techniques. Although neuroimaging has an increasing clinical role, no specific brain abnormality (or other cause) is found in the majority of patients with epilepsy.

Epilepsy can be erroneously diagnosed as the cause of paroxysmal neurological and psychiatric symptoms, and it is important to keep in mind the extensive differential diagnosis (see Box 14.5). A clear description of the circumstances surrounding the episode and the mode of onset is fundamental. The most important differential diagnoses of generalized seizures are vasovagal syncope (commonly associated with involuntary movements, a fact not always appreciated) and cardiac arrhythmias. Hyperventilation (of which the patient is often unaware) and panic attacks frequently produce symptoms similar to complex partial seizures, and may lead to actual loss of consciousness if prolonged. Sudden changes in motor activity, affect, and cognition can occur in schizophrenia.

Factors that together suggest a seizure include abrupt onset, a stereotyped course lasting from many seconds to a few minutes, tongue-biting, urinary incontinence, cyanosis, sustaining injury during the attack, and prolonged post-ictal drowsiness or confusion. However, none of these alone is necessary or sufficient to make the diagnosis. Some forms of frontal lobe epilepsy are particularly likely to be misdiagnosed as psychogenic. If the diagnosis remains uncertain, and attacks are frequent, close observation in hospital, including video recording and EEG telemetry and ambulatory monitoring, may be worthwhile.

Functional non-epileptic attacks (pseudoseizures)

Paroxysmal attacks that can be mistaken for epilepsy but which are not caused by seizures or epileptiform activity in the brain are called *pseudoseizures* or *functional non-epileptic attacks* (Agrawal and Govender, 2011). They can be very difficult to distinguish from epilepsy, and make up about 20% of referrals to epilepsy services. Features that suggest non-epileptic episodes include identifiable psychosocial precipitants, a past history of physical or sexual abuse, a history of psychiatric disorder, an unusual or variable pattern of attacks, occurrence either only in public or only while alone, and the absence of autonomic signs or change in colour during 'generalized' attacks. The patient may be suggestible or betray other evidence of retained awareness during the episode. Complex, purposeful behaviour is more often seen in dissociative states. Video recordings of the attacks (e.g. from smart phones) and ambulatory EEG may be helpful. However, some types of seizure may not be reflected in the surface EEG and, conversely, EEG abnormalities occur in perhaps 3% of healthy individuals. Post-ictal serum prolactin levels are useful in a minority of cases (they are elevated after a generalized seizure), but should not be relied upon to make the distinction.

Psychiatric aspects of epilepsy

Psychiatric comorbidity is common in people with epilepsy, with overall rates increased by at least twofold, and higher among those in specialist care. Many different types of psychiatric disorder are associated with epilepsy, including cognitive, affective, emotional, and behavioural disturbances. They are usually classified according to whether they occur before, during, after, or between seizures (see Box 14.24). Psychiatric comorbidity is a major determinant of quality of life for people with epilepsy, and plays an important part in their risk of premature death (Fazel *et al.*, 2013).

The relationship between epilepsy and psychiatric disorder may reflect any of the following factors:

- a shared aetiology or pathophysiology—for example, temporal lobe pathology appears to predispose to epilepsy and to psychosis
- the stigma and psychosocial impairments associated with epilepsy
- the side effects of antiepileptic drugs.

For reviews of the psychiatric aspects of epilepsy, see Agrawal and Govender (2011) and Lin *et al.* (2012). For review of management, see Kanner (2016).

Pre-ictal disturbances

Increasing tension, irritability, and anxiety and depression are sometimes apparent as prodromata for several hours or even days before a seizure, generally increasing in intensity as the seizure approaches.

Ictal disturbances

Ictal psychiatric disturbances (i.e. those directly related to seizure activity) are common and diverse, as noted above. During seizures, transient confusional states, affective disturbances, anxiety, automatisms, and other abnormal behaviours often occur (especially in partial seizures). On occasion, an abnormal mental state may be the only sign of non-convulsive (complex partial or absence) status epilepticus, and the diagnosis is easily overlooked.

Psychosis may occur as an ictal phenomenon. Clues to this possibility include sudden onset and termination of psychiatric disturbance, olfactory or gustatory hallucinations (especially with partial seizures), a relative lack of first-rank symptoms, and amnesia for the period of the disturbance.

Ictal violence is extremely rare, and crimes committed during epileptic automatisms are probably even rarer, an important medicolegal consideration (Treiman, 1999; see also Chapter 18).

Post-ictal disturbances

Psychiatric disturbances may occur during the hours following a seizure. Psychotic symptoms are seen in 2% of cases (Clancy *et al.*, 2014), and are associated with bilateral and extratemporal seizure foci, long duration of epilepsy, and structural brain lesions. These transient psychoses are distinct from the inter-ictal psychoses described below. Diverse motor, sensory, cognitive, and autonomic dysfunction can also occur and, as with the psychoses, may occur as part of a delirium, or in clear consciousness.

Post-ictal violence is rare, although it is more common than violence during the seizure, and may be secondary to psychotic experiences. Extreme post-ictal violence may be recurrent, stereotyped, and more likely to occur in men, after a cluster of seizures. There is usually amnesia for the episode.

Inter-ictal disturbances

Cognitive impairments

In the nineteenth century it was widely believed, based on experience with institutionalized populations, that epilepsy was associated with an inevitable decline in intellectual functioning. However, it is now established that relatively few people with epilepsy show cognitive changes. When these do occur, they are likely to reflect concurrent brain damage, unrecognized non-convulsive seizures, or the effects of antiepileptic drugs. A few patients with epilepsy show a progressive decline in cognitive function. In such cases, careful investigation is required to exclude an underlying progressive neurological disorder; this is a particular concern in paediatric practice. For review, see Lodhi and Agrawal (2012).

Personality

The historical concept of an 'epileptic personality', characterized by egocentricity, irritability, religiosity, quarrelsomeness, and 'sticky' thought processes, has been discarded. Community surveys indicate that only a minority of patients have serious personality difficulties, and these probably reflect the adverse effects of brain damage on education, employment, and social life, rather than a specific association with epilepsy. It has been suggested that behavioural abnormalities (including hypergraphia) are particularly associated with medial temporal lobe lesions. For a discussion of this subject, see Mellers (2009).

Depression and emotional disorders

Depression and anxiety are common in people with epilepsy, for both biological and psychosocial reasons. The rate of depression is increased almost threefold, with a prevalence of over 20% (Fiest *et al.*, 2013). Many subjects meet the criteria for dysthymia rather than major depression, and the term *inter-ictal dysphoric disorder* is sometimes used. The risk factors for depression in epilepsy are summarized in Box 14.25. The relationship between epilepsy and depression is bidirectional, with depression preceding epilepsy as well as vice versa, and reflecting common pathogenic factors for the two conditions. For review of depression in epilepsy, see Hoppe and Elger (2011).

Inter-ictal psychosis

The nature and prevalence of inter-ictal psychosis has long been controversial, including the fundamental question as to whether the two coexist more or less often than expected. Following the important study by Slater *et al.* (1963), the evidence now supports the view that epilepsy is associated with an increased risk of psychosis, especially a schizophrenia-like presentation. A recent meta-analysis reported a rate of inter-ictal psychosis of 5.2% (Clancy *et al.*, 2014). Religious and paranoid delusions appear to be particularly common, and affect tends to be preserved. Risk factors include complex partial seizures, especially with the focus in the mesial temporal or frontal lobe, a lesion which is prenatal in origin, and possibly in the left hemisphere more than the right one. For review, see Mellers (2009).

Suicide

Suicide and deliberate self-harm are more common among people with epilepsy than in the general population. Although estimates vary markedly, a meta-analysis found an adjusted odds ratio of 3.7 (Fazel *et al.*, 2013). The rate appears to be higher in those with temporal lobe epilepsy, and after surgical treatment for epilepsy (Harris and Barraclough, 1997). Suicide risk factors in epilepsy encompass the same range of risk factors as in the general population (see Chapter 21).

Social aspects of epilepsy

The consequences for quality of life correlate with the severity of the seizure disorder, the presence of structural brain pathology, and with any psychiatric comorbidity. The social implications and stigma attached to a diagnosis of epilepsy can be far-reaching, as is the unpredictability of seizure occurrence. When counselling patients and their families, it is important to be sensitive to these issues and to allay groundless fears and misconceptions. Restrictions on driving are a major burden for many patients, whose livelihood may be at stake. To obtain a UK driving licence, the patient must have had at least 1 year with no seizures while awake, whether or not they are still taking antiepileptic drugs. Those who have seizures only while asleep may hold a licence if this pattern has been stable for at least 3 years.

Sexual dysfunction with reduced libido and impaired performance is common in patients with epilepsy, especially where there is a temporal lobe focus. This is thought to be mainly due to antiepileptic medication, although psychosocial factors are also important, and rarely there may be a direct link to the cause of the seizures.

Epilepsy has been said to be associated with crime and violence. However, there is little evidence for either assertion. In meta-analyses, rates of epilepsy among prisoners

---

Box 14.25 Risk factors for depression in epilepsy

Biological

Family history of mood disorder

Focus in temporal or frontal lobe

Left-sided focus

Psychosocial

Perceived stigma

Fear of seizures

Pessimistic attributional style

Decreased social support

Unemployment

Iatrogenic

Epilepsy surgery

Antiepileptic drugs, especially polypharmacy and high serum levels

were not increased (Fazel *et al.*, 2002), nor was the risk of violence higher in people with epilepsy (Fazel *et al.*, 2009b). The latter result emphasizes that ictal and post-ictal violence, mentioned earlier, are both very rare events.

Treatment of epilepsy

The drug treatment of epilepsy is usually undertaken by general practitioners and neurologists. Here the discussion will be restricted to some key points of psychiatric relevance.

- It is important to distinguish between peri-ictal and inter-ictal psychiatric disorders when planning treatment. For peri-ictal disorders, treatment is aimed at control of the seizures.
- Treatment of inter-ictal psychiatric disorders is usually similar to that in non-epileptic patients, but there are relatively few data demonstrating the efficacy of pharmacological or psychological therapies in this population.
- The potential for psychotropic drugs to worsen the seizure disorder should always be considered, though most drugs are safe at therapeutic doses. Indeed, commonly used antidepressants may in fact be anticonvulsant, contrary to common belief (Kanner, 2016). However, antidepressants can cause seizures at toxic doses. Amongst antipsychotics, first-generation drugs such as haloperidol and fluphenazine have a lower seizure propensity than olanzapine, quetiapine, or clozapine.
- Some antiepileptic drugs can cause a variety of cognitive and psychiatric symptoms, whilst others (such as lamotrigine) are increasingly being used to treat psychiatric disorders.
- There are pharmacokinetic interactions between antiepileptic, psychotropic, and other drugs that can lead to toxicity or subtherapeutic levels. The potential for such interactions should always be checked before prescribing (or withdrawing) medication.

Given these considerations, close liaison between neurologist, psychiatrist, and general practitioner is recommended. For review of drug treatment of psychiatric disorders in epilepsy, see Kanner (2016). For psychosocial aspects of treatment, see Mittan (2009).

Intracranial infections

Many intracranial infections cause cognitive impairment, and effective treatment is available for the majority of them. Unusual infections should always be considered as a cause of otherwise unexplained cognitive and psychiatric symptoms. Encephalitis is described later in this chapter; HIV infection is considered in Chapter 22.

For a review, see Dilley and Fleminger (2009).

Neurosyphilis

Neurosyphilis, a manifestation of the tertiary stage of infection with the spirochaete *Treponema pallidum*, is now rare in western countries. However, increasing numbers of cases have been reported in Eastern Europe and in association with HIV. Because of its protean manifestations, the possibility of neurosyphilis should be considered in all 'neuropsychiatric' patients, especially those with delirium or dementia, and appropriate blood or CSF serological tests ordered. Prior treatment with antibiotics may produce partial and atypical syndromes.

An asymptomatic stage precedes clinical disease with variable latency. Symptomatic neurosyphilis takes three forms.

- *Meningovascular syphilis* appears within 5 years of primary infection. It presents with strokes, or with personality changes, emotional lability, and headache. Dementia may occur subsequently, accompanied by psychotic symptoms.
- *General paresis* (also called *general paralysis of the insane*, or *dementia paralytica*) starts to develop about 20 years after infection. Presentation is with dementia, personality change, dysarthria, and motor symptoms and signs. Affective and psychotic symptoms may be florid, classically with euphoria and grandiose delusions. Discovery of the cause of general paresis was an important landmark in the history of psychiatry, stimulating a search for organic causes of other psychiatric syndromes.
- *Tabes dorsalis* is a degeneration of spinal cord pathways, and is unlikely to present to psychiatrists.

In the early stages, treatment with penicillin reverses the condition, and halts progression later in the illness. If the clinical disease is left untreated, death usually occurs within 5 years.

Brain tumours

Many brain tumours cause psychological symptoms at some stage in their course, and a significant proportion present with such symptoms. Psychiatrists are likely to see patients with slow-growing tumours in 'silent' (especially frontal) areas. These produce psychological effects, but few neurological signs—for example, a frontal meningioma or glioma of the corpus callosum. The nature of the psychological symptoms is influenced by the global effects of raised intracranial pressure, in addition to the tumour location. The rate of tumour growth is also important; rapidly expanding tumours with raised intracranial pressure can present as delirium, whereas slower-growing tumours are more likely to cause chronic cognitive deficits. Focal lesions give rise to a variety of specific neuropsychiatric syndromes; those near the frontal poles typically manifest initially as personality change. Craniopharyngiomas and other tumours around the hypothalamus are also often associated with personality changes and apathy. Cognitive impairment after treatment of brain tumours in children is particularly problematic, especially in those who have received radiotherapy.

For a review, see Mellado-Calvo and Fleminger (2009).

Cognitive impairments in cancer

In addition to the direct effects of brain tumours, neoplasms anywhere in the body can impair cognition via a range of mechanisms (see Box 14.26). Occasionally, such complications are the presenting feature, but usually they arise during treatment, at which time the psychiatrist may be asked for a diagnostic and therapeutic opinion. For a review, see Khasraw and Posner (2010).

Box 14.26 Some causes of cognitive impairment in patients with cancer

Mass effects

Primary and metastatic brain tumours
Haemorrhagic change (especially melanoma, renal-cell carcinoma, choriocarcinoma)

Diffuse infiltration

Gliomatosis cerebri
Carcinomatous and lymphomatous meningitis
En plaque meningioma

Paraneoplastic limbic encephalitis

Anti-NMDA-receptor and other autoantibodies

Metabolic derangements

Hypercalcaemia
Hyponatraemia

Acidosis
Hypoglycaemia

Radiotherapy

Acute and subacute radionecrosis
Radiation thromboangiopathy
Accelerated cerebral atherosclerosis
Radiation leucodystrophy
Second malignancies (especially glioma, meningioma)

Chemotherapy

Metabolic encephalopathies
Opportunistic infections secondary to immuno-suppression (herpes zoster, progressive multifocal leucoencephalopathy)

Other neuropsychiatric syndromes

Multiple sclerosis

Multiple sclerosis is the most common cause of chronic neurological disability in young adults in developed countries. Its consequences for work and relationships may be profound. The disease may be difficult to diagnose early in the course, and physical symptoms are sometimes misinterpreted as psychiatric. Psychiatric symptoms are rarely the presenting feature, but the majority of patients will experience them at some stage, especially fatigue, depression, cognitive impairment, and euphoria (Box 14.27). Such symptoms probably result both directly from the disease process and from the disabilities associated with it. There is a several-fold increase in the risk of suicide.

Depression is more common in multiple sclerosis than in other neurological disorders, with a lifetime risk of 50%. It does not appear to be closely related to the severity of the clinical syndrome or the site of lesions. It is also a side effect of beta-interferon, which is used to treat multiple sclerosis (Feinstein *et al.*, 2014). Both antidepressant and cognitive behaviour therapy approaches can be effective. Cognitive impairment is present in at least 40% of patients from community samples. It may be an early manifestation of the illness, and occasionally

a rapidly progressive dementia occurs. In most cases, however, intellectual deterioration begins later, is less severe, and progresses slowly. Well-practised verbal skills are often preserved despite deficits in problem-solving, abstraction, memory, and learning. Cognitive impairment correlates with total lesion load and degree of callosal atrophy on MRI, and probably reflects axonal loss rather than demyelination per se.

For a review of psychiatric aspects of multiple sclerosis, see Wong *et al.* (2013a).

Encephalitis

Encephalitis is inflammation of the brain parenchyma. The term is sometimes used to apply specifically to a primary viral infection, although encephalitic involvement can also occur as a complication of bacterial meningitis (meningoencephalitis) or a cerebral abscess. Moreover, it is now clear that many cases of encephalitis are not due to infection but have an autoimmune basis, as described below.

The commonest viral cause of encephalitis is Herpes simplex (Sabah *et al.*, 2012). Without treatment, it was often fatal or left devastating consequences. Although intravenous aciclovir provides an effective treatment, it remains a serious condition. In the acute stage, headache, vomiting, and impaired consciousness are usual, and seizures are common. Presentation may be with delirium. The psychiatrist may be involved in initial diagnosis, but is more likely to see chronic complications, which include prolonged anxiety and depression, a profound amnesic syndrome, personality change, or complex partial epilepsy. Other significant types of encephalitis in adults include those produced by arthropod-borne viruses and, especially in the immune compromised, varicella zoster. For review of viral encephalitis, see Dilley and Fleminger (2009).

A major recent development is the realization that many cases of encephalitis are not in fact viral, but are autoimmune in origin. In particular, autoantibodies against various neuronal proteins (especially NMDA glutamate receptors and potassium channels) are now recognized as being a relatively common cause of limbic encephalitis, and often present floridly with delirium and psychosis, as well as with epilepsy and other neurological features (Vincent *et al.*, 2011). Hence they may present to psychiatrists, and liaison psychiatrists

---

Box 14.27 Psychiatric features of multiple sclerosis

Common

Fatigue

Depression

Cognitive impairment

Less common

Euphoria

Pseudobulbar affect

Psychosis

Bipolar disorder

Source: data from Advances in Psychiatric Treatment, 19(5), Wong EKO, Krishnadas R and Cavanagh J, The interface between neurology and psychiatry: the case of multiple sclerosis, pp. 370-377, Copyright (2013a), The Royal College of Psychiatrists.

may also be involved in their management (Barry *et al.*, 2015). These antibodies not only underlie the encephalitis of paraneoplastic syndromes but also occur in the absence of cancer or other known cause. They can also be triggered by Herpes simplex, blurring the distinction between viral and autoimmune forms of the illness. Screening for autoantibodies is now routine in investigation of suspected encephalitis, and positive cases are treated using immunosuppression. Whether antineuronal antibodies can produce psychiatric syndromes (especially a schizophrenia-like psychosis, or narcolepsy) without other evidence of encephalitis remains controversial (see Chapter 11).

An outbreak of *encephalitis lethargica* (also called postencephalitic parkinsonism) was reported in Vienna in 1917 by Von Economo. The condition reached epidemic proportions in the 1920s, and was thought to be related to the influenza pandemic of the time. By the 1930s it had largely disappeared. Parkinsonism was the most disabling complication; personality change with antisocial behaviour, and psychosis, also occurred. In his famous 1973 book *Awakenings,* Sacks gave a vivid description of such cases, and the striking but temporary 'awakening' brought about in some by l-dopa. Current speculation is that the condition may have been caused by anti-NMDA receptor antibodies.

Normal pressure hydrocephalus

The characteristic clinical triad in this condition (Adams *et al.*, 1965) consists of a striking 'gait apraxia' (a broadbased, small-stepped gait with difficulty in initiation) on which supervenes a progressive frontal subcortical syndrome with bradyphrenia and, later, urinary incontinence. Frank dementia is rare. The prevalence is uncertain, but is reported to be 0–6% of cases of late-life dementia in published series. The condition is more common in the elderly, but sometimes occurs in middle life, and in children with congenital abnormalities.

The pathogenesis has been thought to be a block to CSF flow within the ventricular system owing to aqueduct stenosis, or in the subarachnoid space. However, often no cause can be discovered. Ventricular pressure is generally normal or low, although episodes of raised pressure may also occur. Ventricular enlargement out of proportion to the degree of cortical atrophy, often with periventricular signal change, is the hallmark finding on brain imaging.

It is important to differentiate this condition from a degenerative dementia, and from depression with pseudodementia. Cases with a short history and prominent gait disturbance with relative sparing of intellect may be amenable to a neurosurgical shunt procedure to improve the circulation of CSF. However, the outcome is variable and difficult to predict. The presence of hippocampal atrophy on imaging suggests associated Alzheimer's disease, and predicts a poor response to shunting.

For a review, see Finney (2009).

Anoxia, hypoglycaemia, and carbon monoxide poisoning

Anoxia (e.g. due to cardiac arrest), hypoglycaemia, and carbon monoxide poisoning produce similar patterns of brain injury. Cerebral and cerebellar atrophy may occur, and the hippocampus and globus pallidus are particularly vulnerable. Clinical experience suggests that the recovery trajectory is relatively brief compared with traumatic brain injury, and that neurological sequelae are less disabling. Parkinsonism is not infrequent after a latent interval. The commonest cognitive impairment is poor memory. For a review, see Auer (2004).

Carbon monoxide poisoning usually arises from deliberate self-harm by car exhaust fumes, and, more recently, from burning charcoal in the Far East. However, it can also occur accidentally as a result of badly ventilated gas boilers or fires. The prevalence of complications after carbon monoxide poisoning is unclear, with a wide range of figures reported. It is also unclear whether residual symptoms ever occur if the poisoning was insufficient to cause loss of consciousness, although complaints of problems with memory, concentration, fatigue, and headache are common (Ho *et al.*, 2012).

Systemic lupus erythematosus

Systemic lupus erythematosus (SLE) has neuropsychiatric manifestations in about 10% of patients at time of first presentation, and in 20–75% of patients at some stage of the illness. The commonest feature is cognitive dysfunction, affecting all domains of memory, as well as poor attention and concentration, and reduced psychomotor speed. Mood disorder is also common, and psychosis affects up to 8% of cases. SLE is an autoimmune disorder, and anti-NMDA receptor, antiphospholipid, and other antibodies are implicated, together with an inflammatory component. For a review of neuropsychiatric SLE and its treatment, see Hanly (2014).

Secondary or symptomatic neuropsychiatric syndromes

All of the disorders discussed in this chapter so far are either defined by their underlying pathology (e.g. the dementias) or have an undisputed biological basis (e.g. epilepsy). However, by convention, neuropsychiatry also includes disorders that are not usually included in this category (i.e. are 'functional' or idiopathic), but which can on occasion be explained in the same fashion. They are described as *secondary, symptomatic*, or *organic*. ICD-10 and DSM-5 code these disorders in different ways and use differing terminologies (see Table 14.1). As noted earlier, in this book we cover psychiatric disorders secondary to brain diseases in this chapter, whereas those resulting from systemic diseases are covered in Chapter 22. Examples of secondary neuropsychiatric disorders are listed in Table 14.6. See also Lovestone (2009b).

The clinical features of these secondary disorders are generally indistinguishable from those in the equivalent primary psychiatric disorder. Thus recognition of a secondary syndrome depends on the associated features. The following suggest that the disorder is secondary to a physical condition:

- Evidence of cerebral disease, damage, or dysfunction, or of physical disease, known to be associated with one of the listed syndromes.
- A temporal relationship (of weeks or a few months) between the development of the underlying disease and the onset of the psychiatric syndrome.
- Recovery from the psychiatric disorder following removal or improvement of the presumed cause.

Table 14.6 Some causes of symptomatic or secondary psychiatric syndromes

Syndrome	Causes
Psychosis	Temporal lobe disorders, Huntington's disease, basal ganglia lesions, dementias, endocrinopathies, metabolic disorders, cerebral vasculitides, neurosyphilis, limbic encephalitis
Mood disorder	Alzheimer's disease, stroke, head trauma, Parkinson's disease, multiple sclerosis, Huntington's disease, endocrinopathies, metabolic disorders (especially hypercalcaemia), neurosyphilis
Personality change	Frontotemporal dementias, frontal lesions, Huntington's disease, focal basal ganglia lesions, neurosyphilis, prion disease, paraneoplastic limbic encephalitis
Obsessive–compulsive behaviours	Frontotemporal dementias, complex partial seizures, basal ganglia disorders, Rett syndrome

- Absence of evidence suggesting an alternative 'psychological' cause of the psychiatric disorder (e.g. in the case of depression, no evidence of a family history of mood disorder, relevant personality traits, previous episodes of mood disorder, recent life events, etc.).

Further reading

Bang J *et al.* (2015). Frontotemporal dementia. *Lancet*, **386**, 1672–82.

David AS *et al.* (2009). *Lishman's Organic Psychiatry*, 4th edn. Wiley Blackwell, Oxford. (The definitive textbook on neuropsychiatry—an essential reference.)

Yudofsky SC and Hales RE (2010). *Essentials of Neuropsychiatry and Behavioural Neurosciences*, 2nd edn. American Psychiatric Press, Washington, DC. (A shorter American equivalent to 'Lishman'. Includes chapters on the underlying neuroscience.)

CHAPTER 15
Personality and personality disorder

Personality

The term personality refers to those enduring qualities of an individual that are shown in their ways of
behaving in a wide variety of circumstances. We use
it to distinguish between people. Personality differs
from mental disorder. The behaviours that define it
have been present throughout adult life, whereas the
behaviours that define mental disorder differ from the
person's previous behaviour. When we say that mentally ill persons are 'not their normal selves', we are
drawing on our understanding of their personality
and usual behaviour. The distinction is easy to make
when behaviour changes markedly over a short period
of time (as in a manic disorder), but can be difficult
when the changes occur very gradually (as in some
cases of schizophrenia).

The importance of personality

Gaining an understanding of and familiarity with a
patient's personality is important in psychiatry for a
number of reasons. Different personalities predispose
to some psychiatric disorders, and they may colour
the presentation ('pathoplastic' factors). They may also
influence how a patient approaches treatment, and dic-
tate different strategies for establishing and maintaining
a successful therapeutic relationship.

Personality as predisposition

Personality can predispose to psychiatric disorder by
modifying an individual's response to stressful events.
For example, adverse circumstances are more likely to
induce an anxiety disorder in a person who has always
worried about minor problems.

Personality as a pathoplastic factor

Personality can contribute to unusual features of a
disorder, particularly when personality traits become
exaggerated with illness. For example, rumination and
inhibition may be the presentation of depression in an
individual with an obsessional personality. The underlying diagnosis can be obscured if the psychiatrist has not
made an accurate assessment of personality.

Personality in relation to treatment

Personality is an important determinant of a person's approach to treatment. For example, people with obsessional traits may become frustrated and resistant if treatment does not follow their expectations, and anxiety-prone people may discontinue medication prematurely because of concerns about minimal side effects. Some people with a severe disorder of personality, particularly so-called Cluster B disorders (antisocial, borderline, impulsive, histrionic, and narcissistic personality disorders; see below) have often been effectively excluded from services because of the difficult relationships they form with clinicians (see Lewis and Appleby, 1988). This is a significant problem, as there is strong evidence that personality disorder is common in clinical populations, and that people with personality disorders have an increased risk for a range of mental illnesses (Moran, 2002). There has been a concerted move to remedy this, addressed later in this chapter and in Chapter 24.

Patients are often aware of their personalities—they know if they are 'emotional' or 'conscientious' or 'anxious'. Acknowledging this diplomatically (making sure to note the positive aspects as well as the negative ones) and discussing how it may interact with their treatment (and with their life more generally) can be an effective tool in maintaining treatment.

Personality types

A first step in understanding personality is to identify some basic types. Clinicians have generally derived these from a mixture of clinical and common-sense collective experience with several generally recognizable categories, such as a sociable and outgoing type, a solitary and self-conscious type, and an anxious and timid type. Psychologists have adopted a more rigorous scientific approach using personality tests to measure aspects of personality ('traits') such as anxiety, energy, flexibility, hostility, impulsiveness, moodiness, orderliness, and self-reliance. These are then subject to statistical investigations to discover how they cluster into 'factors'.

Although these statistical procedures appear very scientific, their results are determined by the investigators' original hypotheses (which traits they considered important and included in their analyses, and the order in which they included them, etc.). Like diagnoses, these are essentially working hypotheses, which are continuously evolving and should not be treated with too much reverence—their value lies in their utility.

Different investigators have derived different personality factors from such traits. Cattell (1963) identified five factors, whereas Eysenck (1970a) originally proposed only two 'dimensions' (high-level factors), which he labelled extraversion–introversion and neuroticism. Subsequently he added a third dimension, 'psychoticism' (Eysenck and Eysenck, 1976), but his use of the term is rather misleading, denoting coldness, aggressivity, cruelty, and antisocial behaviour.

A five-factor formulation for personality has persisted, although the terms used for the factors have varied. They can be identified as openness to experience (or novelty-seeking), conscientiousness, extraversion–introversion, agreeableness (or affiliation), and neuroticism.

Cloninger (Cloninger *et al.*, 1993) developed an alternative scheme with three 'basic behavioural dispositions' expressed as four basic temperaments (a seven-factor model). The behavioural dispositions are behavioural activation, behavioural inhibition, and behavioural maintenance. Cloninger considered behavioural activation to be associated with the basic temperament of *novelty-seeking*, behavioural inhibition with *harm avoidance*, and behavioural maintenance with *reward dependence*. The fourth basic temperament is *persistence*. Cloninger's scheme also includes three character traits, namely *self-directedness*, *cooperativeness*, and *transcendence*. The various types of personality and personality disorder are constructed from these four basic temperaments and three character traits. Cloninger's scheme includes both inherited differences in brain function and the effects of experience.

These factor schemes of personality have survived despite sustained criticism that they are largely dependent on what was included in the original factor analyses. Zuckerman (2005) has also criticized these theories because they assume an alignment between personality traits and brain systems. In recent years there has been some refinement, with greater emphasis on cognitive factors. A cognitive–adaptive theory has been proposed (Penke and Denissen, 2007), and Mischel has emphasized the dynamic nature of personality in his cognitive–affective system (Mischel *et al.*, 2004). Current texts on personality theory (for example, Matthews and Deary,

2009) are weighty tomes, and those interested in deepening their understanding might be best advised to start by consulting a clinical psychology colleague.

Despite these scientific approaches, clinicians continue to use everyday words to describe the positive and negative features of normal personality. Positive attributes include 'outgoing', 'self-confident', 'stable', and 'adaptable'. Negative attributes include 'sensitive', 'jealous', 'irritable', 'impulsive', 'self-centred', 'rigid', and 'aggressive'.

The origins of personality

The biological basis of personality types

Genetic influences

Everyday observation suggests that children often resemble their parents in personality. Such similarities could be either inherited or acquired through social learning. Three kinds of scientific study have been used to study the inheritance of personality.

Studies of body shape and personality. Different personalities have been linked to body shape ('beware of Brutus, he has a lean and hungry look'). If this were true, the link could be genetic. Kretschmer (1936) described three types of body build—pyknic (stocky and rounded), athletic (muscular), and asthenic (lean and narrow). He suggested that the pyknic body build was linked to the cyclothymic personality type (sociable with variable moods), whereas the asthenic build was related to the 'schizotypal' personality type (cold, aloof, and self-sufficient). Kretschmer's ideas were based on subjective judgements, and were influenced by experience of the 'associated' psychotic disorders (manic-depressive disorder and schizophrenia). Quantitative methods to assess physique and more objective ratings of personality fail to support the link (Sheldon *et al.*, 1940).

Studies of twins. More direct evidence has been obtained from personality tests of monozygotic and dizygotic twins. These suggest that the heritability for traits of extraversion and neuroticism is 35–50% (McGuffin and Thapar, 1992). The heritability of other personality traits is broadly similar.

Molecular genetic studies. Genetic linkage and association studies have revealed a number of loci and genes contributing to personality traits, but the findings remain preliminary (Balestri *et al.*, 2014). It is clear that the genetic predisposition to personality (and its disorders) arises from the cumulative effect of multiple genes, each of very small effect. Some of these genetic influences are shared with those underlying psychiatric disorders, and this overlap likely explains much of the association between them (such as neuroticism with depression).

Childhood temperament and adult personality

Young infants differ enormously in patterns of sleeping and waking, approach or withdrawal from new situations, intensity of emotional responses, and span of attention. These differences, which are described in more detail in Chapter 16, could form the basis for personality development. They do persist into later childhood, but their relationship to adult personality has been difficult to establish.

Childhood experience and personality development

Everyday experience suggests that childhood experience shapes personality (society is built on this premise), but it is not easy to demonstrate it. Experiences that seem relevant are difficult to quantify or even to record reliably, and it is extremely difficult and expensive to conduct prospective studies that span the time period from childhood events to adult personality, although some ongoing studies, such as the Dunedin cohort study in New Zealand, are able to link confirmed early experience and adult states (Poulton *et al.*, 2015). Retrospective studies are easier to arrange, but recall of childhood experiences is unreliable. While scientific data on personality development are sparse, psychodynamic and infant development theories retain considerable influence.

The *Freudian theory* of personality development emphasizes events during the first 5 years of life. Freud proposed that crucial stages of libido development must be accomplished successfully for healthy personality development. Failure or fixation at particular stages explained certain features of adult personality. Freud's explanation is excessively comprehensive and flexible. It can be made to explain almost all personality variation in terms of infantile experience, but its very flexibility makes it impossible to test scientifically. However, it retains enormous intuitive appeal and is widely used both within and outside of psychiatry.

Jung considered personality development to be a life-long process, with 'individuation' as its aim. His theories are particularly valued in disorders of later life. He introduced the terms 'introvert' and 'extrovert'.

Later analysts rejected Freud's exclusive focus on libido development. *Adler* emphasized a struggle for mastery (overcoming the 'inferiority complex'). The 'neo-Freudians' increasingly emphasized social and peer-group factors in personality development.

Erikson extended Freud's schema, using less offputting terms, for the individual developmental challenges. Erikson's eight developmental stages continued right into late adult life and each was presented as a conflict, such as 'trust versus mistrust', 'autonomy versus doubt', that had to be resolved. Erikson emphasizes the importance of adolescence.

Attachment theory

Attachment theory derives from the work of John Bowlby. Although a psychoanalyst, Bowlby's work is based on observation and simple processes that are being subjected to structured testing. Bowlby emphasized the importance of *maternal deprivation* in the development of personality in orphan children just after the second World War. He proposed that a close, reliable relationship was needed for effective attachment and that a '*secure attachment*' promoted health. Alternatives were '*insecure*' or '*anxious*' attachments, which could lead to later problems in forming relationships (Bowlby, 1951). Despite critical examination (Rutter, 1991), attachment theory commands extensive respect, and structured instruments for establishing styles of attachment have been developed, such as the Adult Attachment Interview (van Ijzendoorn, 1995).

The assessment of personality

The assessment of personality is discussed in Chapter 3, but two points need to be emphasized. The first is that the assessment of personality used in everyday life cannot be applied reliably in clinical practice. Normally we assume that current behaviour reflects the person's habitual ways of behaving (their personality), and in general this assumption is correct. This is not the case when we assess patients, because their current behaviour reflects the effects of their illness as well as their personality. A patient's personality can only be judged confidently from reliable accounts of past behaviour, which have been obtained wherever possible from informants as well as from the patient.

Secondly, the assessment instruments developed for personality mentioned earlier (see page 392), although more reliable in healthy individuals, can be misleading in the presence of mental disorder. In addition, they rarely measure the traits that are most relevant to clinical practice. Personality tests, although useful in research, are seldom used in clinical practice. For a review of personality assessment methods, see Clark and Harrison (2001).

The importance of personality assessment

The assessment of personality is important when making decisions about aetiology, diagnosis, and treatment. In aetiology, knowledge of personality helps to explain why certain events are stressful to that patient. In diagnosis, an understanding of personality may explain the presence of unusual features in a disorder that might otherwise cause uncertainty. In treatment, an assessment of personality helps to explain the patient's reaction to their illness and its treatment, and aids the establishment of an effective therapeutic relationship. Personality assessment should be an integral part of every formulation, and not just reserved for those where a personality disorder is suspected.

It is best to record a series of descriptive terms chosen from the features of accepted personality disorders, because the more theoretical personality factors are too general to help the clinician. Examples would be 'sensitive', 'lacking in self-confidence', and 'prone to worry'. Such descriptions help to construct a picture of the unique features of each patient, which is a fundamental element of good clinical practice.

Personality disorder

The concept of abnormal personality

Some personalities are obviously abnormal—for example, paranoid personalities characterized by extreme suspiciousness, sensitivity, and mistrust. However, it is impossible to draw a sharp dividing line between normal and abnormal personalities. Abnormal personalities are in practice recognized because of the *pattern* of their characteristics, but our current classificatory processes in psychiatry demand that we identify *criteria* for inclusion. However, precisely which criteria should be used to make this distinction remain controversial. Two types of criteria have been suggested, namely statistical and social.

According to the *statistical criterion*, abnormal personalities are quantitative variations from the normal, and the dividing line is decided by a cut-off score on an appropriate measure. This approach is attractive, as it parallels that used successfully when defining abnormalities of intelligence, it appears non-judgemental, and it has obvious value in research. However, its usefulness in clinical practice is uncertain.

According to the *social criterion*, abnormal personalities are those that cause the individual to suffer, or to cause suffering to other people. For example, an abnormally sensitive and gloomy personality causes suffering for the individual who has it, and an emotionally cold and aggressive personality causes suffering for others. These criteria are subjective and lack the precision of the first approach, but they serve the needs of clinical practice better and they have been widely adopted.

It is not surprising that it is difficult to frame a satisfactory definition of abnormal personality. The ICD-9 described personality disorders as follows:

Severe disturbances in the personality and behavioural tendencies of the individual, not directly resulting from disease, damage or other insult to the brain, or from another psychiatric disorder. They usually involve several areas of the personality and are nearly always associated with considerable personal distress and social disruption. They are usually manifest since childhood or adolescence and continue throughout adulthood.

ICD-10 emphasizes enduring patterns of behaviour, but the ICD-9 definition is more concise, and still valuable.

The 'personal distress' referred to in ICD-9 may sometimes only become apparent late in life (e.g. when a longstanding supportive relationship is lost). There are usually, although not always, significant problems in occupational and social performance.

It is important to recognize that people with abnormal personalities generally also have favourable traits, which the clinician should always assess. For example, those with obsessional traits are often dependable and trustworthy. Management plans that play to an individual's strengths are more likely to be helpful for them.

Personality change

In some circumstances during adult life there may be a profound and enduring change in personality that is distinct from the temporary changes that may accompany stressful events or illness. This lasting change may result from:

- Injury to or organic disease of the brain.
- Severe mental disorder, especially schizophrenia.
- Exceptionally severe stressful experiences (e.g. those experienced by hostages or by prisoners undergoing torture).

ICD-10 contains categories for each type of change. 'Change in personality due to organic disease of the brain' is classified with the organic mental disorders in section F00, and includes the changes that occur following encephalitis and head injury. In DSM-5 this condition is diagnosed as personality change due to another medical condition.

In ICD-10 the other two forms of personality change listed above are classified in section F60, disorders of adult personality and behaviour. To diagnose 'enduring personality change after psychiatric illness', the change of personality must have lasted for at least 2 years, be clearly related to the experience of the illness, and not have been present before it. 'Enduring personality change after a catastrophic experience' must also have lasted for at least 2 years and have followed a stressful experience that was extreme (e.g. prolonged kidnapping, a terrorist attack, or torture). Victims are commonly hostile, irritable, distrustful, socially withdrawn, and on edge. The condition may follow post-traumatic stress disorder, but is considered distinct from it.

The historical development of ideas about abnormal personality

The concept of abnormal personality is recognized from psychiatry's beginnings at the start of the nineteenth century. The French psychiatrist Philippe Pinel used *manie sans délire* for patients prone to outbursts of rage and violence, but who were not deluded. J. C. Prichard, senior physician to the Bristol Infirmary, suggested a new term, *moral insanity*, which he defined as a:

morbid perversion of the natural feelings, affections, inclinations, temper, habits, moral dispositions and natural impulses, without any remarkable disorder or defect of the intellect or knowing or reasoning faculties, and in particular without any insane delusion or hallucination. (Prichard, 1835)

Prichard's moral insanity included conditions that we would now diagnose as personality disorder. The term 'moral' was then equivalent to our 'social'. The 'moral treatment' developed by the Tuke family in the York Retreat in the 1790s embodied socialization not ethical instruction.

Henry Maudsley used the term more as we would understand an antisocial personality disorder:

having no capacity for true moral feeling—all his impulses and desires, to which he yields without check, are egoistic, his conduct appears to be governed by immoral motives, which are cherished and obeyed without any evident desire to resist them. (Maudsley, 1885)

Julius Koch introduced the term 'psychopathic inferiority', subsequently replaced by personality (Koch, 1891). Emil Kraepelin was at first uncertain how to classify these people, and only adopted the term 'psychopathic personality' in the eighth edition of his textbook, where finally he devoted a whole chapter to it.

Kurt Schneider broadened the concept in 1923 to include markedly depressive or insecure characters. He used 'psychopathic' to cover the whole range of abnormal personality, not just antisocial personality. The term came to have two meanings—a wider meaning of abnormal personality of all kinds, and a narrower meaning of antisocial personality—which has led to subsequent confusion.

In the 1959 Mental Health Act for England and Wales, psychopathic disorder was interpreted narrowly, and in the 1983 Act it was defined as:

a persistent disorder or disability of mind (whether or not including significant impairment of intelligence) which results in abnormally aggressive or seriously irresponsible conduct on the part of the person concerned.

This narrow concept, which emphasized aggressive or irresponsible behaviour, made its inclusion in the original 1959 Act controversial. Consequently, the requirement of 'treatability' as a condition of detention was added exclusively to it, out of all the mental disorders. This distinction was abandoned in the 2007 amendment to the 1983 Mental Health Act (see Chapter 4) because it was perceived to present a barrier to effective treatment.

A recent short-lived development in the United Kingdom was the administrative category of 'dangerous and severe personality disorder (DSPD)'. This refers mainly to men with antisocial personality disorder and a history of serious violent or sexual offending which can be linked to their personality disorder. The evolution of effective treatments for this group has proved elusive and, in any event, changes in the law to permit indeterminate sentences for prisoners who pose persisting serious risks have made the category redundant.

Because the term 'psychopathic personality' is ambiguous, the preferred terms are *personality disorder* and *antisocial personality disorder* to denote the wide and narrow senses, respectively.

The classification of abnormal personalities

General issues

The use of categories

Personality traits are continuously distributed, but the classification of psychiatric disorders uses categories and requires definitions and boundaries. However, the criterion for inclusion (distress to the person or to others) is very imprecise, so cases that fall just short of it (subthreshold cases) are frequent. These subthreshold cases often present clinical problems that are similar to those of definite cases.

Comorbidity

It is not only the boundary between normal and abnormal personality that is imprecise and arbitrary; the boundaries between the different types of personality are also ill defined. This leads to an important divergence of practice between clinical psychiatrists and researchers and some psychologists. Many patients have features contained in the criteria for more than one personality disorder (Fyer *et al.*, 1988). Structured instruments for measuring personality disorder, such as the International Personality Disorder Examination (Loranger *et al.*, 1997), are often used by researchers and psychologists. They permit more than one personality diagnosis to be made in a single patient, and the term 'comorbidity' is used. From a clinical perspective it seems more likely that the patient has a single personality disorder that has features which overlap two of the arbitrary sets of criteria used in the current systems of diagnosis. We would usually diagnose the single personality disorder that best fits the mixed picture and is most useful in understanding and helping the patient in front of us. Comorbidity is used when a patient has both a mental illness and a personality disorder (or more often a mental illness and substance abuse), but makes little clinical sense for personality disorder alone.

Conditions related to personality disorder and classified elsewhere

Cyclothymia and schizotypal disorder were previously classified as personality disorders. In ICD-10 both of these conditions have been removed from the personality disorders and classified instead with the mental disorders (cyclothymia with affective disorders, and schizotypal disorder with schizophrenia). This reflects the fact that these two conditions may begin in adult life and, in the case of schizotypal disorder, evidence from family studies that links it genetically to schizophrenia (see page 399). In DSM-5, cyclothymic disorder is classified with bipolar and related disorders, but schizotypal disorder is retained as a personality disorder. In both classifications, multiple personality disorder is classified with dissociative disorders.

Classification of personality disorders in ICD-10 and DSM-5

In Table 15.1 the classification of personality disorders in ICD-10 is compared with that in DSM-5. The two schemes are broadly similar, but there are some differences.

In DSM-IV, personality disorders were classified on a different 'axis' (Axis II) from mental disorders (which are classified on Axis I). This has been abandoned in DSM-5,

which has a single axis. ICD-10 did not have a separate axis. The personality should still be assessed, and if no personality disorder is present this should be recorded in the formulation.

Grouping into clusters

In DSM-5, but not in ICD-10, personality disorders are grouped into three 'clusters':

1. *Cluster A:* paranoid, schizoid, and schizotypal.
2. *Cluster B:* antisocial, borderline, histrionic, and narcissistic.
3. *Cluster C:* avoidant, dependent, and obsessive–compulsive.

This convention is adopted later in this chapter.

Different names for the same personality disorder

The individual names for personality disorders differ somewhat between the two classifications. This reflects the real uncertainty about their boundaries and also an attempt through renaming to de-stigmatize some disorders. In ICD-10 the term 'dissocial' is used, whereas in DSM-5 the term 'antisocial' (the term used in this book) is used. In ICD-10, the term 'anankastic' is used, whereas 'obsessive–compulsive' is used in DSM-5. In ICD-10, the term 'anxious' is used, whereas 'avoidant' is used in DSM-5.

Conditions that are present in one classification but not the other

Emotionally unstable impulsive personality disorder and enduring personality change not attributable to brain damage or disease are found in ICD-10 but not in DSM-5. Narcissistic personality disorder is included in DSM-5 but not in ICD-10. As noted above, schizotypal personality disorder is classified with schizophrenia in ICD-10 (and named schizotypal disorder), whereas in DSM-5 it is classified as a personality disorder.

Two new radically different approaches to classification

Despite their intuitive appeal and enduring utility the traditional 10 personality diagnoses are criticized for their lack of theoretical underpinning and their unreliability. Two radically different approaches have been proposed to alter this and introduce a more *dimensional* component to diagnosis (Tyrer *et al.*, 2015). DSM-5 trialled an assessment based on severity of impairments and a range of traits. This involved a reduction from ten to six categories—borderline, obsessive–compulsive, avoidant, schizotypal, antisocial, and narcissistic personality disorders. The approach was found to be impractical by clinicians, and so this *hybrid model* was omitted from the main DSM-5, but is included in section III, 'Emerging Measures and Models'.

For ICD-11 a proposal is being considered to abandon the clinical categories and replace it with the diagnosis of personality disorder (present or absent) with different degrees of severity defined. It is not known whether this proposal will be adopted. Only time will tell whether either of these attempts to shift the focus from categories to dimensions will be adopted by clinicians. On past experience it seems unlikely.

Descriptions and diagnostic criteria

This section contains an account of the abnormal personalities listed in ICD-10 and DSM-5 (see Table 15.1). The criteria for diagnosis are lengthy, and differ in wording and emphasis in the two systems. The main common features from the two sets of definitions are given, simplified, or paraphrased where appropriate to give a more general description.

All personality disorder diagnoses must meet the basic criteria for personality disorder summarized from the ICD-10 criteria for research as follows:

- The characteristic and enduring patterns of behaviour differ markedly from the cultural norm and in more than one of the following areas: cognition, affectivity, control of impulses and gratification, and ways of relating to others.
- The behaviour is inflexible, and maladaptive or dysfunctional in a broad range of situations.
- Personal distress is caused to others and/or to self.
- The presentation is stable and longlasting, usually beginning by late childhood or adolescence.
- The behaviour is not caused by another mental disorder, or by brain injury, disease, or dysfunction.

There are several diagnostic instruments for personality disorder, but they are mainly of value in research.

Cluster A personality disorders

Paranoid personality disorder

Such people are suspicious and sensitive (see Box 15.1). They have a marked sense of self-importance, but easily feel shame and humiliation. They are suspicious and constantly on the lookout for attempts by others to deceive or exploit them, which makes them difficult for others to get on with. They have difficulty making friends and avoid involvement in groups. They are usually mistrustful and often jealous. They may appear secretive and self-sufficient to a fault. They take offence easily and see criticism where none was intended.

Suspicious ideas can be so intense that they are mistaken for persecutory delusions. These *sensitive ideas of reference* are considered further in Chapter 12. Paranoid individuals can be resentful and bear grudges, engaging in litigation, often against all advice.

Table 15.1 Classification of personality disorders

	ICD-10	DSM-5
Cluster A	Paranoid	Paranoid
	Schizoid	Schizoid
	(Schizotypal; see text)	Schizotypal
Cluster B	Dissocial	Antisocial
	Emotionally unstable	Borderline
	Impulsive type	
	Borderline type	
	Histrionic	Histrionic
	—	Narcissistic
Cluster C	Anankastic (obsessive–compulsive)	Obsessive–compulsive
	Anxious (avoidant)	Avoidant
	Dependent	Dependent

Source: data from The ICD-10 classification of mental and behavioural disorders: clinical descriptions and diagnostic guidelines, Copyright (1992), World Health Organization; Diagnostic and Statistical Manual of Mental Disorders, Fifth Edition, Copyright (2013), American Psychiatric Association.

Box 15.1 Features of paranoid
personality disorder

Suspicious
Mistrustful
Jealous
Sensitive
Resentful
Bears grudges
Self-important

Schizoid personality disorder

The term 'schizoid' was suggested by Kretschmer (1936), who believed that this type of personality is related to schizophrenia. People with this disorder are emotionally cold, *detached and aloof*, introspective, and prone to engage in excessive fantasy (see Box 15.2). They are unable to express either tender feelings or anger, and show little interest in sexual relationships. When the disorder is extreme they may appear callous. They are generally ill at ease in company, do not form intimate relationships, and show little family feeling. They are seclusive, following a solitary course through life, and often remain unmarried. They show little sense of enjoyment or pleasure in the activities that most people enjoy, which contributes to their separation from others. *Introspective and prone to fantasy*, they are interested in intellectual matters, and have a complex inner world of fantasy, albeit without emotional content.

Schizotypal personality disorder

Schizotypal individuals are socially anxious and behave eccentrically. They can experience cognitive and perceptual distortions, and have oddities of speech and inappropriate emotional responses. This personality disorder

Box 15.2 Features of schizoid
personality disorder

Emotionally cold
Detached
Aloof
Lacking enjoyment
Introspective

appears to be related to schizophrenia, so it is not classified as a personality disorder in ICD-10 (as is the case in DSM-5), but is placed with schizophrenia and called schizotypal disorder (see Chapter 11).

Schizotypal individuals experience *social anxiety* in company, so have difficulty in forming relationships and lack friends and confidants. They feel different from other people and do not fit in. (This is in contrast to schizoid individuals, who are quite content with this situation.) Their *cognitive and perceptual distortions* include ideas of reference (but not delusions), suspicious ideas, odd beliefs, and magical thinking (e.g. belief in clairvoyance, mind reading, and telepathy), and unusual perceptual experiences (e.g. awareness of a 'presence', or experiences bordering on hallucinations). They also show *oddities of speech*, such as unusual constructions, words, and phrasing, as well as vagueness, and a tendency to digression. Their *affective responses are unusual*, and they appear stiff, odd, and constricted in their emotions. Their *behaviour is eccentric*, with odd mannerisms, unusual choices of clothing, disregard of conventions, and awkward social behaviour.

Cluster B personality disorders

This is the group of personality disorders that looms largest in current psychiatric practice. Whereas most personality disorders 'colour' the presentation and management of patients, individuals with cluster B disorders are often referred specifically with a request for treatment of the personality disorder itself.

Antisocial (dissocial) personality disorder

The term 'antisocial' is used in DSM-5 and in this book, whereas 'dissocial' is the term used in ICD-10. Antisocial personality disorder is not simply another term for *delinquency*. People with this disorder show a callous lack of concern for the feelings of others. They disregard the rights of others, act impulsively, lack guilt, and fail to learn from adverse experiences (see Box 15.3). Often their abnormal behaviour is made worse by the abuse of alcohol or drugs. Hervey Cleckley's 1941 book *The Mask of Sanity* (Cleckley, 1964) is a vivid and influential description of this type of personality.

The criteria for diagnosis differ slightly in the two classifications; the following criteria are taken from ICD-10. The DSM-5 criteria include the requirement of conduct disorder before the age of 15 years.

A central feature is a *callous lack of concern for others*. People with antisocial personality disorder may be

Box 15.3 Features of antisocial personality disorder

Callous
Transient relationships
Irresponsible
Impulsive and irritable
Lacking guilt and remorse
Failure to accept responsibility

exploitative and even violent, and their sexual activity lacks tenderness. They may inflict cruel or degrading acts on other people, and their partners may be physically or sexually abused. They may have a *superficial charm*, but their *relationships are shallow and short-lived*. They are *irresponsible and depart from social norms*. They do not obey rules and may repeatedly break the law, often committing violent offences. Their offending typically begins in adolescence.

Such individuals are *impulsive*, rarely plan ahead, and typically have an unstable work record. They take risks, disregarding their own safety and that of other people. They are *irritable*, and when angry sometimes assault others in a violent way. These features of personality are accompanied by a striking *lack of guilt or remorse* and a failure to change their behaviour in response to punishment or other adverse outcomes. They *avoid responsibility*, transferring blame on to other people and rationalizing their own failures. They are often deceitful and irresponsible about finances.

The concept of 'psychopathy' overlaps with antisocial personality disorder. Although it has been dropped from the diagnostic classification, it is still in use in psychology (particularly forensic psychology) and the prison service, and has a very specific meaning. It is generally considered to be a character trait, and is usually assessed using the Hare Psychopathy Checklist-Revised (PCL-R) (Hare, 1991). This distinguishes two factors—violent and impulsive behaviour, and charm and exploitation. The terms 'psychopathy' and 'antisocial personality disorder' are often unhelpfully interchanged, and psychopathy is probably best avoided by general psychiatrists.

Borderline personality disorder

The term 'borderline personality disorder' is a confusing and unsatisfactory one, which reflects its complex history. It was originally used in psychodynamic circles to describe people with a marked 'instability' of presentation, as opposed to a steady neurotic state. The proposed 'border' at that time was with psychosis. Kernberg (1975) described it as involving:

1. Ego weakness with poor control of impulses.
2. 'Primary process' (i.e. irrational) thinking despite intact reality testing.
3. Use of less 'mature' defence mechanisms, such as projection and denial.
4. Diffuse personal identity.

People with borderline personality disorder experience their lives as being dominated by *strong and fluctuating emotions* that often overwhelm them. They strive for affection and intimacy but are regularly disappointed, and may exhaust their partners with the intensity of their emotional demands. They are themselves confused by the strength and *unpredictability of their moods* as they plunge into anger or despair. They are often *insecure in their personal identity* and need reassurance and stability, which they may then find constricting and irritating. *Self-harm* is common (either suicidal attempts, or cutting to release tension). Such self-destructive behaviour can be extreme and may dominate the relationship with care services. *Alcohol and drug abuse* are also common, as they attempt to blunt their distressing emotions. Clinical populations are dominated by relatively young women, although the epidemiological studies challenge this distribution.

When this type of personality disorder was introduced into the classification systems, more objective criteria were developed, but it remains unsatisfactory. The diagnosis was (and still is) almost exclusively applied to young women. This raised the question of whether it was a more culturally determined expression of mood disorder (i.e. depression) filtered through a histrionic (at that time referred to as 'hysterical') personality. The suggestion that it may respond (at least partially) to antidepressants has fuelled this controversy, as has the greater degree of variation over time than in other personality disorders, and the observation that in most patients it seems to resolve.

Not surprisingly, with such uncertainty different names have been adopted in the two classifications—borderline personality disorder in DSM-5 and emotionally unstable personality disorder in ICD-10. The latter is divided into a 'borderline type' and an 'impulsive type'. The diagnostic criteria (slightly abbreviated) are shown in Table 15.2. Several features of the ICD-10 impulsive type are among the criteria for borderline personality disorder in DSM-5.

Borderline personality disorder remains a controversial and contested diagnosis. It was originally entered into DSM-III only after a protracted debate and on the grounds that its utility would be researched. Many people who meet the criteria for borderline personality disorder in DSM-5 also meet the criteria for histrionic, narcissistic, and antisocial personality disorder (Skodol et al., 2002a); the overlap with bipolar disorder is also controversial and can be clinically problematic.

Impulsive personality disorder

This disorder is recognized in ICD-10 as a subtype of emotionally labile personality disorder. It is not included separately in DSM-5, although several of its features match the criteria for borderline personality disorder. The diagnostic criteria are listed in Table 15.2, and three criteria must be met for the diagnosis. People with impulsive personality disorder cannot control their emotions adequately, and are liable to outbursts of sudden unrestrained anger which they subsequently regret. They may use physical violence occasionally, causing serious harm. Unlike people with antisocial personality disorder, they do not generally have other difficulties in relationships.

Histrionic personality disorder

Histrionic personality disorder is included in both ICD-10 and DSM-5, but the criteria are somewhat different. Box 15.4 lists the features that are diagnostic criteria in ICD-10, and also notes the criteria that differ between the two systems.

Self-dramatization is a striking feature, and may include 'emotional blackmail', angry scenes, and demonstrative suicide attempts. These individuals are *suggestible* and easily influenced by others, especially by figures of authority. They *seek attention and excitement*, are easily bored, and have short-lived enthusiasms. They have a *shallow labile affect*. Their emotional life is dramatic and may exhaust others. However, they recover quickly and often cannot understand why others are still upset. They seek intimacy and can be *inappropriately seductive*.

Histrionic individuals are often insecure about their value, and consequently may be *over-concerned with physical attractiveness*. They can appear *self-centred* and vain. They may also have a marked capacity for *self-deception*, being convinced by their own fabrications—however elaborate and improbable these may be—even when other people have seen through them. In its most extreme form, histrionic personality disorder is observed in 'pathological liars' and swindlers. Blanche DuBois in Tennessee Williams' *A Streetcar Named Desire* poignantly portrays the disastrous consequences that such

Table 15.2 Abbreviated criteria for emotionally unstable and borderline personality disorders

ICD-10	DSM-5
Emotionally unstable personality disorder, borderline type	**Borderline personality disorder**
Disturbed or uncertain self-image	Identity disturbance
Intense and unstable relationships	Intense and unstable relationships
Efforts to avoid abandonment	Efforts to avoid abandonment
Recurrent threats or acts of self-harm	Recurrent suicidal behaviour
Chronic feelings of emptiness	Chronic feelings of emptiness
—	Transient stress-related paranoid ideation
Impulsive type	
Impulsive	Impulsive
Liability to anger and violence	Difficulty controlling anger
Unstable capricious mood	Affective instability
Quarrelsome	—
Difficulty maintaining a course of action	—

Source: data from The ICD-10 classification of mental and behavioural disorders: clinical descriptions and diagnostic guidelines, Copyright (1992), World Health Organization; Diagnostic and Statistical Manual of Mental Disorders, Fifth Edition, Copyright (2013), American Psychiatric Association.

a personality can have both for the individual and for those around them.

Narcissistic personality disorder

This personality disorder is listed in DSM-5 but not in ICD-10, where it is one of the disorders coded in the residual category 'Other specific personality disorder'. The DSM-5 criteria are summarized and paraphrased in Box 15.5.

People with this disorder have a grandiose sense of self-importance and are boastful and pretentious. They are preoccupied with fantasies of unlimited success, power, beauty, or intellectual brilliance. They consider themselves special, and expect others to admire them and offer them special services and favours. They feel entitled to the best, and seek to associate with people of

> ### Box 15.4 Features of histrionic personality disorder
>
> Self-dramatization
> Suggestibility
> Shallow labile affect
> Seeks attention and excitement
> Inappropriately seductive
> Over-concern with physical attractiveness
>
> *Note:* DSM-5 has two additional criteria:
>
> - Speech excessively impressionistic
> - Considers relationships to be more intimate than they are

high status. They exploit others and do not empathize with or show concern for their feelings. They envy the possessions and achievements of others, and expect that those individuals will envy them in the same way. They appear arrogant, disdainful, and haughty, and behave in a patronizing or condescending way.

Narcissistic personality disorder carries probably the most pejorative overtones of any of the personality disorder diagnoses. It should be reserved for only the most undeniable examples, and only after you have made sure that the diagnosis is not coloured by personal dislike. On balance it is probably a term to avoid if at all possible, like some older personality terms such as 'immature personality' or 'inadequate personality', which have no place in modern mental healthcare.

Cluster C personality disorders

Avoidant (anxious) personality disorder

DSM-5 uses the term 'avoidant' and in ICD-10 the term 'anxious' is preferred, with 'avoidant' as an accepted alternative. The diagnostic criteria in the two classifications are listed in Box 15.6. Liability to tension is a criterion only in ICD-10.

People with this disorder are *persistently tense*. They feel insecure and lack self-esteem. They feel *socially inferior*, unappealing, and socially inept. They are *preoccupied with the possibility of rejection*, disapproval, or criticism, and worry that they will be embarrassed or ridiculed. They are cautious about new experiences, *avoid risk*, and *avoid social activity*. They have few close friends, but they are not emotionally cold, and indeed crave the social relationships that they cannot manage to attain.

Dependent personality disorder

Box 15.7 lists the diagnostic criteria in ICD-10 and DSM-5. People with this disorder *allow others to take responsibility* for important decisions in their lives. They are *unduly compliant*, but are *unwilling to make direct demands* on other people. They lack vigour and *feel unable to care for themselves*. Lacking self-reliance, they avoid responsibility, and may need *excessive help to make decisions*.

They are often protected by support from a more energetic and determined partner, and may only come to medical attention when the partner leaves or dies.

> ### Box 15.5 Features of narcissistic personality disorder
>
> Grandiose sense of self-importance
> Fantasizes about unlimited success, power, etc.
> Believes himself or herself to be special
> Requires excessive admiration
> Sense of entitlement to favours and compliance
> Exploits others
> Lacks empathy
> Envious of others, and believes that others envy him or her
> Arrogant and haughty

> ### Box 15.6 Features of avoidant (anxious) personality disorder
>
> Feels socially inferior
> Preoccupied with rejection
> Avoids involvement
> Avoids risk
> Avoids social activity
>
> *Note:* DSM-5 has two additional criteria:
>
> Restraint in intimate relationships, due to fear of being shamed or ridiculed

> ### Box 15.7 Features of dependent personality disorder
>
> Allows others to take responsibility
> Unduly compliant
> Unwilling to make reasonable demands
> Feels unable to care for himself or herself
> Fear of being left to care for himself or herself
> Needs excessive help to make decisions
>
> *Note:* Three additional criteria are used in DSM-5. They can be summarized as follows:
>
> - Experiences difficulty in initiating projects
> - Goes to excessive lengths to obtain support
> - Urgently seeks a supportive relationship

> ### Box 15.8 Features of obsessive–compulsive (anankastic) personality disorder
>
> Preoccupied with details, rules, etc.
> Inhibited by perfectionism
> Over-conscientious and scrupulous
> Excessively concerned with work and productivity
> Over-conscientious, scrupulous, and inflexible in ethics and morals
> Unable to discard worthless objects
> Reluctant to delegate tasks or work with others
> Miserly
> Rigidity and stubbornness

Obsessive–compulsive personality disorder

DSM-5 uses the term 'obsessive–compulsive personality disorder' whereas ICD-10 uses the term 'anankastic' (originated by Kahn, 1928). Kahn used this term to avoid the implication that this personality disorder is linked to obsessive–compulsive disorder. Box 15.8 lists the diagnostic criteria in ICD-10 and DSM-5.

These individuals are *preoccupied with details and rules*, order, and schedules. They have an *inhibiting perfectionism* that makes ordinary work a burden as they are immersed in endless detail. They may lack imagination and fail to take advantage of opportunities. However, they usually have high moral standards, are often *excessively conscientious*, and may be rather judgemental. They can appear humourless and ill at ease when others are enjoying themselves.

These people lack adaptability to new situations. They are generally *rigid and inflexible*, avoiding change and preferring a familiar routine. They can be *stubborn and controlling* and generally thrifty, sometimes to the point of being miserly. They may hoard objects and money. They may be *pedantic and unduly concerned with social conventions*. They can also be particularly troubled by *excessive doubt and caution*, leading to indecision.

Affective personality disorders

Some people have lifelong disorders of mood regulation. They may be persistently gloomy (depressive personality disorder) or habitually in a state of inappropriate elation (hyperthymic personality disorder). A third group alternates between these two extremes (cycloid or cyclothymic personality disorder). These types of personality have been described for many years, and are readily recognized in clinical practice. In both ICD-10 and DSM-5 they are classified under disorders of mood and not under disorders of personality. In ICD-10 they are classified under 'persistent mood (affective) states' (cyclothymia or dysthymia), and in DSM-5 under bipolar and related disorders. Nevertheless, it is useful to describe them briefly here.

People with *depressive personality disorder* always seem to be in low spirits. They have a persistently gloomy and pessimistic view of life, and may brood about their misfortunes and worry unduly. They have little capacity for enjoyment and are dissatisfied with their lives. Some are irritable and bad-tempered.

People with *hyperthymic personality disorder* are habitually cheerful and optimistic, and exhibit a striking zest for living. If they have these traits to a moderate degree, they are often highly effective and successful individuals whom we envy. However, if the traits are more pronounced they can show poor judgement and irritate those around them.

People with *cyclothymic personality disorder* alternate between the extremes of depressive and hyperthymic states described above. This instability of mood is much more disruptive than either of the persisting conditions. People with this disorder are periodically extremely cheerful, active, and productive, at which times they take on additional commitments in their work and social lives. When their mood changes they become gloomy and defeatist, and with reduced energy levels they now find their newly acquired obligations a burden.

Rates of personality disorder in the clinic and the general population

Clinical population rates

For a psychiatrist, the more important question is how frequently personality disorder will be encountered in their clinical practice. Prevalence rates vary more for personality disorder than for mental illnesses both in clinic and in population surveys because of diagnostic uncertainty. A series of studies have investigated this, and the 16 largest and most rigorous studies were summarized by Zimmerman *et al.* (2008). Zimmerman's review showed that much higher rates were found in structured assessments, at around 40%. Rates of personality disorder in those in contact with mental health services have been estimated at 40% for UK community mental health teams (CMHTs; Newton-Howes *et al.*, 2010) or 50% internationally for outpatient attendees (Beckwith *et al.*, 2014). Rates are even higher for prison populations (Fazel and Danesh, 2002). Among primary care consultations in the UK, the rate is as high as 30% (Moran *et al.*, 2000).

However, we know that rates in the clinic and rates in the general population are likely to be very different. Treatment seeking by individuals with personality disorder is powerfully affected by the existence of a comorbid mental illness (Kessler *et al.*, 1999).

General population rates

Epidemiological research into personality disorders in the general population began with the development of standardized instruments using DSM-III criteria. Studies require large samples because the prevalence rates of some personality disorders are low. It is also difficult to identify personality disorder reliably in community surveys without access to informants. Data come mainly from studies in the USA, the UK, and Germany, and from a recent World Health Organization (WHO) mental health survey review (Huang *et al.*, 2009). The most extensive data come from 10 epidemiological studies in the USA and four in Europe cited by Huang *et al.* (2009). The prevalence rates for any personality disorder from these studies range from 4% to 16%. Only one survey was international, sampling seven countries across five continents (Huang *et al.*, 2009). This found a point prevalence of 6.1%, lowest in Europe (2.4%) and highest in North and South America (7.6% USA, 7.9%

Table 15.3 Median prevalence rates of personality disorders in epidemiological surveys

Personality cluster	Personality disorder category	Number of studies (*n*)	Median prevalence rate (%)
Cluster A	Paranoid	13	1.6
	Schizoid	13	0.8
	Schizotypal	13	0.7
Cluster B	Antisocial	24	1.5
	Borderline	15	1.6
	Histrionic	12	1.8
	Narcissistic	10	0.2
Cluster C	Obsessive–compulsive	13	2.0
	Avoidant	13	1.3
	Dependent	12	0.9
	Passive–aggressive	8	1.7

Source: data from Guzzetta F and de Girolamo G, Epidemiology of personality disorders. In: Gelder M et al, eds. New Oxford Textbook of Psychiatry, 2nd edn, pp. 881–6, Copyright (2009), Oxford University Press.

Colombia). In contrast to clinic populations, personality disorder is at least as common in men as women (Coid *et al.*, 2006) and it is as common in ethnic minority as in host populations (Crawford *et al.*, 2012). Rates appear to be higher in urban populations (Torgesen *et al.*, 2001).

Estimates of the prevalence of the various types of personality disorder from the review by Guzzetta and de Girolamo (2009) are shown in Table 15.3. In these studies, sample sizes ranged from 200 to 1600. Some of these estimates have a substantial range, reflecting among other sources of variation the use of different assessment instruments. The rates of some disorders vary between men and women. Antisocial personality disorder is more common among men (estimated ratios range between 2.1 and 7.1). Although borderline and histrionic personality disorders are clinically reported more frequently in women, this was not consistently confirmed in epidemiological studies.

Structured assessment instruments have high reliability but may have more questionable validity. Certainly they seem to generate more positives than most clinicians would expect, and the absolute rates should be treated with some caution. However, the relatively primitive state of personality disorder theory and assessment may explain much of this variation. The surprising findings of remarkably high rates of remission in personality disorder when using these instruments may indicate that they should be treated cautiously. However, there is a growing belief among personality disorder researchers that their lifelong nature has been overstated (Tyrer, 2015; Newton-Howes *et al.*, 2015).

Aetiology

General issues

The causes of personality disorder are uncertain, and this is an area in which hypotheses are many and research findings varied. The two major areas are genetic factors and various kinds of early life experience. Some personality disorders have been linked aetiologically with the psychiatric disorders that they resemble. The state of evidence for each of these three general issues will be considered with the individual personality disorders.

The study of the influence of *early life experiences* is made difficult by the long interval between these experiences and the diagnosis of personality disorder in adult life. Psychodynamic theories linking childhood experience and personality are hard to test, but have been influential.

Most clinicians accept that there are causal links between childhood experience, personality, and personality disorder. It is agreed good practice to assess childhood experiences and to use common-sense judgement to decide whether any of these may have influenced the personality. For example, extreme and repeated rejection by the parents may explain low self-esteem in adult life. Retrospective studies present obvious problems, but prospective studies are now becoming available. For example, independently documented gross physical neglect or abuse or sexual abuse in childhood has been shown to be associated with cluster B personality disorders (Johnson *et al.*, 1999). Different causes have been suggested for the various personality disorders so they will be considered separately. Important, representative research evidence is cited below but the reader should not lose sight of the overall picture that aetiology in this group of disorders is very unclear.

Antisocial personality disorder

Genetic causes

The much quoted early twin studies by Lange (1931) and Rosanoff *et al.* (1934) were concerned with probands with repeated conviction for criminal offences rather than antisocial personality disorder as such, so their relevance is uncertain. More recent twin studies have confirmed the heritability of antisocial behaviour in adults, and have shown that genetic factors are more important in adults than in antisocial children or adolescents where the shared environmental factors dominate (Lyons *et al.*, 1995).

One gene contributing to antisocial behaviour is monoamine oxidase A (*MAOA*); a common low-activity *MAOA* genetic variant predisposes to adult antisocial behaviour in men, especially in those who experienced early adversity—an example of a gene–environment interaction (Byrd and Manuck, 2014).

Cadoret (1978) found that adoptees separated at birth from a parent who had displayed persistent antisocial behaviour had higher rates of antisocial personality disorder than did adoptees whose biological parents were not antisocial. Antisocial personality disorder was diagnosed more often in men than in women, although the women had an increased rate of what was then diagnosed as hysteria (and is probably closer to the current diagnosis of borderline personality disorder). Cadoret suggested that hysteria (borderline personality disorder) is an expression in women of the same genetic endowment that causes antisocial personality disorder in men. Similar findings were reported in an earlier study by Crowe (1974). Data linkage studies from Sweden confirm the genetic contribution to sexual offending by demonstrating the association between rates and degree of relationship (Långström *et al.*, 2015).

Cerebral pathology and cerebral maturation

As some brain-injured patients show aggressive behaviour, minor degrees of brain injury have been sought as a cause of antisocial personality. However, there is no convincing evidence to support this idea. MRI studies have found reduced prefrontal grey matter (Raine *et al.*, 2000), and reduced amygdala volume may be linked to the characteristic lack of empathy (Blair, 2003).

5-Hydroxytryptamine and aggression

Abnormalities in brain 5-hydroxytryptamine (5-HT) neurotransmission have been reported in patients with impulsive and aggressive behaviour, and low levels of the 5-HT metabolite 5-hydroxyindoleacetic acid (5-HIAA) have been found in the cerebrospinal fluid of subjects who have committed acts of unpremeditated violence (Linnoila and Virkkunen, 1992). In addition, more recent studies have found abnormalities in 5-HT-mediated neuroendocrine function and brain 5-HT$_{2A}$-receptor availability *in vivo* in people with high trait aggressiveness (Coccaro *et al.*, 2010; Rosell *et al.*, 2010). It has been suggested that the same abnormalities may be relevant to personality disorders that are characterized by impulsive behaviour, particularly in the presence of prefrontal deficits (Dolan *et al.*, 2002; New *et al.*, 2004).

Developmental theories

Separation. In a much-quoted early study, Bowlby (1944) studied 44 'juvenile thieves' and concluded that separation of a young child from their mother could lead to antisocial behaviour and failure to form close relationships. This work stimulated much research into the effects of separating children from their mothers (see page 425), introduced radical changes into aspects of social and paediatric care, and has given rise to attachment theory. Not all separated children are affected adversely, and the effects of separation depend on many factors, including the child's age, the previous relationship with the mother and father, and the reasons for separation. Rutter (1972) showed that *parental marital disharmony* partly accounts for the association between separation and antisocial disorder in sons.

Social learning in childhood. Scott (1960) proposed four ways in which antisocial behaviour could develop through social learning:

1. Growing up in an antisocial family.
2. Lack of consistent rules in the family.
3. Overcoming other problems (e.g. aggressive behaviour to hide feelings of inferiority).
4. Poor ability to sustain attention, and other impediments to learning.

There is evidence for some of these factors. Antisocial personality disorder is associated with physical abuse and with violent parenting without consistently applied rules (Pollock *et al.*, 1990), and with low IQ and large family of origin (Farrington *et al.*, 1988). The main value of Scott's proposal is in providing a framework for the assessment.

Childhood behaviour problems and antisocial personality. A 30-year follow-up study of children attending a child guidance clinic found an association between behaviour problems in childhood and antisocial personality disorder in adult life (Robins, 1966). Only a minority of those even with serious antisocial behaviour in childhood became persistently antisocial in adult life, but *most* of the adults with antisocial personality disorder had behaviour problems in childhood. The association was stronger if in childhood there was more than one kind of antisocial behaviour, and if antisocial acts were repeated. Stealing among boys and sexual delinquency among girls were especially likely to be followed by antisocial behaviour in adult life. Early conduct problems have been shown to predict antisocial personality independently of associated adverse family and social factors (Hill, 2003), hence the requirement for a history of conduct disorder for the diagnosis of antisocial personality disorder in DSM-5.

Paranoid personality disorder

Little is known about the causes of this disorder. Some investigators have reported that paranoid personality disorder is more frequent among first-degree relatives of probands with schizophrenia than among the general population (Kendler *et al.*, 1985), but others have not confirmed this finding (see Chapter 11).

Schizoid personality disorder

The cause of this disorder is unknown. It does not appear to be closely related genetically to schizophrenia

(Fulton and Winokur, 1993). The psychoanalyst Melanie Klein outlined what she called the 'paranoid–schizoid position' (Klein, 1952). This was an early developmental phase before infants could sustain a clear understanding of their mother as an individual who came and went (the 'depressive position', so called because the infant could then miss the mother). Klein's views were not intended to explain either paranoid or schizoid disorders, although they are often quoted as such, but rather to emphasize the importance of the mother–child relationship more than she thought Freud had done.

Schizotypal personality disorder

This is more frequent among biological relatives of individuals with schizophrenia than among adopted relatives or controls (Kendler *et al.*, 1981). A review of 17 structural imaging studies of people with this personality disorder found brain abnormalities that were similar in most ways to those in people with schizophrenia (Dickey *et al.*, 2002). Similarly, there is strong evidence for a genetic contribution, with heritability scores of 0.35–0.81 in twin studies (Ji *et al.*, 2006; Kendler *et al.*, 2006, 2007). These findings suggest that this personality disorder may be a milder form of schizophrenia, or that the two are related in some other way.

Borderline personality disorder

There is now an impressive volume of research into biological factors in borderline personality disorder (New *et al.*, 2008), and some evidence for the importance of genetic factors. Twin studies show heritability scores of 0.65–0.76 (Torgersen *et al.*, 2000; Ji *et al.*, 2006). First-degree relatives of patients with borderline personality disorder are 10 times more likely to be treated for borderline personality disorder or 'similar personality disorder' (Loranger *et al.*, 1982). Some of the genes and loci associated have begun to be identified (Lubke *et al.*, 2014). A wide range of imaging studies have implicated subtle grey matter changes in prefrontal and limbic regions, as well as functional dysregulation of the cortico-limbic circuitry involved in emotional regulation (Ruocco *et al.*,

2013). A recent ligand binding and PET imaging study has suggested that there are abnormalities in opioid regulation in the same brain regions (Prossin *et al.*, 2010).

It is becoming accepted that it may be more fruitful to study the genetics of personality traits (e.g. dysregulation of affect and poor impulse control) than the personality disorders themselves (Siever *et al.*, 2002). Psychodynamic theories propose a disturbed relationship with the mother at the stage of individuation of the child (Kernberg, 1975), and people with a borderline personality are more likely to report that they experienced physical and sexual abuse in childhood (Berelowicz and Tarnopolsky, 1993).

Histrionic personality disorder

There have been few objective studies of the causes of this personality disorder. The genetics have not been studied with standardized methods of assessment, and the few reported investigations have yielded inconsistent findings (McGuffin and Thapar, 1992). Freud's views of the role of the Oedipus complex and the failure of mature intimacy leading to oversexualized relationships are impossible to test, but may help when dealing with histrionic individuals.

Obsessional personality disorder

Obsessional personality appears to have a substantial genetic aetiology (Murray and Reveley, 1981), although its nature is unknown. Psychoanalytic explanations were initially influential, but have now faded even within psychotherapy circles.

Anxious–avoidant, dependent, and passive–aggressive personality disorders

The genetics of these personality disorders have not been specifically studied, and their causes remain unknown at present.

The course of personality disorder

Personality disorders are defined as lifelong conditions, so little change would be expected with time. There is little reliable evidence about their outcome, other than

for borderline personality disorder and, to a lesser extent, antisocial personality disorder. The results of those studies that have been conducted make surprising reading.

Much of the influential work comes from the USA and uses repeated assessment according to DSM-IV criteria for personality disorder diagnosis or for personality disorder traits. Overall, this work indicates that personality disorder is much less stable than had previously been believed. Skodol (2008) concludes that, of studies conducted in the DSM-III era, over 50% of patients subsequently failed to meet personality disorder criteria over time. In this review of four large naturalistic studies, two reported changes in personality traits and two reported changes in diagnoses. All of them showed marked improvements; for example, a 48% reduction in personality disorder traits between 15 and 22 years of age (Cohen *et al.*, 2005) and a reduction in the number of individuals continuing to meet the diagnostic criteria for borderline personality disorder are outlined below. Newton-Howes *et al.* (2015) cite several studies of change in personality and personality disorder in adult and even late-adult age. However, in the face of such figures it is difficult not to question the validity of the measures. A judgement has to be made as to whether they are genuinely measuring what we understand by personality.

Borderline personality disorder. The outcome is very varied, suggesting that it may not be a single entity, or could in fact be a questionable one (Skodol *et al.*, 2002b). In the most influential outcome study, the McLean Hospital follow-up (Zanarini *et al.*, 2006), 290 patients with borderline personality disorder were interviewed using the SCID II (First *et al.*, 1997) every 2 years for 10 years. A total of 88% achieved 'remission' over this time period, 39% by 2 years, a further 22% by 4 years, a further 22% by 6 years, and so on. Those who still showed a borderline personality disorder more often had comorbid substance abuse or a history of childhood sexual abuse. A high rate of suicide has been found in some studies (8.5% in the study by Stone *et al.*, 1987), raising the suspicion of an atypical affective disorder.

Aggressive and antisocial personality disorders. Clinical impressions indicate that minor improvement may take place slowly, especially in aggressive and antisocial behaviour ('psychopathy burns out'). In the study by Robins and Regier (1991), about one-third of people with persistent antisocial behaviour in early adult life improved later, as judged by the number of arrests and contacts with social agencies. However, they still had problems in relationships, as shown by hostility towards partners and neighbours, as well as an increased rate of suicide. There is a problem of circularity here in that *criminality is one of the features of antisocial personality disorder in DSM-5* (although not in ICD-10), and not all antisocial personality disorder patients identified in community studies (Regier *et al.*, 1990) have problems with the law, and not all criminals meet the criteria for antisocial personality disorder (Hare, 1983; Coid and Ullrich, 2010). Whether antisocial personality disorder improves significantly over time is the subject of conflicting evidence. Robins and Regier (1991) reported a high rate of remission in the third and fourth decades of life, whereas Rutter and Rutter (1993) emphasized its stability. The view that such patients 'burn out' may reflect a reduction in help-seeking rather than late maturing.

Much less is known about the longer-term outcome in the other personality disorders. The overwhelming clinical impression is that borderline personality disorder is distinguished from the other disorders by its apparent variability. However, in the longitudinal studies using structured assessments there is also a high level of remission for other personality disorders. For instance, in a collaborative multi-site study of 668 DSM-IV-diagnosed personality disorder patients in the USA (Skodol *et al.*, 2005), remission occurred in 38% of those with obsessive–compulsive personality and 23% of those with schizotypal personality disorder within 2 years.

Mehlum *et al.* (1991) reported a 3- to 5-year follow-up of schizotypal personality disorder in which the outcome was worse than borderline personality disorder. 'Cluster C' personality disorders (see page 402) seem to have a better outcome than the other groups.

Treatment

There is little hard evidence on the treatment of personality disorder (Bateman *et al.*, 2015) and most of the available data are concentrated on the two dominant cluster B disorders, borderline and antisocial, and the latter mainly conducted with incarcerated offenders. It is not surprising that research is limited. This is a patient group that is hard to engage in either treatment or research; the core features, such as functional disability and disturbed relationships, are much harder to operationalize and measure than traditional symptoms; comorbidity complicating the picture is the norm rather than the exception.

Most of the studies that have been conducted utilize the epiphenomena of the disorders as outcome. In borderline personality disorder self-harm and readmissions to hospital, while in antisocial personality disorder most commonly reduced aggression in the short term and reduced offending in the longer term are used as outcome measures. Despite (or perhaps because of) the variation in the manifestations of personality disorder reported in studies using structured assessments (Skodol *et al.*, 2005), no trials have demonstrated changes to core features such as social functioning or sense of identity. If treatments reduce some of the disruptive and distressing aspects of these disorders that is an important and worthwhile achievement.

Despite the poverty of evidence, national guidelines have been published in the UK for the management of both these disorders (NICE, 2009b; Gabbard, 2007) and the emphasis is firmly on psychosocial interventions with the use of drugs restricted to symptomatic management of crises. For the practising psychiatrist this focus on cluster B disorders makes sense. Cluster A disorders—the schizoid, eccentric, and often socially withdrawn group—rarely seek help, and the cluster C disorders—the anxious and obsessional—seek help for comorbidity, rarely for the direct consequences of their personality disorder.

The management of personality disorders

Assessment

As well as establishing a diagnosis of personality disorder, the *strengths and weaknesses* of the individual should be assessed. Strengths are important, because treatment should build on favourable features as well as attempting to modify unfavourable ones. The patient's *circumstances* should be assessed.

One of the most important services that a psychiatrist can provide for a personality-disordered patient is an honest yet diplomatic sharing of their understanding of what is going on. Most patients have recognized that they have a problem of some kind and may be quite realistic about what psychiatrists have to offer. They may only have come to the psychiatric services because others have suggested it. An opportunity to talk through the strengths and weaknesses of their habitual responses can help an individual to put their characteristic behaviour patterns in perspective and perhaps find less damaging strategies for dealing with difficulties. It can also avoid the development of unrealistic expectations of what others can do, which could otherwise lead to unproductive dependency. Regular attendance at outpatient clinics when there is in reality nothing that can be done can seem benign and compassionate, but it carries a strong misleading message both for the patient and for others who relate to them.

Supportive therapy

Psychological support has been the mainstay of treatment of people with personality disorder. For some, modest but useful progress can be achieved by having a secure point of reference and a sense of being taken seriously over a period of months or, sometimes, years. Support may be provided by a member of the psychiatric team or, if the person has broken the law, by a probation officer. The dangers of this rather 'paternalistic' approach are increasingly being recognized, and supportive psychotherapy is probably best restricted to fairly senior staff, as it is difficult to do well and has a number of pitfalls.

General aims of management

Although there has been some progress in the treatment of personality disorders, management still consists largely of helping people to find a way of life that conflicts less with their character. Whatever approach is used, the aims should be modest and considerable time should be allowed to achieve them. A trusting and confiding relationship is the basis of treatment. However, care should be exercised to avoid excessive dependency. Group treatment can sometimes be a way of lessening dependency and increasing social learning.

Often more than one professional is involved in the care of these patients. This can be risky, and close collaboration is needed to avoid inconsistencies of approach. Many of these patients react badly to changes in staff, which may re-enact painful losses, rejections, or separations in their earlier life. One consistent, albeit limited relationship, may be a much better learning experience than a range of contacts, no matter how skilled they are.

The overall plan should include attempts to help the patient to have less contact with situations that provoke difficulties, and more opportunity to develop assets in their personality. They should be encouraged to take an active part in planning their care, and the reasons for decisions should be explained clearly and discussed fully. Helping them to avoid adding to their problems by misusing drugs or alcohol is essential. Even if no major improvement is achieved, this approach may stabilize the situation until some fortuitous change in the patient's life brings about improvement.

Choice of psychotherapy. Psychodynamic or cognitive psychotherapy may be explored when the patient is well motivated and enough stability has been achieved to enable them to focus on the treatment. The approach will depend on the type of personality disorder, on local availability, and on the patient's own preference.

Choice of medication. Medication plays only a small part in the treatment of personality disorders. It should not be the first choice, and when it is prescribed it should be part of a wider plan that embraces psychological and social care. Anxiolytic medication should be used with special caution because of the risk of dependency. Antidepressants are used mainly for associated mood disorder—a common reason for the worsening of the emotional and behavioural problems associated with the personality disorder. The use of antidepressants in borderline personality disorder is discussed below. Antipsychotics are occasionally useful to reduce aggressive behaviour.

Organization of services. People with personality disorder can be cared for by a single practitioner, who integrates the psychological, pharmacological, and social aspects of treatment, calling on specialist help when needed. This makes it easier for the practitioner to understand and help with relationship problems, and it emphasizes the essential unity of the person's diverse problems. However, it can be difficult to sustain when the personality disorder is severe. Alternatively, care can be provided by a community team, with a key worker who coordinates the contributions of other team members. Since the publication of the Department of Health paper, *Personality Disorder: No Longer a Diagnosis of Exclusion* (National Institute for Mental Health in England, 2003) in the UK, specialist teams have been established specifically for the treatment of personality disorder. Their configuration varies enormously, but a form of therapeutic day programme based on therapeutic community principles (Bateman, 1999), and often incorporating principles of mentalization, is commonly the central feature (Bateman and Fonagy, 2009). For a review of services for patients with personality disorder, see Bateman and Tyrer (2004b).

Progress

Progress is often achieved as a series of small steps by which the person gradually moves closer to a satisfactory adjustment. Setbacks are common, but they can be used constructively, as it is at these times that the patient is most likely to be willing to confront their problems. Although therapists should try long and hard to help patients with personality disorder, they should recognize that some people may not benefit.

The management of Cluster A and C disorders

The type of personality disorder is not always a good guide to the choice of effective treatment. Nevertheless, some associations have been described, mainly on the basis of clinical experience, and these will be considered here before outlining the approach to borderline and antisocial disorders.

Patients with *paranoid personality disorder* do not engage well with treatment because they are touchy and suspicious. Patients with *schizoid personality disorder* avoid close personal contact, and often drop out after a few sessions of treatment. If they can be persuaded to continue they tend to intellectualize their problems and question the value of their treatment. The therapist should try to help these people to become more aware of their problems and respond to them in ways that cause fewer difficulties. For both disorders progress is slow and the results are limited. Exploratory psychotherapy is unlikely to succeed, and medication is generally unhelpful.

Paranoid personality traits and experiences have become the focus of recent research into the possibility of intervening early in psychosis. Studies in virtual reality laboratories have been used to identify them and tailored forms of cognitive behaviour therapy are being tested as possible approaches (Freeman and Garety, 2014).

Patients with *obsessional personality disorder* do not respond well to psychotherapy. Unskilled treatment can lead to excessive morbid introspection, which leaves the person feeling worse rather than better. Treatment should be directed towards avoiding situations that increase difficulties, and developing better ways of coping with stressful situations. Patients often seek help during an associated depressive disorder, and it is important to identify and treat this comorbid condition.

Patients with *avoidant (anxious) personality disorder* generally have low self-esteem, and fear disapproval and criticism. They can be helped by a therapeutic relationship in which they feel valued and able to reconsider their perception of themselves. As with obsessional personality disorder, the possibility of a comorbid depressive disorder that requires treatment should be considered.

Patients with *dependent personality disorder* are usually helped more by problem-solving counselling, in which they are encouraged to take increasingly more responsibility for themselves. Medication should be avoided unless there is an associated depressive disorder.

Borderline personality disorder

Little is achieved by arguing about the nosological coherence of borderline personality disorder—its contested history and boundaries and, least of all, its misleading name. Borderline is the personality disorder that calls for a response from psychiatry and psychiatrists. It is in the nature of the disorder that management has to be negotiated—patients will inevitably exert a considerable influence on the choice of treatment, and all psychiatrists, irrespective of their interests, are likely to have to manage them. While the main body of research is into sophisticated daycare units based on either mentalization or dialectic behaviour therapy (DBT; see below), not all patients can have access to these nor will all of them accept this approach. As a consequence, virtually every form of psychotherapy or social therapy has responded with adaptations and strategies (Bateman *et al.*, 2015).

In many parts of the world psychoanalytical approaches are still pursued in outpatient or office-based practice, although focused more firmly on transference issues (Clarkin *et al.*, 1999). Cognitive behaviour therapists focus more on schemas (the underlying assumptions patients make rather than exclusively on automatic thoughts) (Davidson, 2000). Short-term integrative therapies such as cognitive analytical therapy (Clarke *et al.*, 2013) have specified adaptations for borderline patients. The two most influential adaptations have been in behaviour therapy, with the development of dialectical behaviour therapy (Linehan 1993; Linehan *et al.*, 1991), and in psychodynamic therapy, with

mentalization (Bateman and Fonagy, 2004; Bateman and Fonagy, 2009).

Dialectical behaviour therapy

DBT is an intense form of psychotherapy that includes individual sessions, group sessions, and, optimally, daycare. It was developed by the psychologist Marsha Linehan to help people reduce harmful behaviours, such as self-harm, suicidal thinking, and substance abuse. The approach aims to increase emotional and cognitive regulation by awareness of triggers and assessing coping skills to apply. Linehan has more recently acknowledged that her life was dominated by such behaviours and that finding some effective treatment was vital for her own functioning. It includes an eclectic mix of therapies, with cognitive behaviour therapy to increase emotional regulation plus mindfulness to increase awareness, and some pretty blunt confrontation. The treatment is outlined in Chapter 24.

Mentalization

The residential therapeutic communities developed after the second World War to help individuals with personality disorder were aimed at those with antisocial personality disorder but contained many with what would now be recognized as borderline personality disorder. They are described in Chapter 24 and, because of an absence of evidence for their effectiveness and their cost, are no longer a feature of mental health care (although they are still influential in prisons and drug treatment units). However, day units based broadly on therapeutic community principles have evolved for the treatment of borderline personality disorder. What distinguishes them is their focus on 'mentalization' (Bateman and Fonagy, 2004; Bateman and Fonagy, 2009). Essentially, this involves helping the patient become more fully aware of their thoughts and feelings rather than acting on them without reflection.

Mentalization day hospitals vary, but all usually include both individual and group work, and their approach is summarized in Box 15.9. For the many patients unable or unwilling to attend such units, principles of 'generalist' management have evolved (Gunderson and Links, 2014; Bateman and Krawitz, 2013), and are summarized in Box 15.10.

Antisocial personality disorder

Most treatment programmes are delivered by forensic psychologists in the prison service and comprise schema-based cognitive behaviour therapy, often in groups. Few psychiatrists feel they have much to offer in

> **Box 15.9 Five common characteristics of evidence-based treatments for borderline personality disorder**
>
> 1. Structured (manual-directed) approaches to prototypic borderline personality disorder problems
> 2. Patients are encouraged to assume control of themselves (i.e. sense of agency)
> 3. Therapists help connections of feelings to events and actions
> 4. Therapists are active, responsive, and validating
> 5. Therapists discuss cases, including personal reactions, with others

> **Box 15.10 Proposed characteristics for a generalist approach to treating borderline personality disorder**
>
> 1. Treatment providers have previous experience with borderline personality disorder
> 2. Supportive (i.e. encouraging, advisory, and educational)
> 3. Focus on managing life situations (not on the in-therapy interactions)
> 4. Non-intensive (i.e. once per week, with additional sessions as needed)
> 5. Interruptions are expected; consistent regular appointments are optional
> 6. Psychopharmacological interventions are integrated; group or family interventions are encouraged when necessary

the treatment of antisocial personality disorder beyond identifying it and exploring its consequences with the patient and family.

Pharmacotherapy

NICE guidance (2009b) advises against the use of medication unless a clear comorbid disorder (e.g. major depression) is present, whereas the American Psychiatric Association has considered targeted pharmacotherapy an important adjunct (Oldham *et al.*, 2001). This is not always possible in practice, and a meta-analytical review by Lieb *et al.* (2010) concluded that there was some evidence, albeit limited, that antipsychotic drugs and anticonvulsant mood stabilizers could have beneficial effects on aspects of borderline personality disorder, such as affective instability, impulsive dyscontrol, and cognitive perceptual symptoms. Nevertheless, it does not appear likely that current drug treatments are able to modify core borderline symptomatology, including fear of abandonment, feelings of emptiness, and identity disturbance.

Ethical problems

Stigma and patient involvement

From the early ideas of moral insanity to the present time, the concept of personality disorder has been linked to a moral judgement. People who are told that they have a disordered personality believe there is something inadequate about who they are. This can be entrenched by some professionals' attitudes, and by the difficulty that people with personality disorder experience in accessing psychiatric and other services. Once the diagnosis has been made it tends to stick and to affect the person's subsequent care, as well as the way that other people think of them over the longer term. For this reason, many clinicians are reluctant to make the diagnosis.

This situation is changing, and the policy document, *Personality Disorder: No Longer a Diagnosis of Exclusion* (National Institute for Mental Health in England, 2003), highlighted the need for all psychiatrists to engage with personality-disordered individuals. The existence of a personality disorder is associated with increased rates of other psychiatric disorders. Even if psychiatrists do not believe that they can change the patient's personality, that is no reason not to treat the associated problems. This renewed interest has also led to the establishment of specific psychotherapeutic teams and services for personality-disordered patients. These services are very varied in their form (reflecting the absence of strong evidence for specific treatments), but, as mentioned above, many of them are centred around a psychodynamic day service (Bateman and Krawitz, 2013).

Further reading

Gelder MG *et al.* (eds) (2009). Section 4.12: Personality disorders. In: MG Gelder, NC Andreasen, JJ López-IborJr and JR Geddes (eds.) *The New Oxford Textbook of Psychiatry*. Oxford University Press, Oxford. (The seven chapters in this section provide a comprehensive review of personality disorder.)

Schneider K (1950) *Psychopathic Personalities* (trans. MW Hamilton). Cassell, London. (A classic text of great importance in the development of ideas about personality disorder.)

CHAPTER 16

Child psychiatry

Introduction

A significant proportion of 'adult' mental illness starts before the age of 18 years. There are also specific psychiatric disorders of childhood. These factors attest to the importance of properly assessing child development, identifying early signs of mental illness, and instituting effective treatment. The period of childhood is relatively brief, yet the developmental tasks a child needs to perform are considerable, including learning a broad range of skills, developing physically and cognitively, and managing the social and peer environment with adequate communication skills and emotional control. Mental illness can impact on the developmental tasks of childhood and potentially negatively impact on a child's developmental trajectory for the rest of their life, if, for example, it means that a child might have such low self-esteem that they are not able to make friends at school or perform badly in school achievement tests and not pursue higher education.

The practice of child psychiatry differs from that of adult psychiatry in a number of important ways.

- *Children are usually dependent on an adult to help them access services.* They seldom initiate the consultation and are usually brought by a parent, or another adult, who has concerns about some aspect of the child's cognitive, emotional, or behavioural development. Whether a referral is sought depends on the attitudes and tolerance of these adults, and how they perceive the child's behaviour. Healthy children may be brought to the doctor by overanxious and solicitous parents or teachers, while in other circumstances severely disturbed children may be left to themselves.

- *The child's difficulties may reflect the problems of other people*—for example, parental physical or mental illness.

- *The child's stage of physical and cognitive development must be considered* when deciding what is abnormal. For example, repeated bedwetting may be normal in a 3-year-old child but is abnormal in a 7-year-old. In addition, the child's response to life events changes with age. Thus separation from a parent will affect children in different ways across their childhood.

- *Children are generally less able to express themselves in words.* For this reason, evidence of disturbance often comes from observations of behaviour made by parents, teachers, and others. These informants may give differing accounts, in part because children's behaviour varies with their circumstances, and in part because the various informants will likely have different beliefs about the parameters of normal and abnormal behaviour. For this reason, informants should be asked for specific examples of any problem they describe, and asked about the circumstances in which it has been observed.

- The vast majority of children attend *schools* which are found across the world with variable sizes, resources, philosophies, and impacts. They can play an important role in the overall development of children and can also be areas of great academic and social stress for children. Furthermore, schools offer a location for accessing children for prevention and treatment of mental illness.

- *The emphasis of treatment is different.* Medication is used considerably less in the treatment of children than in the treatment of adults, and is usually started by a specialist rather than the family doctor. Instead, there is more emphasis on psychological interventions, working with the parents and the whole family, reassuring and retraining children, and coordinating the efforts of others who can help children, especially at school. Thus multidisciplinary working is even more important in child psychiatry than in adult psychiatry. Consequently, treatment is usually provided by a team that includes at least a psychiatrist, psychiatric nurses, a psychologist, and potentially also those trained in other therapies, social care, or occupational therapy.

- Ethical considerations can make participation of children in research complicated, and so the evidence base, particularly on pharmacological interventions, is limited for children.

The first part of this chapter is concerned with a number of general issues concerning psychiatric disorder in childhood, including its frequency, causes, assessment, and management. The second part of the chapter contains information about the principal syndromes encountered in the practice of child and adolescent psychiatry. The chapter does not provide a comprehensive account of child psychiatry. It is an introduction to the main themes for psychiatrists who are undertaking specialist general training. It is expected that they will follow it by reading a specialist text such as one of those listed under Further reading on page 484. Intellectual disability among children is considered in Chapter 17, but the reader should remember that many aspects of the study and care of children with intellectual disability are similar to those described in this chapter.

Normal development

The practice of child psychiatry calls for some knowledge of the normal process of development from a helpless infant into an independent adult. To judge whether any observed emotional, social, or intellectual functioning is abnormal, it has to be compared with the corresponding normal range for the age group. This section gives a brief and simplified account of the main aspects of development that concern the psychiatrist. A textbook of paediatrics should be consulted for details of these developmental phases (for example, see Kliegman *et al.*, 2015).

The first year of life

This is a period of rapid motor, sensory, and social development, and includes the first stages of language development. Three weeks after birth, the baby smiles at faces, selective smiling appears by 6 months, fear of strangers by 8 months, and anxiety on separation from the mother shortly thereafter.

Bowlby (1980) emphasized the importance of a general process of attachment of the infant to the parents, and of more selective emotional bonding. Although bonding to the mother is most significant, important attachments are also made to the father and other people who are close to the infant. Other studies have shown the reciprocal nature of this process and the role of early contacts between the mother (or other carers) and the newborn infant in initiating bonding. Attachment and bonding are discussed further on page 425.

By the end of the first year, the child should have formed a close and secure relationship with the mother or other close carer. There should be an ordered pattern of sleeping and feeding, and weaning onto solid food has usually been accomplished. Infants will be able to point at objects and things they want. Children will have begun to learn about objects outside themselves, simple causal relationships, and spatial relationships. By the end of the first year, they enjoy making sounds and may say 'mama', 'dada', and perhaps one or two other words.

Year two

This too is a period of rapid development. Children begin to wish to please their parents, and appear anxious when they disapprove. They explore their environment more through play and with increasing mobility, as most will be walking by the time they are 18 months. They also begin to learn to control their behaviour. By now, attachment behaviour should be well established. *Temper tantrums* occur, particularly if exploratory wishes are frustrated. These tantrums do not last long, and should lessen as the child learns to accept constraints. They learn to point at things that they want others to observe out of interest. By the end of the second year the child should be able to put two or three words together as a *simple sentence*.

Preschool years (2–5 years)

This phase brings a further increase in intellectual abilities, especially in the complexity of language. Social development occurs as children learn to live within the family. They begin to identify with the parents and adopt their standards in matters of conscience. Social life develops rapidly as they learn to interact with siblings, other children, and adults. Temper tantrums continue, but diminish and should disappear before the child starts school. Attention span and concentration increase steadily. At this age, children are very curious about the environment and ask many questions.

In children aged 2–5 years, fantasy life is rich and vivid. It can form a temporary substitute for the real world, enabling desires to be fulfilled regardless of reality. Special 'transitional' objects such as teddy bears or pieces of blanket can become important to the child. They appear to comfort and reassure the child, and help them to sleep.

Children begin to learn about their own *identity*. They realize the differences between males and females in appearance, clothes, behaviour, and anatomy. Sexual play and exploration are common at this stage. According to psychodynamic theory, at this stage defence mechanisms develop to enable the child to cope with anxiety arising from intolerable emotions. These defence mechanisms have been described on page 137.

During these years the most common mental health presentations to primary care services include difficulties in feeding and sleeping, as well as clinging to the parents (separation anxiety), temper tantrums, oppositional behaviour, and minor degrees of aggression. As described below, these should be referred to mental health services if they are persistent and interfere with the child's ability to develop physically or interact socially in their family or with peers.

Middle childhood

By the age of 5 years, children should have a clearer understanding of their identity, and their position in the family. They learn to cope with school, and to read, write, and begin to acquire numerical concepts. The teacher becomes an important person in children's lives. At this stage children gradually learn what they can achieve and what their limitations are. Conscience and standards of social behaviour develop further. According to psychoanalytical theory, *defence mechanisms* develop further while psychosexual development is quiescent (the latent period).

Common problems in middle childhood

The common problems in this age group include fears, nightmares, minor difficulties in relationships with peers, disobedience, and fighting.

Adolescence

Adolescence is the growing-up period between childhood and maturity, and is also a sensitive period in the development of the brain. Adolescence is a time of significant neuroplasticity—where the nervous system adapts its structure and function in response to environmental demands, experiences, and physiological changes (Fuhrmann *et al.*, 2015). Among the most obvious features are the physical changes of puberty. The age at which these changes occur is quite variable, usually taking place between 11 and 13 years in girls, and 13 and 17 years in boys. The production of sex hormones precedes these changes, starting in both sexes between the ages of 8 and 10 years. An adolescent has increased awareness of personal identity and individual characteristics. At this age, young people become self-aware, are concerned to know who they are, and begin to consider where they want to go in life. They can look ahead, consider alternatives for the future, and feel hope and despair. Some experience emotional turmoil and feel alienated from their family, but such experiences are not universal.

Peer group influences become more prominent, and close friendships often develop, especially among girls. Membership of a group is common, and this can help the adolescent in moving towards autonomy. Adolescence brings a marked increase in sexual interest and activity. At first, tentative approaches are made to the opposite sex. Gradually these become more direct and confident.

How far and in what way sexual feelings are expressed depends greatly on the standards of society, the behaviour of the peer group, and the attitudes of the family.

Common problems in later childhood and early adolescence

Common problems among children aged from 12 to 16 years include fluctuating mood and also persistent low mood, a range of different anxiety problems, difficulties in relationships with peers, disobedience and rebellion, including truancy, experimenting with illicit substances, fighting, and stealing. Schizophrenia and bipolar disorder may have their onset in this age group, but are uncommon.

Developmental psychopathology

In child psychiatry it is important to adopt a developmental approach for three reasons.

- *The stage of development determines whether behaviour is normal or pathological.* For example, as noted above, bedwetting is normal at the age of 3 years but abnormal at the age of 7 years.
- *The effects of life events differ as the child develops.* For example, infants aged under 6 months can move to a new carer with little disturbance, but children aged 6 months to 3 years of age show great distress when separated from a familiar carer, because an attachment relationship has been formed. After the age of 3 years, attachment bonds are still strong but the child's ability to understand and to use language can reduce the effect of a change of care-taker provided that it is arranged sensitively.
- *Psychopathology may change as the child grows older.* Anxiety disorders in childhood tend to improve as the child develops, depressive disorders often recur and continue into adult life, conduct disorders can continue into adolescence as aggressive and delinquent behaviour, and also commonly as substance abuse— a problem that is less common in younger children. These changes and continuities are sometimes related as much to changes in the environment as to developmental changes in the child.

The psychopathology of individual disorders will be discussed later in the chapter. Here some general issues regarding childhood psychopathology are summarized.

The influence of genes. Susceptibility genes have been identified for a few disorders, namely autism, attention-deficit disorder (ADHD), and specific reading disorder.

However, for most disorders, the amount of variance explained by identified genes is not great, suggesting multiple genes of small effect. The importance of epigenetics and interactions between genes and the environment also plays a key role as many neurodevelopmental disorders display remarkable syndromal overlap despite large genetic differences (heterogeneity) (Kiser *et al.*, 2015).

The influence of the environment. Factors in the environment may predispose to or precipitate disorders, and they may also maintain them. They may also protect from the effects of other causative agents—for example, the risk of depression in adulthood as a consequence of poor parental care in childhood is reduced by the experience of a caring relationship with another person. This experience is not protective against all causative factors—for example, a caring relationship does not reduce the risk of depression in adulthood following child abuse (Hill *et al.*, 2001). Furthermore, genetic and environmental factors interact, making certain exposures more likely to occur, or affecting their expression. For example, genes influence the personality traits of irritability and impulsiveness that lead to the repeated breakdown of relationships.

The dividing line between normal and abnormal. The common childhood disorders are at the extreme end of a continuum with normal behaviour. Despite this, we study them using a categorical system because decisions about treatment require 'yes or no' answers. To form a category, a cut-off point has to be decided, and this is often arbitrary. Children who fall just below the cut-off point—and hence outside the diagnostic group—can nevertheless have problems and need help. For example, some adolescents who fall below the threshold for depressive disorder have significant psychosocial impairment, and even mild depressive symptomatology can be associated with poor academic performance (Pickles *et al.*, 2001).

Continuities and discontinuities. Some symptoms and behaviour problems in childhood are associated with problems in adulthood, and might make an adult up to six times more likely to have adverse outcomes; for example, with increased prevalence of substance misuse and suicidality when they become young adults (Copeland *et al.*, 2015). In addition, overactivity and difficulties in behavioural management at the age of 3 years are associated with offending in adult life.

Parent–child interactions. Maternal behaviour affects the child, but children also elicit behaviours from their parents. For example, a mother is likely to be less responsive to an infant who does not respond to cuddling and play than to a sibling who is responsive to her. Her lack of responsiveness may then affect the infant, thus increasing the difficulty with attachment.

Most of these issues are also relevant to psychopathology in adults, and are considered further in Chapter 5.

Classification of psychiatric disorders in children and adolescents

Both DSM-5 and ICD-10 contain a scheme for classifying the psychiatric disorders of childhood. Disorders of adolescence are classified partly with this scheme, and partly with the categories used in adult psychiatry.

Seven main groups of childhood psychiatric disorders are generally recognized by clinicians. The terms used in this book for the seven groups are listed below, with some alternatives shown in parentheses:

- adjustment reactions
- autism spectrum disorders (ASD)
- specific developmental disorders
- conduct (antisocial or externalizing) disorders
- attention-deficit hyperactivity disorders
- emotional (internalizing) disorders
- symptomatic disorders.

Many child psychiatric disorders cannot be classified in a satisfactory way by allocating them to a single category. Therefore multiaxial systems have been proposed. ICD-10 has six axes:

1. Clinical psychiatric syndromes.
2. Specific delays in development.
3. Intellectual level.
4. Medical conditions.
5. Abnormal social situations.
6. Level of adaptive functioning.

DSM-5 has removed the multiaxial component of diagnosis used in DSM-IV and instead places emphasis on both diagnostic criteria and *clinical case formulation*. In the latter, a clinical summary of the social,

psychological, and biological factors that contribute to the development of a mental disorder is incorporated, as well as a measure of clinical significance, which is a proxy for individual distress and/or impairment (Harris 2014).

The DSM-5 and ICD-10 classifications for child psychiatric disorders are shown in Table 16.1. (In this book, intellectual (learning) disability in childhood is considered in Chapter 17.) Both schemes are complicated, so only the main categories are shown in Table 16.1. In DSM-5 many of the disorders of childhood have been removed from a more generic 'infancy, childhood and adolescence section' present in DSM-IV and integrated into the chapter relevant to that specific disorder. The chapters are then organized and presented in chronological fashion, with diagnoses most applicable to infancy and childhood listed first. The disorders are similar in the two diagnostic systems, but the changes in DSM-5 mean that the overlap is less than was previously the case. Furthermore, DSM-5 has included two new disorders: social communication disorder (SCD) and disruptive mood dysregulation disorder (DMDD). For more information on the DSM-5 classification of neurodevelopmental disorders see Harris (2014).

Several DSM-IV categories are now are subsumed into larger lifespan chapters in DSM-5, including 'Feeding and eating disorders', 'Elimination disorders', and 'Disruptive, impulse-control and conduct disorders'. In ICD-10, eating and elimination disorders are classified with sleep disorders under 'Other behavioural and emotional disorders'.

For further information about classification in child psychiatry, see Scott (2009a).

Epidemiology

Behavioural and emotional disorders are common in childhood. Estimates vary according to the diagnostic criteria and other methods used, but it appears that rates

in different developed countries are similar. Moreover, the rates of emotional and behavioural disorders in low- and middle-income countries are similar to those

Table 16.1 **Classification of main childhood psychiatric disorders**

DSM-5	ICD-10
Neurodevelopmental disorders with onset in the developmental period Autism spectrum disorders Attention-deficit hyperactivity disorders Intellectual disability/intellectual developmental disorder	**F8 Disorders of psychological development** Pervasive developmental disorders Specific developmental disorders of scholastic skills
Communication disorders	Specific developmental disorders of speech and language
Motor disorders Tic disorders	Specific developmental disorder of motor function
	F9 Behavioural and emotional disorders with onset usually occurring in childhood and adolescence
	Hyperkinetic disorders
	Conduct disorders
	Mixed disorders of conduct and emotions
	Emotional disorders with onset specific to childhood
	Tic disorders
Other disorders of infancy, childhood, and adolescence	Other behavioural and emotional disorders with onset usually in childhood and adolescence (includes elimination disorders and feeding disorders)

Source: data from The ICD-10 classification of mental and behavioural disorders: clinical descriptions and diagnostic guidelines, Copyright (1992), World Health Organization; Diagnostic and Statistical Manual of Mental Disorders, Fifth Edition, Copyright (2013), American Psychiatric Association.

in high-income ones. In the UK, the prevalence of child psychiatric disorder in ethnic minority groups has usually been found to be similar to that in the rest of the population. The few exceptions are mentioned later in this chapter.

A landmark study was carried out more than 40 years ago on the Isle of Wight in the UK. The study was concerned with the health, intelligence, education, and psychological difficulties in all the 10- and 11-year-olds attending state schools on the island—a total of 2193 children (Rutter *et al.*, 1970a). In the first stage of the enquiry, screening questionnaires were completed by parents and teachers. Children identified in this way were given psychological and educational tests and their parents were interviewed. The 1-year prevalence rate of psychiatric disorder was about 7%, with the rate in boys being twice that in girls. The rate of emotional disorders was 2.5%, and the combined rate of conduct disorders together with mixed conduct and emotional disorders was 4%. Conduct disorders were four times more frequent among boys than girls, whereas emotional disorders were more frequent in girls, in a ratio of almost 1.5:1.

There was no correlation between psychiatric disorder and social class, but prevalence increased as intelligence decreased. It was also associated with physical disability and especially with evidence of brain damage. In addition, there was a strong association between reading difficulties and conduct disorder. A subsequent study using the same methods was conducted in an inner London borough (Rutter *et al.*, 1975). Here the rates of all types of disorder were twice those in the Isle of Wight.

Overall rates of psychiatric disorder. The results of these early studies have been broadly confirmed in subsequent investigations, using standard diagnostic criteria, conducted in the UK (Meltzer *et al.*, 2000), in New Zealand (Fergusson *et al.*, 1993), and in the Great Smoky Mountains in the USA (Costello *et al.*, 1996). For example, in the UK study, ICD-10 disorders were present in about 10% of the over 10,000 children aged 5–15 years assessed. The most common problem was conduct disorder (5%), closely followed by emotional disorders (4%), while 1% were rated as hyperactive. The less common disorders (autism, tic disorders, and eating disorders) were present in about 0.5% of the population.

A systematic review and meta-analysis of worldwide prevalence of mental disorders in children and adolescents reported a pooled prevalence of mental disorders worldwide of 13% (Polanczyk *et al.*, 2015). The prevalence of anxiety disorder was 7%, depressive disorder was 3%, ADHD 3%, and any disruptive disorder (including conduct disorder and oppositional defiant disorder) was 6% (Figure 16.1).

Rates in adolescence. Evidence about adolescence was provided originally by a 4-year follow-up of the Isle of Wight study (Rutter *et al.*, 1976b). At the age of 14 years, the 1-year prevalence rate of significant psychiatric disorder was about 20%. Prevalence estimates in subsequent studies vary somewhat, but most broadly confirm the original findings, with rates between 15% and 20%. However, there are some minor differences over time. In the UK, for example, there is evidence of a substantial increase in conduct and emotional problems in adolescents over the past two decades (Collishaw *et al.*, 2004, 2010). The most recent National Comorbidity Study in US adolescents showed that, for adolescents, anxiety disorders are the most common condition (31%), followed by behaviour disorders (19%), mood disorders (14%), and substance use disorders (11%) (Merikangas *et al.*, 2010). The overall prevalence of disorders with severe impairment and/or distress was 22% (11% mood; 8% anxiety; 9% behaviour). The median age of onset for disorders was earliest for anxiety (6 years) followed by

11 years for behaviour, 13 years for mood, and 15 years for substance use disorders.

Variations with gender and age. Before puberty, disorders are more frequent overall among males than among females; after puberty, disorders are more frequent among females. Particular disorders also vary in frequency according to gender and age (see Table 16.2).

Other sources of variation. In the middle years of childhood, rates of psychiatric problems differ between areas of residence, being twice as high in urban areas (about 25%) as in rural areas (about 12%) (Rutter, 1975). Subsequent studies have confirmed these earlier findings and helped to categorize risk factors that increase the likelihood of mental, emotional, and behavioural disorders into six domains (Greenberg *et al.*, 2015):

1. Child: e.g. self-regulation problems.
2. Family: quality of parent–child attachment.
3. Peer: isolation.
4. Demographic: family income and family structure/parental relationship.
5. School: school climate.
6. Community/policy: neighbourhood policy and crime rates.

Comorbidity. Studies using DSM criteria find high rates of comorbidity between childhood disorders. For example, in the National Comorbidity study, 40%

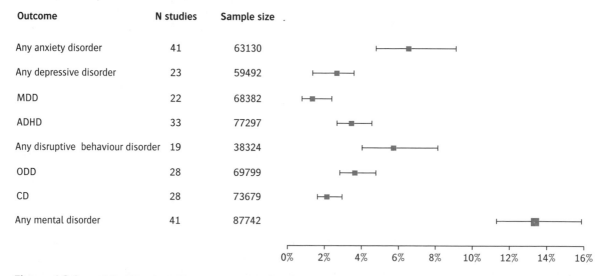

Figure 16.1 Worldwide pooled prevalence estimates of mental disorder in childhood and adolescence. MDD, Major depressive disorder; ADHD, attention-deficit hyperactivity disorder; ODD, oppositional defiant disorder; CD, conduct disorder.

Table 16.2 Comparative frequency of childhood psychiatric disorders in males and females

More frequent in males	Equal	More frequent in females
Autism spectrum disorders	Depression before puberty	Depression (postpubertal)
Specific developmental disorders	School refusal*	Anxiety disordersSpecific phobia
ADHD	Selective mutism	Eating disorders
Oppositional and conduct disorders		Deliberate self-harm
Juvenile delinquency*		
Nocturnal enuresis—in older children		
Tic disorders		
Suicide		
Disorders which usually begin after puberty:		
Depressive disorders, mania, psychosis, agoraphobia and panic disorder, eating disorders, substance abuse, deliberate self-harm and suicide, and juvenile delinquency		

* Juvenile delinquency and school refusal are descriptive terms, not diagnoses.

of those with a disorder had a comorbid condition (Merikangas *et al.*, 2010). As in adulthood, this could be because one disorder predisposes to another, or because they have common predisposing factors, or because the classification system has gone too far in identifying, as distinct disorders, patterns of behaviour that can occur in more than one condition.

For a review of the psychiatric epidemiology of childhood and adolescence, see Costello and Angold (2009).

Outcomes of child and adolescent mental illness

Mild symptoms and behavioural or developmental problems are usually short-lived. However, conditions severe enough to be diagnosed as psychiatric disorders often persist for years. Thus in the Isle of Wight study, 75% of children with conduct disorder and 50% of those with emotional disorders at age 10 years were still affected by these problems 4 years later (Rutter *et al.*, 1976b).

The *prognosis* for adult life of psychiatric disorder in childhood has been investigated in a number of longitudinal studies. Whilst separation anxiety rarely persists into adulthood, many of the other anxiety disorders do persist into adulthood, and rates of full remission for generalized anxiety disorder and panic disorder are both low (Costello and Maughan, 2015). Social anxiety disorder and agoraphobia, which rarely has onset before adolescence, can persist for many years and have low

remission rates if left untreated. The course of depression can present with a persistent pattern and, because there seems to be significant overlap with anxiety disorders, longitudinal studies often place both anxiety and depression together as 'emotional disorders'. Studies have shown that children who have early episodes of emotional disorders are at increased risk into adulthood and that about half of those with depression in youth will have an adult episode of a depressive or anxiety disorder (Costello and Maughan, 2015). For example, in a study in the US, child or adolescent depression doubled the risk of depression in early adulthood, and those most at risk in adulthood had multiple adolescent episodes (Rohde *et al.*, 2013). A family history of emotional disorders and the presence of comorbid difficulties are associated with risk of recurrence, while a positive emotional style, family bonding and good parent–child relationships may be protective against the likelihood of developing adult depressive disorders (Costello and Maughan, 2015).

A substantial proportion of children with ADHD remain relatively impaired into adulthood. In one study of participants followed from the age of 6–12 years into their forties, 22% continued to meet full diagnostic criteria for ADHD and a further 10% met reduced symptom criteria (Klein *et al.*, 2012). However, most conduct disorder remits into adult life, although a small proportion of children with disruptive behaviour problems go on to show severe antisocial difficulties well into adult life. For adolescents with substance use disorders, the consensus is that 75% will perform fairly normally as adults—with completion of secondary school and supportive psychosocial environments being the best predictors of more positive outcomes (Costello and Maughan, 2015).

These examples show that continuities in psychiatric disorder between childhood and adulthood can be *homotypic* (where the same disorder persists over time) or *heterotypic* (where later disorders are of an apparently different kind). Although half of those who have had a diagnosable disorder in childhood will be free of their initial child difficulties by adulthood, they are still more likely to be in the more impaired groups on measures of later physical health, education and income, social and family functioning, and avoidance of crime.

Aetiology

In discussing the causes of child psychiatric disorders, the principles are similar to those described in Chapter 5 on the aetiology of adult disorders. Most childhood disorders are likely to emerge from a complex interaction between emerging neurodevelopmental vulnerabilities and aspects of the child's prenatal and postnatal environment (Johnson *et al.*, 2015). There is also a developmental aspect; children mature psychologically and socially as they grow up, and their disorders reflect this maturation. In the following paragraphs, four interacting groups of factors will be considered briefly. These are heredity, temperament, physical impairment with special reference to brain damage, and environmental factors in the family and society. All aspects of aetiology are discussed more fully in Thapar *et al.* (2015).

Genetic factors

Children with psychiatric problems often have parents who suffer from a psychiatric disorder. Environmental factors account for a substantial part of this association. However, population-based twin studies indicate that there is a significant genetic contribution to some psychiatric disorders, especially to ASD, hyperactivity, and anxiety disorders (with a heritability of around 40%). Genetic studies are considered further when the aetiology of particular childhood psychiatric disorders is described later in this chapter. Here, we consider some general matters concerned with the interpretation of the results of genetic studies. Methods of genetic investigation are discussed on page 102. Examples of genetic findings in child psychiatry are given at relevant points in this chapter, especially in the sections on autism and hyperactivity, where genetic research has produced some relevant findings (see page 446). Some general points about the interpretation of genetic studies are shown in Box 16.1.

Temperament and individual differences

Many years ago, Thomas *et al.* (1968) conducted an influential longitudinal study in New York. They found that certain *temperamental factors* detected before the age of 2 years predisposed to later psychiatric disorder. In the first 2 years, one group of children ('difficult children') tended to respond to new environmental stimuli by withdrawal, slow adaptation, and an intense behavioural response. Another group ('easy children') responded to new stimuli with a positive approach, rapid adaptation, and a mild behavioural response. This second group was less likely than the first to develop behavioural disorders later in childhood. The investigators thought that these early temperamental differences were determined both genetically and by environmental factors.

More recent studies have confirmed an association between temperamental styles and subsequent childhood psychopathology. For example, *behavioural inhibition* predicts later anxiety disorders, while *low positive affect* has been linked to the development of depression. Perhaps unsurprisingly, children characterized by difficulties with self-control and high levels of irritability are more likely to be diagnosed subsequently with disruptive behaviour problems, including conduct disorder (Caspi and Shiner, 2008).

Brain disorders

Although serious physical disease of any kind can predispose to psychological problems in childhood, those affecting the brain, such as traumatic injury, epilepsy, infections, tumours, neurodegenerative, or other conditions, are the most important risk factors. This relationship was first noted in the original Isle of Wight study (see above), with about 7% of physically healthy

Box 16.1 Interpreting the results of genetic studies of childhood psychiatric disorders

Phenotype and genotype. Although standard diagnostic criteria are valuable in research, the results of this research show that diagnostic categories generally do not map closely onto the genetic factors in aetiology. For example, the phenotype of autism spectrum disorders includes some kinds of developmental language disorder, while the phenotype of Gilles de la Tourette syndrome (Chapter 14) seems to extend to obsessional thinking and behaviour.

Comorbidity. Many children have symptoms that qualify for more than one psychiatric diagnosis—for example, depressive disorder and conduct disorder, or depressive disorder and eating disorder. It is not clear whether this overlap arises because one disorder predisposes to another, or because they are two manifestations of the same genetic predisposition.

Polygenic effects and environmental influences. The hereditary factors of importance in child psychiatry are largely polygenic. As in adulthood, these multiple genes interact with psychosocial factors, and genetic investigations may include estimates of environmental factors.

Indirect effects. Genes may exert their effects through factors such as intelligence and temperament, which in part determine whether certain situations are experienced as stressful.

Shared and non-shared environment. Analyses of population genetic data divide the variance into genetic, shared environmental, and non-shared environmental factors (see page 102). Twins, full siblings, and half-siblings are increasingly used as comparison groups in studies and, although these sibling comparison groups are assumed to be similar in many aspects of 'shared' environment, this assumption has limitations, especially in the interpretations of the impact of the non-shared environment. For example, a shared environment can affect different children in different ways, and this effect then appears in the analyses as 'non-shared environment'.

children aged 10–11 years classified as having psychiatric problems, compared with about 12% of physically ill children of the same age, and 34% of children with brain disorders (Rutter *et al.*, 1976b). The high prevalence in the latter group was not explained by the adverse social factors known to be associated with the risk of brain disorder. Many other studies have since confirmed that psychiatric problems are more likely to result from 'brain disorders' than physical disorders that do not include the brain.

Children with brain injury are more likely to develop psychiatric disorder if they encounter adverse psychosocial influences of the kind that provoke psychiatric disorder in children without brain damage.

Maturational changes and delayed effects

The effects of brain lesions are more complex in childhood than in adult life because the brain is still developing. This has two consequences:

- *Greater capacity to compensate.* The immature brain is more able than the adult brain to compensate for localized damage—it has greater *plasticity*. For example, even complete destruction of the left hemisphere in early childhood can be followed by normal development of language.
- *Delayed effects.* Early damage may not be manifested as a disorder until a later stage of development when the damaged area takes up some key function. It is well established that brain injury at birth may not result in seizures until many years later. It has been suggested that there may be similar delays in the behavioural consequences of brain injury.

The consequences of head injury in childhood

Head injury is a common cause of neurological damage in childhood. The form of the consequent disorder is not very specific, partly because the effects of head injury are seldom localized to one area of the brain. Common consequences of severe injury are intellectual impairment and behaviour disorder. The former is proportional to the severity of the injury, but the relationship of behaviour disorder to the injury is less direct.

Epilepsy as a cause of childhood psychiatric disorder

The relationship between epilepsy and psychiatric disorder in adults is considered on page 379. In childhood there is a strong association between recurrent seizures and psychiatric disorder. As in adult life, the causal relationship may be of four kinds:

- The brain lesion causing the epilepsy may also cause the psychiatric disorder.
- The psychological and social consequences of recurrent seizures may cause the disorder.

- The effects of epilepsy on school performance may cause the disorder.
- The drugs used to treat epilepsy may cause the disorder through their side effects.

The *site and the type of epilepsy* appear to be generally less important, apart from the fact that temporal lobe epilepsy seems to be associated with psychological disorder. The age of onset of seizures also determines the child's response to epilepsy. For a review of the influence of brain injury and epilepsy on psychopathology, see Heyman *et al.* (2015).

Environmental factors

The effect of life events

The concept of *life events* (see page 98) is useful in child psychiatry as well as adult psychiatry. Life events may predispose to or provoke a disorder, or protect against it. Events can be classified by their severity, their social characteristics (e.g. family problems, or the death of a parent), or their general significance—for example, exit events (i.e. separations) or entrance events (i.e. additions to a family by the birth of a sibling). The way in which stressful life events contribute to childhood psychiatric disorders is not well understood but, as in adults, the psychological impact of such events is influenced by factors such as temperament, cognitive style, and previous life experience.

It is important to note that life events often occur in a setting of chronic stress, which may itself play a causal role in the precipitation of psychiatric disorder. Also, in children, as in adults, there are important differences in the liability of individuals to experience negative life events. This may be a reflection of societal factors such as poverty and discrimination, but the behaviour of individuals can also shape life experience in important ways. For example, children with conduct disorder have a substantially increased risk of experiencing negative life events (Scott *et al.*, 2015a).

Family influences

As children progress from complete dependence on others to independence, they need a stable and secure family background with a consistent pattern of emotional warmth, acceptance, help, and constructive discipline. *Prolonged separation* from or *loss* of parents can have a profound effect on psychological development in infancy and childhood. Poor relationships in the family may have similar adverse effects, and overt conflict between the parents seems to be especially important.

Maternal deprivation and attachment

The much quoted work of Bowlby (1951) led to widespread concern about the effects of 'maternal deprivation'. Bowlby suggested that prolonged separation from the mother was a major cause of juvenile delinquency. Although this suggestion has not been confirmed, it was an important step towards his idea that attachment is a crucial stage of early psychological development. Attachments are formed in the second 6 months of life, and adaptive attachments are characterized by an appropriate balance between security and exploration. Bowlby proposed that infants derive, from their experiences of attachment, internal models of themselves, of other people, and of their relationships with others. He proposed further that these internal models persist through later childhood into adult life, and that they influence self-concept and relationships. Thus children whose caregivers are loving, sensitive to their child's needs, and consistent in their responses are likely to grow up with self-esteem and able to form loving and trusting relationships.

Bowlby's ideas have been generally supported by studies in which attachment has been measured in infancy and in later years. Attachment has usually been measured at around 6–18 months of age using the Strange Situation Procedure (Ainsworth *et al.*, 1978), which evaluates the infant's response to separation from, and subsequent reunion with, the mother or other attachment figure. In this test, the response to the initial separation appears to be determined more by temperament than by attachment, and it is the response to reunion that is used to measure attachment. Other measures of attachment have been developed for older children. Using such tests, attachments have been divided into one secure and three insecure types:

- *Secure:* present in about 60% of infants, and associated with caregiving that is sensitive and responsive to the child's needs.
- *Avoidant*: present in about 15%, and associated with caregiving that is rejecting or intrusive.
- *Disorganized:* present in about 15%, and associated with caregiving that is unpredictable or frightening.
- *Resistant–ambivalent*: present in about 10%, and associated with caregiving that is inconsistent or lacking.

Studies of older children indicate that the type of attachment develops early in life and tends to be stable thereafter, although it is modified to some extent by changing life circumstances. Securely attached children generally do better than those with insecure attachments. Insecure attachments are associated not only with the factors mentioned above, but also with maternal depression, maternal alcoholism, and child abuse. Of the three types of insecure attachment, the disorganized type is the best predictor of future difficulties, especially externalizing problems.

The effect of separation. Bowlby's original studies of the effects of separation on young infants have been broadly confirmed, but it has become clear that the effects depend on many factors, including:

- the age of the child at the time of separation
- the previous relationship with the carers
- the reasons for the separation
- how the separation was managed
- the quality of care during the separation.

The impact of adverse caregiving environments: the more extreme caregiving abnormalities include a severe lack of stimulation and interaction with the infant/child, inconsistent experiences of the caregiver by the child, and a lack of emotionally invested caregiving. In DSM-5 two separate disorders are described relating to children who have experienced adverse caregiving. These are reactive attachment disorder (RAD) and disinhibited social engagement disorder (DSED), and are discussed below on page 439.

Family risk factors

Family risk factors for psychiatric disorder in childhood are multiple and cumulative. The risk increases in children of families with severe marital or other relationship conflict, low social status, large size or overcrowding, paternal criminality, and parental psychiatric disorder. The risk is also increased in children who are placed in care away from the family.

Protective factors

Protective factors reduce the rate of psychiatric disorder associated with a given level of risk factors. Protective factors include good parenting, strong affectionate ties within the family, including good sibling relationships, sociability, and the capacity for problem-solving in the child, and support outside the family from individuals, or from the school or church (Jenkins *et al.*, 2015).

Child-rearing practices

Some patterns of child-rearing are clearly related to psychiatric disturbance in the child, particularly those that involve verbal or physical abuse and scapegoating. Sexual abuse is another important risk factor (Glaser *et al.*, 2015).

Effects of alternative childcare

Working parents entrust part of the care of their children to other people. In general, the use of alternative childcare does not appear to be a major risk factor for psychiatric disorder, although multiple features of the nature of care need to be assessed. For example, high-quality care with sufficient individual attention can result in improved development of cognitive, social, and language skills. Generally, however, exposure to a large amount of alternative care correlates with increased levels of behavioural problems reported subsequently by teachers (Belsky *et al.*, 2007).

Effects of parental mental disorder

Some disorders are especially common in adults during the childbearing years, such as depression, anxiety, eating disorders, and alcoholism, and these are associated with an increased risk of psychological disturbances in children. The impacts are likely to be different depending on the developmental stage of the child. Perinatal mental illness in particular has been shown to have long-term effects reaching into early adulthood, and may manifest as emotional or behavioural difficulties, insecure or disorganized attachment, lower levels of cognitive development, as well as impaired physical growth and development (Stein, 2014). Antenatal depression and anxiety have also been associated with later childhood disturbances. Whether these arise through genetic confounds, through exposure to mental health disorders in the postnatal period, or through direct effects on fetal development remains unclear (see Chapter 22). Children of parents with depression or anxiety have a markedly increased rate of behaviour problems (such as conduct disorder at school age), and are at increased risk of depression and anxiety disorders. Paternal depression in particular has been shown to be associated with increased risk of behavioural problems in the early years of life. The causes are complex and are likely to be both genetic and environmental. An important mediator of the effect of parental depression on children is parenting. For example, this has been demonstrated for depressed mothers, where attachment to the infant is impaired by lower levels of warmth and responsiveness. Importantly, the effects of parental mental health disorders on children are not inevitable and are moderated by socioeconomic status, education, and the chronicity of the parental disorder.

Mothers who misuse alcohol or drugs. Children of such mothers suffer from a series of disadvantages, which are related not only to the effects of drug taking on the development of the fetus and the mother's care of the child, but also to features of the mother's personality that led her to take drugs, and to social problems associated with the substance misuse. For a review, see Greenfield *et al.* (2010).

Effects of parental separation

There are often two main effects of childhood parental separation (including divorce): economic difficulties and exposure to interpersonal conflict. The children of divorced parents have more psychological problems than the children of parents who are not divorced, but it is not certain how far these problems precede the divorce and are related to conflict between the parents, the behaviour of one or both parents that contributed to the decision to divorce, and the changes in family relationships that accompany remarriage or cohabitation following the divorce. Distress and dysfunction in the children are greatest in the year after the divorce; after 2 years these problems are still present but are generally less severe than those of children who remain in conflictual marriages. In a review, parental divorce was associated with multiple negative outcomes among children and, although evidence for a causal effect of divorce on children was reasonably strong, effect sizes were small in magnitude. Children showed a substantial degree of variability in outcomes following parental divorce, with some children declining, others improving, and most not changing at all (Amato and Anthony, 2014).

Death of a parent

In children, the response to the death of a parent varies with age, but data from two large cohorts show that parental death is associated with multiple negative outcomes in children (Amato and Anthony, 2014). Children aged below 4–5 years do not have a complete concept of death as causing permanent separation. Such children react with despair, anxiety, and regression to separation, however caused, and their reaction to bereavement is no different.

Children aged 5–11 years have an increasing understanding of death. They usually become depressed and overactive, and may show disorders of conduct. Some have suicidal thoughts and ideas that death would unite them with the lost parent. Suicidal actions are infrequent. In children over the age of 11 years, the response is increasingly similar to that of adults (see page 427).

Bereavement may have long-term effects on development, especially if the child was young at the time of the parent's death, and if the death was sudden or violent. Outcomes probably depend largely on the effects of the bereavement on the surviving parent. Most studies of bereavement in children have been concerned with the death of a parent; few have concerned the death of a sibling. For a review, see Black and Trickey (2009).

Social and cultural factors

Although the family is undoubtedly the part of children's environment that has most effect on their development, wider social influences are also important, particularly as a cause of conduct disorder. In the early years of childhood, these social factors act indirectly through their influence on the patterns of family life. As the child grows older and spends more time outside the family, they have a direct effect as well. These factors have been studied by examining the associations between psychiatric disorder and type of neighbourhood and school.

Effects of neighbourhood

Rates of childhood psychiatric disorder are higher in areas of social disadvantage. For example, as already noted above (see page 420), the rates of both emotional and conduct disorder were found to be higher in a poor inner-London borough than on the Isle of Wight. The important features of inner-city life may include lack of play space, inadequate social amenities for older children and teenagers, exposure to violence, overcrowded living conditions, and lack of community involvement.

Effects of school

Children spend more time in school than in any other institutional structure, and the importance of the school environment has long been recognized in child development and promoting mental health in the children and teachers at a school (Fazel *et al.*, 2014a). Schools can play an important role in a number of areas for the child—from academic attainment to social and peer relationships, as well as physical and moral development. It has long been known that rates of child psychiatric referral and delinquency vary between schools. These differences persist when allowance is made for differences in the neighbourhoods in which the children live. It seems that children are less likely to develop psychiatric problems in a school in which teachers praise, encourage, and give responsibility to their pupils, set high standards, and organize their teaching well. Factors that do not seem to affect rates of psychiatric disorder include the size of the school and the age of its buildings. There are some school-specific factors that can impact on children's mental health that will be discussed below: bullying and teacher–pupil relationships.

Bullying often takes place within the school context and is prevalent across schools in both high-, low-, and middle-income countries—a UK survey showed that over 45% of children have been bullied and experienced peer victimization. Both bullies and victims of bullying are at risk for psychiatric problems in childhood and beyond. Olweus (2013) uses three key criteria (intentionality, some repetitiveness, and imbalance of power) to define bullying or peer victimization: a student is exposed, repeatedly and over time, to negative actions on the part of one or more other students. This definition emphasizes intentionally negative or aggressive acts that are carried out repeatedly and over time. It also assumes a certain imbalance of power or strength, with students who are exposed to negative actions having difficulty defending themselves. With the advent of cyberbullying these criteria remain broadly similar.

A number of meta-analyses have shown convincingly that being involved in bullying, either as a bully, a victim, or a bully–victim, with some regularity is not a harmless and passing school problem. Rather, such involvement can result in serious long-term consequences and adjustment problems for all groups; these are of a different nature, manifesting as depression and other internalizing problems for the victims and as criminality/antisocial behaviour and other externalizing problems for the bullies (Olweus, 2013).

It seems that around 2–8% of children are bullied once or more a week. They may be divided into a passive group, who are insecure and anxious and withdraw when attacked, and a provocative group, who are themselves aggressive either directly or by getting others into trouble. The bullies are more often boys than girls; boys are more likely to be physically aggressive, whereas girls are more likely to exclude their victims or campaign against them. Children who were bullied around the age of 5 years were found to exhibit a greater risk of emotional problems and disruptive behaviours at 2-year follow-up (Arseneault et al., 2006). Bullying in older children has important associations with self-harm, violent behaviour, and psychotic symptoms (Arseneault et al., 2010). Adult psychiatric outcomes of school-aged bullying have been reported in the Great Smoky Mountain study. This showed that both victims and those who were bullies and victims had elevated rates of young adult psychiatric disorders and family hardships (Copeland et al., 2013). Victims had a higher prevalence of agoraphobia, generalized anxiety, and panic disorder. Bully–victims were at increased risk of young adult depression, panic disorder, and suicidality in males. Bullies were also at risk for antisocial personality disorder.

It must also be noted that many interpersonal challenges with peers are exacerbated by social media contact, and cyber-bullying that takes place through social media has been reported as a significant new method through which to victimize other peers (Kowalski et al., 2014). Its use and effects should be explored with young people, although many victims of cyber-bullying also experience traditional bullying within the school context, and levels of cyber-bullying are seen to reduce following strategies to reduce traditional bullying.

Relationship with teachers: poor relationships between students and teachers are a predictor of the onset of childhood psychiatric disorder and of low attainment (Fazel et al., 2014a). Furthermore, difficulties with behavioural management can negatively affect teacher–pupil relationships and the classroom environment, and might impact on the mental health of both teacher and child.

Psychiatric assessment of children and their families

The aims of assessment are to obtain a clear account of the presenting problem, to find out how this problem is related to the child's past development and present life in its psychological and social context, and to plan treatment for the child and the family.

The psychiatric assessment of children differs in several ways from that of adults, which was described in Chapter 3.

- *A more flexible approach.* With children it is often difficult to follow a set routine, so a flexible approach to interviewing is required, although it is still important that information and observations are recorded systematically.

- *Interviewing of family members.* Parents or other carers should be asked to attend the assessment interview, and it is often helpful to have other siblings present.

- *Information from schools.* Time can be saved by asking permission to obtain information from teachers before the child attends the clinic. This information should be concerned with the child's behaviour in both structured and unstructured settings at school and their educational attainments.

Child psychiatrists vary in their methods of assessment. All agree that it is important to see the family together at some stage to observe how they interact. Some psychiatrists do this before seeing the patient alone, while others do it afterwards. It might be easier to better engage some adolescents if initially seen on their own, but this might not help with other adolescents and so must be decided on a case by case basis. With younger children the main informants are usually the parents, but children over the age of 6 years should usually be seen on their own at some stage. In the special case of suspected child abuse, the interview with the child is particularly important. Whatever the problem, the parents should be made to feel that the interview is supportive and does not undermine their confidence.

Interviewing the parents

Parents are likely to be anxious, and some fear that they may be blamed for their child's problems. Time should be taken to put them at ease and explain the purpose of the interview. They should then be encouraged to talk spontaneously about the problems before systematic questions are asked. The methods of interviewing are similar to those used in adult psychiatry (see Chapter 3). The items to be included in the history are listed in the Appendix to this chapter. As in adult psychiatry, an experienced interviewer will keep the complete list in mind, while focusing on those items that are relevant to the particular case. It is important to obtain some developmental history, specific examples of general problems, to elicit factual information, and to assess feelings and attitudes.

Interviewing and observing the child

Younger children may not be able or willing to express their ideas and feelings in words, therefore observations of their behaviour and interactions during the interview are especially important. With very young children, drawing and the use of toys may be helpful. With older children, it may be possible to follow a procedure similar to that used with adults, provided that care is taken to use words and concepts appropriate to the child's age and background. Standardized methods of observation and interviewing have been developed mainly for research purposes.

Starting the interview. It is essential to begin by establishing a friendly atmosphere and winning the child's confidence, and asking what they like to be called. It is usually appropriate to begin with a discussion of neutral topics such as pets, favourite games, or birthdays, or current school information—such as which class they are in and which subjects they like—before turning to the presenting problem.

Techniques of interviewing. When a friendly relationship has been established, the child can be asked about the problem, their likes and dislikes, and their hopes for the future. It is often informative to ask what they would request if they were given three wishes or, with older children, to ask them for three goals they would like to achieve following their contact with mental health services. Younger children may be given the opportunity to express their concerns and feelings in paintings or play. Children can generally recall events accurately, although not always in the correct sequence. They are more suggestible than adults, and, when asked a question, are used to trying to give the answer that the adult has in mind—as they might, for example, in school. Therefore it is particularly important not to use leading questions when interviewing, and not to suggest actions or interpretations to a child who is being observed while painting or at play.

Behaviour and mental state. The items to be noted are listed in the Appendix to this chapter (see page 483). Children who are brought to see a psychiatrist may appear silent and withdrawn at the first meeting; this behaviour should not be misinterpreted as evidence of depression.

Developmental assessments. By the end of the interview an assessment should have been made of the child's stage of development relative to other children of the same age.

For further information and advice about interviewing and communicating with children, see Bostic and Martin (2009).

Interviewing the family

A family interview can contribute to the assessment of the interactions between family members, but it is not necessarily a good way to obtain factual information. The latter is generally more effectively obtained in interviews with the parents or other family members on their own. Of the various aspects of family interaction, the psychiatrist will usually be most interested in discord and disorganization, which are the features most closely associated with the development of psychiatric disorder. Patterns of communication between family members are also important.

It is usually best to see the family at the first assessment or soon after this, before the interviewer has formed a close relationship with the young patient, or with one of the parents, as this may make it more difficult to interview the other family members or could jeopardize the early therapeutic relationship between the therapist and child.

The interviewer could begin by asking 'Who would be the best person to tell me about why we are here/ your difficulties?' If one family member monopolizes the interview, another member should be asked to comment on what has been said. A useful question to stimulate discussion is 'How do you think that your partner (daughter, son) would see the problem?' The interviewer can then ask the partner (daughter, son) how they in fact see the problem. As an alternative, family members who are present can be asked what they think an absent member would think about the issues.

While observing the family's ways of responding to these and other questions, the interviewer should consider the following:

● Who is the spokesperson for the family?

● Who seems most worried about the problem?

● What are the alliances within the family?

● What is the hierarchy in the family? For example, who is most dominant?

● How well do the family members communicate with one another?

● How do they seem to deal with conflict?

Psychological assessment

Measures of intelligence and educational achievement are often valuable. If mental development and achievement are inconsistent with chronological or mental age, or with the expectations of parents or teachers, this may indicate a generalized or specific disorder of development or may indicate a source of stress in disorders of other kinds. Some of the more commonly used procedures are listed in Table 16.3. For further information, see Charman *et al.* (2008).

Other information

The most important additional informants are the primary care practitioners and the child's teachers. Teachers can describe classroom behaviour, educational achievements, and relationships with other children. They may also make useful comments about the child's family and home circumstances. It is often helpful for a member of the mental health team to observe the child at school as well as visit the home. This visit can provide useful information about material circumstances in the home, the relationship of family members, and the pattern of their life together.

Table 16.3 Notes on some psychological measures in use with children

Intelligence tests	
Stanford-Binet test, 5th edition	Tests verbal and non-verbal intelligence from 2 years to adulthood
Wechsler Intelligence Scale for Children (WISC IV)	Provides a profile of specific verbal and performance ability as well as IQ for children aged 6–14 years; widely used and well standardized; cannot be used for IQ below 40. Translated into several languages
Wechsler Pre-School and Primary Scale of Intelligence	A version of WISC for use with children aged 3–7 years
British ability scales	One for age 2–6 years, the other for age 6–18 years, covering six areas: speed of information processing; reasoning; spatial imagery; perceptual matching; short-term memory; and retrieval and application of knowledge. Analysis can be general or specific
Social development assessments	
Bayley scales of infant and toddler development, 3rd edition	Standard tasks scored on mental, motor, and behaviour scales and compared with normsUseful measure of infant development from ages 1 month to 3½ years
Other developmental assessment	
Denver developmental screening test, 2nd edition	General developmental screening test from birth to 6½ years. Identifies delays in personal and social development, fine and gross motor development, and language skills. For use only as a screen to identify those needing further assessment

Physical examination

If the child has not been examined recently by the general practitioner, an appropriate physical examination may be needed to complete the assessment. What is appropriate depends on the nature of the problem, but it will often be concerned with evidence of conditions that might affect the brain. Therefore the first step is to observe the child's appearance, coordination, and gait, at rest and during play. A basic physical examination may follow, with emphasis on the nervous system. If abnormalities are found or suspected, the opinion of a paediatrician or paediatric neurologist may be needed.

Ending the assessment

At the end of the assessment the psychiatrist should explain to the parents—and to the child, in terms appropriate to their age—the result of the assessment; they could at this point agree goals for any treatment plan. Psychiatrists should explain how they propose to inform and work with the general practitioner, and seek consent to contact other people involved with the child, such as teachers or social workers. Throughout, the psychiatrist should encourage questions and discussion.

Formulation

A formulation can be helpful when summarizing key issues. It usually starts with a brief statement of the *current problem*. The *diagnosis and differential diagnosis* are discussed next. The diagnosis can be recorded as per the ICD-10 within a multiaxial framework, ensuring that broader developmental and environmental factors are recorded (as discussed above). *Aetiology* is then considered, with attention to predisposing, precipitating, and perpetuating factors. The *developmental stages* of the child should be noted (if this has not already been done in the multiaxial diagnostic system), as well as any particular strengths and achievements. An assessment of the problems and the strengths of the family is also recorded. Any further assessments should be specified, a *treatment plan* drawn up, and the *expected outcome* recorded.

Court reports

Psychiatrists may be asked to prepare court reports in relation to children. These reports are usually undertaken by specialists in child psychiatry; therefore only an outline will be given here. If general psychiatrists are

required to prepare such a report, they should ensure that they are thoroughly aware of the relevant legislation, ask advice from a colleague with relevant special experience, and read a more detailed account of the requirements for court reports.

Courts concerned with children obtain evidence from several sources, including social workers, probation officers, community nurses, psychologists, and psychiatrists. In their reports, psychiatrists should focus on matters within their expertise, including:

- The child's age, stage of development, and temperament, and the relevance of these to the case.
- Whether the child has a psychiatric disorder.
- The child's own wishes about their future, considered in relation to their age and understanding.
- The parenting skills of the carers, how far they can meet the child's needs, and other relevant aspects of the family.

While focusing on these matters, the psychiatrist should also be prepared to provide information about the following issues:

- The child's physical, emotional, and educational needs.
- The likely effect on the child of any possible change of circumstances (e.g. removal from home, or living with one or other parent after a divorce).
- Any harm that the child has suffered or is likely to suffer.

The *wishes of the child* should be considered in relation to their age and ability to understand the present situation and possible future arrangements, and to relevant factors in the present situation—for example, some abused children can maintain strong attachments to the abuser.

Parenting skills are judged partly on the basis of the history and reports of other people. They are also judged on direct observations of the interactions between the parents and the child, including the parents' attachment to the child, their sensitivity to cues from the child, and their ability to meet the child's needs.

The report is similar in structure to a court report for an adult, and is presented under the headings shown in Box 16.2.

Children as witnesses

A child's evidence is important in cases of suspected abuse, and occasionally in other kinds of case, such as witnessed assault on another family member. When seeking such evidence, the interviewer should be aware of certain points about children's memory and the factors that can influence their accounts.

Memory varies with age, as do the verbal skills required to describe what has been remembered. Children below the age of 3 years seldom have the cognitive and other capacities to produce an account that can be presented in a court of law. Children above the age of 3 years can produce detailed and accurate memories, although they may not be able to describe them clearly without some prompting.

Most children above the age of 6 years can use straightforward grammar and syntax adequately, but their vocabulary is limited and they may be confused by complicated questions. Also, children of this age may expect that an adult who asks a question already knows the right answer, as this is how they learn (e.g. 'How many flowers did you see in the picture?') Consequently, they *may agree with leading questions* asked by an adult or, when they cannot remember, make up an answer in the hope that it will be the one that is wanted by the questioner. A further problem is that young children do not have an accurate sense of the sequencing and timing of events. Finally, the events that children are asked to recall when they are questioned as witnesses are usually frightening and experienced in a state of emotional arousal. Memories of such events are often incomplete, although the recalled fragments may be detailed and vivid.

> **Box 16.2 Topics to be addressed in a court report about a child**
>
> - The qualifications of the writer
> - Who commissioned the report, and what questions were asked
> - What written information was available, and who was interviewed
> - A summary of the findings from the interview (it is not necessary to repeat information contained in social enquiry reports)
> - The writer's interpretation of the information from the interviews and written material
> - In the light of the findings, comments on the options before the court, remembering always that it is for the court and not the psychiatrist to determine which option is selected
>
> Thompson and Pearce (2009) suggest the use of the following principles when evidence is obtained from a child:
>
> - Allow the child to talk freely, asking as few questions as possible.
> - Obtain the evidence as soon as possible after the event, and whenever possible before any counselling has taken place.
> - Try to complete the account on the first occasion, as subsequent accounts are likely to be less accurate.
> - Be aware that the greater the pressure to remember, the less accurate the account is likely to be.

Psychiatric treatment for children and their families

This section is concerned with the general features of treatment for children. Aspects of treatment that are specific to individual disorders are discussed later in the sections concerned with those disorders.

The role of the primary care team

General practitioners and other members of the primary care team spend much of their time in advising parents about children, but they refer only a small proportion of these children to a child psychiatrist or a paediatrician. General practitioners are more likely to refer children with the following to a paediatrician, some of whom will be working in teams with psychological support:

- developmental difficulties
- physical symptoms with a probable psychological cause
- psychological complications of physical illness.

They are more likely to refer emotional, attentional, and conduct disorders to a child psychiatrist. Most of the disorders that are referred are similar to those that they already manage but often with a greater element of functional or educational impairment or are impacting on family and peer relationships. Often these referrals will be precipitated by parents or school involvement.

The psychiatric team

Way of working. Although psychiatrists, psychologists, psychotherapists, family therapists, nurses, occupational therapists, and social workers have special skills, when working in a child psychiatry team they do not confine themselves to their traditional professional role. Instead, they adopt whatever role is most likely to be helpful in the particular case, as they do when working in a community team caring for adults.

The team usually adopts a *family-centred approach*, and it liaises closely with other professionals involved with the child or the family. These professionals include paediatricians, members of child health and social services, teachers, and other school-based professionals. Since many childhood problems are evident at school, or lead to educational difficulties, the child's teachers usually need to be involved in some way. They may need advice about the best way to support the child or manage disturbed behaviour in the classroom, changes that may be needed in the child's school timetable, or remedial teaching that may be required. Occasionally a change of school is indicated.

In the following sections, brief accounts are given of the main kinds of treatment. In the second part of the chapter, information is given about the management of specific disorders. Additional information about treatment in child psychiatry can be obtained from one of the textbooks listed at the end of this chapter.

Medication

Drugs have a limited place in child psychiatry, primarily because of the potential effects that medication might have on the developing brain but also because the evidence base for pharmacological therapies is particularly limited. The main indications for medication are in the treatment of depression, severe anxiety disorders, ADHD, sleep disorders, psychosis, obsessional disorders, and tic disorders. In all cases, dosages should be checked carefully in the manufacturer's literature or a standard reference book, making sure that the dose is correct for the child's age and body weight.

Psychological treatment

Psychological aspects of management

Whatever the plan of management, children benefit from a *warm, secure, and accepting relationship* with the therapist. The security of this relationship helps the child to express their feelings and to find alternative ways of behaving. For younger children, play with toys can help to establish the relationship and provide a medium through which they can express their problems and feelings more effectively than they can with words.

At first, children often perceive the therapist as an agent of the parents, and might expect the therapist to share their attitudes. Children should feel accepted in their own right, and not criticized. However, they should not be allowed to feel that anything they do will be approved. It is often advisable to delay discussion of the presenting problems until the child's confidence has been gained by talking about neutral subjects that interest them.

More commonly utilized psychological treatments in psychiatric clinics include behavioural interventions, cognitive behaviour therapy, systemic family therapy, and psychodynamic psychotherapy, although the evidence base for all of these is poor for pre-adolescents (Forti-Buratti *et al.*, 2016).

Cognitive behaviour therapy

Behavioural methods have several applications in child psychiatry. They can be used to encourage new behaviour by positive reinforcement and modelling. This is often done by first rewarding behaviour that approximates to the desired behaviour (*shaping*), and then giving reinforcement in a more discriminating way. For example, in children with ASD, shaping has been used for behavioural problems such as temper tantrums and refusal to go to bed- by reinforcing behaviours that are more closely aligned with the desired behaviour. Punishment is not used in shaping behaviour because its effects are temporary and it is ethically unacceptable. Instead, efforts are made to identify and remove any factors in the child's environment that are reinforcing unwanted behaviour. It is often found that undesired behaviour is being *reinforced unwittingly* by extra attention given to the child when the behaviour occurs. If the child is ignored at such times and attended to when their behaviour is more normal, beneficial changes often take place. More specific forms of behaviour therapy are available for enuresis (see page 468) and phobias (see page 179). *Social skills training* in a group or in individual sessions may be used for children who have difficulty in relationships with other children and adults. The methods generally resemble those used with adults (see Chapter 24: Psychological Treatments).

Cognitive therapy is useful for older children, who can describe and learn to control the ways of thinking that give rise to symptoms and problem behaviours. Older children and adolescents with anxiety disorders, depressive disorders, and eating disorders can be treated with the techniques originally devised for adults. Special techniques have been developed for children with aggressive behaviour (see page 458).

For a review of the efficacy of cognitive behaviour therapy in childhood and adolescent anxiety and depression, see James *et al.* (2013) and Graham (2009).

Psychodynamic therapies

Most psychodynamic approaches for children are based on the methods of Anna Freud and Melanie Klein. Reviews have generally concluded that, although many outcome studies have methodological flaws, the better investigations indicate that dynamic psychotherapy is rather more effective than no treatment across a range of common mental disorders (Abbass *et al.*, 2013). However, psychodynamic therapy has not been shown to produce better results than those of counselling or cognitive behaviour therapy. Consequently, long-term, analytically based, psychodynamic therapies are now used infrequently in the UK, although group therapy and creative therapies (e.g. play therapy and art therapy) continue to be provided for selected children with severe and enduring difficulties. For a more positive assessment of the value of psychodynamic therapies for children, see Fonagy and Target (2009).

Parent training

Parent training is used for a range of child psychiatric problems, and includes improving the skills of parents who have some difficulties and want help with parenting skills, as well as those who abuse or neglect their children and those with low intelligence. It is also used to assist parents of children with behaviour problems that require special parenting skills—for example, the parents of children with conduct disorder or ADHD. Most research has been with parents of children who are oppositional or defiant or have conduct disorders. Parent training can be carried out with an educational approach, in which skills of general importance are taught, or with a behavioural approach, in which the specific problems of the particular parent and child are analysed and corrected. In the behavioural approach, use may be made of video-recorded vignettes showing desirable and undesirable parental responses to children's behaviour. These responses are discussed with the parents of a particular child, or with a group of parents. Whatever approach is adopted, it is important to take account of the stage of development of the child, and of the changing needs of children of different ages.

Studies of the behavioural training of parents have now firmly established the effectiveness of this approach in improving parenting skills and parent–child relationships, and reducing antisocial behaviour in children. For example, for groups often considered as 'hard to treat'

for reasons of social disadvantage or psychopathology, parenting interventions can improve child behaviour. For families with very complex needs, such as those in the child protection system, the evidence is more promising than for other interventions. Parenting programmes delivered as part of school-based programmes tend to have small effects on children's behaviour in school. Research is now focusing on which families can benefit and the long-term effects. For a review of parent training programmes, see Scott *et al.* (2015b).

Family therapy

This is a specific form of treatment to be distinguished from the general family approach to treatment described above. In family therapy, the symptoms of the child or adolescent are viewed as an expression of malfunctioning of the family, which is the primary focus of treatment. Several approaches have been used, based on behavioural or psychoanalytical, interpersonal or structural theories. These kinds of therapy are described on page 703. In practice, most therapists adopt an eclectic approach.

The *indications* for family therapy are still debated, but there is general agreement that it can be used appropriately when:

- the child's symptoms are judged to be part of a disturbance of the whole family
- individual therapy is not proving effective
- family difficulties have arisen during another kind of treatment.

The *contraindications* to family therapy are that the parents' relationship is breaking up, or the child's problems do not seem to be closely related to family function.

The best evidence for effectiveness is for structural and behavioural forms of family therapy, where benefits have been shown in youth offending, substance misuse, and eating disorders. For a comprehensive review of family interventions, see Eisler *et al.* (2015).

Internet-based therapies

In recent years there has been a rise in different technologies that children and adolescents can access through home computers and tablets or smartphones that can either supplement or provide treatment for a range of mental disorders. There has been a rise in 'applications' or 'apps' that can be utilized via a variety of interfaces. Internet-based or computerized cognitive behaviour therapy has shown some positive effects for symptoms of depression and anxiety for those over the age of 12 years, but not in younger populations (Pennant *et al.*, 2015).

Social work

Social workers play an important role in the care of children with psychiatric disorders, and of their families. In the UK they have statutory duties with regard to the protection and safeguarding of children who are at risk within the family, and who require special care or special supervision. They help parents to improve their skills in caring for their children, and to solve problems with finances or accommodation. Social workers carry out family assessments and family therapy, and may also provide individual counselling for the child and members of the family. They can play a key role when the relationships around an adolescent break down and the adolescent might need to find alternative accommodation and/or educational provision.

Occupational therapy

Occupational therapists can play a valuable part in assessment of the child's development, in psychological treatment, and in devising measures to improve parent–child interaction. They work both in day-patient and inpatient units, and in the community. They work closely with teachers in both assessing and providing therapeutic activities for children, in particular those with neurodevelopmental disorders.

Special education

Children who are attending outpatient clinics, and the much smaller number who are day-patients or inpatients, often benefit from additional educational arrangements. Special teaching may be needed to restore confidence, and to remedy delays in writing, reading, and arithmetic, which is common among children with conduct disorders as well as those with specific developmental disorders. For further information about special education and the issue of integration with 'mainstream' teaching, see Howlin (2008).

Substitute care

Residential care

There are two main reasons for residential care in children. The first is for those with profound intellectual and neurodevelopmental disorders, to provide for their physical, social, and educational needs; the second is for children who have been maltreated or have significant emotional and behavioural problems with symptoms that result from, or are maintained by, a severely unstable home environment or extreme parental rejection. The rest of this section will discuss the needs of this second group. For this second group, residential care has a long history in the provision of services and is an umbrella term, capturing various forms of residentially based living arrangements, from small group homes to large institutions, across three service systems—social services/child welfare, mental health, and juvenile justice. These care settings can provide therapeutically planned behavioural health interventions to unrelated youth with a wide range of problems in a 24-hour structured and multidisciplinary care environment. Children who are considered for residential placement often present with severely disordered behaviour and might have a number of psychiatric diagnoses, including conduct disorders and emerging personality disorders as well as breakdown in their educational provision.

Removal of a child from their primary caregivers should be considered only after every practical effort has been made to improve the circumstances of the family. Residential care may be provided in a foster home, a children's home (in which a group of about 10 children live in circumstances as close as possible to those of a large family), or a residential school. Residential care, other than fostering, is seldom arranged for children under 5 years of age, because of the need to try and ensure attachment to a primary caregiver. In general, children in residential care are a population particularly vulnerable to physical and sexual abuse. They have high rates of psychosocial problems in later childhood and in adult life, hence there is international consensus about the need to avoid prolonged stays in residential care. Residential care is associated with adult criminal convictions, depression, and low self-efficacy. Evidence of the abuse of children placed within care provides a reminder of the need to ensure good training and supervision of the staff of children's homes and residential schools.

For a review of residential care, see Ijzendoorn *et al.* (2015).

Fostering and adoption

Foster care may be of three kinds:

- *Short-term emergency care*—for example, when a caregiver is ill or when the parents of an autistic child need respite.
- *Medium-term care*, which may be followed by a return home—for example, if the caregiver is receiving

treatment for problems that led to neglect or abuse of the child.

- *Long-term care*, in which the child remains until they are adopted or able to live independently.

Children in foster care have better outcomes than those in residential care, but children in long-term foster care have more problems than children who have been adopted. It is difficult to determine to what extent these problems are related to experiences before fostering, and to what extent they are due to the lesser security of fostering as opposed to adoption. Problems seem to be greater when the fostered child has experienced prenatal exposure to substances, is older, and when children in the fostering family are of the same age as the fostered child. Children in foster care usually retain some contact with their biological parents, but it is not helpful to the child to have sporadic and distressing contacts. For a review of fostering, see Ijzendoorn *et al.* (2015).

Adoption is the process whereby the parenting of a child is transferred from that person's biological or legal parent/s to another person, and it is usually intended to mark a permanent change in status, legally recognized as such. Adoption practices can be open or closed. If open, then there remains an opportunity for contact with biological parents; closed adoption is when the identities of the biological parents, biological kins, and adoptee identities are not disclosed, although the transmittal of non-identifying information such as medical history can be allowed. It is generally understood that a lack of openness can be detrimental to the psychological well-being of adoptees and so closed apotion is becoming less prevalent.

Adoptions can occur between related family members or unrelated individuals. Unrelated adoptions may occur through the following routes:

- *Private domestic adoptions:* under this arrangement, charities and other organizations bring together, from within the same country, prospective adoptive parents and children to be placed.
- *Foster care adoption:* this is an adoption of a child who is initially placed in foster care.
- *International adoption:* this is the placing of a child for adoption outside that child's country of birth. Different countries have different laws regarding international adoptions. Research following international adoptions from severely deprived institutional settings has helped to elucidate the long-effects of early deprivation and to try to address the emotional, cognitive, social, and physical sequelae. For a review of international adoption, see Julian (2013) and Kumsta (2015).

- *Embryo adoption:* this is the donation of embryos (usually remaining after another couple have completed *in vitro* fertilization (IVF) treatments) to another individual or couple, followed by the placement of those embryos in the woman's uterus to facilitate pregnancy.

Given the range of different types of adoption and also the different reasons leading to a child being adopted as well as experiences prior to and the child's age at adoption, the psychological impacts of adoption can either be minimal or widespread. The areas most commonly raised are those around loss and grief for biological parents, identity development (which can be more difficult for an adopted child), and poor self-esteem. For a review of adoption in children and its psychological impact, see Cohen *et al.* (2015).

Intensive treatments

Intensive community services and inpatient care are essential components of the provision of child psychiatry, particularly for those children more severely disturbed and at risk of self-harm, suicide, or at risk of causing harm to others. Intensive community services form an increasingly important level of care between outpatient and inpatient services. Child psychiatric inpatient units require easy access to paediatric advice, adequate space for play, easy access to schooling, and an informal design that still allows close observation. There should be some provision for mothers to stay with their younger children.

Admission for inpatient treatment is usually arranged for any of three reasons:

- *Severity:* when the disorder is too severe to treat in any other way—for example, more violent behaviours, extreme mood disorders (both depression and mania), difficult-to-treat psychosis, severe pervasive developmental disorder, and life-threatening anorexia nervosa.
- *Observation:* when the diagnosis is uncertain.
- *Separation*: inpatient treatment can provide a necessary period away from a severely disturbing home environment and an assessment of the child is needed outside of this environment.

The high financial costs of inpatient units have contributed to expansion of other types of intensive services, but whether these can improve clinical outcomes and reduce numbers of admissions, length of stay, and costs still needs to be determined. *Day-hospital treatment* for children provides many of the advantages of inpatient care without removing them from home. Unless there is any danger that the child may be abused, remaining at home has the advantage that relationships with other family members are maintained. Daycare can relieve the family from some of the stressful effects of managing a child with severe behavioural disturbance or eating problems.

Increasingly, intensive community-based support is provided for children and adolescents with severe problems. Such support requires a well-staffed and experienced team of professionals with an 'assertive-outreach' approach (see page 785). Although such services are valuable, they do not remove the need for inpatient provision. For a review of the provision of intensive treatments in child and adolescent psychiatry, see James *et al.* (2015).

Review of syndromes

The review of syndromes begins with the problems encountered in *preschool children. Specific and pervasive developmental disorders* are described next. An account is then given of *the main psychiatric disorders of childhood*, in the order in which they appear in the major systems of classification. Other psychiatric disorders of childhood are described next, before a brief account of the disorders of adolescence (which are generally similar to those of either childhood or adulthood). The chapter ends with a discussion of *child abuse*.

Problems of preschool children and their families

It has already been noted that in the preschool years children are learning several kinds of social behaviour, although it should be noted that children are also shaped by culturally regulated customs, child-rearing practices, and belief systems. Preschool children are acquiring sphincter control. They are learning how to behave at mealtimes, to go to bed at an appropriate time, and to control angry feelings. They are also becoming less dependent. Most of these behaviours are learned within the family. The psychiatric problems of preschool children centre around these behaviours, and they often reflect factors in the family and caregiving environment as well as factors in the child. Many psychological problems at this age are brief, and can be thought of as variants in normal development. Most are treated in primary care and by paediatricians. The more serious problems may be referred to child mental health teams.

Prevalence

In a much quoted study, Richman *et al.* (1982) studied 705 families with a 3-year-old child in a London borough. The most frequent abnormalities of behaviour in these children were bedwetting at least three times a week (present in 37%), wetting by day at least once a week (17%), overactivity (14%), soiling at least once a week (13%), difficulty in settling at night (13%), fears (13%), disobedience (11%), attention-seeking (10%), and temper tantrums (5%).

Whether these behaviours are reported as problems depends on the attitudes of the parents as well as on the nature, severity, and frequency of the behaviour. Richman *et al.* overcame this difficulty by making their own ratings of the extent of problems. They based this assessment on the effects on the child's wellbeing and the consequences for the other members of the family. They used common-sense criteria to decide whether the problems were mild, moderate, or severe. In total, 7% of 3-year-olds in their survey had behaviour problems of marked severity and 15% had mild behaviour problems. The behaviours most often rated as problems were *temper tantrums, attention-seeking,* and *disobedience.*

Subsequent epidemiological surveys employing more modern diagnostic criteria have also found significant rates of psychological problems in preschool children. Pooling a number of predominantly US epidemiological surveys, Egger and Angold (2006) concluded that about 15% of preschool children had a psychiatric problem. More recent surveys with samples from outside the US have lower prevalence rates of around 7%, with ADHD and depressive disorders more common in boys than girls. More emotional and behavioural disorders were seen in children whose parents did not live together and in those of low socioeconomic status. The most common disorders are *ADHD, oppositional disorders, emotional disorders, and anxiety disorders*; comorbidity among disorders is common (Wichstrøm *et al.*, 2012).

Some common problems of preschool children

Temper tantrums and disruptive behaviours

Temper tantrums are among the most common childhood behaviour problems and approximately 5–7% of children between 1 and 3 years of age have temper tantrums lasting at least 15 minutes three or more times per week. They are extreme episodes of frustration or anger, with mood and behaviour returning to normal between tantrums. Only persistent or very severe tantrums are abnormal. Children often have temper tantrums to get something they want, to avoid something they do not want to do, or to seek parental attention. They are more likely to occur when the child is tired, hungry, ill, or frustrated. The immediate effect can be an unwitting reinforcement by excessive attention and inconsistent discipline on the part of the parents. Tantrums may persist if parents have emotional problems of their own, or because the relationship between them is unsatisfactory.

Temper tantrums can be difficult to stop once they start, and so identifying triggers and potential causes and preventing tantrums is important. During a tantrum it is usually best to try and remain calm and to respond kindly with firm and consistent setting of limits. In treatment it is first necessary to discover why the parents have been unable to set limits in this way. They might need to be helped with any problems of their own and advised how to respond to the tantrums.

Sleep problems

The most common sleep difficulty is *wakefulness at night*, which is most frequent between the ages of 1 and 4 years and is reported by around 20–30% of parents. About 20% of children of this age take at least an hour to get to sleep or are wakeful for long periods during the night. Bedtime struggles and middle of the night wakings are not only a source of sleep disruption for children and their parents, but can also be a source of conflict and negative emotion among family members. When wakefulness is an isolated problem and not very distressing to the family, it is enough to reassure the parents that it is likely to improve. If sleep disturbances are severe or persistent, two possible causes should be considered. First, the problems may have been made worse by various comorbidities (emotional disorders, autism, ADHD) or physical illness. Secondly, they may have been exacerbated by the parents' excessive concern and inability to reassure the child.

If no medical or psychiatric disorder is detected, the reasons for the parents' concerns should be sought and dealt with as far as possible. Some parents overstimulate their child in the evening, or unwittingly reinforce crying in the night by taking the child into their own bed. A behavioural approach to these problems is generally helpful. Other sleep problems, such as *nightmares and night terrors*, are common among healthy toddlers, but they seldom persist for long. They are discussed on page 329. For a review of sleep problems and interventions in children, see Harvey *et al.* (2015).

Feeding problems

Normal feeding and eating depends on the successful integration of a range of physical functions and interpersonal relationships during early development, therefore a minor disruption in one or more of these areas can result in a feeding problem in infants and early childhood. Common disturbances include delayed development of feeding/eating skills, difficulty managing or tolerating foodstuffs, and reluctance or refusal to eat based on taste, texture, and other sensory factors. Minor food fads and food refusal are common in preschool children, but do not usually last long. In a minority, however, the behaviour is severe or persistent, although not accompanied by signs of poor nourishment. When this happens it might be because the parents are overattentive and this might unwittingly reinforce the child's behaviour. Feeding problems become 'Feeding disorders of infancy and childhood' when the problems are persistent (over 1 month in duration) and are associated with significant failure to gain weight (Bryant-Waugh, 2010).

Treatment is directed to the parents' management of the problem. They should be encouraged to ignore the feeding problem and refrain from offering the child special foods or otherwise attempting to do anything unusual to persuade him or her to eat. Instead, the child should be offered a normal meal and left to decide whether to eat it or not.

Pica

Pica is the diagnostic term for the eating of items that are generally regarded as inedible, such as soil, paint, or paper. It is often associated with other behaviour problems and is inappropriate to the child's developmental level. Cases should be investigated carefully because some are due to brain damage, autism, or intellectual disability. It can also co-occur with other mental disorders, such as schizophrenia, but for a diagnosis of pica it must present as severe enough to warrant independent clinical attention. Otherwise, treatment consists of common-sense precautions to keep the abnormal items of diet away from the child. Pica usually diminishes as the child grows older. For further discussion see Pica section in Chapter 13.

Disorders associated with adverse caregiving

As explained above, children's *attachments to their parents* vary in their security, and they may vary between caregivers—for example, being insecure with one parent but secure with the other. Attachment disorders are more extreme variations from the norm, and do not correspond exactly to any of the types of insecure attachment described earlier (see page 425). They are *pervasive*, affecting all relationships. They start before the age of 5 years and are associated with grossly abnormal caregiving.

In DSM-5 two separate disorders are described relating to children who have experienced adverse caregiving. The first is *reactive attachment disorder* (RAD), where there is an absence of attachment behaviour secondary to social neglect. These children have the developmental capacity to form attachments, and these disorders are very responsive to enhanced caregiving. For example, in children from Romanian orphanages who had experienced extreme deprivation, the signs of RAD diminished or disappeared once children were placed in families and received adequate care—with best outcomes if they were removed before 2 years of age (Zeanah *et al.*, 2015). The second disorder is *disinhibited social engagement disorder* (DSED), in which the child lacks appropriate reticence with unfamiliar adults and violates socially sanctioned boundaries. Compared with RAD, children with DSED are usually more functionally impaired, have difficulties with close relationships and more need for special education, and have a poorer outcome.

Assessment and treatment of the problems of preschool children

Assessment. Usually the information is largely obtained from the parents. The assessor seeks to discover whether the problem is primarily in the child or related to difficulties in the primary caregiver, other potential attachment figures, or the entire family. The problem behaviour is assessed, together with the child's general level of development, and the functioning of the family.

Treatment. Apart from the particular points already mentioned under the specific disorders, treatment includes advice for the parents (and, if necessary, for other family members) about relevant aspects of child-rearing. There is little systematic evidence about the value of treatment, although parenting interventions are the best established approaches, and have some benefit even where the underlying condition has a strong genetic basis. It may be helpful to arrange for the child to spend part of the day away from the family in a playgroup or nursery school, provided that the care offered is of high quality. Specially adapted cognitive approaches can be helpful for emotional and anxiety disorders.

Specific developmental disorders

DSM-5 and ICD-10 both contain categories for specific developmental disorders, which are circumscribed developmental delays that are not attributable to another disorder or to lack of opportunity to learn (see Table 16.4).

It is debatable whether these conditions should be classified as mental disorders at all, since many children who meet the criteria have no other signs of psychopathology. Developmental learning, communication, and motor problems can affect children throughout development, influencing their lives and personalities, and can therefore have long-term implications for children's emotional and regulatory development, affecting their transitions into adulthood. Some of these disorders, when detected and treated early, can be remediated successfully. Others are chronic, and compensatory skills must be taught. In ICD-10, these developmental disorders are divided into specific developmental disorders of *scholastic skills, speech and language, and motor function*. In DSM-5, the same disorders are called *learning disorder, communication disorders, and motor skill disorder*, respectively.

Specific developmental disorders of scholastic skills are divided further into specific reading disorder, specific spelling disorder, and specific arithmetic disorder.

Specific learning disorders

Reading disorder

In DSM-5, reading disorder is grouped with other learning disorders. Previously, the disorders of reading, writing, or arithmetic were considered selective or specific impairments, but it is increasingly apparent that they can frequently co-occur with each other and with other communication impairments, attention disorder, and developmental coordination disorders. Significant advances have been made in understanding the nature and causes of children's reading difficulties, especially through better elucidation of the cognitive models involved. There are two different, but commonly occurring, reading disorders in children: dyslexia and reading comprehension disorder.

Dyslexia

Dyslexia refers to a difficulty in learning to decode, leading to poor appreciation of the spelling patterns of words and their pronunciation. Therefore, children with dyslexia can have difficulties accurately reading aloud and with spelling. It is usually diagnosed because the child has serious *delay in learning to read*, evident from the early years of schooling, which is sometimes preceded by delayed acquisition of basic language skills. *Writing and spelling are impaired*, and in older children these problems may be more obvious than the reading problems. Errors in reading and spelling include omissions, substitutions, or distortions of words, slow reading, long hesitations, and reversals of words or letters. There may

Table 16.4 Specific learning disorders

DSM-5	ICD–10
Specific learning disorder	**Specific developmental disorders of scholastic skills**
Reading disorder	Specific reading disorder
Disorder of written expression	Specific spelling disorder
Mathematics disorder	Specific disorder of arithmetic skills
Learning disorder not otherwise specified	Mixed disorder of scholastic skills
Communication disorders	**Specific developmental disorders of speech and language**
Speech sound disorder	Specific speech articulation disorder
Language disorder	Expressive language disorder
	Receptive language disorder
	Acquired aphasia with epilepsy
Child-onset fluency disorder	Stuttering (coded under behavioural disorders)
Social (pragmatic) communication disorder	
Motor disorders	
Developmental coordination disorder	Specific developmental disorder of motor function

Source: data from The ICD-10 classification of mental and behavioural disorders: clinical descriptions and diagnostic guidelines, Copyright (1992), World Health Organization; Diagnostic and Statistical Manual of Mental Disorders, Fifth Edition, Copyright (2013), American Psychiatric Association.

be associated emotional problems, but development in other areas is not affected. Of note: the DSM-5 uses the term specific learning disorder (SLD) to describe a number of different disorders of language and not the term dyslexia; the SLDs are considered a type of neurodevelopmental disorder.

Estimates of the presence of dyslexia in English-speaking countries range from 3% to 10% in school-aged children, with more boys referred than girls and higher numbers in urban versus rural populations and in those with English as a second language. Typically the spelling difficulties in people with dyslexia are more resistant to remediation than their reading difficulties.

Those with specific reading difficulties are more often male and are more likely to have minor neurological abnormalities, and to come from socially disadvantaged homes. Sensory impairments are common; for example, some auditory processing tasks, especially frequency discrimination, present in up to 30–40% of children with dyslexia.

For a review of dyslexia, see Peterson and Pennington (2015).

Reading comprehension impairment

Children with *reading comprehension impairment* show a contrasting pattern, where they are able to read aloud accurately but have difficulty understanding what they have read. These children present less frequently to services as they often go unnoticed. It might be quite common, as some studies have suggested up to 5% of secondary school pupils have this disorder. They might experience higher-level language difficulties, including problems with inferencing and with figurative language use. Much of the clinical profile has similarities with that seen in ADHD.

Aetiology of reading disorders

Reading is a complex skill that depends on more than one psychological process and is learned in several stages; its aetiology is varied and depends on genetic and environmental factors. It is not surprising, therefore, that no single cause has been identified for reading disorders. The predominant cognitive explanation of dyslexia is that it arises from a phonological deficit—a problem in processing the speech sounds of spoken words. Phonological skills provide the support for verbal short-term memory and, more broadly, the learning of verbal information. This theory does not necessarily account for all the reading problems encountered in dyslexia. Another theory focuses on naming speed measured by rapid automatized naming tests (RAN), where tasks involve the rapid naming of familiar objects, colours, etc. Performance in RAN can be a good marker of those who will go on to have reading problems. RAN might link into the verbal mapping that is critical to learning how to read. A model that can be useful in clinical practice is one that explains how children first use visual methods when learning to read; they learn the appearance of whole words, and cannot decipher new words. The next stage of learning is alphabetical; children become able to decode new words from the sounds associated with the letters. In the final stage, reading becomes automatic and flexible in combining visual and alphabetical methods.

Genetic causes. The frequent occurrence of reading disorder in other family members suggests a genetic cause, and the family patterning suggests that there is not a single mode of inheritance but a range of genetic and molecular mechanisms contributing to the different disorders. For example, rare protein-coding mutations in the *FOXP2* transcription factor gene can cause severe problems with sequencing sounds, while risk variants of small-effect sizes in many genes (e.g. *CNTNAP*1, *ATP2C2*, and *CMIP*) are associated with commoner forms of language impairment (Graham and Fisher, 2013).

Neurological causes. Although the majority of children do not show any structural brain abnormalities, early neurodevelopmental abnormalities appear to be involved. Right prefrontal brain mechanisms seem to be involved and may be critical for reading improvement in dyslexia. Children with cerebral palsy and epilepsy have increased rates of specific reading disorder. Another suggestion is that there is a *disorder of brain maturation* affecting one or more of the skills required in reading. This explanation is consistent with the following findings: difficulty in visual scanning, confusion between right and left, and general improvement with age.

Social factors. The environment plays a critical role in shaping a child's reading development, and parental educational level and range of vocabulary at home may reflect differences in amount and quality of literacy-related activities delivered to children at home. For example, parental teaching of print concepts has been shown to be associated with better reading outcomes.

Assessment and treatment

Children with reading disorders are rarely referred to a child psychiatrist unless such difficulties have contributed to emotional and behavioural difficulties. However, it is easy to miss a disorder in a child with mental health problems. It is important to identify the disorder early. *Assessment* is carried out by an educational or clinical psychologist using an individually administered standardized test of reading accuracy and comprehension. *Treatment* is predominantly in educational methods, and there is strong evidence to support the effectiveness of phonological interventions (developing phonological awareness, alphabet knowledge, early decoding skills). There is less evidence for interventions to help reading fluency problems that might persist once the basic decoding skills are mastered in children, but repeated oral reading programmes can help to improve reading fluency. There is less evidence for reading comprehension impairment; however, many sessions of individual teaching or small group teaching can help. If there are additional medical or behavioural problems, these will require separate intervention. If there are behavioural

problems secondary to frustration caused by the reading difficulty, they may lessen as reading improves; others may need separate attention. For more information on educational interventions for children's specific learning difficulties, see Hulme *et al.* (2015).

Prognosis

The prognosis varies with the severity of the condition. Even among children with a mild problem in mid-childhood, only about 25% achieve normal reading skills by adolescence. Very few with severe problems in mid-childhood overcome them by adolescence. Although there is insufficient evidence to be certain what happens to these people as adults, those with substantial difficulties in adolescence seem likely to retain them. Specific reading difficulties are common in adults with antisocial behaviour.

For a review of reading disorders, see Snowling *et al.* (2015).

Mathematics disorder (specific arithmetic disorder)

Mathematics disorder is a DSM-5 term that is under the category of specific learning disorders, whilst *specific arithmetic disorder* is used in ICD-10. It is also known as *dyscalculia*. Mathematics disorder has typically been defined as a difficulty in learning mathematics that is out of line with other aspects of a child's development (particularly IQ). Problems include failure to understand simple mathematical concepts, failure to recognize numerical symbols or mathematical signs, difficulty in carrying out arithmetic manipulations, and inability to learn higher level mathematical skills such as geometry and algebra. These problems are not due simply to lack of opportunities to learn, and are evident from the time of the child's first attempts to learn to count. Although it causes less severe difficulties in everyday life than reading difficulties, mathematics disorder can lead to secondary emotional difficulties when the child is at school.

Epidemiology. The incidence reported in several studies lies between 1.3% and 6%, and the disorder frequently co-occurs with specific reading difficulties (Snowling *et al.*, 2015).

Aetiology. This is less well understood than reading difficulties as less is known about the mechanisms of mathematical skills and their development. Mathematical skills depend on a complex interplay between non-verbal and verbal cognitive systems, and are likely to result from a number of cognitive deficits, including impairments in an abstract approximate number sense system located in the parietal brain areas and verbal systems that interact with this system. Twin studies suggest a significant genetic influence.

Assessment. This is usually based on the arithmetic subtests of the Wechsler Intelligence Scale for Children (WISC) and the Wechsler Adult Intelligence Scale (WAIS), and on specific tests.

Treatment. There is a growing evidence base for interventions, but these remain much fewer than for reading deficits. The studies suggest that elements, including remedial intensive teaching utilizing a variety of techniques and concrete materials, and practice in counting and number skills, can greatly benefit children with these deficits. Without treatment the condition appears to persist over several years of follow-up. For a review, see Hulme *et al.* (2015).

Disorders of communication, speech, and language

Communication is the transmission of information (a message) using a common signalling system, and language is a form of communication that humans have developed to assist in communication. Language is a complex formal system that makes use of sounds and words in rule-governed ways to convey an infinite number of meanings. Language can take a variety of forms—it can be written or conveyed using manual signs—however, the most widely used form for expressing language is through speech (Norbury *et al.*, 2015). The process by which language is acquired is complex, and is still not fully understood.

Children vary widely in their achievement of speech and language. Half of all children use words with meanings by about 12 months of age, and 97% do so by 21 months. Half of all children form words into simple sentences by 23 months. Vocabulary and complexity of language develop rapidly during the preschool years. Specific language impairment appears to be a relatively common disorder, with estimates of around 7% in kindergarten children; there are high levels of comorbidity with reading disorders, motor coordination, general learning disorders, and ADHD. It is also associated with psychiatric problems because it can be a sign of a common brain abnormality and also because language disorder impairs social interaction and education.

Causes of speech and language disorder

The causes of language impairment remain poorly understood. Children appear to have pronounced problems in word learning (vocabulary knowledge), grammar learning, and phonology. A minority might have another primary disorder, such as is *intellectual disability*, hearing problems, *cerebral palsy*, and *ASD*; it is important to detect whether another primary disorder is also present. *Social deprivation* can cause mild delays in speaking or add to the effects of the other causes. There is a genetic contribution, with mutations in a gene called *FOXP2* causing some cases of severe language disorder (Peterson, 2015).

Classification

The classification differs in some ways between ICD-10 and DSM-5. ICD-10 uses the title 'specific developmental disorders of speech and language', whereas DSM-5 has the wider title 'communication disorders'. Three disorders appear in both classifications, although with some differences in nomenclature.

- Speech sound disorder (in DSM-5) or specific speech articulation disorder (in ICD-10).
- Language disorder (DSM-5) or expressive language disorder and receptive language disorder (ICD-10).
- Childhood onset fluency disorder (DSM-5) or stuttering (coded under behavioural disorders in ICD-10).

ICD-10 (but not DSM-5) has a fourth category of 'Acquired aphasia with epilepsy', and DSM-5 has a new category of 'Social (pragmatic) communication disorder' (see Table 16.4).

Speech sound disorder (specific speech articulation disorder)

In this condition, accuracy in the use of speech sound is below the level appropriate for the child's mental age, but language skills are normal. Errors in making speech sounds (phonemes) are normal in children up to the age of about 4 years, but by the age of 7 years most speech sounds should be normal. By age 12 years nearly all speech sounds should be made normally. Children with specific speech articulation disorder make errors of articulation so severe that it is difficult for others to understand their speech. Speech sounds may be omitted or distorted, or other sounds substituted. When assessing speech production, appropriate allowance should be made for regional accents and dialects. The sounds most often affected are those that develop later in the normal sequence of development (l, r, s, z, th, and ch for English speakers).

Prevalence. This depends on the criteria used to determine when speech production is abnormal; a rate of 2–3% has been cited among 6- to 7-year-olds, reducing with older age to approximately 1% in all school-aged children (Norbury *et al.*, 2015).

Aetiology and treatment. Because the disorder tends to run in families, a genetic influence has been assumed, but for the majority no specific cause is identified. The best prognosis is for those who receive intervention in the preschool or primary grades, with most being able to achieve speech normalization by age 8 years. Speech therapy can be helpful if the articulation disorder problem is an isolated problem without, for example, associated hearing loss or cognitive impairment.

Language disorder

Language disorders are persistent difficulties in the acquisition and use of language across modalities, and may involve comprehension or production deficits in one or more of the following: 1) vocabulary (word knowledge and use); 2) sentence structure (the ability to put words and word endings together to form sentences based on rules of grammar); and 3) discourse (the ability to use vocabulary and connect sentences to explain or describe a topic or have a conversation). The disorders in language therefore follow these three areas.

- *Disorders of vocabulary*. These children are slow to acquire their first words and they often have limited vocabulary. They tend to rely on non-specific words such as 'thingie' and have difficulty learning words with multiple or abstract meanings.
- *Grammar and morphology*. Language development varies considerably among normal children, but the absence of single words by 2 years of age, and use of word combinations delayed from 2½–4 years of age signifies abnormality. Signs at later ages include restricted vocabulary, shorter utterances, and immature grammatical usage. For example, in English children might have difficulty adding endings to words to denote a different tense (help*ed*). Non-verbal communication, if impaired, is not affected as severely as spoken language, and the child makes efforts to communicate.
- *Discourse*. Some children speak rapidly and with an erratic rhythm such that the grouping of words does not reflect the grammatical structure of their speech. This abnormality, which is known as *cluttering*, is classified in ICD-10 (with stammering) among other behavioural disorders of childhood but is not included in DSM-5.

Prevalence. The prevalence of language disorder depends on the method of assessment; a rate of 1–5% of children has been proposed (Norbury *et al.*, 2015).

Prognosis. Children with language comprehension deficits can be resistant to change and are likely to require ongoing support for their language. It is

reported that about 50% of the children who meet the DSM-5 criteria develop normal speech by adulthood, while the rest have longlasting difficulties. The prognosis is worse when the language disorder is severe, and when there is a comorbid condition, such as conduct disorder.

Treatment. This mainly involves specialist speech and language therapists and special education provision; for example, focusing on developing vocabulary and narrative skills. Psychiatrists may be involved when there is a comorbid disorder, and may need to advise the parents about the child's rights for special education.

For a review of language disorder, see Norbury *et al.* (2015).

Acquired epileptic aphasia (Landau Kleffner syndrome)

In this rare disorder, a child whose language has so far developed normally loses both receptive and expressive language but retains general intelligence. There are associated EEG abnormalities, nearly always bilateral and temporal, and often with more widespread disturbances. Most of the affected children develop seizures either before or after the change in expressive language. The disorder generally starts between 3 and 9 years of age, usually over a period of several months but sometimes more rapidly.

About 20% of cases are caused by mutations in the *GRIN2A* gene, which codes for a subunit of the NMDA glutamate receptor (Lesca *et al.*, 2013). The *prognosis* is variable; about two-thirds of children are left with a receptive language deficit, but the other third recover completely. Treatment of the seizures does not always lead to improvement in language.

Assessment of speech and language disorders

Early investigation is essential both to determine the nature and severity of the speech and language disorder and to exclude mental retardation, deafness, cerebral palsy, and pervasive developmental disorder. The speech-producing organs should be examined. It is particularly important to detect deafness at an early stage.

Parents can give some indication of the child's speech and language skills, especially if they complete a standardized inventory. With younger children it may be necessary to rely on this information, but children from the age of about 3 years can be tested by a standard test of language appropriate to the child's age. If possible, such a test should be carried out by a speech therapist or a psychologist specializing in the subject.

Motor learning disorder

Some children have delayed motor development, which results in clumsiness in school work or play. In ICD-10, this condition is called specific developmental disorder of motor function. It is also known as clumsy child syndrome or specific motor dyspraxia. The child can carry out all normal movements, but coordination is poor. Children are late in developing skills such as dressing, walking, and feeding. They tend to break things and are poor at handicrafts and organized games. They may also have difficulty in writing, drawing, and copying. IQ testing usually shows good verbal but poor performance scores.

These children are sometimes referred to a psychiatrist because of secondary emotional disorder. An explanation of the nature of the problem should be given to the child, the family, and the teachers. Special teaching may improve confidence. It may be necessary to exempt the child from organized games or other school activities that involve motor coordination. There is usually some improvement with time. For further information, see Hulme *et al.* (2015).

Social (pragmatic) communication disorder

The introduction of this category of disorder in DSM-5 is predominantly as a result of changes to the diagnostic criteria for ASD (see below). This category is used for children with persistent difficulties in the social use of verbal and non-verbal communication. Four key areas of deficit need to be present for a diagnosis: using communication for social purposes (greetings); changing communication to match context or needs of the listener; following rules for conversation (turn-taking); and understanding what is not explicitly stated and non-literal or ambiguous meanings. These children must not meet diagnostic criteria for ASD (no repetitive behaviours and restrictive interests), although similarities might be evident between the two groups; they also must not have intellectual and language impairments that cause these deficits (Norbury *et al.*, 2015). As this is a new disorder, there is not yet clear evidence for interventions, although speech and language therapy focusing on communication needs is the usual intervention provided.

Autism spectrum disorders

ASD, or the ICD-10 term *pervasive developmental disorder*, refers to a group of disorders characterized by *abnormalities in communication and social interaction* and by *restricted repetitive activities and interests*. These abnormalities occur in a wide range of situations. Usually development is abnormal from infancy, and most cases are manifested before the age of 5 years.

Six conditions are included under this rubric in ICD-10 (see Table 16.5), whilst DSM-5 has made a new class of ASD, uniting four previously separate conditions to reflect scientific consensus that there is probably a single condition with different levels of symptom severity in two core domains; this will be utilized in this section as the main descriptive category unless stated otherwise. ASD now encompasses the previous DSM-IV and current ICD-10 autistic disorder, Asperger syndrome, childhood disintegrative disorder, and pervasive developmental disorder not otherwise specified. ASD is characterized by: 1) deficits in social communication and social interaction; and 2) restricted repetitive behaviours, interests, and activities (RRBs). As both components are required for diagnosis of ASD, social communication disorder is diagnosed if no RRBs are present (see above). Furthermore, two other disorders are classified in ICD-10: atypical autism and overactive disorder with mental retardation and stereotyped movements, whilst Rett's syndrome has been removed from DSM-5 but remains in ICD-10. The information for this section has been drawn from Le Couteur *et al.* (2015).

Clinical characteristics

ASD is used to denote impairments in reciprocal social communication and a tendency to engage in repetitive stereotyped patterns of behaviours, interests, and activities. ASD is a neurodevelopmental disorder that arises from atypical brain development, so core features are often present in early childhood, although they may not always be apparent.

In both DSM-5 and ICD-10, three main categories of abnormality are important for diagnosis. They reflect the features highlighted in Kanner (1943), who first described the syndrome:

- abnormalities of social development
- abnormalities of communication
- restriction of interests and behaviour.

The clinical presentation is remarkably diverse and is variable both between individuals and in the same individual at different ages (see Box 16.3).

In childhood many individuals have an apparent history of early regression or lack of progress. Some of the earliest social communication symptoms are difficulties in joint attention, eye contact, lack of intention to communicate with others, lack of socially imitative play, and fascination with sensory stimuli.

Abnormalities of social development. The child is unable to form warm emotional relationships with people (autistic aloneness) and might not respond to their parents'

Table 16.5 Autism spectrum disorders

DSM-5 Autism spectrum disorder	ICD-10 Pervasive developmental disorder
Autism spectrum disorder	Childhood autism
	Rett's syndrome
	Other childhood disintegrative disorder
	Overactive disorder with mental retardation and stereotyped movements
	Asperger syndrome
Social communication disorder	Atypical autism Pervasive developmental disorder not otherwise specified

Source: data from The ICD-10 classification of mental and behavioural disorders: clinical descriptions and diagnostic guidelines, Copyright (1992), World Health Organization; Diagnostic and Statistical Manual of Mental Disorders, Fifth Edition, Copyright (2013), American Psychiatric Association.

affectionate behaviour by smiling or cuddling. Instead, they appear to dislike being picked up or kissed. They are sometimes no more responsive to their parents than to strangers, and do not show interest in other children. There can be little difference in their behaviour towards people and inanimate objects. A characteristic sign is gaze avoidance—that is, the absence of eye-to-eye contact.

Abnormalities of communication. Speech may develop late or never appear. Occasionally, it develops normally until about the age of 2 years and then disappears in part or completely. This lack of speech is a manifestation of a severe cognitive defect. As children with ASD grow up, about 50% acquire some useful speech, although serious impairments usually remain, such as the misuse of pronouns and the inappropriate repeating of words spoken by other people (echolalia). Some children are talkative, but their speech can be repetitive monologue rather than a conversation with another person.

The cognitive defect also affects *non-verbal communication and play*, as the child might not take part in the imitative games of the first year of life, and later they do not use toys in an appropriate way. They show little imagination or creative play.

Restriction of interests and behaviour. Obsessive desire for sameness is a term often applied to children with ASD stereotyped behaviour, and to their distress if there is a change in the environment. For example, some children

insist on eating the same food repeatedly, on wearing the same clothes, or on engaging in repetitive games. Some are fascinated by spinning toys. Odd behaviour and mannerisms are common. Some children carry out odd motor behaviours such as whirling round and round, twiddling their fingers repeatedly, flapping their hands, or rocking. Others do not differ obviously in motor behaviour from normal children.

Other features. Children with ASD may suddenly show anger or fear without apparent reason. They may be overactive and distractible, sleep badly, or soil or wet themselves. Some injure themselves deliberately. About

Box 16.3 Clinical clues for autistic spectrum disorders

In preschool children:
- delay or absence of spoken language
- not responsive to other people's feelings
- lack of pretend play or social play
- unable to share pleasure
- does not point out objects to another person
- unusual or repetitive hand and finger mannerisms
- unusual reactions to sensory stimuli

In school-age children:
- persistent echolalia
- reference to self as 'you', 'she', or 'he' beyond 3 years
- unusual vocabulary for child's age
- tendency to talk freely only about specific topics
- inability to join in play of other children (occasionally disruptive)
- easily overwhelmed by social and other stimulation
- extreme reactions to invasion of personal space
- difficulty managing change

In adolescent children:
- socially 'naïve', not as independent as peers
- speech peculiarities
- difficulty making and maintaining peer friendships
- preference for highly specific, narrow interests or hobbies, or may enjoy collecting, numbering, or listing
- strong preferences for familiar routines
- problems using imagination

Reproduced from Progress in Neurology and Psychiatry, 19(6), Ellison-Wright Z and Boardman C, Diagnosis and management of ASD in children and adolescents, pp. 28-32, Copyright (2015), with permission from John Wiley & Sons.

25% of autistic children develop *seizures*, usually about the time of adolescence.

Intelligence level. Cognitive difficulties are very common, and some form of intellectual disability is identified in 25–50% of individuals with ASD, with the most common pattern being poor language and social comprehension but with relative strengths—'splinter skills'—in visuospatial abilities. Among high functioning individuals (those likely to fall under the ICD-10 Asperger's syndrome), the opposite pattern may occur, or there may be pragmatic difficulties with the social use of communication. Some children show areas of ability despite impairment of other intellectual functions, and in some cases they have exceptional but restricted powers of memory or mathematical skill. Some children with higher functioning often develop intense circumscribed interests that can be seen in typically developing children but are pursued in a solitary, non-social manner.

Although there is a tendency for core behaviours to improve over time, some may persist and cause difficulties in the long term. Those affected can have difficulties with independent living, motor coordination, sensory sensitivities, sleep and eating problems, mental health difficulties, and behaviours that place themselves and others at risk.

Epidemiology

A prevalence rate for ASD of around 1% in high-income and lower in low- and middle-income countries has been reported in systematic reviews (Le Couteur *et al.*, 2015). It is unclear if there has been a true increase in prevalence or if the increase in rates is as a result of recent increase in public awareness of ASD, broadening of the diagnostic criteria, and more clinicians having a better understanding of the disorder. Whilst previously, classification systems had discouraged diagnoses of comorbid disorders, now ASD can be diagnosed alongside ADHD, Down syndrome or fragile X syndrome. A rapid increase in prevalence was observed when legislation determined that children with ASD could access special schools, and there is some increase in 'diagnostic substitution', with children with 'intellectual disability' now being diagnosed with ASD. The *prevalence* of ASD is much higher in boys than in girls, with a ratio as high as 5–6 to 1, but it is unclear if ASD is under recognized in higher functioning females. A large surveillance study across the US (Baio, 2012) showed that approximately 1 in 42 boys and 1 in 189 girls had ASD, with non-Hispanic white children the group with highest prevalence. Of children with ASD, 31% were classified as having IQ scores in the range of intellectual disability (IQ ≤70), 23% in the borderline range (IQ = 71–85), and

46% in the average or above average range of intellectual ability (IQ >85). The proportion of children classified in the range of intellectual disability differed by race/ethnicity, with, for example, significantly greater prevalence among non-Hispanic white children than non-Hispanic black children.

Risk factors and possible aetiology

ASD has a strong genetic basis. The heritability of ASD in the population is around 90%. The rate of ASD is about 25 times higher in siblings of affected children than in the general population. The genetic architecture of ASD is complex. Like most psychiatric syndromes, the genetic predisposition in many cases results from the combination of multiple common polymorphisms of small effect. There are also copy number variants (CNVs) that are rare but confer a larger risk, and some cases that are caused by specific gene mutations or chromosomal abnormalities (Box 16.4). These cases can be identified by genetic testing (Ellison-Wright and Boardman, 2015). Evidence is steadily accumulating that the highly heterogenous and functionally diverse set of ASD genes identified so far converges on a smaller set of specific molecular pathways or brain circuits—possibly contributing to aberrant synaptic *pruning*. For a review of the genetics of ASD, see de la Torre-Ubieta *et al.* (2016).

Neuroimaging studies have also provided useful insights into the neural substrates underlying ASD and the pathological changes that occur in the brain. They indicate that the brain matures along an atypical trajectory. This leads to differences in neuroanatomy, functioning, and connectivity within the wider neural systems that probably mediate autistic symptoms and traits (Ecker *et al.*, 2015).

Various risk factors have been identified; for example, a sibling with autism (reflecting a genetic predisposition), birth defects, including cerebral palsy, gestational age less than 35 weeks, and maternal use of valproate in pregnancy. As noted earlier, ASD can also occur in a range of genetic disorders such as fragile X, muscular dystrophy, neurofibromatosis, and tuberous sclerosis; since autistic features are not invariable in these conditions, they may also be viewed as being as risk factors for ASD rather than specific genetic causes of it.

Other potential risk factors include obstetric complications—although it is not clear whether these are a true risk factor or represent an outcome associated with a primary abnormality in the fetus. Other environmental causes being explored include immune dysfunction, with studies showing a variety of peripheral and central immune changes, including T cell dysfunction and microglial and astroglial activation. Altered gene expression is also implicated, with differences in two modules of coexpressed genes being observed in the brain in autism. The first module, related to synaptic function and neuronal projection, was underexpressed, whereas the second module, which was enriched for immune genes and glial markers, was overexpressed. These data support the view that synaptic dysfunction as well as immune dysregulation are important in the pathogenesis of ASD.

Socioeconomic status might influence ASD, as risk is increased for children with mothers born abroad, with the risk for low-functioning autism peaking when migration occurred around the time of pregnancy. Different mechanisms can be proposed to explain these results, such as the high level of maternal stress or low immunity regarding common infections. Four reviews have suggested that both maternal and paternal age are risk factors for autism, with paternal age perhaps playing a more significant role—this might be because of a high frequency of point mutations, gene imprinting effects, genetic changes in sperm cells, *de novo* CNVs, or epigenetic influences that may increase risk of autism in the offspring (Le Couteur *et al.*, 2015).

Exposure to drugs and toxins may increase autism risk. Prenatal exposure to valproate is a recognized risk factor for ASD, especially in the first trimester of pregnancy; children exposed in utero to valproate have an eightfold increased risk for ASD (Christensen *et al.*, 2013). Use of selective serotonin reuptake inhibitors (SSRIs) during pregnancy has also been suggested to modestly increase the risk of ASD, but data are weak. Lastly, exposure to toxins, especially pesticides, may increase ASD risk (for review, see Rossignol *et al.*, 2014).

Finally, there have been a number of other associations by the public, media, and scientific community proposed about possible causes of ASD, involving speculation about mechanisms, including immunological causes (infections or vaccinations such as MMR), and exposure to mercury in tooth fillings. There is, however, a lack of scientifically valid evidence to support any of these theories. A proposed association between increased rates of autism in children whose mothers took SSRIs in pregnancy is likely to be confounded by the more general association between depression in mothers and increased rates of autism in their children.

For a summary of risk factors for ASD, see Chaste and Leboyer (2012).

Cognitive and emotional processes

Identifying and understanding the cognitive profile of ASD is likely to play an important role in

---

> ### Box 16.4 Genetic architecture of autism spectrum disorders
>
> **In terms of inheritance pattern**
>
> *Complex*—additive risk from multiple genes
>
> *Autosomal recessive* (e.g. Smith–Lemli–Opitz syndrome)
>
> *Autosomal dominant* (e.g. Timothy syndrome; tuberous sclerosis complex)
>
> *X-linked* (e.g. fragile X syndrome; Duchenne muscular dystrophy)
>
> **In terms of mechanism**
>
> Single nucleotide polymorphisms
>
> Copy number variation (CNV; e.g. 16p11.2 duplication; *NRXN1* deletion)
>
> Chromosomal translocation (e.g. Phelan–McDermid syndrome)
>
> Trinucleotide repeat expansion (e.g. fragile X syndrome)
>
> Adapted from Nature, 22(4), de la Torre-Ubieta L *et al.*, Advancing the understanding of autism disease mechanisms through genetics, pp. 345-361, Copyright (2016), with permission from Nature Publishing Group.

---

understanding the underlying brain systems and structures involved in this very heterogenous disorder. The more prominent theoretical models include: theory of mind (ToM) executive dysfunction and weak central coherence (WCC).

Theory of mind. This theory attempts to identify a basic psychological disorder in ASD. By the age of 4 years, normal children are able to form an idea of what others are thinking. As an example, consider a normal child who watches while another normal child is first shown the location of a hidden object and is then sent out of the room while the object is moved to a new hiding place. The child who has remained in the room will conclude that the child who left temporarily will expect the object to be in the original position when he returns to the room. A child with ASD tends to lack this appreciation of what another child is likely to be thinking. In the example, a child with ASD is likely to say that the child who left the room will think that the object has been moved to its new place. It is not certain how specific to ASD is this difficulty in appreciating what others know and expect, nor how central it is to the psychopathology. In any case, its cause is not known.

Impairment of frontal lobe executive functions involved in planning and organization, resulting in perseveration and poor self-regulation, and impaired ability to extract high-level meaning from diverse sources of information, has been hypothesized to contribute to the ASD profile, but this might be more related to atypical cognitions in ASD rather than executive function deficits. The *weak central coherence (WCC) theory* tries to explain how, in autism, a 'local processing bias' explains the enhanced performance of children with autism on some neurocognitive tasks and could explain the 'islets of ability' that are commonly observed in individuals with ASD. For a review of cognitive phenotypes in autism, see Charman *et al.* (2010) and Le Couteur *et al.* (2015).

Differential diagnosis

ASD represents a broad phenotype with differing levels of impairment, but the presentation must be distinguished from the following:

- Neurodevelopmental disorders (e.g. language disorders).
- *Communication disorder*, which differs from ASD in that the child usually responds normally to people and has good non-verbal communication.
- *Intellectual disability*, in which responses to other people are more 'normal' than those of a child with ASD. A child with ASD has more impairment of language relative to other skills than is found in an intellectually disabled child of the same age.
- Mental and behavioural disorders (similar to those comorbid with ADHD; see below).
- Conditions in which there is developmental regression (Rett syndrome).
- *Deafness*, which can be excluded by appropriate tests of hearing.

Furthermore, it is important to be aware that certain disorders are more likely to occur with ASD, such as ADHD, depression, anxiety, and conduct disorder/challenging behaviours.

For a review of differential diagnosis and comorbidity in ASD, see Matson and Williams (2013).

Prognosis

Longitudinal studies have found ASD to be a stable diagnosis. However, at follow-up, usually a couple of years later, a systematic review has demonstrated the diagnostic stability of ASD diagnosis ranging from 53% to 100% of children studied (Woolfenden *et al.*, 2012). There is wide variation in outcome, with between <5% and 25%

having a very good outcome from childhood to adult. For example, around 10–20% of children with childhood autism begin to improve between the ages of about 4 and 6 years, and are eventually able to attend an ordinary school and obtain work. A further 10–20% can live at home, but cannot work and need to attend a special school or training centre, and remain very dependent on their families and/or support services. The remainder, at least 60%, improve little and are unable to lead an independent life; many need long-term residential care. Those who improve may continue to show language problems, emotional coldness, and odd behaviour. As noted already, a substantial minority develop epilepsy in adolescence.

Overall, for many individuals there is gradual reduction in autistic symptoms and improvement in adaptive ability over time but there is marked variability in individual outcomes. The major predictors of better outcomes are higher IQ and presence of useful speech at age 5 years. Periods of transition can be particularly difficult, such as becoming an adolescent and then becoming an adult, where at times functioning can be seen to deteriorate. This may coincide with development of comorbid anxiety and mood disorders.

Assessment

Assessment should be concerned with more than the diagnosis of autism. Therefore an ASD-specific developmental history, ASD observational assessments, and standardized individual assessments should be undertaken. The following additional factors need to be considered:

- cognitive level
- language ability
- communication skills, social skills, and play
- repetitive or otherwise abnormal behaviour
- stage of social development in relation to age, mental age, and stage of language development
- associated medical conditions (e.g. comorbid epilepsy)
- psychosocial factors, including the needs of the family.

Individual ASD assessments (through direct interaction and observation) often use an ASD-specific tool such as the Autism Diagnostic Observation Schedule (ADOS), the Diagnostic Interview for Social and Communication Disorders (DISCO), the Development, Dimensional and Diagnostic Interview (3di), or the Child Autism Rating Scale (CARS). For a review of the diagnosis and assessment of autism, see Le Couteur *et al.* (2015).

Management

The key aspect of management for a child with ASD is to have an individualized approach informed by the specific strengths and difficulties of the child, which also manages the changing developmental needs and goals of the child. The management will often need to consider a number of key areas, which include reducing the core symptoms and behaviours of ASD, enabling individuals to achieve their potential, treating comorbid or co-occurring problems, including difficulties encountered by caregivers, and supporting the family through education and specific evidence-based approaches. These are summarized below, but see Le Couteur *et al.* (2015) for a more detailed description.

Management of abnormal behaviour: psychosocial and behavioural interventions: early intensive behavioural intervention (EIBI) is the most studied preschool intervention and along, with a number of other, predominantly behaviourally informed interventions, has been shown to improve short-term outcomes for preschool children (Tonge *et al.*, 2014). These interventions include strategies for parents, teachers, and carers to improve joint attention skills and reciprocal communication, often through interactive play and action routines. There are fewer studies on older children, and the quality of evidence is poorer, but social skills training and peer-mediated social communication interventions show some promise. Overall, the social communication programmes may help address social isolation (Kendall *et al.*, 2013), but there is little evidence, to date, for interventions to treat the core features of restricted, repetitive behaviours or sensory sensitivities.

Other interventions: it is important to note that many different therapeutic interventions have been tried, but, as with those addressing the core features above, there is insufficient evidence to support their use at present. These include sensory integration therapy, auditory integration therapy, visual therapies, music therapies, and restricted diets or dietary supplementation. For example, the gluten-free casein-free diet (GFCFD) is the most frequently implemented restrictive dietary intervention, but there remains a lack of evidence for its use. There is, however, some evidence that vocational programmes can increase employment success for some individuals with ASD. There are no drugs licensed to treat the core ASD syndrome. Potential treatments based on the underlying genetic and neural mechanisms are under active investigation (Sahin and Sur, 2015).

Identification and treatment of co-occurring mental health problems: as described above, children with ASD have higher rates of other mental health problems, including ADHD, oppositional defiant disorder, obsessive–compulsive disorder (OCD), anxiety disorders, and mood disorders. Most clinical guidelines recommend implementing evidence-based interventions for these disorders, with necessary modifications to meet the needs of the person with ASD. For example, cognitive behaviour therapy for children with anxiety disorders can help if they have good verbal and cognitive capacity, as can family and school-based interventions for those with ADHD. The response rate for stimulant medication for ADHD is, however, lower for a child with ASD when compared to a child without ASD. Similarly, there is little good evidence to support the use of SSRIs for OCD, mood, and anxiety disorders, although these might be commonly used in practice. There is some evidence to support the use of antipsychotic medication to ameliorate associated symptoms of aggression and irritability, but these should be used with caution, starting at low doses and used for short periods only. As with most management of psychological problems, focusing on the factors that can increase risk of developing problems is likely to be important. For children with ASD these will include understanding sensory sensitivities, changing circumstances, physical or mental illness, exploitations, and bullying at school.

Educational issues: depending on the level of cognitive and verbal skills of the child, there has been a move across the globe to try and include children with ASD within mainstream schools, although some children with ASD will require special educational environments and, if the difficulties are so severe that the child cannot stay in the family, residential schooling is necessary. In some cases, the educational and residential needs of children with ASD can be provided through the services for the intellectually disabled. Older adolescents may need vocational training. There is no evidence for the effectiveness of different educational environments but, for those children with better functioning, education will need to ensure that both culturally valued skills are learned as well as specific skills and social understanding.

Family support: the family of a child with ASD may experience increased parental and family stress, psychological difficulties, and poorer quality of life. There are, however, few evidence-based interventions that have been shown to help, and the general principles of interventions should be the management of behaviours that challenge (National Institute for Health and Care Excellence, 2013c). The family might need prompt assessment of their child's needs and easy access to appropriate educational and other provisions. Although doctors may be able to do little specifically to help the child, they must not withdraw from the family, who need continuing support as well as support for their efforts to help the child and to obtain help from educational and social services. Some parents request genetic counselling, and it seems that the risk of a further child with ASD is about 3%. Many parents find it helpful to join a voluntary organization in which they can meet other parents of children with ASD and discuss common problems.

Rett syndrome

Rett's disorder (or Rett's syndrome) is a rare X-linked condition that occurs almost exclusively in girls. The reported prevalence is about 1 per 10,000 girls. After a period of normal development in the first months of life, head growth slows and over the next 2 years there is arrest of cognitive development and loss of purposive skilled hand movements. Stereotyped movements develop, with hand-clapping and hand-wringing movements. Ataxia of the legs and trunk may develop. Interest in the social environment diminishes in the first few years of the disorder, but may increase again later. Expressive and receptive language development is severely impaired and there is psychomotor retardation. Some patients develop severe intellectual disability.

The disorder is caused by sporadic mutations in the *MeCP2* gene, located on the X chromosome. These mutations interfere with the normal roles of *MeCP2* in epigenetic regulation of brain development. For a review, see Lyst and Bird (2015).

Childhood disintegrative disorder

Childhood disintegrative disorder (ICD-10; also known as *Heller's disease*) is a rare condition that begins after a period of normal development usually lasting for more than 2 years. It is unclear how far this is distinct from childhood autism and hence it is included in the DSM-5 under ASD. There is a marked loss of cognitive functions, abnormalities of social behaviour and communication, and unfavourable outcome. The child loses motor skills and bowel or bladder control. The condition may arrest after a time, or progress to a severe neurological condition with worsening symptoms.

Asperger syndrome, atypical autism, and pervasive developmental disorder not otherwise specified

Asperger syndrome remains in the ICD-10 but not in DSM-5. It denotes a group of children with ASD who have no cognitive or language retardation although speech may be stilted. They are therefore often able to attend mainstream schools as their functioning within education can be good, although social and communication difficulties can persist as per other children with

ASD. The term atypical autism (in ICD-10) denotes a residual category for pervasive developmental disorders that resemble ASD but do not meet the diagnostic criteria for any of the syndromes within this group. The prevalence of these cases varies according to the criteria adopted, but most investigations show that they are more common than the ICD-10 diagnosis of autism itself (Fombonne, 2009). The relationship between these cases and those that meet the criteria for the other syndromes within the group of pervasive developmental disorders is poorly understood.

For review of Asperger syndrome, see Barahona-Corrêa and Filipe (2016),

Attention-deficit hyperactivity disorder

ADHD is the second most common psychiatric disorder of childhood. Although about one-third of children are described by their parents as overactive, and 5–20% of school children are so described by teachers, these reports encompass a continuum of behaviour ranging from normal high spirits to a severe and persistent disorder. This overactivity often varies in different situations. The norms of childhood behaviour therefore encompass a spectrum of behaviour that is often culturally determined and therefore it is important to ensure that ADHD denotes the functionally impairing, persistent end of the spectrum. ADHD is the term that is most commonly used and comes from the DSM-5 criteria, where symptoms need to be present from the main categories of inattention and hyperactivity and impulsivity. The term hyperkinetic disorder denotes a more severe form of the disorder and is used in ICD-10 (as below). For a summary of ADHD, see Verkuijl *et al.* (2015).

Clinical features

The core features of ADHD are inattention, hyperactivity, and impulsivity. These features are pervasive, occurring across situations, although they can vary somewhat in different circumstances, so that parents and teachers may give rather different accounts of the child's behaviour.

Children with the disorder are often *reckless and prone to accidents*. They may have *learning difficulties*, which result in part from *poor attention and lack of persistence with tasks*. Many develop minor forms of antisocial behaviour as the condition continues, particularly disobedience, temper tantrums, and aggression. These children are often socially disinhibited and can cause disruption both at home and in the classroom. They can be susceptible to bullying or can be easily influenced to do 'silly' things. Mood fluctuates, but low self-esteem and depressive mood are common.

Restlessness, overactivity, and related symptoms often start before school age. Sometimes the child was overactive as a baby, but more often significant problems begin when the child starts to walk; they are constantly on the move, interfering with objects and exhausting their parents.

Diagnostic criteria

In both ICD-10 (hyperkinetic disorder) and DSM-5 (ADHD) the cardinal features for the diagnosis of the disorder are impaired attention, hyperactivity, and impulsiveness starting in childhood and lasting for at least 6 months to a degree that is maladaptive and inconsistent with the developmental level of the child. However, the two systems differ in the details of the criteria for diagnosis and there is a greater emphasis on symptoms rather than impairment in the DSM-5 categorization. DSM-5 also has more information on diagnoses in older children and, for example, if over 16 years, then fewer symptoms are required for a diagnosis.

- ICD-10 requires that the symptoms started before 6 years of age, whereas DSM-5 specifies that they started before 12 years of age.
- ICD-10 requires both hyperactivity and impaired attention, whereas DSM-5 requires either inattention, or hyperactivity and impulsiveness.

The result of these differences is that children who meet the ICD-10 criteria are more severely impaired than those who meet the DSM-5 criteria.

In ICD-10 the disorder can be further classified as a disturbance of activity and attention, or as hyperkinetic conduct disorder. The latter term is used when criteria for both hyperkinetic disorder and conduct disorder are met. (The provision is made because the presence of *associated aggression, delinquency, or antisocial behaviour* is associated with a poorer outcome; see below.)

Comorbidity and associated conditions. About 50% of children with ADHD meet diagnostic criteria for other conditions as well, principally oppositional defiant disorder, conduct disorder, depressive disorder, or anxiety disorder. Specific learning difficulties and poor motor coordination are also commonly present. Estimations vary substantially for prevalence rates of ASD in children with ADHD, but have been estimated at 20–50%.

Epidemiology

Estimates of the prevalence of ADHD vary according to the criteria for diagnosis.

The 2010 Global Burden of Disease Study found that worldwide point prevalence rates of childhood ADHD were 2.2% in males and 0.7% in females (Erskine *et al.*, 2013). However, the diagnosis rates of and treatment approaches to ADHD vary worldwide,

For example, two studies, from the US and UK, explored parent-reported ADHD diagnosis 'ever' made. The US study reported a 42% increase in ADHD diagnoses from 2003 to 2011, with 8.8% having a current diagnosis of ADHD. The UK study reported a prevalence of 1.7%, with no evidence of an increase between 1999 and 2009. Overall, 6.1% of children in the US receive drugs for ADHD, in contrast with an estimated 0.7% in the UK (Verkuijl *et al.*, 2015).

Aetiology

ADHD is due to both heritable and non-heritable factors, and there is much evidence suggesting a disorder of higher cognitive executive function related to abnormalities of neurotransmission in the prefrontal cortex and associated subcortical structures.

Neurological findings. Signs suggesting neurodevelopmental impairment or delay are found in children with hyperkinetic disorder—for example, clumsiness, language delay, and abnormalities of speech. Although these signs are generally associated with birth complications, they could result from factors acting at an earlier stage of development of the brain. The disorder can also occur as a consequence of severe traumatic brain injury.

Neuroimaging studies. Recent studies have shown a reduction in volume and cortical thickness in certain areas of the brain, especially the grey matter of the basal ganglia. These changes are associated with ADHD and are possibly related to a delay in brain maturation (Rubia, 2012). Other studies have shown functional and structural abnormalities in areas involved in self-organization, including the prefrontal and striatal regions, as well as the cerebellum. There is also evidence for white matter disruption and disordered anatomical and functional connectivity between these various brain regions. For a review, see Hart *et al.* (2014).

Genetic studies. Investigations of family members, twins, adopted children, and monozygotic and dizygotic twins all suggest that genetic factors are important, with heritability estimates of about 70–80%. Compared with controls, probands with ADHD have more first-degree relatives with the same disorder. There is also a much higher concordance for monozygotic than for dizygotic pairs. Adoption studies show that the biological parents of children with ADHD are more likely to have had the same or a related disorder than are the adoptive parents. Molecular genetic studies have made limited progress in revealing the risk genes. Both common and rare variants are implicated, and genes affecting the dopamine system have been identified in some studies. Some of the genetic risk likely interacts with environmental factors, such as maternal smoking, to influence ADHD risk. For review, see Martin *et al.* (2015).

Other factors. A number of other factors have been shown to be associated with ADHD; these include early psychosocial adversity (demonstrated by studies of children raised in extreme deprivation), maternal alcohol and substance misuse during pregnancy, low birth weight, prematurity, nutritional deficiencies, and exposure to environmental toxins.

Prognosis

Inattention and impulsiveness often persist into adult life whilst overactivity usually lessens gradually as the child grows older, especially when it is mild and not present in every situation; it often ceases by puberty. About 50% of the cases diagnosed in childhood retain the full diagnosis in adolescence. The prognosis for any associated learning difficulties is less good, whilst antisocial behaviour has the worst outcome. When *the overactivity is severe*, and is accompanied by *learning failure* or *low intelligence*, the prognosis is poor and the condition may persist into adulthood, as antisocial disorder and drug misuse rather than as continued hyperactivity.

By adulthood most patients will no longer meet the full criteria for ADHD or hyperkinetic syndrome, but the majority will retain some functional impairment. Although this would suggest that the incidence of the disorder should be low in adulthood, surveys have indicated rates of about 4%, suggesting the presence of additional cases that were not detected during childhood or might commence in adulthood—a late-onset ADHD. Furthermore, the diagnostic criteria in DSM-5 has reduced the number of symptoms required for adults, potentially increasing the rate of detection of ADHD in adults. Adults with ADHD can experience more opportunities to 'live with' the disorder as they no longer need to attend school with its associated institutional demands and can potentially choose career paths more suited to their work patterns and needs. However, many describe procrastination, poor motivation, and mood lability, while irritability, inattention, and poor organization can lead to problems with both work and social relationships. Comorbid mood disorders and substance misuse are common. Studies of psychostimulants and atomoxetine show a similar clinical response to that seen in children. For a review of ADHD in young adulthood, see Agnew-Blais *et al.* (2016) and for the assessment and treatment of adults with ADHD, see Janakiraman and Benning (2010).

Treatment

Psychosocial interventions. Overactive children exhaust their parents, who often need support as they might have had feelings of being judged by other parents or teachers for not being able to control their child's behaviour for a number of years. Educational interventions to support teachers are also important, and special education provision may be needed. Psychosocial interventions are often recommended in guidelines as a first step but with more severe cases this is usually combined with stimulant medication. Although the evidence base for most psychosocial interventions is limited, parent training, social skills training, cognitive training, and specific classroom interventions have all been studied. Behavioural interventions often include parent, child, and school-based elements, and seem to be most effective in combination with medication.

Parent training for ADHD is commonly utilized, although it has a weak evidence base. It is usually group-based and focuses on making unwanted behaviours for the child explicit, clarifying family rules, and anticipating potentially difficult times in the day, such as transition times. Cognitive behavioural training for children with ADHD might have some benefit for those with comorbid anxiety or depressive disorders. Interventions to assist children with ADHD in the classroom, including advice for teachers, can provide some positive effects.

Dietary advice. A minority of children with ADHD might benefit from free fatty acid supplementation, and some parents who suspect their children's behaviour is affected by the food they eat have observed improvements following the elimination of certain foods after following a strict elimination diet. The restriction of artificial food colourants can also help a minority of children with ADHD.

Medication. Drugs can improve the three core symptoms of inattention, overactivity, and impulsivity, and should be tried if there is severe restlessness and attention deficit, and where parent training and psychological approaches have not proved effective. There are two main groups of clinically effective drugs for ADHD: stimulants and others. *Stimulant drugs* increase available central dopamine and noradrenaline, and it is thought that these actions underlie their therapeutic effects. The most commonly prescribed medication is *methylphenidate*, which can be prescribed in short- or long-acting preparations. Dexamphetamine is also used. The dosage should be related to body weight, following the manufacturers' instructions and advice about contraindications.

The potential short-term benefits of stimulant treatment are decreased restlessness, reduced aggressiveness, and, sometimes, improved attention. These effects do not usually diminish with time, but it has not been shown that they are associated with better long-term outcome. The *side effects* include irritability, depression, insomnia, and poor appetite, with resultant height and weight impacts. Tics may be made worse. As medication may be needed for many months, and some children take it for years, careful monitoring is essential. Some parents are understandably reluctant to agree to long-term drug treatment for their children. In such cases it can be helpful to give the drugs for a trial period so that the benefits and disadvantages can be assessed for a particular child. The drug may be stopped from time to time in an attempt to minimize side effects and to confirm that medication is still needed.

The noradrenaline reuptake inhibitor, *atomoxetine*, has also been licensed for the treatment of hyperkinetic syndrome and ADHD. Common adverse effects of atomoxetine include nausea, abdominal pain, loss of appetite, and sleep disturbance. Rarely (about 1 in 50,000 patients treated), severe liver damage can occur. Although atomoxetine has the theoretical advantage of lacking psychostimulant properties, experience with its use is necessarily limited compared with that for methylphenidate and studies show that, although it is effective, methylphenidate has better outcomes. It may be more suitable in patients with comorbid tic disorders, which are often worsened by stimulant treatment. It can also be used in those who have not responded to stimulant treatment, or who are poorly tolerant of it.

In clinical trials, short-term symptomatic and functional benefits of stimulants have been shown in about two-thirds of children, although the long-term benefits are uncertain. It therefore seems best to reserve drug treatment for more severe cases that have not responded to other treatment.

For recent clinical guidelines for drug treatment of ADHD, see Bolea-Alamañac *et al.* (2014). For a review of the assessment and treatment of children with ADHD, see Sonuga-Barke *et al.* (2015), and for guidance in both children and adults, see the National Institute for Health and Care Excellence (2016).

Oppositional and conduct disorders

Oppositional defiant disorder (ODD) and conduct disorders (CDs) are characterized by *antisocial behaviours* outside of socially acceptable norms and often intrude on other people's expectations or rights. They form the largest single group of psychiatric disorders in older children and adolescents. For review, see Blair *et al.* (2014).

Clinical features

The essential feature of both ODD and CD is persistent abnormal conduct that is more serious than ordinary childhood mischief. The abnormal behaviours centre around *defiance, aggression, and antisocial acts*. The upset, disruption, and costs inflicted on the family, peer group, schools, and wider society can be considerable.

In the preschool period, oppositional defiant behaviour usually manifests as defiant and aggressive behaviour in the home, often with overactivity. The behaviours include disobedience, temper tantrums, physical aggression towards siblings or adults, and destructiveness. In later childhood, CD is manifested in the home as stealing, lying, and disobedience, together with verbal or physical aggression. Later, the disturbance often becomes evident outside as well as inside the home, especially at school, as truanting, delinquency, vandalism, and reckless behaviour, or as alcohol or drug abuse. Antisocial behaviour among teenage girls includes spitefulness, emotional bullying of peers, and running away.

In children older than 7 years, persistent stealing is abnormal. Below that age, children seldom have a real appreciation of other people's property. Many children steal occasionally, so that minor or isolated instances need not be taken seriously. A small proportion of children with CD present with sexual behaviour that incurs the disapproval of adults. In younger children, masturbation and sexual curiosity may be frequent and obtrusive. Frequent unprotected sex and pregnancy may be a particular problem in adolescent girls. Fire-setting is rare, but is obviously dangerous (see page 520).

To constitute ODD and CDs, these behaviours have to be more persistent than a reaction to changing circumstances, such as adjusting to the arrival in the family of a new step-parent. There is no sharp dividing line between these disorders and ordinary bad behaviour; instead there is a continuum on which diagnostic criteria define a cut-off point. The cut-off defines the most severe cases that have the worst outcome and are most in need of help. Much of this help is social or educational, but psychiatrists have an important role in identifying comorbid disorders and arranging multidisciplinary care.

Classification

Both ICD-10 and DSM-5 include ODD/CD, which are characterized by a repetitive pattern of antisocial behaviour. In ICD-10 ODD is a subtype of CD, whilst in DSM-5 it is a separate entity. ODD is usually a diagnosis given to younger children, whilst CD is typically given to older children and teenagers. The criteria are almost identical in the two systems. ODD requires four from a list of eight symptoms to be present for at least 6 months and CD requires the presence of three symptoms from a list of 15, with a duration of at least 12 months. The criteria are closely similar in the two systems of classification.

CDs vary widely in their clinical features, and so ICD-10 has four subdivisions of CD—socialized conduct disorder, unsocialized conduct disorder, CDs confined to the family context, and ODD. Of note, DSM-5 has two other disorders that may overlap: intermittent explosive disorder (which can only be diagnosed after age 6), and a new disorder, disruptive mood dysregulation disorder (DMDD). Although DMDD has been explicitly introduced to prevent overdiagnosis and medication for bipolar disorder, it appears to have considerable overlap with ODD.

Prevalence

The overall prevalence of ODD and CD together varies between 5% and 10%, with much variability attributed to diagnostic criteria and methods utilized in studies. ODD/CD makes up about half of all child and adolescent psychopathology, and ODD is commoner in younger children whilst CD is commoner in adolescents. There is fairly good agreement on rates of 5–8% in general longitudinal surveys where multiple informants have been used (Scott *et al.*, 2015b). ODD is about twice as common in boys than in girls but this ratio rises for CD, with rates that are 3–7 times more common in boys than in girls. There is also a strong socioeconomic contributor to prevalence, with those having the lowest socioeconomic status experiencing five times greater prevalence than those in the highest groups. Rates are also highest in children that have been maltreated, brought up in residential care, transferred to foster care, and in those with intellectual disability. Furthermore, prevalence has shown to have increased considerably over the second half of the twentieth century.

Aetiology

Many different factors influence the development of ODD/CD and, although some risks are intercorrelated, being subject to more risk factors has a cumulative effect, worsening outcomes. The importance of the parenting/family environment and the complex interplay this might have with individual temperaments and differential responses to environments and interventions is an area of interesting current research. The aetiological factors can be divided into individual-level influences and family-level influences, although, as indicated above, the relationship between the two can be close.

Individual-level influences

Genetic factors. It has become clear that, for some subtypes, there is a strong genetic contribution to CD/ODD. CD clusters in families. There is a highly heritable trait of liability to externalizing disorders in general (CD, ODD, and ADHD), but shared environmental factors are also important in the aetiology of CD. For example, genetic contribution is higher for antisocial behaviour in the presence of inattention and hyperactivity, callous unemotional traits, or high levels of physical aggression, but where these factors are absent, the genetic contribution is low. There is evidence that a variant of the *monoamine oxidase-A (MAOA) gene* predisposes to CD, but only when combined with adverse factors in the child's environment such as child maltreatment. If genetic factors are involved, it is not known whether they exert their effect by influencing temperament or in some other way. For review, see Kendler *et al.* (2013).

Pregnancy and perinatal complications: maternal alcoholism during pregnancy has been associated with CD, but this might be mainly because of the effect on the developing child's IQ.

Temperament: several studies have shown associations between early temperament and later conduct problems, with traits such as negative emotionality, poor emotional regulation, inattention, and restlessness usually identified. It seems likely that a 'difficult' temperament becomes more likely to lead to disruptive behaviour problems when it interacts with a harsh and inconsistent parenting style (Bornovalova *et al.*, 2014).

Brain functioning: there is some evidence of abnormalities in the paralimbic system involved in motivation and affect, with limbic structures and the amygdala as well as the lateral orbital and ventromedial prefrontal cortices affected. Furthermore, children with conduct problems have been consistently shown to have poor executive functions—compromising their ability to achieve goals successfully through appropriate, effective actions. Children with brain damage and epilepsy are more prone to CD, as they are to other psychiatric disorders.

Language, IQ, and educational attainment: low IQ and low school achievement are important predictors of ODD/CD and delinquency. In a study of twins aged 13 years, low IQ of the child predicted conduct problems independent of social class and the IQ of the parents (Goodman, 1995). Children who struggle to assert themselves verbally may attempt to gain control of social exchanges using aggression. Low IQ can contribute to academic difficulties, which can impact on self-esteem and there is a higher likelihood of school being perceived as an unrewarding environment. This low school attainment then adds to the probability of ODD/CD developing.

Family-level influences

These are important, as quality of parenting, along with gender, is the strongest predictor of antisocial behaviour in most studies CDs are commonly found in children from *unstable, insecure, and rejecting families living in deprived areas*. Antisocial behaviour is frequent among children from broken homes, those from homes in which family relationships are poor, and those who have been in residential care in their early childhood. CDs are also related to adverse factors in the wider social environment of the neighbourhood and school (Scott *et al.*, 2015b).

Child-rearing practices and attachment: there is ample evidence that ODD/CD is associated with less than optimal parenting practices, characterized by harsh, inconsistent discipline, low warmth and involvement, and high criticism (Scott *et al.*, 2015b). The reasons and processes by which these behaviours develop have been postulated and include the negative reinforcement trap—where a parent responds to mildly oppositional behaviour with a prohibition that might then cause the child's behaviour to escalate until the parent backs off, teaching the child that if he becomes more aggressive then he is more likely to get his way. Of note, insecure attachment, particularly of the disorganized type, is strongly associated with antisocial behaviour. Children with ODD/CD come in disproportionate numbers from poor families, and this might be because poor circumstances can affect parenting quality, which in turn affects child behaviour.

Child maltreatment and exposure to interparental conflict and violence: associations between physical abuse and conduct problems are well established and, although some child conduct presentations might increase the likelihood of experiencing corporal punishment (smacking, spanking), when it comes to injurious physical maltreatment of children, the effects this has on their later likelihood of CD are strong. In addition, children exposed to domestic violence between adults are more likely themselves to become aggressive.

Other influences beyond the family: there are important peer influences—with studies showing how children with ODD/CD have more negative interchanges with other children. They are more likely to be rejected by peers, making it more likely that they associate with deviant peers. Peer influences to antisocial behaviour are most evident in adolescence. There are also important school effects, as children with ODD/CD are more likely to attend schools with high delinquency rates, at

which there are high levels of distrust between teachers and students, low pupil commitment to school, and unclear rules. Not only, as mentioned above, do children with ODD/CD come disproportionately from poor families but they also come from neighbourhoods that are more likely to be inner-city areas with high disorganization and high residential mobility.

For a review of the aetiology of conduct disorder, see Scott *et al.* (2015b).

Prognosis

The long-term outcome of CD varies considerably with the nature and extent of the disorder. In an important study, Robins (1966) found that almost 50% of people who had attended a child guidance clinic for CD in adolescence showed some form of antisocial behaviour in adulthood. Subsequent studies have shown that this is most likely to be violent offending, heavy drug usage, teenage pregnancy, leaving school without qualifications, and receiving state benefits. No cases of sociopathic disorder were found in adulthood among those with diagnoses other than CD in adolescence.

Follow-up of conduct-disordered children cared for in children's homes and of controls led to similar conclusions. About 40% of the conduct-disordered children had antisocial personality disorder in their twenties, and many of the rest had persistent and widespread social difficulties below the threshold for diagnosis of a personality disorder. Where CDs first *present* in adolescence, the prognosis is better, with about 80% no longer demonstrating significant antisocial behaviour in adulthood (Scott *et al.* (2015b) (see Box 16.5). As individuals get older their offending does reduce considerably, especially by the time they are in their forties, but their overall 'life failure' rates—as determined by multiple indices, remains high. Their general health outcomes are also worse.

Management

Mild CDs often subside without treatment other than common-sense advice to the parents. For more severe disorders, treatment for the child is often combined with treatment and social support for the family. Any coexisting disorders (e.g. ADHD, depression) should be treated. There is no convincing evidence that any treatment affects the overall long-term prognosis. Nevertheless, some short-term benefits can often be achieved, and in some cases adverse family factors can be modified in a way that could improve prognosis. Some families are difficult to help by any means, especially where there is material deprivation, with chaotic relationships, and poorly educated parents.

Parent training programmes. These programmes are the mainstay of treatment of ODD/CD and use behavioural principles (see page 434). Parents are taught how the child's antisocial behaviour may be reinforced unintentionally by their attention to it, and how it may be provoked by interactions with members of the family. Parents are also taught how to reinforce normal behaviour by praise or rewards, and how to set limits on abnormal behaviour—for example, by removing the child's privileges, such as an hour less time to play a game. Parents in some programmes are also trained how to read with their children, thus tackling other influences for the child's behaviour. As aids to learning, parents are provided with written information and video recordings showing other parents applying behavioural procedures. For a review of parent training programmes, see Scott *et al.* (2015a).

Anger management. Young people who are habitually aggressive have been shown to misperceive hostile intentions in other people who are not in fact hostile. They also tend to underestimate the level of their own aggressive behaviour, and choose inappropriate behaviours rather than more appropriate verbal responses. *Anger management programmes* seek to correct these ideas by teaching how to inhibit sudden inappropriate responses to angry feelings—for example, children say to themselves 'Stop! What should I do?' They also learn how to *reappraise the intentions* of other people and use socially acceptable forms of self-assertion.

Other methods. Remedial teaching should be arranged if there are associated reading difficulties. Medication is of value if there is a comorbid disorder such as ADHD. There is increasing use of atypical antipsychotics to target reactive aggression; however, the evidence that this is effective is modest and might best be considered when there is poor emotional regulation characterized by prolonged rages. If used, they should only be considered as a short-term intervention.

Interventions in school. There is growing interest in how schools can try and develop interventions to help address the effects of ODD/CD in their classrooms. A number of interventions have been developed that are mainly preventive programmes, including promoting social and emotional learning. They are often delivered by teachers to all children and include proactive strategies focusing on positive behaviours, with effective instructions given to children alongside effective behavioural management. As yet, the evidence base for these interventions, as well as the use of teaching assistants, in classrooms is poor.

> ### Box 16.5 Factors that predict poor outcome in children with conduct disorder
>
> **In the young person**
> - Early onset (before age 8 years)
> - Severe, frequent, and varied antisocial behaviours
> - Hyperactivity and attention problems
> - Low IQ
> - Pervasiveness (at home, in school, and elsewhere)
>
> **In the family**
> - Parental criminality and alcoholism
> - High hostility/discord focused on the child
> - Harsh inconsistent parenting
> - Low income
>
> **In the wider environment**
> - Economically deprived area
> - Ineffective schools
>
> Reproduced from Scott S, Oppositional and conduct disorders, In: Thapar A. *et al.*, Rutter's Child and Adolescent Psychiatry, 6th edn., pp. 913-931, Copyright (2015), with permission from John Wiley & Sons.

Forensic child psychiatry and juvenile delinquency

Forensic psychiatry is predominantly associated with children's interactions with the juvenile justice system, and can include the assessment and management of mentally disordered offenders or those at risk of offending, and issues such as mental competency, fitness to testify, victimization, and child custody disputes. This section will focus on the young offender, with the term juvenile delinquent often used to denote a young person who has broken the law and has been found guilty of an offence that would be categorized as a crime if committed by an adult. In most countries, the term applies only to a young person who has attained the age of criminal responsibility (at present 10 years in the UK, but this varies widely in other countries). Thus delinquency is not a psychiatric diagnosis but a legal category. The term 'children in conflict with the law' is gaining increasing popularity. However, juvenile delinquency may be associated with psychiatric disorder, especially conduct disorder. For this reason, it is appropriate to interrupt this review of the syndromes of child psychiatry to consider juvenile delinquency.

The majority of adolescent boys, when asked to report their own behaviour, admit to offences against the law, and about 20% are convicted at some time. Most offences are against property. In England in 2009, young people aged between 10 and 17 years committed about 200,000 detected offences of sufficient gravity to result in a court disposal. The largest category (about 42,000 offences) was for theft and handling stolen goods, although violence against the person was a close second (about 38,000 offences). Many fewer girls than boys are delinquent, although the ratio has fallen from 11:1 to 4:1 over the past decades (Youth Justice Board, 2011). About 75% of those with three or more convictions as juveniles go on to offend as adults (Farrington, 2002).

Delinquency is sometimes equated with conduct disorder. This is wrong, for, although the two categories overlap, they are not the same. Many delinquents do not have conduct disorder (or any other psychological disorder). Equally, many of those with conduct disorder do not offend. Nevertheless, in an important group, persistent law-breaking is preceded and accompanied by abnormalities of conduct, such as *truancy, aggressiveness, and attention-seeking*, and by *poor concentration*.

Causes

The causes of juvenile delinquency are complex and overlap with the causes of conduct disorder. The causes are reviewed briefly here, with many of the findings coming from the Cambridge Study in delinquent development which has followed up 411 males from age 8 to 50 years; for a more detailed account, see Young *et al.* (2015).

Social factors. Delinquency is related to low social class, poverty, poor housing, bullying, and poor education. There are marked differences in delinquency rates between adjacent neighbourhoods that differ in these respects. Rates also differ between schools. Many social theories have been put forward to explain the origins of crime, but none offers a completely adequate explanation.

Family factors. Many studies have found that crime and interpersonal violence runs in families (Frisell *et al.*, 2011). For example, about 50% of boys with criminal fathers are convicted, compared with 20% of those with fathers who are not criminals. The reasons for this are poorly understood, but they may include poor parenting and shared attitudes to the law (Farrington and Welsh, 2008).

Although delinquency is particularly common among those who come from broken homes, this seems to be largely because separation often reflects family discord in early and middle childhood. Other family factors that are correlated with delinquency are large family size and child-rearing practices, including erratic discipline and harsh or neglecting care.

Factors in the child. Genetic factors appear to be less significant among the causes of delinquency than in the more serious criminal behaviour of adulthood (see page 515). (The role of genetic factors in conduct disorder is considered above.) There are important associations between delinquency and a range of neurodevelopmental disorders (Hughes, 2012), with prevalence rates in those with delinquent behaviours of 23–32% of intellectual disability, 43–57% of specific learning disability, 15% of ASD, and ADHD in 11–30% (Hughes 2012; Young *et al.*, 2015).

Assessment

When the child is seen as part of an ordinary psychiatric referral and the delinquency is accompanied by a psychiatric syndrome, the latter should be assessed in the usual way. It is important to be aware that there is a high prevalence of mental disorder among juvenile offenders and it is important to screen for anxiety, depression, and suicidal risk in particular. A thorough assessment is often needed, as a juvenile offender can present with a broad range of needs and risks, requiring information from collateral sources, clear notes, clear risk assessments, and management plans. Sometimes the child psychiatrist is asked to see a delinquent specifically to prepare a court report. In these circumstances, as well as making enquiries among the parents and teachers, it is essential to consult any social worker or probation officer who has been involved with the child.

Psychological testing of intelligence and educational achievements can be useful. Other factors to be taken into account are listed in Box 16.6. The form of the report is similar to that described earlier in this chapter and in Chapter 18: Forensic psychiatry. It should include a summary of the history and present mental state together with recommendations about treatment.

Risk of violence among adolescents

The term violence encompasses a wide range of acts, from slapping to homicide with or without weapons (Young *et al.*, 2015). It is useful to distinguish between planned and reactive aggression. Planned aggression (also called instrumental or proactive) is classically associated with low anxiety and psychopathic traits, whilst reactive aggression is associated with angry outbursts, mood dysregulation, and disorders such as ADHD. There are now a number of tools that can assist in assessing adolescent violence, including the Structured Assessment of Violence Risk in Youth (SAVRY; Borum *et al.*, 2005) and, for sexually harmful behaviour, the Juvenile Sex Offender Assessment Protocol II (J-SOAP-II; Prentky and Righthand, 2003).

Interventions for juvenile offenders

In this section we consider interventions that are intended to reduce the chances of further offending, often falling under the risk-need-responsivity (RNR) model, which focuses on the prediction of risk and classification of offenders for treatment. For juvenile offenders with psychiatric disorders, including conduct disorders, mood disorders, ADHD, substance misuse and dependence, and intellectual disability, the treatment of these disorders should be a core aspect of care; treatment follows the principles described elsewhere in this chapter. The range of interventions developed for juvenile offending can be conceptualized within a public health framework and is listed in Box 16.7 and described in more detail in Young *et al.* (2015).

Psychiatrists who treat juvenile offenders need to understand the legal system in the country in which they work. The legal responses usually include a warning not to offend again, a fine, the requirement that the parent or guardian take proper control, supervision by a social worker, a period at a special centre, or an order committing the child to the care of the local authority. Since delinquent behaviour is common, mainly not serious, and is often a temporary phase, it is generally appropriate to treat first offences with minimal intervention coupled with firm disapproval. The same applies to minor offences that are repeated. A more vigorous response is required for more serious, recurrent delinquency. For this purpose a *community-based programme* is usually preferred, with the main emphasis on improving the family environment, reducing harmful peer group influences, helping the offender to develop better skills for solving problems, and improving educational and vocational accomplishments. In the UK, such a programme has been introduced by the setting up of Youth Offending Teams. When this approach fails, custodial care may be considered.

The main aim of the law as it applies to children and adolescents is treatment rather than punishment. There has been extensive criminological research to determine the effectiveness of the measures used. The general conclusions are not encouraging, although not surprising since, as explained above, delinquency is strongly related

---

> ### Box 16.6 **Assessment of young offenders**
>
> #### The offence
> - Nature and seriousness
> - Characteristics of victim
> - Motive
> - Role in the group, if others are involved
> - Attitude to the offence and the victim
>
> #### Other problem behaviours
> - Other offences (number, nature, and whether detected/convicted)
> - Violence
> - Self-harm
> - Cruelty to children or animals
> - Fire-setting
>
> Adapted from Goodman R and Scott S, Child and Adolescent Psychiatry, 3rd edn., Copyright (2012), with permission from John Wiley & Sons.

---

to factors external to the child, including family disorganization, antisocial behaviour among the parents, and poor living conditions. The risks of reconviction are greater among children who have had any court appearance or period of detention than among children who have committed similar offences without any official action having been taken (Farrington and Welsh, 2008).

Of the many approaches to the treatment of juvenile offending, a few are described below, but the evidence base remains poor for most of the interventions.

- *Structured programmes following cognitive behavioural models as well as problem-solving skills training.* These can focus on teaching social skills, anger management, and problem-solving. An additional component, attributional retraining, helps to correct cognitive distortions whereby delinquent youths readily perceive threat and hostility even in neutral interpersonal situations.

- *Multisystemic therapy.* This consists of an intensive set of integrated interventions across multiple systems in the young person's life, following nine treatment principles, including family therapy, helping the young person to find non-delinquent friends, personal development (including assertiveness training), improving family problem-solving skills, liaison with teachers, and coordination of other involved agencies.

- *Multidimensional treatment foster care*. The young person lives in a foster home, away from delinquent friends, for about 6 months and learns better life skills. There are high levels of clinical support, daily contact, and points systems for rewards alongside clear consequences for negative behaviour. At the same time, the family are taught the skills needed to respond to the young person more effectively.

Studies of these and other approaches indicate the need to match the type of treatment to the needs of the particular offender. Some seem to respond better to authoritative supervision, others to more permissive counselling. However, it is not yet possible to provide any satisfactory guidelines for matching treatment and offender. See Young *et al.* (2015) for a review of forensic aspects of child and adolescent psychiatry.

Box 16.7 Interventions for youth offending

Primary prevention

Parenting programmes
Preschool programmes
Daycare programmes
School programmes
Cognitive skills training
Peer programmes
Community programmes
Situational crime prevention

Secondary prevention

Family-focused therapies
Mentoring
Therapeutic foster care
Safeguarding of children
Treatment of parental substance misuse

Tertiary prevention

Cooperation between police, social services, and mental health
Intensive supervision and surveillance
Assertive treatment of mental disorder
Restorative justice
Victim support

Anxiety disorders

Anxiety disorders are the most common mental disorders of childhood. Fear and anxiety play important roles in functioning and have major evolutionary significance, and therefore it is important for a clinician to distinguish between normal anxiety and anxiety disorders in childhood. This distinction is usually made when the symptoms are impairing function and/or cause marked avoidance and significant distress. In ICD-10, anxiety disorders in childhood are classified as 'Emotional disorders with onset specific to childhood' (see Table 16.6). DSM-5 classifies all childhood and adult anxiety disorders together in the 'Anxiety disorders' section, although it has placed obsessive–compulsive disorder and post-traumatic stress disorder in new sections for each. Only ICD-10 has a diagnosis of sibling rivalry disorder, whilst this is included in 'Relational disorders' in DSM-5.

Prevalence

Anxiety disorders are the most common mental disorders in childhood and are more frequent in girls than boys. They are associated with significant impairment, with phobias and separation anxiety disorders the most common in childhood and social anxiety becoming more prominent in adolescence. Surveys of the general population suggest overall prevalence rates of anxiety disorders in children of around 5–10%, with age and cultural factors possibly influencing the rates, which, in individual studies, can range from 1% to 24% (Pine *et al.*, 2015).

Anxiety at different ages

The nature and manifestations of anxiety change as the child grows older. Infants pass through a stage of fear of strangers. During the preschool years, separation anxiety and fears of animals, imaginary creatures, and the dark are common. In early adolescence these fears are replaced by anxiety about social situations and personal adequacy. Anxiety disorders in childhood resemble these normal anxieties and follow the same developmental sequence, although they are more severe and more prolonged. In later adolescence, rates of generalized anxiety disorder and panic disorder start to increase. Comorbidity is common in childhood anxiety disorders, especially with other types of anxiety disorders.

Aetiology

The main factors that have been studied in the aetiology of anxiety disorders concern the interlinked issues of the child's temperament, genetic influences, and the family social environment, including parenting behaviours. Family aggregation and genetic studies indicate raised vulnerability to anxiety in offspring of adults with the disorder (e.g. the temperamental style of behavioural inhibition, or information processing biases). Environmental factors are also important; these include adverse life events and exposure to negative information or modelling. Both mothers and fathers are likely to be key, although not unique, sources of such influences, particularly if they are anxious themselves. Some parenting behaviours associated with child anxiety, such as overprotection, may be elicited by child characteristics, especially in the context of parental anxiety, and these may serve to maintain an anxiety disorder in the child. Emerging evidence emphasizes the importance of taking the nature of child and parental anxiety into account and of considering bidirectional influences. For a review of aetiology see Murray *et al.* (2009).

Prognosis

Longitudinal surveys of anxiety disorders highlight how most affected children will be free of anxiety disorders in adulthood. Anxiety disorders in childhood do, however, predict later major depression in some samples. In studies of adults with anxiety disorders, the majority had childhood anxiety disorders, therefore they do increase risk of later disorders. Anxiety may also have greater long-term impact in females. For a summary of relevant studies, see Pine *et al.* (2015).

Management

Early detection and treatment of childhood anxiety disorders can prevent substantial impairment over the course of a child's development and accumulation of functional disability. Early treatment may also prevent later development of adult psychiatric illness and impaired development and accumulated functional disability. Family education and training can reduce reinforcement of anxiety and avoidance, but parents with their own anxiety disorders or other psychopathology may need separate treatment. Existing studies support a number of pharmacological and psychotherapeutic treatments for childhood anxiety disorders. Both cognitive behaviour therapy and SSRIs are effective treatments for separation, generalized, and social anxiety disorders in children and adolescents, although non-pharmacological interventions are usually used in the first instance. Combination treatment with SSRIs and cognitive behavioural therapy has been found to be more effective than either treatment alone (Mohatt *et al.*, 2014; James *et al.*, 2013; Reynolds *et al.*, 2012).

Table 16.6 Anxiety disorders in childhood

DSM-5	ICD–10
Anxiety disorders	**F93 Emotional disorders with specific onset in childhood**
Separation anxiety disorder	Separation anxiety disorder of childhood
Specific phobia	Phobic anxiety disorder of childhood
Social anxiety disorder (social phobia)	Social anxiety disorder of childhood
Generalized anxiety disorder	
Relational disorders Sibling relational disorder	Sibling rivalry disorder
Obsessive–compulsive and related disorders	*Other anxiety disorders* Obsessive–compulsive disorder
Trauma- and stressor-related disorders	
Post-traumatic stress disorder	Post-traumatic stress disorder

Source: data from The ICD-10 classification of mental and behavioural disorders: clinical descriptions and diagnostic guidelines, Copyright (1992), World Health Organization; Diagnostic and Statistical Manual of Mental Disorders, Fifth Edition, Copyright (2013), American Psychiatric Association.

Separation anxiety disorder

Separation anxiety disorder is a fear of separation from people to whom the child is attached that is clearly greater than the normal separation anxiety of toddlers or preschool children, or persists beyond the usual preschool period, and is associated with significant problems of social functioning. The onset is before the age of 6 years. The diagnosis is not made when there is a generalized disturbance of personality development.

Clinical picture

While separation anxiety is part of normal early-child development, children with this disorder are excessively anxious when separated from parents or other attachment figures, and are unrealistically concerned that harm may befall these persons or that they will leave the child. They may refuse to sleep away from these persons or, if they agree to separate, may have disturbed sleep with nightmares. They cling to their attachment figures by day, demanding attention. Anxiety is often manifested as physical symptoms of stomach ache, headache, nausea, and vomiting, and may be accompanied by crying, tantrums, or social withdrawal. Separation anxiety disorder is one cause of school refusal (see page 467).

Epidemiology

Community surveys suggest that rates of separation anxiety disorder are about 5% among 7- to 11-year-old boys and girls (Pine *et al.*, 2015).

Aetiology

Separation anxiety disorder is sometimes precipitated by a *frightening experience*. This may be brief (e.g. admission to hospital) or prolonged (e.g. conflict between the parents). In some cases separation anxiety disorder develops in children who react with excessive anxiety to a large number of everyday stressors and who are therefore said to have an *anxiety-prone temperament*. Sometimes the condition appears to be a response to anxious or overprotective parents.

Prognosis

The disorder often improves with time, but may worsen again when there is a change in the child's routine, such as a move of school. Some cases progress to generalized or other anxiety disorders in adult life.

Treatment

Account should be taken of the whole range of possible aetiological factors, including stressful events, previous actual separation, an anxiety-prone temperament, and the behaviour of the parents. Stressors should be reduced, if possible, and children should be helped to talk about their worries. It is more important to involve the family, helping them to understand how their own concerns or overprotection affect the child, and to find ways of making the child feel more secure. Anxiolytic drugs may be needed occasionally when anxiety is extremely severe, but they should be used for short periods only. When separation anxiety is worse in particular circumstances, the child may benefit from the behavioural techniques used for phobias, as described in the next section.

Phobic anxiety disorder

This diagnosis for children corresponds to specific phobia for adults (see page 171). Minor phobic symptoms are common in childhood. They usually concern animals, insects, the dark, school, and death. The prevalence of more severe phobias varies with age. Severe and persistent fears of animals usually begin before the age of 5 years, and nearly all have declined by the early teenage years, but a minority, probably about 10%, persist into adult life.

Most childhood phobias improve without specific treatment provided that the parents adopt a firm and reassuring approach. For phobias that do not improve, simple behavioural treatment can be combined with reassurance and support. The child is encouraged to encounter feared situations in a graded way, as in the treatment of phobias in adult life (see page 170).

Social anxiety disorder of childhood

This term is used in ICD-10 to describe disorders starting before the age of 6 years in which there is anxiety with strangers greater or more prolonged than the fear of strangers that normally occurs in the second half of the first year of life. Children with this condition tend to have an inhibited temperament in infancy. These children are markedly anxious in the presence of strangers and avoid them. The fear, which may be mainly of adults or of other children, interferes with social functioning. It is not accompanied by severe anxiety on separation from the parents.

Treatment resembles that of other anxiety disorders of childhood.

Sibling rivalry disorder

This category is listed in ICD-10 for children who show *extreme jealousy* or other signs of rivalry in relation to a sibling, starting during the months following the birth of that sibling. The signs are clearly greater than the emotional upset and rivalry common in such circumstances, and they are persistent and cause social problems. When the disorder is severe there may be hostility and even physical harm to the sibling. The child may regress in behaviour—for example, losing previously learned control of bladder or bowels—or act in a way appropriate for a younger child. There is usually opposition to the parents and behaviour intended to obtain their attention, often with temper tantrums. There may be sleep disturbance and problems at bedtime. In treatment, parents should be helped to divide their attention appropriately between the two children, to set limits for all children, and to help the child to feel valued.

Post-traumatic stress disorder

Although not included in ICD-10 among the anxiety disorders with onset usually in childhood, post-traumatic stress disorder (PTSD) can occur in children. The clinical picture resembles that of the same disorder in adult life (see page 142), with disturbed sleep, nightmares, flashbacks, and avoidance of reminders of the traumatic events. Developmental factors can play an important role in the presentation of PTSD, and so children may also present with behavioural problems, developmental regression, physical symptoms, and more generalized fears.

Aetiology

As in adults, the cause is an encounter with an exceptionally severe stressor—for example, those encountered by children experiencing natural and man-made disasters, war, physical or sexual abuse, violence to self and others, and serious or life-threatening injury or illness. As with adults, cases after vehicle and other accidents are more common than after the less frequent major disasters. Estimates of PTSD in children who have been exposed to potentially traumatic events are around 16% (Alisic *et al.*, 2014). The prevalence of PTSD appears to vary with a number of factors, such as the gender and age of the child or adolescent, type of trauma, frequency and severity of exposure, and the amount of time since the traumatic event. Children and adolescents who have undergone complex trauma defined by repeated or chronic trauma, which is often of an interpersonal nature and begins early in life, may demonstrate different responses to children and adolescents who have undergone other forms of trauma, and therefore may respond differently to different therapies for PTSD.

Prognosis

Exposure to trauma in childhood is associated with a broad range of adverse psychiatric outcomes in adulthood. Longitudinal studies have shown that 15–30% of children with PTSD can continue to suffer from the disorder in adulthood, in addition to generalized anxiety disorders, substance misuse disorders, depression, and suicidality (Yule *et al.*, 2015).

Management

Treatment resembles that for adults (see page 145). The most studied treatments include trauma-focused cognitive behaviour therapy (TF-CBT)—for which there is the greatest evidence base—as well as eye-movement desensitization and reprocessing (EMDR), narrative exposure therapy (NET), and supportive counselling (Gillies, 2013).

Obsessive–compulsive disorder

OCDs are increasingly recognized in childhood and, although previously thought to be rare, are now seen to be a common cause of distress for children and adolescents. As with the disorder in adults, OCD is characterized by the presence of obsessions (unwanted, repetitive, or intrusive thoughts) and compulsions (unnecessary repetitive behaviours or mental activities). OCD is a complex disorder, as there are clear continuities and discontinuities of the disorder with normal development. Of note, several related forms of *repetitive behaviour*

are common, particularly between the ages of 4 and 10 years. These repetitive behaviours include preoccupation with numbers and counting, the repeated handling of certain objects, and hoarding. Normal children commonly adopt rituals such as avoiding cracks in the pavement or touching lampposts. These behaviours cannot be called compulsive because the child does not struggle against them. The preoccupations and rituals of OCD are more extreme than these behaviours of healthy children, and take up an increasing amount of the child's time—for example, re-checking schoolwork many times, or frequently repeated hand washing. OCD is also associated with certain neurological disorders, such as Tourette's disorder, and there is increasing evidence that there might also be some subgroups of OCD unique to child populations (Rapoport *et al.*, 2015).

Clinical features

OCD typically develops in late childhood and early adolescence. Obsessional disorders in childhood generally resemble those in adulthood (see page 184). Most children have a combination of obsessions and rituals and commonly present with washing *rituals*, followed by repetitive actions and checking. Obsessional thoughts are most often concerned with contamination, accidents, or illness affecting the patient or another person, and concerns about orderliness and symmetry. The content of symptoms often changes as the child grows older. The obsessional symptoms may be provoked by external cues such as unclean objects. Children with obsessional symptoms usually try to conceal them, especially outside the family. Obsessional children often involve their parents by asking them to take part in the rituals or give repeated reassurance about the obsessional thoughts.

Aetiology

OCD in childhood reflects a similar combination of biological and psychological factors, with both genetic and environmental influences, as in adult-onset OCD.

Genetic factors are suggested as OCD is a highly heritable disorder, particularly when it has childhood onset. The concordance rate in monozygotic twins (about 80%) is significantly more than that of dizygotic twins (about 40%). Family studies find a 10-fold increase in rates of OCD among relatives of children with OCD, compared to a doubling of rates of OCD among relatives of those with adult-onset OCD. The genetic contribution to OCD is increased when there is a comorbid tic disorder (Rapoport *et al.*, 2015).

Neural basis. The conceptual model of OCD links the endless repetitive thoughts and actions of OCD with uncontrolled activity of parallel, discrete loops within the brain. These loops are postulated to connect the basal ganglia, prefrontal cortex, and thalamus. Another model of OCD views the disorder as a result of the over-activation of a system designed to monitor performance completion, leading to a constant feeling that the action is 'not just right' which then creates a need to correct perceived mistakes.

Autoimmune factors. The association with Sydenham's chorea, which is thought to be an autoimmune disorder following group A beta-haemolytic streptococcal infection, has led to the description of a subtype of childhood-onset OCD with similar aetiology. The condition is known as *paediatric autoimmune neuropsychiatric disorder associated with streptococcal infection (PANDAS)*. See Rapoport *et al.* (2015) for a review of aetiology.

Epidemiology

The overall prevalence of OCD in young people up to 18 years of age is around 1–3%, with males having an earlier age of onset and therefore higher prevalence rates in child as compared to adult populations. Rates are much lower in young children and rise exponentially with age (Flament and Robaey, 2009).

Associated disorders

Severe and persistent obsessional thoughts and compulsive rituals in childhood are often accompanied by other anxiety and depressive symptoms. The patterns of comorbidity among childhood-onset OCD are similar to adult-onset, with tic disorders (30%), major depression (26%), and specific developmental disabilities (17%) the most common. Simple phobias, ADHD, conduct disorder, and separation anxiety disorders also occur.

Prognosis

OCD in childhood has a *generally poor prognosis*, persisting in almost half of cases, and 50% of adults with OCD report that their symptoms started in childhood. The poorest outcomes are predicted by earlier age of onset, comorbid psychiatric illness, and poor initial response to treatment. OCD patients with tics or Tourette's have a waxing and waning course, and, although tics can often improve after age 10 years, OCD symptoms can continue for several more years.

Management

The first step is to inform the child, the parents, and the teachers about the disorder and allow time for discussion of the implications. When obsessional symptoms occur as part of an anxiety or depressive disorder, treatment is directed to the primary disorder. True obsessional disorders of later childhood are treated along similar lines to the same disorder in adults (see page 189), with *cognitive behavioural methods, medication,* or a *combination of the two.* The cornerstone of psychological therapies for children with OCD is exposure and response prevention (ERP). A hierarchy of increasingly intense anxiety-provoking situations that trigger obsessional thinking is constructed, and subjects are exposed gradually to these situations and encouraged to refrain from engaging in compulsive behaviours. They are taught relaxation and anxiety management techniques to help them in this process. Whatever the treatment, it is important to involve the family, and about 30% of children will not respond to treatment.

Both SSRIs and clomipramine are more effective than placebo, but are associated with side effects. In the UK, sertraline and fluvoxamine are licensed for the treatment of OCD in people under 18 years of age, and, although clomipramine is well studied, it is now rarely used as, in adults, the symptoms are reduced but not removed by this treatment. In one trial with children and adolescents with OCD, treatment with sertraline gave a remission rate of 20%, which is modest but worthwhile when compared with the placebo rate of 4%. In the same trial, the remission rate with cognitive behavioural treatment was about 40%, and that with combined treatment was over 50% (Pediatric OCD Treatment Study Team, 2004). As OCD is frequently a chronic disorder, long-term maintenance therapy is often needed.

Somatoform and related disorders

Children with a psychiatric disorder often complain of *somatic symptoms* which do not have an underlying physical cause. These complaints include abdominal pain, headache, and limb pains. Most of these children are treated in primary care. The minority who are referred to specialists are more likely to be sent to paediatricians than to child psychiatrists.

Chronic fatigue syndrome

Chronic fatigue syndrome (CFS), which is described on page 641, usually occurs after puberty. It is associated with severe mental and physical fatigue that is not alleviated by rest, coupled with significant disability. Its prevalence has been estimated at around 0.1–2% of child and adolescent populations, with two-thirds estimated to be female and those with CFS having high rates of psychiatric comorbidity, predominantly anxiety and depressive disorders. The strongest evidence regarding aetiology in younger populations is that the Epstein–Barr virus is associated with an increased risk of CFS. There is some evidence for certain personality traits, with excessive conscientiousness, rigidity, fearful behaviour, and sensitivity being reported more frequently in young people with CFS (Lievesley *et al.*, 2014).

The principles of treatment resemble those for the treatment of the disorder in adults (see page 643). Cognitive behaviour therapy, similar to that used for adults, has been found to be effective in adolescents with a framework that conceptualizes how inactivity can contribute to maintaining fatigue alongside other related behavioural vicious cycles (Garralda *et al.*, 2015). Often it is best for treatment to be carried out jointly by a paediatrician and a psychiatrist or clinical psychologist, and a good collaborative relationship with the family is essential. Although the longer-term prognosis for fatigue is relatively favourable, the short-term effects on school performance can have serious consequences.

Recurrent abdominal pain

Childhood recurrent abdominal pain is one of the most common medical complaints of childhood, with no organic pathology identified in the majority of cases. It affects approximately 10% of children, and is a common reason for presentation to primary care services and referral to a paediatrician. In many cases, the abdominal pain is associated with headache, limb pains, and sickness, some of which are related to anxiety, some to 'masked' depressive disorder, and some to stressful events. Treatment is similar to that for other emotional disorders. Follow-up suggests that 25% of cases severe enough to require investigation by a paediatrician develop adult depression, generalized anxiety disorder, or unexplained physical symptoms.

Conversion disorders

Conversion disorders (or conversion and dissociative disorder in ICD terminology) are described on page 648. They are more common in adolescence than in childhood, both in individual patients and in the rare epidemic form of the disorders. In childhood, symptoms are usually mild and they seldom last long. The most frequent symptoms include paralyses, abnormalities of gait, and inability to see or hear normally. As with adults, organically determined physical symptoms are sometimes misdiagnosed as conversion disorder when the causative physical pathology is difficult to detect and stressful events coincide with the onset of the symptom. For this reason, the diagnosis of conversion disorder should be made only after a careful search for organic disease.

Epidemiology

Conversion disorders are relatively rare, with most cases diagnosed after age 7 years; the incidence increases with age and has a female preponderance. Incidence rates have been reported of 1.3–4.2 per 100,000, although some studies in India and Turkey have reported higher prevalence rates, suggesting an influence of culture and ethnicity on aetiology.

Management

Conversion and other somatoform disorders should be treated as early as possible, before secondary gains (see page 648) accumulate. The psychiatrist and paediatrician should work closely together and with the family and school. Unnecessary physical investigation should be avoided. Treatment is directed mainly at reducing any stressful circumstances and encouraging the child to talk about the problem. Symptoms may subside with these measures, or management comparable to that used for conversion disorder in adults may be needed (see page 649), with graded physiotherapy and behavioural methods. The majority will improve on follow-up but almost a third will develop a new psychiatric disorder in this time.

For a review of child somatoform and related disorders see Garralda *et al.* (2015).

Mood disorders

Depression

Major unipolar depression is a significant global health problem, with the highest incident risk being during adolescence. A depressive illness during this period is associated with negative long-term consequences, including suicide, additional psychiatric comorbidity, interpersonal relationship problems, poor educational performance, and poor employment attainment well into adult life (Cousins and Goodyer, 2015).

It is normal for healthy children to experience low mood or feel depressed in response to distressing circumstances—for example, when a parent is seriously ill or a grandparent has died. Some, including those experiencing grief, may also lose interest, concentrate poorly, and eat and sleep badly. In adolescence, depressive mood may be less immediately obvious than anger, alienation from parents, withdrawal from social contact with peers, underachievement at school, substance abuse, and deliberate self-harm. This section will cover clinical depression and not normal variations in mood or depressive symptoms that are part of another disorder, such as anxiety or conduct disorder. Although there are many similarities with adult depression, the treatment implications are very different. For a review of childhood depression, see Brent and Maalouf (2015) and Thapar *et al.* (2012).

Clinical picture

The clinical picture of major depression in childhood and adolescence is in most ways similar to that in adults, but can be easily missed. Irritability can be a common feature in adolescents. Young children might not express guilt in an adult way, and may have difficulty in describing feelings of sadness. Furthermore, their sleep may not be disturbed in the ways found among adults with depressive disorder and they might complain of symptoms such as unexplained abdominal pains, headache, anorexia, and enuresis. However, while these latter symptoms can be the first to be brought to medical attention, their investigation should include the possibility of a depressive disorder. When this is done, history-taking and mental state examination will reveal persistent sadness, anhedonia, irritability, and other symptoms typical of depressive disorder (Luby *et al.*, 2003).

Epidemiology

Depressive symptoms are more common in adolescence than in childhood. Estimates of the prevalence of major depressive disorder give figures of less than 1% in prepubertal children, with an equal male to female ratio. The picture changes dramatically following puberty, with a 1-year prevalence of around 4%, with females at a greater risk with a 2:1 ratio of females to males. These prevalence estimates can vary according to instrument used, population studied, and duration investigated (Thapar *et al.*, 2102).

Aetiology

There are many individual, family, and social risks for child and adolescent depression that are strongly correlated and might also impact on continuing and later adversities. The causes of depressive disorder in childhood appear to be similar to those of depressive disorder in adulthood; however, in adolescence, major pubertal, and brain and cognitive maturation processes take place and are likely to have an influence on the aetiology and/or impact of depression. The increased risk of depression in women correlates with endocrinological/pubertal changes rather than chronological age (Joinson *et al.*, 2011). The heritability of major depression in adolescents is greater than that in younger children. As in children, genes could act indirectly—for example, through interaction with life events in the family or

elsewhere. Negative cognitive biases and increased cortisol secretion have also been identified as risk factors. For a description of the different models of depression and its neurobiology, see Brent and Maalouf (2015) and Table 16.7.

Genetic factors. Genetic factors appear similar in nature and magnitude as in adult depression (see Chapter 9). No individual genes have been identified, although the *5-HTTLPR* variant is reportedly associated with early-onset depression in the presence of serious life events, peer victimization, or child maltreatment—an example of a gene–environment interaction (Caspi *et al.*, 2010).

Neurobiology. This is described in detail in Brent and Maalouf (2015). Current models include the potential role of cortisol in the hypothalamic–pituitary–adrenal (HPA)-stress system, its link with the prefrontal cortex, and the increased sensitivity of female brains to psychosocial stressors.

Other causes. Negative *life events* often precede the onset of depressive disorder in children, as they do in adults. *Temperament* also seems to be important, especially the tendency to react intensely to environmental stimuli.

Management

General measures. Any distressing circumstances and stressors should be reduced as far as possible, while the child is helped to talk about their feelings. The possibility of depression in the parents should be considered, and treated if necessary. With school-age children, the management plan should involve the teachers to help them to understand the effect of depression on the child's performance, and to help to identify and reduce any stressors at school, including bullying. The nature of the disorder is explained to the parents and, in terms appropriate to their age, to the child. This explanation, and the approach to possible stressors, should take full account of culture and ethnicity.

Psychological treatment. If depression does not improve with the above measures, a specific psychological treatment should be considered. Cognitive therapy, interpersonal therapy, and brief family therapy can be used, although most of the evidence for their efficacy is from trials with older children and adolescents.

Medication. When a child has failed to respond to psychosocial measures and psychological treatment, or if the depressive disorder is severe at the outset, drug treatment can be considered. For depressive disorders, SSRIs have been shown to have clinical benefit for the treatment of moderate to severe depression, while tricyclic antidepressant drugs have not shown significant

Table 16.7 Aetiology of depressive disorder in childhood

Vulnerability factors for depression		Environmental risk factors	
Genetic	See text below	*Parental depression and family discord*	Negative impact of maternal depression possibly mediated by family discord and expressed emotion directed towards the child
Cognitive distortion and rumination	Biased attention to negative emotional cues along with rumination can influence the onset of depression	*Child maltreatment*	Potent risk factor for the onset and recurrence of depression
Emotion regulation	If difficulties in emotional regulation, less able to shift attention away from negative cues in environment and possibly related to growth of children's depressive symptoms	*Peer victimization*	Higher rates of depression in both bullies and their victims; can have longlasting effects
Behavioural disorders and irritability	Increased rates in children with ADHD as well as their parents	*Sexual minority status*	3× higher risk of depression
Sleep	Sleep deprivation leads to increased mood lability and greater attention to negative emotional cues	*Bereavement*	3× increased risk; greatest risk immediately after the bereavement and if a past history of depressive symptomatology
Comorbid medical illness	Poor physical health associated with depression	*Resilience*	Higher IQ

Adapted from Brent D and Maalouf F, Depressive disorders in childhood and adolescence, In: Thapar A. *et al.*, Rutter's Child and Adolescent Psychiatry, 6th edn., pp. 874–892, Copyright (2015), with permission from John Wiley & Sons.

benefit over placebo in depressed adolescents (Cousins and Goodyer, 2015; National Institute for Health and Clinical Excellence, 2005d). Of the SSRIs, a network meta-analysis has demonstrated that fluoxetine is the only antidepressant currently considered to have a favourable risk–benefit ratio (Cipriani *et al.*, 2016), with another meta-analysis quoting a number needed to treat of 10 (Bridge *et al.*, 2007). Clinicians should look for the emergence or exacerbation of suicidality on starting medication, especially with SSRIs and venlafaxine, and therefore prescribing decisions in these circumstances are best made by a specialist in child psychiatry. The potential benefits and adverse effects are examined in each case, and discussed with the carers and, in appropriate terms, with the child. The information should include warning about the delay between starting medication and improvement, and dangerous side effects, including *worsening ideas of and behaviour around self-harm*. If an antidepressant is prescribed, it should be

for a child or adolescent with a confirmed diagnosis of moderate or severe depression, closely monitored, especially in the first few weeks, and it should, if possible, be combined with some form of psychological treatment.

In the Treatment for Adolescents with Depression (TADS) study, sponsored by the US National Institute for Mental Health (NIMH), 439 depressed adolescents were randomly allocated to fluoxetine, pill placebo, cognitive behaviour therapy, or a combination of fluoxetine and cognitive behaviour therapy. After 12 weeks of treatment, response rates for pill placebo (34%) and cognitive behaviour therapy (43%) were significantly less than for fluoxetine alone (61%) and the combination treatment (71%). By 18 weeks, the response to cognitive behaviour therapy (65%) was similar to that found with fluoxetine alone (69%), while the response to combination treatment was now 85%. As noted above, fluoxetine treatment was associated with an *increased risk of suicidal ideation and self-harm* relative to placebo, but this increase was not seen in patients in whom fluoxetine was combined with cognitive behaviour therapy (March and Vitiello, 2009). The TADS study supports the view that the best treatment for moderate to severe depression in adolescence is a *combination of fluoxetine and cognitive behaviour therapy.*

Psychological treatments. A network meta-analysis has shown that *interpersonal therapy* and *cognitive behaviour therapy* should be considered as the most effective psychotherapies for depression in children and adolescents (Zhou *et al.*, 2015).

Prognosis

As with adult depression, child and adolescent depression tends to be *chronic and recurrent*, although 60–90% will remit within 1 year; 50–70% will develop subsequent depressive disorders within 5 years. There is an increased risk of depression in adulthood, and chronic depression in childhood is also associated with *educational underachievement* and *interpersonal difficulties.*

Bipolar disorder

In the past two decades there has been a marked increase in knowledge about childhood-onset bipolar disorder. It can be one of the most impairing childhood psychiatric illnesses, with significant morbidity and mortality. Mania is generally thought to be extremely uncommon before puberty, although there have been significant recent diagnostic changes giving rise to estimates of bipolar disorder in paediatric populations of about 1%.

The diagnostic criteria for making a diagnosis are similar to those in adults and are described in Chapter 10. Recent changes in DSM-5 have helped to clarify some of the more complex issues involved in diagnosis. These include a clearer distinction between the prominence of irritability in childhood presentation of mania compared to other disorders such as generalized anxiety disorder, ASD, and ADHD. In the new classification of childhood bipolar disorder, irritability has to be present at the same time as some of the 'B symptoms' of mania, such as decreased need for sleep. The second key area that helps distinguish mania from the overactivity of ADHD involves the presence of these five symptoms: elation, grandiosity, hypersexuality, flight of ideas/increased goal-directed activity, and decreased need for sleep.

The most significant departure in the DSM-5 classification is the introduction of a new category of 'disruptive mood dysregulation disorder' (as described on page 453), which is now a key differential diagnosis to consider. DMDD, as distinguished from childhood bipolar disorder, involves chronic, severe, irritability characterized by frequent temper outbursts out of proportion to the situation and child's developmental level, and a persistently irritable or angry mood. A longitudinal perspective is very important to ensure the presence of different episodes to help confirm a diagnosis.

Children with bipolar disorder tend to cycle more frequently than adults and are more likely to have an impairing illness with symptoms much of the time. Their treatment requires a complex approach to meet the complex needs of the disorder, with targeted pharmacotherapy and psychotherapy. Most of the treatment data comes from adult studies. For mania, second-generation antipsychotic medications have the strongest efficacy data in young people with bipolar disorder. However, as with the treatment of psychosis, there are significant side effects, such as substantial weight gain and metabolic syndrome. Risperidone, aripiprazole, and quetiapine have all been licensed by the Food and Drug Administraiton (FDA) to treat mania or mixed states in 10–17-year-olds. There is some support for the use of lithium in childhood bipolar disorder, and weakest support for the therapeutic efficacy of antiepileptic drugs. The treatment of depression associated with bipolar disorder in childhood is poorly studied, although the data suggests that adolescents with bipolar disorder spend considerable time suffering from symptoms of depression and anxiety. There is some suggestion that the risk of manic induction on antidepressant treatment is higher in prepubertal children than in older adolescents.

For a full review of bipolar disorder in childhood, see Leibenluft *et al.* (2015).

School refusal

School refusal is not a psychiatric disorder but a pattern of behaviour that can have many causes. It is convenient to consider it at this point in the chapter because of its association with *anxiety and depressive disorder*. School refusal is one of several reasons for repeated absence from school. Physical illness is the most common. A small number of children are deliberately and repeatedly kept at home by parents to help in the home or for other reasons. Others are *truants* who could go to school but choose not to, often as a form of rebellion, and usually without their parents' knowledge. Finally, school refusers stay away from school but with parents' knowledge; they experience emotional distress at the prospect of attending school and their parents often try to get them to attend school (Maynard *et al.*, 2015).

Epidemiology

Temporary absences from school are extremely common, but the prevalence of school refusal is around 1–2% of the general population and up to 15% of those referred to mental health services.

Clinical picture

At times, the first sign to the parents that something is wrong is the child's sudden and complete refusal to attend school. More often there is an increasing reluctance to set out, with signs of unhappiness and anxiety when it is time to go. These children often complain of somatic symptoms of anxiety such as headache, abdominal pain, diarrhoea, sickness, or vague complaints of feeling ill. These complaints occur on school days but not at other times. Some children appear to want to go to school, but become increasingly distressed as they approach it. The final refusal can arise in several ways. It may follow a period of gradually increasing difficulty of the kind just described. It may appear after an enforced absence for another reason, such as a respiratory tract infection. It may follow an event at school such as a change of class. It may occur when there is a problem in the family such as the illness of a grandparent to whom the child is attached. Whatever the sequence of events, the child is extremely resistant to efforts to return them to school, and their evident distress makes it hard for the parents to insist that they go.

Almost 50% of school refusers referred to clinics have a diagnosable anxiety disorder, including separation anxiety disorder, specific phobias, social phobia, generalized anxiety disorder, and panic disorder with agoraphobia.

Aetiology

School refusal is a complex problem that is determined by a broad range of risk factors that interact with each other and change over time. The risk factors involve individual, family, school, and community factors. Individual factors include behavioural inhibition, fear of failure, low self-efficacy, and physical illness. The family factors can include separation and divorce, parental mental illness, overprotective parenting style, and dysfunctional family interactions. School factors include bullying, physical education lessons, transition to secondary school, while community factors can include increasing pressure to achieve academically and inadequate support services (Maynard *et al.*, 2015). Separation anxiety is particularly important in younger children. In older children there may be a true school phobia, i.e. a specific fear of certain aspects of school life, including travel to school. Some fear bullying, or failure to do well in class. Other children have no specific concerns, but feel generally inadequate and depressed. Some older children have a depressive disorder.

Prognosis

In the absence of treatment most youth with school refusal continue to display problematic school attendance and emotional distress, leading to short- and long-term adverse consequences. Studies of the longer prognosis of school refusal show that, of those with more severe problems, between a third and a half have emotional problems and others will have poorer social adjustment and limited social contacts. The impact on families can also be great.

Treatment

Except in the most severe cases, arrangements should be made for an early return to school. There should be discussion with the schoolteachers, who should be asked about the child's problems, asked how they can help the child to catch up with missed education, and advised how to manage any difficulties that may arise when the child returns. By the time that help is sought, parents often have difficulty in pressuring the child to go to school. Psychosocial treatments for children with school refusal typically incorporate both cognitive and behavioural interventions. There are a number of manualized cognitive behaviour therapy interventions and all involve individual treatment, some level of parental involvement, consultation with school staff, and between-session tasks. Graded exposure to school attendance is commonly advocated, and many manuals incorporate problem-solving training with the young person and family work on communication and problem-solving. For a review of psychosocial interventions, see Maynard *et al.* (2015).

Other childhood psychiatric disorders

Functional enuresis

Functional enuresis is the repeated involuntary voiding of urine occurring after an age at which continence is usual (see below), in the absence of any identified physical disorder. Enuresis may be nocturnal (bedwetting) or diurnal (daytime wetting), or both. Most children achieve daytime and night-time continence by 3 or 4 years of age. Nocturnal enuresis is often referred to as primary if there has been no preceding period of urinary continence. It is called secondary if there has been a preceding period of urinary continence.

Nocturnal enuresis can cause great unhappiness and distress, particularly if the parents blame or punish the child. This unhappiness may be made worse by limitations imposed by enuresis on activities such as staying with friends or going on holiday.

Epidemiology

Estimates of prevalence vary, depending on the definition and method of assessment. In the UK, the prevalence of nocturnal enuresis occurring once a week or more is about 10% at 5 years of age, 4% at 8 years, and 1% at 14 years. Similar figures have been reported from the USA. Nocturnal enuresis occurs more frequently in boys. Daytime enuresis has a lower prevalence and is more common in girls than in boys. More than 50% of daytime wetters also wet their beds at night (Butler, 2008).

Aetiology

Nocturnal enuresis occasionally results from physical conditions, but more often appears to be caused by delay in the maturation of the nervous system, either alone or in combination with environmental stressors. There is some evidence for a *genetic contribution*; about 70% of children with enuresis have a first-degree relative who has been enuretic. Also, concordance rates for enuresis are twice as high in monozygotic as in dizygotic twins (Butler, 2008). Some family influences include exposure to family adversity and stress in early childhood, parenting style, and difficulties in toilet training—either due to child temperamental factors, parental factors, or a combination of both.

Although most enuretic children are free from psychiatric disorder, the proportion with psychiatric disorder is greater than that of other children and it can be associated with low self-esteem if prolonged. There is evidence that early childhood difficult temperament (problems adapting to change, high intensity, and negative mood) and behaviour problems (conduct problems, hyperactivity, and low levels of prosocial behaviour) are risk factors for later bedwetting (Joinson *et al.*, 2015). Enuresis is more frequent in large families living in overcrowded conditions. Stressful events are associated with the onset of secondary enuresis. Rigid or other particular kinds of training have not been shown to improve outcomes.

Assessment

A careful history and appropriate physical examination are required to determine if the enuresis is primary or secondary and to exclude undetected physical disorder, particularly urinary infection, diabetes, or epilepsy, and to assess possible precipitating factors and the child's motivation. A question should be asked about faecal soiling. The child should be screened for other psychiatric disorders and a history taken to determine if any difficult or distressing events might have contributed to the presentation.

Management

Primary care and paediatric services usually treat these disorders. Any physical disorder should be treated. If the enuresis is functional, an explanation should be given to the child and the parents that the condition is common and the child is not to blame. It should be explained to the parents that punishment and disapproval are inappropriate and unlikely to be effective. The parents should be encouraged to reward success without drawing attention to failure, and not to focus attention on the problem. Many younger enuretic children improve spontaneously soon after being given an explanation of this kind, but those over 6 years of age are likely to need more active measures.

The next step is usually advice about restricting fluid before bedtime, voiding at daytime intervals and/or before bedtime, taking the child during the night to the toilet, and the use of star charts to reward success.

Enuresis alarms. Children who do not improve with these simple measures may be treated with an *enuresis alarm* with high reported success rates. Modern alarms consist of a detector pad attached to the night clothes, and an alarm buzzer carried in a pocket or on the wrist. When the child begins to pass urine the detector is activated and the alarm sounds. The child turns off the alarm, gets up to complete the emptying of the bladder, and changes their pyjamas and sheets, with help from the parents if needed. The method requires about 6–8 weeks of treatment, and, if carried to completion, is effective within a month in about 70–80% of cases, although about a third relapse within 1 year. It seems that children with associated psychiatric disorder do less well than the rest.

Medication. The synthetic antidiuretic hormone *des-amino-D-arginine vasopressin (desmopressin)* has been used in the treatment of nocturnal enuresis in children over 5 years of age. It can be administered as a tablet or in a nasal spray. In one clinical trial, about 50% of the enuretic children treated with intranasal hormone became dry, and good results have been reported for an oral preparation. However, patients relapse when treatment is stopped. Side effects of the oral preparation include rhinitis and nasal pain; other side effects are nausea and abdominal pain. For this reason it is often used for temporary relief at important times—for example, during an overnight stay with friends. It is also possible to use desmopressin in conjunction with the enuresis alarm to speed the acquisition of bladder control. Imipramine and anticholinergic agents have also been used. For guidelines for the treatment of enuresis, see Walle *et al.* (2012).

Faecal soiling

At the age of 3 years, 6% of children are still soiling themselves with faeces at least once a week; at 7 years the figure is 1.5%. By the age of 11 years, the figure is only 1% once a month or more. Soiling is three times more frequent in boys than in girls (Butler, 2008).

The term *encopresis* is used, but in two senses. In its wider sense it is a synonym for faecal soiling. In its narrower sense it denotes the repeated deposition of formed faeces in inappropriate places, including the underclothes. Because of this ambiguity, the term faecal soiling is used here.

Children who soil their clothes for any reason may feel ashamed, deny what has happened, and try to hide the dirty clothing.

Aetiology

Faecal soiling has several causes.

- *Constipation with overflow* is a common cause. Constipation has many causes, but common ones are a low-fibre diet, pain on defaecation (due, for example, to an anal fissure), or refusal to pass faeces as a form of rebellion. Hirschsprung's disease is an uncommon but important cause. Soiling results when, after prolonged constipation, liquid faeces leak round the plug of hard faeces in the rectum.

- *Fear of using the toilet.* Occasionally children who have no pain on passing faeces fear sitting on the toilet for other reasons—for example, because they believe that some harmful creature lives there. Shy or bullied children may fear going to the toilet at school.

- *Failure to learn bowel control.* This can occur in children with intellectual disability or children of normal intelligence whose training has been inconsistent or inadequate.

- *Stress-induced regression.* Children who have recently learned control may lose it as a result of a highly stressful experience, such as sexual abuse.

- *Rebellion.* Some children appear to defaecate deliberately in inappropriate places, and some children smear faeces on walls or elsewhere. Usually the family has many social problems, and often the child has other emotional or behavioural difficulties. The act appears to be a form of aggression towards the parents/carers, although this intention is usually denied by the child.

Treatment

Treatment depends on the cause. The first step is to check for chronic constipation, and if it is present, to treat the cause. For this, joint assessment with a paediatrician may be needed. Even when constipation is not the main cause, it may require treatment as a secondary problem. It is generally managed with a combination of laxatives and behavioural interventions aimed at re-establishing normal bowel habits, including short periods (less than 5 minutes) of toilet sitting after meals, self-initiated toileting, and self-management of cleanliness. A child who is fearful of the toilet should be reassured sympathetically. Inadequate toilet training may be improved using behavioural techniques, including achievable targets, and star charts or other rewards, together with help for the parents. Stress-induced regression usually disappears when the child has been helped to overcome the trauma. Soiling as rebellion is more difficult to treat, as it is generally part of wider social and psychological difficulties, which may require intensive and prolonged help. If outpatient treatment fails in these cases, or in those owing to inadequate or unsuitable training, the child may respond to behavioural management in hospital. If the child is admitted, the parents need to be closely involved in the treatment to avoid relapse when the child returns home.

Prognosis

Whatever the cause, it is unusual for encopresis to persist beyond the middle teenage years, although associated problems may continue. When treated, most cases improve within a year.

For a review of faecal soiling, see Butler (2008).

Selective mutism

In this condition, sometimes called *elective mutism*, a child consistently refuses to speak in certain social situations, although they do so normally in others. Usually speech is normal in the home but lacking at school. There is evidence that, although these children are able to speak in some situations, they do have lower scores on standardized measures of language than their peers. These children often have a comorbid anxiety disorder, usually social phobia, and so in DSM-5 this condition has now been placed with the anxiety disorders. The condition usually begins between 3 and 5 years of age, after *normal speech has been acquired*. Although reluctance to speak is not uncommon among children starting school, clinically significant elective mutism is rare, probably occurring in about 1 per 1000 children.

Assessment is difficult because the child often refuses to speak to the psychiatrist, so that diagnosis depends to a large extent on the parents' and other informant accounts. When questioning the parents, it is important to ask whether speech and comprehension are normal at home. Treatment approaches aim to lower the anxiety that a child has for speaking in certain situations and increase the contexts in which the child may speak comfortably. In general behavioural treatments, cognitive behaviour therapy and/or play therapy will be the first choice of intervention. Selective mutism is persistent, with a remission rate of only 58% 13 years after first referral and high rates of phobia and social anxiety, as well as increased risk for depression and substance misuse in unresolved cases (Norbury *et al.*, 2015).

Stammering

Stammering (or 'child-onset fluency disorder' in DSM-5) is a disturbance of the rhythm and fluency of speech. It may take the form of repetitions of syllables or words, or of blocks in the production of speech. This may be accompanied by excessive tension, struggle behaviour, and secondary mannerisms such as eye-blinking or arm movements. Stammering is four times more frequent in boys than in girls. It is usually a brief problem in the early stages of language development, although prognosis after age 7 years is more guarded. However, 0.3%–1% of children suffer from stammering after they have entered school.

The cause of stammering is not known, although many theories exist. It seems unlikely that all cases have the same causes. Over 60% have a concurrent speech and language disorder, with the most common being speech sound disorder. Genetic factors, brain damage, and anxiety may all play a part in certain cases, but do not seem to be general causes. Stammering is not usually associated with a psychiatric disorder, even though it can cause embarrassment and distress. Most children improve whether treated or not. Many kinds of psychiatric treatment have been tried, including psychotherapy and behaviour therapy, but none has been shown to be effective. The usual treatment is speech therapy, and four classes of intervention are used: fluency shaping, stuttering modification, use of electronic devices, and parent-implemented techniques. For a summary see Norbury *et al.* (2015).

Tic disorders

Tic disorders, including *Gilles de la Tourette* syndrome, are considered on page 376.

Dementia

Dementing disorders are extremely rare in childhood. They result from organic brain diseases such as lipidosis, leucodystrophy, or subacute sclerosing panencephalitis. Many of the causes are genetically determined and may affect other children in the family. The prognosis is usually poor, and many cases are fatal.

Psychosis and early-onset schizophrenia

Psychotic symptoms are relatively common in young people, especially in childhood. Prevalence is higher in younger (9–12 years) compared to older (13–18 years) children, although they are rare before 9 years of age. For example, in a systematic review of population-based studies the prevalence of psychotic symptoms was 17% among children aged 9–12 years and 7.5% among adolescents aged 13–18 years (Kelleher *et al.*, 2012). In a UK population cohort, up to 14% of 12-year-olds had 'non-clinical psychotic symptoms', with higher levels in those from low socioeconomic status families and with low IQ (Horwood, 2008). Experience of the psychotic symptoms seemed to be similar to those of adult psychosis, but only 3% met strict phenomenological criteria for adult psychotic disorders. In another cohort, Polanczyk *et al.* (2010) confirmed that a significant minority of 12-year-olds in the community self-report hallucinations (most commonly) and delusions. In addition, these symptoms were associated with many of the same risk factors and correlates as adult schizophrenia, including genetic, social, neurodevelopmental, home-rearing, and behavioural risks. Therefore, psychotic symptoms in childhood are often a marker of an impaired developmental process and should be actively assessed. Psychotic symptoms generally occur in the context of other childhood psychiatric problems, indicating that it is worthwhile to ask all preadolescent psychiatric patients about hallucinations and delusions. Even if the psychotic symptoms are not themselves impairing, they are associated with important risk factors, such as chaotic household, maternal negativity, and physical maltreatment, and with behavioural problems, such as early tobacco use and self-harm, that should be a focus of attention.

For those at the most severe end of the spectrum, early-onset schizophrenia, starting in childhood or adolescence is accepted to be clinically and biologically continuous with the adult disorder. The most prominent differences are that the early-onset form of schizophrenia is often more severe, has a greater association with early neurodevelopmental difficulties, and has poorer treatment response. There may also be a higher proportion of cases attributable to CNVs (see Chapter 12). The whole range of symptoms that characterize schizophrenia in adulthood may occur, and in both DSM-5 and ICD-10 the criteria for diagnosis in children are the same as those used in adults; there is no separate category of childhood schizophrenia. It is highlighted in DSM-5 that, if other communication disorders of childhood are present where disorganized speech and negative symptoms are also present, a diagnosis of schizophrenia should be made only if prominent hallucinations or delusions are also present for at least 1 month. Schizophrenia in adolescence is more common in boys than in girls. Before symptoms of schizophrenia appear, many of these children experience non-specific behavioural changes, social withdrawal, and declining school performance. The prognosis may be good for a single acute episode with florid symptoms, but for the majority, early-onset schizophrenia runs a chronic course and is especially poor when the onset is insidious.

Effective *treatments* are less well established for early-onset schizophrenia than for adult populations, and include antipsychotic medications combined with psychoeducational, psychotherapeutic, and educational interventions. For children, adolescents, and young adults, the balance of risk and benefit of antipsychotics appears less favourable than in adults (Stafford *et al.*, 2015). Studies suggest that many young people with early-onset schizophrenia do not respond adequately to available *antipsychotic drugs* and are vulnerable to adverse events, particularly metabolic side effects (McClellan and Stock, 2013). In recent years there has been a growing emphasis on early detection and intervention, with intervention in those with 'at-risk mental states', but especially to minimize the duration of untreated psychosis in child and adolescent populations, as these populations often have long periods of untreated psychotic symptoms (Fraguas *et al.*, 2014).

For review of childhood schizophrenia, see Driver *et al.* (2013).

Gender dysphoria

These disorders are discussed in detail in Chapter 13. This field, and the classification of these disorders, has changed dramatically over the last few years. Although some children might prefer to dress in the clothes of and to play with the toys of the other gender, often referred to previously as effeminacy in boys or tomboyishness in girls, the gender dysphorias in children are associated with a strong desire to be of the other gender or an insistence that he or she is the other gender. For a review see Zucker *et al.* (2015).

Suicidal behaviour and self-harm

Self-harm and suicide are major public health problems in adolescents, with rates of self-harm being high in the teenage years and suicide being the second most common cause of death in young people worldwide. Important contributors to self-harm and suicide include genetic vulnerability and psychiatric, psychological, familial, social, and cultural factors. The effects of media and contagion are also important. Prevention of self-harm and suicide needs both universal measures aimed at young people in general and targeted initiatives focused on high-risk groups. There is little evidence of effectiveness of either psychosocial or pharmacological treatment, with particular controversy surrounding the usefulness of antidepressants. Restriction of access to means for suicide is important.

These issues are discussed in Chapter 21. For a full account, see Hawton *et al.* (2012).

Psychiatric aspects of physical illness in childhood

The associations between physical and psychiatric disorders in children resemble those in adults (see Chapter 22). There are three main groups to consider; these are children with:

- psychiatric manifestations of medical illnesses and treatments or adjustment to their medical illness;
- psychiatric disorders presenting with physical symptoms without an identified underlying organic cause—for example, abdominal pain;
- physical complications of psychiatric disorders—for example, eating disorders.

In this section we consider only some problems specific to childhood. For more information on psychiatric aspects of somatic disease in children, see Pinsky *et al.* (2015).

The impact of childhood physical illness
Psychiatric manifestations of medical illness

Children with medical illnesses serious enough to warrant hospitalization are at increased risk for emotional disorders, with estimates of psychological distress in children and adolescents varying from 20% to greater than 35% and estimates of those with chronic illnesses ranging from 10% to 30% (Pinsky *et al.*, 2015). Those that impact on the central nervous system, such as epilepsy and cerebral palsy, pose additional risks. Other factors associated with poor psychological adjustment to chronic medical conditions include physical disability and brain dysfunction, pain frequency, younger age, poverty, single-parent family, and increased psychological symptoms in the parents. There is evidence that a child's psychiatric illness may affect the physical disease process, not only by influencing adherence and lifestyle, but also by producing psychophysiological changes. For instance, children with diabetes mellitus are at greater risk for depressive disorders, and those who have comorbid depression are at increased risk for treatment non-adherence and repeated hospitalization as well as disease-related complications (e.g. diabetic retinopathy) (DeMaso et al., 2009).

Non-adherence to medical treatments is common across conditions, with estimates ranging from 50% to 80%; the factors contributing to poor adherence are many, but include the medication regimen, family systems, denial, psychiatric illness, and relationships with medical providers. *Asthma* is the most common chronic illness of childhood and it is important when treating a child with asthma to understand the factors that affect adherence, delineate common psychosocial stresses that may act as triggers for asthma attacks, and teach stress management skills to improve adherence and decrease morbidity. At the other extreme, childhood *cancer* is rare but also presents numerous challenges to adaptation and development, although most studies show that childhood cancer survivors adapt well following treatment. Psychological support is particularly beneficial at the more stressful times, with these often being at the time of diagnosis, the onset of treatment, and treatment completion, as well as, for some, dealing with any late effects of cancer and its treatment—such as any effects on sexual maturation that might have been affected by chemotherapy or relapse. Challenges to psychosocial adaptation often include persistent pain, persistent debilitating side effects of treatment such as nausea, alteration in body image, school disruptions, compromised peer relationships, and family stresses and conflicts.

There is evidence that cognitive behavioural therapy has positive effects in the treatment of symptoms of depression and anxiety in children who have chronic physical illness (Bennett et al., 2015). There are growing psychological medicine or psychiatry-liaison services working in general hospital settings, and mental health services integrating with the general or specialist medical teams can provide enhanced models of care for children with medical illnesses and work closely as part of the team contributing to the management of often complicated needs.

Effect on parents

The effects on parents are greater when the child's physical illness is *chronic or disabling*. Their response depends on factors such as the nature of the physical disorder, the temperament of the child, the parents' emotional resources, and the circumstances of the family. The parents may experience a sequence of emotional reactions like those of bereavement, and their marital and social lives may be affected. Most parents develop a warm, loving relationship with a physically disabled child and cope successfully with the difficulties. A few manage less well; they may have unrealistic expectations, or they may be rejecting or overprotective. The support of a multidisciplinary team and, if needed, respite options for care are important for families. It is important also to ensure that the brothers and sisters of children with medical illnesses do not feel neglected, irritated by restrictions on their social activities, or resentful of having to spend so much time helping in the case of a child with greater physical and emotional needs. Although some studies have shown more emotional and behavioural disturbances in siblings than would be expected by chance, most siblings manage well, and some even benefit through increased abilities to cope with stress and to show compassion for others.

Children in hospital

It is important to prepare children for admission by explaining in appropriate terms what will happen, and by introducing to them the members of staff who will care for them and, if possible, to visit the hospital or treatment area in advance. Once admitted, many hospitals appreciate the importance of ensuring a family member can stay with their child, and, depending on each particular situation, let them stay overnight in the same room with them or sleep in facilities on or close to the hospital. The wider family and friends should be able to visit frequently and, where appropriate, primary carers can take part in the care of the child. Many hospitals have educational facilities attached or associated with them as children who have prolonged hospital stay, and are well enough, might benefit from educational input—not only to distract them whilst in hospital but also to make the adjustment back into school easier as they will not have to catch up on quite as much missed work. For issues to consider in the very unwell or when a child dies in hospital, see Pinsky et al. (2015).

Special considerations for adolescent populations

Adolescence and young adulthood are the years in which an individual establishes the social, cultural, emotional, educational, and economic resources to maintain their health and wellbeing across the life course (Patton *et al.*, 2016). It is a dynamic period of brain development, with significant changes taking place within neural systems. Early adolescence (10–14 years) is biologically dominated by puberty and the effects of the rapid rise in pubertal hormones on body morphology and sexual and brain development. Adolescence is a time of remodelling of the brain's reward system. Psychologically it is characterized by low resistance to peer influences, low risk perception, often leading to increases in risk-taking behaviour, and poor self-regulation. School and family environments are critical social contexts during this period. In late adolescence (15–19 years) pubertal maturation continues and the brain continues to be extremely developmentally active, particularly in the development of the prefrontal cortex and the increased connectivity between brain networks. During this phase many adolescents develop greater executive functioning and also increased autonomy. When making decisions, adolescents seek out and are more influenced by exciting, arousing, and stressful situations compared with adults.

In many low- and middle-income settings adolescent males and females might start to work, get married, and have children, whilst in high-income countries, education continues into mid or late adolescence, and responsibilities come later. Adolescents are expected both to conform to the rules of society and to become more independent and develop restraints on their own behaviour. Many of the problems of adolescence relate to conflicts between these two expectations, or to the rejection of the rules of society. Although such problems are sometimes conspicuous, they are not inevitable.

Epidemiology of psychiatric disorder in adolescence

Although psychiatric disorders are only slightly more common in adolescence than in the middle years of childhood, the pattern of disorder is closer to that of adults. In a UK survey, Meltzer *et al.* (2000) found that, between the ages of 11 and 15 years, 13% of boys and 10% of girls had a psychiatric disorder. Both *emotional disorders* and *conduct disorder* were more frequent than in childhood, and occurred with approximately the same frequency.

Clinical features of psychiatric disorders of adolescence

There are no specific disorders of adolescence. Nevertheless, special experience and skill are required to apply the general principles of psychiatric diagnosis and treatment to patients at this time of transition between childhood and adult life. It can be difficult to distinguish psychiatric disorder from the normal emotional reactions of the teenage years. The clinical features of adolescent depression, anxiety, psychosis, and other disorders are discussed under the relevant sections in this chapter. A few specific disorders not included elsewhere and important to mention are now included below.

Eating disorders

Problems with *eating* and *weight* are common in adolescence. They are discussed in Chapter 13, to which the reader is referred, as they closely resemble the same conditions in adulthood. It is particularly important to involve the parents and perhaps other family members in the treatment of an adolescent patient with eating disorder. Systemic family therapy has been shown to be of value for anorexia nervosa in adolescents. For a review, see Bryant-Waugh (2015).

Alcohol and substance use disorders

Substance use disorders are among the most prevalent psychiatric disorders in those aged 9–21 years and in children and adolescents are similar to those in adulthood, as described in Chapter 20. The number with substance use disorders rises rapidly in adolescence, peaks around age 20 years, and has a declining incidence after age 25 years. However, adolescent substance use disorders often persist into adulthood and those persisting further become leading causes of adult deaths. There is considerable country-to-country variability in substance use; a 36-country average of rates showed that in 16-year-olds, on average around 87% had 'ever' used alcohol, 54% cigarettes, and 17% cannabis. Substance use patterns also shift over time as well as new, abusable substances appearing and becoming more readily available via online sources.

Excessive drinking is common among adolescents, especially among those with conduct disorder. Most adolescent heavy drinkers seem to reduce their drinking as they grow older, but a few progress to more serious drinking problems in adulthood. Prevention programmes have been developed, but there is little evidence for their effectiveness.

Occasional *drug taking* is common in adolescence, and is often a group activity. Cigarette smoking and the use of cannabis and 'ecstasy' are especially frequent. Solvent abuse is largely confined to adolescence, and is usually of short duration. Abuse of drugs such as amphetamines, barbiturates, opiates, and cocaine is less common but more serious, as most drug-dependent adults will have experimented with these drugs during adolescence. There is a strong association between conduct disorder in childhood and drug taking in adolescence.

Most adolescents experiment with drugs for short periods and do not become regular users. Those who persist in taking drugs are more likely to come from discordant families or broken homes, to have failed at school, and to be members of a group of persistent drug users. Feelings of alienation and low self-esteem may also be important.

Since regular drug taking starts less often in adulthood than in adolescence, and the developing brain is likely to be more vulnerable to the deleterious effects of substance misuse, the limitation of drug taking among adolescents is an important aim. One approach is the application of appropriate psychosocial interventions in young people at high risk of drug misuse (see page 470 and National Institute for Health and Clinical Excellence, 2007). See Crowley et al. (2015) for an account of substance misuse by adolescents.

Assessment of adolescents

Special skills are needed when interviewing adolescents to know which approach might be best for that particular person. In general, young adolescents require an approach similar to that used for children, while for older adolescents it is more appropriate to employ the approach used with adults. It must always be remembered that a large proportion of adolescents attending a psychiatrist do so somewhat unwillingly, and also that most have difficulty in expressing their feelings in adult terms. Therefore psychiatrists must be willing to spend considerable time establishing a relationship with their adolescent patients. To do this, they must show interest in the adolescents, respect their points of view, and talk in terms that they can understand. As in adult psychiatry, it is important to collect systematic information and describe symptoms in detail, but with adolescents the interviewer must be prepared to adopt a more flexible approach to the interview.

It is usually better to see the adolescent before interviewing the parents. In this way, it is made clear that the adolescent is being seen as an independent person. Later, other members of the family may be interviewed, and sometimes the family may be seen as a whole. As well as the usual psychiatric history, particular attention should be paid to information about the adolescent's

functioning at home, in school, or at work, and about their relationships with peers. Relevant physical examination should be carried out unless this has already been done by the doctor who made the referral.

Services for adolescents

The proportion of adolescents in the population who are seen in psychiatric clinics is less than the proportion of other age groups. Of those referred, some of the less mature adolescents can be helped more in a child psychiatry clinic. Some of the older and more mature adolescents are better treated in a clinic for adults. Nevertheless, for the majority the care can be provided most appropriately by a specialized adolescent service, provided that close links are maintained with child and adult psychiatry services and with paediatricians.

There are variations in the organization of these units and the treatment that they provide, but most combine individual and family psychological treatment with the possibility of drug treatment for severe disorders. Most units accept outpatient referrals not only from doctors but also from senior teachers, social workers, and the courts. When the referral is non-medical, the general practitioner should be informed and the case discussed. All adolescent units work with schools and social services. Inpatient facilities are usually limited in extent, so it is important to agree with social services what kinds of problems need admission to a health service unit and which should be cared for in residential facilities provided by social services (in the UK). Reasons for admission to a health service inpatient unit include the following:

- severe or very unusual mental symptoms requiring that the person's mental state be observed carefully, investigations carried out, or treatment monitored closely;
- behaviour that is dangerous to the self or to others, and that is due to psychiatric disorder.

When dangerous behaviour relates to personality and circumstances and not to illness, a hospital unit is not more effective than secure residential accommodation, and the behaviour of such adolescents may be stressful for others with mental disorders. For a review of the organization of mental health services for children and adolescents, see Wolpert (2009).

Child maltreatment

The World Health Organization definition states that child maltreatment includes:

'all forms of physical and/or emotional ill treatment, sexual abuse, neglect or negligent treatment or commercial or other exploitation, resulting in actual or potential harm to the child's health, survival, development or dignity in the context of a relationship of responsibility, trust or power.'

Over the past decade the concept of child maltreatment and abuse has therefore been widened to include the overlapping categories of *physical abuse (non-accidental injury), emotional abuse, sexual abuse,* and *neglect.* (Table 16.8).

Most of the literature on child abuse refers to high-income countries; however, abuse of children is prevalent throughout the world, although it can take different forms such that in low- and middle-income countries other causes and risk factors are involved. For example, there might be greater numbers of children in low-income countries exposed to physical violence and corporal punishment, growing up without a primary caregiver for reasons ranging from parental illness (such as HIV/AIDS) to migrant labour where parents have to leave home to find employment, and child labour and trafficking. A UK community survey found that nearly one in five children experience some forms of maltreatment and that children who have experienced one form of maltreatment are 2–3 times more likely to experience other forms of maltreatment and to be victimized by other perpetrators over time (Danese *et al.*, 2015). The term *safeguarding* is increasingly used to denote the consideration of and care needed for children who are either at risk of or who have a past or current history of child maltreatment; the term also encompasses ensuring that they come to least harm and are protected.

The term *fetal abuse* is sometimes applied to behaviours that are detrimental to the fetus, including physical assault and the taking by the mother of substances that are likely to cause fetal damage. *Fabricated and induced illness (or Munchausen syndrome by proxy)* is the name given to apparent illness in children, which has been fabricated by the parents, and to conditions induced by parents—for example, by giving medication or other substances when not indicated (see page 644).

Aetiology

There are many interacting causes for child maltreatment (see Box 16.8). Although several risk factors show a statistical association with child maltreatment, no single risk factor is either necessary or sufficient for maltreatment to occur. The most useful way to frame the many risks is to consider them in a multilevel model, with individual, family, and community factors considered alongside appreciating the bidirectional nature of the child–adult interaction and how this might influence maltreatment.

The environment. Child maltreatment is more frequent in neighbourhoods in which family violence is common, schools, housing, and employment are unsatisfactory, and there is little feeling of community.

The parents. Factors associated with child maltreatment include young age of parents, impaired capacity for empathy, low education, psychiatric disorder and/or substance misuse, social isolation, family dysfunction, and a criminal record. If a parent has a psychiatric disorder, it is most often a personality disorder. Many parents give a history of having themselves suffered abuse or deprivation in childhood, and the parental relationship is marked by conflict and sometimes violence. Although physical abuse is more common in families with other forms of social pathology, it is certainly not limited to such families.

The children. Risk factors include younger age, especially under age 5 years, and other factors associated with increased child vulnerability, including prematurity, physical, and intellectual disabilities, chronic illness, and those with either a more difficult temperament or a more dependent relationship with carers.

Table 16.8 **National Institute of Health and Care Excellence guidelines on recognition of child maltreatment**

Emotional abuse	Age-inappropriate behaviour, aggression, body-rocking, eating and feeding difficulties, encopresis, wetting, dissociation, cutting, and other forms of self-harm
Physical abuse	Abrasions, teeth marks, bruises, burns and scalds, cuts, eye injuries, fractures, intra-abdominal injuries, oral injuries, petechiae, retinal haemorrhage, subdural haemorrhage
Sexual abuse	Anal symptoms and signs, anogenital injuries, dysuria, genital symptoms and signs, sexualized behaviour, pregnancy
Neglect	Abandonment, failure to thrive, lack of supervision, poor hygiene, persistent infestations, poor medication adherence

Adapted from Danese and McCrory, Child maltreatment, In: Thapar A. *et al.,* Rutter's Child and Adolescent Psychiatry, 6th edn., pp. 364–376, Copyright (2015), with permission from John Wiley & Sons.

Physical abuse (non-accidental injury)

Estimates of the prevalence of physical abuse of children vary according to the criteria used. Most studies report prevalence rates of physical abuse in childhood in the range 5–15%, depending on how this is defined, with lower rates of significant violence.

Clinical features

Parents may bring an abused child to the doctor with an injury said to have been caused accidentally. Alternatively, relatives, neighbours, school staff, or other people may become concerned and report the problem to police, social workers, or voluntary agencies. The most common forms of injury are multiple bruising, burns, abrasions, bites, torn upper lip, bone fractures, and subdural or retinal haemorrhages. Some infants are smothered, often with a pillow, and the parents might report an apnoeic attack. Suspicion of physical abuse should be aroused by the pattern of the injuries, a previous history of suspicious injury, a vague or inconsistent account of the way in which injuries came about; an account that is inconsistent with the nature and extent of injury, delay in seeking help, and incongruous parental reactions. The psychological characteristics of abused children vary, but include fearful responses to the parents, other evidence of anxiety or unhappiness, and social withdrawal. Such children often have low self-esteem, may avoid adults and children who make friendly approaches, and may be aggressive.

Assessment and management

Doctors and others involved in the care of children should always be alert to the possibility of physical abuse. They need to be particularly aware of the risks to children who have some of the characteristics described above, or who are being cared for by parents with the predisposing factors listed. It is important for professionals to receive regular child protection training to be aware of the different ways these children might present, especially as the majority are thought to be missed by health services, and also of the heightened needs of these children.

Doctors who suspect abuse should refer the child to hospital and inform a paediatrician or casualty officer of their suspicions. The paediatrician will usually take a careful history, documenting the information in as much detail as possible, and also perform a thorough physical examination. For further information about the physical examination, see a textbook of paediatrics. In the hospital emergency department,

> ### Box 16.8 Risk factors for child maltreatment
>
> #### The parent(s)
>
> Young age
> Low education or intelligence
> Social isolation/no one to provide help
> Breakdown of relationship with partner
> Poor parenting skills: lack of awareness of child's needs, harsh punishment, little reward; unrealistic expectations of child
> Experience of maltreatment as a child
> Criminal record
> Impaired emotional regulation
> Psychiatric problems: depression, substance abuse, personality disorder
>
> #### The child
>
> Factors leading to weak attachment to the parents: prematurity, health problems including disability
> Separation from mother during early life (e.g. in neonatal unit)
> Difficult temperament, cries a lot
>
> #### The environment
>
> Problem neighbourhood: high levels of family and community violence, problem schools, high unemployment
> Large family size or single parent
> Non-biological transient carers in the home
> Poverty
> Little feeling of community

inpatient admission should be arranged for all children in whom non-accidental injury is suspected. If possible, social services should become involved early and the doctor's concerns should be discussed with the parents, and in any case they should be told that admission is necessary to allow further investigations. If the parents refuse admission, it may be necessary in England and Wales to apply to a magistrate for a Place of Safety Order; similar action may be appropriate in other countries. During admission, assessment must be thorough and include formal photographs of injuries (of a quality that could be used in court if needed, so this can often be through the medical illustration departments of the hospital) and full skeletal survey radiography. Radiological examination may show evidence of previous injury or, occasionally, of bone abnormalities such as osteogenesis imperfecta. A CT scan may be needed if subdural haemorrhage is suspected.

Once it has been decided that non-accidental injury is probable, the first priority is to establish the child's safety. The procedures involved will vary according to the administrative arrangements in different countries. In the UK, the Social Services Department is responsible for child protection and should be notified; police departments also often get involved. It may be decided to put the child's name on a child abuse register, thereby giving the Social Services Department responsibility for visiting the home and checking the problem regularly.

In some cases, the risk of returning the child to their parents is too great, and separation is required. If the parents do not agree to separation, a *care order* can be sought by the Social Services Department. If the abuse is severe, prolonged, or permanent, separation may be necessary and the parents may face criminal charges. Because there are known cases of injury or death in children who have been returned to their parents, it is vitally important that the most careful assessment is undertaken before physically abused children are returned to their family. Countries vary in the requirements and procedures for reporting and monitoring possible physical abuse in children, and readers should familiarize themselves with the arrangements that exist in the area in which they work.

Prognosis

Children who have been subjected to physical abuse are at high risk of further problems. For example, the *risk of further severe injury is probably around 10–30%*, and occasionally the injuries are fatal, therefore a priority in the intervention is to try to prevent any recurrence of maltreatment. Abused children are likely to have subsequent high rates of physical disorder, delayed development, and learning difficulties. There are also increased rates of behavioural and emotional problems in later childhood and adulthood, even when there has been earlier therapeutic intervention. As adults, many former victims of abuse have difficulties in rearing their own children. The outcome is better for abused children who can establish a good relationship with an adult (often from outside the family), and who have dispositions that include sociability and academic competence.

Emotional abuse

The term emotional abuse usually refers to *persistent neglect or rejection sufficient to impair a child's development*. However, the term is sometimes applied to gross degrees of overprotection, verbal abuse, or scapegoating, which impair development. Emotional abuse often accompanies other forms of child abuse.

Emotional abuse has various effects on the child, including failure to thrive physically, impaired psychological development, and emotional and conduct disorders. Diagnosis depends on observations of the parents' behaviour towards the child, which may include frequent belittling or sarcastic remarks about them during the interview. One or both parents may have a disorder of personality, or occasionally a psychiatric disorder. The parents should be interviewed separately and together to discover any reasons for the abuse of this particular child—for example, the child may fail to live up to their expectations, or may remind them of another person who has been abusive to one of them. The parents' mental state should be assessed.

Management

In treatment, the parents should be offered help with their own emotional problems and with their day-to-day interactions with the child. It is often difficult to persuade parents to accept such help. If they reject help and if the effects of emotional abuse are serious, it may be necessary to involve social services and to consider the steps described above for the care of children suffering physical abuse. The child is likely to need individual help.

Child neglect

Child neglect is the failure to provide necessary care. It can take several forms, including emotional deprivation, neglect of education, physical neglect, lack of appropriate concern for physical safety, and denial of necessary medical or surgical treatment. These forms of neglect may lead to physical or psychological harm, including poor academic performance and disturbed behaviour.

Child neglect is more common than physical abuse, and it may be detected by various people, including relatives, neighbours, teachers, doctors, or social workers. Child neglect is associated with adverse social circumstances, and is a common reason for a child to need to be taken into foster care or other living arrangements.

Non-organic failure to thrive and deprivation dwarfism

Paediatricians recognize that some children fail to thrive when there is no apparent organic cause. For these children their calorific intake is insufficient to maintain growth; this is usually associated with emotional deprivation, psychological abuse, or both. The child is usually under the fifth centile for weight and height, and the rate of weight gain is less than expected for age. Nonorganic failure to thrive (NOFTT) is most frequent under 3 years of age; in older children it has been referred to as psychosocial short stature syndrome (PSSS).

Clinical picture

NOFTT is caused by the deprivation of food and close affection. In the children who are seen in the psychiatric service, there is usually evidence of problems in the parent–child relationship since the child's early infancy; these include rejection and, in extreme cases, expressed hostility towards the child. There may be physical or sexual abuse as well. The infant who is failing to thrive may present with recent weight loss, persistently low weight, or reduced height. There may be cognitive and developmental delay. The infant may be irritable and unhappy, or, in more severe cases, lethargic and resigned. There is a clinical spectrum ranging from infants with mild feeding problems to those with all of the severe features described above. If food and care are provided, the infant usually grows and develops quickly.

PSSS or 'deprivation dwarfism'. These children have abnormally short stature, unusual eating patterns, retarded speech development, and temper tantrums. Although short in stature, the child may be of normal weight. Emotional and behavioural disorders occur, and there may be cognitive and developmental delay with impairment of language skills. These children have low self-esteem and are commonly depressed. There is usually a history of deprivation or of psychological maltreatment. Away from the deprived environment, these children eat ravenously.

Management

When treating either syndrome, the first essential is to ensure the child's safety, which may require admission to hospital. Subsequently, some children can be managed at home, but others need to be moved to alternative living arrangements, including foster care. Some parents can be helped to understand their child's needs and to plan for them; other parents are too hostile to be helped. If help is feasible, it should be intensive and should probably focus on changing patterns of parenting. It is unusual for the parents to be psychiatrically ill. Home-based intervention programmes may improve treatment effects, particularly in cognitive and behavioural domains.

Prognosis

With both syndromes, the prognosis for early cases is relatively good (Rudolf and Logan, 2005). However, some children have to be placed permanently in foster care because family patterns are resistant to change. In a positive emotional setting the abnormal behaviour is usually lost quickly and mental development follows physical growth.

Sexual abuse

The term *sexual abuse* refers to the involvement of children in sexual activities which they do not fully comprehend and to which they cannot give informed consent, and which violate generally accepted cultural rules. The term covers various forms of sexual contact with or without varying degrees of violence. The term also covers some activities that do not involve physical contact, such as posing for pornographic photographs or films. The abuser is commonly known to the child and is often a member of the family (*incest*). A minority of children are abused by groups of paedophiles (sex rings).

Epidemiology

Child sexual abuse is highly prevalent around the globe, and differentiating between types of abuse is important to obtain meaningful estimates of prevalence. A review collating results from other studies estimated prevalence rates of sexual abuse and separated abuse into four different types. For non-contact abuse (inappropriate sexual solicitation, indecent exposure) the rates were estimated at 17% for males and 31% for females; for contact abuse (fondling, touching, kissing) the rates were 6% for males and 13% for females; for forced intercourse (oral, vaginal, anal, and attempted) the rates were 3% for males and 9% for females; and for mixed sexual abuse (more than one type of abuse occurring) the rates were for 8% males and 15% for females (Barth *et al.*, 2013). Females therefore have a twofold or threefold risk compared to males to be sexually abused in childhood, and about one in ten women is confronted with this experience. Children with disabilities are more likely to be victims of sexual abuse.

The majority of children know their abuser, usually because they are in their family, or occasionally because they have been befriended as part of a grooming process. The majority of abusers are male (85–95%) and stepfathers are overrepresented. The extent of sexual abuse by women is not known; a few carry out abuse in conjunction with a man, and those that abuse alone are more likely to abuse boys. Sexual abuse by children and adolescents, mostly boys, has become widely recognized and is no longer considered an acceptable variant of childhood or adolescent sexual development. Sixty per cent of contact sexual abuse reported by children in the UK was perpetrated by other children and young people under the age of 18 years (Glaser *et al.*, 2015). Many adult abusers report the onset of their abusive activities in adolescence.

Clinical features

The presentation of child sexual abuse depends on the type of sexual act and the relationship of the offender to the child. Children are more likely to report abuse when the offender is a stranger. It might come to light when a child talks about it to a friend, relative, or teacher, or it is suspected on the basis of less specific indicators described below. Spontaneous and intentional disclosures are likely to be credible. Specific indicators include age-inappropriate sexualized behaviour, rarer genital physical signs, sexually transmitted diseases, and pregnancy in a young girl, especially when the identity of the father is not clear. Non-specific indicators include sudden onset of unexplained difficulties in a previously untroubled child, such as distractibility, educational deterioration, social isolation, aggressiveness, low self-esteem, marked unhappiness, disturbed sleep and nightmares, fearfulness, and separation anxiety. Depression, running away, deliberate self-harm, and drug and alcohol misuse may arise later (Glaser *et al.*, 2015). There may also be physical symptoms in the urogenital or anal area, pregnancy, and behavioural or emotional disturbance. When abuse occurs within the family, marital and other family problems are common.

Effects of sexual abuse

Childhood sexual abuse is a significant risk factor for mental health disorders in childhood, adolescence, and adulthood as well as having effects on physical health.

Effects in childhood and adolescence: not all children will develop difficulties and some will only develop them later, but a wide range of difficulties, which may not appear immediately, has been found with considerable effect sizes: depression, anxiety, PTSD, self-harm, low self-esteem, conduct disorder, bulimia, promiscuity, and sexual victimization of other children. It may lead to unwanted pregnancy. The worst prognosis is for children younger than 7 years when the abuse takes place and also in those who have negative self-attributions about the abuse, including self-blame and shame, children who have experienced penetration in the abuse and those who have depressed parents.

Effects in adulthood are significant and have been estimated to contribute to around 13% of all adult psychopathology. For example, in an Australian study, 23% of adult survivors of childhood sexual abuse required long-term mental health services as compared with 7% of a comparison population (Cutajar *et al.*, 2010). The effects include depressed mood, low self-esteem, self-harm, difficulties in relationships, and sexual maladjustment in the form of either hypersensitivity or sexual inhibition. The effects of abuse are generally greater when the abuse has involved physical violence and penetrative intercourse. Some of the long-term effects may be related to the events surrounding the disclosure of the abuse, including any legal proceedings, and to other problems in the family, such as neglect of the children and sexual deviance or substance abuse. Nevertheless, even when these other factors are controlled for, sexual abuse in childhood seems to be associated with psychiatric disorder later in life, especially with *depressive disorders, anxiety disorders*, and *personality disorders* (Glaser *et al.*, 2015).

Aetiology

Sexual abuse of children occurs in all socioeconomic groups, and studies have shown no ethnic differences in rates. Although socioeconomic status is unrelated to the incidence of childhood sexual abuse, there is an overrepresentation of low socioeconomic groups in clinic samples (Glaser *et al.*, 2015). There are several preconditions that make sexual abuse more likely. In the abuser, these include deviant sexual motivation, impulsivity, a lack of conscience, and a lack of external restraints (e.g. cultural tolerance); in the child, they include a vulnerability by virtue of age, disability, social isolation, and previous sexual abuse, which can be identified and preyed upon by abusers.

Assessment

It is important to be ready to detect sexual abuse and to give serious attention to any complaint by a child of being abused in this way. When abuse has been established, it is important to assess whether it is likely to continue if the child remains at home and, if so, how dangerous it is likely to be. It is also important not to make the diagnosis without adequate evidence, and this requires social investigation of the family as well as psychological and physical examination of the child.

The child should be interviewed sympathetically and encouraged to describe what has happened. Drawings or toys may help younger children to give a description, but great care must be taken to ensure that they are not used in a way that suggests to the child events that have not taken place. Young children can recall events accurately, but they are more suggestible than adults. Interviewing is difficult, and, whenever possible, it should be carried out by a child psychiatrist or social worker with special experience. See Jones (2009) for further advice on interviewing.

In the UK, responsibility for child protection rests with social services, to whom suspicions of abuse and actual abuse must be reported. Multidisciplinary involvement, often including the police and the judicial system, is usually needed to establish whether abuse has taken place and what the appropriate response should be. As with the physical abuse, the first priority is to protect the child and other children who might be at risk. The arrangements vary in different countries, and readers should find out how they apply in the country in which they are working.

Management

The initial management and the measures to protect the child are similar to those for physical abuse (see Box 16.9), including a decision about separating the child from the family. There are particular difficulties involved in intervening with families in which sexual abuse has occurred. These include a marked tendency to deny the seriousness of the abuse and other family problems, and in some cases deviant sexual attitudes and behaviour of other family members, possibly including other children. Not all children require therapy; however, a minimum requirement is for the child to have an appropriate narrative about their abuse and to have access to an identified person who believes the child and is able to listen to the child supportively and uncritically. Several meta-analyses have found large to moderate effect sizes for psychotherapy, group therapy, and cognitive behaviour therapy combined with supportive, psychodynamic, or play therapy.

The treatment of child and adolescent abusers requires coordinated multidisciplinary support with child protection services. Cognitive behaviour therapy individually and in groups has been used, as has structured group work.

Ethical and legal problems in child and adolescent psychiatry

As well as the ethical and legal problems related to the treatment of adults and which are discussed in Chapter 4 and elsewhere, the following issues are particularly likely to arise in the care of children with psychiatric disorders.

Conflicts of interest

In general, *the interests of the child take precedence over those of the parents*. This principle is most obvious, and most easily followed, in cases of child abuse. In other cases, the decision is more difficult—for example, when a depressed mother is neglecting her child and is likely to become more depressed if substitute care is arranged. Such problems can usually be resolved by discussion with the parents, and between the professionals who are caring for the child and for the parent.

Confidentiality

The care of children often involves collaboration between medical and social services, and sometimes with teachers. Different agencies may have different policies about the confidentiality of records, and doctors should take account of these differences when deciding what information to disclose.

Consent

In each country, the law decides an age below which the child is deemed not to have capacity and so parents give consent on behalf of the child. Below this age, the

---

Box 16.9 Steps in the assessment and management of child sexual abuse

1. Suspicion and recognition; referral to child protection services (often social services and police).
2. Establish whether immediate protection is needed.
3. Plan investigation: interagency discussion, interview child, medical examination, family assessment.
4. Initial multiagency child protection meeting.
5. Investigation and draw up protection plan.
6. Plan implementation and review.
7. Legal proceedings.
8. Therapeutic work.

Reproduced from Glaser D, Child sexual abuse, In: Thapar A. *et al.*, Rutter's Child and Adolescent Psychiatry, 6th edn., pp. 376-389, Copyright (2015), with permission from John Wiley & Sons.

child's assent should be obtained, if possible, as this will aid treatment, but if the child refuses the parents can decide. This problem arises, for example, when an adolescent under the legal age of consent refuses treatment for anorexia nervosa. The parents can also refuse treatment; however, their right to do so is linked to their duty to protect the child. In cases in which the parents' refusal appears not to be in the interests of the child, countries generally have provisions for a decision by a court of law.

Some of the complexities of English law can be mentioned briefly to illustrate the problems that have to be resolved in all legal systems. A fuller account of these and other issues is given by Hale *et al.* (2015). Readers are advised to find out for their respective countries the age at which a 'minor' can consent to their own treatment and the rights of parents when it comes to treatment.

In English law, the age from which people are judged legally capable of giving or refusing consent is 18 years. However, English law recognizes that most of those aged between 16 and 18 years have the capacity to give consent to receive treatment, and allows them to do so without the need for consent by a parent. The position is less clear when a 16- or 17-year-old does not consent to treatment, but it is probably the case that the parents' consent is sufficient. The decision in each case is likely to depend on the consequences of refusal; the more severe these are, the more likely it is that a court would accept that the child's refusal can be overridden by the parents. Further complexities arise with children under 16 years of age, some of whom are competent to give consent to certain treatments. There is no general

assumption of competence at this age, and it has to be established in the individual case, but, if it is established, the minor can give consent.

The question arose most notably with regard to the provision of contraception without the additional consent of a parent. In the *Gillick case* it was ruled that, in English law, a sufficiently competent minor could consent without the need to obtain the consent of the parent (now called *Gillick competence* and related *Fraser guidelines*). It is probable, however, that with certain more invasive and risky treatments, the consent of a parent could be legally necessary, as well as clinically desirable. If a minor under the age of 16 years refuses treatment, this can be overruled by the parents if refusal is likely to result in harm. A final complexity concerns the definition of a parent. This problem arises, for example, when the person accompanying the child is not the person recognized by the law as having parental responsibility. For example, in English law, a father who is not married to the mother does not automatically have legal responsibility.

Consent for research poses similar problems for patients below the legal age of consent. In most countries, parents consent on behalf of their children, and they may find it difficult to balance the risks to the child against the benefits, which are usually not to their child but to other children who might be treated for the same condition in the future. It is important that children, however, give their assent to the research and that they are able to discuss the issues and any concerns they might have, including with a person other than the individual who is requesting the consent (e.g. a nurse in their usual clinic).

Appendix: Basic elements in child and adolescent psychiatric assessments

The format and extent of an assessment will depend on the nature of the presenting problem and the age of the child. The role of the parental history and information from other sources, including education and other carers, will be important in child psychiatry. The following scheme is adapted from Leckman et al. (2015), which should be consulted for further information.

1 Reason for referral: why this child and why now? Nature, frequency, and severity of presenting problem(s). Situations in which it occurs. Provoking and ameliorating factors. Stresses thought by parents to be important. Need to use this initial time to build therapeutic relationship and also gauge opinions on potential treatment options.

2 Child's strengths, talents, and interests, and environmental supports.

3 Presence of other comorbid problems or complaints.

   (a) Physical. Headaches, stomach ache. Hearing, vision. Seizures, faints, or other types of episodes.

   (b) Eating, sleeping, or elimination problems.

   (c) Relationships with other children. Special friends. Experience of bullying or negative experiences with peers (including on social media).

   (d) Level of activity, attention span, concentration.

   (e) Mood, energy level, sadness, misery.

   (f) Response to frustration. Temper tantrums.

   (g) Antisocial behaviour. Aggression, stealing, truancy.

   (h) Educational attainments, attitude to school attendance.

   (i) Sexual interest and behaviour.

   (j) Any other symptoms, tics, etc.

4 Family history, current structure, and functioning (construct genogram).

   (a) Parents. Ages, occupations. Current physical and emotional state. History of physical or psychiatric disorder. Whereabouts of grandparents. Quality of parental relationship. Sharing of attitudes over child's problems. Quality of parent–child relationship. Positive interaction: mutual enjoyment. Parental level of criticism, hostility, rejection.

   (b) Siblings. Ages, presence of problems.

   (c) Home circumstances: sleeping arrangements.

   (d) Overall pattern of family relationships. Alliance, communication. Exclusion, scapegoating. Intergenerational confusion.

5 Developmental, educational, and medical history, including possible traumatic events and current level of development (can include review of birth and paediatric records, education evaluations).

   (a) Pregnancy issues, delivery, and state at birth, early mother–child relationship, postpartum depression, early feeding patterns. Milestones. Obtain exact details only if outside range of normal.

   (b) Language: comprehension, complexity of speech.

   (c) Spatial ability.

   (d) Motor coordination, clumsiness.

   (e) Past illnesses and injuries. Hospitalizations.

6 Personal history.

   (a) Early temperamental characteristics. Easy or difficult, irregular, restless baby and toddler.

   (b) Separations lasting a week or more. Nature of substitute care.

   (c) Schooling history. Ease of attendance. Educational progress.

   (d) Use of social media/screen time: how much, which sites, bad experiences online.

   (e) Gender preference and sexual identity.

7 Mental state examination

   (a) Appearance. Signs of dysmorphism. Nutritional state. Evidence of neglect, bruising, cuts, etc.

   (b) Activity level. Involuntary movements. Capacity to concentrate.

   (c) Mood. Expression of signs of sadness, misery, anxiety, tension.

   (d) Rapport, capacity to relate to clinician. Eye contact. Spontaneous talk. Inhibition and disinhibition.

   (e) Relationship with parents. Affection shown. Resentment. Ease of separation.

   (f) Habits and mannerisms.

   (g) Presence of delusions, hallucinations, thought disorder.

   (h) Level of awareness. Evidence of minor epilepsy.

8 Physical and neurological examination of child—only indicated if concern of presence of any genetic, medical, metabolic, endocrine, or neurological disorders that may impact the child's course of illness and treatment; or conduct as a baseline before treatment.

  (a) Note any facial asymmetry.

  (b) Eye movements. Ask the child to follow a moving finger and observe eye movement for jerkiness, incoordination.

  (c) Finger–thumb apposition. Ask the child to press the tip of each finger against the thumb in rapid succession. Observe clumsiness, weakness.

  (d) Copying patterns. Drawing a man.

  (e) Observe grip and dexterity in drawing.

  (f) Jumping up and down on the spot.

  (g) Hopping.

  (h) Hearing. Capacity of child to repeat numbers whispered 2 metres behind them.

Further reading

Goodman R and Scott S (2012). *Child and Adolescent Psychiatry*, 3rd edn. Wiley-Blackwell, Oxford. (A concise introduction to the subject.)

Megitt C (2012). *Child Development: An illustrated guide: birth to 19 years*, 3rd edn. Pearson Education Canada. (An accessible source of information about child development.)

Thapar A, Pine D, Leckman, J *et al.* (eds) (2015). *Rutter's Child and Adolescent Psychiatry*, 6th edn. Blackwell, Oxford. (An established, comprehensive work of reference.)

CHAPTER 17

Intellectual disability (mental retardation)

Introduction

This chapter is concerned with a general outline of the features, epidemiology, and aetiology of intellectual disability, the organization of services, and, more specifically, with the psychiatric disorders that affect these people. Intellectual disability refers to a developmental disability presenting in infancy or the early childhood years, although in some cases it cannot be diagnosed until the child is older than 5 years of age, when standardized measures of developmental skills become more reliable and valid (Moeschler *et al.*, 2014).

Many of the psychiatric problems of children with intellectual disability are similar to those of children of normal intelligence; an account of these problems is given in Chapter 16.

Terminology

Over the years, several terms have been applied to people with intellectual impairment from early life. In the nineteenth and early twentieth centuries, the word 'idiot' was used for people with severe intellectual impairment, and 'imbecile' for those with moderate impairment. The special study and care of such people was known as the field of *mental deficiency*. When these words came to carry stigma, they were replaced by the terms *mental* *subnormality* and *mental retardation*. The terms *mental handicap* and *learning disability* have also been widely used, but now the term *intellectual disability* is generally preferred and has been adopted in DSM-5 (and is used in this chapter). However, the term mental retardation is still used in ICD-10, and, along with learning disability, is employed in many countries. Moreover, in the USA the term learning disability is generally applied to dyslexia and similar forms of specific disability, rather than to intellectual disability.

Intellectual disability is sometimes divided into *syndromic* and *non-syndromic* forms. *Syndromic intellectual disability* refers to the presence of additional medical or behavioural features (which allow a 'syndrome' to be diagnosed); if not, the term *non-syndromic intellectual disability* is used.

The development of ideas about intellectual disability

A fundamental distinction, first made by Esquirol in 1845, is drawn between general intellectual impairment starting in early childhood (*intellectual disability*) and intellectual impairment developing later in life (*dementia*). Complementing these two categories, *acquired brain injury (ABI)* is the term used to describe individuals who develop an intellectual disability after birth, either because of trauma (e.g. following a head injury) or that may be non-traumatic (e.g. because of a brain tumour).

Early in the twentieth century, Binet's tests of intelligence provided quantitative criteria for ascertaining intellectual disability. These tests also made it possible to identify lesser degrees of the condition that might not be obvious otherwise. Unfortunately, it was widely assumed at the time that people with such lesser degrees of intellectual impairment were socially incompetent and required institutional care.

Similar views were reflected in the legislation of the time. For example, in England and Wales the Idiots Act of 1886 made a simple distinction between idiocy (more severe) and imbecility (less severe). In 1913, the Mental Deficiency Act added a third category for people who 'from an early age display some permanent mental defect coupled with strong vicious or criminal propensities in which punishment has had little or no effect'. As a result of this legislation, people of normal or near normal intelligence were admitted to hospital for long periods simply because their behaviour deviated from the values of society.

Although in the past the use of social criteria clearly led to abuse, it is unsatisfactory to define intellectual disability in terms of intelligence alone. Social criteria must

be included, since a distinction must be made between people who can lead a normal or near-normal life and those who cannot. DSM-5 places intellectual disability in the broader category of neurodevelopmental disorders and defines intellectual disability as involving 'impairments of general mental abilities that impact adaptive functioning in three domains, or areas'. These domains determine how well an individual can cope with everyday life and include communication and social skills, personal independence, and school/work functioning. The disorder is considered chronic and often co-occurs with other mental conditions like depression, attention-deficit hyperactivity disorder (ADHD), and autism spectrum disorder (ASD).

Having defined the disorder with a focus on adaptive functioning and ability to meet developmental and sociocultural standards, it is subdivided by severity levels according to adaptive functioning into mild, moderate, severe, and profound categories, placing some weight on standardized IQ testing. The categories broadly map onto the ICD-10 subtypes that are made according to IQ: mild (IQ 50–70); moderate (IQ 35–49); severe (IQ 20–34); profound (IQ below 20).

The original World Health Organization (WHO) classification of impairment, disability, and handicap is useful when considering the problems of people with intellectual disability. (The WHO now employs a more positive terminology, with *activity* replacing 'disability', and *participation* replacing 'handicap'.) The impairment is of the central nervous system, and the disability (or limitation of activity) is in learning and acquiring new skills. The extent to which impairment leads to disability (limits activity) depends, in part, on experiences in the family and at school, and on the correction of associated problems such as deafness. The final stage, namely handicap (or limited participation), depends on the degree of disability and on other factors such as the support that is provided.

Educationalists use other terms, and these too differ between countries. In the UK, the term is *special educational needs*, whereas in the USA mild, moderate, and severe cognitive impairment is most commonly used, with 90% of the children with intellectual disability falling in the mild category, which approximately equates to an IQ lying between 55 and 70.

Epidemiology of intellectual disability

Level of IQ is a key criterion in defining intellectual disability, with IQ tests designed to be normally distributed with a mean of 100 and a standard deviation of 15. In

DSM-5 intellectual disability is considered to be approximately two standard deviations or more below the population, which equals an IQ score of about 70 or below, approximately 2.3% of the population (Simonoff *et al.*, 2015). Placing the diagnostic criteria on both IQ and adaptive functioning allows for considerable individual differences in presentation and diagnosis, as these differences can be within syndromes and dependent on family functioning and levels of engagement with activities of daily living; therefore the boundaries between the categories of mild, moderate, and severe intellectual disability are not firmly fixed. A current estimate for the UK is 9–14 in 1000 children, and 3–8 in 1000 adults (Cooper and Smiley, 2009).

Variability in apparent prevalence rates is due partly to experimental factors such as methods of ascertainment and definition, but also reflects genuine differences across time and place. In recent years, the *incidence* has fallen substantially, because of the improvement in preventable prenatal and perinatal causes of severe intellectual disabilities. However, the *prevalence* has not fallen, and in fact is expected to rise by over 10% by 2020. The preserved or increasing prevalence despite reduced incidence reflects two factors. First, people with intellectual disability, particularly those with Down's syndrome, are living longer. This has also affected the age distribution of people with severe intellectual disability, so that the

numbers of adults have increased. Secondly, improvements in maternal and neonatal care, especially those born extremely premature (below 32 weeks' gestation) are resulting in a growing number of children with intellectual disability, especially those in the severe and profound categories, who have survived significant events.

A further important point regarding the prevalence of intellectual disability was made by Tizard (1964), who drew attention to the distinction between 'administrative' prevalence and 'true' prevalence. He defined the former as 'the numbers for whom services would be required in a community which made provision for all who needed them'. In practice, the term usually means the number with needs who are known to the service providers. It is estimated that less than 50% of all such people require special provision. Administrative prevalence is higher in lower socioeconomic groups and in childhood, when more patients need services. It falls after the age of 16 years because there is continuing slow intellectual development and gradual social adjustment.

The clinical features of the individual syndromes that cause intellectual disability and the epidemiology of psychiatric disorders for those with intellectual disability are covered later in the chapter.

Clinical features of intellectual disability

The most frequent manifestation of intellectual disability is uniformly low performance on all kinds of intellectual tasks, including learning, short-term memory, the use of concepts, and problem-solving (see Table 17.1). Specific abnormalities may lead to particular difficulties. For example, lack of visuospatial skills may cause practical difficulties, such as inability to dress, or there may be disproportionate difficulties with language or social interaction, both of which are strongly associated with behaviour disorders. Among children with intellectual disability, the common behaviour problems of childhood tend to occur when they are older and more physically developed than children in the general population, and the problems last for longer. Such behaviour problems usually improve slowly as the child grows older, but may be replaced by problems that start in adulthood.

Mild intellectual disability (IQ 50–70)

People with mild learning disability account for about 85% of those with learning disability. Usually their appearance is unremarkable and any sensory or motor

deficits are slight. Most people in this group develop more or less normal language abilities and social behaviour during the preschool years, and their learning disability may never be formally identified. In adulthood, most people with mild learning disability can live independently in ordinary surroundings, although they may need help in parenting and coping with family responsibilities, housing, and employment, or when under unusual stress.

Moderate intellectual disability (IQ 35–49)

People in this group account for about 10% of those with learning disability. Many have better receptive than expressive language skills, which is a potent cause of frustration and behaviour problems. Speech is usually relatively simple, and is often better understood by people who know the patient well. Many make use of simplified signing systems such as Makaton sign language. Activities of daily living such as dressing, feeding, and attention to hygiene can be acquired over time, but other activities of daily living, such as the use of money

Table 17.1 Features of mild, moderate, and severe/profound intellectual disability

	Mild	Moderate	Severe/profound
IQ range	69–50	49–35	<35
Percentage of cases	85%	10%	5%
Ability to self-care	Independent	Need some help	Limited
Language	Reasonable	Limited	Basic or none
Reading and writing	Reasonable	Basic	Minimal or none
Ability to work	Semi-skilled	Unskilled, supervised	Supervised basic tasks
Social skills	Normal	Moderate	Few
Physical problems	Rare	Sometimes	Common
Specific cause discovered	Sometimes	Often	Usually

and road sense, generally require support. Similarly, supported employment and residential provision are the rule.

Severe intellectual disability (IQ 20–34)

It is difficult to estimate IQ accurately when the score is below 34 because of the difficulty in administering the tests in a valid manner to individuals in this group. Estimates suggest that people with severe learning disability account for about 3–4% of the learning disabled. In the preschool years their development is usually greatly slowed. Eventually many people can be helped to look after themselves under close supervision, and to communicate in a simple way—for example, by using objects of reference. As adults they can undertake simple tasks and engage in limited social activities, but they need supervision and a clear structure to their lives.

Profound intellectual disability (IQ below 20)

People in this group account for 1–2% of those with intellectual disability. Development across a range of domains tends to be around the level expected of a 12-month-old infant. Accordingly, people with profound intellectual disability are a highly vulnerable group who require considerable support and supervision, even for simple activities of daily living.

Physical disorders among people with intellectual disability

People with intellectual disabilities experience a greater variety and complexity of physical health problems than the rest of the population, but may not complain of feeling ill, nor be able to articulate their symptoms, and conditions may be noticed only because of changes in behaviour. The prevalence of obesity among young people with intellectual disability is almost double that of the general population and it is unclear if this is because of mealtime behaviours and/or infrequent physical activity (Segal 2016). Clinicians should be aware of the associations between certain intellectual disability syndromes and physical illness (e.g. Down's syndrome;

see page 497), and that people with an intellectual disability are more likely to die prematurely. A UK review of deaths of over 200 people with intellectual disabilities showed that nearly a quarter were younger than 50 years when they died, and the median age at death was 64 years—for males 13 years younger and for females 20 years younger than the median age of death for the general population. Contributory factors to the premature deaths included poor health care and living in inappropriate accommodation (Heslop *et al.*, 2014). With the exception of people with severe and multiple disabilities or Down's syndrome, the life expectancy of this group now more closely approximates to that of the general population. Middle and old age, which until 30 years ago were not recognized in this population, are now important parts of the life course of these individuals. Older adults with intellectual disabilities form a small but significant and growing proportion of older people in the community (Coppus, 2013).

Sensory and motor disabilities and incontinence are the most important physical disorders in people with intellectual disability. People with severe intellectual disability (especially children) usually have several of these problems. Only one-third are continent, ambulant, and without severe behaviour problems. Around 25% are highly dependent on other people. Among those with mild intellectual disability, similar problems occur, but less frequently. Nevertheless, they are important because they determine whether special educational programmes are needed. Sensory disorders add an important additional obstacle to normal cognitive development. Motor disabilities include spasticity, ataxia, and athetosis. Ear infections and dental caries are common in this population.

Epilepsy is a frequent and clinically important problem in intellectual disability. Around 22% of people with intellectual disability have a history of epilepsy, compared with 5% in the general population (Robertson *et al.*, 2015). The prevalence increases with the severity of intellectual disabilities, with lifetime history of epilepsy estimated to be 12% in people with Down's syndrome, 15% in mild to moderate intellectual disability, and 30% in severe and profound intellectual disability. The risk appears higher among those with additional neurological diagnoses, such as cerebral palsy and those with ASD. Epilepsy is also more commonly associated with fragile X syndrome, tuberous sclerosis, Angelman syndrome, and Rett syndrome, while certain epilepsy syndromes, such as West syndrome and Lennox–Gastaut syndrome, are more common among people with intellectual disability. The proportion of epilepsy cases that are drug-resistant is also greater among people with intellectual disability. Of particular concern is the incidence of *sudden unexplained death in epilepsy (SUDEP)*, which is estimated to be 1 in 295 per year in the intellectual disability population, compared with 1 in 1000 per year in epilepsy patients in the general population.

For a review of the aetiology, diagnosis, and treatment of epilepsy in intellectual disability, see Iivanainen (2009).

Psychiatric disorders among people with intellectual disability

In the past, psychiatric disorder among the learning disabled was often viewed as different from that seen in people of normal intelligence. One view was that people with intellectual disability did not develop emotional disorders. Another view was that they developed these disorders, but that the causes were biological rather than psychosocial. It is now generally agreed that people with intellectual disability experience psychiatric disturbances similar to those that affect the general population. However, the symptoms are sometimes modified by low intelligence, and may not be easily recognized or communicated. Therefore, when diagnosing psychiatric disorder among people with intellectual disability, more emphasis may have to be given to behaviour and less to reports of mental phenomena than is usually the case.

For reviews of psychiatric disorders in intellectual disability, see Einfeld *et al.* (2011) and Dosen (2009), and for a review of their clinical assessment, see Holland (2009) and Volkmar *et al.* (2014). Here we outline their epidemiology and clinical characteristics. Their assessment and treatment are covered later in the chapter.

Epidemiology and features of psychiatric disorder in people with intellectual disability

Among people with intellectual disability, published rates of psychiatric disorder vary widely, because of methodological limitations in studies with case ascertainment, detection, and definition. Early studies primarily had the selection bias of including mainly people from institutions. Although more recent studies have included people from the community, it is difficult, if not impossible, to detect all adults with intellectual disability, particularly those with mild disability. The diagnostic criteria used in different studies have also varied—some used screening instruments, while others used structured diagnostic instruments. In addition, studies have varied in terms of whether they included behaviour disorders in the count of psychiatric disorders. Having noted these caveats, recent surveys report a prevalence of 16–45% among adults with intellectual disability (Cooper and Smiley, 2009; Morgan *et al.*, 2008). Studies in children with psychiatric disorders demonstrate a high prevalence of intellectual disability, with estimates that 50% of children with ASD have intellectual disability and 15–20% of children with ADHD having intellectual disability (Einfeld *et al.*, 2011; Simonoff *et al.*, 2007). Other disorders with higher rates in individuals with intellectual disability include schizophrenia, bipolar disorder, and dementia. Behavioural problems are particularly common, especially hyperactivity, stereotypies, and self-injury (Deb *et al.*, 2001).

In general, the aetiology of psychiatric disorders in intellectual disability is similar to that in the general population, in that they result from a complex and non-deterministic combination of biological, psychological, and social factors. However, there are some specific factors that add additional risk and complexity to the incidence and detection of psychiatric disorders. Although the direction of effects can be difficult to unpick, intellectual disability and psychiatric disorders might have shared genetic and other risk factors; they might result from medical adversities that affect the brain (e.g. epilepsy, cerebral palsy); they might come from environments of increased family psychosocial adversity; and the intellectual disability itself might impact on the individual's capacity to communicate, understand their environment, and respond flexibly to various situations (Simonoff *et al.*, 2015). Some of these factors are summarized in Table 17.2. Furthermore, the complexity of the presentation of psychiatric disorders

in those with intellectual disability reflecting the often behavioural, medical, and neuropsychiatric components of an individual's specific intellectual disability contributes to why a psychiatrist is often a key member of the multidisciplinary team helping to manage the needs of someone with an intellectual disability experiencing difficulties.

Psychotic disorders

The epidemiological studies available suggest an increased prevalence of psychotic disorders among individuals with intellectual disability. Schizophrenia affects 3–4% of people with intellectual disability, compared with less than 1% in the general population (Deb *et al.*, 2001). The overlap between the two conditions largely reflects shared genetic factors. Clinically, delusions may be less elaborate than in patients with schizophrenia of normal intelligence, hallucinations may have a simpler content, and thought disorder is difficult to identify. When IQ is less than 45, it is difficult to make the diagnosis with any certainty. Furthermore, some of the symptoms of underlying brain damage, such as stereotyped movements and social withdrawal, may wrongly suggest schizophrenia, so a comparison of current with previous behaviour is always valuable.

The diagnosis of schizophrenia should be considered as one of several possibilities when intellectual or social functioning worsens without evidence of an organic cause, and especially if any new behaviour is odd and out of keeping. When there is continuing doubt, a trial of antipsychotic drugs is sometimes appropriate. The principles of treatment of schizophrenia in people with intellectual disability are the same as those for patients of normal intelligence (see Chapter 11); however, as

Table 17.2 Summary of factors in those with intellectual disability associated with psychiatric illness

Biological	Psychological	Social
Genetic syndromes ('behavioural phenotypes')	Coping style	Living circumstances
Epilepsy	Self-esteem	Daily structure and routine
Autism spectrum disorder	Social comparison	Social support
ADHD		
Physical illness		
Medication		

Adapted from Woodbury-Smith M, Hollins S, Psychiatric illness and disorders of intellectual development: a dual diagnosis. In: Woodbury-Smith, M, Clinical Topics in Disorders of Intellectual Development, Copyright (2015), with permission from The Royal College of Psychiatrists.

with all pharmacological interventions in those with intellectual disability it is important to be aware that often lower therapeutic doses are needed and titration should be slower.

Mood disorder

The rate of depressive disorders is estimated to lie between 3% and 6%—slightly higher than that of the general population (Davies and Oliver, 2014). However, people with intellectual disability are less likely to complain of mood changes or to express depressive ideation. Diagnosis has to be made mainly on the basis of an appearance of sadness, changes in appetite and sleep, and behavioural changes of retardation or agitation. Severely depressed patients with adequate verbal abilities may describe hallucinations or delusions. Of note, depressive disorder occurs commonly in association with Down's syndrome during late adolescence and early adulthood, independent of life events (Collacott et al., 1998). Mania has to be diagnosed on the basis of hyperactivity and behavioural signs of excitement, irritability, or nervousness.

The differential diagnosis of mood disorder in people with intellectual disability includes thyroid dysfunction, which is especially prevalent in people with Down's syndrome, and grief (Brickell and Munir, 2008).

The rate of suicide in people with moderate and more severe intellectual disability is lower than in the general population. The rate of deliberate self-harm is less certain, because it is difficult to decide patients' intentions and their knowledge of the likely effects of the injurious behaviour.

The principles of treatment of mood disorders are the same as those for people of normal intelligence (see Chapter 9).

Anxiety disorders and related conditions

Adjustment disorders are common among people with intellectual disability, occurring when there are changes in the routine of their lives. Anxiety disorders are also frequent, especially at times of stress, and social anxiety is often seen in individuals with fragile X syndrome (Cordeiro et al., 2010). Obsessive–compulsive disorders are also found. Conversion and dissociative symptoms are sometimes florid, taking forms that can be interpreted in terms of the patient's understanding of illness. Somatoform disorders and other causes of functional somatic symptoms can result in persistent requests for medical attention. Treatment is usually directed mainly to bringing about adjustments in the patient's environment, and reassurance. Counselling, at an appropriate level of complexity, can also be helpful.

Eating disorders

Overeating and unusual dietary preferences are frequent among people with intellectual disability. Abnormal eating behaviours, including *pica* (Chapter 13), are not uncommon, but classical eating disorders appear to be less common than in the general population. Overeating and obesity are features of Prader–Willi syndrome (see below).

Personality disorder

Personality disorder is difficult to diagnose among people with intellectual disability. In this population there is a considerable overlap between the diagnosis of behavioural disturbance and that of personality disorder (Reid and Ballinger, 1987). Sometimes the personality disorder leads to greater problems in management than those caused by the intellectual disability itself. The general approach is as described on page 409, although with more emphasis on finding an environment to match the patient's temperament, and less on attempts to bring about change through self-understanding.

Delirium and dementia

Delirium. This may occur as a response to infection, medication, and other precipitating factors. As in people of normal intelligence, delirium in people with intellectual disability is more common in childhood and in old age than at other ages. Disturbed behaviour due to delirium is sometimes the first indication of physical illness. Delirium may also occur as a side effect of drugs (especially antiepileptics, antidepressants, and other psychotropic medication).

Dementia. As the life expectancy of people with intellectual disability increases, dementia in later life is becoming more common. Alzheimer's disease is particularly common among people with Down's syndrome (see page 501), but dementia is also more commonly in other elderly intellectually disabled people, with a prevalence of 18.3% in those over the age of 65 years, making it 2–3 times more common in this population (Strydom et al., 2009). Prevalence rates do not differ between mild, moderate, and severe intellectually disabled groups. Dementia in people with intellectual disability may initially present with seizures, or with the usual progressive decline in intellectual and social functioning, which has to be distinguished from conditions such as depression and delirium.

Disorders that are usually first diagnosed in childhood and adolescence

Many of the disorders in this category are more frequent in children with intellectual disability than in the general population, and they are more likely to continue into adulthood. It is important to be aware that relatively specific developmental disorders of scholastic skills, speech, and language and motor function may occur alongside more global intellectual disability.

Autism spectrum disorder and attention-deficit hyperactivity disorder

Hyperactive behaviour and autistic-like behaviour are frequent symptoms of intellectual disability. In addition, the diagnoses of ASD and ADHD are more common for those with intellectual disability than among the general population. There is a particular comorbidity between intellectual disability and ASDs, probably reflecting an overlap in their aetiology, especially with regard to genetic factors (Mefford *et al.*, 2012).

Abnormal movements

Stereotypes, mannerisms, and rhythmic movement disorders (including head banging and rocking) occur in about 40% of children and 20% of adults with severe intellectual disability. Repeated self-injurious behaviours are less common but important. There is a specific association with Lesch–Nyhan syndrome, in which the biting away of the corner of a lip is common. Prader–Willi syndrome is strongly associated with a pattern of self-injury where patients pick at their skin.

Behaviour that challenges

The term *behaviour that challenges* (or *problem behaviour*) is used to describe problematic behaviour that is relatively specific to intellectual disability and is associated with neurodevelopmental disorders such as ASD. It describes behaviour of an intensity or frequency sufficient to impair the physical safety of a person with intellectual disability, to pose a danger to others, or to make participation in the community difficult (Simonoff *et al.*, 2015). Those who present with behaviour that challenges are often marginalized, stigmatized, disempowered, and excluded from mainstream society as it often provokes punitive or restrictive responses (Banks *et al.*, 2007). It is probable that around 20% of intellectually disabled children and adolescents, and 15% of intellectually disabled adults have some form of behaviour that challenges. The causes of such behaviour are listed in Box 17.1. Whenever possible, the primary cause should be understood and treated. It is essential that the behaviour is understood in the context of that individual and their environment, and therefore any intervention must address the person, environment, and the interaction between the two. The person might be expressing unhappiness in their current

> ### Box 17.1 Causes of behaviour that challenges
>
> Physical: pain, discomfort, malaise
>
> Psychiatric and neuropsychiatric disorder: mood disorders, psychosis, anxiety, obsessive–compulsive disorders, ADHD, dementia
>
> Psychological trauma: reaction to abuse or loss; or wish to escape an unpleasant situation
>
> Communication difficulties: hearing loss, unclear communication, insufficient vocabulary or means of expression, difficulties understanding communication of others
>
> Phenotype-related behaviours: Prader–Willi syndrome, Lesch–Nyhan syndrome, Williams syndrome
>
> Understimulation or overstimulation
>
> Desire for attention or other reward
>
> Side effects of medication

environment and the complexities of assessment might require a comprehensive and multidisciplinary assessment, including a functional assessment of behaviour, underlying medical and organic factors, psychological/psychiatric factors, communication, and social/environmental factors.

Intervention should be delivered in a person-centred context and a framework of positive behavioural support. This can include proactive and reactive strategies, psychotherapy, communication, positive programming, physical and/or medical, and psychopharmacological. For more information see Banks *et al.* (2007) and Emerson and Einfeld (2011). Behavioural treatment (see page 510) is the most widely used treatment. Behaviour that challenges is more likely to be encountered in the family home, in small-scale community settings, or in environments that are poorly organized and unable to respond well to the needs of the person. Therefore the response of those in their environment is key and, as these interventions are often provided in the places where the behaviour usually appears, competency-based training and professional support is often required for carers but, in severe cases, a residential unit might be needed.

Sleep disorders

Impaired sleep is common in people with intellectual disability, with prevalence estimates ranging from 9% to

34% (van de Wouw *et al.*, 2012). Serious sleep difficulties, such as obstructive sleep apnoea, excessive daytime sleepiness, and parasomnias, have a reported prevalence of 9%, and can be a source of considerable distress. Furthermore, sleep disorders may be associated with subsequent challenging behaviours and a worsening of cognitive impairment. The high rate of sleep disorders is accounted for by five factors:

- Coexisting damage to brain structures that are important for the sleep–wake cycle.
- Epileptic seizures that start during sleep.

- Epilepsy-related sleep instability that disrupts sleep architecture.
- Structural abnormalities in the upper respiratory tract causing sleep apnoea (particularly common among people with Down's syndrome).
- Poor sleep hygiene.

Treatment follows the usual principles of identifying and treating the cause, and non-pharmacological interventions such as improving sleep hygiene (see Chapter 13). Melatonin may have a role if medication is indicated (Braam *et al.*, 2009).

Other clinical aspects of intellectual disability

Sex, relationships, and parenthood

Most people with intellectual disability develop sexual interests in the same way as other people. Yet although people with intellectual disability are encouraged to live as normally as possible in other ways, sexual expression is usually discouraged by parents and carers, and sexual feelings may not even be discussed.

In the past, sexual activity of people with intellectual disability was strongly discouraged because it was feared that they might produce disabled children. It is now known that many kinds of severe intellectual disability are not inherited, and that those which are inherited are often associated with infertility. Another concern is that people with intellectual disability will not be good parents. Some studies have shown that low parental intellectual capacity can negatively impact child outcomes, while other studies indicate that child development approaches population norms (Collings and Llewellyn, 2012). Parents will be best able to care for a child successfully if they are strongly supported, especially with behavioural interventions such as teaching parenting skills (Wilson *et al.*, 2014). Social exclusion, bullying, and stigma are commonplace for children raised by intellectually disabled parents, and they are at high risk of being removed from parental care (Collings and Llewellyn, 2012).

It is especially important to consider issues of capacity and ability to consent to sexual relationships if a person with an intellectual disability becomes involved in such a relationship. These issues should be considered carefully in each case, and contraception made available where appropriate. Some intellectual disability teams run groups to help people who wish to find a partner.

Individuals in these groups are assessed carefully to create a safe environment, which is essential for those who are vulnerable.

Sexuality

There is little published literature on the sexual wellbeing of people with intellectual disabilities. Carers may regard people with intellectual disabilities as being more childlike and not as sexual beings, and restrict their access to sexual health information and services. Protective attitudes may be linked to the fact that people with intellectual disabilities have been vulnerable to abuse, and parents may fear that sexual knowledge exacerbates this vulnerability. Some people with intellectual disability have a childlike curiosity about other people's bodies, which can be misunderstood as sexual. Some expose themselves without fully understanding the significance of their actions. This is usually best dealt with by behavioural interventions or with specialized group therapy for those who are more able. Promising approaches have been developed to sex and relationships education, starting early and using innovative methods, and to sexual health services, adapted to allow additional time, address specific fears, and ensure accessible communication (Talbot *et al.*, 2010).

Maltreatment and abuse

There is a strong association between disability (physical and intellectual) and child maltreatment, and children are therefore significantly more likely to experience abuse than their non-disabled peers, more so if they have communication difficulties and behavioural disorders (Stalker and McArthur, 2012). Furthermore, a proportion of children with intellectual disability are raised in families characterized by the factors that are associated in the general population with the maltreatment of children, but there is no convincing evidence that sexual or physical abuse is more frequent in families with an intellectually disabled child. Instead, the sequelae of abuse are often found in people with intellectual disability who were brought up in an institution.

There is also evidence to suggest that abuse is often underreported in disabled children. This might be for a number of reasons, including difficulty communicating, perceived threat, fears of being separated from family, and tolerance of abuse to be accepted or receive rewards or affection. When abuse has occurred, it may lead to psychological problems concurrently and later in life which are similar to those experienced by any other victim of such abuse—for example, depression and post-traumatic stress disorder. However, because of difficulty in emotional expression and communication, such disorders may present with challenging behaviours in situations with which the individual associates past abuse.

Growing old

Several problems arise more frequently as people with intellectual disability live longer, other than just the emergence of dementia and physical health problems (Hubert and Hollins, 2006). When the parents are the carers, they may find care increasingly burdensome as they grow old. Such parents are often concerned about the future of their child when they have died, yet can be reluctant to arrange alternative care while they are still alive.

The older person with intellectual disability also faces special challenges. If their parents die first, they face problems of bereavement. The isolation felt by many bereaved individuals may be increased because other people are not sure how to offer comfort, and because the intellectually disabled person may be excluded from the ritual of mourning and other supports that might be needed at this time. These bereaved people should be helped to come to terms with the loss, using the principles that apply generally to grief counselling, but choosing appropriately simple forms of communication, such as life story work, memory boxes, using photographs, storytelling, art work, and films to help them explore loss in constructive ways (McEvoy, 2016).

Effects of intellectual disability on the family

When a newborn child is found to be disabled, many parents can be distressed. Feelings of rejection are common, but seldom last for long, and are replaced by feelings of loss of the hoped-for normal child. Frequently the diagnosis of intellectual disability is not made until after the first year of life, and the parents then have to change their hopes and expectations for the child. They can experience prolonged depression, guilt, shame, or anger, and have difficulty in coping with the many practical and financial problems. A few reject their children, some become overinvolved in their care, sacrificing other important aspects of family life, while others seek repeatedly for a cause to explain the intellectual disability. Most families eventually achieve a satisfactory adjustment, although the temptation to overindulge the child can remain. However well they adjust psychologically, the parents might still be faced with the prospect of prolonged dependence, frustration, and social difficulties. If the child also has a physical disability, these difficulties can be increased.

There have been several studies on the effect of a child's intellectual disability on the family. In an influential study, Gath (1978) compared families who had a child with Down's syndrome at home and families with a normal child of the same age. She found that most families with an intellectually disabled child had adjusted well and were providing a stable and enriching environment for their child(ren), although the other siblings were at some disadvantage because of the time and effort devoted to the disabled child. These findings have been supported by subsequent research reinforcing that families do best under conditions of high social support and low financial hardship (McConnell *et al.*, 2014). Furthermore, services that facilitate improved functioning in activities of daily living and assist the families in accessing suitable family supports have the potential to influence family quality of life positively (Foley *et al.*, 2014). Teams specializing in services for children with intellectual disability often offer a support service or support groups for siblings.

As the parents grow older, many fear for the future of their now adult disabled son or daughter. They need advice about ways in which they can arrange additional help when they become unable to provide the support that they gave when they were younger, and about ways of helping their son or daughter to remain in the family home after they have died.

For a review of the effects of intellectual disability on the family, see Gath and McCarthy (2009).

Criminal justice system

People with mild intellectual disability have higher rates of criminal behaviour than the general population (see also Chapter 18, page 518). The causes of this excess are multiple, but influences in the family and social environment are often important. Impulsivity, suggestibility, vulnerability to exploitation, and desire to please are other reasons for involvement in crime, alongside an increased likelihood in being detected. Compared with the general population, intellectually disabled people who commit offences are more likely to be detected and, once apprehended, may be more likely to confess. Among the more serious offences, arson and sexual offences (usually exhibitionism) are said to be particularly common.

Of note, people with intellectual disability may be suggestible and may therefore give false confessions, so particular care should be taken when questioning them about an alleged offence. In the UK, police interrogation should accord with the Police and Criminal Evidence Act, which requires the presence of an appropriate adult to ensure that the person with intellectual disability understands the situation and the questions. Once an intellectually disabled person has been convicted, psychiatric supervision in a specialized forensic intellectual disability unit and specialized education may be needed. They are also more likely to be the victims of crime and are perceived to be poor witnesses.

Aetiology of intellectual disability

In a classic study of the 1280 mentally retarded people living in the Colchester Asylum, Penrose (1938) found that most cases were due not to a single cause but to a hypothesized interaction of multiple genetic and environmental factors. This conclusion still broadly applies, especially for mild intellectual disability. Conversely, a specific cause for severe intellectual disability is increasingly often found. Table 17.3 lists the main categories of intellectual disability aetiology, and some examples of each.

Genetic factors are a major cause of intellectual disability. IQ is heritable (with estimates of 30–50%; Deary *et al.*, 2009), and intellectual disability is in this respect just the tail end of the normal distribution of intelligence in the population (indeed, by definition, 2% of people are expected to have an IQ of less than 70). This aspect of genetic predisposition to intelligence reflects the cumulative effects, and interactions, of a large number of genes, most of which have yet to be identified. In addition, a specific chromosomal or genetic defect can be the necessary and sufficient cause of a person's learning difficulty. These include Down's syndrome and fragile X syndrome, the two commonest causes of intellectual disability. It has recently been estimated that over 1000 genes underlie intellectual disability; the majority have yet to be discovered.

The crude division of intellectual disability into cases where a specific cause can be found, and those where it reflects multiple, largely 'non-specific' causes, parallels the categorization into either 'subcultural' (later sociocultural) or 'pathological' mental retardation (as it was then called) made by Lewis (1929).

At a mechanistic level, the types of genetic abnormality that cause intellectual disability are diverse (see Box 17.2) and can be because of chromosomal abnormalities, X-linked disorders, autosomal dominant and recessive disorders, as well as copy number variants (duplications and deletions) of chromosomal regions. (See Chapter 5 for an introduction to genetics.) The clinical features of the major genetic causes of intellectual disability are listed in Table 17.4, with additional details given in the text for Down's syndrome and fragile X syndrome. For a review of the genetic causes of intellectual disability, see Vissers *et al.* (2016).

Environmental factors are conveniently divided into prenatal, perinatal, and postnatal factors, reflecting the time at which they are believed to have occurred. The relative importance of environmental factors varies according to setting. For example, they are more significant in low- and middle-income countries and where health care provision or general health are poorer, and they may be affected by local factors (e.g. areas of low iodine predispose to congenital hypothyroidism). Social as well as biological factors should be considered in the environmental category. Even though the evidence remains inconclusive, it is notable that low intelligence is related to, and predicted by, psychosocial factors such as lower social class, poverty, and an unstable family environment (Sameroff *et al.*, 1987). Some non-genetic causes of intellectual disability are summarized in Table 17.5.

Note also that aetiology of intellectual disability is sometimes defined in terms of an accompanying physical characteristic, such as hydrocephalus, microcephaly, or cerebral dysgenesis. Finally, the descriptive category of *inborn errors of metabolism* encompasses multiple different syndromes, mostly due to a single gene disorder affecting an enzyme that is important in a particular biochemical pathway. They include urea cycle disorders and lysosomal

Table 17.3 **The types of causes of intellectual disability**

Genetic category	Examples
Chromosomal disorders	
Trisomies	Down's syndrome, Edward's syndrome
Other aneuploidies	Turner's syndrome (XO), Klinefelter's syndrome (XXY)
X-linked	Fragile X syndrome, Coffin–Lowry syndrome
Copy number variation	Angelman syndrome (some cases), velocardiofacial syndrome, cri du chat
Single gene disorders	
Autosomal dominant	Neurofibromatosis, tuberous sclerosis
Autosomal recessive	Phenylketonuria, Tay–Sachs disease, Hurler's syndrome
X-linked	Rett syndrome
Mitochondrial disorders	
Complex (non-Mendelian) disorders	
Environmental causes	
Prenatal	
Infection	Rubella, toxoplasmosis, syphilis
Toxins	Fetal alcohol syndrome, lead poisoning
Maternal	Pre-eclampsia, placental insufficiency
Nutritional	Iodine deficiency, severe malnutrition
Immune	Rhesus incompatibility
Perinatal	
Obstetric complications	Brain injury, cerebral palsy
Complications of prematurity	
Postnatal	
Infection	
Injury	
Impoverished environment	
Miscellaneous	
Hydrocephalus	
Microcephaly	
Spina bifida	
Inborn errors of metabolism	Mucopolysaccharidoses, Lesch–Nyhan syndrome
Idiopathic	

Box 17.2 The genetic basis of intellectual disability

Genetic factors of various kinds underlie intellectual disability. (See also page 102 for an introduction to relevant genetic concepts and terminology.)

Chromosomal abnormalities. An abnormal number of chromosomes (*aneuploidy*) invariably causes intellectual disability. *Trisomy* refers to possession of an extra copy of a chromosome; the classic example is trisomy 21 (Down's syndrome). Absence of an autosome is not compatible with life, but an absence (or excessive number) of a sex chromosome is, and produces a variable phenotype in which mild intellectual disability is common (e.g. XO, Turner's syndrome).

Intellectual disability is 25% more common in boys, and Lehrke (1972) was the first to suggest that this might be due to X chromosome-linked causes. This suggestion has proved to be largely correct, with fragile X syndrome being the commonest disorder, but many others have been identified as well. *X-linked intellectual disability* is a collective term used to describe these disorders. Their clinical picture can be particularly complex (e.g. in terms of girls being affected, and the severity of the phenotype).

Copy number variations (CNVs) were introduced in Chapter 5. They comprise *deletions* and *duplications* of part of a chromosome. Note that we have two copies of each autosomal chromosome, one from each parent, and only one is affected, hence the more precise term *hemideletion*. Occasionally, the clinical picture depends upon which parental chromosome is affected, via a process called *imprinting*. For example, in chromosome 15q 11–13, the parental origin of the deletion determines whether Prader–Willi (paternal) or Angelman syndrome (maternal) is present. Some parts of the genome are 'hotspots' for deletions and rearrangements, such as the q11 band of chromosome 22, which causes velocardiofacial syndrome (Box 11.10). The tips of the chromosomes (telomeres) also seem to be particularly vulnerable, with *subtelomeric deletions* thought to cause 5–10% of 'idiopathic' intellectual disability. Cumulatively, CNVs represent the commonest cause of intellectual disability.

Single gene disorders are those attributed to a defect limited to a single gene, and where the identity of the gene, and often the causative mutation within it, is known. This category includes most *inborn errors of metabolism*. Single gene disorders can be dominant or, more commonly, recessive, and can be autosomal or X-linked.

Note that these points illustrate that genetic factors do not in fact fall into discrete categories, but are more like a spectrum of causality. Thus the size of the abnormality can be anything from a whole chromosome to a CNV to a mutation in a single nucleotide. Similarly, the impact of the genetic variation can range from being the sole cause of the syndrome through to acting as a minor risk factor. Since many of the genetic deficits arise *de novo* (i.e. are spontaneous mutations) in the individual (owing to an error during gametogenesis, fertilization, or early development), they blur the distinction between genetic (in the sense of inherited) and environmental causes.

For review, see Vissers *et al.* (2016).

---

storage disorders, which in turn include mucopolysaccharidoses (e.g. Hurler's syndrome), sphingolipidoses (e.g. Tay–Sachs disease), and others (e.g. phenylketonuria). For a comprehensive review, see Scaglia (2014).

Overall, it is estimated that prenatal (genetic and environmental) factors cause 50–70% of intellectual disability, with 10–20% originating perinatally, and 5–10% originating postnatally; the proportions, and the causes within each category, depend on the population being studied. For reviews of the aetiology of intellectual disability, see Kaski (2009), and Reichenberg *et al.* (2016).

Down's syndrome

Down's syndrome, first described by Langdon Down in 1866, is a frequent cause of intellectual disability,

occurring in 1 in about every 650 live births. It is most commonly caused by an additional chromosome 21 (95% of cases), chromosomal translocation causing partial trisomy (in approximately 4% of cases), or chromosomal mosaicism (in approximately 1% of cases). It is more frequent in children of older women, occurring in about 1 in 2000 live births to mothers aged 20–25 years, and 1 in 30 live births to those aged 45 years or over. Improvements in the antenatal screening process (maternal serum testing and, later, measurement of fetal nuchal translucency) has led to an increase in the number of terminations of pregnancy due to Down's syndrome. However, the incidence is stable, reflecting how the older average age of mothers increases the risk of having a child with Down's syndrome (Morris and Alberman, 2009).

Table 17.4 **Notes on some genetic causes of intellectual disability**

Syndrome	Aetiology*	Clinical features	Comments**
Chromosome abnormalities and copy number variants			
Down's syndrome	Trisomy 21	See text	
Fragile X syndrome	See text	See text	
Edwards's syndrome	Trisomy 18	Growth deficiency, abnormal skull shape and facial features, clenched hands, rocker-bottom feet, cardiac and renal abnormalities	Rare. Early death common
Cri du chat	Deletion of chromosome 5p, mostly sporadic	Microcephaly, hyperteleorism, typical cat-like cry, failure to thrive	1 in 35,000. ID often severe. Hyperactivity. Early death common
Prader–Willi syndrome	70% due to deletion of paternal 15q11; the rest are due to inheriting two copies of the same region of maternal chromosome 15	Floppy infants. Small stature, hypogonadal. Excessive appetite, leading to obesity. Daytime sleepiness. Delayed motor milestones and speech difficulties. Skin-picking	1 in 40,000. ID usually mild or moderate
Angelman syndrome	Overlaps with Prader–Willi syndrome. Deletions and mutations affect *UBE3A* gene on 15q11	Ataxia, hypotonia and epilepsy. Small head, hook nose, characteristic face and wide mouth. 'Happy puppets'— jerky movements, episodic paroxysmal laughter, sociable	1 in 10,000. Severe to profound ID with absence of speech. Hyperactivity
22q deletion syndrome (velocardiofacial syndrome, di George syndrome)	Deletion involving chromosome 22q11; 10% inherited and 90% spontaneous	Variable. Cardiac deficits, characteristic facial appearance with flat nose and cleft palate, short stature, long thin fingers	1 in 2000. ID variable, mild ID to borderline IQ typical. Poor social interactions with autistic features and ADHD. 25% develop schizophrenia-like disorders in adolescence (Box 11.10)
Williams syndrome (idiopathic infantile hypercalcaemia)	Deletion of 7q11, affecting elastin gene. Most cases are sporadic	Distinctive facies with 'elfin' appearance, small stature, with harsh, brassy voice. Supravalvar aortic stenosis common, failure to thrive	1 in 1500. Most have moderate ID, delayed but preserved language skills. Superficially sociable but lacks social flexibility and often anxious
Inborn errors of metabolism			
Phenylketonuria	Autosomal recessive, causing lack of liver phenylalanine hydroxylase. Commonest inborn error of metabolism	Lack of pigment (fair hair and blue eyes), retarded growth, associated epilepsy, microcephaly, eczema, and hyperactivity	1 in 10,000. Detectable by neonatal screening of blood or urine; treated by removing phenylalanine from diet early in life
Galactosaemia	Autosomal recessive, deficiency of one of three enzymes involved in galactose metabolism (GALT)	Presents following introduction of milk into diet; failure to thrive, hepatosplenomegaly, cataracts	Very rare. Detected by neonatal screening. Intellectual disability usually mild, if treated (by galactose-free diet)

Table 17.4 Continued

Syndrome	Aetiology[*]	Clinical features	Comments[**]
Hurler's syndrome (mucopolysaccharidosis type I (MPS I)	Autosomal recessive, affecting α-L-iduronidase, causing accumulation of dextran and heparin sulphate	Grotesque features, protuberant abdomen, hepatosplenomegaly, cardiac abnormalities	Rare. Death before adolescence. MPS II (Hunter syndrome) and MPS III (Sanfilippo syndrome) are milder
Lesch–Nyhan syndrome	X-linked mutation of *HGPRT* gene, leading to enzyme defect affecting purine metabolism. Excessive uric acid production and excretion	Severe self-injurious behaviour, compulsive biting of fingers and lips. Development of spastic cerebral palsy and choreoathetoid movements.	Almost all are normal at birth but then develop low–mild ID. Very rare. Diagnosed prenatally or postnatally, carrier screening possible. Death in early adult life
Smith–Magenis syndrome	Deletion of chromosome 17p11.2, affecting the *RAI1* gene. Usually sporadic	Broad flat face, brachycephaly, hypoplasia, short stature, hoarse voice, peripheral neuropathy	Severe ID often with speech delay. Engaging personalities but severe self-injurious behaviour, tantrums, and sleep disturbance
Other single gene disorders			
Neurofibromatosis 1 (von Recklinghausen's syndrome)	Autosomal dominant, but 50% of cases are spontaneous mutations. Caused by neurofibromin gene at 17q11	Neurofibromata, vitiligo, café au lait spots. Astrocytomas and meningiomas	1 in 3000. Intellectual disability in 50%
Tuberous sclerosis (epiloia)	Autosomal dominant, but variable penetrance and many cases sporadic. Caused by two genes: *TSC1* (hamartin) on 9q, and *TSC2* (tuberin) on 16p	Epilepsy, adenoma sebaceum on face, white skin patches, shagreen skin, retinal phakoma, subungual fibromata, multiple renal and other tumours	1 in 7000. ID usually mild. Autism and other psychiatric disorders common
Duchenne muscular dystrophy	X-linked recessive; dystrophin gene on Xp21	Males. Progressive muscle weakness, including respiratory and cardiac muscles	1 in 4000. 25% have ID. Verbal IQ lower than performance IQ. Depression and anxiety common
Rett syndrome	*MeCP2* gene mutation at Xq28	Females affected (lethal in males). Epilepsy, compulsive hand-wringing movements, agitation	1 in 10,000. Normal early development, abnormalities beginning end of first year, leading to progressive intellectual disability with death common by adolescence (see Chapter 16)
Cornelia de Lange syndrome	50% of cases due to mutation in *NIPBL* gene; other genes include *SMC1A, HDAC8, RAD21*, and *SMC3*. All affect the cohesin complex, which plays a role in early growth	Typical facial features, including low anterior hairline and arched eyebrows, long eyelashes. Prenatal and postnatal growth retardation. Ptosis, myopia, microcephaly, GOR 60%	Typically severe ID but variable IQ. Self-injurious behaviour, Communication impaired

[*] Numeral refers to chromosome number. p, short arm; q, long arm. [**]ID: intellectual disability; GOR, gastro-oesophageal reflux.

Table 17.5 Some non-genetic causes of intellectual disability

Syndrome	Aetiology	Clinical features	Comments
Infection			
Rubella	Viral infection in first trimester	Cataract, microphthalmia, deafness, microcephaly, congenital heart disease	If mother infected in first trimester, 10–15% infants are affected
Cytomegalovirus	Intrauterine infection	Brain damage; only severe cases are apparent at birth	60% of survivors have intellectual disability
Toxoplasmosis	Protozoal infection of mother	Hydrocephaly, microcephaly, cerebral calcification, renal problems, hepatosplenomegaly, epilepsy	Variable
Congenital syphilis	Syphilitic infection of mother	Many die at birth; variable neurological signs, 'stigmata' (Hutchinson's teeth and rhagades)	Uncommon since routine testing of pregnant women
Other			
Hydrocephalus	Sex-linked recessive; inherited developmental abnormality, e.g. atresia aqueduct, Arnold–Chiari malformation, meningitis, spina bifida	Rapid enlargement of head. In early infancy, symptoms of raised CSF pressure; other features depend on aetiology	Mild cases may arrest spontaneously; may be symptomatically treated by CSF shunt; intelligence can be normal
Microcephaly	Recessive inheritance, irradiation in pregnancy, maternal infections	Features depend upon aetiology	Intellectual disability usually severe
Cerebral palsy	Perinatal brain damage; strong association with prematurity	Spastic (common), athetoid, and ataxic types; variable in severity	Majority are below average IQ; athetoid are more likely to be of normal IQ
Hypothyroidism (cretinism)	Iodine deficiency or (rarely) atrophic thyroid	Appearance normal at birth; abnormalities appear at 6 months; growth failure, puffy skin, lethargy	Now rare in UK; responds to early thyroxine replacement
Fetal alcohol syndrome		Facial dysmorphology—thin upper lip, low-dset ears, growth retardation, microcephaly	1 in 3000, depending on criteria. Intellectual disability usually mild, or moderate. Hyperactivity and irritability
Hyperbilirubinaemia	Haemolysis, rhesus incompatibility, and prematurity	Kernicterus (choreoathetosis), opisthotonus, spasticity, convulsions	Prevention by anti-rhesus globulin; treatment by exchange transfusion

The clinical picture consists of a number of features, any one of which can occur in a person without Down's syndrome. Four features together are generally accepted as strong evidence for the syndrome. The most characteristic signs are listed in Box 17.3. IQ is generally between 20 and 50, but in 15% of individuals it is above 50. Mental abilities usually develop fairly quickly in the first 6 months to 1 year of life, but then increase more slowly. Children with Down's syndrome are often described as loveable and easy-going, but there is wide individual variation. Emotional and behaviour problems are less frequent than in forms of retardation associated with clinically detectable brain damage.

> ### Box 17.3 Features of Down's syndrome
>
> Moderate or severe intellectual disability
>
> Placid temperament
>
> Physical features
>
> - Slanted eyes and epicanthic folds
> - Small mouth with furrowed tongue
> - Flat nose
> - Flattened occiput
> - Stubby hands, fingers, and single transverse palmar crease
> - Hypotonia with hyperextensibility of joints
>
> Associated medical problems
>
> - Cardiac anomalies, especially septal defects
> - Gastrointestinal abnormalities
> - Atlantoaxial instability
> - Susceptibility to infection
> - Impaired hearing
>
> Increased risk of leukaemia, hypothyroidism, and autoimmune disorders
>
> Increased risk of adolescent and early adult depression

In the past, the infant mortality of Down's syndrome was high, but with improved medical care survival into adulthood is usual, and about 25% of people with Down's syndrome now live beyond 50 years of age. Although longevity in people with Down's syndrome has improved appreciably, age-specific risk for mortality is still considerably increased, with many body systems exhibiting signs of premature or accelerated ageing. This may be due to both genetic and epigenetic factors (Zigman 2013).

Aetiology

In 1959, Down's syndrome was found to be associated with the chromosomal disorder of trisomy (three chromosomes instead of the usual two). About 95% of cases are due to trisomy 21. These cases result from failure of disjunction during meiosis, and are associated with increasing maternal age. The risk of recurrence in a subsequent child is about 1 in 100. The remaining 5% of cases of Down's syndrome are attributable either to translocation involving chromosome 21 or to mosaicism. The disorder leading to translocation is often inherited, and the risk of recurrence is about 1 in 10. Mosaicism occurs when non-disjunction takes place

during any cell division after fertilization. Normal and trisomic cells occur in the same person, and the effects on cognitive development are particularly variable.

Although trisomy 21 is one of the most widespread genetic causes of intellectual disability, it is still poorly understood. Down's syndrome pathology is assumed to be due primarily to the increased 'dosage' of genes, and thus increased production of the proteins that they encode. This probably also accounts for the frequent early onset of Alzheimer's dementia, with approximately 80% of individuals with Down's syndrome developing Alzheimer's disease pathology by 40 years of age (Box 14.11; see Ballard et al., 2016 for review).

Fragile X syndrome and X-linked intellectual disability

Fragile X syndrome is the second most common specific cause of intellectual disability after Down's syndrome, and is the most common inherited cause. It occurs in around 1 in 4000 males and in a milder form in about 1 in 6000 females. It accounts overall for about 10% of those with intellectual disability. The condition was so named because the X chromosome is 'fragile' when lymphocytes from affected individuals are cultured without sufficient folic acid.

As shown in Box 17.4, there are a number of characteristic but highly variable clinical features, none of which is diagnostic, including enlarged testes, large ears, a long face, and flat feet. Psychological features include abnormalities of speech and language, social anxiety, autistic behaviour and other social impairments, disorders of attention and concentration, and hyperactivity.

The inheritance of the condition, and the characteristics of carriers, are unusual and complex. Fragile X syndrome is caused by an amplified CGG repeat sequence in the *FMR1* gene, which leads to silencing of the gene and thus an absence of FMR1 protein. FMR1 regulates genes involved in synaptic function and plasticity, and the syndrome is thought to arise because the lack of FMR1 interferes with the action of these other genes. Some of these genes are now therapeutic targets for fragile X syndrome, notably the metabotropic glutamate receptor mGluR5, but as yet there are no established treatments. Folic acid is ineffective. For review of fragile X syndrome, see Bagni et al. (2012).

It is now realized that fragile X is one of a family of X-linked causes of intellectual disability, which together occur in up to 1 in 600 boys, account for about 16% of cases of male intellectual disability, and underlie the male excess of the condition. For review, see Lubs *et al.* (2012) and Bagni *et al.* (2012). However, these disorders can also affect girls; an extreme example is Rett syndrome (see Table 17.4 and Chapter 16), which only affects girls, probably because it is lethal to male embryos. Note: All features are particularly variable.

Assessment and classification of psychiatric conditions in people with intellectual disability

Assessment of a person with suspected intellectual disability can be different to those with normal intelligence, especially when the person has communication and cognitive difficulties affecting their emotional, perceptual, and thought-related experiences Volkmar *et al.* (2014). The assessment is directed towards five main areas:

- the cause and severity of the disorder
- intellectual and social skills development
- associated medical conditions
- associated psychiatric disorders
- assessment of needs.

A multiaxial classification is available to record some of this information, the DC-LD (Diagnostic Criteria for Psychiatric Disorders for Use with Adults with Learning Disabilities) (Royal College of Psychiatrists, 2001), namely:

Axis I: Severity of intellectual disability

Axis II: Cause of intellectual disability

Axis III: Psychiatric disorders:

    Level A: Developmental disorders

    Level B: Psychiatric illness

    Level C: Personality disorders

    Level D: Problem behaviours

    Level E: Other disorders.

This system helps to ensure that all of the key components are considered and recorded. It also highlights the fact that the assessment is both about characterizing the intellectual disability and its consequences, and also about making a specific diagnosis, where possible, as to its aetiology.

Severe intellectual disability is usually diagnosed in infancy, especially as it is often associated with detectable physical abnormalities or with delayed motor development. Some people with intellectual disability have specific developmental disorders— that is, impairment of specific functions greater than would be expected from the general intellectual level (see Chapter 16). The clinician should be cautious when diagnosing less severe intellectual disability on the basis of delays in development. Although routine examination of a child may reveal signs of developmental delay, suggesting possible intellectual disability, confident diagnosis often requires specialist assessment. Milder forms of intellectual disability often present when the child attends school, and can include non-attendance at school, low academic achievements, and immature interests and behaviour.

Full assessment involves several stages, including history-taking, examination of the mental state, physical examination, genetic and other laboratory investigations, developmental testing, functional behavioural assessment, analysis of the interactions between the disabled person and the family and the social support systems, and other aspects of adjustment. Each of these stages will be considered in turn. Although this section is concerned mainly with the assessment of children, similar principles apply to assessments later in life.

For reviews of the assessment of intellectual disability, see Holland (2009) and Eng *et al.* (2013).

History-taking

In the course of obtaining a full history, particular attention should be given to any family history suggesting an inherited disorder, and to any difficulties or abnormalities in the pregnancy or the delivery of the child. Dates of passing developmental milestones should be ascertained. A full account of any behaviour disorders should be obtained. Details of any associated medical conditions, such as congenital heart disease, epilepsy, and cerebral palsy, should be documented.

Mental state examination

The approach should be flexible. Many people with intellectual disability attend and concentrate poorly. Therefore the interview may need to be carried out rather informally while the person is engaged intermittently in some other interest. Questions should be simplified to take account of each person's receptive language and developmental level. Behavioural observations by family, friends, and carers are often more helpful than the observations that the assessor is able to make. Clinical assessment can also be supplemented by using standardized scales for the assessment of psychopathology, adapted for use in patients with intellectual disability.

Physical examination

A systematic physical examination should include noting the child's overall appearance, looking for dysmorphic features and other physical signs suggestive of specific disorders (see Tables 17.3 and 17.5, and Boxes 17.3 and 17.4). Head circumference should be recorded. The parents' appearance may also be worth noting. Neurological examination is important and should include particular attention to impairments of vision and hearing.

As in the assessment of patients of normal intelligence, it is important to find out the person's previous baseline state before concluding that an item of current behaviour is evidence of a psychiatric disorder. Some longstanding behaviours, such as stereotyped

---

Box 17.4 Features of fragile X syndrome

More common in males

Caused by *FMR1* gene mutation

Intellectual disability

- Variable from mild to profound
- Increases late in childhood
- Performance IQ affected more than verbal IQ
- Poor attention and concentration
- Speech repetitive, lacking themes or content ('litany speech')

Behavioural features

- Autistic features common

Physical features

- Large, protruding ears
- Long face with high-arched palate
- Flat feet
- Lax joints
- Soft skin
- Large testes (after puberty)
- Mitral valve prolapse

---

movements or social withdrawal, may resemble and be mistaken for symptoms of schizophrenia or other psychiatric disorders—so-called *diagnostic overshadowing* (Reiss and Szyszko, 1983). However, an increase in a longstanding behaviour may be the first, and sometimes the only, evidence of psychiatric disorder—so-called *baseline exaggeration* (Sovner and Hurley, 1989).

Genetic and laboratory investigations

As many cases of intellectual disability, especially moderate and severe forms, are caused by a specific chromosomal or genetic abnormality, genetic investigations are a major component of assessment. For example, at the time of writing, chromosomal microarray (CMA) is considered a first-tier genetic test, especially if a causal diagnosis is not known (Moeschler *et al.*, 2014). A clinical geneticist can provide up-to-date information about the conditions for which screening is available and the cytogenetic and molecular genetic methods in use (since both are evolving rapidly) (see Vissers *et al.*, 2016), as well as help with the interpretation of test results, and sharing the information with the family and addressing their questions. Genetic investigations are also critical in preventative screening for intellectual disability.

Depending on the clinical suspicion, and informed by knowledge of the common causes of intellectual disability, a range of blood tests to detect inherited metabolic and endocrine disorders, and brain imaging, may also be indicated. Close involvement with a paediatrician or paediatric neurologist is recommended.

Developmental assessment

This assessment is based on a combination of clinical experience and standardized methods of measuring intelligence, language, motor performance, and social skills. Although the IQ is the best general index of intellectual development, it is not reliable in the very young or among people who have severe to profound degrees of intellectual disabilities.

Tests used in developmental assessment

Standardized assessment instruments are widely used for screening, diagnosing, and assessing the severity of disorders of psychological development (Carr *et al.*, 2016). Many require special training for correct administration, but some do not. The choice of test is important because many neuropsychological tests are too difficult to perform on some people with intellectual disability. The type of test is also important. There are norm-referenced tests such as the Wechsler Adult Intelligence

Scale (WAIS) and other IQ measures, criterion-referenced tests that apply to particular skills without reference to population norms, tests of adaptive behaviour in social settings, and assessments of behavioural functioning. An abbreviated version of the WAIS, called the Wechsler Abbreviated Scales of Intelligence (WASI) (Psychological Corporation, 2004), is now available. Another quick useful method is the use of a Picture Vocabulary Test or another non-verbal test, such as Raven's Progressive Matrices. Other commonly used instruments are summarized in Table 17.6 and include general, adaptive functioning, intelligence, language, and other aspects of development. All have good reliability and validity.

Functional behavioural assessment

The functional assessment of behaviour involves an assessment of events before, during, and immediately after the behaviour takes place. It is based on observations reported by family, carers, and members of the clinical team. It is concerned with abilities related to self-care, and social abilities, including communication, sensory motor skills, and social relationships. Sometimes key behaviours are counted and recorded on paper or using a palmtop computer.

Assessment of social interaction and adjustment

This assessment is concerned with the interaction between the person with intellectual disability and the individuals closely involved in their care. It is also concerned with opportunities for learning new skills, making relationships, and achieving more choice. If the person with intellectual disability has reasonable language ability, it is usually possible to obtain much of the information from him or her. If language ability is less well developed, the account has to be obtained mainly from informants. It is particularly important to obtain a complete description of any change from the usual pattern of behaviour. It is often appropriate to ask parents, teachers, or care staff to keep records of behaviours such as eating, sleeping, and general activity so that problems can be identified and quantified. The assessor should keep in mind the possible causes of psychiatric disorder outlined above, including unrecognized epilepsy.

Assessment of needs

As the diagnostic assessment progresses, the likely needs of the patient require careful consideration, too, as these will form the basis of the care package and management plan to be implemented. The needs assessment brings together the social, emotional, and health needs of the person, and takes into account their views and wishes as well as those of their significant others. This approach, sometimes termed 'person-centred planning', is now integral to most intellectual disability services (Robertson *et al.*, 2007).

A modification of the Camberwell Assessment of Need, known as CANDID (Camberwell Assessment of Need for Adults with Developmental and Intellectual Disabilities), is available for use in adults with intellectual disability.

Follow-up assessments

Once intellectual disability has been diagnosed, regular reviews are required. For children, these are usually carried out by a multidisciplinary child health team together with teachers and social workers. The child psychiatrist liaises with the team, and has a particular role where the child has emotional, behavioural, or other psychiatric problems. When the child reaches school-leaving age, a thorough review is important. This should assess the need for further education, the prospects for employment and independent living, and the need for ongoing specialist physical and psychological healthcare. Adults with intellectual disability need to be assessed regularly to make sure that their care remains appropriate; an intellectual disability psychiatrist will usually contribute to these multidisciplinary reviews.

The care of people with intellectual disability

A historical perspective

Current arrangements for care are best understood in a historical context (Thomson, 1998), which usefully begins in the early nineteenth century. At this time

there were numerous reports of improved forms of care, notably by Itard, physician-in-chief at the Asylum for the Deaf and Dumb in Paris, who attempted to train a 'wild boy' found in Aveyron in 1801. This child was thought to have grown up in the wild, isolated from human beings. Itard made great efforts to educate the boy but, after persisting for 6 years, he concluded that the training had failed. Nevertheless, his work had important and lasting consequences, for it led others to try educational methods. These methods were developed, for example, by Seguin, director of the School for Idiots at the Bicêtre in Paris, who in 1842 published the *Theory and Nature of the Education of Idiots*. Seguin believed that the intellectually disabled had latent abilities which could be encouraged by special training, involving physical exercise, moral instruction, and graded tasks. These ideas were taken up in other countries, particularly Switzerland and Germany, with the opening of institutions that attempted to train their pupils and thereby enable them to live as independently as possible, while recognizing that many would need long-term care.

At the end of the nineteenth century, several influences led to a more custodial approach. These influences included the development of the science of genetics, the eugenics movement, the measurement of intelligence, and a general decrease in public tolerance of abnormal behaviour. In England and Wales, such ideas were reflected in the Mental Deficiency Act 1913, which empowered local authorities to provide for the confinement of the 'intellectually and morally defective', and imposed upon the authorities a responsibility to provide training and occupation. In the years that followed, the total number of people of this kind in institutions rose from 6000 in 1916 to 50,000 in 1939, and remained at high levels well into the postwar period.

In the 1960s the need for reform was recognized in several high-income countries, prompted in part by the changes away from institutions and towards community care that had already been effected in general psychiatry. Campaigning by groups of parents, and public concern about the generally—and in some instances scandalously—poor conditions in which people with intellectual disabilities were housed, was also important. Surveys of hospitals for the 'retarded' showed that the mean IQ of their patients was over 70, and thus many residents had only mild intellectual disability and did not need hospital care. At around the same time it was shown that training was beneficial in intellectual disability across the severity range (O'Connor, 1968), and that there was an advantage to providing residential care in small homely units (Tizard, 1964).

It is now recognized in many high-income countries that people with intellectual disability should be integrated into and included by society as far as possible. However, there have been divergent views about the best way to achieve greater integration. In the UK, resources have been inadequate and progress has been slow. In the USA, deinstitutionalization was carried out more quickly, with both successes and failures.

The current predominant principle of care is *normalization*, an idea that was developed in Scandinavia in the 1960s. This term refers to the general approach of providing a pattern of life as near normal as possible. Normalization implies that almost all people with intellectual disability will live in the community, participating in normal activities and relationships, making choices, and having full social opportunities. Children are brought up whenever possible with their families, and adults are encouraged to live as independently as is feasible. For the few who need special social and health care, accommodation and activities are designed to be as close as possible to those of family life. The concept of normalization has been further developed in the USA and elsewhere, and includes specialist educational and other help to enable people to achieve their full potential. Increasingly, disabled people are organizing themselves into advocacy groups, and those who are unable to speak for themselves about the services have advocates speak for them. A recent systematic review confirmed the better outcomes of community-based services compared with institutional care (Kozma et al., 2009).

General provisions

The precise model for the care of people with intellectual disability in a community matters less than the level of detail in which it is planned and the enthusiasm with which it is carried out. Good planning requires both an estimate of the needs of the population to be served, and a summation of individual assessments of those identified, as each person has individual needs. To achieve this, local case registers and linked developmental records are needed.

The general approach to care is educational and psychosocial, together with appropriate psychiatric interventions for mental health problems. The family doctor and paediatrician are mainly responsible for the early detection and assessment of intellectual disability. The multidisciplinary team providing continuing health care benefits by including psychiatrists, psychologists, speech therapists, nurses, occupational therapists, and physiotherapists. Volunteers and self-help groups for carers can play a valuable part. In the UK, residential provisions for people with intellectual disability are from several sources, including the education service, health service, social services, and voluntary organizations.

Table 17.6 Commonly used instruments for developmental assessment

Vineland Adaptive Behaviour Scale This scale measures adaptive behaviour across the life-course and assesses four domains: communication, daily living skills, socialisation and motor skills.	**Autism Behaviour Checklist (ABC)** This questionnaire is completed by the parent or other carer. It is a reliable indicator of problems in the area of autism and delay in social development and easy to administer.
The British Ability Scales and Differential Ability Scales These scales measure a range of functions and educational attainments (spelling, arithmetic, reading), and can be used to calculate an overall IQ.	**The Disability Assessment Scale** This scale focuses on autistic and related social developmental, language disorders, and behavioural problems.
ABAS (Harrison and Oakland, 2000) The ABAS assesses adaptive behaviours within the domains of: communication, functional academics, health and safety, self.	**British (Peabody) Picture Vocabulary Test** A test of language comprehension, suitable for non-speaking children. The test booklet is largely pictorial and the age range covered is 3–19 years. Although professional training is not required, the test is used mainly by psychologists and speech therapists.
The Portage Guide to Early Education This assessment has been adopted for use internationally. It provides a broad developmental assessment including socialization, self-help, language, and cognitive and motor domains. Only a brief period of training is required. The test requires the active involvement of parent or other carer.	**Reynell Scales of Language Development** These scales assess comprehension and expressive language in the age range 1 month to 6 years. The test is of particular use with non-verbal children.
Griffiths mental development scales For 2 to 8 years of age. Consists of subscales of: locomotor, personal-social, language, hand-eye coordination, performance and practical reasoning.	**Developmental, Dimensional and Diagnostic Interview** This is a parental autism interview that measures both symptom intensity and comorbidity across the full range of the autistic spectrum.
Bayley scales of infant development (Bayley III; Bayley, 2005). Children are assessed in the five key developmental domains of cognition, language, social-emotional, motor and adaptive behaviour. Validated for 1–42 months.	**Wechsler Intelligence Scale for Children (WISC-IV) and for adults (WAIS-IV)** Gives a full scale IQ and measures cognitive functioning within four domains of verbal comprehension, perceptual reasoning, processing speed and working memory. The WISC-IV is validated for use between 6–16 years; the WAIS-IV for 16–90 years.

For a review of services for intellectual disability, see Bouras and Holt (2009), and for a practical guide to their organization, see Bernard and Turk (2009).

Specific services

The main elements in a comprehensive service for people with intellectual disability are as follows:

- the prevention and early detection of intellectual disability
- regular assessment of the intellectually disabled person's attainments and disabilities

- advice, support, and practical measures for families
- provision for education, training, occupation, or work
- housing and social support to maximize self-care
- medical, nursing, and other services for those who require these forms of help as outpatients, day-patients, or inpatients
- psychiatric and psychological services.

Preventive services

Primary prevention consists of genetic counselling, the education of pregnant women (and the population in general) about behaviours that may put the fetus at risk, early detection of fetal abnormalities during pregnancy, and good obstetric and perinatal care. *Secondary prevention* aims to prevent the progression of disability by either medical or psychological means. The latter includes 'enriching' education and early attempts to reduce behavioural problems. In high-income countries, there remains considerable scope for reduction of the genetic causes of severe intellectual disability, but it is unlikely that it will be possible to affect the incidence of mild intellectual disability significantly. In low- and middle-income countries, the incidence of intellectual disability could be substantially reduced by general measures to improve the health of mothers during pregnancy, and by better perinatal care. For a review, see Kaski (2009).

Genetic screening and counselling

These measures begin with an assessment of the risk that an intellectually disabled child will be born. Such an assessment is based on study of the family history, on knowledge of the genetics of conditions that give rise to intellectual disability, and on awareness of the possibilities for genetic screening. The risks of screening are explained to the parents, who are encouraged to discuss them. Most parents seek advice only after a first abnormal child has been born. Those who seek advice before starting to have children usually do so because there is a person with intellectual disability in the family. A positive diagnosis of an abnormality leading to termination or, indeed, a false-positive result of screening causes considerable distress. It is important, therefore, that those involved in screening are alert to psychological issues and have the appropriate counselling skills. Close liaison with a clinical geneticist is recommended, given the rapid developments in the indications for screening, the methods used, and the significant ethical and counselling issues involved.

Prenatal care

Prenatal care begins even before conception, with immunization against rubella for women who lack immunity, and advice on diet, alcohol, smoking, and folic acid supplementation.

Prenatal diagnosis overlaps with genetic screening, which is becoming available for an increasing number of conditions with the aim of providing information to those at risk of having abnormal children, reassurance to others, and appropriate treatment of affected infants through early diagnosis. Maternal blood tests, ultrasound scanning, fetoscopy, chorionic villus sampling, and amniocentesis can reveal chromosomal abnormalities, most open neural tube defects, and about 60% of inborn errors of metabolism. Amniocentesis carries a small but definite risk, and so is usually offered only to women who have carried a previous abnormal fetus, women with a family history of congenital disorder, and those with significant risk that the fetus they are carrying will have a serious condition or abnormality.

Rhesus incompatibility is now largely preventable. Sensitization of a rhesus-negative mother can usually be avoided by giving anti-D antibody. An affected fetus can be detected by amniocentesis and treated if necessary by exchange transfusion. For pregnant women with diabetes mellitus, special care can improve the outlook for the fetus. Further information about these aspects of care can be found in textbooks of obstetrics and paediatrics.

Postnatal prevention

In the UK, all infants are routinely tested for phenylketonuria, and testing for hypothyroidism and galactosaemia is becoming increasingly common. Screening for elevated levels of lead has been advocated, especially in areas where they are known to be high. Intensive care units and improved methods of treatment for premature and low-birthweight infants can prevent intellectual disability in some who would previously have suffered brain damage. However, these methods also enable the survival of some disabled children who would otherwise have died.

Help for families

As noted earlier, having a child with intellectual disability can have a major emotional and practical impact on the family, and support is needed for the family from the time that the diagnosis is first made (Gath and McCarthy, 2009). It is not enough to give worried parents a full explanation on just one occasion. They may need to hear the explanation several times before they can absorb all of its implications. Adequate time must be allowed to explain the prognosis, indicate what help can be provided, and discuss the part that the parents can play in helping their child to achieve his or her full potential. Community paediatricians, health visitors, and sometimes clinical geneticists are usually involved in this process.

Thereafter, the parents need continuing support as there is good evidence for promoting child development with parent-sensitive responsiveness (Guralnik, 2016). When the child starts school, the parents should be kept informed about progress, and feel involved in the planning and provision of care. They should be given help with practical matters, such as daycare during school holidays, babysitting, or arrangements for family holidays. In addition to practical assistance, the parents might need continuing psychological support, which may be provided as a programme for the whole family.

Families are likely to need extra help when their child reaches puberty or leaves school. Making the transition from child to adult services is often extremely stressful. Both respite day and overnight care can be required to relieve carers and to encourage the intellectually disabled person to become more independent.

Education, training, and occupation

One aspect of the policy of normalization is that children with intellectual disability should be educated as far as possible within inclusive preschool settings and mainstream schools. The extent to which this is done varies in different countries and also in different regions of the same country.

Compensatory education is intended to provide optimal conditions for the mental development of the disabled child. An early example was the Head Start programme in the USA, which provided extra education for deprived children, including nursery schooling and attempts to teach specific skills. Many of the results were disappointing, and it was followed by a more intensive programme with similar aims, carried out in Milwaukee (Garber, 1988). Skilled teachers taught children living in slum areas with mothers who had a low IQ (less than 75). This additional education started at 3 months of age and continued until the child reached school age. At the same time, the mothers were trained in a variety of domestic skills. These children were compared with children of the same age from similar families who had not received these interventions. At the age of four and a half, the trained children had a mean IQ 27 points higher than that of the controls. This study can be faulted because the selection of children was not strictly random, and because some of the changes in test scores could have been due to practice. Nevertheless, the main findings probably stand—substantial effort by trained staff can produce worthwhile improvement in children of low intelligence born to socially disadvantaged mothers. Overall, it seems that early interventions can be effective, especially if they are family-centred. However, many uncertainties remain about the components and the delivery of such help.

Research has consistently shown the improved cognitive and social outcomes for children with intellectual disability, if educational interventions are commenced early and, if possible, in inclusive play group or nursery classes (Guralnick, 2016). When school age is reached, the least disabled children can be supported within mainstream classes and, if needed, attend remedial classes. Others need to attend special educational programmes for children with intellectual disabilities. It is still not certain which intellectually disabled children benefit from ordinary schooling. Education in an ordinary school offers the advantages of more normal social surroundings, social integration, and the expectation of progress, but it may have the disadvantage of a lack of special teaching skills and equipment. Also, the methods of teaching that emphasize self-expression are inappropriate for some children with intellectual disability, who need special teaching of language and communication. Another advantage of educating disabled children in ordinary schools is that other pupils appreciate that their integration into society is the norm.

Before intellectually disabled children leave school, they need reassessment and vocational guidance. The resources and opportunities available to young people with intellectual disability have an unfortunate tradition of being inadequate and not meeting their complex needs; this is exacerbated by many accepting limited aspirations set for them by themselves and others (Talbot *et al.*, 2010). Most young people with mild intellectual disability are able to take normal jobs or enter sheltered employment. Adults with severe disability are likely to transfer to adult day centres, which should provide a wide range of activities if the abilities of each attender are to be developed as much as possible.

Residential care

It is now widely accepted that parents should be supported in caring for their intellectually disabled children at home. If care is too heavy a burden for the parents because of their other family commitments, the child with intellectual disability should, if possible, be placed in another family. Adults should be supported in ordinary housing, or placed with a family, or in suitable lodgings, or in a small residential group home. Staff need to encourage the residents to develop their social skills and to live as normally as possible.

Medical services

People with intellectual disability should have the same access to general and specialist medical services as other citizens, but they require extra support if they are to obtain full benefit. This care is usually obtained from the ordinary medical services and this arrangement can work well, provided that doctors and nurses are sufficiently aware of how to deal with a person with intellectual disability, and have the time and resources to do so. Families and carers are helped when care is coordinated by a single person, so that they do not receive conflicting advice. Specialist nurses have a particularly important role in such coordination. Shared care between neurologists and psychiatrists can improve outcomes for some patients—for example, in the diagnosis and treatment of epilepsy.

People with intellectual disability have increased health needs and it is therefore generally recommended that annual health checks be performed. This helps to screen for treatable conditions and improve their quality of life, as well as preventing early death.

Psychiatric services

Psychiatric care is an essential part of a comprehensive community service for people with intellectual disability. In some countries it is provided by generic mental health services, but in the UK it is generally provided by staff who specialize in the care of people with intellectual disability. The psychiatrist with such a specialism forms part of a wider intellectual disability team, consisting of intellectual disability nurses, psychologists, and social workers. Once known to the team, the patient may access the psychiatrist in the event of psychiatric disorders or behaviours that are challenging. Some psychiatrists with specialist intellectual disability training may also diagnose, treat, and manage epilepsy, although, as noted above, a neurologist may also be involved in this and in other neurological aspects of management.

Treatment of psychiatric disorder and behavioural problems

Psychiatric disorder in people with intellectual disability usually comes to notice through changes in behaviour. It should be remembered, however, that behavioural change can also result from physical illness or from stressful events, both of which should be carefully excluded. In the most disabled, and especially those with sensory deficits, behavioural disturbance may be due to understimulation and frustration owing to the inability to communicate wishes and needs. Once the cause is clear, the treatment follows. Physical illness should be treated promptly, stressful events reduced if possible, or a more stimulating environment provided when appropriate. If the disturbed behaviour results from a psychiatric disorder, the treatment is similar in most ways to that for a patient of normal intelligence with the same disorder. Carers are often involved in behavioural assessment and treatment methods, and it is important to support them adequately.

The most serious and persistent disorders occasionally require hospital admission for more intensive behavioural management, which may be combined with pharmacotherapy.

Medication

The indications for psychotropic drugs are generally the same as for patients of normal intelligence, and the full range of such medication should be available for the intellectually disabled. However, the psychiatrist has particular responsibility for organizing effective ongoing monitoring, including regular physical examination. The latter is especially important for patients with severe communication impairments who cannot describe adverse effects. Also, neurologically impaired patients may develop adverse effects at lower doses and suffer from oversedation, delirium, and extrapyramidal symptoms. Antipsychotic and benzodiazepine drugs are often useful in the short-term control of behaviour problems, generally at much lower doses than would be prescribed in the general population. There are few controlled trials of the efficacy and tolerability of antipsychotic drugs in the longer-term treatment of abnormal behaviour. None the less, clinical experience suggests that severely behaviourally disturbed patients who do not respond to psychosocial interventions sometimes benefit from prolonged use of medication with frequent monitoring of its effects and adjustment of dosage. For a review, see Bramble (2011).

Antiepileptic drug treatment is frequently required, given the prevalence of epilepsy in intellectual disability (see page 489). Special care is needed to select a drug and dosage that controls seizures without causing unwanted effects. The older antiepileptic drugs sometimes cause oversedation and cognitive blunting, and newer drugs, such as sodium valproate, are usually preferred. Because of the problem of drug resistance, second-line and combination therapies may be required, and involvement of an epilepsy specialist is recommended. For a review of the management of epilepsy in intellectual disability, see Iivanainen (2009).

Psychological treatment

Although limited understanding of language sets obvious limitations to the use of psychotherapy, it can be useful in some settings. More able patients can benefit from a modified or simplified approach, and psychological therapies are a key intervention for people with an intellectual disability when experiencing distress. Although the evidence base is small, some of the key psychological therapies currently used include behaviour therapy, cognitive behaviour therapy, psychodynamic psychotherapy, systemic family therapy, and a range of arts therapies (Talbot *et al.*, 2010). Cognitive therapies can be attempted with some patients with higher levels of verbal ability, although the most useful psychological treatment takes the form of behavioural therapies. These may be, and are, used for a wide variety of problems (e.g. challenging behaviour in a wide variety of patient abilities). Some intellectual disability nurses take a special interest in such therapies, and some psychologists are extensively trained in the area. Counselling for parents is an important part of treatment. If more formal family therapy is undertaken, families generally prefer structural approaches, which address the problems and solutions that are relevant to them. Some children with profound intellectual disability can be helped by the use of play and sensory stimulation to encourage developmental advances.

Behaviour modification

Behavioural methods are helpful to people with severe intellectual disability as some of the methods do not require language, and can be used to encourage basic skills such as washing, toilet training, and dressing. These are also discussed above in the section 'Behaviours that challenge' with Positive Behaviour Supports a prominent intervention. Often parents and teachers are taught to carry out the training so that it can be maintained in the patient's everyday environment. If the problem is an undesired behaviour, a search is made for any environmental factors that seem regularly to provoke it or reinforce it (functional analysis). If possible, these environmental factors are changed and carers helped to avoid rewarding the behaviour. At the same time, alternative adaptive responses are reinforced. Aggressive behaviour is sometimes dealt with by so-called 'time-out', in which the person is ignored or secluded until the behaviour subsides. However, techniques that employ negative reinforcement should not be used (Banks *et al.*, 2007). If the problem is an insufficiency of some socially desirable behaviour, attempts can be made to reinforce such behaviour with material or social rewards, if necessary by 'shaping' the final behaviour from simpler components. Reward should be given immediately after the desired behaviour has taken place (e.g. using the toilet). For training in skills such as dressing, it is often necessary to provide modelling and prompting in the early stages, and to reduce them gradually later.

Ethical and legal issues in intellectual disability

Normalization, autonomy, and the conflict of interests

The policy of normalization has encouraged intellectually disabled people to live as near normal lives as possible. This policy can create conflicts between the interests of the intellectually disabled person and those of others, such that it may be difficult to balance the interests of the disabled person with those of their carer(s) and other family members. Normalization can also produce unintended effects. For example, it requires that intellectually disabled children should be educated in ordinary schools whenever possible. However, in secondary schools, children with special needs were found to be bullied three times more often than other children (Whitney *et al.*, 1994). It could be argued that it is in the immediate interests of an individual child to be educated in a special school where he or she is less likely to be bullied, whereas the long-term interests of intellectually disabled children as a group may be advanced more by a policy of education in ordinary schools while making strenuous efforts to eradicate bullying.

Normalization also leads to practical ethical questions about sexual activity, contraception, and parenting, as mentioned earlier. The social inclusion of people with intellectual disability includes being able to participate in social networks, having friends, holding membership of clubs, and being able to travel.

Consent to treatment

Many people with severe intellectual disability are unable to give informed consent, and it is essential to be aware of local legislation and practice. In the UK, these issues are covered by the Mental Capacity Act (see Chapter 4), under which the practitioner is required to try to explain the nature of the procedure in a way that the patient can understand. If the patient is deemed to lack capacity, steps should be taken to help the person understand through assistive methods. The least restrictive option in keeping with the best interests of the intellectually disabled person should be pursued, usually through the involvement of a person closely involved in their care and who knows them well (Kelly, 2015). An advocate may also be involved. If there is doubt and inpatient admission is being sought, it is good practice to discuss matters with the local Mental Capacity Act office and hold a 'best interests' meeting. Discussing the case with an experienced practitioner is also helpful.

Seriously ill patients who refuse potentially life-saving treatments can prove difficult to deal with in general medical settings. If the patient is sufficiently impaired as not to understand the nature of the choice that they face and there is a medical emergency, a Mental Capacity Act assessment should be completed by the medical team. If there is time, it may be necessary to refer the case for review in court—for example, when the question of termination of pregnancy has to be decided.

Consent to research

Consent to research requires the ability to understand information, to use the information rationally, to appreciate the consequences of situations, and to decide between alternatives (see Chapter 4). The assessment of these abilities among the intellectually disabled has been described by the American Psychiatric Association (1998). Any individual who has agreed to take part in research should understand that they can withdraw consent if they wish, a point that should be explained with particular care (Arscott et al., 1998). In general, no research should be undertaken involving people who cannot consent, unless the same research cannot be successfully carried out without involving these people. It is important to remember that individuals with intellectual disability vary in their capacity to provide informed consent. Some may be able to provide verbal rather than written consent. Some may need sign language, pictures, or written information in simple language and a large font size. For some the proposal may have to be discussed repeatedly. It is also good practice to have agreement with the carers and the multidisciplinary team members. In every case the research should follow strictly the relevant research governance criteria and, in the UK, the Mental Capacity Act (see Chapter 4).

Further reading

Bhaumik S et al. (2015). The Frith Prescribing Guidelines for Adults with Learning Disability, 3rd edn. Wiley-Blackwell, Chichester.

Emerson E and Einfeld SL (2011). Challenging Behaviour, 3rd edn. Cambridge University Press, Cambridge.

Gelder MG, Andreasen NC, López-Ibor JJ Jr, and Geddes JR (eds) (2009). Part 10: Intellectual disability. In: The New Oxford Textbook of Psychiatry, 2nd edn. Oxford University Press, Oxford. (The nine chapters in this part of the textbook provide a systematic account of the subject written for the general psychiatrist.)

Hassiotis A et al. (2009). Intellectual Disability Psychiatry: a practical handbook. John Wiley & Sons, Chichester.

CHAPTER 18

Forensic psychiatry

Introduction

Chapter 4 covered general legal and ethical issues in the practice of medicine and psychiatry. This chapter is concerned with other aspects of psychiatry and the law covered by the term *forensic psychiatry*, which is used in two ways.

1. Narrowly, it is applied to the branch of psychiatry that deals with the assessment and treatment of mentally abnormal offenders.

2. Broadly, the term is applied to all legal aspects of psychiatry, including the civil law and laws regulating psychiatric practice.

Forensic psychiatrists are concerned with both of these issues. In addition, they also assess risk and treat people with violent behaviour who have not committed an offence in law. They have a growing role in the assessment and treatment of victims.

Offenders with mental disorders constitute a minority of all offenders, but they present many difficult problems for psychiatry and the law. These include *legal issues*, such as the relationship between the mental disorder and the crime, which may affect the court's determination of responsibility, and *practical clinical questions*,

such as whether an offender needs psychiatric treatment, and finding the appropriate setting for that treatment.

The psychiatrist therefore needs knowledge not only of the law but also of the relationship between particular kinds of crime and particular kinds of psychiatric disorder. Mental health services form only a small part of the social and legal response to criminal deviance. The psychiatrist who is working with offenders needs to be able to liaise with others in the criminal justice system, such as lawyers, prison staff, and probation officers. Concepts of deviance, guilt, and legality are influenced by legal, political, and social factors, as well as by clinical issues.

In reading this chapter it is important to be aware of the very large differences between countries and jurisdictions, with substantial national variations in epidemiology, definitions of crime, legal practice, and the role of the psychiatrist. Readers need to be aware of legal issues and procedures in their jurisdiction. In the following account, the situations and procedures in the UK (and more especially England and Wales) are used as examples to illustrate general themes. Ethical issues are summarized in Box 18.1.

> ### Box 18.1 Ethical issues in forensic psychiatry
>
> The principal ethical issues relate to 'boundary problems'. The psychiatrist and others involved need to be clear about accountability to legal authorities, etc., rather than to the individual who is being assessed and treated. This applies to a variety of activities:
>
> 1. *Preparation of medicolegal reports.* In the UK, the responsibility of the psychiatrist is to the Court rather than to the patient or their legal representative.
> 2. *Assessment of risk.* Assessment of the risk to others may be paramount.
> 3. *Voluntary and compulsory treatment.* The primary reason for treatment may involve decreasing the risk of harm to others.

General criminology

There is an extensive literature on criminology and many theories of the causes of crime; interested readers are referred to criminology textbooks (see Maguire *et al.*, 2012). Most theories have emphasized the sociological aspects of crime and deviance, particularly social and economic causes of crime in the family, peer group, and subculture. These include poverty, poor schooling, and unemployment. Predisposing social and individual factors are often interrelated, so simple conclusions are rarely possible. However, social causes are widely considered more important than individual factors such as genetics and psychological traits. Despite this, most correctional and forensic mental health programmes rely on psychological risk factors to encourage, for example, the development of coping skills (Dowden *et al.*, 2003).

Prevalence

International data indicate a steady reduction in crime, particularly violent crime, over the past two decades. Prevalence figures must be viewed cautiously because much criminal behaviour goes unrecorded by the police. This is especially true of violence within the home, such as rape, child abuse, or partner battering. Crime surveys probably provide more accurate figures. Data from the British Crime Survey are shown by the curve in Figure 18.1. Property offences are the most common type of crime, but forensic mental health services are most likely to be involved with crimes of interpersonal violence.

National differences

There are large national differences in the rates and patterns of crime (United Nations Office on Drugs and Crime,

2010). Within Europe, overall crime rates in the UK are lower than those in the Netherlands but higher than those in the Scandinavian countries. Crimes of assault are more common in the USA and Australia. National statistics are affected by local legislation, the recording of crimes, and by the conduct of legal proceedings.

Gender

Crime is predominantly an activity of young men. In England and Wales, 50% of all indictable offences are committed by males aged under 21 years, and 25% by those under 17 years. Men represent at least 80% of offenders (Monahan, 1997), and, in most western countries, male prisoners outnumber female prisoners by 30:1. This gender difference is reflected in forensic mental health services, where the majority of patients are male.

Ethnicity

Ethnic minority groups are usually overrepresented in prisoner populations (Hassan *et al.*, 2011). Minority groups are more likely to be poor, unemployed, and living in poor housing, all of which are risk factors for crime. Consequently, they are overrepresented in forensic patient populations (Kaye and Lingiah, 2000).

The high rates of arrests and convictions in ethnic minority groups may also reflect discrimination at all stages of the criminal justice system—from stop and search through to trial and sentencing.

Victims

Most property crime is committed against strangers, but most serious interpersonal violence (rape, homicide, or child abuse) is committed by offenders known to the

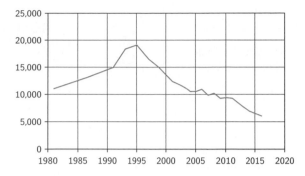

Figure 18.1 Crimes reported to the British Crime Survey by the public during the period 1981–2016. The y axis shows numbers of crimes in thousands.

victim. Women are exposed to sexual violence from men in both developed and developing countries. Women and children are particularly at risk in developing countries during armed conflicts, where about 70% of casualties are non-combatants (Kennedy Bergen *et al.*, 2005).

Victims of crime tend to be disadvantaged groups living in poorer parts of urban communities, so the mentally disordered are more likely to be victims of crime, and the risk is further increased as a consequence of their illness (Hart *et al.*, 2012).

Causes of crime

Criminal behaviour (crime) needs to be distinguished from rule-breaking behaviour. Not all rule-breaking or socially unacceptable behaviour is criminal, nor is all criminal behaviour violent. In fact, the vast majority is not, so general theories of the causes of crime will not necessarily address the causes of violence. Aggressive behaviour is not always violent, as it can be constrained by social rules. Violence is aggressive behaviour that transgresses social norms, as in street fighting as opposed to, for example, boxing.

Many factors determine whether an individual is aggressive in a particular situation. These include personality, the immediate social group, the behaviour of the victim, disinhibiting factors such as alcohol or drugs, general environmental factors such as noise and social pressure, physiological factors such as fatigue, hunger, and lack of sleep, and the presence of mental abnormality.

Genetic and physiological factors

Early *studies of twins* suggested that concordance rates for criminality were substantially greater in monozygotic twins than in dizygotic twins (Lange, 1931). Results from well over 100 behavioural genetics

studies with different designs—including twin studies, studies of twins reared apart, and adoption studies—have converged on the conclusion that antisocial and aggressive behaviour have a considerable genetic basis. Estimates of the variance that is attributable to genetics vary, but several meta-analyses estimate heritability at between 40% and 60%, broadly consistent between genders and ethnicities (Glenn and Raine, 2014).

The gender difference in offending has raised the question of the influence of either the Y chromosome or testosterone levels on offending. However, there is little evidence that *chromosomal or hormonal abnormalities* are causally associated with criminal behaviour or aggression. As was noted in Chapter 15, low brain 5-HT function has been associated with impulsive aggression. There is evidence that individuals with sociopathic personalities have longstanding neuropsychological deficits, particularly in executive processes (Raine *et al.*, 2005).

Psychosocial factors

Individual psychological development interacts with social factors and cultural values to make offending more likely (see Box 18.2). Rule-breaking and antisocial behaviour often starts in childhood or early adulthood:

- Follow-up studies of delinquent young people show that early patterns of antisocial behaviour are likely to persist into adulthood.
- Delinquency is associated with harsh parenting and poverty.
- Exposure to physical abuse or neglect in childhood significantly increases the risk of violent offending in later life, for both men and women (Rutter, 2005).

The association between childhood adversity and violence may have several mechanisms. Abused and neglected children may have a heightened perception of threat from others. They may have decreased capacities to form successful interpersonal relationships owing to either decreased empathy for others or reduced capacity for self-awareness. Alternatively, they may have a decreased capacity to manage arousal or regulate anger or anxiety arising from excessive exposure to fear experiences. It is also possible that children and parents simply share genetic factors that impair affect regulation or the ability to empathize. However, it is always important to consider the impact of resilience or vulnerability factors, such as temperament (Rutter, 2005).

Psychiatric causes

A small but important group of offenders exhibit criminal behaviour that seems to be partly explicable by specific psychological or psychiatric abnormalities. This group particularly concerns the psychiatrist, and is discussed in the next section.

> ### Box 18.2 Psychosocial risk factors for offending
>
> #### Individual and family factors
>
> Prenatal and perinatal influences—birth complications, maternal rejection, fetal neurological maldevelopment, maternal nicotine and alcohol consumption
> Hyperactivity and impulsivity
> Low intelligence
> Punitive parenting style—poor supervision, harsh discipline, rejection
> Teenage mothers
> Parental conflict—separations
> Criminal parents
> Large family size
>
> #### Social factors
>
> Socioeconomic deprivation
> Peer influences
> School influences
> Community influences
>
> Source: data from Farrington D P, Psychosocial causes of offending. In: Gelder MG, Andreasen NC, Lopez-Ibor JJ and Geddes J (eds.), The New Oxford Textbook of Psychiatry, Copyright (2009), Oxford University Press; Nature Reviews Neuroscience, 15(1), Glenn A L and Raine A, Neurocriminology: implications for the punishment, prediction and prevention of criminal behavior, pp. 54–63, Copyright (2014), Nature Publishing Group.

The association between mental disorder and crime

Frequency

The association between mental disorder and violence has been repeatedly demonstrated. Fazel *et al.* (2009a) conducted a systematic review of violence and schizophrenia and other psychoses. This meta-analysis of 20 studies, including 18,423 individuals, found that schizophrenia and other psychoses were associated with violence (especially homicide). However, this risk was mediated by comorbid substance abuse, and was the same for individuals with substance abuse without psychosis. The increased risk of violent offending in both men and women with a diagnosis of affective psychosis could be accounted for by alcohol and substance misuse. Alcohol and substance misuse by themselves are associated with a substantially increased risk of violent offending, as is personality disorder (see Table 18.1; Johns, 2009).

Research on the prevalence and association of mental disorder in prisoners has recognized limitations:

- Not all criminals are brought to trial and found guilty.
- Not all criminals go to prison (potential sampling bias).
- Mentally disordered offenders may be diverted away from courts and prisons, or they may not be prosecuted.

Table 18.1 Relative risk estimates of violent crime from the Danish Birth Register

Disorder	Male	Female
Schizophrenia spectrum disorder	4.8	13.7
Affective disorders	3.5	4.3
Learning difficulties	1.7	—
Personality disorders	5.7	7.9

Reproduced from Psychological Medicine, 45(11), Stevens H et al, Post-illness-onset risk of offending across the full spectrum of psychiatric disorders, pp. 2447–2457, Copyright (2015), with permission from Cambridge University Press.

The proportion of prisoners with mental disorders is higher than the proportion of the general population with such disorders (Ogloff, 2009). In a meta-analysis of 62 psychiatric surveys of prisoners, Fazel and Danesh (2002) found that about one in seven had a treatable psychiatric illness (see Table 18.2). A larger number suffer from antisocial personality disorder. Hassan *et al.* (2011) surveyed the mental health of over 3000 prisoners on admission and found up to 17% with mental illness and over half with drug or alcohol misuse.

The nature of the association

A causal relationship between mental disorder and crime is difficult to show empirically, especially if the type of crime is not defined. The finding that mentally disordered individuals are overrepresented in prison does not necessarily mean that their mental disorder caused them to offend. Nor is criminal law-breaking an indicator in itself of mental disorder, no matter how heinous or bizarre the behaviour.

Only a small minority of all people who commit violent acts have serious mental illness such as psychosis. Swedish national registers linking hospital admissions and criminal convictions over 13 years demonstrated a population-attributable risk fraction of 5.2% (i.e. only 5% of convictions were accounted for by individuals with severe mental illness). This attributable risk

Table 18.2 Meta-analysis of 62 psychiatric surveys of prisoners

Disorder	Male (%)	Female (%)
Psychosis	4	4
Major depression	10	12
Antisocial personality	65	42

fraction was higher in women across all age bands. In women aged 25–39 years, it was 14.0%, and in those aged 40 years or over, it was 19.0% (Fazel and Grann, 2006). In a more recent Swedish register study, Fazel *et al.* (2014a) showed that, within 5 years of their first diagnosis of schizophrenia, 10.7% of men and 2.7% of women were convicted of a violent offence. The vast majority of patients with psychotic illnesses are no more dangerous than members of the general population. There is no evidence that homicidal behaviour is becoming more common in people with mental illness—indeed, it appears to have been declining since the early 1970s (Large *et al.*, 2008).

For a review of the association between psychiatric disorder and offending, see Thomson and Darjee (2009) (see also Box 18.3).

Specific psychiatric disorders

Substance dependence and crime

There are close relationships between substance abuse and crime, which have substantially affected legislation, enforcement, and national policies (Grann and Fazel, 2004).

Alcohol and crime are related in three important ways:

1. Alcohol intoxication may lead to charges related to public drunkenness or to driving offences.
2. Intoxication reduces inhibitions and is strongly associated with crimes of violence, including murder.
3. The neuropsychiatric complications of alcoholism may also be linked with crime.

Offences may be committed during alcoholic amnesias or 'blackouts'. Blackouts are periods of several hours or days, which the heavy drinker cannot recall, although at the time they appeared normally conscious to other people and were able to carry out complicated actions. However, the association is complex, and social factors related to drinking may be as important as alcohol itself. For a review, see Johns (2009).

Intoxication with drugs may lead to criminal behaviour, including violent offences. Drug misusers, especially those who are dependent on heroin and cocaine, commit repeated offences against both property and people to fund their drug habit. Some of the offences involve violence. Rates of drug abuse are increased among prisoners, and many succeed in obtaining drugs in prison. Involvement in criminal activity and with other criminals may lead to drug usage. For a review of the relationship between drug dependence and crime, see Johns (2009).

> ### Box 18.3 Psychiatric disorder and offending
>
> - People with psychotic disorders are more likely than members of the general public to acquire convictions for violent or other crimes (by factors of approximately 4 and 10, respectively).
> - This increased likelihood is altered in strength by local factors such as crime rate and sociodemographic variables.
> - Antisocial personality disorder and substance misuse disorders have stronger associations with offending than does psychotic illness.
> - A combination of psychiatric disorders (particularly when one of them is substance misuse disorder) may
>
> be more relevant than any single category of psychiatric disorder.
> - Most offending by those with psychiatric disorder is minor in nature; violence, when it occurs, is likely to be targeted at a family member.
>
> Source: data from Thomson L and Darjee R, Associations between psychiatric disorder and offending. In: Gelder MG, Andreasen NC, Lopez-Ibor JJ and Geddes J (eds.), The New Oxford Textbook of Psychiatry, pp. 1917–26, Copyright (2009), Oxford University Press; Journal of the American Academy of Psychiatry and the Law, 34(4), Mullen PE et al, Assessing and managing the risks in the stalking situation, pp. 439–50, Copyright (2006), American Academy of Psychiatry and the Law.

Intellectual disability

There is no evidence that most criminals are of markedly low intelligence. However, reduced intellectual ability is an independent predictor of offending (Holland *et al.*, 2002).

People with learning disabilities may commit offences because they do not understand the implications of their behaviour, or because they are susceptible to exploitation by others. Property offences are the most common, but sexual offences are overrepresented, particularly indecent exposure by males (Perry *et al.*, 2002). The exposer is often known to the victim and therefore the rate of detection is high. There is also an association between learning disability and arson (Taylor *et al.*, 2002).

Mood disorder

Depressive disorder is sometimes associated with shoplifting. Severe depressive disorder may rarely lead to *homicide*. The depressed person may be deluded, for example, that the world is too dreadful to live in, and they consequently kill their family members to spare them. Suicide often follows. A mother suffering from postpartum disorder may sometimes kill her newborn child or her older children. Rarely, a person with severe depressive disorder may commit homicide because of a persecutory belief—for example, that the victim is conspiring against them. Occasionally, ideas of guilt and unworthiness lead depressed patients to confess to crimes that they did not commit.

Manic patients may spend excessive amounts of money on expensive objects, such as jewellery or cars, that they cannot pay for. They may be charged with fraud, theft, or false pretences. They are also prone to irritability and aggression, which may lead to offences of violence, although this is seldom severe.

Schizophrenia and related disorder

Psychotic illnesses may be associated with violence, especially when paranoid symptomatology is present, or the patient also has a substance abuse problem. Violence may occur because the offender is frightened, and self-control may be reduced by the presence of the psychotic state. Any state in which paranoid psychotic symptoms feature carries an increased risk of violent behaviour.

Epidemiology

Epidemiological studies have strongly suggested that schizophrenia is associated with an increased risk of both violent and non-violent offending (Fazel *et al.*, 2014a). This risk is substantially increased by substance misuse, but the proportion of violent crime attributable to schizophrenia is low. A number of clinical risk factors for violence in schizophrenia have been proposed, including the following:

- fear and loss of self-control associated with non-systematized delusions
- irresistible urges
- instructions from hallucinatory voices (command hallucinations)
- dual diagnosis, particularly substance misuse
- a strong negative affect (e.g. depression, anger, agitation).

Coid *et al.* (2013) found that six out of 32 types of delusions generated anger in the patient and, of these, three (persecution, being spied on, and conspiracy) resulted in increased risks of violence. Risk assessment is discussed on page 534. Violent threats made by patients with psychosis should be taken very seriously (especially in those with a history of previous violence). Most serious violence occurs in those already known to psychiatrists, particularly if there is an identifiable victim.

Post-traumatic stress disorder

Post-traumatic stress disorder (PTSD) may be related to offending in three ways:

- PTSD patients may abuse drugs and alcohol.
- PTSD is associated with increased irritability and decreased affect regulation.
- PTSD patients may rarely experience dissociative episodes involving violence, especially in circumstances resembling their original trauma. This is often hard to determine retrospectively.

PTSD has increasingly been the basis for psychiatric defences to homicide, especially in the US. It has also been advanced for battered women with a history of prolonged trauma, in whom occasional acts of retaliatory violence are not uncommon.

Morbid jealousy

The syndrome of morbid (pathological) jealousy (see Chapter 12) may be associated with several of the above diagnoses. It has been identified in 12% of 'insane' male and 3% of 'insane' women murderers. It is particularly dangerous because of the risk of the offence being repeated with another partner. It may sometimes be difficult to distinguish morbid jealousy from extreme possessiveness or control over women's behaviour, which may be accompanied by violence.

Organic mental disorders

Delirium is occasionally associated with criminal behaviour, usually because of the associated confusion or disinhibition. Diagnostic problems may arise if the mental disturbance improves before the offender is examined by a doctor.

Dementia is sometimes associated with offences, although crime is otherwise uncommon among the elderly, and violent offences are rare. Violent and disinhibited behaviour may also occur after a *head injury* (Fazel *et al.*, 2009b) and be difficult to distinguish from PTSD.

Epilepsy

The association between epilepsy and crime is complex and poorly understood. It has been widely believed that the risk of epilepsy is greater in prisoners than in the general population, but a meta-analysis of seven studies did not find this (Fazel *et al.*, 2002), and a longitudinal study found that, after adjusting for familial confounding, epilepsy was not associated with increased risk of violent crime (Fazel *et al.*, 2011a). Violent behaviour

associated with EEG abnormalities in the absence of clinical epilepsy is unlikely to indicate a causal relationship (Fazel *et al.*, 2009b). *Epileptic automatisms* may, very rarely, be associated with violent behaviour and subsequent criminal proceedings. Violence is more common in the post-ictal state than ictally.

Impulse control disorders

DSM-5 contains a category 'Disruptive impulse-control and conduct disorders', which includes speculative conditions relevant to forensic psychiatry—intermittent explosive disorder, pyromania, and kleptomania. In ICD-10 these conditions are classified under abnormalities of adult personality and behaviour as 'habit and impulse disorders'. Whatever the clinical value of such classifications, none of these conditions has been established as a separate diagnostic entity.

Intermittent explosive disorder

This term is used to describe repeated episodes of seriously aggressive behaviour out of proportion to any provoking events and not accounted for by another psychiatric disorder (e.g. antisocial personality disorder, substance abuse, or schizophrenia). The aggression may be preceded by tension, followed by relief, followed by remorse. The condition is rare, and many psychiatrists doubt whether it is a distinct psychiatric disorder.

Pathological gambling

Pathological gambling, 'gambling disorder', was included with impulse control disorders in DSM-IV but has been moved to 'Substance-related and addictive disorders' in DSM-5 (Grant *et al.*, 2013; Petry, 2010). Gambling is pathological when it is repeated frequently and dominates the person's life, and persists when the person can no longer afford to pay their debts. The person lies, steals, defrauds, or avoids repayment to continue the habit. Family life may be damaged, other social relationships may be impaired, and employment put at risk. Pathological gamblers demonstrate a range of cognitive distortions, such as *magnification of gambling skill, superstitions, temporal telescoping, predictive skill*, and obviously *selective memory* (Hodgins *et al.*, 2011). Treatments using cognitive behaviour therapy (CBT) and family therapy have received some support. Gamblers Anonymous is widely used but has not been carefully evaluated. Because of the reclassification of gambling disorder with addictions, various trials have been conducted with opioid receptor antagonists and indicate some modest benefits (Hodgins *et al.*, 2011).

Pathological gamblers have an intense urge to gamble, which is difficult to control. They are preoccupied with thoughts of gambling, much as a person dependent on alcohol is preoccupied with thoughts of drink. Increasing sums of money are gambled, either to increase the excitement or in an attempt to recover previous losses. If gambling is prevented, the person becomes irritable and even more preoccupied with the behaviour.

Similarities with the behaviour of people who are dependent on drugs have led to the suggestion that pathological gambling is itself a form of addictive behaviour. Brain imaging studies of pathological gamblers show abnormalities in mesolimbic reward pathways similar to those in drug dependence (Goudriaan *et al.*, 2004).

The prevalence of pathological gambling is not known. The explosive growth in internet gambling, smartphone gambling apps, and TV spot-betting have undoubtedly increased the risks. There is currently considerable governmental pressure to reduce the spread of online betting and betting shops and so limit the potential losses with gambling machines. It is probably more frequent among males. Most gamblers seen by psychiatrists are adults, but there is concern that young people are increasingly being involved, usually with gambling machines in amusement arcades. For a review of pathological gambling, see Moran (2009).

Pyromania

Pyromania refers to repeated episodes of deliberate fire-setting, which are not carried out for identifiable reasons such as monetary gain, to conceal a crime, as an act of vengeance, or as a consequence of hallucinations or delusions. Impaired judgement resulting from intoxication, dementia, or mental retardation excludes the diagnosis of pyromania, as does antisocial personality disorder, a manic episode, or

(among children or adolescents) a conduct disorder. Prins (2009) reviews arson and observes that the rates have more than doubled over the past 40 years, that women are increasingly the perpetrators and that repeat offending is more common. Like many authorities he doubts that pyromania is a specific disorder and is better considered as a symptom. In the rare condition of pyromania, the act of fire-setting is preceded by tension or arousal, followed by relief. People with pyromania have a preoccupation with fires and fire-fighting, and enjoy watching fires. They may plan the offence in advance, taking no account of the danger to other people.

Kleptomania

Kleptomania refers to repeated failure to resist impulses to steal objects that are not needed, either for use or for their monetary value. The impulses are not associated with delusions or hallucinations, or with motives of anger or vengeance. Before stealing there is increased tension, which the stealing relieves. The diagnosis is excluded by associated antisocial personality disorder, a manic episode, or (among children or adolescents) a conduct disorder, or when the stealing results from sexual fetishism. The objects stolen may be of little value and may be hoarded, thrown away, or later returned to the owner. The patient knows that the stealing is unlawful, and may feel guilty and depressed after the immediate pleasurable sensations that follow the act.

Kleptomania occurs more often among women. Associations with anxiety and eating disorders have been described. It may be sporadic, or persist for years despite repeated prosecutions. The diagnosis depends entirely on accused individuals' descriptions of their own motives and is therefore viewed with some scepticism.

Specific offender groups

Female offenders

Women are more law-abiding than men. Shoplifting accounts for 50% of all their convictions, and violent and sexual offences are uncommon.

Men and women are treated differently by the criminal justice system. Women are sentenced more leniently for similar offences, and they are more likely to be viewed as 'sick'. Psychiatric disorder is frequent among women admitted to prison, with personality disorder and substance misuse being especially common (Fazel

and Danesh, 2002), and self-harm before and during imprisonment is also common (Jenkins *et al.*, 2005).

Young people

National crime statistics indicate that a significant proportion of crime is conducted by those under the age of 18 years, or 'juveniles'. In the UK the rates appear to be declining but not in the US (Ministry of Justice, 2015; National Center for Juvenile Justice, 2014). In Scotland, for example, in the year 2000, 34% of young people (aged 12–15 years) reported committing a criminal offence in the previous year, compared with 22% in 1992 (Scottish Executive Central Research Unit, 2002). Where a young person is violent, the victim is often well known to them, commonly a family member. Serious violence by young people and children is rare, and the individuals involved have frequently been the recipients of violence themselves, both within and outside their families (Hamilton *et al.*, 2002). Data from the American National comorbidity study explored the relationship between crime and psychiatric disorders in those under 18 years of age (Kendell *et al.*, 2014). They showed that there was a high prevalence of crime, with 18.4% of those with a psychiatric disorder before the age of 18 years reporting a crime and arrest history. Conduct disorder, alcohol use disorders, and drug use disorders had the greatest odds.

Ethnic minorities

Some ethnic groups are overrepresented in both the criminal justice system and forensic psychiatric services. Non-white prisoners are more likely to receive diagnoses of mental illness rather than personality difficulties. Those with African Caribbean origin have higher rates of imprisonment in the UK, but lower rates of psychiatric morbidity despite an excess of African Caribbeans in secure hospitals (Coid *et al.*, 2002).

Psychiatric aspects of specific crimes

The following sections are concerned with the types of offences that are most likely to be associated with psychological factors. These are crimes of violence, sexual offences, and some offences against property.

Crimes of violence

Violence among mentally abnormal offenders is more strongly associated with personality disorder than with major mental illness. It is particularly common in people with antisocial personality traits who misuse alcohol or drugs, or who have marked paranoid or sadistic traits. It is often part of a persistent pattern of impulsive and aggressive behaviour, but it may be a sporadic response to stressful events in 'over-controlled' personalities.

Homicide

Rates of total homicide and stranger homicide have increased in the UK between 1973 and 2003, but rates committed by people with mental illness have remained static (Appleby *et al.*, 2015). Stranger homicides by the mentally ill have fallen somewhat since 2006, constituting 7% of all such homicides (Appleby *et al.*, 2015). Thus the proportion of homicides committed by the mentally ill has fallen in the era of community care.

Normal and abnormal homicide

Mental disorders may count as mitigation for an individual charged with murder, reducing the charge to manslaughter. Homicide can be divided according to the legal outcome into *normal* (murder or common-law manslaughter) and *abnormal* (insane murder, suicide murder, diminished responsibility, or infanticide).

Normal homicide accounts for half to two-thirds of all homicides in the UK, as in other western countries, including the USA, where the rate is much higher. It is most likely to be committed by socially disadvantaged young men. In the UK, the victims are mainly family members or close acquaintances. In countries with high homicide rates, a greater proportion of killings are associated with robbery or sexual offences. Sexual homicide may result from panic during a sexual offence. Alternatively, it may be a feature of a sadistic killing, sometimes committed by a shy man with bizarre sadistic and other violent fantasies.

Abnormal homicide accounts for one-third to half of all homicides in the UK. It is usually committed by older people. The victims of abnormal homicide are often family members. The most common psychiatric diagnoses are psychoses, substance use disorder, and personality disorder (Fazel and Grann, 2004). Depressive disorder can also be involved, especially in those who kill themselves afterwards. Homicide by women is much less frequent than that by men, but is nearly always 'abnormal'.

A large proportion of all murderers are under the influence of alcohol at the time of the crime, and drug misuse is also an important factor.

Multiple homicide

Multiple murders are rare, although they attract great public attention. They include:

- Individuals without mental illness who kill several people at once, sometimes a family killing which is often followed by suicide. Paranoid and grandiose character traits are common (Mullen, 2004).

- Killings attributable to a psychotic illness in which the killer aims to save himself or his family from a perceived threat.
- Serial killings that take place over a period of time. These may be 'normal' (e.g. killings by terrorists) or 'abnormal' (e.g. psychotic, or motivated by sexual sadism or necrophilia).

Homicide followed by suicide

Homicide followed by suicide accounts for about 50 deaths in the UK annually, while in the USA the comparable figure is 1000–1500 (Chiswick, 2000). Barraclough and Harris (2002) studied 180 victims and 147 perpetrators in the UK, and found that 80% of the incidents involved one victim and one perpetrator, 88% exclusively involving members of the same family. Around 75% of the victims were female, and 85% of the perpetrators were male, whose victims were nearly always current or previous female partners and their children. The victims of female perpetrators were predominantly their children.

Parents who kill their children

Around 25% of all victims of murder or manslaughter in the UK are under the age of 16 years, and babies under the age of 1 year are at the highest risk of all age groups (Breslin and Evans, 2004). Most children are killed by a parent who is mentally ill, usually the mother. The classification of child murder is difficult, but useful categories are mercy killing, psychotic murder, and, most common, killing resulting from battering or neglect (D'Orban, 1979).

Infanticide

A woman who kills her child may be charged with murder or manslaughter. English law recognizes a special category, infanticide, where the child is under 12 months of age. Infanticide is treated as manslaughter with less harsh penalties. The English legal concept of infanticide is unusual, requiring only that the woman's mind was disturbed as a result of birth or lactation, not that the killing was a consequence of her mental disturbance.

Fewer than five cases a year are recorded in the UK. Infants are most at risk on the first day of life, and the relative risk decreases steadily to that of the general population by 1 year. Fathers are slightly more likely to be recorded as the prime suspect over time and receive more severe sentences. Puerperal psychosis is a relatively infrequent cause of homicide, and depression is a factor in some cases. Later infant homicides are usually due to fatal child abuse. Infanticide has been associated with early motherhood.

Family homicide

Homicides can be distinguished by the relationship between perpetrator and victim. Most serious violence takes place within the family (25% of homicide victims are aged under 16 years, 80% killed by their parents). Around 50% of female victims are wives or partners, and the rest are often friends or relatives.

Domestic violence

Domestic violence accounts for about 25% of all violent incidents recorded by the British Crime Survey, about one million incidents annually in England and Wales, about two-thirds against women. Most batterers do not have either a diagnosable mental disorder or a criminal history. However, heavy drinking is common.

Some people are violent only within their family, while others are also violent outside. Violence in the family can have long-term deleterious effects on the psychological and social development of the children and on the mental health of the partner. Violence in the family also affects children and elderly relatives (page 551). Any of these forms of violence may rarely result in homicide.

Alertness to possible domestic violence is required not only in accident and emergency departments, but also in primary care and in obstetric and paediatric clinics. Intervention is difficult and raises ethical issues (see Box 18.4).

> ### Box 18.4 Ethical and legal issues: domestic violence
>
> Confidentiality is especially important because of the risk of retaliation by the abuser.
>
> Careful records are essential, including documentation of the injuries. Written consent should be obtained for photographs.
>
> Specialist advice should be sought about providing practical and other help to those who wish to end the relationship.
>
> Where the risk of serious violence is believed to be very high, disclosure to the police and other authorities to provide protection needs to be carefully planned with the maximum collaboration with the victims.

Violence towards partners

Violence by men towards their female partners is much more frequent than violence by women towards their male partners. It is physically more serious and is more often reported. Most 'wife batterers' are men with aggressive personalities, while a minority are violent only when psychiatrically unwell, usually with a mood disorder. Other common features among these men are morbid jealousy and heavy drinking. Such men may have suffered violence in childhood, and often come from backgrounds in which violence is frequent and tolerated. Behaviour by the victim may contribute to or provoke (but never justify) violence. This is difficult to assess if only the perpetrator is interviewed but, when battering is possibly a 'joint' problem, may be more difficult to stop. Repetitive battering, especially motivated by jealousy, is a real risk factor for homicide. The impacts of intimate partner violence to any children in the household must always be considered (Gonzalez *et al.*, 2014).

Sexual offences

Sexually violent offences

In the UK, sexual offences account for less than 1% of all indictable offences recorded by the police. Although only a small proportion of these are referred to psychiatrists they account for a significant number of assessments. Most sexual offences are committed by men.

Sexual offenders are generally older than other offenders. Reconviction rates are generally lower but recidivist sexual offenders are extremely difficult to manage (see Box 18.5). In the UK, Part 1 of the Sex Offenders Act 1997 requires those convicted or cautioned for relevant sex offences to be kept by police on the Sex Offender Register.

The most common sexual offences are indecent assault against women, indecent exposure, and unlawful intercourse with girls aged under 16 years. Some sexual offences do not involve physical violence (e.g. indecent exposure, voyeurism, and most sexual offences involving children), but others, such as rape, may involve considerable violence. The nature and treatment of non-violent sexual offences are discussed in Chapter 13; only their forensic aspects are considered here. For a review, see Gordon and Grubin (2004) or Hucker (2009).

> **Box 18.5 Some factors associated with increased risk of reoffending in sex offenders**
>
> - Previous criminal history
> - Higher number of sexual offences and more than one type of sexual offence
> - Being a childhood victim of sexual abuse
> - Violent sexual fantasies
> - Negative attitudes to women
> - Belief that victims consent to or enjoy the act
> - Choice of location and occupation to facilitate access to victims
> - Use of sadomasochistic or paedophilic pornography
> - Substance misuse
> - Treatment non-compliance
>
> Source: data from Advances in Psychiatric Treatment, 10(1), Gordon H and Grubin D, Psychiatric aspects of the assessment and treatment of sex offenders, pp. 73–80, Copyright (2004), The Royal College of Psychiatrists.

Sexual abuse of children

The age of consent varies in different countries. In England and Wales it is illegal to have any sexual activity with a person aged under 16 years, and this accounts for over 50% of all reported sexual offences. Underreporting is probable, particularly within families. Severity varies from mild indecency to seriously aggressive behaviour, but the large majority do not involve violence.

Offenders may or may not be paedophilic. *Paedophiles* are defined as having a primary sexual interest in pre-pubertal children. They are almost always male, either homosexual or heterosexual, and usually abuse children not previously well known to them. Paedophiles are rarely mentally ill. Victims are often prepared ('groomed') over a long period of time, increasingly via the internet. Some paedophiles may seek work in occupations where they will have access to children who will be left in their care. Cultural tolerance of paedophilia is now negligible, and high profile 'historical abuse' investigations are taking place worldwide, focusing on the church, childrens' homes, and the entertainment industry.

It is difficult to classify paedophiles, but the following groups have been recognized:

- the timid and sexually inexperienced
- the learning disabled

- those who have experienced normal sexual relationships but prefer sexual activity with children
- a predatory group who may use violence. In rare cases, paedophile sexual activities end in murder.

However, not all child sex offenders are paedophiles thus defined. A significant majority do not have a primary sexual interest in children. Many have 'normal' heterosexual histories and may be involved in such relationships at the time when they offend. Paedophilic child sex offenders typically are strangers to children, or else have gained opportunistic access through their chosen work or social activities. However, the majority of child sex offending is carried out by men (usually), who have some familial relationship to the child. Most commonly these are stepfathers or other male members of the extended family circle, who are typically not primary paedophiles.

The prognosis is difficult to determine. Among those who receive a prison sentence, the recidivism rate is about one in three. An important minority progress to violent sexual offences, so psychiatrists may be asked to give an opinion on their dangerousness.

Assessment

Usually, the perpetrator and the victim are assessed by different people. When trying to decide whether an offence is likely to be repeated or to progress to more serious offences, the psychiatrist should first consider the depositions and the victim's statement to gain available information about the following:

- The duration and frequency of the particular sexual activity in the past (remembering that paedophiles often deny their offending).
- The offender's predominant sexual preferences; exclusively paedophile inclinations and behaviour indicate a greater risk of repetition. Older paedophiles are less likely to be aggressive.

The interviews should determine:

- The offender's previous sexual history.
- Whether alcohol or drugs played any part in the offence, and, if so, whether the person is likely to continue to use them.
- Whether there are any feelings of regret or guilt.
- Any stressful circumstances associated with the offence (and the likelihood that these will continue).
- The degree of access to children.

- Evidence of any psychiatric disorder or relevant personality features.

Treatment

Treatment is directed towards any associated psychiatric disorder. Direct treatment of the sexual behaviour is difficult. Group therapy run jointly by mental health and probation services may be helpful, as is individual and group support provided by some charities. A recent systematic review showed some effect of group CBT to reduce reoffending at 1 year (number needed to treat [NNT] = 6) (Kenworthy *et al.*, 2004), but, despite enormous investment in prison services, there is little strong evidence of effect. The use of antiandrogens such as cyproterone and medroxyprogesterone has also been advocated, but their use is associated with many adverse effects and ethical issues.

Indecent exposure

This is the legal term for the offence of exposing the genitals to other people. It is applied to all forms of exposure; exhibitionism is by far the most frequent form, but exposure may also occur as an invitation to intercourse, as a prelude to sexual assault, or as an insulting gesture. *Exhibitionism* is the medical name for the behaviour of those who gain sexual satisfaction from repeatedly exposing to the opposite sex. In England and Wales, indecent exposure is one of the most frequent sexual offences, usually by men aged between 25 and 35 years with no history of psychiatric disorder or other criminal behaviour. Occasionally it is associated with compulsive disorder or substance misuse. Despite this, exhibitionism is listed as a psychiatric disorder in both DSM-5and ICD-10. A proportion of offenders are repeat recidivists, and may proceed to more serious sexual violence.

Indecent assault

The term indecent assault refers to a wide range of behaviour, from attempting to touch a stranger's buttocks to sexual assault without attempted penetration. The psychiatrist is most commonly asked to give a psychiatric opinion on adolescent boys and on men who have assaulted children. Although many adolescent boys behave in ways that could be construed as 'indecent', more serious indecent behaviour is associated with aggressive personality, ignorance, lack of social skills, and, occasionally, learning difficulties. Treatment depends on the associated problems.

Stalking

The lay term 'stalking' is usually taken to mean the repeated, unwanted, and intrusive targeting of a particular victim with following and other harassment. It implies an intensive preoccupation with the victim. The scope of behaviour is wide, and includes:

- following the victim
- communication by telephone, mail, and electronic communication
- ordering goods and services in the victim's name
- aggression and threats, including violence, damage to property, and false accusations.

Most stalkers are men, and most victims are women. The victims invariably suffer severe distress. Management requires cooperation between forensic psychiatrists and the criminal justice system in assessing risks, treating any associated psychiatric disorder (e.g. erotomania), and protecting and treating the victim. For a review, see Mullen *et al.* (2009) (also see Chapter 12).

Rape

In English law, a man commits rape if:

- He has unlawful sexual intercourse (whether vaginal or anal) with a woman or man who at the time of the intercourse does not consent to it.
- At the time he knows that the victim does not consent to the intercourse, or he is reckless as to whether they consent to it.

Most jurisdictions define rape in terms of the lack of consent of the victim. Not all jurisdictions recognize male rape or sexual assault. Some countries (such as the USA) additionally define lack of consent by age—so-called 'statutory rape'. English law is among the few that recognize rape within marriage.

Rape varies in the degree of violence used, and the extent to which it is mainly to exert control, or exciting in its own right. Most rapists are married or in partnerships, and over half fail to perform sexually during the assault. Rapists frequently have previous non-sexual violent convictions.

Stranger rape is rare and most rapists know their victims. Stranger rapes are more likely to be physically violent and involve the use of weapons, whereas rapists who know their victims may not need to use physical threats. Most rapes take place in the home (see Box 18.6).

Epidemiology

Rape and other forms of sexual aggression towards women are probably much more frequent than reported (see Box 18.6). Only one-third of reported rapes are proceeded with by the police, and only one-third of those proceeded with will be heard at a higher court. Even

> **Box 18.6 Sexual assault of women: findings from the British Crime Survey of 2000**
>
> - About 1% of women said that they had been subject to some form of sexual victimization in the past year.
> - In total, 0.4% of women (leading to an estimate of 61,000 victims in the UK) said that they had been raped in the previous year.
> - Current partners (at the time of the attack) were responsible for 45% of rapes. Strangers were responsible for a minority (8%) of attacks.
> - Around 18% of sexual assaults were reported to the police.
>
> Source: data from Myhill A and Allen J, Rape and Sexual Assault of Women: the extent and nature of the problem. Findings from the British Crime Survey. Home Office Research Study 237, Copyright (2002), Home Office.

then, the alleged rapist has only a one in three chance of being convicted, and this is most likely where the rape fits the stereotype of stranger rape. Victims of acquaintance rape (often rightly) assume that they will not be believed.

The prevalence of male rape is unknown and even then it is likely that many male rapes go underreported, as male victims may be reluctant to come forward. As in rape of females, it often aims to degrade or dominate the victim. Rapists of males tend to be violent heterosexual men. It has been suggested that rape is associated with gender identity problems in the rapist.

Causes

Most explanations of rape are sociocultural in terms of cultural attitudes to women, and social constructions of male and female gender roles. Men who are violent towards women often have rigid and conservative views of their role. Rapists frequently blame their victims for the attack (e.g. 'She deserved it because she was flirting with X'). That the victim is often an acquaintance, and in 20% of cases may have some engagement in events leading up to the offence, should not be interpreted as consent or voluntary participation. There is little evidence for the frequently expressed view that rape victims encourage the rape or change their minds after having sex.

Rape has been found in population studies to be associated with severe mental illness, and the proportion of all sexual crimes that were committed by patients psychiatrically hospitalized at some point in their lifetimes is 20% (Fazel *et al.*, 2007). Sexual behaviour may be associated with disinhibition as part of a manic or other psychotic illness, substance abuse comorbidity, or paranoid delusions in psychotic states. Evidence of current substance abuse is found in over 50% of rapists. Often both rapist and victim will have been using drugs or alcohol, as many rape scenarios begin in social situations. Some men who commit rape, homicide, or other violent offences have considerable sexual problems or suffer sexual jealousy, which contribute to their dangerousness. A small group of men obtain sexual pleasure from sadistic assaults on unwilling partners (Novak *et al.*, 2007).

Prognosis

In the UK, most rapists serve only half their sentence in prison, and are then released on licence to be supervised by the probation service. The reconviction rate is 30%. The prison service offers psychological treatment to rapists as part of the Sex Offender Treatment Programme (SOTP) in prisons, but data to date suggest that little improvement occurs in individuals on this programme (Marques *et al.*, 2005). Adding to the evidence base is made difficult by the constant evolution of the SOTP programme, so that effective comparisons and systematic reviews are problematical. In a broader review of treatments for sex offenders, there is evidence for several individual interventions, but this is usually supported by small studies and few with effective randomization (Schmucker and Lösel, 2008).

Child abduction

Child abduction is rare. A child may be abducted by one of the parents, by a man with a sexual motive, or by an older child. Babies are usually abducted by women. Their motives are to achieve comfort, or to manipulate another person, or may occur on impulse in psychiatrically disturbed women. Fortunately, most stolen babies are well cared for and are found quickly.

Offences against property

Shoplifting

The vast majority of shoplifting, like other theft, is carried out by people without any mental disorder. Many adolescents admit to occasional shoplifting. Both observational studies and the reports of huge losses from shops suggest that shoplifting is common among adults (including shop staff).

A minority of shoplifters suffer from psychiatric disorders. Depressive disorders are most common, but various other psychiatric diagnoses can be associated with shoplifting (Lamontagne *et al.*, 2000). Patients with any type of mental illness, especially those with substance abuse problems, may steal because of economic necessity. Patients with disinhibiting conditions may be more likely to steal impulsively, and patients with eating disorders may steal food. In other conditions, shoplifting may result from distractibility—for example, in organic mental disorders, when the person is confused or forgetful, and during panic attacks when the person may run out of the shop without paying.

The assessment of a person charged with shoplifting is similar to that for any other forensic problem. If the accused has a depressive disorder at the time of the examination, the psychiatrist should try to establish whether the disorder was present at the time of the offence or developed after the charge was brought. The legal question most often posed is whether the accused had the intention to steal, and if a mental condition could have affected that intention.

Arson

Arson is regarded extremely seriously, because it can result in great damage to property and threatens life. Most arsonists are males. Although the courts refer many arsonists for psychiatric assessment, the psychiatric literature on arson is small. Certain groups can be recognized:

- Fire-setters who are free from psychiatric disorder and who start fires for financial or political reasons, or for revenge; they are sometimes referred to as *motivated arsonists*.
- So-called *pathological fire-setters*, who suffer from learning difficulties, mental illness, or alcoholism; this group accounts for about 10–15% of arsons.
- A group that meet the DSM-5 criteria for *pyromania* (see page 520). These individuals (who sometimes join conspicuously in firefighting) obtain intense satisfaction and relief of tension from fire-setting.
- Those with psychotic illness (Anwar *et al.*, 2009).

Soothill *et al.* (2004) found at follow-up that 10% were re-convicted for arson, but over 50% for offences of other kinds. A person convicted of arson a second time is at much greater risk of committing further offences. The factors associated with an increased risk of repetition include:

- antisocial personality disorder
- learning difficulties
- persistent social isolation
- fire-setting for sexual gratification or relief of tension.

The scope for psychiatric intervention is limited. Management of arsonists within hospital requires a secure setting and close observation.

Children also present with fire-setting. Sometimes it represents extreme mischievousness in psychologically normal children, at times it is a group activity, and sometimes it arises from psychiatric disturbance, most commonly conduct disorder (Martin *et al.*, 2004). The recurrence rate in the following 2 years is reported to be less than 10%.

Psychiatric aspects of being a victim of crime

It is only relatively recently that criminology and society have paid attention to the role and needs of victims (Mezey and Robbins, 2009). General population surveys indicate that being a victim of crime is frequent, and is related to geographical area, gender, age, and social habits. Much violence, especially sexual and domestic assaults, goes unreported. Young men are particularly at risk of personal violence, whereas women are more likely to suffer domestic and sexual violence. In the UK, around one-sixth of assaults on Asians and Afro-Caribbeans are believed to be racially motivated.

The response of the victim is important in determining whether an offence is reported to the police and whether charges are brought.

Psychological impact

Childhood abuse and experience of violence during childhood may have major consequences in adulthood. *Adult* crime victims are at risk of a variety of early and late psychological problems. These include the immediate distress following the crime, and the subsequent distress associated with the investigation and court hearings. PTSD is frequently reported. These consequences are more common and severe immediately after the crime, but they may persist for many years.

Types of crime

Murder

Relatives of victims experience feelings of isolation and shame, and an inability to share their distress that is greater than in other kinds of bereavement. The bureaucracy and delay of legal processes increases anger and feelings of isolation.

Rape

Rape victims may suffer long-term psychological effects (Mezey and Robbins, 2009). Recent research has shown very high levels of intrusive thoughts and other post-traumatic symptoms in the week following rape. Serious distress may also be experienced by the partners and families of rape victims.

In many countries, including the UK, crisis intervention centres staffed by multidisciplinary teams have been set up for rape victims. Police practice has significantly improved, and there is now more sensitive handling of rape cases.

Burglary and robbery

Although the consequences are less severe than those following violent crime, they can include adjustment disorder and PTSD. Victims may become excessively preoccupied with security.

Terrorist crimes

There are increasing reports of terrorist crimes, including shootings, bombings, and hostage-taking, and all note severe immediate distress. PTSD and other psychiatric consequences only become persistent in a minority of cases.

Management

Critical incident debriefing as a routine treatment is not helpful (Raphael and Wilson, 2000). Clinical judgement is needed in assessing the severity and persistence of psychological problems to determine whether victims require specific psychological help.

Support for victims of crime may be available within the community. In the UK, the Home Office funds the national Victim Support schemes, which routinely contact victims of crime to offer support, and a service is also available to support crime victims appearing at the Crown Court. However, these services rely on volunteers, who may not be able to offer long-term help and who cannot offer specialist psychiatric intervention. Voluntary groups, such as Rape Crisis, offer support to victims of sexual assault. Compensation is available to crime victims from the Criminal Injuries Compensation Board, and psychiatrists may be asked to provide reports in relation to claims for compensation for psychological distress.

Specialist services

Specialist psychiatric assessment and treatment services acquire particular experience of the problems suffered by victims. These may be provided within normal community services, specialized trauma clinics, or designated units such as rape clinics.

Routine psychiatric care

Assessment of routine referrals to psychiatric services should include enquiry about experiences of being a victim, as this may be important in both aetiology and planning treatment.

The role of the psychiatrist in the criminal courts

Mental state, intention, and responsibility

Most jurisdictions require evidence of *guilty intention* for an offender to be convicted. Psychiatrists are therefore most often asked to provide opinions about whether a psychiatric illness affects the accused's intent to commit the crime. The underlying principle is that no one should be regarded as culpable unless they were able to control their own behaviour and to choose whether to commit an unlawful act or not. In determining guilt, it is necessary to consider the mental state at the time of the act, and especially intention (*mens rea*). This means the person perceives and intends that their act will produce unlawful consequences. Three other forms of intent need consideration.

1. *Recklessness*. The deliberate taking of an unjustifiable risk when the consequences can be foreseen but are not avoided.
2. *Negligence*. Bringing about a consequence which a 'reasonable and prudent' person would have foreseen and avoided.
3. *Accident* (or 'blameless inadvertence').

The key issue is whether the accused had the mental capacity to form the intention, or whether mental disorder might have affected that capacity. Sometimes it will be beyond psychiatric expertise or evidence to answer this question. Asked to give an opinion on these matters, the psychiatrist should liaise closely with the lawyers.

Children

In most jurisdictions, the age of the accused is thought to affect their capacity to form the intent to commit crime. Most jurisdictions exclude children under a certain age from criminal prosecution; for example, in English law, children under 10 years of age are excluded because they are deemed incapable of forming criminal

intent. The Latin term for this is *doli incapax*. Children between the ages of 10 and 14 years may be convicted if there is evidence of *mens rea* and that the child knew that the offence was legally or morally wrong. The English age for legal responsibility is lower than in most other European states, and is likely to be raised in the near future.

Competence to stand trial

This issue may arise in relation to any charge. Most jurisdictions require that a defendant must be in a fit condition to defend themselves. In English law, the issue is called 'fitness to plead' and may be raised by the defence, the prosecution, or the judge. It cannot be decided in a magistrates' court, but only by a jury.

It is necessary to determine how far the defendant can:

- understand the nature of the charge
- understand the difference between pleading guilty and not guilty
- instruct counsel
- challenge jurors
- follow the evidence presented in court.

A person may be suffering from severe mental disorder but still be fit to stand trial.

If an individual is found not fit to plead, the court will hold a 'trial of the facts' to determine whether the individual carried out the offence. If the offence is not serious, the court may make an order directing the offender to have treatment, often as an outpatient. In cases where the offence is serious, or carries a mandatory penalty (e.g. murder), the court will direct the offender to be detained in hospital indefinitely. If the person should become fit to plead, they may be returned to court for a trial. Detention after being found unfit to plead (or legally insane) operates in the same way as detention accompanied by a restriction order.

Legal insanity (not guilty by reason of insanity)

This defence may also be raised to any charge. It is argued that the defendant lacked *mens rea* for the charge because they were 'legally insane'. This term has nothing to do with diagnostic terms or classifications such as ICD-10 or DSM-5. Legal insanity is defined in different ways in different jurisdictions. It usually results in the defendant being admitted for treatment in hospital, as opposed to being sent to prison. In some jurisdictions, a 'not guilty by reason of insanity' verdict may result in more lenient sentencing.

In English law, insanity is defined in law by the McNaughton Rules, after the famous case of Daniel McNaughton, who in 1843 shot and killed Edward Drummond, the Private Secretary to the then Prime Minister, Sir Robert Peel. In the trial at the Old Bailey, a defence of insanity was presented on the grounds that McNaughton had suffered from delusions that he was being persecuted by spies. His delusional system gradually focused on the Tory Party, and he decided to kill their leader, Sir Robert Peel. McNaughton was found not guilty on the grounds of insanity, and was admitted to Bethlem Hospital. Because this was such a contentious decision, rules were provided for guidance. It must be clearly proved that, at the time of committing the act, the accused was:

labouring under such a defect of reason, from disease of the mind, as not to know the nature and quality of the act he was doing, or, if he did know it, that he did not know what he was doing was wrong.

Several other common law jurisdictions (including some states in the USA and Australia) have used this as the basis for their own definitions of legal insanity. Critics argue that the rules are too narrow, and that few mentally ill offenders would fulfil these criteria. Indeed, McNaughton himself may not have fulfilled them. In some countries, the insanity defence is widely used, especially in crimes of violence such as homicide. In English law, the alternative defence of diminished responsibility is more usual.

Diminished responsibility

Some jurisdictions include the concept of diminished responsibility. In this an individual's blameworthiness may be reduced (rather than removed) by virtue of having a mental illness. In English law, it is *only* available in relation to the charge of murder, and is defined as follows:

where a person kills or is party to a killing of another, he shall not be convicted of murder if he was suffering from such abnormality of mind (whether arising from a condition of arrested or retarded development of mind or any inherent causes or induced by disease or injury) as substantially impaired his mental responsibility for his acts and omissions in doing or being party to the killing.

There are several difficulties with this definition. 'Abnormality of mind' does not fit any diagnostic category but is basically anything which a 'reasonable man' would call abnormal. It has been widely interpreted. Successful pleas have been based on conditions such as 'emotional immaturity', 'mental instability', 'psychopathic personality', 'reactive depressed state', 'mixed emotions of depression, disappointment, and exasperation', and 'premenstrual tension'.

The relationship between abnormality of mind and responsibility is also unclear, and psychiatrists have no special expertise in this area. Most legal commentators argue that the finding of responsibility is for the jury to decide, not a matter of expert evidence. Nevertheless, psychiatrists are frequently asked to comment on this issue.

Assessment

Most defendants who are charged with murder undergo extensive psychiatric assessment, often by a specialist in forensic psychiatry but sometimes by a general psychiatrist. Defence lawyers often seek independent psychiatric advice. It is good practice for the doctors involved, whether engaged by prosecution or defence lawyers, to discuss the case together. Disagreement is unusual. Copies of the reports are distributed to the judge and to the prosecution and defence lawyers. Similar arrangements apply to other offences in which a psychiatric opinion is required.

If the psychiatric evidence is accepted by the court, supporting diminished responsibility, the defendant will be convicted of manslaughter rather than murder. In some jurisdictions, diminished responsibility may protect the convicted offender from the death penalty.

In the UK, offenders who are convicted of manslaughter in this way may be detained in hospital under the Mental Health Act. If the offence is particularly dangerous, and the offender presents a risk to the public, the court may impose a restriction order, requiring the Home Office to agree discharge.

Infanticide is a particular form of manslaughter charge, which can only be brought against women who have killed their newly born children (under 1 year old). If there is psychiatric evidence to show that the woman was mentally ill at the time of the killing, she will be found guilty of infanticide rather than murder. If the court makes a hospital order, a restriction order is rarely applied. This is a rare example of the English law formally recognizing the existence of psychiatric illness, namely postpartum psychosis, as relevant to the commission of an offence.

Absence of intention (automatism)

It is sometimes argued that the defendant lacked intention altogether (technically, the absence of *mens rea*) and this is referred to as *automatism*. The paradigm example is acts committed while sleepwalking. Automatism is difficult to determine retrospectively, and the defence is now rarely used, although it played a significant role in nineteenth-century psychiatry's development. With patients who abuse alcohol or drugs, it may be argued that because they were 'intoxicated' they had no intention to commit the crime. The law on intoxication is complicated, and specialist legal advice should be sought.

Fitness to be punished

In those jurisdictions that have corporal or capital punishment, psychiatrists may be asked to assess offenders to determine whether they are mentally well enough to be punished. In addition to assessment, psychiatrists may be asked to treat offender patients to make them fit to be punished or executed. Clearly it is unethical for psychiatrists to be involved in such procedures.

Other psychiatric issues that may be relevant to the criminal court

Amnesia

Over one-third of those charged with serious offences, especially homicide, report some degree of amnesia for the offence and inadequate recall of what happened. It has been argued, unsuccessfully, that loss of memory should be regarded as evidence of unfitness to plead. The factors most commonly associated with claims of amnesia are *extreme emotional arousal*, alcohol abuse and *intoxication*, and *severe depression*. Amnesia has to be distinguished from malingering, but there appear to be instances of true amnesia for offences, just as there is impaired recall by victims and witnesses. Moreover, the

factors associated with amnesia are similar in offenders and victims. In the absence of a relevant neuropsychiatric disorder, the presence of amnesia is unlikely to be accepted as having any legal implications.

False confessions

False confessions to criminal deeds are sometimes made, but their frequency is unknown. Gudjonsson (1992) suggested that there are three main types of false confession:

1. Voluntary.
2. Coerced–compliant.
3. Coerced–internalized.

Voluntary confessions may arise from a morbid desire for notoriety, from difficulty in distinguishing fact from fantasy, from a wish to expiate guilt feelings, or from a desire to protect another person. Coerced–compliant confessions result from forceful interrogation, and are usually retracted subsequently. Coerced–internalized confessions are made when the technique of interrogation undermines the suspect's own memories and recollections, so that they come to believe that they may have been responsible for the crime. Factors that make a person more likely to make a false confession include a history of substance abuse, head injury, a bereavement, current anxiety, or guilt.

The assessment of possible false confessions is difficult. It requires a thorough review of the circumstances of arrest, custody, and interrogation, as well as an assessment of the personality and the current mental and physical state of the suspect. Clinical psychologists can carry out a neuropsychological assessment and, in some cases, an assessment of suggestibility.

False accusations

Occasionally there are reports of individuals who claim to be the victims of a crime that has not occurred, and who make false accusations. Examples are accusations of rape and also of stalking (Pathé *et al.*, 1999). Legal and clinical experience suggests such cases are uncommon, and that accusers frequently have severe personality and other problems.

The treatment of offenders with mental disorder

General issues

The *assessment* needs to include as much information as possible from a variety of sources, including, if possible, the general practice notes. Relatives may not be the most

reliable informants, particularly if they are victims of interpersonal violence. Careful attention must be paid to both mental illness and personality disorders, as well as histories of substance misuse, which are extremely common.

Forensic psychiatric treatment usually involves treating general psychiatric conditions in specialized settings, such as secure treatment units or hospitals. It may also involve involuntary outpatient care (Swanson *et al.*, 2000). Treatment planning involves not only the appropriate medications, but also organization of appropriate psychological interventions. This is particularly important for forensic patients with severe personality disorders. Management of such patients requires specialist training for staff and support by forensic psychotherapists. It also depends upon introducing evidence-based psychiatric care into forensic practice. Many forensic patients have personality disorder; the general principles of management are described in Chapter 15 (see also Bateman *et al.*, 2015).

Settings of treatment

After conviction, an offender may be treated on either a compulsory or voluntary basis. In the UK, special treatment for mentally abnormal offenders is, in principle, provided by the Home Office (the prison medical service and the probation service) and by the Department of Health (high secure hospitals, specialist forensic services, and general psychiatry services). There has been a lack of research in forensic psychiatry, which means that the evidence base for effective treatment is slender. For a general review of the organization of forensic psychiatric services, see Taylor and Dunn (2009).

Much work with offenders is carried out by general psychiatrists, who assess patients and prepare court reports. General psychiatrists as well as forensic psychiatrists treat offenders who have been given non-custodial sentences. Forensic psychiatrists work in separate units and undertake specialized assessment and court work. In many places there are community forensic services to provide assessment and treatment, and the management of the boundary with general services is subject to ongoing controversy (Dawson and Burns, 2016). Forensic psychiatrists may work to provide care for patients who need security in ordinary psychiatric hospitals.

The mentally abnormal in prison

About one-third of sentenced prisoners have a psychiatric disorder and 4% have a psychosis (Fazel and Danesh, 2002), although more recent surveys using structured diagnoses find higher rates, with up to 10% classified with psychotic illnesses (Hassan *et al.*, 2011). Most of these disorders can be treated in prison, but a few offenders need transfer to a hospital (see Box 18.7).

The care of mentally disordered prisoners has come under intense scrutiny in recent years. The increase in

> **Box 18.7 Reasons for hospital transfer of prisoners with psychiatric disorder**
>
> - Psychosis
> - Failure to improve with medical treatment in prison
> - Refusal to have treatment for serious psychiatric illness
> - Life-threatening self-harm
> - Risk of abuse

prison suicides (Fazel *et al.*, 2011b) (when that in the general population is falling), plus the transfer of prison health care to the NHS in the UK, have highlighted the issue. Prison medical services have to provide psychiatric care under extremely difficult conditions, and a substantial increase in psychiatric input to prisons is needed. A few prisons offer psychological treatment, usually for personality disorders and sexual offences, as a main part of their work. Grendon Underwood in England is a long-established specialist prison for such treatments. A recent initiative in the UK established four special units in prisons and high secure hospitals to treat prisoners/patients with severe personality disorder (see below, dangerous severe personality disorder [DSPD]). While effectively discontinued, the initiative has generated a pathway within prisons for the care of such individuals. Although there is an undoubted need for psychiatric care within prisons, the benefits should be weighed against any encouragement for courts to send the mentally abnormal to prison rather than hospital.

Offenders in hospital

Most jurisdictions allow for the detention of mentally abnormal offenders in secure psychiatric settings. In England and Wales, a convicted offender may be committed to hospital for compulsory psychiatric treatment under a Mental Health Act hospital order. There is also provision in law for a prisoner to be transferred from prison to a psychiatric hospital. Hospital orders may have no time limit, whereas most prison sentences are of fixed length. The length of stay in a psychiatric hospital may be shorter than a prison sentence, or it may be longer. Prisoners cannot be treated against their will in prisons.

Special hospitals and secure units in the UK

In the UK, detention of mentally abnormal offenders may be in a local psychiatric hospital, a medium security unit, or a maximum secure hospital ('special hospital'). In England, the first special provision for the criminally insane was made in 1800, when a criminal wing was established at the Bethlem Hospital. In 1863, Broadmoor, the oldest of the special hospitals, opened under the management of the then Home Office. There are now four high-security special hospitals in England and Wales for patients who require such high levels of security.

The detention of patients in special hospitals is usually for an indeterminate duration. For those with mental illness (mostly schizophrenia), the length of detention is determined by the severity or chronicity of the psychiatric disorder, rather than by the nature of the offence. By contrast, for patients suffering from psychopathic disorder, the main determinant of length of stay is the assessment of the future risk of offending.

The closure of the larger mental hospitals in the UK has had unforeseen consequences for the care of mentally abnormal offenders. There is less physical security in the new psychiatric wards and hospitals, and less willingness by hospital staff and other patients to tolerate severely disturbed behaviour. Allied with shorter admission practices, it has become increasingly difficult to arrange admission to hospital for offenders, particularly those who are severely disturbed. Two alternative provisions have been developed:

1. Well-staffed secure areas in ordinary psychiatric hospitals in which the less dangerous of these patients can be treated.

2. Special secure units associated with psychiatric hospitals, to provide a level of security intermediate between that of an ordinary hospital and a special hospital (medium-secure units).

Dangerous severe personality disorder units

The notion of DSPD is an administrative category based on clinical diagnosis and risk assessment. It was introduced in England in 1999 as a response to two pressing problems of public safety. The first was offenders coming to the end of their sentences with a persisting serious risk of violence. The second was that psychiatrists would not detain severely personality-disordered individuals because they judged there to be no evidence of their 'treatability'. Treatability was, uniquely, required in the 1983 Mental Health Act for personality disorder but not for mental illness stemming from the original 1959 Act.

Four pilot units were established—two in prisons and two in high secure hospitals. They reflected the context of decreased public tolerance of risk of violent crime, improved standardized risk assessment, establishment of CBT programmes for sexual and violent offenders (McGuire, 2008), and international experience from the Netherlands and Canada (Maden, 2007). The criteria for admission were very prescriptive, requiring a violent crime, a clear personality disorder, and an established link between the personality disorder and the crime.

In practice, the units have proved difficult to staff and utilize fully, and the introduction of indefinite sentencing has removed much of their *raison d'être*. The hospital units are already closed, and the prison units are revising their remit and practice.

Treatment in the community

Offender patients may not pose sufficient risk, or be sufficiently ill, to require treatment in hospital. Courts may also use non-custodial sentences in which the offender patient may receive support from the probation service as well as psychiatric treatment. On occasion, psychiatric treatment may be made a condition of probation, with which the offender must agree to comply.

The psychiatric treatment provided for a mentally abnormal offender is similar to that for a patient with the same psychiatric disorder who has not broken the law. It is often difficult to provide psychiatric care for offenders with chronic psychiatric disorders who commit repeated petty offences, move around, and often become homeless. In the past many would have been long-stay patients in a psychiatric hospital.

The management of violence in health care settings

Violent incidents are not confined to patients with forensic problems, but this is a convenient place to consider their management. Although not frequent, violent incidents in hospitals are increasing. The reasons for this increase appear to include the following:

- changes in mental health policies emphasizing dangerousness as a reason for admission
- overcrowding
- lack of sufficiently experienced staff
- increased use of illegal drugs.

All psychiatrists should be familiar with how to manage incidents of violence in inpatient settings. Prior education and training are essential, and the National Institute for Health and Clinical Excellence (2005c and 2015) has provided guidelines (see Figure 18.2). It is important that staff have a clear policy for managing incidents of violence and are trained to implement it. Such a policy calls for attention to the design of wards, arrangements for summoning assistance, and suitable training of staff.

When violence is threatened or actually occurs, staff should be available in adequate numbers, and emergency medication such as intramuscular lorazepam and haloperidol should be unobtrusively available. The emphasis should be on the prevention of violence (see Box 18.8).

Potentially dangerous people can often be calmed by sympathetic discussion or reassurance, preferably given by someone whom they know and trust. It is important not to challenge the patient but inappropriate to reward

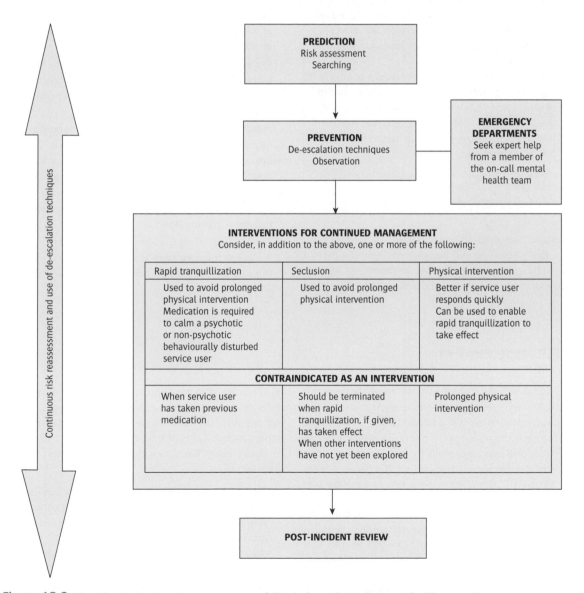

Figure 18.2 Algorithm for the short-term management of disturbed or violent behaviour in health care settings.

Source: data from NG10: Violence and aggression: short-term management in mental health, health and community settings, Copyright (2015), National Institute for Health and Care Excellence.

> ### Box 18.8 De-escalation techniques used to prevent violence
>
> - If a service user becomes agitated or angry, one staff member should take the primary role in communicating with them. That staff member should assess the situation for safety, seek clarification with the service user, and negotiate to resolve the situation in a non-confrontational manner.
> - Use emotional regulation and self-management techniques to control verbal and non-verbal expressions of anxiety or frustration (for example, body posture and eye contact) when carrying out de-escalation.
> - Use a designated area or room to reduce emotional arousal or agitation and support the service user to become calm. In services where seclusion is practised, do not routinely use the seclusion room for this purpose because the service user may perceive this as threatening.
>
> Source: data from National Institute for Health and Care Excellence, Copyright (2015).

violent or threatening behaviour by making concessions. Every effort should be made to allow the patient to withdraw from confrontation without loss of face. The use of medication should be followed by appropriate monitoring (for advice about the use of medications in emergencies, see Chapter 25).

After an incident has occurred, the clinical team should meet to consider the following issues.

- *The future care of the patient.* For mentally disordered patients, there should be a review of the drugs prescribed and their dosage. When violence occurs in a person with a personality disorder, medication may be required in an emergency, but it is usually best to avoid maintenance medication. Other measures include trying to reduce factors that provoke violence, or providing the patient with more constructive ways of managing tension, such as taking physical exercise or asking a member of staff for help.

- *Supportive psychological interventions.* These may be required for patients or staff who have been the victims of a violent assault (see the earlier section on victims of crime).

- *Whether the police should be informed.* It should not be forgotten that such assaults may be criminal. Opinion has moved to a preference for involving the police more often, although they are often reluctant to press charges.

- *The possible effect on the whole patient group.* Other patients may need support whether or not they were present at the incident.

- *The need for changes in the general policy of the ward.* A violent incident may enable lessons to be learned that are applicable in a general way to ward policies and procedures.

Risk assessment

The change to community care has made both minor criminality and rare violent offences more conspicuous, and has resulted in increased public disquiet. Psychiatric services need the resources to minimize difficulties and to identify and manage serious threats of violence. For a review of dangerousness and risk, see Buchanan (2008). The psychiatrist may need to assess risk in everyday psychiatric practice and also in forensic work.

In everyday practice, careful risk assessment may be required so that the most appropriate steps can be taken in the interests of the patient and of other people. Risk of serious harm to others is an important consideration for compulsory detention in hospital.

In forensic work, the court may ask about the defendant's dangerousness, so that a suitable sentence can be passed. The psychiatrist may also be asked to comment on offenders who are being considered for release from institutions. In both situations there is an ethical conflict between the need to protect the community and respect for the rights of the offender.

There have been two broad approaches to risk assessment.

1. Clinical psychiatrists have tried to identify factors associated with dangerousness in an individual patient (see Box 18.9). While general predictors of violence (e.g. past violence, antisocial personality disorder, substance misuse) are helpful, they lack specificity in identifying particular individuals at risk (Fazel *et al.*, 2012).

2. Actuarial methods have been used to predict future criminal behaviour among offenders and psychiatric patients. In general, the low correlations between

Box 18.9 Factors associated with dangerousness

Male gender

History

One or more previous episodes of violence
Repeated impulsive behaviour
Evidence of difficulty in coping with stress
Previous unwillingness to delay gratification
Antisocial traits and lack of social support
History of conduct disorder

The offence

Bizarre violence
Lack of provocation
Lack of regret
Continuing major denial

Mental state

Morbid jealousy
Paranoid beliefs plus a wish to harm others
Deceptiveness
Lack of self-control
Threats to repeat violence
Attitude to treatment, poor compliance

Circumstances

Provocation or precipitant likely to recur
Alcohol or drug misuse
Social difficulties and lack of support

predicted and observed behaviour have meant that they have been unhelpful for making individual predictions. Recent instruments have an improved predictive accuracy, but may be more useful in predicting those *not likely to be violent* than those who are (Fazel *et al.*, 2012).

There are no fixed clinical rules for assessing risk, but there are recognized basic principles. A thorough review should be conducted of the history of previous violence, the characteristics of the current offence and the circumstances in which it occurred, and the mental state of the individual (see Figure 18.3). When making the review, it is helpful to consider the following key factors:

- whether any consistent pattern of behaviour can be discerned
- whether any circumstances have provoked violence in the past and are likely to occur again in the future
- whether there is any good evidence that the defendant is willing to change their behaviour
- whether there is likely to be any response to treatment (see Figure 18.3).

Of these predictors, the most useful is a history of past violence (Buchanan, 2008).

Particular difficulties may arise in the assessment of dangerousness in people with antisocial personality or learning disabilities, who may be poorly motivated.

Another difficult problem is presented by the person who threatens to commit a violent act such as homicide. Here the assessment is much the same as for suicide threats but with a lower threshold for intervention. The psychiatrist should ask the individual about their intent, their motivation, and the potential victim, and should make a full assessment of the person's

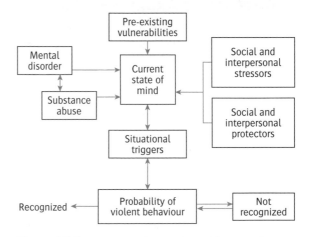

Figure 18.3 Schematic representation of the issues that should be considered when assessing the probability of violent behaviour.

Source: data from Mullen P and Ogloff RP, Dangerousness, risk and the prediction of probability. In: Gelder MG, Andreasen NC, López-Ibor JJ Jr and Geddes JR (eds), The New Oxford Textbook of Psychiatry, 2nd edn, Copyright (2009), Oxford University Press.

mental state. Some patients who make threats can be helped by outpatient support and treatment, but sometimes hospital admission is required if the risk is high. It may be necessary to warn potential victims or the police.

It is good practice for the psychiatrist to discuss their evaluation of dangerousness with other colleagues, including other psychiatrists, general practitioners, social workers, and the individual's relatives.

The psychiatric report

A psychiatric report prepared for a major criminal charge is an important document, and should be based on a full psychiatric and social assessment. It is essential that the psychiatrist reads all of the depositions by witnesses, statements by the accused, and any previous medical notes and social reports. Family members should be interviewed. When evidence about previous offences is not admissible (as is the case in English law) the psychiatrist's report should not include these facts. This may cause problems for the psychiatrist, whose opinion is often based in large part on the offender's previous behaviour. The writing of the court report follows the format described in Box 18.10, and should include an assessment of the person's mental state at the time of the alleged offence, and of their fitness

to plead. The involvement of the psychiatrist at various stages of the legal process in England and Wales is shown in Table 18.3.

The role of the psychiatrist in relation to the court

The psychiatrist's role is to draw on their special knowledge *to help the court*. They should not attempt to tell the court what to do. In the UK, the duty of the expert medical witness is to the court as a whole; they are not expected to be partisan. It is sometimes hard for psychiatrists to appreciate that they must remain neutral and not provide evidence to order that supports the party instructing them. This is particularly

---

Box 18.10 Some headings for a court report

- A statement of the *psychiatrist's full name, qualifications,* and *present appointment* (and, in England and Wales, whether they are approved under Section 12 of the Mental Health Act).
- Where and when the interview was conducted and whether any third person was present.
- *Sources of information,* including documents that have been examined.
- *Family and personal history of the defendant/plaintiff.* Usually this does not need to be given in great detail, particularly if a social report is available to the court. The focus should be on information that is relevant to the diagnosis and disposal.
- *Present mental state.* Only the salient positive findings should be stated, and negative findings should be omitted. A general diagnosis should be given in the terms used in the old 1983 Mental Health Act (mental illness, mental impairment, or psychopathic disorder). A more specific diagnosis can then be given, but the court will be interested in a broader

categorical statement rather than the finer nuances of diagnosis.
- *Mental state at the time of the relevant events.* This is often a highly important issue, especially in criminal cases, and yet it can be based only on retrospective speculation. The assessment can be helped by accounts given by eye witnesses who saw the offender at the time of the crime or soon afterwards. A current psychiatric diagnosis may suggest the likely mental state at the time of the crime. For example, if the accused suffers from chronic schizophrenia or a chronic organic mental syndrome, the mental state may well have been the same at the time of the crime as at the examination. However, if the accused suffers from a depressive disorder (now or recently) or from an episodic disorder such as epilepsy, it is more difficult to infer the mental state at the material time. Even if it is judged that the defendant was suffering from a mental disorder, a further judgement is needed as to their *mens rea* at the time of the crime.
- *Conclusions.* A summary of the key findings.

Table 18.3 The involvement of psychiatrists in the stages of the UK legal process

Stage I Arrest	Stage II Pre-trial	Stage III At the trial	Stage IV After the trial
Removal to a place of safety (police station, hospital, for medical examination)	Court report Remand for inpatient assessment or treatment	Special problems: fitness to plead, diminished responsibility	Treatment under hospital orders or guardianship
Assessment after arrest Court diversion schemes	Transfer from prison for assessment	Advice about subsequent management	Transfer from prison Decisions about release Treatment in the community

difficult because most psychiatrists use their clinical skills to establish rapport with individuals on whom they are preparing a report, and they experience a desire to advocate for them.

The psychiatrist should be aware that the court will see the report and that it may be read out in open court. Reports that are commissioned and paid for by lawyers are the property of the court.

The assessment

When conducting a psychiatric assessment on a person who is accused of a crime or who has been convicted of an offence, some key points should be kept in mind.

1. Prepare as thoroughly as possible before the interview. Have a clear idea of the purpose of the examination, and particularly about any question of fitness to plead. Obtain details of the present charge and past convictions, together with copies of any statements made by the defendant and witnesses. Study any available reports of the defendant's social history; during the subsequent interview go through this report with the defendant and check its accuracy.

2. Begin by explaining the source of the referral and why it was made. You should explain that their opinion may be given in court and that *they are under no obligation to answer any of your questions* if they choose not to do so.

3. Make detailed notes, recording any significant comments in the defendant's own words. At some stage in the interview (not necessarily at the start), the alleged crime should be discussed. The defendant may or may not admit guilt, but the psychiatrist is not obliged to comment on this.

4. Take a detailed history of any physical illnesses, paying particular attention to neurological disorders, including head injury and epilepsy.

5. Obtain a careful history of previous psychiatric disorder and treatment. Make a full examination of the present mental state. Special investigations should be requested if appropriate. If the defendant's intelligence level is under question, a clinical psychologist should make a separate assessment.

6. If possible, obtain further information from relatives and other informants. If the defendant is remanded in custody, the staff may have long periods of contact with the prisoner and may be able to provide particularly useful information.

Preparing the report

The preparation of a court report will be affected by the circumstances of the case, and the instructions given by solicitors. Court reports for civil and criminal cases may be very different. A possible outline is shown in Box 18.10. For further details, see O'Grady (2009).

When preparing a court report, the psychiatrist should remember that it will be read by people with a non-medical background. Therefore the report should be written in simple English and should avoid the use of jargon. If technical terms are used, they should be defined as accurately as possible. The report should be concise.

Advice on medical treatment

One of the psychiatrist's main functions is to give an opinion on whether psychiatric treatment is indicated. The psychiatrist should make sure that any recommendations on treatment are feasible, if necessary by consulting colleagues, social workers, or others. If hospital treatment is recommended, the court should be informed whether or not a suitable placement is available.

The assessment of risk is important here (see page 534). The psychiatrist should not recommend any form of disposal other than treatment. However, the court often welcomes respectfully worded comments on the suitability of possible sentences, particularly in the case of young offenders.

The psychiatrist appearing in court

The psychiatrist appearing in court should be fully prepared and should have well-organized copies of all reports and necessary documents. It is helpful to speak to the lawyer involved beforehand to clarify any points that may be raised in court. When replying to any questions in court, it is important to be brief and clear, to restrict the answers to the psychiatric evidence, and to avoid speculation. A number of expert witness training programmes are available, which may be useful for psychiatrists who often give expert evidence.

Further reading

Gelder MG *et al.* (eds) (2009). Part 11: Forensic psychiatry. In: MG Gelder, NC Andreasen, JJ Lopez-Ibor, and J Geddes (eds.) *The New Oxford Textbook of Psychiatry*. Oxford University Press, Oxford pp. 1895–2014.

Hart C *et al.* (2012). A UK population-based study of the relationship between mental disorder and victimization. *Social Psychiatry & Psychiatric Epidemiology*, **47**, 1581–90.

CHAPTER 19
Psychiatry of the elderly

Introduction

Older people with mental health problems present particular challenges to the practice of old age psychiatry and the organization of its services. They are often physically as well as mentally frail, and this affects presentation and course. On the other hand, they have the advantage of a rich history to tell and a lifetime's experience of responding to fortune and adversity. Dementia comprises a substantial part of the clinical practice.

When considering psychiatric disorder in the elderly, the clinician must be able to collect and integrate information from a variety of sources, and produce a management plan that takes account of physical and social needs, as well as psychological ones. This plan is likely to involve the cooperation of several professionals. It is in this clinical complexity that much of the challenge and fascination of old age psychiatry lies.

This chapter deals with the psychiatry of old age, with two important exceptions, both of which were covered in Chapter 14:

- delirium (see page 351)
- the clinical features, aetiology, and investigation of dementia (see page 356).

Normal ageing

Demographics

In 1993, 6% of the world's population was over 65 years of age. However, in higher income countries the proportion was about 14%, while in low- and middle-income countries it was 4%. The latter have higher birth rates, but the life expectancy at birth is substantially lower than in higher income countries—60 years, compared with 73 years. In the UK, life expectancy at birth has increased from 41 years in 1840 to 46 years in 1900, 69 years in 1950, and 80 years in 2011.

Table 19.1 shows that the difference in age structure of the population is changing, and Table 19.2 shows that the proportion of older people in low- and middle-income countries is increasing much faster than it is in higher income countries. Although some psychiatric disorders become less common (see Figure 19.1), the prevalence of dementia increases rapidly with age (see below), and all countries face the increasing problem of managing large numbers of cognitively impaired older people.

Table 19.1 Percentage change in the world population during the period 1975–2000

Age (years)	Total	Percentage change during the period 1975–2000	
		Developed countries	Less developed countries
<15	57.6	20.2	72.6
15–24	41.8	8.6	50.0
25–34	56.5	4.2	75.0
35–44	72.2	16.9	95.0
45–54	74.5	33.2	104.2
55–64	64.5	30.5	86.7
65–74	68.9	33.2	104.2
75–79	84.3	53.4	121.2
≥80	91.7	64.7	138.0

Source: data from United Nations, Copyright (2010).

Physical changes in the brain

The weight of the human brain decreases by approximately 5% between the ages of 30 and 70 years, by a further 5% by the age of 80 years, and by another 10–20% by the age of 90 years. As well as these changes, the ventricles enlarge and the meninges thicken. MRI studies show a complex temporal and spatial profile of changes affecting both grey and white matter, with volume reductions prominent in the hippocampus, frontal cortex, and cerebellum (Caserta *et al.*, 2009).

There is some loss of neurons, although this is regionally selective and much less marked than was formerly believed, and reductions in synapses appear to be more important. The cytoplasm of some neurons contains a pigment, lipofuscin. The ageing brain also tends to accumulate senile plaques and neurofibrillary tangles, but with a more restricted distribution and smaller numbers than in Alzheimer's disease (see Chapter 14). Neurofibrillary tangles are usually limited to neurons in the hippocampus and entorhinal cortex, while senile plaques can also occur in the neocortex and amygdala. Similarly, a small proportion of brains from healthy old people contain Lewy bodies. For reviews of the neuropathology of normal ageing, see Yankner *et al.* (2008).

Ageing itself is thought to reflect genomic changes (e.g. acquired damage to DNA or its epigenetic regulation), mitochondrial damage (caused in part by disorders of calcium regulation and to free radicals), and alterations in some growth factor and signalling pathways, together with the accumulation of multiple random (stochastic) changes. For a review of the biology of ageing, see Bittles (2009).

Table 19.2 Percentage of the population aged 60 years or over, 65 years or over, and 80 years or over by gender

Major areas and regions	Age 60 years or over			Age 65 years or over			Age 80 years or over		
	Total	Male	Female	Total	Male	Female	Total	Male	Female
Worldwide	10.8	9.7	11.9	7.5	6.6	8.4	1.5	1.1	1.9
More developed regions	21.4	18.7	23.9	15.8	13.2	18.2	4.2	2.9	5.5
Less developed regions	8.5	7.9	9.1	5.7	5.2	6.2	0.9	0.7	1.1
Least developed countries	5.1	4.7	5.5	3.3	3.0	3.6	0.4	0.3	0.5

Source: data from United Nations, Copyright (2010).

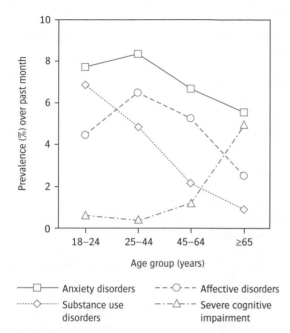

Figure 19.1 Prevalence of mental disorders across age groups: data are 1-month prevalence rates from the Epidemiologic Catchment Area Study using DSM-III criteria.

Reproduced from Jorm AF, The ageing population and the epidemiology of mental disorders among the elderly. In: MG Gelder, NC Andreasen, JJ López-Ibor Jr and Geddes JR, (eds.), The New Oxford Textbook of Psychiatry, Copyright (2000), with permission from Oxford University Press.

The neuropsychology of ageing

Assessment of cognitive function in the elderly is complicated by the frequent presence of physical ill health, notably sensory deficits, and by the need carefully to distinguish normality from the earliest phase of dementia.

Longitudinal studies suggest that intellectual function, as measured by standard intelligence tests, shows a significant decline only in later old age. A characteristic pattern of change occurs, with psychomotor slowing and impairment in the manipulation of new information. By contrast, tests of well-rehearsed skills such as verbal comprehension show little or no age-related decline.

Short-term memory, as measured by the digit span test, for example, does not change in the normal elderly. Tests of working memory show a gradual decrease

in capacity, so that the elderly perform significantly less well than the young if attention has to be divided between two tasks or if the material has to be processed additionally in some way. The elderly can usually recall remote events of personal significance with great clarity. Despite this, their long-term memory for other remote events shows a decline. Overall, there appears to be a balance between losses in flexible problem-solving, and the benefits of accumulated wisdom derived from experience. For a review, see Anderson (2008).

As well as these cognitive and motor changes, there are alterations in personality and attitudes, such as increasing cautiousness and rigidity.

Physical health

In addition to a general decline in functional capacity and adaptability with ageing, chronic degenerative conditions are common. As a result, the elderly consult their family doctors frequently and occupy over 50% of all hospital beds. These demands are particularly large in those aged over 75 years. Medical management is made more difficult by the presence of more than one disorder and by sensory and motor disabilities, as well as by an increased risk of side effects of treatment.

Social circumstances

For most people, ageing brings with it profound changes in social circumstances. Retirement affects not only income but also social status, time available for leisure, and social contacts. Loss of income is a serious problem facing many older people, and financial problems were the commonest worry reported in a large European survey of people over 65 years of age.

Social isolation is a fact of life for many older people, especially in higher income countries. In the UK and the USA, about one-third of those over 65 years of age were living alone in 1993, compared with 7% in Chile and 3% in China. However, for many older people, living alone is not seen as a problem. Many older people see family, friends, and neighbours regularly, and provide as much support as they receive.

Epidemiology of psychiatric disorders in the elderly

Kay *et al.* (1964) conducted the first systematic prevalence study of psychiatric disorder among older people

in the general population, including those living at home as well as those living in institutions, in an area of Newcastle upon Tyne, in northern England. The findings (see Table 19.3) have been broadly replicated in subsequent surveys, taking into account changes in diagnostic criteria (e.g. inclusion of depression in their category of neurosis), and the problems of case finding. For example, a large French population study of people aged 65 years or over found a point prevalence of 14% for anxiety disorder, 11% for phobia, 3% for major depression, and 1.7% for psychosis, using an interview to make DSM-IV diagnoses (Ritchie *et al.*, 2004). These figures mask the significant changes in the prevalence and proportions of disorders at different stages of old age, as shown by a large Swedish study (Skoog, 2004), summarized in Table 19.4.

Other surveys have shown a high prevalence of psychiatric disorder among older people in sheltered accommodation and in hospital. One-third of the residents in old people's homes have significant cognitive impairment. In general hospital wards, between one-third and half of the patients aged 65 years or over have some form of psychiatric illness.

It has often been reported that general practitioners are unaware of many of the psychiatric problems among older people living in the community. Moreover, the presentation of such disorders to general practitioners and mental health services is determined as much by social factors as by a change in the patient's mental state. For example, there may be a sudden alteration in the patient's environment, such as illness of a relative, or bereavement. Sometimes an increasingly exhausted or frustrated family decides that they can no longer continue to care for their elderly relative.

As in younger people, there are gender differences in the prevalence, presentation, and course of some psychiatric disorders, and in treatment needs (Lehmann, 2003).

Table 19.3 Prevalence of psychiatric disorder in people over 65 years of age

Disorder	Prevalence (%)
Dementia (severe)	5.6
Dementia (mild)	5.7
Neurosis and personality disorder	12.5
Manic depression	1.4
Schizophrenia	1.1
Any disorder	26.3

Source: data from British Journal of Psychiatry, 110(465), Kay DWK, Beamish P and Roth M, Old age mental disorders in Newcastle-upon-Tyne: 1: a study in prevalence, pp. 146–58, Copyright (1964), The Royal College of Psychiatrists.

For a review of the epidemiology of psychiatric disorders in the elderly, see Henderson and Fratiglioni (2009).

Dementia

Although there are references in classical literature, dementia in the elderly has been recognized by modern medicine since the French psychiatrist Esquirol described *démence sénile* in 1838. Emil Kraepelin distinguished dementia from psychoses due to other organic causes such as neurosyphilis, and divided it into presenile, senile, and arteriosclerotic forms. In an important study, Roth (1955) showed that dementia in the elderly differed from affective disorders and paranoid disorders in its poorer prognosis.

Reflecting its growing contribution to the global burden of disease, there has been extensive research on the prevalence of dementia, and several meta-analyses (see Tables 19.5 and 19.6). A recent systematic review reported a global prevalence of 5–7% in those aged 60 or older, corresponding to about 36 million people; this number is predicted to double every 20 years, with over 70% of cases being in low- or middle-income countries by 2050 (Prince *et al.*, 2013). The prevalence of dementia rises continuously in old age, approximately doubling every 5 years, reaching 45% in those aged 95 or older (Alexander *et al.*, 2015). Equally, these figures illustrate that half of the oldest old still remain cognitively intact. Moreover, there is now strong evidence that the age-adjusted incidence of dementia is decreasing; the decline is unexplained, and not attributable solely to reductions in vascular risk factors (Matthews *et al.*, 2013; Satizabal *et al.*, 2016).

As discussed in Chapter 14, the commonest causes of dementia are Alzheimer's disease, vascular dementia, and dementia with Lewy bodies, with frequent coexistence of the features of more than one disorder.

Delirium

Delirium and its many causes were discussed in Chapter 14. Age is also a major risk factor. For example, in the community, rates of delirium rise from 1–2% to at least 14% in those over 85 years of age (Rahkonen *et al.*, 2001). Elderly patients in hospital are at particular risk, with about one-third experiencing an episode of delirium (see Chapter 14).

Mood disorder

Despite the focus on dementia in the elderly, depressive disorders are considerably more common. A systematic

Table 19.4 **Changing prevalence of psychiatric disorders with age among the elderly**

Age (years)	Number	Dementia[*]	Depression	Anxiety disorders	Psychotic disorders
70	392	2	6	6	1
75	303	5	6	4	2
79	206	11	11	3	3
85	494	31	13	10	5

[*] Moderate or severe.

Figures are percentage values.

Adapted from Acta Psychiatrica Scandinavica, 109(1), Skoog I, Psychiatric epidemiology of old age: the H70 study—the NAPE lecture 2003, pp. 4–18, Copyright (2004), with permission from John Wiley & Sons.

review of community-based studies found an average prevalence of clinically relevant depression of 13.5% for those aged 55 years or over, of which 9.8% was classed as minor and 1.8% as major. Prevalence was higher in women and among older people living in adverse circumstances (Beekman *et al.*, 1999). Consistent with these data, a large European collaborative study found rates of 9–14% for clinically significant depression in the elderly and 1–4% for major depression (Copeland *et al.*, 1999). Amongst the over-75s, the prevalence of major depression is about 7%, and 17% for all depressive disorders (Luppa *et al.*, 2012). The figures show that many depressed older people do not meet the criteria for major depression, but are instead variously labelled as having minor depression, dysthymia, or subthreshold depression. However, this does not diminish its clinical significance, as these cases have a similar morbidity and course to those of patients who meet the criteria for major depression (Beekman *et al.*, 2002).

Rates of depression in the elderly depend on the setting. Koenig and Blazer (1992) reported rates of 0.4–1.4% in the community, 5–10% among medical outpatients, 10–15% among medical inpatients, and 15–20% among nursing home patients. These variations probably reflect the frequent comorbidity of depression in the elderly with other psychiatric (Devanand, 2002) and physical (Huang *et al.*, 2010) disorders. However, not all physical disorders show the same association; rates of depression are clearly increased with cardiac and pulmonary disease, but not with gastrointestinal disease (Huang *et al.*, 2010). The physical comorbidities may also contribute to the increased mortality rate, especially from cardiac events (Penninx *et al.*, 1999), found in older people with depression. Elderly prisoners have particularly high rates of depression (Fazel *et al.*, 2001).

Table 19.5 **Prevalence and incidence of dementia in different populations**

	Prevalence at age ≥60 years (%)	Incidence per 1000 individuals	Number of people with dementia in 2001	Predicted increase in proportion with dementia during the period 2001–2040
Western Europe	5.4	8.8	4.9 million	2-fold
North America	6.4	10.5	3.4 million	2.7-fold
Latin America	4.6	9.2	1.8 million	3.9-fold
China	4.0	8.0	6 million	3.4-fold
India and South Asia	1.9	4.3	1.8 million	3.1-fold
Africa	1.6	3.5	0.5 million	2.3-fold
Combined values	3.9	7.5	24.3 million	2.3-fold

Adapted from Lancet, 366(9503), Ferri CP et al, Global prevalence of dementia: a Delphi consensus study, pp. 2112–17, Copyright (2005), with permission from Elsevier.

Table 19.6 Prevalence of dementia at different ages in European populations

Age (years)	Prevalence
60–65	0.15 (0–2.3)
65–70	1.2 (0–3.4)
70–75	3.6 (1.3–5.9)
75–80	7.6 (5.2–10.0)
80–85	13.4 (10.6–16.1)
85–90	21.3 (18.1–24.6)
90–95	31.2 (27.7–35.6)
>95	44.7 (39.8–49.6)

Values are percentages, with 95% confidence interval in brackets.

Reproduced from Journal of Alzheimer's Disease, 48(2), Alexander M et al, Age-stratified prevalence of mild cognitive impairment and dementia in European populations: a systematic review, pp. 355–369, Copyright (2015), with permission from IOS Press, Inc.

The high prevalence of depressive disorder masks the fact that first episodes become less common after the age of 60 years and rare after the age of 80 years. Similarly, though bipolar disorder remains a prevalent disorder in the elderly (Sajatovic *et al.*, 2015), first episodes of mania are rare, and an organic cause (e.g. secondary to steroids) should always be suspected (Richards and Curtice, 2011). C-reactive protein is elevated prior to the onset of late-onset bipolar disorder, suggesting that inflammation may play a role (Wium-Andersen *et al.*, 2016).

The incidence of suicide, especially in men, increases steadily with age (see Chapter 21), and suicide in the elderly is usually associated with depressive disorder (Waern *et al.*, 2002).

Anxiety disorders

In general practice, Shepherd *et al.* (1966) found that, after the age of 55 years, the incidence of new cases of neurosis (i.e. anxiety disorder) declined. However, the frequency of consultations with the general practitioner for neurosis did not fall—presumably as a result of chronic or recurrent cases. Subsequent larger population surveys have largely confirmed this view, although prevalence and incidence figures differ markedly between studies, depending on the case definitions employed. For example, in a study from Liverpool, 1-month prevalence rates for 'caseness' for neurotic disorders were less than 1% in men and less than 2% in women over 65 years of age, whereas 'subcase' rates were about 20% in both sexes. In a 3-year follow-up, this corresponded to an incidence rate of 4.4 per 1000 per year. For a review, see Lindesay (2008).

Schizophrenia-like disorders

Schizophrenia has an estimated prevalence of 0.1–0.5% in those aged 65 or older, with 20–25% of these having an onset after aged 40 years (Cohen *et al.*, 2015).

Schizophrenia-like and paranoid disorders with their first onset in old age have been a longstanding source of debate and terminological confusion, as discussed in Chapter 11, with the terms *paraphrenia* and *late paraphrenia* still commonly used. There are no good data on prevalence.

Principles and practice of old age psychiatry

Having surveyed the epidemiological landscape, in this section we outline the principles and practice of old age psychiatry, in terms of service organization, assessment, treatment, and legal issues. The remainder of the chapter describes the specific features and treatments of the individual psychiatric disorders of old age.

Organization of services

An international consensus statement defined the essential elements of a mental health service for older people as follows (Wertheimer, 1997):

- primary health care team
- specialist old age psychiatry team
- inpatient unit
- rehabilitation
- daycare
- availability of respite care
- range of residential care facilities
- family and social supports
- liaison with geriatric medicine
- education of health care providers about the needs of older people with psychiatric problems

research, especially into epidemiological issues, and evaluation of services.

The 'team' concept is highlighted as being the key to effective provision of care, with multidisciplinary involvement being the norm. However, beyond these broad points of consensus, national policies have differed considerably in terms of the development of services and how they are implemented. In the USA, emphasis has been placed on care in hospitals and nursing homes. In Europe, Canada, and Australasia, there has been varying emphasis on social policies to provide care in the community and sheltered accommodation. In this section, services in the UK will be described as an example. Health, social, and voluntary services will be described separately, although good care depends on close collaboration at all levels, from strategic planning to the coordinated provision of care for each individual patient. Reflecting this need, health and social services, and their budgets, are now usually integrated in the UK.

A National Dementia Strategy, 'Living well with dementia' was launched in England and Wales in 2009 (Department of Health, 2009), with three key steps:

1. Ensure better knowledge about dementia and remove stigma.
2. Ensure early diagnosis, support, and treatment for people with dementia and their families and carers.
3. Develop services to better meet changing needs.

The strategy remains in place, and dementia remains high on the political agenda. There are no research data regarding the extent to which the goals of the strategy have yet been achieved.

For review of old age psychiatry services, see Dening (2013).

Health services

Primary care

The general practitioner has a central role in assessment and management of the problems of mentally ill older people. In many instances, the general practitioner, together with other health professionals in the primary care team and community health services, assesses and manages patients without referring them to a specialist. However, as already mentioned, general practitioners do not detect all of the psychiatric problems of the elderly at an early stage (Mitchell *et al.*, 2011), nor do they always provide all of the necessary long-term medical supervision. These problems may be due to lack of awareness of the significance of psychiatric illness among the elderly, or to reliance on a traditional service model in which doctors respond to requests from

patients rather than seeking out their problems. Some old age psychiatry services will only accept referrals from a general practitioner, but, increasingly, referrals may be accepted directly from any source, although liaison with the general practitioner will always be important.

Old age psychiatry services

The organization of psychiatric services varies in different localities, as it reflects the local styles of service providers, local needs, and the extent of provision for this age group by general psychiatric services, as well as national policies. Nevertheless, there are some general principles of planning.

- The aims should be to maintain the elderly person at home for as long as possible, to respond quickly to medical and social problems as they arise, to ensure coordination of the work of those providing continuing care, and to support relatives and others who care for the elderly person at home.
- There should be close liaison with primary care, other hospital specialists who may be involved, social services, and voluntary agencies.
- A multidisciplinary approach should be adopted with a clinical team that may include psychiatrists, psychologists, community psychiatric nurses, occupational therapists, and social workers. Some members of the team should expect to spend more of their working day in patients' homes and in general practices than in the hospital.
- Issues of mental capacity should always be borne in mind, and the relevant legislation adhered to (see page 77).
- It is important that the care provided by different agencies is coordinated. In the UK the Care Programme Approach (CPA) is intended to improve coordination by making a single person, the key worker or 'care coordinator', responsible for ensuring that appropriate assessment, care planning, and review take place (see Chapter 26).

The contributions of the various parts of an old age psychiatry service will now be considered. In England and Wales, severe financial constraints and the reorganization of the NHS to move control of budgets to general practitioners mean that the description of services for older people are rapidly changing and will no doubt change further over the lifetime of this edition of this book. Although the basic principles and components of care may not change radically, the relative availability of these components may do so, and readers will need to familiarize themselves with local conditions.

Domiciliary psychiatric care. Assessment and treatment commonly takes place in the patient's own home. This is more convenient for the patient, and offers a more relevant and realistic assessment of the difficulties facing the patient and their carers. Assessment is often undertaken by a member of the community mental health team who has a clinical background in nursing, occupational therapy, or social work. This person may become the patient's care coordinator, able to take an overview of their health and social needs, and who can liaise between different agencies, including primary care and specialist services. Care coordinators may assess referrals from general practitioners, monitor treatment in collaboration with general practitioners and the psychiatric services, and take part in the organization of home support for older people with dementia.

Outpatient clinics. Although assessment at home is desirable, outpatient clinics are convenient for the assessment and follow-up of mobile patients. In recent years, *memory clinics* have been developed in most areas for the specialist assessment and treatment of patients with memory problems (Kelly, 2008). In the UK, these clinics provide information, advice, and support to patients and their carers; they also initiate medication used to treat dementia, which can be prescribed subsequently in primary care.

Day hospitals and day centres. Although some treatments can be provided at home, others may require the patient to attend a day hospital, where a high level of stimulation and social interaction can also be provided. In the 1950s, day care began in geriatric hospitals. A few years later the first psychiatric day hospitals for the elderly were opened. Psychiatric day hospitals should provide a full range of diagnostic services and offer both short-term and continuing care for patients with functional or organic disorders, together with support for relatives. Currently, daycare is more often provided by day centres rather than day hospitals. These centres combine health and social care elements, very often with the financial and practical involvement of voluntary organizations, such as the Alzheimer's Society. Day centres provide an important and cost-effective component of the services available for the elderly with psychiatric problems. All daycare-based arrangements depend crucially on adequate transport facilities.

Inpatient units. Inpatient teams should be able to provide multidisciplinary assessment and treatment of patients with severe disorders. In addition to psychiatrists and psychiatric nurses, these teams may include occupational therapists, psychologists, speech and language therapists, physiotherapists, social workers, healthcare assistants, and others. There is substantial variation in different areas both in the composition of teams and in whether patients with functional illnesses are cared for separately from or together with those with organic disorders.

Geriatric medicine. There is inevitably some overlap in the characteristics of patients treated by units for geriatric medicine and those treated in psychiatry units; both are likely to treat patients with dementia. However, in the geriatric medicine setting the primary concern is likely to be with a patient's physical health; in old age psychiatry units the predominant problem usually relates to behaviour, personality, or comorbid mental illness (e.g. depression). Earlier concern that many patients were 'misplaced' and therefore received poor treatment, stayed too long in hospital, and had an unsatisfactory outcome has not been confirmed by research. Optimal placement depends on the relative predominance of behavioural and physical problems. Medical and psychiatric teams need to cooperate closely if all patients are to receive appropriate treatment. Geriatric medicine units are usually found in acute general hospitals, wherein the increasing availability of liaison psychiatry expertise helps to integrate medical and psychiatric treatments.

Long-term care. In some countries, many elderly psychiatric patients are still treated in the wards of psychiatric hospitals. However, the nature of the care provided is more important than the type of institution in which it is given. The basic requirements are opportunities for privacy and the use of personal possessions, together with occupational and social therapy. Provided that these criteria are met, long-term hospital care can be the best provision for very disabled patients. In the UK, long-term care is now almost entirely provided outside hospital in residential and nursing homes. There is an active debate on how long-term care should be funded. The Dilnot Report in 2011 recommended that, once a certain funding contribution ('cap') had been reached by a particular individual, their social care costs should be free. The recommendations of this report are to be implemented in 2017, but the details remain uncertain. In England and Wales, the Care Act (2014) enshrines in law the duty of local authorities to provide appropriate assessment and support for social care needs. However, the provision, availability, and costs incurred by individuals differ considerably in different parts of the UK. Further changes are also to be anticipated as personal health budgets are introduced into the NHS.

Social services

Domiciliary services

In addition to medical services, domiciliary services include home helps, meals at home, laundry, telephone, and emergency call systems. In the UK, local authorities both provide and commission these services; they also support voluntary organizations and encourage local initiatives such as good-neighbour schemes and self-help groups. Increasing financial pressures on local authorities, and rising demand from the increasing number of elderly people, mean that all services are under constant threat. The last decade has also witnessed a major shift in provider for these services, with the majority being from private or voluntary organizations.

Residential and nursing care

Older people may need a variety of social service accommodation, ranging from entirely independent housing through sheltered housing schemes, where there may be some communal provision, often including access to a warden, to residential or nursing homes where there are staff available at all times. There is a need for special housing for the elderly that is conveniently sited and easy to run. Ideally, the elderly should be able to transfer to more sheltered accommodation if they become more disabled, without losing all independence or moving away from familiar places.

In residential homes, the needs of residents for help with personal care can be met by health care assistants, whereas in nursing homes more skilled nursing care is available with a greater proportion of staff with a higher level of training. Some, but not all, nursing homes specialize in the care of older people with mental disorders.

In the UK, local social services are responsible for providing residential homes and other sheltered accommodation. However, many independent organizations and charities also provide residential homes for older people and play an increasing and substantial role.

Voluntary and third sector services

Voluntary agencies play a large and increasing role in the provision of facilities and support for patients, their families, and carers. Previously the task for NHS services was to ensure that their contributions were integrated with health and social service provisions. As their role has increased, they may be set to play a dominant role in this area. Any discussion of service provision for elderly

mentally ill patients must acknowledge the major part played by informal carers.

Carers

In the present context, carers are unpaid relatives, neighbours, or friends who look after older people at home. These informal carers provide substantially more care to older people than do the statutory services, and their role in the overall provision of care should not be underestimated. Most informal carers of older people are (in descending order of frequency) partners, daughters, or sons. About twice as many women as men are informal carers, and about 50% of all informal carers are themselves elderly.

Several studies have shown that patients suffering from dementia place the greatest stress on carers (Pinquart and Sörensen, 2003). Incontinence, behavioural disturbance at night, and aggression are the most distressing problems for carers, both practically and emotionally. The degree of strain imposed on these committed individuals (who are themselves often elderly and with their own health problems) is often undeclared and easily underestimated. Caregiver symptoms lessen when the patient has moved to permanent residential care (Gaugler *et al.*, 2009).

Accurate assessment of carers' needs is important and, in the UK, social services now have a statutory responsibility to provide this, where requested. Box 19.1 summarizes the key recommendations made by Levin (1997). Time should be spent with carers, giving advice and

---

Box 19.1 Support for carers of elderly patients with dementia

Early identification of dementia

Comprehensive medical and social assessment of identified cases

Timely referrals between agencies

Continuing reviews of each patient's needs, and back-up for carers

Active medical treatment for any intercurrent illness

Provision of information, advice, and counselling

Regular help with household and personal care tasks

Regular breaks for carers (e.g. daycare and respite care)

Appropriate financial support

Permanent residential care when this becomes necessary

discussing their problems. Such support can help families to avoid some of the frustration and anxiety involved in caring for elderly relatives. Published guides available on the internet are also useful. Other practical help can ease the burden; for example, carer support groups, additional support at home (e.g. laundry or meal services), daycare, respite care, or holidays designed to be suitable for people with dementia. The assessment of need and carer support may often have to be multidisciplinary; both community psychiatric nurses and care managers (social workers) play essential roles in coordinating these services, supporting relatives, and providing direct nursing care.

The best evidence for an effective treatment to support carers is for an eight-session, manual-based coping intervention. This was shown to improve mood and anxiety significantly over a 2-year period, and to be cost-effective (Livingston *et al.*, 2014a). However, such interventions are not widely available.

Psychiatric assessment in the elderly

The principles and basic purpose of assessment of older people are not substantially different from those for all other patients (Chapter 3). Assessment is intended to establish a diagnosis, to develop the best possible plan of care, and to inform the prognosis. However, there are differences of emphasis and process.

- The assessment is likely to take longer, requiring more than one interview, and with a greater reliance on informants. In the assessment of suspected dementia, an informant is essential to complete the history and to verify the extent to which the impairments are affecting the patient's capabilities and safety. Time will also be required to administer cognitive rating scales.

- The assessment is likely to include assessment of the wider psychosocial situation, taking into account not only the patient's needs but also those of carers, dependents, and other individuals who are involved. This is particularly relevant for the patient with moderate or severe dementia.

- The physical examination and laboratory investigations play a greater role, because of the higher prevalence of organic disorders as a cause of psychiatric symptoms in the elderly. The psychiatric assessment may also bring coincidental medical problems to light which require investigation or referral.

For a review of psychiatric assessment in the elderly, see Jacoby (2009).

The referral

It is important to establish at the outset what prompted the referral, and what the referrer hoped to gain from it. This may well require information to be collected even before the patient is seen, not least to establish the most useful way to approach the assessment. In any one case, each person involved in the patient's care may have different, and possibly conflicting, expectations and needs.

Informants

Many old people seen by psychiatrists are unable to give complete or reliable information about themselves. Frequently there is a partner or other close relative living with the patient, but in other cases it may be necessary (with consent) to talk to neighbours, friends, or relatives living away from the patient, to build up a picture of the patient's personality and past history. Most patients will already be well known to their general practitioner or to other health professionals, and it is always worth consulting them.

Where to assess the patient

In the UK, most old age psychiatrists prefer to assess patients in their own homes. This enables much essential 'real-life' information about the patient's ability to function at home to be gained (e.g. ability to make a cup of tea, or recognize relatives in family photographs). It also avoids the patient appearing excessively disorientated simply because of the disturbing effect of having to travel to a hospital for assessment in an unfamiliar environment. Furthermore, it makes it easier to interview other members of the family, and to assess the level of support from neighbours or outside carers, who may be available at the patient's home during the assessment. For review of home assessment in old age psychiatry, see Ng and Atkins (2012).

Old age psychiatrists may also be asked to assess patients on general hospital wards, for example because the admission may have revealed, or exacerbated, underlying cognitive (or other) difficulties. Although this provides less information about the patient's circumstances, it makes close liaison with the hospital team possible. Conditions on hospital wards are often unfavourable for a quiet, private interview. It is important to spend time reading the notes carefully, talking to nursing and other staff, and then requesting the use of an office or side room in which to see the patient. Even if the family or other carers cannot be present, it may be possible to telephone them. Similar principles apply to assessment in residential and nursing homes.

Increasingly, patients with early cognitive impairments are offered assessments in a *memory clinic*. This offers the advantages of a systematic and detailed assessment, and enables relevant further investigations and follow-up to be arranged as efficiently as possible. It is also the vehicle by which drugs to treat dementia are prescribed in the NHS.

The assessment

The information that is required about the medical and psychiatric history is the same as in younger patients. However, it may be necessary to piece it together from accounts given by the patient and by other informants. It is particularly important to obtain a clear medical history and to determine the patient's past and present medication.

During the mental state examination, assessment of cognitive function has particular significance, especially for those in whom memory impairment is apparent or suspected. This assessment requires a range of clinical questions and observations, supplemented by one or more of the questionnaires available for this purpose (see Chapter 3), such as the Mini-Mental State Examination (MMSE) or Montreal Cognitive Assessment (MoCA).

As physical problems are extremely common, the psychiatrist will often need to examine the patient (especially if this has not been done recently by the general practitioner), including a neurological examination. Laboratory investigations are important for patients on admission, and in all others with significant psychiatric disorder (for investigation of dementia, see Chapter 14).

Finally, the assessment process includes assessments of risk, and of the needs of the carer(s), discussed above, as most older people with psychiatric disorders live in their own homes and are cared for by family members or, occasionally, by good neighbours or friends.

Psychiatric treatment in the elderly

As with assessment, the principles of psychiatric treatment in the elderly resemble those for other adults, but the greater age of these patients does require one to bear in mind three issues that have an impact upon treatment (Oppenheimer, 2009).

- Elderly patients are likely to have multiple problems. Psychiatric, physical, and social difficulties usually coexist to some extent. 'Treatment' may thus include a broad range of interventions beyond those normally associated with psychiatry—for example, antibiotics for a urinary tract infection, or liaison with a district nurse or dietitian. These complex treatment needs are reflected in the multidisciplinary nature of services, described above, and require careful planning and integration of treatment provision.

- Clear boundaries between normality and disease are rare. This poses challenges for treatment thresholds and service provision.

- Lack of competence (capacity) is common, due to cognitive impairment. There is an increasing focus on how (lack of) competence should be assessed and responded to. The question of capacity underlies a range of ethical and legal issues in which old age psychiatrists become involved (see below).

Physical treatments

The efficacy of psychotropic drugs is generally not affected by age, and elderly patients should not be denied effective drug treatment, especially for depressive disorders. However, prescribing in the elderly requires particular caution, for two main reasons.

- The incidence of unpleasant or dangerous side effects is high, and can produce delirium and other psychiatric disorders. Most problems arise with drugs used to treat cardiovascular disorders (antihypertensives, diuretics, and digoxin) and those that act on the central nervous system (antidepressants, hypnotics, anxiolytics, antipsychotics, and antiparkinsonian drugs). These problems arise because of differences in pharmacokinetics with ageing, and the greater number of drugs that older people are prescribed, which increases the likelihood of harmful interactions. There is particular concern about the use of antipsychotics in dementia, especially Lewy body dementia (see page 368).

- Compliance with treatment may be compromised in those who live alone, who have poor vision, or who are forgetful or confused.

Given these factors, the following points should be borne in mind when prescribing for the elderly person with a psychiatric disorder.

- Start with a low dose, increase slowly, and expect the final dose to be considerably lower than in younger patients. The main exceptions to this are the selective serotonin reuptake inhibitors (SSRIs), for which comparable doses are used.

- All medication should be reviewed regularly, and kept to a minimum. Before starting a drug in the elderly, it is good practice to state clearly in the notes the reason for the decision (including, for example, the score on a depression rating scale), and the criteria by which the effects of the treatment will be assessed. If good evidence of efficacy is not achieved, medication should be gradually withdrawn.

- The drug regimen should be as simple as possible. Medicine bottles should be labelled clearly, and memory aids, such as packs containing the drugs to be taken on a single day with daily dose requirements, should be provided. If possible, drug-taking should be supervised.

Electroconvulsive therapy

Electroconvulsive therapy (ECT) remains one of the most effective and valuable treatments for serious depressive disorder in the elderly (see below). Advanced age is not a contraindication. However, attention should be paid to the physical health of all elderly patients undergoing this treatment, and frail patients should be assessed by an experienced anaesthetist before receiving ECT.

Psychological treatment

In all patients, supportive therapy with clearly defined aims can be helpful, including joint sessions with the patient's partner or carer.

In patients who have no cognitive impairment, the specific psychological therapies that are used in younger individuals remain appropriate for the same range of disorders and with similar expectations of success. In particular, cognitive and behavioural interventions for mood and anxiety disorders are effective, and are often preferred by the patient. Family or systems therapy, although not widely available, is advocated as it explicitly recognizes the patient in their social context (Jacoby, 2009). Psychodynamic psychotherapy is less appropriate for the elderly and is seldom used, although cognitive analytic therapy has been found useful.

Even mild cognitive impairment militates against the use of most of the common psychological therapies, as it is likely to prevent the patient from understanding or implementing the treatment (Oppenheimer, 2009). However, a range of specialized psychological and behavioural interventions (e.g. reminiscence therapy) are becoming widely used in this group, with the benefits targeted as much at the carer as at the patient.

For a review of psychological treatment in the elderly, see Wilkinson (2013).

Psychosocial treatments

Some patients can achieve independence through measures designed to encourage self-care and domestic skills, and to increase social contacts. For those living at home, a domiciliary occupational therapist may be able to give useful advice on environmental or other modifications that will help the patient to live more independently. More severely impaired patients who are living in institutional care can benefit from an environment in which individual needs and dignity are respected, and each person retains some of their personal possessions. Further psychosocial interventions of this kind are discussed in the section on treatment of dementia.

Legal, financial, and ethical issues

Both the law and ethical principles apply as much to the elderly as to younger people, and these issues are discussed in Chapter 4. However, certain legal and ethical issues that are relevant in psychiatry have particular relevance to the elderly (see Box 19.2), for several reasons:

- The nature of the common illnesses from which they suffer, especially dementia, which compromises their competence to make decisions and give consent.

Box 19.2 Ethical and legal issues in the elderly

Confidentiality in relation to information from carers

Confidentiality of information about financial circumstances

Consent to treatment

- Capacity to consent to physical and psychological treatment
- Advance directives
- Decisions 'not to treat'

Damaging behaviour

Management of financial affairs

- Nominating another to take responsibility (Power of Attorney)
- Procedures to enable others to take responsibility

Entitlement to drive a vehicle

Consent to participate in research

- Problems arising from increasing age and frailty (e.g. driving).
- The greater likelihood and proximity of death, which gives greater urgency to issues such as testamentary capacity (Posener and Jacoby, 2008) and advance directives.

In the UK, many of these issues are governed by the Mental Capacity Act 2005.

Financial affairs

Older people, particularly those with mental disorders, may have difficulty in managing their financial affairs. In the UK, if the issues are relatively simple—for example, involving only a state pension and benefits—the person can request that someone else, known as an appointee, collects these benefits on their behalf. Alternatively, while the person still has mental capacity to understand what is involved, they can grant a Lasting Power of Attorney in favour of one or more others. The attorney then has authority to carry out any financial transaction on behalf of that person. If the donor of the power subsequently becomes mentally unable to manage their own affairs, the attorney may continue to do so on their behalf (in the UK, provided the arrangement is registered with the Court of Protection). Sometimes a person becomes mentally incapable of managing their affairs without having made any formal arrangement for someone else to act on their behalf. Under these circumstances, an application supported by medical evidence of incapacity may be made to the Court of Protection for a deputy to be appointed to manage the patient's affairs.

Under the Mental Capacity Act an attorney can also make proxy health and welfare decisions on behalf of an incompetent person. This requires that the person was competent to donate that Power of Attorney before subsequently becoming incompetent. The Mental Capacity Act introduced a new power, the Advance Decision to Refuse Treatment (ADRT), which allows an agreed proxy to make decisions that are binding even where they will result in death. Because of the gravity of this power, it must be written and witnessed and confirm the competence of the patient at the time at which it is arranged (see Chapter 4). The ADRT can be overridden by the Mental Health Act.

Driving

A common practical problem is the inability of older patients, especially those with dementia and Parkinson's disease, to drive safely. As with other disorders, doctors generally have an obligation, which overrides confidentiality, to inform the authorities responsible for the provision of driving licences if patients decline to do so themselves. In practice, older people often make the decision to stop driving anyway, or are persuaded to do so by relatives. For review, see Wilson and Pinner (2013).

Abuse and neglect of the elderly

Abuse and neglect of the elderly by family members, carers, or acquintances, raises the importance of safeguarding awareness for all health care professionals working with the elderly. Its psychiatric relevance arises in part from the finding that people with dementia are particularly likely to be abused.

Elder abuse

This term refers to actions by a carer or other trusted person that cause harm or create a serious risk of harm to an elderly person (whether or not harm is intended), or to failure by a caregiver to satisfy the elderly person's basic needs or protect them from harm. The term 'elder maltreatment' is also used.

Five forms of elder abuse are recognized—physical, psychological, sexual, financial, and neglect. Prevalence rates of 2–10% are reported, with a higher risk if:

- the abused person has dementia
- the carer and the abused person live together
- the abused person is socially isolated (e.g. lacks close friends)
- the carer has a psychiatric disorder or misuses alcohol
- the carer is heavily dependent (e.g. financially) on the person who is being abused.

Elder abuse is associated with an increased mortality rate compared with that for matched older people, and with other adverse outcomes, ranging from depression to placement in a nursing home.

Although there is now widespread awareness of the problem, and of the need to identify elder abuse and respond to it, there is no evidence about the effectiveness of interventions. At present, a range of measures are used, such as increased social support, respite care, relationship counselling, and carer education programmes. Legal approaches (e.g. guardianship, law enforcement agencies) may also be necessary.

For a review of elder abuse, see Lachs and Pillemer (2015).

Clinical features and treatment of psychiatric disorders in the elderly

Depressive disorder in the elderly

Clinical features

There is no clear distinction between the clinical features of depressive disorders in the elderly and those in younger people, but some symptoms are more striking in the elderly. Post (1972) reported that one-third of depressed elderly patients had severe retardation or agitation. A recent meta-analysis confirmed these findings, and also reported that hypochondriasis and somatic symptoms were more common, whereas guilt and loss of libido were less common than in younger adults (Hegeman *et al.*, 2012). Depression itself is sometimes not conspicuous in the elderly and may be masked by other symptoms, particularly hypochondriacal complaints, and so depressive disorder should always be considered when the patient presents with symptoms of this kind. Psychotic depression in the elderly also differs in some respects from psychotic depression in younger adults, with a greater overall severity and more prominent hypochondriacal delusions (Gournellis *et al.*, 2014).

Depressive pseudodementia

Some retarded depressed patients, especially the elderly, present with '*pseudodementia*'—that is, they have conspicuous difficulty with concentration and remembering, but careful clinical testing shows that there is no major defect of memory. Differentiation of these patients from those with early dementia is important and can be difficult. Moreover, the distinction is complicated by evidence that depressive pseudodementia is a strong predictor of subsequent dementia (Saez-Fonseca *et al.*, 2007). Features that suggest depressive pseudodementia include the following:

- The patient's complaint of memory disturbance tends to be greater than the informant's account of memory problems in everyday life.
- Depressive symptoms that pre-dated the memory difficulties.
- 'Don't know' responses and poor involvement with neuropsychological tests (these features are characteristic).
- A personal or family history of mood disorder.

Aetiology

The aetiology of depressive disorders of first onset in late life broadly resembles the aetiology of similar disorders at younger ages, with biological, psychological, and social influences (Fiske *et al.*, 2009). Twin studies and genome-wide profiling show a comparable genetic contribution to that of depression occurring earlier in life (Demirkan *et al.*, 2013).

It might be expected that the loneliness and hardship of old age would be important predisposing factors for depressive disorder. Surprisingly, there is no convincing evidence for such an association. Indeed, Parkes *et al.* (1969) even found that the association between bereavement and mental illness no longer held in the aged.

The major difference in aetiology for depression in late life is related to vascular factors. First noted by Post (1972), it has become the prominent hypothesis since Alexopoulos *et al.* (1997) coined the term '*vascular depression*'. There is now diverse evidence for a multifaceted and bidirectional relationship between late-life depression and vascular disease. Meta-analysis shows that cardiovascular disease, diabetes, stroke, and a composite vascular risk score are all significant risk factors for depression in the elderly, but hypertension, smoking, and dyslipidaemia are not (Valkanova and Ebmeier, 2013). Biological mechanisms include findings that the neuropathological basis of the white matter hyperintensities that are frequently seen in late-life depression on MRI scans reflects focal areas of ischaemia and infarction, with effects on brain connectivity. Inflammation is also thought to be a contributory factor. For review see Taylor *et al.* (2013).

Differential diagnosis

As noted above, it is sometimes difficult to distinguish between depressive pseudodementia and dementia, and this problem is compounded by the fact that depression may occur during the course of dementia. It is essential to obtain a detailed history from other informants and to make careful observations of the patient's mental state and behaviour using the differentiating features listed earlier. Psychological testing can be a useful adjunct, but it requires experienced interpretation and it usually adds little to skilful clinical assessment. At times, dementia and depressive illness coexist. If there is real doubt, a trial of antidepressant treatment may be appropriate. Other aspects of the differential diagnosis are similar to those for depressive disorder in younger people.

Treatment

The principles of the treatment of depressive disorder are the same as for younger adults, as described in Chapter 9, and should follow current guidelines (Cleare *et al.*, 2015). Effective treatments thus exist, but often they are not implemented, both because cases are not diagnosed and because interventions are not offered (Park and Unutzer, 2011). Guidelines for managing late-life depression in primary care have been produced (Baldwin *et al.*, 2003). With elderly patients it is especially important to be aware of the risk of suicide. Any intercurrent physical disorder should be thoroughly treated.

Antidepressants are as effective as in younger people. The drugs should be used cautiously, perhaps starting with half the normal dosage and increasing this slowly in relation to side effects and response. SSRIs are preferred to tricyclic antidepressants because of their lower propensity to cause side effects and cardiotoxicity. Potential interactions with other drugs that are being taken by the patient must also be noted, and may influence the choice of antidepressant (Spina and Scordo, 2002). For patients who do not respond to the maximum tolerated dose of an antidepressant, it may be necessary to use a combination of drugs, as in younger patients, or to combine medication with psychological treatment (Cooper *et al.*, 2011).

As with medication, psychological interventions show similar efficacy in the elderly, and are often preferred by patients, but their availability is very limited (Simon *et al.*, 2015). There is evidence that, within this setting, the outcome is improved by models of collaborative care in which specialists provide some input, and care is supplemented by education about depression and medication (Park and Unutzer, 2011).

ECT is appropriate for depressive disorder with severe and distressing agitation, suicidal ideas and behaviour, life-threatening stupor, or failure to respond to drugs. Concerns that ECT is dangerous or ineffective in elderly patients are unwarranted; in fact, remission rates are favourable (Rhebergen *et al.*, 2015).

After recovery, expert guidelines suggest that full-dosage antidepressant medication should be continued for at least 12 months for a first episode in the elderly, and proportionately longer for subsequent episodes. Indefinite continuation has also been advocated (see Cleare *et al.*, 2015).

For a review of the depression in the elderly and its management, see Unutzer (2007).

Course and prognosis

In his classic study, Post (1972) described depression in the elderly as following the rule of threes—a third recover, a third remain the same, and a third deteriorate and become 'chronic invalids'. Later studies have generally found a similar, if not poorer, outcome. For example, in a 6-year longitudinal study of 277 elderly depressed people, Beekman *et al.* (2002) found that 32% had a severe, chronic course, 44% had a fluctuating course, and only 23% achieved substantial remissions. The natural history of depression in old age has implications for its management (see below).

Factors that are believed to predict a good prognosis for depression in old age include the following:

- onset before the age of 70 years
- short duration of illness
- good previous adjustment
- the absence of disabling physical illness
- good recovery from previous episodes
- religiosity (self-reported faith, or belonging to a religious group).

Poor outcome is associated with the severity of the initial illness, the presence of organic cerebral pathology, poor compliance with treatment, and severe life events during the follow-up period. As discussed in Chapter 21, the risk of suicide remains high in older people with depression, especially men.

Depression and dementia. As well as the finding mentioned earlier that depressive pseudodementia increases the risk of dementia several years later, there is now strong evidence that a history of depression in late life (Diniz *et al.*, 2013) and at younger ages (da Silva *et al.*, 2013) approximately doubles the risk of developing dementia, including Alzheimer's disease and vascular dementia. The mechanism for the association between depression and dementia is not known. The use of statins may decrease the risk of dementia in late-onset depression (Yang *et al.*, 2015).

Bipolar disorder in the elderly

Broadhead and Jacoby (1990), in the first prospective study of mania in old age, found that the clinical picture was the same as in younger patients, but that a depressive episode immediately after the manic episode occurs more frequently. Mixed affective episodes may be somewhat more common than in younger patients. As with depression, a history of bipolar disorder appears to increase the risk of dementia (da Silva *et al.*, 2013).

Management of bipolar disorder in the elderly follows the principles described in Chapter 10 for younger patients (Goodwin *et al.*, 2016). Lithium prophylaxis remains valuable, but blood levels should be monitored with particular care and kept at the lower end of the therapeutic range (0.4–0.6 mmol/l). For a review, see Sajatovic *et al.* (2015).

Anxiety disorders in the elderly

In later life, anxiety disorders are seldom causes for referral to a psychiatrist, although this may be largely because of non-presentation by patients and lack of recognition or referral by general practitioners. It does not reflect their rarity in the population, as shown by the epidemiological data reviewed earlier in the chapter.

Symptoms of anxiety disorders among the elderly are often non-specific, with features of both anxiety and depression. Hypochondriacal symptoms may be prominent. As in younger patients, the possibility that anxiety symptoms are secondary to an underlying depressive episode should always be actively considered before the diagnosis is made. Personality disorder is a predisposing factor, while physical illness and life events such as retirement or a change of accommodation may act as precipitants. A first onset of panic attacks in an elderly person should always prompt a search for an underlying physical or depressive disorder.

The approach to treatment is similar to that for anxiety disorders in younger adults, with a preference for psychological and behavioural interventions. In practice, medication is often prescribed first-line, and should be done cautiously. For review, see Goncalves and Byrne (2012).

Schizophrenia-like disorders in the elderly

Schizophrenia usually begins in early adulthood (see Chapter 11), but new-onset cases after the age of 60 years, although uncommon, are well recognized. This section will focus on the features that characterize such cases compared with schizophrenia of younger onset. It also highlights some issues that affect the management of all patients with schizophrenia as they become elderly (sometimes called 'graduates'). The complicated terminology in this area has been covered earlier in this chapter (and see Box 11.4), and reflects the longstanding view that these cases are, to some extent, clinically different from earlier-onset cases.

For review of late-onset schizophrenia, see Brunelle *et al.* (2013). For a review of schizophrenia in the elderly, see Cohen *et al.* (2015).

Clinical features

Although the core symptoms and overall clinical profile are very similar to those of younger-onset cases, the relative prominence of some features does differ (see Box 19.3). Of these, the extreme rarity of thought disorder and negative symptoms in the elderly is the most

---

> **Box 19.3 Features characteristic of late-onset compared with early-onset schizophrenia**
>
> **Symptoms that are more common**
> Visual, tactile, and olfactory hallucinations
> Third-person, running commentary, and derogatory auditory hallucinations
> Persecutory delusions
>
> **Symptoms that are less common**
> Formal thought disorder
> Affective flattening and blunting
> Negative symptoms
>
> **Other features**
> Female predominance
> No clear genetic loading
> Association with sensory deficits and social isolation
> Less premorbid educational and psychosocial impairment
> Less working memory and verbal learning impairment
> Much lower antipsychotic doses required

---

striking. A similar generalized cognitive impairment is seen regardless of age of onset, but late-onset cases show somewhat milder deficits, especially in working and verbal memory. However, it should also be noted that a history of schizophrenia is associated with a threefold increase in risk of dementia at age 65 years, with a lesser but still significant increased risk at older ages (Riisgaard *et al.*, 2015).

Course and prognosis

There are no contemporary data on the course or outcome of schizophrenia with onset in old age. There is no good evidence that it heralds or progresses to dementia.

Differential diagnosis

Compared with younger-onset schizophrenia, there is a greater likelihood that an elderly patient presenting with psychotic symptoms has an organic psychosis of some kind. Therefore all elderly patients who present with a first onset of schizophrenia-like features should be assessed carefully to exclude a delirium, dementia, or organic psychosis due to a neurological or medical disorder such as neurosyphilis, HIV, or neoplasm (see Chapter 14). As in younger patients, schizophrenia must also be distinguished from other psychiatric disorders in which psychotic symptoms occur, notably delusional disorder or affective psychosis. Such distinctions may be particularly difficult if the patient presents with persecutory beliefs but no other clear symptoms, and if there is a history suggestive of paranoid personality traits. For those in whom visual hallucinations are an isolated symptom, consider Charles Bonnet syndrome (see page 555).

Aetiology

Familial aggregation is much less common than in earlier-onset schizophrenia, which suggests that there is a smaller genetic predisposition. There is no familial association with neurodegenerative or cerebrovascular disorders. Brain imaging changes are similar in nature and magnitude to those described in younger-onset schizophrenia. Unlike late-life depression, rates of white-matter hyperintensities are not increased. A role for sex hormones in the aetiology of late-onset schizophrenia has been proposed, based upon the female predominance (which approaches 3:1), but there is little direct evidence for this. Schizoid or paranoid personality traits are common in older people who develop late-onset psychotic disorders (Kay *et al.*, 1976). Deafness is also a risk factor.

Treatment

Antipsychotic medication is the mainstay of treatment of late-onset schizophrenia, as in younger patients. However, much lower doses (10–20% of a 'normal' dose) are often sufficient. This is not just a reflection of the age of the patient, as higher doses are typically needed for earlier-onset cases when they reach the same age. Another reason for cautious use of antipsychotic medication is that the risk of tardive dyskinesia appears to be considerably greater than in younger patients, although this may be independent of age at onset of illness (Liddle, 2013). Atypical antipsychotics probably have a lower risk of tardive dyskinesia than do typical antipsychotics in this age group, but recent concerns that they may increase cerebrovascular events in the elderly must be taken into account (see page 558). Cognitive and other psychological interventions may reduce disability, as in earlier-onset cases, although there is little direct evidence for this (Schimming and Harvey, 2004).

Management of schizophrenia in the elderly must also focus due attention on the complex medical and social needs of many patients; services are often fragmentary and inadequate, in part because of the emphasis on younger patients (Cohen *et al.*, 2015).

Personality disorder in the elderly

As discussed in Chapter 15, some personality traits and disorders attenuate with age, while others remain or become exaggerated. A meta-analysis found that the prevalence of personality disorder in people over 50 years of age was 7–10% (Abrams and Horowitz, 1996), somewhat lower than in younger adults. The decline is mainly attributable to a decline in Cluster B personality disorders, whereas obsessive–compulsive and schizoid characteristics may become more prominent (Debast *et al.*, 2014). Schizoid or paranoid traits may become accentuated by the social isolation of old age, sometimes to the extent of being mistaken for a delusional disorder or schizophrenia. Criminal behaviour is unusual, with only 1.7% of men in England and Wales who are found guilty of indictable offences being aged 60 years or older (Fazel *et al.*, 2001).

For a review of personality disorder in the elderly, see Oppenheimer (2013).

Other psychiatric syndromes of the elderly

Senile squalor syndrome

Senile squalor syndrome, also known as *Diogenes' syndrome*, is characterized by severe neglect of self and surroundings, domestic squalor, and social withdrawal and isolation. *Syllogomania* (the hoarding of rubbish) also occurs. It may be precipitated by stressful life events, and is associated with a high mortality after hospital admission. Other causes of self-neglect must be excluded, notably dementia, psychosis, or severe depression. The person usually stubbornly refuses all offers of help, and it is difficult to decide when to intervene using compulsory powers.

For a review, see Pavlou and Lachs (2006).

Charles Bonnet syndrome

Charles Bonnet syndrome refers to the occurrence of visual hallucinations without any other features of psychosis, dementia, or delirium. The syndrome is important, as misdiagnoses, especially of psychosis, resulting in inappropriate treatments have been reported. It is named after a Swiss philosopher who described the case of his own grandfather in 1760. The syndrome is particularly common in older people with failing eyesight, in whom there is a prevalence of 10–15%. It is usually thought to involve direct damage to the visual system. It is said to occur in up to 3.5% of referrals to old age psychiatrists.

The visual hallucinations are well formed, elaborate, vivid, and perceived in external space. They may be transient or persistent, and either variable in content or stereotyped. They have no personal meaning for the patient. Although they meet most of the criteria for true hallucinations, patients usually retain some insight into their unreality, and can often make the image disappear by closing their eyes.

The condition tends to improve if vision is restored, or when total blindness occurs. There is no specific treatment. It has been suggested that the syndrome may be an early indication of dementia, but this is unproven (Russell and Burns, 2014).

For a review, see Jacob *et al.* (2004).

Treatment of dementia

The clinical, epidemiological, and aetiological features of dementia were described in Chapter 14, and its epidemiology was discussed earlier in this chapter. Here its management will be covered. First the treatment of the behavioural and psychological disturbances of dementia, for which non-pharmacological and pharmacological strategies are used, will be discussed. Then the pharmacological treatment of Alzheimer's disease and some other specific dementias for which drugs are becoming available will be considered.

For an overview of the management of dementia, see Cullum (2013).

Treatment of behavioural and psychological symptoms of dementia

A spectrum of behavioural changes and psychological symptoms occurs during the course of dementia, as described in Chapter 14 and summarized in Box 19.4. These features affect the majority of sufferers at some stage of the illness, although the overall prevalence and frequency of individual features vary according to the type of dementia. The behavioural and psychological symptoms cause considerable problems for carers, and their management can be difficult. There is increasing concern about the inappropriate use of medication, yet there is a shortage of evidence-based non-pharmacological alternatives. For review, see Kales *et al.* (2015).

Before any treatment is considered, careful assessment is required, and attention should be paid to the following points:

- The nature of the problem behaviour(s) should be clearly identified, including its duration, severity, and any suspected causative or modifying factors. Rating scales may be useful (see Box 14.8). Examples of remediable causal factors include urinary tract infections,

constipation, and pain. The latter is often overlooked as a cause of agitation, and adequate analgesia may not be provided (Corbett *et al.*, 2012). Pain in dementia may be due to concurrent physical problems (e.g. leg ulcers, arthritis), or it may be part of the disease process.

- A mental state examination is needed to determine whether the behaviour can be explained in terms of an underlying psychopathology (e.g. whether there is evidence of psychotic symptoms, low mood, or anxiety). If this examination, together with the history

---

Box 19.4 Behavioural and psychological symptoms of dementia

Behaviours

Agitation
Shouting
Wandering
Apathy
Inappropriate sexual behaviour
Impaired sleep

Symptoms

Delusions
Hallucinations
Depression
Anxiety

Contributory factors

Constipation
Pain
Superimposed delirium
Sensory deficits

and other observations, supports a diagnosis (e.g. of psychosis, depression, or delirium), it will probably influence the treatment plan. On other occasions, however, no such diagnostic evidence may be forthcoming, in which case the behaviour is dealt with on its merits.

- The natural history is that behavioural and psychological symptoms of dementia fluctuate and often last for less than 3 months (Hope *et al.*, 1999). Any treatment, especially if drugs are used, should reflect this fact. Regular reassessment and trials of medication withdrawal should be an integral part of the management plan.

- Behavioural changes in dementia are usually problems for the carer rather than for the patient. This reality should be borne in mind when treatment decisions are made, especially as informed consent is often not possible because of the patient's cognitive impairment.

Non-pharmacological treatment of behavioural and psychological symptoms

If a behaviour or symptom is deemed, following assessment, to be sufficient to require treatment, a hierarchical approach should be employed. The first approach is to treat any underlying remediable cause, as outlined above. If the problem persists, the next approach should be based on modification of the patient's environment, or a behavioural or psychological intervention, the choice of which will be influenced by the nature of the problem, the severity of the dementia, the setting, and the resources and expertise available. Medication should be reserved for those patients in whom such approaches prove unsuccessful.

Many types of intervention are used (Box 19.5), as reviewed in Patel *et al.* (2014), but there are few randomized controlled trials. Evidence is strongest for an effect on agitation of person-centred care, communication skills training, dementia care mapping, and music therapy, but aromatherapy and light therapy did not demonstrate efficacy (Livingston *et al.*, 2014b). For a review of strategies for use in primary care, see Robinson *et al.* (2010).

Drug treatment of behavioural and psychological symptoms

High rates of prescribing of psychotropic drugs in dementia, largely to control behavioural problems, have been reported in nursing homes and other institutions. However, the evidence shows that medication has at most a modest effect and, in the case of antipsychotics,

---

> ### Box 19.5 Non-pharmacological interventions for behavioural and psychological symptoms of dementia
>
> **Sensory stimulation**
> Music therapy
> Aromatherapy (e.g. lavender oil)
> Bright light therapy
> Massage/touch
> White noise
>
> **Behavioural management**
> Differential reinforcement
> Stimulus control
>
> **Social contact**
> One-to-one interaction
> Pet therapy
>
> **Person-centred care**
> Dementia care mapping
> Exercise
> Structured activity programmes
> Environmental modifications
> Wandering areas
> Carer education and support

---

is associated with considerable morbidity and an excess mortality, as noted below. Reflecting these increasing concerns, medication for behavioural problems and psychological symptoms in dementia should not be contemplated until:

- A full assessment has been conducted.
- Any aggravating physical and environmental factors have been addressed.
- Non-pharmacological strategies have been attempted. In a randomized trial, Fossey *et al.* (2006) showed that enhanced psychosocial care led to a significant reduction in the prescribing of medication for nursing home residents with dementia.

Box 19.6 summarizes the drug treatments currently used for behavioural problems in dementia (Ballard and Corbett, 2013). A recent trial showed citalopram to be effective for agitation in Alzheimer's disease, but at the expense of a worsening of cognition and QTc interval prolongation, emphasizing that drug treatment in this area requires a

> ### Box 19.6 Daily doses of drugs used to treat behavioural and psychological symptoms of dementia
>
> #### For mild agitation
> Trazodone 50–100 mg
> Benzodiazepines, e.g. lorazepam 0.5–4 mg
> SSRIs, e.g. citalopram 10–20 mg
> Carbamazepine 50–300 mg
> Sodium valproate 250–1000 mg
> Rivastigmine (for Lewy body dementia) 1.5–6 mg
>
> #### For severe agitation with psychosis
> Quetiapine 25–200 mg
> Risperidone 0.5–3 mg
> Olanzapine 2.5–10 mg
>
> #### For depression
> SSRI, as above
> Mirtazapine 15–45 mg
>
> #### For severe behavioural problems
> Consider haloperidol in small doses (0.5–4 mg), for a limited time
>
> Reproduced from British Medical Journal, 338, Burns A, Illiffe S, Dementia, b75, Copyright (2009), with permission from BMJ Publishing Group Ltd.

careful consideration of risks and benefits (Þorsteinsson et al., 2014). The combination of dextromethorphan and quinidine is another potential treatment, which appears to be well tolerated (Ballard et al., 2015).

Antipsychotics

Despite their widespread use, robust evidence for the efficacy of antipsychotics in the behavioural problems associated with dementia is limited to the short-term (6–12 weeks) treatment of aggression (Seitz et al., 2013). They can often be withdrawn without any deterioration in behavioural problems. Moreover, their limited benefits must be set against the significant risk of extrapyramidal side effects, postural hypotension, tardive dyskinesia, metabolic syndrome, and the many other side effects of antipsychotics to which the elderly are prone (Schneider et al., 2006). The increasing concern about the use of antipsychotics in dementia is enhanced by three other serious potential risks.

- They are associated with a dose-related increased mortality risk (Maust et al., 2015) and increased risk of stroke (Mehta et al., 2010).
- Antipsychotics can precipitate an irreversible and sometimes fatal syndrome of parkinsonism, impaired consciousness, and autonomic disturbance, notably in patients with dementia with Lewy bodies.
- Antipsychotics may hasten cognitive decline (McShane et al., 1997), an observation confirmed in a randomized trial of quetiapine (Ballard et al., 2005). The mechanism involved is unknown, but may relate to antimuscarinic actions.

These concerns apply to atypical and typical antipsychotics. In consequence, current UK guidelines recommend that antipsychotics should not be used in dementia unless the patient's problems are severe, associated with either psychotic symptoms or serious distress, or the behaviour poses a danger of physical harm. Comparable warnings and restrictions are also in force elsewhere, and have led to a fall in prescribing rates (Kales et al., 2011). However, many older people, especially those in nursing homes, continue to be prescribed these drugs (Shah et al., 2011). Antipsychotics should be used rarely, if ever, in dementia with Lewy bodies. Assessment for vascular risk factors is advised because of the risk of stroke. As older people are more sensitive to antipsychotics, treatment should always start with a low dose, which is increased slowly, and the effects should be monitored regularly (Uchida et al., 2009). The choice of antipsychotic should be based on the side effect risk profile, with particular attention to extrapyramidal and anticholinergic effects and sedation.

Cholinesterase inhibitors and memantine

These drugs were developed to treat the cognitive symptoms of Alzheimer's disease. They are used to treat behavioural problems and psychological symptoms of dementia, too, in part because of the increasing concern about antipsychotics. However, they have limited efficacy against these aspects of dementia. A recent meta-analysis was inconclusive (Rodda et al., 2009), and they are not recommended for routine clinical practice (Ballard and Corbett, 2013), although they do have a role in behavioural disturbances occurring in dementia with Lewy bodies (Stinton et al., 2015).

Other drugs

A range of other drugs are also used, as illustrated in Box 19.6, based upon limited evidence. For depression in dementia, antidepressants show equivocal efficacy (Modrego, 2010).

Drug treatment of Alzheimer's disease

Treatment of behavioural and cognitive symptoms continues to be the most important element of therapy of dementia. However, pharmacological treatment of Alzheimer's disease itself is now available using cholinesterase inhibitors and memantine, and a range of other drugs are under investigation. For clinical practice guidelines for the use of antidementia drugs, see O'Brien *et al.* (2017).

Cholinesterase inhibitors

A loss of acetylcholine was the first neurochemical abnormality of Alzheimer's disease to be discovered, and led to the development of cholinesterase inhibitors as the first effective treatments for the disease. They now have an important role in clinical practice, and their discovery was responsible for bringing a new therapeutic optimism to old age psychiatry. They work by decreasing the enzymatic breakdown of acetylcholine and thus increase its availability at the synapse; some of the drugs may also enhance activity at nicotinic cholinergic receptors. However, their efficacy is limited, they do not alter the disease process, and the magnitude of their clinical benefit, as well as their cost-effectiveness, has been controversial, reflected in the UK by shifts in their availability within the NHS (see below).

The first cholinesterase inhibitor was tacrine, but its use was limited by hepatotoxicity. The drugs currently available are donepezil, rivastigmine, and galantamine. All of these are approved for use in mild to moderate Alzheimer's disease, based upon trial data showing beneficial effects, relative to placebo, on cognitive function (usually measured on the cognitive portion of the Alzheimer's Disease Assessment Scale, ADAS-Cog) and on global functioning (assessed with the Clinician Interview-Based Impression of Change scale with carer input, CIBIC-Plus). The size of the effect is relatively modest—for example, benefits of about 3 points on the ADAS-Cog (range of scores, 0–70), and 0.4 on the CIBIC-Plus (range of scores, 1–7). As disease progression averages about 7 points on the ADAS-Cog per year, cholinesterase inhibitors may be viewed as delaying progression by about 6 months. In other words, the drugs roughly double the likelihood of a patient improving by 4 ADAS-Cog points. The efficacy of the three drugs is similar.

Given the inexorable progression of dementia, and the limitations of rating scales alone, an alternative and attractive way to view medication efficacy is in terms of whether it reduces the percentage of patients who 'clinically deteriorate'. Clinical deterioration can be defined as cognitive decline, plus a decline in activities of daily living, plus a decline in global functioning. Using these criteria, donepezil significantly reduces clinical worsening (from 30% on placebo to 14% on donepezil) over a 24-week period, with a greater proportional benefit among patients with milder dementia (MMSE >18, from 21% to 7%) (Wilkinson *et al.*, 2009).

Side effects of cholinesterase inhibitors are common and can be troublesome. They include nausea, vomiting, diarrhoea, muscle cramps, insomnia, bradycardia, syncope, and fatigue. Their occurrence can be reduced by starting with a low dose, taking the drug with meals, and increasing the dose slowly. If a patient does not respond to, or cannot tolerate, a cholinesterase inhibitor, a trial of a different one is worthwhile (O'Brien *et al.*, 2017).

Current UK practice is that treatment with a cholinesterase inhibitor should be instituted in memory clinics by a specialist, following a formal assessment of the patient, from which the diagnosis of Alzheimer's disease is made, and its severity established as mild or moderate, using the MMSE and other cognitive scales. The response should be assessed 2–4 months later, and the drug continued only if the MMSE score has not declined, together with evidence of global or behavioural improvement. In those who show this initial response, the drug should continue as long as the MMSE score remains above 12, taking into account the patient's overall condition and global functioning. However, the benefits of treatment may continue beyond that point (Howard *et al.*, 2012). Decisions to stop medication are also complicated by some evidence that this is followed by an accelerated cognitive decline, such that within months the patient returns to the expected level of functioning had treatment never been given.

Memantine

Memantine is an N-methyl-D-aspartate (NMDA)-type glutamate receptor antagonist. The rationale for its use in Alzheimer's disease is that neurotoxicity mediated via the NMDA receptor might contribute to the disease process (Danysz and Parsons, 2012).

Randomized controlled trials have shown that memantine benefits cognition and function in moderate to severe Alzheimer's disease; its efficacy is modest, but it is better tolerated than cholinesterase inhibitors (Matsunaga *et al.*, 2015a). Applying the concept of clinical worsening mentioned with regard to cholinesterase inhibitors, memantine significantly reduces the risk compared with placebo (11% versus 21%) (Wilkinson and Andersen, 2007). Combining memantine and a cholinesterase inhibitor has equivocal benefits and is not currently recommended (Howard *et al.*, 2012; Matsunaga *et al.*, 2015b).

In the NHS, memantine can be prescribed for patients with severe Alzheimer's disease, and for those with moderate Alzheimer's disease who cannot tolerate cholinesterase inhibitors.

Other drugs

As discussed in Chapter 14, exposure to hormone replacement therapy, non-steroidal anti-inflammatory drugs, and statins have all been associated with lower rates of Alzheimer's disease. Each of these drug classes has therefore been used to treat the condition, but without benefit. Vitamin E has uncertain efficacy. None of these drugs are recommended for clinical practice (O'Brien *et al.*, 2017).

Extracts from the leaves of the maidenhair tree, *Ginkgo biloba*, have long been used in China as a remedy for various diseases. A recent meta-analysis suggests some efficacy, and it is well tolerated (Tan *et al.*, 2015).

Novel treatment approaches

Treatments currently under development for Alzheimer's disease are intended to modify the disease process, and thereby produce greater and more persistent benefits than the drugs that are being used at present.

The evidence that β-amyloid is central to the Alzheimer's disease process (see Box 14.11) has led to this molecule and its biochemical pathways being the key treatment targets of current research. Three main approaches are being used:

- Drugs to inhibit the enzymes (*secretases*) by which β-amyloid is formed from its precursor molecule.
- Drugs to prevent aggregation of β-amyloid.
- Immunization strategies that target β-amyloid.

The other main therapeutic target is tau and its phosphorylation (Iqbal *et al.*, 2016; see page 364); there is also emerging interest in novel types of anti-inflammatory therapies (Heppner *et al.*, 2015). To date, none of these strategies have produced clear positive results in clinical trials; one reason may be that the trials need to be carried out in patients at an earlier, ideally presymptomatic, phase of the illness (Langbaum *et al.*, 2013). For review of current treatment research in Alzheimer's disease, see Anand *et al.* (2014) and Scheltens *et al.* (2016).

Drug treatment of other dementias

There are no drugs currently licensed for any other common dementia. However, several of the approaches that are being used in Alzheimer's disease are also being applied in these disorders, and some are mentioned in dementia treatment guidelines (O'Brien *et al.*, 2017).

Vascular dementia

There have been few randomized trials of treatment for vascular dementia. Cholinesterase inhibitors and memantine are of little benefit and they are not recommended for use. Similarly, there are insufficient data to support routine use of the calcium channel blockers, cerebrolysin, or huperzine A (a natural cholinesterase inhibitor derived from a Chinese herb). Currently, treatment of vascular dementia remains limited to control of the cardiovascular risk factors, such as cholesterol and blood pressure, that are thought to underlie the condition. However, there is no good evidence that this is effective at preventing onset of dementia. For a review of management of vascular dementia, see O'Brien and Thomas (2015).

Dementia with Lewy bodies

Cholinesterase inhibitors have moderate effectiveness in dementia with Lewy bodies and in Parkinson's disease dementia (Wang *et al.*, 2015). The evidence is strongest for rivastigmine, which also has some beneficial effects on behavioural symptoms. This is valuable given the toxicity of antipsychotic drugs in this patient group. Memantine is minimally effective. For a review, see Stinton *et al.* (2015).

Other dementias

In *frontotemporal dementia*, no treatments have been shown to improve cognition or behavioural symptoms; cholinesterase inhibitors are not effective and may worsen the behavioural symptoms (Bang *et al.*, 2015). No treatments are known for the dementia of *Huntington's disease*, although a range of drug interventions for its psychiatric and motor components are available (Videnovic, 2013).

Finally, despite much interest in delaying the onset of dementia, there are no drug treatments effective for *mild cognitive impairment* (Cooper *et al.*, 2013), but aerobic exercise, mental activity, and reduction of cardiovascular risk factors are recommended (Langa and Levine, 2014).

Further reading

Dening T and Thomas A (2013). *Oxford Textbook of Old Age Psychiatry*, 2nd edition. Oxford University Press, Oxford.

Gelder MG *et al.* (eds) (2009). Section 8: The psychiatry of old age. In: *The New Oxford Textbook of Psychiatry*. Oxford University Press, Oxford.

CHAPTER 20

The misuse of alcohol and drugs

Introduction

The presentation of alcohol and drug misuse is not limited to any particular psychiatric or indeed medical specialty. Alcohol and drug use may play an important part in all aspects of psychiatric practice, and is relevant, for example, to the assessment of a patient with acute confusion on a medical ward, a suicidal patient in the accident and emergency department, an elderly patient whose self-care has deteriorated, a troubled adolescent, or a disturbed child who may be inhaling volatile substances.

The phrases 'substance use disorders' (DSM-5) or 'disorders due to psychoactive drug use' (ICD-10) are used to refer to conditions arising from the misuse of alcohol, psychoactive drugs, or other chemicals such as volatile substances. In this chapter, problems related to alcohol will be discussed first under the general heading of alcohol use disorders. Problems related to drugs and other chemicals will then be discussed under the general heading of other substance use disorders.

Classification of substance use disorders

The two classification systems, DSM-5 and ICD-10, use broadly similar categories for substance use disorders, but group them in different ways. Both schemes recognize intoxication and withdrawal states. ICD-10 has separate categories for 'harmful use' and 'dependence'. In contrast, DSM-5 has a single category of 'use disorder', which is rated on a continuum from mild to severe depending on the number of features present; there is therefore no separate category for 'drug dependence'. ICD-10 also recognizes drug-induced psychotic states and amnestic states, while in DSM-5 these are coded with the psychiatric disorders with which they share phenomenology; thus an alcohol-induced psychotic disorder would be classified under 'Schizophrenia spectrum and other psychotic disorders'. These and some additional categories are shown in Table 20.1.

In both diagnostic systems the first step in classification is to specify the *substance or class of substance* that is involved (see Table 20.2); this provides the primary diagnostic category. Although many drug users take more than one kind of drug, the diagnosis of the disorder is made on the basis of the most important substance used. Where this judgement is difficult or where use is chaotic and indiscriminate, ICD-10 has a category, 'disorder due to multiple drug use', which may be employed. Then the relevant disorder listed in Table 20.1 is added to the substance misused. In this system any kind of disorder can, in principle, be attached to any drug, although in practice certain disorders do not develop with individual drugs; for example, hallucinogens do not have a recognized withdrawal syndrome.

Table 20.1 Substance-related disorders

DSM-5	ICD-10
Intoxication	Intoxication
Use disorder	Harmful use
	Dependence syndrome
Withdrawal	Withdrawal state
Delirium[*]	Withdrawal state with delirium
Psychotic disorders[*]	Psychotic disorder
Neurocognitive disorder[*]	
Amnestic disorder[*]	Amnestic syndrome
Mood disorders[*]	Residual and late-onset psychotic disorder
Anxiety disorders[*]	Other mental and behavioural disorders
Sexual dysfunctions[*]	
Sleep disorders[*]	
[*]Classified under related psychiatric disorder	

Source: data from The ICD-10 classification of mental and behavioural disorders: clinical descriptions and diagnostic guidelines, Copyright (1992), World Health Organization; Diagnostic and Statistical Manual of Mental Disorders, Fifth Edition, Copyright (2013), American Psychiatric Association.

Table 20.2 Classes of substances

DSM-5	ICD-10[*]
Alcohol	Alcohol
Stimulants	Other stimulants, including caffeine
Caffeine	
Cannabis	Cannabinoids
Cocaine	Cocaine
Hallucinogens (phencyclidine and other)	Hallucinogens
Inhalants	Volatile solvents
Tobacco	Tobacco
Opioids	Opioids
Sedatives, hypnotics, or anxiolytics	Sedatives or hypnotics
Other	Multiple drug use

[*] The order of entries in the classification has been amended to show parallels with DSM-5.

Source: data from The ICD-10 classification of mental and behavioural disorders: clinical descriptions and diagnostic guidelines, Copyright (1992), World Health Organization; Diagnostic and Statistical Manual of Mental Disorders, Fifth Edition, Copyright (2013), American Psychiatric Association.

ICD-10 also has a specific category, 'residual and late-onset psychotic disorder', which describes physiological or psychological changes that occur when a drug is taken but then persist beyond the period during which a direct effect of the substance would reasonably be expected to be operating. Such categories might include 'hallucinogen-induced flashbacks' and 'alcohol-related dementia'.

Definitions in DSM-5 and ICD-10

Intoxication

Both DSM-5 and ICD-10 provide definitions of *intoxication*. In both systems, intoxication is considered to be a transient syndrome due to recent substance ingestion that produces clinically significant psychological and physical impairment. These changes disappear when the substance is eliminated from the body. The nature of the psychological changes varies with the individual as well as with the drug—for example, some people when intoxicated with alcohol become aggressive, while others become maudlin.

Use disorder, harmful use, and dependence

The terms 'use disorder' in DSM-5 and 'harmful use' in ICD-10 refer to maladaptive patterns of substance use that impair health in a broad sense. As noted above in ICD-10 there is a distinction between 'harmful use' and the more serious condition of 'dependence', whereas in DSM-5 the concept of 'use disorder' covers the range of severity of substance use. The latter includes features associated with drug dependence in ICD-10, such as the experience of 'pharmacological tolerance' and 'withdrawal', a 'sense of compulsion to take the substance' and 'neglect of alternative goals and interests' (Table 20.3 and Box 20.1). Thus in ICD-10 it is possible to meet criteria for harmful use without meeting those for dependence, but the presence of dependence always implies harmful use.

Tolerance

This is a state in which, after repeated administration, a drug produces a decreased effect, or increasing doses are required to produce the same effect.

Table 20.3 Criteria for harmful use and dependence (ICD-10)

Harmful use	Dependence
A. A pattern of psychoactive substance use that is causing damage to health; the damage may be to physical or mental health	**A.** Diagnosis of dependence should be made if three or more of the following have been experienced or exhibited at some time during the last year:
	(1) A strong desire or sense of compulsion to take the substance
	(2) Difficulties in controlling substance-taking behaviour in terms of its onset, termination, or levels of use
	(3) Physiological withdrawal state when substance use has ceased or been reduced, as evidenced by either of the following: the characteristic withdrawal syndrome for the substance, *or* use of the same (or closely related) substance with the intention of relieving or avoiding withdrawal symptoms
	(4) Evidence of tolerance, such that increased doses of the psychoactive substance are required to achieve effects originally produced by lower doses
	(5) Progressive neglect of alternative pleasures or interests because of psychoactive substance use and increased amount of time necessary to obtain or take the substance or to recover from its effects
	(6) Persisting with substance use despite clear evidence of overtly harmful consequences (physical or mental)

Source: data from The ICD-10 classification of mental and behavioural disorders: clinical descriptions and diagnostic guidelines, Copyright (1992), World Health Organization.

Withdrawal state

This refers to a group of symptoms and signs that occur when a drug is reduced in amount or withdrawn, which last for a limited time. The nature of the withdrawal state is related to the class of substance used. Sometimes the pharmacological properties of substances allow for *cross-tolerance*; for example, benzodiazepines can be used to stave off alcohol dependence.

Box 20.1 Substance use disorder in DSM-5

DSM-5 captures all the symptoms associated with harmful use and dependence in ICD-10. However, there is no separate category for 'dependence' in DSM-5 and the extent of the substance use disorder is decided by the number of symptoms endorsed out of a total of 11 (mild, 2–3 symptoms; moderate, 4–5 symptoms; severe, 6 or more symptoms). The symptoms cover the following areas:

- Use of the substance in greater amounts and for longer than was initially intended, with concomitant problems in cutting down use, often associated with craving.
- The substance and the energies needed to obtain it gradually take over more and more of the person's life despite the harm this causes to other interests, roles, activities, and relationships.
- Substance use continues despite knowledge of the harm being done to the physical and psychological health of the person. This can include the physical safety of the person and/or that of others to whom the person owes responsibility.
- The presence of pharmacological tolerance and withdrawal symptoms.

Source: data from Diagnostic and Statistical Manual of Mental Disorders, Fifth Edition, Copyright (2013), American Psychiatric Association.

Alcohol-related disorders

Terminology

Alcoholism. In the past, the term *alcoholism* was generally used in medical writing. Although the word is still widely used in everyday language, it is unsatisfactory as a technical term because it has more than one meaning. It can be applied to habitual alcohol consumption that is deemed excessive in amount according to some arbitrary criterion, and it may also refer to damage, whether mental, physical, or social, resulting from such excessive consumption. In a more specialized sense, alcoholism may imply a specific disease entity that is supposed to require medical treatment. However, to speak of an alcoholic often has a pejorative meaning, suggesting behaviour that is morally bad. For most purposes it is better to use four terms that relate to the ICD-10 classification outlined above.

1. *Excessive consumption of alcohol.* This refers to a daily or weekly intake of alcohol that exceeds a specified amount (see below). Excessive consumption of alcohol is also known as *hazardous drinking. Harmful drinking* is a term used to describe levels of hazardous drinking at which damage to health is very likely.

2. *Alcohol misuse.* This refers to drinking that causes mental, physical, or social harm to an individual. However, it does not include those with formal alcohol dependence.

3. *Alcohol dependence.* This term can be used when the criteria for a dependence syndrome listed in Table 20.3 are met.

4. *Problem drinking.* This term is applied to those in whom drinking has caused an alcohol-related disorder or disability. Its meaning is essentially similar to alcohol misuse, but it can also include drinkers who are dependent on alcohol.

At this point it is appropriate to examine the moral and medical models of alcohol misuse.

The moral and medical models

According to the *moral model*, if people drink too much, they do so of their own free will, and if their drinking causes harm to them or their family, their actions are morally bad. The corollary of this attitude is that public drunkenness and associated criminal activity should be punished. In many countries this is the official practice; public drunks are fined, and if they cannot pay the fine they go to prison. Many people now believe that this approach is too harsh and unsympathetic. Whatever the humanitarian arguments, there is little practical justification for punishment, since there is little evidence that it influences the behaviour of dependent drinkers. However, it is possible that social disapproval could play a role in dissuading non-dependent drinkers from excessive consumption.

According to the *medical model*, a person who misuses alcohol is *ill* rather than wicked. Although it had been proposed earlier, this idea was not strongly advocated until 1960, when the physiologist and alcohol researcher, E. Morton Jellinek (1890–1963), published an influential book, *The Disease Concept of Alcoholism*. The disease concept embodies three basic ideas.

1. Some people have a specific vulnerability to alcohol misuse.

2. Excessive drinking progresses through well-defined stages, at one of which the person can no longer control their drinking.

3. Excessive drinking may lead to physical and mental disease of several kinds.

One of the main consequences of the disease model is that attitudes towards excessive drinking become more humane. Instead of blame and punishment, medical treatment is provided. The disease model also has certain disadvantages. By implying that only certain people are at risk, it diverts attention from some important facts. First, anyone who drinks regularly for a long time may become dependent on alcohol. Secondly, the best way to curtail the misuse of alcohol may be to limit consumption *in the whole population*, and not just among a predisposed minority. Thirdly, it may suggest that excessive drinking, at least initially, is not a product of a personal choice.

Perhaps a useful way to resolve these two approaches is to apply the moral model to excessive drinking in the population in the hope of decreasing the number of people who put themselves at risk of alcohol-related disability. However, once dependence has occurred, with its attendant loss of control over drinking, a medical approach may be more appropriate.

Excessive alcohol consumption

In many societies the use of alcohol is sanctioned and even encouraged by sophisticated marketing techniques. Therefore the level of drinking at which an individual is considered to demonstrate excessive alcohol consumption is a somewhat arbitrary concept, which is usually defined in terms of the level of use associated with significant risk of alcohol-related health and social problems. It is usually expressed in units of alcohol consumed per week. For example, in the UK, government advice published in 2015 suggests that men and women should not regularly drink more than 14 units a week and that those drinking towards the higher end of this range should spread their drinking over 3 days or more. These limits are lower than those previously recommended (3–4 units a day for men and 2–3 units a day for women).

If the concept of excessive alcohol consumption is to be understood and accepted, it is necessary to explain the units in which it is assessed. In everyday life, this is done by referring to conventional measures such as pints of beer or glasses of wine. These measures have the advantage of being widely understood, but they are imprecise because both beers and wines vary in strength (see Table 20.4). Alternatively, consumption can be measured as the amount of alcohol (expressed in grams). This measure is precise and useful for scientific work, but is difficult for many people to relate to everyday measures.

For this reason, the concept of a *unit of alcohol* has been introduced for use in health education. A unit can be related to everyday measures because it corresponds to half a pint of beer, one moderately-sized glass of table wine, one conventional glass of sherry or port, and one single bar measure of spirits. It can also be related to average amounts of alcohol (see Table 20.4). Thus on this measure a can of beer (450 ml) contains nearly 1.5 units, a bottle of table wine contains about 12 units, a bottle of spirits contains about 30 units, and 1 unit is about 8 g of alcohol. The increase in strength of wine and beer over the past two decades has made many of these calculations difficult. Wine sold in the UK now contains an average of 12–14% alcohol, and sometimes more. To compound matters, the size of wine glass used in most restaurants has increased from 125 ml to 175 ml, so that an average serving in a restaurant or public house is equivalent to a minimum of 2 units.

Table 20.4 Alcohol content of some beverages

Beverage	Approximate alcohol content (%)	Grams of alcohol per conventional measure	Units of alcohol per conventional measure (approximate)
Beer and cider			
Ordinary beer	3	16 per pint	2 per pint
		12 per can	1.5 per can
Strong beer	5.5	32 per pint	4 per pint
		24 per can	3 per can
Extra-strong beer	7	40 per pint	5 per pint
		32 per can	4 per can
Cider	4	24 per pint	3 per pint
Strong cider	6	32 per pint	4 per pint
Wine and spirits			
Table wine	10–14	10 per glass	1.5 per glass
		70 per bottle	12 per bottle
Fortified wines (sherry, port, vermouth)	13–16	8 per measure	1 per measure
		120 per bottle	15 per bottle
Spirits (whisky, gin, brandy, vodka)	32–40	8–12 per single measure	1–1.5 per measure*
		240 per bottle	30 per bottle

* Somewhat larger measures are used in Scotland and Northern Ireland (12 grams).

Epidemiological aspects of excessive drinking and alcohol misuse

Epidemiological methods can be applied to the following questions concerning excessive drinking and alcohol misuse.

1. What is the annual per capita consumption of alcohol for a nation as a whole, and how does this vary over the years and between nations?

2. What is the pattern of alcohol use of different groups of people within a defined population?

3. How many people in a defined population misuse alcohol?

4. How does alcohol misuse vary with such characteristics as gender, age, occupation, social class, and marital status?

Unfortunately, we lack reliable answers to these questions, partly because different investigators have used different methods of defining and identifying alcohol misuse and 'alcoholism', and partly because excessive drinkers tend to be evasive about the amount that they drink and the symptoms that they experience.

Consumption of alcohol in different countries and at different times

In the UK, the annual consumption of alcohol per adult (calculated as absolute ethanol consumption) doubled between 1960 and 2000, rising from about 4 litres to over 8 litres. Consumption in western Europe has generally been higher than this, particularly in France and Luxembourg. High levels of consumption are also seen in the former Soviet Union and Eastern Europe, while in the Eastern Mediterranean and in Muslim countries consumption is much less.

Recent changes in the UK can be usefully considered in a historical perspective. For example, in Great Britain, between 1860 and 1900 the annual consumption of alcohol was about 10 litres of absolute alcohol per head of population over 15 years of age. It then fell until the early 1930s, reaching about 4 litres per person over 15 years of age per annum. Consumption then increased slowly until the 1950s, when it began to rise more rapidly, reaching a peak in about 2005. Over the past few years there has been a small but continuing drop in annual consumption; however, the average annual amount drunk in 2014 was still about twice what it was in the 1950s (see Figure 20.1).

Drinking habits in different groups

Surveys of drinking behaviour generally depend on self-reports, a method that is open to obvious errors. Enquiries of this kind have been conducted in several countries, including the UK and the USA. Such studies show that the highest reported consumption of alcohol is generally among *young men* who are *unmarried*,

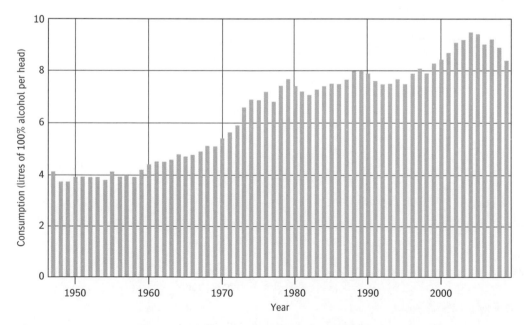

Figure 20.1 Average annual consumption of alcohol in the UK between 1947 and 2009.
Source: data from BBPA Statistical Handbook, Copyright (2010), British Beer and Pub Association.

separated, or divorced. However, over the past 15 years drinking by women has increased.

Based on population estimates in 2013 in the UK, 15% of men and 20% of women had drunk no alcohol in the past year, while just over 60% drank at levels with low risk of harm. The remainder—that is about a quarter of the adult population—drank at levels that could be considered to represent *harmful use.* In 2013 about 40% of school pupils aged 7–11 said that they had drunk alcohol at least once; this figure is less than that reported in 2003 (61%) (Health and Social Care Information Centre, 2015).

The prevalence of alcohol misuse

This can be estimated in three ways—from hospital admission rates, from deaths from alcoholic cirrhosis, and by surveys of the general population.

Hospital admission rates

These give an inadequate measure of prevalence, because a large proportion of excessive drinkers are not admitted to hospital.

- In the UK during the period 2012–2013 there were just over 1,000,000 hospital admissions where an alcohol-related disease, injury, or condition was the primary reason for hospital admission or a secondary diagnosis.
- In the UK in 2012 there were over 6000 deaths directly related to alcohol use (see Alcohol Concern, 2016).

Deaths from alcoholic cirrhosis

About 10–20% of people who drink alcohol excessively develop *cirrhosis of the liver*, and there are correlations in a population between rates of liver cirrhosis and mean alcohol consumption. Therefore deaths from cirrhosis can be used as a means of estimating rates of alcohol misuse. For example, in the UK in 2012, over 60% of deaths directly related to alcohol were caused by cirrhosis. UK deaths from cirrhosis have risen 20% over the past 10 years while declining in many other European countries (Alcohol Concern, 2016).

General population surveys

One method of ascertaining the rate of alcohol misuse in a population is by seeking information from general practitioners, social workers, probation officers, health visitors, and other agencies who are likely to come into contact with heavy drinkers. Another approach is the community survey, in which samples of people are asked about the amount they drink and whether they experience symptoms. For example, the National Survey Comorbidity Replication in the USA found a 1-year prevalence rate for DSM-IV alcohol abuse of 3.1%, while the prevalence of alcohol dependence was 1.3% (Kessler *et al.*, 2005b). A more recent USA population study using the more liberal 'alcohol use disorder' criteria of DSM-5 found a 1-year prevalence of 13.9% (Grant *et al.*, 2015). The Psychiatric Morbidity Survey in England, reporting 6-month prevalences, classified 24% of adults living in households as hazardous drinkers, and 6% as alcohol-dependent (although 5% of these individuals were classified as having 'mild' dependence) (McManus *et al.*, 2009). Over time there are significant individual fluctuations in alcohol consumption, with a substantial proportion of people moving from hazardous drinking towards safer drinking, while others move into the hazardous drinking category.

Surveys based on households are likely to miss certain groups at high risk of alcohol misuse and dependence. The British Psychiatric Morbidity Survey sampled separately from homeless populations and from those in institutions such as prisons. Among people living in night shelters or sleeping rough, 40% were found to drink more than 50 units of alcohol a week, and about 35% of those sleeping rough were estimated to have severe alcohol dependence (Gill *et al.*, 1996).

Alcohol misuse and population characteristics

Gender

Rates of alcohol misuse and dependence are consistently higher in men than in women, but the ratio of affected men to women varies markedly across cultures. In western countries, about three times as many men as women suffer from alcohol misuse and dependence, but in Asian and Hispanic cultures a higher ratio of men to women are affected. In the Psychiatric Morbidity Survey in England the rate of hazardous drinking among white men (36%) was more than twice as high as that among white women (16%), while the rate among South Asian men (12%) was four times higher than that among South Asian women (3%) (McManus *et al.*, 2009). However, perhaps because of changing social attitudes, the gap between men and women with regard to excessive drinking seems to be narrowing in many western countries. This is of concern because studies indicate that women are more susceptible than men to many of the damaging effects of alcohol (see below).

Age

Early use of alcohol is an important determinant of later use. A cross-sectional survey of over 10,000 US adolescents showed that 15.1% met criteria for lifetime abuse of alcohol with the median age at onset of 14 years (Swendsen *et al.*, 2012). We have seen that the heaviest drinkers are men in their late teens or early twenties. In most cultures the prevalence of alcohol misuse and dependence is lower in those aged over 45 years.

Religion, culture, and ethnicity

The followers of certain religions which proscribe alcohol (e.g. Islam, Hinduism, and the Baptist Church) are less likely than the general population to misuse alcohol. It is also worth noting that the non-Caucasian population in the UK and the USA are less likely to drink excessively than the Caucasian population, and therefore have a lower rate of alcohol-related disorders. In some instances, the low consumption of alcohol in a particular ethnic group may be due to a *biologically determined lack of tolerance* to alcohol. For example, some Asian populations with a particular variant of the isoenzyme of aldehyde dehydrogenase experience flushing, nausea, and tachycardia owing to accumulation of acetaldehyde when they drink alcohol. Such individuals are likely to be at reduced risk of excess drinking and the consequent development of alcohol-related disorders (Hurley and Edenberg, 2012).

Occupation

The risk of alcohol misuse is much increased among several occupational groups. These include chefs, kitchen porters, bar workers, and brewery workers, who have easy access to alcohol, executives and salesmen who entertain on expense accounts, actors and entertainers, seamen, and journalists. Doctors have been said to have an increased risk of harmful drinking, but whether this is in fact the case has been questioned. However, doctors do have higher rates of prescription drug misuse, and treatment programmes for both this problem and alcohol-related disorders may be difficult to institute (Marshall, 2008).

Alcohol dependence and alcohol withdrawal

Patients are described as *alcohol-dependent* when they meet the ICD-10 criteria for dependence described in Table 20.3. The presence of *withdrawal phenomena* is not necessary for the diagnosis of dependence, and a substantial minority of individuals who meet the dependence criteria do not experience any withdrawal phenomena when their intake of alcohol decreases or stops. However, about 5% of dependent individuals experience severe withdrawal symptomatology, including *delirium tremens* and *grand mal seizures*.

Course of alcohol misuse and dependence

Vaillant (2003) described a 60-year follow-up of 194 men who had exhibited *misuse of alcohol* at some point in their adult life. By the age of 70 years, over 50% of the cohort had died and about 20% were abstinent. Around 10% were drinking in a controlled way, while a further 10% continued to misuse alcohol. In a number of individuals alcohol misuse had apparently persisted for decades without remission, death, or progression to formal dependence. However, for *alcohol-dependent* men, periods of controlled drinking were invariably followed by a return to a pattern of alcohol dependence. Attendance at Alcoholics Anonymous was the best predictor of good outcome. This study suggests that the prognosis of alcohol misuse is very variable. However, once an individual has become alcohol-dependent the prognosis is poor unless abstinence can be maintained.

Trim *et al.* (2013) carried out a follow-up study of 129 men aged between 28 and 33 years, who were diagnosed initially with an alcohol use disorder. Over the next 20 years, 60% of the sample showed remission at some point and in 45% the remission was sustained. Predictors of a good response included a diagnosis of *alcohol misuse* rather than *dependence* as well as a lower drinking frequency and the receipt of a structured treatment for the alcohol problem soon after the onset of the disorder. This supports the view that a diagnosis of *alcohol dependence* carries a poor prognosis, and also suggests a longer-term benefit for specific treatment early in the course of the condition.

The alcohol withdrawal syndrome

Withdrawal symptoms occur across a spectrum of severity, ranging from mild anxiety and sleep disturbance to the life-threatening state known as *delirium tremens*, a specific form of delirium (Chapter 14) that is described further below. The symptoms generally occur in people who have been drinking heavily for years and who maintain a high intake of alcohol for weeks at a time. The symptoms follow a drop in blood alcohol concentration. They characteristically appear on waking, after the fall in concentration has occurred during sleep. *Dependent drinkers* often take a drink on waking to stave off withdrawal symptoms. In most cultures, *early-morning drinking* is diagnostic of dependency. With the increasing need to stave off withdrawal symptoms during the day, the drinker typically becomes secretive about the amount consumed, hides bottles, or carries them in a pocket. Rough cider and cheap strong beers may be drunk regularly to obtain the most alcohol for the minimum cost.

The earliest and commonest feature of alcohol withdrawal is acute tremulousness affecting the hands, legs, and trunk ('the shakes'). The sufferer may be unable to sit still, hold a cup steady, or fasten buttons. They are also agitated and easily startled, and often dread facing people or crossing the road. Nausea, retching, and sweating are frequent. Insomnia is also common. If alcohol is taken, these symptoms may be relieved quickly; otherwise they may last for several days (see Box 20.2).

As withdrawal progresses, *misperceptions* and *hallucinations* may occur, usually only briefly. Objects appear distorted in shape, or shadows seem to move; disorganized voices, shouting, or snatches of music may be heard. Later there may be *epileptic seizures*, and finally, after about 48 hours, *delirium tremens* may develop.

Other alcohol-related disorders

The different types of damage—*physical, psychological*, and *social*—that can result from alcohol misuse are described in this section. A person who suffers from these disabilities may or may not be suffering from *alcohol dependence* but will certainly meet criteria for *harmful use* (ICD-10) or *alcohol use disorder* (DSM-5).

Physical damage

Excessive consumption of alcohol may lead to physical damage in several ways. First, it can have a direct toxic effect on certain tissues, notably the brain and liver. Secondly, it is often accompanied by poor diet, which may lead to deficiency of protein and B vitamins. Thirdly, it increases the risk of accidents, particularly head injury. Fourthly, it is accompanied by general neglect, which can lead to increased susceptibility to infection.

Gastrointestinal disorders

Gastrointestinal disorders are common, notably liver damage, gastritis, peptic ulcer, oesophageal varices, and acute and chronic pancreatitis. Damage to the liver, including fatty infiltration, hepatitis, cirrhosis, and

---

hepatoma, is particularly important and is occurring at younger ages. For a person who is dependent on alcohol, the risk of dying from liver cirrhosis is almost 10 times greater than the average. However, only about 10–20% of alcohol-dependent people develop cirrhosis.

Nervous system

Alcohol also damages the nervous system. Neuro-psychiatric complications are described later; other neurological conditions include *peripheral neuropathy, epilepsy*, and *cerebellar degeneration*. The last of these is characterized by unsteadiness of stance and gait, with less effect on arm movements or speech. Rare complications are optic atrophy, central pontine myelinolysis, and Marchiafava–Bignami syndrome. The latter condition results from widespread demyelination of the corpus callosum, optic tracts, and cerebellar peduncles. Its main features are dysarthria, ataxia, epilepsy, and marked impairment of consciousness; in the more prolonged forms, dementia and limb paralysis occur. *Head injury* is also common in alcohol-dependent people.

Cardiovascular system and other general medical conditions

Alcohol misuse is associated with *hypertension* and increased risk of *stroke*. Paradoxically, low to moderate alcohol consumption (up to about 10 units a week) appears to have modest cardiovascular protective effects (O'Keefe *et al.*, 2014). Alcohol use, even at low levels, has been linked to the development of certain cancers, notably of the mouth, pharynx, oesophagus, liver, and breast.

Other physical complications of excessive consumption of alcohol are too numerous to detail here. Examples include anaemia, myopathy, episodic hypoglycaemia, haemochromatosis, cardiomyopathy, vitamin deficiencies, and tuberculosis. They are described in textbooks of medicine, such as the *Oxford Textbook of Medicine* (Warrell *et al.*, 2010).

Alcohol misuse in women

Studies suggest that women progress more rapidly than men to problem drinking, and tend to suffer the medical consequences of alcohol use after a shorter period of exposure to a smaller amount of alcohol. As well as the expected medical complications noted above, female drinkers also show elevated rates of breast cancer and reproductive pathology, including amenorrhoea, anovulation, and possibly early menopause.

Damage to the fetus

There is evidence that drinking alcohol in pregnancy can lead to a number of fetal abnormalities estimated to

---

> ### Box 20.2 Symptoms and signs of acute alcohol withdrawal
>
> Anxiety, agitation, and insomnia
>
> Tachycardia and sweating
>
> Tremor of limbs, tongue, and eyelids
>
> Nausea and vomiting
>
> Seizures
>
> Confusion and hallucinations
>
> Reproduced from British Medical Journal, 330(7483), Ritson B, Treatment for alcohol-related problems, pp. 139–41, Copyright (2005), with permission from BMJ Publishing Group Ltd.

affect around 2% of people in high income countries, of which *fetal alcohol syndrome* is the most severe. This consists of a syndrome of *facial abnormality, small stature, low birth weight, low intelligence, and overactivity*. Fetal alcohol syndrome is associated with clearly excessive alcohol use during pregnancy. However, subsequent research has suggested that even moderate or low levels of alcohol consumption at this time can have adverse effects on childhood behavioural, cognitive, and physical development, and the 'safe limit' for alcohol consumption during pregnancy (if such a level exists) is not known. Current advice from the UK Department of Health is that women should avoid alcohol during pregnancy. For a review of the prevalence and characteristics of fetal alcohol syndrome, see May *et al.* (2014).

Mortality

People with a low level of alcohol consumption (about 1 unit daily) have decreased mortality rates compared with non-drinkers; however, it has been suggested that this apparently protective effect is mainly attributable to confounding lifestyle factors (Knott *et al.*, 2015). Not surprisingly, however, the mortality rate is increased in those who misuse alcohol. Follow-up investigations have studied mainly middle-aged men drinking excessively, in whom overall mortality is at least twice the expected rate, and mortality in women who drink excessively appears to be substantially higher than this (Harris and Barraclough, 1998). In England it has been estimated that over 6000 deaths a year are *directly* attributable to the medical consequences of alcohol misuse (Alcohol Concern, 2016). Of course, alcohol must contribute *indirectly* to many more deaths from causes such as accidents. At a global level, the World Health Organization has estimated that alcohol causes 1.8 million deaths annually (about 3.2% of all deaths).

Psychiatric disorders

Alcohol-related psychiatric disorders fall into four groups:

- intoxication phenomena
- withdrawal phenomena
- toxic or nutritional disorders
- associated psychiatric disorders.

Intoxication phenomena

The severity of the symptoms of alcohol intoxication correlates approximately with the blood alcohol concentration. As noted above, there is much individual variation in the psychological effects of alcohol, but certain reactions, such as lability of mood and belligerence,

are more likely to cause social difficulties. At high doses, alcohol intoxication can result in serious adverse effects, such as falls, respiratory depression, inhalation of vomit, and hypothermia.

The *molecular mechanisms* that underlie the acute effects of alcohol are unclear. An influential view has been that alcohol interacts with neuronal membranes to increase their fluidity—an action also ascribed to certain anaesthetic agents. This action gives rise to more specific changes in the release of a range of neurotransmitters, leading to the characteristic pharmacological actions of alcohol. For example, the pleasurable effects of alcohol use could be mediated by release of dopamine and opioids in the mesolimbic forebrain, while the anxiolytic effects could reflect facilitation of brain gamma-aminobutyric acid (GABA) activity (Lingford-Hughes *et al.*, 2010).

The term *idiosyncratic alcohol intoxication* has been applied to marked maladaptive changes in behaviour, such as aggression, occurring within minutes of taking an amount of alcohol insufficient to induce intoxication in most people (with the behaviour being uncharacteristic of the affected individual). In the past, these sudden changes in behaviour were called pathological drunkenness, or *mania à potu*, and the descriptions emphasized the explosive nature of the outbursts of aggression. However, there is doubt as to whether behaviour of this kind really is induced by small amounts of alcohol. The term 'idiosyncratic alcohol intoxication' does not appear in DSM-5 or ICD-10.

Memory blackouts or *short-term amnesia* are frequently reported after heavy drinking. At first the events of the night before are forgotten, even though consciousness was maintained at the time. Such memory losses can occur after a single episode of heavy drinking in people who are not dependent on alcohol. If they recur regularly, they indicate habitual excessive consumption. With sustained excessive drinking, memory losses may become more severe, affecting parts of the day or even whole days.

Withdrawal phenomena

The general withdrawal syndrome has been described earlier under the heading of alcohol dependence. Here we are concerned with the more serious psychiatric syndrome of *delirium tremens*. Delirious states are described generally in Chapter 14, but delirium tremens is discussed here because of its prevalence and mortality, and its somewhat different treatment.

Delirium tremens occurs in people whose history of alcohol misuse extends over several years. Following alcohol withdrawal there is a dramatic and rapidly changing picture of disordered mental activity, with clouding of consciousness, disorientation in time and place, and impairment of recent memory. Perceptual disturbances include misinterpretations of sensory stimuli and vivid hallucinations, which are usually visual but sometimes occur in other modalities. There is severe agitation, with restlessness, shouting, and evident fear. Insomnia is prolonged. The hands are grossly tremulous and sometimes pick up imaginary objects; truncal ataxia may occur. Autonomic disturbances include sweating, fever, tachycardia, raised blood pressure, and dilatation of pupils. Dehydration and electrolyte disturbance are characteristic. Blood testing shows leucocytosis and impaired liver function.

The condition lasts for 3 or 4 days, with the symptoms characteristically being worse at night. It often ends with deep prolonged sleep from which the patient awakens with no symptoms and little or no memory of the period of delirium. Delirium tremens carries a *significant risk of mortality* and should be regarded as a medical emergency.

Neurological damage

Neurological syndromes include *Korsakov's psychosis* and *Wernicke's encephalopathy* (see also Chapter 14). In the past, the term 'alcoholic dementia' was widely used, but it remains unclear whether this is a discrete category (Ridley *et al.*, 2013); most cases of dementia in people with a history of alcohol misuse are probably attributable to Alzheimer's disease and other common forms of dementia. Instead, the above conditions are now often referred to collectively as '*alcohol-related brain damage*', covering the spectrum of cognitive impairments (Jauhar *et al.*, 2014).

In this respect, it is worth noting that cognitive impairments in severe alcohol use disorders often have a *multifactorial aetiology*, which can include effects of head injury, vascular changes, and metabolic and nutritional impairments as well as direct alcohol neurotoxicity. The neurotoxicity of alcohol is magnified by concomitant thiamine deficiency, which is common in heavy drinkers. However, even young heavy drinkers can exhibit evidence of neuropsychological impairments; for example, in executive function (Jauhar *et al.*, 2014).

Attention has also been directed to the related question of whether chronic alcohol misuse can cause structural brain atrophy. Both computerized tomography (CT) scanning and magnetic resonance imaging (MRI) have shown that excess alcohol consumption is associated with *enlarged lateral ventricles*. Furthermore, MRI scans have shown focal deficits, with *loss of grey matter* in both cortical and subcortical areas. Subcortical changes are more likely to be found in patients with Korsakov's syndrome. White matter changes are also common in heavy drinkers, and studies using diffusion tensor imaging indicate that there is demyelination, particularly in tracts linking limbic system and prefrontal cortex.

Many of the changes noted above occur in patients without obvious neurological disturbance, although, as noted above, psychological testing usually reveals deficits in cognitive function. The changes in brain structure and cognitive impairment that are seen in excessive drinkers remit to some extent with cessation of alcohol use. However, some abnormalities can still be detected after long periods of abstinence. For a review of alcohol-related brain damage, see Jauhar *et al.* (2014).

Associated psychiatric disorder

Personality deterioration. As the patient becomes increasingly concerned with the need to obtain alcohol, interpersonal skills and attention to their usual interests and responsibilities may deteriorate. These changes in social and interpersonal functioning should not be confused with personality disorder, which should be diagnosed only when the appropriate features have been clearly present prior to the development of alcohol dependence.

Mood and anxiety disorders. The relationship between alcohol consumption and mood is complex. On the one hand, some depressed and anxious patients drink excessively in an attempt to improve their mood. On the other hand, excess drinking may induce persistent depression or anxiety. People with a history of alcohol dependence have a fourfold increased risk of experiencing subsequent *major depression*, and the risk remains elevated even in those who are no longer drinking. The risk of experiencing an *anxiety disorder* is also significantly increased, but to a somewhat lesser extent (Anthenelli, 2010).

Suicidal behaviour. Suicide rates among people with alcohol use disorders are much higher than those among individuals who do not misuse alcohol. Conner and Duberstein (2004) identified a number of risk factors for suicidal behaviour among people with alcohol dependence, including *impulsivity, negative affect,* and *hopelessness*. Suicide among alcohol misusers is discussed further in Chapter 21. Here it is worth noting that suicide in young men is associated with a high rate of substance misuse, including alcohol misuse.

Pathological jealousy. Excessive drinkers may develop an overvalued idea or delusion that their partner is being unfaithful. This syndrome of pathological jealousy is described in Chapter 12.

Alcoholic hallucinosis. This is characterized by *auditory hallucinations*, usually involving voices uttering insults or threats, which occur in clear consciousness. The patient is usually distressed by these experiences, and appears anxious and restless. The hallucinations are not due to acute alcohol withdrawal, and can indeed persist after several months of abstinence. There has been considerable controversy about the aetiology of the condition. Some follow Kraepelin and Bonhoffer in regarding it as a rare organic complication of alcoholism; others follow Bleuler in supposing that it is related to schizophrenia. More recent reviewers have concluded that alcoholic hallucinosis is an alcohol-induced organic psychosis, which is distinct from schizophrenia and has a good prognosis if abstinence can be maintained (Mann and Kiefer, 2009).

In both DSM-5 and ICD-10, 'alcoholic hallucinosis' is subsumed under the heading of 'substance-induced psychotic disorder'.

Social damage

Family problems

Excessive drinking is liable to cause profound social disruption, particularly in the family (Box 20.3). Marital (or other relationship) and family tension is virtually inevitable. The divorce rate among heavy drinkers is high, and the partners of men who drink excessively are likely to become anxious, depressed, and socially isolated. The partners of 'battered wives' frequently drink excessively, and some women who are admitted to hospital because of self-poisoning blame their partner's drinking. The home atmosphere is often detrimental to any children present, because of quarrelling and violence, and a drunken parent provides a poor role model. Children of heavy drinkers are at risk of developing emotional or behavioural disorders, and of performing poorly at school.

Work difficulties and road accidents

At work, the heavy drinker often progresses through declining efficiency, lower-grade jobs, and repeated dismissals to lasting unemployment. There is also a strong association between road accidents and alcohol misuse. The strength of the association varies between countries. For example, in 2006, the proportion of fatal traffic accidents involving alcohol was about 17% in the UK, whereas the corresponding figures for France and Germany were about 27% and 11%, respectively. Whether these figures are attributable to real cross-national differences in the role of alcohol in traffic fatalities, or whether they are due to variations in 'legal' alcohol limits for driving, methods of data collection and definition, is not certain (Assum and Sørensen, 2010).

Crime

Excessive drinking is also associated with crime, mainly petty offences such as larceny, but also with fraud, sexual offences, and crimes of violence, including murder. Studies of recidivist prisoners in England and Wales have shown that many had serious drinking problems before imprisonment. It is not easy to determine to what extent alcohol causes the criminal behaviour and to what extent it is part of the lifestyle of the criminal. In addition, there is a link between certain forms of alcohol misuse and *antisocial personality disorder*.

The causes of excessive drinking and alcohol misuse

Despite much research, surprisingly little is known about the causes of excessive drinking and alcohol dependence. At one time it was believed that certain people were particularly predisposed, either through personality or due to an innate biochemical anomaly. Nowadays this simple notion of specific predisposition is no longer held. Instead, alcohol misuse is thought to result from a

---

Box 20.3 Medical and social consequences of excessive alcohol consumption in the UK

1. Annual alcohol-related costs of crime and public disorder are £7.3 billion, workplace costs are £6.4 billion, and health costs are £1.7 billion.

2. Up to one-third of all accident and emergency attendances involve alcohol.

3. Around 2.9 million (6%) of the adult population are dependent on alcohol.

4. Around 47% of victims of violence believe that their assailant was under the influence of alcohol.

5. Alcohol is involved in 30–60% of child protection cases. Up to 1.3 million children are adversely affected by family drinking.

Source: data from Prime Minister's Strategy Unit, Copyright (2003).

variety of interacting factors, which can be divided into individual factors and those in society.

Individual factors

Genetic factors

Most genetic studies of alcoholism have investigated individuals with evidence of alcohol dependence. If less severe diagnostic criteria are involved—for example, fairly broadly defined alcohol misuse—the relative genetic contribution is somewhat less. However, it is well established that alcohol dependence aggregates in families, and twin studies show a higher concordance in monozygotic than dizygotic twins, with an estimated heritability of about 50% (Bienvenu *et al.*, 2011).

Support for a genetic explanation also comes from investigations of adoptees. A number of studies have indicated a higher risk of alcohol misuse and dependence in the adopted-away sons of alcohol-dependent biological parents than in the adopted-away sons of non-alcohol-dependent biological parents. Such studies suggest a genetic mechanism, but they do not indicate its nature.

Adoption studies in Sweden led to the suggestion that there are two separate kinds of alcohol dependence, which have been called *type 1* and *type 2* (Cloninger *et al.*, 1988). Type 2 alcoholism is strongly genetic, predominantly occurs in males, has an early age of onset, and is associated with criminality and sociopathic disorder in both adoptee and biological father. By contrast, type 1 alcoholism has a later age of onset, is only mildly genetic, and occurs in both men and women. Subsequent typologies of alcohol dependence have become more complex, but continue to include a group of alcohol-dependent people with early age of onset and sociopathic disorder. In others, however, an early age of onset of alcohol dependence is associated not with sociopathic traits but with high levels of *anxiety-related symptoms* (Leggio *et al.*, 2009).

If a genetic component to aetiology were to be confirmed, it would still be necessary to discover the mechanism. The latter might be biochemical, involving the metabolism of alcohol or its central effects, or psychological, involving personality. In addition, it is important to note that a predisposition to misuse alcohol and develop dependence *will only be expressed* if a person consumes excessive amounts of alcohol. Here non-genetic familial factors are likely to play a major role.

Genes for alcohol dependence risk. Allelic association studies have focused in particular on genes that affect alcohol metabolism because, as we have already seen, people with impaired activity of the alcohol-metabolizing enzyme, aldehyde dehydrogenase, have unpleasant reactions when they consume alcohol, and are therefore at significantly lower risk of alcohol dependence. At a molecular level, a point mutation in the gene for a form of aldehyde dehydrogenase (*ALDH2*) renders the enzyme inactive; this mutation is less common in people with alcohol dependence. Subsequent linkage analyses have confirmed that mutations in the genes that code for aldehyde dehydrogenase protect against harmful drinking (Hurley and Edenberg, 2012). However, such mutations are rare in people of European ancestry.

Other candidate genes have included the *dopamine* D_4 *receptor* and the *GABA receptor*, and some associations with alcohol dependence have been reported. However, attempts at replication have yielded inconsistent findings. Similarly, genome-wide association studies (GWAS) have not generally provided reliable indications of relevant genes, although the effect of genes coding for alcohol metabolizing enzymes on the risk of alcohol dependence was confirmed (Hart and Kranzler, 2015).

Other biological factors

The *sons of men with alcohol dependence* are at increased risk of developing alcohol dependence themselves, and a number of studies have attempted to find biological abnormalities that may antedate and predict the development of alcohol dependence in these individuals. A variety of impairments have been described, including diminished performance on cognitive tasks, particularly *executive function*, and an abnormal P300 visual evoked response, which is a measure of visual information processing. There is also reasonably consistent evidence that sons of alcohol-dependent men are *less sensitive* to the acute intoxicating effects of alcohol. Presumably, if people experience less subjective responses to alcohol, they may tend to drink more, thus putting themselves at risk of developing alcohol dependence. There is also evidence that young heavy drinkers have lesser subjective and neural responses to alcohol than light drinkers, but whether this diminished effect represents a vulnerability factor or results from alcohol tolerance is unclear (Gilman *et al.*, 2012).

Learning factors

Alcohol use. Children tend to follow their parents' drinking patterns, and from an early age boys tend to be encouraged to drink more than girls. Non-genetic familial factors appear to be important in determining levels of alcohol use. Nevertheless, it is not uncommon to meet people who are abstainers although their parents drank heavily. In addition, the risk of children of alcohol-dependent parents developing alcohol use disorders is apparently little influenced by whether their parents are currently drinking or not. This suggests that *modelling of drinking behaviour* does not contribute substantially to the increased risk in the children.

Reward dependence. It has also been suggested that learning processes may contribute in a more specific way to the development of alcohol dependence. Thus the ability of alcohol to increase pleasurable feelings and decrease anxiety could lead to behavioural reinforcement, particularly in people who for physiological or social reasons overemphasize the positive effects of alcohol while ignoring its negative consequences. Recent formulations that combine biochemical and cognitive approaches emphasize the role of dopamine release in mesolimbic pathways in mediating incentive learning. In this way drugs such as alcohol, which increase dopamine levels in this brain region, stimulate motivational behaviours that are focused on the need to secure further drug supplies. These behaviours may eventually evade conscious control, and become difficult to extinguish (Lingford-Hughes *et al.*, 2010).

Personality factors

Little progress has been made in identifying personality factors that contribute to alcohol misuse and dependence. In clinical practice it is common to find that excessive alcohol consumption is associated with chronic anxiety, a pervading sense of inferiority, or self-indulgent tendencies. However, many people with personality problems of this kind do not resort to excessive drinking or become alcohol dependent. Other surveys have emphasized the role of personality traits that lead to risk-taking and novelty-seeking. It seems likely that these characteristics apply to those with antisocial personality disorder, who are known to be at increased risk of misusing alcohol and developing alcohol dependence. However, the majority of alcohol-dependent people do not have an antisocial personality disorder.

Childhood factors

We have seen that genetic factors are involved in the tendency of alcohol dependence to run in families, but the estimated heritability (about 50%) leaves much room for environmental factors. Childhood exposure to potentially traumatic events, particularly emotional abuse, predisposes to alcohol misuse in adulthood, and there is also a role for associated factors such as family disruption, poverty, and social isolation (Shin *et al.*, 2015). It is, of course, likely that alcohol dependence in a parent will contribute towards the latter.

Psychiatric disorder

Alcohol misuse is commonly found in conjunction with other psychiatric disorders, and sometimes appears to be secondary to them. For example, some patients with *depressive disorders* use alcohol in the mistaken hope that it will alleviate low mood. Those with anxiety disorders, particularly *panic disorder* and *social phobia*, who use alcohol to relieve anxiety are also at risk. In other cases alcohol misuse appears to *precede* another psychiatric disorder, suggesting that heavy alcohol consumption itself can act as an aetiological factor, perhaps in a person who is predisposed through genetic and other environmental factors to develop the specific psychiatric condition.

A national epidemiological survey of alcohol-related disorders carried out in the USA found that 55% of patients with alcohol dependence had a coexisting lifetime psychiatric disorder. The majority of this comorbidity was with *mood disorders* (40%), *anxiety disorders* (32%), and *antisocial personality* (14%) (Kandel *et al.*, 2013). Similar findings were reported by Grant *et al.* (2015), who drew attention to the high comorbidity between alcohol and other drug use disorders. Clinically, alcohol misuse is also seen in patients with *schizophrenia*. (The treatment of patients with severe mental illness and comorbid substance misuse is discussed on page 590).

Alcohol consumption in society

There is now general agreement that rates of alcohol dependence and alcohol-related disorders are correlated with the *general level of alcohol consumption* in a society. Previously it had been supposed that levels of intake among excessive drinkers were independent of the amounts taken by moderate drinkers. In 1956, however, the French demographer, Sully Ledermann, challenged this idea, proposing instead that the distribution of consumption within a homogeneous population follows a logarithmic normal curve. If this is the case, an increase in the average consumption must inevitably be accompanied by an increase in the number of people who drink an amount that is harmful.

Although the mathematical details of Ledermann's work have been criticized, there are striking correlations between average annual alcohol consumption in a society and several indices of alcohol-related damage among its members; for example, rates of liver cirrhosis. For this reason, it is now widely accepted that the proportion of a population that drinks excessively is largely determined by the average alcohol consumption of that population.

What then determines the average level of drinking within a nation? Economic, formal, and informal controls must be considered. The *economic control* is the price of alcohol. There is now ample evidence from the UK and other countries that the real price of alcohol (i.e. the price relative to average income) profoundly influences a nation's drinking habits. Furthermore, heavy drinkers as well as moderate drinkers reduce their consumption when the tax on alcohol is increased. For example, modelling the effect of a statutory minimum price for alcohol on consumption in England showed overall a modest reduction; however, the model predicted a more striking decrease in harmful drinking by people on low incomes, where the health gains would be greatest (Holmes *et al.*, 2014).

The main *formal controls* are the licensing laws, but these do not seem to influence drinking behaviours in a consistent way when comparisons are made between different countries. *Informal controls* are the customs and moral beliefs in a society that determine who should drink, in what circumstances, at what time of day, and to what extent. Some communities appear to protect their members from alcohol misuse despite the general availability of alcohol. For example, alcohol-related problems are uncommon among Jewish people even in countries where there are high rates in the rest of the community.

Recognition of alcohol misuse

Detection

Only a small proportion of alcohol misusers in the community are known to specialized agencies. When special efforts are made to screen patients in medical and surgical wards, around 10–30% are found to misuse alcohol, with the rates being highest in accident and emergency wards. It has been estimated that, of the 2.9 million people in the UK who are dependent on alcohol, only about 6% a year receive treatment. There are probably several reasons for this, including lack of help-seeking by users, limited availability of specialist alcohol services, and underidentification of alcohol misuse by health professionals (National Institute for Health and Clinical Excellence, 2011a).

Screening questionnaires

Alcohol misuse may go undetected because patients conceal the extent of their drinking. However, doctors and other professionals often do not ask the right questions. It should be a standard practice to ask all patients (medical, surgical, and psychiatric) about their alcohol consumption. Brief screening questionnaires can be helpful—for example, the CAGE questionnaire, which consists of the following four questions.

- Have you ever felt you ought to *Cut down* on your drinking?
- Have people *Annoyed* you by criticizing your drinking?
- Have you ever felt *Guilty* about your drinking?
- Have you ever had a drink first thing in the morning (an *'Eye-opener'*) to steady your nerves or get rid of a hangover?

Two or more positive replies are said to identify alcohol misuse. Some patients will give false answers, but others find that these questions provide an opportunity to reveal their problems. Overall the CAGE has a good sensitivity but only modest specificity (Mitchell *et al.*, 2014). An alternative is the AUDIT, a 10-item structured interview developed by the World Health Organization for screening for both currently harmful and potentially hazardous drinking. It shows good sensitivity and specificity, can identify mild dependence, and is probably the most useful screening questionnaire for clinicians and researchers in primary care (see Box 20.4).

Scores for each question range from 0 to 4, with the first response for each question scoring 0, and the last response scoring 4. For questions 9 and 10, which only have three responses, the scoring is 0, 2, and 4.

People who score in the range 8–15 should receive a brief intervention based on their risk for developing alcohol-related harm. Those who score 16–19 need a brief intervention and regular monitoring, including referral to specialist alcohol services if heavy drinking continues. Those who score in the range 20–40 should receive an early specialist referral and, depending on the severity of physical dependence, community or inpatient detoxification and other treatments (Pilling *et al.*, 2011).

General 'at-risk' associations

The next requirement is for the doctor to be suspicious about 'at-risk' associations. In general practice, alcohol misuse may come to light as a result of problems in the patient's primary relationship and family, at work, with finances, or with the law. The alcohol misuser is likely to have many more days off work than the moderate drinker, and repeated absences on a Monday should arouse strong suspicion. The high-risk occupations (see 'Occupation' above) should also be borne in mind.

Medical 'at-risk' associations

In hospital practice, the alcohol-dependent patient may be noticed if they develop withdrawal symptoms after admission. Florid delirium tremens is obvious, but milder forms may not be recognized as such, or instead considered to be delirium of another cause—for example, pneumonia or postoperative. In both general and

---

Box 20.4 AUDIT questionnaire: screen for alcohol misuse

1. How often do you have a drink containing alcohol?
   - Never
   - Monthly or less
   - 2–4 times a month
   - 2–3 times a week
   - 4 or more times a week
2. How many standard drinks containing alcohol do you have on a typical day when drinking?
   - 1 or 2
   - 3 or 4
   - 5 or 6
   - 7 to 9
   - 10 or more
3. How often do you have six or more drinks on one occasion?
   - Never
   - Less than monthly
   - Monthly
   - Weekly
   - Daily or almost daily
4. During the past year, how often have you found that you were not able to stop drinking once you had started?
   - Never
   - Less than monthly
   - Monthly
   - Weekly
   - Daily or almost daily
5. During the past year, how often have you failed to do what was normally expected of you because of drinking?
   - Never
   - Less than monthly
   - Monthly
   - Weekly
   - Daily or almost daily

6. During the past year, how often have you needed a drink in the morning to get yourself going after a heavy drinking session?
   - Never
   - Less than monthly
   - Monthly
   - Weekly
   - Daily or almost daily
7. During the past year, how often have you had a feeling of guilt or remorse after drinking?
   - Never
   - Less than monthly
   - Monthly
   - Weekly
   - Daily or almost daily
8. During the past year, have you been unable to remember what happened the night before because you had been drinking?
   - Never
   - Less than monthly
   - Monthly
   - Weekly
   - Daily or almost daily
9. Have you or someone else been injured as a result of your drinking?
   - No
   - Yes, but not in the past year
   - Yes, during the past year
10. Has a relative or friend, doctor or other health worker been concerned about your drinking or suggested that you cut down?
    - No
    - Yes, but not in the past year
    - Yes, during the past year

Reproduced from The Alcohol Use Disorders Identification Test: Guidelines for Use in Primary Care, Copyright (2001), with permission from the World Health Organization.

---

hospital practice, at-risk factors include physical disorders that may be alcohol-related. Common examples are gastritis, peptic ulcer, and liver disease, but others, such as neuropathy and seizures, should be borne in mind. Repeated accidents should also arouse suspicion.

Psychiatric at-risk associations include anxiety, depression, erratic moods, impaired concentration, memory lapses, and sexual dysfunction. Alcohol misuse should be considered in all cases of deliberate self-harm.

Drinking history

If any of the above factors raise suspicion of alcohol misuse, the next stage is to take a comprehensive drinking history (see Box 20.5). This should be done sensitively, with understanding that the patient may have difficulty in giving a clear history. The clinician should aim to build up a picture of what and how much the patient drinks throughout a typical day—for example, when and where they have the first drink of the day. Patients should be asked how they feel if they go without a drink for a day or two, and how they feel *on waking*. This can lead on to enquiries about the typical features of dependence and the range of physical, psychological, and social problems associated with it.

To gain an idea of the duration of alcohol problems, key points in the history may include establishing when the patient first began *drinking every day*, when they began drinking *in the mornings*, and when, if ever, they first experienced *withdrawal symptoms*. It is useful to ask about periods of abstinence from alcohol, what factors helped to maintain this state of affairs, and what led to a resumption of drinking. This can lead on to enquiries about past attempts at treatment.

It is necessary to obtain a clear understanding of the patient's own view of their drinking behaviour, because there are a number of possible treatment goals. In this situation the *patient's attitude* to their problems plays a key role in deciding which approaches are likely to be most beneficial (see the section on motivational interviewing, below).

Laboratory tests

Several laboratory tests can be used to detect alcohol misuse, although none gives an unequivocal answer. This is because the more sensitive tests can give 'false-positive' results when there is disease of the liver, heart, kidneys, or blood, or if enzyme-inducing drugs such as anticonvulsants, steroids, or barbiturates have been taken. However, abnormal values point to the possibility of alcohol misuse. The most useful tests are listed in Box 20.6.

The treatment of alcohol misuse

Early detection and treatment

Early detection of excessive consumption of alcohol and alcohol misuse is important because treatment of established cases is difficult, particularly when dependence

is present. Many cases can be detected early by general practitioners, physicians, and surgeons when patients are seeking treatment for another problem (see Box 20.7).

Brief intervention

General practitioners are well placed to provide early treatment of alcohol problems, and they are likely to know the patient and their family well. It is often effective if the general practitioner gives simple advice in a frank, matter-of-fact way, but with tact and understanding.

Brief interventions generally involve simple education and advice about safe levels of alcohol consumption. The aim is to promote safer drinking, rather than abstinence. Generally, brief interventions lead to modest reductions in alcohol consumption over the next few years, and are the best initial approach for a person whose alcohol consumption exceeds safe limits. However, whether the beneficial effects of brief motivational interviewing or

> **Box 20.7 Approach to treatment of alcohol misuse**
>
> - Raise awareness of problem
> - Increase motivation to change
> - Support and advice
> - Withdraw alcohol (or controlled drinking)
> - High-intensity psychological treatments
> - Alcoholics Anonymous
> - Medication (disulfiram, acamprosate, naltrexone)

> **Box 20.8 Motivational interviewing**
>
> - Express empathy
> - Avoid arguing; don't be judgemental
> - Detect and 'roll with' resistance
> - Point out discrepancies in the patient's history
> - Raise awareness about the contrast between the substance user's aims and behaviour

lifestyle counselling are greater than the simple completion of an AUDIT questionnaire followed by feedback has been questioned (Luty, 2015a). It is, however, agreed that brief interventions are not effective for people with severe drinking problems, particularly those who are alcohol-dependent.

Motivational interviewing

Patients with problems of alcohol misuse, particularly those detected by screening methods, may be unsure whether or not to engage in treatment programmes. An appropriate interviewing style, particularly during the first assessment, can help to persuade the patient to engage in a useful review of their current pattern of drinking.

Confrontation is avoided in *motivational interviewing*, and a less directive approach is taken, during which patients are helped to assess the balance of the positive and negative effects of alcohol on their lives. The clinician can help in this exercise by providing feedback to the patient about the personal risks that alcohol poses both to them and to their family, together with a number of options for change. The aim of motivational interviewing is to persuade the patient to argue their own case for changing their pattern of substance use (see Box 20.8).

For an explanation of the origin of motivational interviewing and a description of the relevant techniques, see Treasure (2004).

Treatment plans for more established alcohol misuse and dependence

For patients who have significant alcohol-related disorders, particularly alcohol dependence, treatment generally needs to be more intensive. Any intervention should be preceded by a full assessment, and should include a drinking history and an appraisal of current medical, psychological, and social problems. Other important issues concern the *use of other drugs* (including

those bought over the counter) and an *assessment of cognitive function* with, for example, the Mini-Mental State Examination (MMSE).

An intensive and searching enquiry often helps the patient to gain a new recognition and understanding of the problem, and this is the basis of treatment. As noted above, however, it is important to avoid confrontation, as this will only alienate someone who is likely to have very mixed feelings about the prospect of life without alcohol. It is usually desirable to involve the patient's partner in the assessment, both to obtain additional information and to give the partner an opportunity to unburden their feelings.

A mutually agreed treatment plan should be worked out with the patient (and their partner if appropriate). There should be specific goals, and the patient should be required to take responsibility for realizing these. The goals should deal not only with the drinking problem, but also with any accompanying problems with regard to the patient's health, marriage, or other relationship, job, and social adjustment. In the early stages they should be short-term and achievable—for example, complete abstinence for 2 weeks. In this way the patient can be rewarded by early achievement.

Longer-term goals can be set as treatment progresses. These will be concerned with trying to change factors that precipitate or maintain excessive drinking, such as tensions in the family. When drawing up this treatment plan, an important decision is whether to aim for total abstinence or limited consumption of alcohol (*controlled drinking*).

Total abstinence versus controlled drinking

The disease model of alcoholism proposes that an alcohol-dependent person must become totally abstinent and remain so, as a single drink would lead to relapse. Alcoholics Anonymous have made this a tenet of their approach to treatment.

The issue of abstinence versus controlled drinking remains unresolved. A prevalent view is that controlled drinking may be a feasible goal for people whose alcohol misuse has been detected early, and who are not dependent or physically damaged. Abstinence is a better goal for dependent drinkers and others who have attempted controlled drinking unsuccessfully. If controlled drinking is to be attempted, the doctor should give the patient clear advice about safe levels (see 'Excessive alcohol consumption' above).

Withdrawal from alcohol

For patients with dependence syndrome, withdrawal from alcohol is an important stage in treatment and should be managed carefully. In less severe cases, withdrawal may take place at home provided there is adequate support and clinical monitoring (see Box 20.9). This should involve daily assessment by the general practitioner, practice nurse, or specialist alcohol worker to check the patient's physical state and supervise medication (see Box 20.10). In uncomplicated cases, withdrawal symptoms usually resolve within 4–6 days. However, any patient who is likely to have severe withdrawal symptoms, especially if there is a history of delirium tremens or seizures, should be admitted to hospital. The Severity of Alcohol Dependence Questionnaire (SADQ) can be useful for estimating the likely severity of alcohol dependence and thereby gauging the amount of difficulty that the patient might encounter during withdrawal. A SADQ score of more than 30 is an indication for inpatient detoxification. Other indications for residential detoxification are *very high alcohol consumption* (over 30 units daily), *concomitant benzodiazepine misuse,* and significant *medical or psychiatric comorbidity* (National Institute for Health and Clinical Excellence, 2011a).

The extensive research on pharmacological treatment for alcohol withdrawal has been systematically reviewed by Lingford-Hughes *et al.* (2012). The most important concern is the prevention of major complications of withdrawal, such as seizures or delirium

---

> **Box 20.10 General management of alcohol detoxification**
>
> 1. Explanation of the process to the patient and their family
> 2. The patient should stay off work and rest. They should not drive
> 3. The patient should take plenty of fluids but avoid caffeinated drinks
> 4. Daily visit by health professional
> 5. Maintain abstinence
> 6. Reducing course of benzodiazepines over 5–7 days (see text)

---

tremens. Treatment with benzodiazepines is usually the most suitable choice.

Benzodiazepines differ in their duration of action (see Chapter 25). Although the longer-acting compounds may carry the risk of oversedation in the elderly or in those with significant liver disease, they also have the advantage of smoother withdrawal and generally better relief of withdrawal symptoms. *Chlordiazepoxide* is often used. A typical outpatient regimen would start with 20–30 mg four times daily, reducing and stopping over a period of 5–7 days. In more severe cases, particularly in inpatients, higher doses are commonly used. If convulsions occur, the dose of benzodiazepine should be reviewed and increased if necessary. Administration of a benzodiazepine that is well absorbed parenterally (e.g. lorazepam) may be useful to relieve severe acute withdrawal, although oral medication can usually be resumed promptly. In home-based withdrawal it is helpful for a family member or friend to supervise the medication.

Carbamazepine has also been found to be effective in the treatment of alcohol withdrawal, and although not often used in the UK, it is a good alternative to the use of a benzodiazepine. There is no added benefit from using carbamazepine and a benzodiazepine together.

Clomethiazole was frequently used in the management of alcohol withdrawal in the past, but is no longer recommended because of its toxicity when combined with alcohol and its danger in overdose. It is occasionally used for the most severe withdrawal states, where intensive inpatient medical monitoring is available, but there is no clear advantage compared with adequate doses of a benzodiazepine.

Antipsychotic drugs lower the seizure threshold and are less effective than benzodiazepines in preventing

---

> **Box 20.9 Considerations before alcohol detoxification**
>
> 1. What are the medical risks?
> 2. What setting is appropriate?
> 3. What does the patient want from detoxification?
> 4. What kind of aftercare is needed to help to maintain abstinence?

delirium. They are sometimes used to reduce agitation during alcohol withdrawal, but use of adequate doses of a benzodiazepine is a safer strategy. Antipsychotic drugs may be required occasionally, however, in patients with delusions that do not respond to benzodiazepines. In these circumstances, combination of antipsychotic treatment with benzodiazepines would be expected to attenuate the pro-convulsive effects of the antipsychotic drug.

Vitamin supplements, particularly thiamine, should also be given to prevent the Wernicke–Korsakoff syndrome. Parenteral thiamine should be given to patients at high risk (i.e. those with alcohol dependence and a poor diet). In the treatment of delirium tremens or Wernicke's encephalopathy, thiamine treatment should always precede glucose administration.

Psychological treatment

As noted above, *provision of information and advice* about the effects of excessive drinking is an important first stage in treatment. The information given should relate to the specific problems of the individual patient, including both those that have already occurred and those that are likely to develop if drinking continues. The technique of *motivational interviewing* can be useful (see Box 20.8).

More specialized, high-intensity psychological treatments are appropriate if the drinking problem is more serious, particularly in cases of alcohol dependence. Several treatment approaches have been employed, although there is significant overlap between the different therapies (see Box 20.11). Important features of successful psychological approaches include the use of *behavioural techniques*, which require drinkers to take some action themselves, as well as the involvement of a *partner* and the drinker's *wider social network*. There are also important roles for *education* and the improvement of *social and interpersonal skills*, as these relate to alcohol misuse.

It may be helpful, for example, to identify situational or interpersonal triggers that cause the patient to drink excessively, and then to plan and rehearse new methods of coping with these situations. This is an important part of *relapse prevention*. The use of *cue exposure* to alcoholic drinks, without subsequent consumption, may also lessen the risk of subsequent relapse when the patient has to contend with the ready availability of alcohol in social settings. It is important for the patient to appreciate that a *lapse* in drinking behaviour does not have to progress to a full-blown *relapse*. Many patients who misuse alcohol have general deficiencies in problem-solving skills, and appropriate training may help to reduce relapse rates. If the patient is in a relatively stable relationship with a partner, *cognitive behavioural relationship*

therapy can produce improvements in both drinking behaviour and relationship adjustment.

For a review of psychological treatments for problem drinking, see National Institute for Health and Clinical Excellence (2011a).

Pharmacological treatments to help to maintain abstinence

A number of different kinds of medication have been employed to help people to abstain from drinking or to experience less drinking-related harm. Medications are not regarded as 'stand-alone' treatments and, when used in the management of drinking problems, should be combined with an appropriate psychosocial intervention (see Lingford-Hughes *et al.*, 2012, and Box 20.12).

Disulfiram (Antabuse) acts by blocking the oxidation of alcohol so that acetaldehyde accumulates. Some patients find it useful because the anticipation of an unpleasant reaction acts as a deterrent to impulsive drinking. The reaction includes facial flushing, throbbing headache, hypotension, palpitations, tachycardia, and nausea and vomiting. In vulnerable patients, cardiac arrhythmias and collapse may occur.

The main contraindications to the use of disulfiram are a history of heart failure, coronary artery disease, hypertension, psychosis, and pregnancy. The patient should be given clear verbal and written instructions, together with a list of alcohol-containing substances to be avoided. Common side effects are drowsiness, bad breath, nausea, and constipation. Disulfiram is given in a single dose of 800 mg on the first day of treatment, reducing over 5 days to 100–200 mg daily.

The efficacy of disulfiram depends on compliance. The treatment is likely to be more successful if a partner or health worker is able to supervise its use, perhaps in the context of a structured treatment such as cognitive behavioural relationship therapy. However, the unsupervised use of disulfiram is not considered to be an effective approach (Luty, 2015b).

Acamprosate (calcium acetyl homotaurinate) appears to suppress the urge to drink in response to learned cues, and can produce modest but useful reductions in drinking behaviour in alcohol-dependent individuals. It is believed to act by stimulating GABA-inhibitory neurotransmission and decreasing the excitatory effects of glutamate. The effects of acamprosate have not been consistent across studies. For example, a large trial in the United States (COMBINE) showed no increased benefit in measures of drinking behaviour when acamprosate was combined with cognitive behaviour therapy compared with cognitive behaviour therapy alone (Anton *et al.*, 2006). However, a meta-analysis of 19 randomized

> ## Box 20.11 High-intensity psychological therapies for alcohol-focused specialist treatment
>
> **Community reinforcement approach**. A broad range of treatments, with the overall aim of changing the drinker's social environment so that sobriety is rewarded. Components include training in communication skills, problem-solving, and assertive drink refusal. Relationship therapy and promotion of relapse prevention are also offered. Disulfiram with monitored compliance is frequently used.
>
> **Social behaviour and network therapy**. Use of the drinker's social network to help to modify their drinking and maintain change. Facilitation of communication within the network and the agreement of common goals with the drinker. Use of pleasant social activities as an alternative to drinking.
>
> **Behavioural self-control training**. Main use is to control drinking rather than to achieve abstinence. Can be used in groups, individually, or in a self-help format. Key components include setting drinking limits, development of methods to control drinking rate, drink refusal skills training, and self-reward for successful behaviours that replace drinking.
>
> **Coping and social skills training**. Can be used in a group or individual format. Improves relationships by building up interpersonal skills, and uses cognitive emotional coping for mood regulation. Coping skills training enhances
>
> activities of daily living and facilitates dealing with stressful life events and the impact of alcohol-related cues that prompt drinking.
>
> **Cognitive behavioural relationship therapy**. Based on social learning theory. Uses behavioural contracting, communication skills training, and behavioural rehearsal with the drinker and their partner. Particularly appropriate in cases where the drinking problem and relationship difficulties exacerbate each other.
>
> **Cue exposure**. Based on Pavlovian conditioning theory, and views craving for alcohol as a conditioned response to specific environmental cues. Aims to 'extinguish' conditioned responses and ameliorate craving by presenting relevant cues in the absence of the reinforcing effect of alcohol. Not used as a 'stand-alone treatment'.
>
> **Relapse prevention**. Difficult to define because it is a goal of treatment rather than a specific treatment modality. Based on cognitive behavioural techniques, and involves training in social skills and coping and behavioural rehearsal. An important component of many other approaches.
>
> Source: data from Raistrick D, Heather N and Godfrey C, Review of the Effectiveness of Treatment for Alcohol Problems, Copyright (2006), National Treatment Agency for Substance Misuse.

trials showed that, over a 2-year follow-up, acamprosate significantly increased the abstinence rate, with a relative risk of 0.83 (95% CI, 0.77–0.88) (National Institute for Health and Clinical Excellence, 2011a).

The usual dose of acamprosate is two tablets (333 mg each) three times daily with meals. In lighter patients (<60 kg), four tablets daily are recommended. Acamprosate is not metabolized in the liver and is excreted by the kidney. It is therefore unlikely to cause drug interactions. Adverse effects include diarrhoea and, less frequently, nausea, vomiting, and abdominal pain. Skin rashes may occur, as can fluctuations in libido.

Naltrexone. The opioid antagonist, *naltrexone*, is believed to block some of the reinforcing effects of alcohol and in this way decrease the likelihood of relapse after detoxification. Not all trials have found a significant benefit over placebo. In the COMBINE study, the best effects on drinking behaviour were shown by participants who received both naltrexone and cognitive

behaviour therapy (Anton *et al.*, 2006). A meta-analysis of 27 randomized trials showed that, over a 12-month follow-up, naltrexone significantly increased rates of abstinence, with a relative risk of 0.83 (95% CI, 0.75–0.91), an effect very similar to that of acamprosate (National Institute for Health and Clinical Excellence, 2011a). Common side effects of naltrexone treatment include nausea, vomiting, headache, dizziness, and weight loss.

Nalmefene, like naltrexone, is an orally active opioid antagonist. Nalmefene has been studied in patients who drink heavily but who do not have severe alcohol dependence with withdrawal symptoms. In this group, given with psychosocial support, nalmefene produces modest reductions in total alcohol consumption and number of days of heavy drinking over the following 6 months. National Institute for Health and Clinical Excellence has recommended nalmefene as a potential treatment for men who drink more than 45 units of alcohol a week and

> **Box 20.12 National Institute for Health and Clinical Excellence (NICE) guidance on the management of harmful drinking and alcohol dependence**
>
> 1. For harmful drinking and mild dependence offer a high-intensity psychological treatment (see Box 20.9).
> 2. For those drinking over 15 units of alcohol a day and/or scoring 15–30 or more on the SADQ* test, offer community-based assisted withdrawal, or inpatient treatment if there are safety concerns.
> 3. After successful withdrawal for patients with moderate or severe alcohol dependence, consider offering acamprosate or oral naltrexone in combination with a high-intensity psychological treatment that promotes relapse prevention.
>
> * Severity of Alcohol Dependence Questionnaire.
>
> Source: data from the National Institute for Health and Care Excellence, Copyright (2014).

women drinking more than 35 units a week. However, whether the benefits of nalmefene in this population are *clinically significant* has been questioned (Palpacuer *et al.*, 2015). The most common side effects of nalmefene are similar to those of naltrexone, namely nausea, vomiting, dizziness, headache, and insomnia.

Topiramate is an anticonvulsant drug which in randomized trials has been shown to benefit drinking outcomes in terms of reductions in days of heavy drinking and harmful drinking consequences, as well as improving quality of life (Lingford-Hughes *et al.*, 2012). The adverse effects of topiramate, however, can be troublesome, and include paraesthesia, anorexia, headache, abdominal pain, sleep disturbance, and cognitive impairment.

Antidepressant medication may be useful in patients who experience persistent symptoms of major depression after detoxification. However, tricyclic antidepressants are not recommended because of potentially serious adverse reactions, including cardiotoxicity and death following overdose. There is no evidence that antidepressants are helpful in patients with alcohol use disorders who are not depressed. Indeed, selective serotonin reuptake inhibitors (SSRIs) appear to worsen the outcome in Cloninger type 2 alcohol dependence (early age of onset, positive family history, impulsive/antisocial personality traits) (Lingford-Hughes *et al.*, 2012).

For a systematic review of the pharmacotheray of alcohol use disorders, see Jonas *et al.* (2014).

Other agencies concerned with drinking problems

Alcoholics Anonymous (AA) is a self-help organization founded in the USA by two alcoholic men, a surgeon and a stockbroker. It has since extended to most countries of the world. Members attend group meetings, usually twice-weekly, on a long-term basis. In crisis they can obtain immediate help from other members by telephone. The organization works on the firm belief that abstinence must be complete. At present there are about 1200 groups in the UK.

Alcoholics Anonymous is based on a number of fundamental principles, known as the 'Twelve Steps', to which members adhere. It does not appeal to all problem drinkers because the meetings involve an emotional confession of problems, and because of the evangelical, quasireligious nature of the twelve-step approach. However, the organization is of great value to some problem drinkers, and anyone with a drink problem should be encouraged to try it.

A treatment approach similar to that provided by Alcoholics Anonymous, coupled with encouragement to attend Alcoholics Anonymous meetings, was one of the psychological therapies employed in Project MATCH (see below). In general, all of the treatments that were employed appeared to be roughly equal in efficacy. However, patients with fewer psychiatric problems at entry tended to have a better outcome with the Alcoholics Anonymous type of treatment.

Al-Anon is a parallel organization that provides support for the partners of excessive drinkers. Alateen has a similar role for their teenage children.

Non-statutory agencies are voluntary bodies that provide a range of services, including advice for problem drinkers and their families, counselling, and help with occupational and social activities for those who have recovered.

Hostels are intended mainly for homeless problem drinkers. They provide rehabilitation and counselling. Usually abstinence is a condition of residence.

Results of treatment

In a famous controlled trial involving 100 male alcoholics, Edwards (1977) compared simple advice with intensive treatment that included introductions to Alcoholics Anonymous, medication, repeated interviews, counselling for their wives, and, where appropriate, inpatient treatment as well. The advice group received a 3-hour assessment together with a single session of counselling with the partner present. The two groups were well matched. After 12 months there was no significant difference between them with regard to drinking behaviour, subjective ratings, or social adjustment.

Similar findings with regard to drinking behaviour were reported by Chick *et al.* (1988), who found that at a 2-year follow-up there was no difference in stable abstinence rates between alcohol-dependent patients who received a minimal treatment intervention, consisting mainly of advice, and those who were offered a broad range of therapies, including inpatient care and group therapy. However, the group that was offered the broad range of therapies suffered *less alcohol-related harm*, particularly in relation to family life.

Some have argued that abstinence rates by themselves do not provide a useful measure of treatment outcome. For example, although the patient may still be drinking, the amount consumed may decrease. This can be associated with a reduction in aspects of alcohol-related harm, as shown by the study by Chick *et al.* (1988). From this viewpoint, harm reduction, even where the individual continues to drink, is a worthwhile achievement. The principles of the harm reduction approach have been applied to the misuse of other substances (see below).

The effectiveness of structured psychological treatments was studied by Project MATCH, a large randomized controlled trial of three psychological treatments for patients with alcohol problems (Project MATCH Research Group, 1997). The three treatments studied were a cognitive behavioural intervention, a brief motivational enhancement therapy, and a treatment that aimed to help patients to make use of the 'twelve-step' philosophy of Alcoholics Anonymous. The main aim of the study was to attempt to find patient characteristics that predicted response to particular treatments. There were no important differences between the treatments, and few strong correlations were found between effectiveness and patient characteristics. However, in general the outcome was favourable, and the authors concluded that structured psychological treatments of various kinds were helpful in the management of alcohol misuse. In fact, the *brief motivational enhancement therapy* was generally as effective as the two more intensive psychological treatments.

Consistent with this, the UK Alcohol Treatment Trial (UKATT), which was conducted at several UK centres, found that *motivational enhancement therapy* was just as effective as *social network therapy* in decreasing alcohol consumption and alcohol dependence. However, at a 1-year follow-up the effects of treatment were fairly modest. For example, relative to baseline levels, average alcohol consumption on a drinking day fell from 27 units to 19 units, and the number of days on which patients abstained from alcohol rose from 30% to 45% (UK Alcohol Treatment Trial Research Team, 2005).

The guidelines from the National Institute for Health and Clinical Excellence (2011a) recommend that patients with alcohol dependence, once withdrawn from alcohol, should be offered a psychological intervention that matches their needs and social situation (Box 20.11), together with either naltrexone or acamprosate. If neither of these are suitable and the patient is committed to the goal of abstinence, disulfiram can be offered if supervision is available.

There are likely to be factors within the patient that will predict a good response to a number of different kinds of treatment. There is some disagreement as to what these factors are, but the following generally predict a better prognosis regardless of which treatment is used:

- Good insight into the nature of the problems.
- Social stability in the form of a fixed abode, family support, and ability to keep a job.
- Ability to control impulsiveness, to defer gratification, and to form satisfactory emotional relationships.

For reviews of the effectiveness of a broad range of treatment approaches for alcohol use disorders, see Luty (2015a, 2015b) and the National Institute for Health and Clinical Excellence (2011a).

Prevention of alcohol misuse and dependence

In seeking to prevent excessive drinking and alcohol-related disorders, two approaches are possible. The first is to improve the help and guidance available to the individual, as already described. The second is to introduce social changes that are likely to affect drinking patterns in the population as a whole (see Box 20.13). It is this second group that we are concerned with here. Consumption within a population might be reduced by four methods:

1. *The pricing of alcoholic beverages.* Putting up the price of alcohol would probably reduce consumption within the population. Based on a systematic review, Wagenaar *et al.* (2010) predicted that doubling alcohol taxes in the USA would reduce direct alcohol-related mortality by 35%, traffic fatalities by 11%, and violent crime by 2%.

2. *Controls on advertising.* Controlling or abolishing the advertising of alcoholic drinks might be another preventive measure. It is unclear how far advertising

> **Box 20.13 Some recommendations by the Academy of Medical Sciences (2004) for decreasing alcohol-related harm in the UK**
>
> - Increase taxes on alcohol to restore its affordability relative to income to that obtaining in the early 1970s
> - Reduce the duty-free allowance of alcohol for travellers
> - Review advertising and promotion of alcoholic drinks, particularly to young people
> - Improve medical research on the damaging effects of alcohol
>
> - Inform the public and encourage debate about the extent of alcohol-related harm
> - Reduce the statutory blood alcohol concentration for drivers from 80 mg/100 ml to 50 mg/100 ml. Impose a zero statutory blood alcohol level for young drivers up to the age of 21 years.

encourages the use of particular brands of alcohol rather than overall consumption. However, in the UK, annual expenditure on alcohol advertising and promotion is over £800 million. There is an accepted link between alcohol advertising and consumption, particularly in young people (Stockings *et al.*, 2016). Alcohol marketing now makes extensive use of digital media, which will enhance the impact of advertising in young people.

3. *Controls on sale.* Another preventive measure might be to control sales of alcohol by limiting hours or banning sales in supermarkets. Although relaxation of restrictions has been shown to lead to increased sales of alcohol in some countries, it does not follow that increased restrictions would reduce established rates of drinking. However, there is evidence that a higher minimum age for legal drinking is associated with a decrease in alcohol consumption and fatal car accidents in young drivers (McCartt *et al.*, 2010). There is concern about the heavy drinking associated with nightlife culture in many UK cities.

4. *Health education.* It is not known whether education about alcohol misuse is effective. Little is known about how attitudes are formed or changed. Although education about alcohol would seem to be desirable, it cannot be assumed that classroom lectures or mass media propaganda alter attitudes. In general, there is little convincing evidence that such approaches are effective. Interventions focusing on the family, designed to improve parenting skills and child–parent relationships, may be more beneficial; for example, by delaying the age at which children start drinking (Stockings *et al.*, 2016).

Other substance use disorders

Under this heading we shall consider the use and misuse of substances other than alcohol. Although these substances include agents such as volatile substances (inhalants), the general term *drug* will be employed because it is in common use. In this discussion the term *misuse* will be applied to what is classified as 'harmful use' in ICD-10 and 'use disorder' in DSM-5 (see Table 20.1 and Box 20.1).

Epidemiology

Illicit drug use

The 2009 National Survey on Drug Use and Health in the USA found that 8.7% of the population aged 12 years or over had used an illicit substance in the past month (Substance Abuse and Mental Health Services Administration, 2010). Use was highest in unemployed people in the 16–25-year age range. The most commonly used illicit drug was *cannabis*, with a slight majority of illicit drug takers (58%) using cannabis only. The Psychiatric Morbidity Survey reported that, in England, 9.2% of adults had taken an illicit drug in the past year, most commonly cannabis (7.5%) (McManus *et al.*, 2009). Use was higher in men (12.0%) than in women (6.7%). Among males, drug use was highest in black men (21.8%) and lowest in South Asian men (3.5%). In women the highest rate of drug use was in white women (6.8%), with South Asian women reporting the lowest rate (0.8%). Highest rates of drug use in the last year were seen in men aged 25–34 years (28.9%) and women aged 16–24 years (21.9%). About 4% of the UK population had used at least one *Class A drug* (opiate, cocaine, lysergic acid diethylamide [LSD], or injected stimulant) in the previous year (see Box 20.14).

The European School Survey Project on Alcohol and Other Drugs (2011) surveyed drug use in 15- to 16-year-olds in 37 European countries. On average, 21% of boys and 15% of girls had tried illicit drugs at least once in their lifetime. Again, cannabis was by far the most commonly used drug. The country with the most frequent cannabis use was the Czech Republic (42%), while those with the lowest use were Albania and Bosnia (4%). The UK had the fifth highest rate (25%). However, there was a 16% decrease in illicit drug use in teenagers in the UK between 1995 and 2011.

Drug misuse and dependence

Little is known for certain about the *prevalence* of different types of drug misuse and drug dependence. In the UK, information comes from two main sources—*criminal statistics* (mainly based on offences involving the use and misuse of illicit drugs) and *community surveys*.

The Psychiatric Morbidity Survey reported that in England the prevalence of drug dependence during the previous 12 months was 4.1% (5.4% of men and 2.3% of women). Most of the dependence was on cannabis

(3.4%). The highest frequency was in the 16–24-year age group (McManus *et al.*, 2009). Rates of drug dependence are much higher among the homeless population and those in prison. For example, the British Psychiatric Morbidity Survey found that 24% of people who were sleeping rough met the criteria for drug dependence. Among remand prisoners, 51% of men and 54% of women reported dependence on drugs before coming into prison, whereas, among sentenced prisoners, 43% of men and 41% of women reported drug dependence (Gill *et al.*, 1996; Singleton *et al.*, 2003).

The National Comorbidity Survey Replication in the USA (Kessler *et al.*, 2005b) found rather lower 12-month rates of drug dependence (0.4%), and the rate of drug abuse was 0.8%. It is difficult to know whether the differences between the UK and the USA in reported rates of drug dependence are real variations in incidence or might instead reflect differences in how the presence of drug dependence is assessed.

Rates of drug misuse and dependence are higher in disadvantaged areas of large cities. Adolescents are at risk, particularly around school-leaving age. A high proportion of attenders at drug-dependence clinics in large cities are unemployed, with few stable relationships, and leading disorganized lives. However, many young drug users remain in employment and apparently regard their drug taking as part of normal recreational activity for their particular peer group.

Causes of drug misuse

There is no single cause of drug misuse. It is generally argued that four factors are important:

- availability of drugs
- a vulnerable personality
- an adverse social environment
- pharmacological factors.

The widespread availability of illicit drugs means that occasional use in a young person can no longer be regarded as abnormal behaviour. However, about 10% of those who experiment with drugs will go on to develop problems with them (Robson, 2009). Once drug taking has started, personal, social, and pharmacological factors play a role in determining misuse and dependence. Studies of the aetiology of misuse of substances other than alcohol are still at an early stage. For example, it is unclear whether similar risk factors predict misuse of a range of substances, including alcohol, or whether there is some specificity in the mechanisms, which leads certain individuals to misuse particular substances.

Availability of drugs

Drugs involved in misuse can be obtained in three main ways:

1. *Legally without prescription*—nicotine and alcohol are obvious contemporary examples, and in the nineteenth century much dependence on opioids resulted from taking freely available remedies containing morphia.

2. *By prescription from doctors*—in the first part of the twentieth century much of the known dependence on opioids and barbiturates in western countries was due to drugs obtained from this source; latterly, *benzodiazepine dependence* was often acquired in this way. Currently, there is concern about growing misuse of drugs prescribed to relieve chronic pain, such as *opiates and gabapentin*.

3. *From illicit sources* ('street drugs').

Personal factors

Of those who experiment with drugs, the users who go on to develop problems appear to have some degree of personal vulnerability before they begin taking drugs. They may live in disrupted families and have started taking drugs at a relatively young age. Associated behaviours include a poor school record, truancy, or delinquency. Traits such as sensation seeking and impulsivity are also common. Many of those who misuse drugs report depression and anxiety, but it is seldom clear whether these are the causes or the consequences of drug misuse and dependence. Some give a history of mental illness or personality disorder in the family. Genetic factors are strongly implicated in a variety of drug use *disorders*, but less so in drug use itself. This suggests that drug use in general is largely dependent on factors such as availability and social environment, but that genes contribute to the propensity to develop harmful use and dependence (Bienvenu *et al*., 2011).

Social environment

The risk of drug misuse is greater in societies that condone drug use of one kind or another. Within the immediate group, there may be social pressures for a young person to take drugs to achieve status. Thus drug use by individuals is influenced by substance use by their peers or parents. There are also links between drug misuse and indices of social deprivation, such as unemployment and homelessness (Gill *et al*., 1996).

Pharmacological factors

Use, misuse, and dependence

Many individuals use drugs without misusing them, and not all drug misusers become drug-dependent. Therefore it is useful to study the biological mechanisms underlying drug use, misuse, and dependence separately. Drugs are used and misused because they have the ability to serve as *positive reinforcers*—that is, they increase the frequency of behaviours that lead to their use. Drugs act as positive reinforcers because they cause positive subjective experiences such as euphoria or a reduction in anxiety.

Neurobiological mechanisms

An important neurobiological substrate that mediates reinforcing effects is the midbrain dopamine system, the cell bodies of which originate in the ventral tegmental area and innervate the forebrain, particularly the ventral striatum. It has been proposed that these dopamine pathways form part of a physiological reward system and it is of interest therefore that at least some drugs of abuse, particularly stimulants and alcohol, increase dopamine release in the ventral striatum. This suggests that activation of midbrain dopamine pathways may be a important property of some drugs that have a propensity to be used and misused. Whether such a mechanism can account for reinforcing effects of other misused drugs, such as cannabis, is less clear (see Nutt *et al*., 2015).

Although this hypothesis may explain in part the social use of particular drugs, it does not account for the misuse of drugs in some circumstances. Presumably this is a consequence of interactions between the pharmacological properties of the drug, the biological disposition and personality of the user, and the social environment. Current neurobiological formulations of drug dependence suggest that the switch from controlled drug taking to compulsive use (misuse and dependence) is associated with a lessening of *prefrontal 'reflective' processes* and a corresponding increase in *striatal activity* which underpins more habitual behaviours. These changes might explain the ability of repeated drug administration in some people to 'hijack' executive behaviour almost exclusively to serve the needs of the drug habit, and the poor judgement and decision-making shown by people with substance dependence. Learning and conditioning factors are likely to be important in this context. It has been suggested that lower levels of dopamine receptor availability in the midbrain, which is itself associated with the trait of novelty-seeking, would make an individual more likely to attribute salience to drug-related cues and thereby more likely to engage in drug misuse.

Neurobiology of tolerance and dependence

The phenomena of tolerance and withdrawal are believed to be a result of *neuroadaptive changes* in the brain. These are part of a homeostatic process that counteracts the acute pharmacological effects that occur when a drug is administered. For example, many drugs that are misused for their anxiolytic and hypnotic properties (e.g. barbiturates, benzodiazepines, and alcohol) have, among their acute pharmacological effects, the ability to enhance brain GABA function. During continued treatment with these agents, adaptive changes occur in GABA- and benzodiazepine-receptor sensitivity that tend to offset the effect of the drugs to facilitate GABA neurotransmission. Such an effect could account for the phenomenon of tolerance, with the result that an individual needs to take more of the drug to produce the same pharmacological effect.

If the drug is abruptly discontinued, persistence of the adaptive changes in receptor function could lead to a sudden decline in GABA activity. In fact, many of the clinical features of withdrawal from anxiolytic drugs, such as anxiety, insomnia, and seizures, can be explained on the basis of diminished brain GABA function. Such an effect can also explain the well-known phenomenon of cross-tolerance between anxiolytics and hypnotics and alcohol, which makes it possible, for example, to treat alcohol withdrawal with a benzodiazepine.

Similar kinds of adaptive changes have been proposed to account for the tolerance and withdrawal phenomena that are seen with other drugs of misuse. For example, while acute administration of opioids decreases the firing of noradrenaline cell bodies in the brainstem, tolerance of this effect occurs during repeated treatment, probably because of adaptive changes in the sensitivity of opioid receptors. If opioids are now abruptly withdrawn, there is a sudden increase in the firing of noradrenaline neurons and in the release of noradrenaline in terminal regions. Increased noradrenergic activity may account for several of the clinical features of acute opioid withdrawal, including sweating, tachycardia, hypertension, and anxiety. These studies have led to the use of the noradrenaline autoreceptor agonists, clonidine and lofexidine, in the management of opioid withdrawal (Lingford-Hughes *et al.*, 2010).

Although the positive reinforcing actions of drugs are considered to be the major factor in promoting drug use, withdrawal effects are likely to play an important part once drug taking is established, because they are invariably unpleasant, and individuals are likely to try to prevent them by taking more of the drug. This 'negative reinforcement' may complete the transition from *impulsive* to *compulsive* drug use.

It is also worth noting that for many months following the cessation of a clear-cut withdrawal syndrome, dependent individuals may experience a sudden intense desire to consume the drug. Often particular psychological and social stimuli that were previously associated with drug use may trigger intense craving associated with symptoms resembling a withdrawal state. It has been proposed that a single exposure to the drug during this period may rapidly lead to a full relapse to drug dependence—the so-called *reinstatement effect*. An analogous effect has been shown in previously drug-dependent animals, where a single priming dose of the drug concerned can lead to a full recovery of drug-seeking behaviours that had previously been extinguished.

For a review of the brain mechanisms involved in drug misuse and their implications for treatment, see Lingford-Hughes *et al.* (2010).

Adverse effects of drug misuse

Drug misuse has many undesirable effects, both for the individual and for society.

Physical health

Drug misuse can lead people to neglect their health, in addition to the direct physical consequences of the substance itself. These are discussed in more detail under the heading of individual drugs.

Intravenous drug use poses particular health risks. This practice is very common with opioid use, but barbiturates, benzodiazepines, amphetamines, and other drugs

---

Box 20.15 Some consequences of intravenous drug misuse

Local

Vein thrombosis
Infection of injection site
Damage to arteries

Systemic

Bacterial endocarditis
Hepatitis B and C
HIV infection
Accidental overdose

may be taken in this way. Intravenous drug use has important consequences, which include both local and general effects (see Box 20.15).

The most serious complications of intravenous drug use include *HIV infection* and *hepatitis*. Rates of HIV infection among drug users in the UK are lower than those found in some other European countries, and some attribute this to the vigorous harm reduction policies in the UK (methadone prescribing, needle exchanges, and education for drug users). However, hepatitis C is a major concern, as preliminary studies suggest that this infection has a prevalence of 50–80% among UK users who inject drugs. Rates of hepatitis B are lower but still significant (30–50%). Accidental drug overdose can occur by any route, but there is a far higher risk of death from heroin overdose when the intravenous route is used.

Substance dependence in women

Substance misuse treatment services, including those for alcohol-related disorders, may not be designed to meet the special needs of women, because existing treatment models have been developed for men. Clinicians need to take into account factors such as the following:

● social and parenting responsibilities
● possible history of victimization and sexual abuse
● social barriers to obtaining medical care
● the availability of female therapists.

Drug misuse in pregnancy and the puerperium

It is not uncommon for drug misusers to have limited contact with health care services until late into pregnancy; this can occur because of limited ability to access services, fear of the possible consequences, and the difficulties of addressing dependence issues. Drug use in pregnancy increases the health risks to both mother and fetus. When drugs are taken in early pregnancy, there is a risk of increased rates of fetal abnormality. Opioids may directly decrease fetal growth. When drugs are taken in late pregnancy, the fetus may become dependent on them. The risk of fetal dependence is high with heroin and related drugs, and after delivery the neonate may develop serious withdrawal effects that require skilled care.

If the mother continues to take drugs after delivery, the safeguarding needs of the infant will need to be considered, usually with close monitoring by a care team to support the family and ensure the needs of the infant are being met. Intravenous drug use may lead to infection of the mother with HIV or other conditions that can affect the fetus. Engagement in treatment and good antenatal care reduce the risks to both mother and baby.

For a review of problem drug use in women, see Greenfield *et al.* (2010).

Psychiatric comorbidity

There is a strong association between substance misuse and psychiatric comorbidity (often described as *dual diagnosis*). For example, people with substance misuse often have additional diagnoses of personality disorder, depression, and anxiety. Sometimes symptoms of mood disturbance may be a direct result of drug use. For example, people who use stimulants can experience depression, particularly during periods of acute withdrawal.

In other cases the relationship is more complex, with premorbid psychiatric disorder interacting with substance misuse. Thus patients with primary psychiatric disorders such as schizophrenia, bipolar disorder, and sociopathic personality disorder frequently misuse alcohol and illicit drugs. This practice increases the morbidity of the underlying disorder and heightens the risk of violence and self-harm. There is debate about the best ways of delivering treatment services to such patients, but as yet there is little firm evidence to provide guidance. The general consensus is that an integrated service, where the same clinical team deals with both psychiatric and substance misuse disorders, is likely to be the best approach. However, implementing such a service model poses challenges.

Social consequences of drug misuse

There are three reasons why drug misuse can lead to undesirable social effects.

1. Chronic intoxication may affect behaviour adversely, leading to unemployment, motoring offences, accidents, and family problems, including neglect of children.

2. Illicit drugs are generally expensive, so the user may steal or sell sexual favours to obtain money.

3. Drug misusers often keep company with one another, and those with previously stable social behaviour may be under pressure to conform to a group ethos of antisocial or criminal activity.

The economic costs of problem drug use in the UK have been estimated to be around £15 billion annually (British Medical Association, 2013) (see Box 20.16).

Diagnosis of drug misuse

It is important to diagnose drug misuse early, at a stage when dependence may be less established and behaviour patterns less fixed, and the complications of intravenous

Box 20.16 Social costs of drug misuse in the UK

Users: premature death, physical and mental illness, low educational achievement, unemployment

Families: adverse effect on children, poverty, and deprivation

Others: victims of dangerous driving, victims of crime, victims of assault

Community: criminal activity related to drug dealing, environmental impoverishment, health and crime risks to community

Industry: sickness absence, theft in the workplace, productivity losses, costs of security

Public sector: health care expenditure, criminal justice expenditure, social services care and benefits

use may not have developed. Before describing the clinical presentations of the different types of drugs, some general principles will be given. The clinician who is not used to treating people who misuse drugs should remember that they are in the unusual position of trying to help a patient who may be attempting to deceive them. Patients who are misusing heroin may overstate the daily dose to obtain extra supplies for their own use or for sale to others. Furthermore, many patients take more than one drug but may not say so. It is important to try to corroborate patients' accounts of the amounts that they are taking by asking detailed questions about the duration of drug taking, and the cost and source of drugs, by checking the story for internal consistency, and by external verification whenever possible.

Physical signs

Certain physical signs lead to the suspicion that drugs are being injected. These include needle tracks and thrombosis of veins, especially in the antecubital fossa, wearing garments with long sleeves in hot weather, and scars. Intravenous drug use should be considered in any patient who presents with subcutaneous abscesses or hepatitis.

Behavioural signs

Behavioural changes may also suggest drug misuse. These include absence from school or work, and occupational decline. Dependent people may also neglect their appearance, isolate themselves from former friends, and adopt new friends in a drug culture. Minor criminal offences, such as petty theft and prostitution, may also be indicators.

Medical presentation

Dependent people may come to medical attention in several ways. Some declare that they are dependent on drugs. Others conceal their dependency, and ask for controlled drugs for the relief of pain such as renal colic or dysmenorrhoea. It is important to be particularly wary of such requests from temporary patients. Others present with drug-related complications, such as cellulitis, pneumonia, hepatitis, or accidents, or for the treatment of acute drug effects, overdose, withdrawal symptoms, or adverse reactions to hallucinogenic drugs. A few are detected during an admission to hospital for an unrelated illness.

Taking a drug history

When taking a drug history (see Box 20.17) from a patient who is misusing drugs, the doctor should ask the patient to describe their drug use the previous day and also to describe a *typical drug-using day* (which drug, how often, and which route of use). A typical week can be described if drugs are not used every day. The doctor should ask about craving, withdrawal symptoms, and other features of the dependence syndrome, such as increased tolerance of the drug and the priority of drug-seeking over other duties and pleasures. The patient should be asked specifically about *risky behaviour*, such as dangerous injecting (into the groin or neck or infected injection sites), and sharing injection equipment.

A *chronological history* of the development of use of *each drug taken* can then be obtained. Useful milestones can include the first use of the drug, when the patient began to use the drug daily, when withdrawal

Box 20.17 Drug-using history

- Typical drug-using day or week
- Types and quantities of drugs taken (including alcohol and nicotine)
- Symptoms experienced when drugs are unavailable
- Tolerance and primacy of drug habit
- Risky behaviour
- Developmental history of drug misuse
- Abstinence and relapse triggers
- Medical and social complications
- Psychiatric and forensic history

symptoms were first experienced, and when the patient first injected drugs. A history of sharing injection equipment will be important when estimating the risk of HIV or hepatitis.

If patients have had periods of abstinence, it is useful to ask which influences helped them to achieve this and what factors led to relapse. A history of complications should include adverse effects of the drug itself, as well as complications of the route of administration. Any history of accidental overdose should also be elicited. The patient should be asked about family, occupational, and legal problems. Any past history of treatment should be elicited. There are several possible goals in the treatment of drug misusers. Abstinence is one, but safer drug use (*harm reduction*) may be a more realistic aim for many. It is therefore important to obtain patients' views about their drug use and the changes that they would like to make.

Laboratory diagnosis

Whenever possible, the diagnosis of drug misuse should be confirmed by laboratory tests. Urine testing is most commonly used, as it is easier and less invasive than blood testing. Immunoassay kits are available that are able to measure a wide range of misused agents in a single urine sample with a reasonably long timeframe of detection (Table 20.5). However, saliva has the advantage that samples can readily be obtained under supervision and are therefore less easily tampered with. It should be remembered that these 'point of care' tests are for purposes of screening and, if inconsistent with the clinical history, a confirmatory laboratory test using

Table 20.5 Detection of illicit substances in urine

Drug	Time limit for detection
Amphetamines and analogues	2 days
Buprenorphine and metabolites	8 days
Methadone (maintenance dosing)	7–9 days
Morphine	2 days
Codeine, dihydrocodeine	2 days
Cannabinoids (single use)	3–4 days
Cannabis (daily use)	20 days

Reproduced from Advances in Psychiatric Treatment, 16(5), Abraham A, Luty J, Testing for illicit drug use in mental health services, pp 369–379, Copyright (2010), with permission from The Royal College of Psychiatrists.

a chromatographic approach should be requested. One issue is that 'false-positive' urine tests for illicit substances can be produced by prescribed psychotropic medication through cross-reactions. For a review see, Abraham and Luty (2010).

Prevention, treatment, and rehabilitation: general principles

Prevention

Because treatment is difficult, considerable effort should be given to prevention. For many drugs, important preventive measures such as restricting availability and lessening social deprivation depend on government, not medical, policy. However, the reduction of overprescribing by doctors is important, especially with regard to *benzodiazepines* and other *anxiolytic drugs* and *opiates*.

Although education programmes by themselves do not seem to be effective in prevention, it is important that information about the dangers of drug misuse should be available to young people in the school curriculum and through the media. Another aspect of prevention is the identification and treatment of family problems that may contribute to drug taking. Family therapy and parental skills training are able to decrease the uptake of illicit drugs in young people (Stockings *et al.*, 2016).

Some young people are particularly vulnerable to drug misuse. This includes those who have been in care, those who are homeless, and those who are not in school due to either truancy or exclusion. Identification of young people at risk of drug misuse should be followed by specific psychosocial interventions that are designed to divert them away from drug use (National Institute for Health and Clinical Excellence, 2007).

Treatment

Motivation and change

When drug misuse has already begun, treatment is more effective if it is given before dependence is established. At this stage, as at later stages, the essential step is to motivate the patient to control their drug taking. This requires a combination of advice about the likely effects of continuing misuse, and help with any concurrent psychological or social problems. The techniques of motivational interviewing (Treasure, 2004) (see Box 20.8) may be useful here. The *stages of change model* described by Prochaska and DiClemente (1986) can help the clinician to encourage motivation effectively (see Box 20.18).

Box 20.18 Stages of change model

Pre-contemplation

Misuser does not believe that there is a problem, although others recognize it

Contemplation

Individual weighs up the pros and cons and considers that change might be necessary

Decision

The point is reached where a decision is made to act (or not to act) on the issue of substance misuse

Action

Individual chooses a strategy for change and pursues it

Maintenance

Gains are maintained and consolidated. Failure may lead to relapse

Relapse

Return to previous pattern of behaviour

However, relapse may be a positive learning experience, with lessons for the future

Aims of treatment

The ultimate aim of treatment of the drug-dependent patient is a good personal and social adjustment in the absence of drug use. However, drug withdrawal (or detoxification) by itself has no effect on long-term outcome, so this process should be part of a wider treatment programme. If withdrawal cannot be achieved, continued prescribing of certain drugs (e.g. opioids) may be considered as part of a *harm reduction programme*. In addition, psychological treatment and social support are required. The general principles of treatment will be outlined below, and later sections of the chapter will consider treatment specific to individual drugs.

Treatment setting

In the UK, drug misusers are treated in a number of different settings, and there is increasing variation in the way that care is delivered locally. A model of *shared care* in which drug misusers are managed jointly by the GP and specialist services is being replaced by a system with a wider range of care providers. For example, treatment can be given by the GP supported by a nurse or drugs worker from the voluntary sector. In secondary care and in specialized drug treatment services, patients continue to be managed by a multidisciplinary team using the key worker system. Inpatient care is provided in psychiatric hospitals, in psychiatric units in general hospitals, or in a small number of specialist inpatient units. Individual counselling, group therapy, and therapeutic communities are provided by a variety of charitable organizations. All doctors in the UK who are treating drug misusers for their drug problems should provide information on the standard form to their local Regional Drug Misuse Database. Contact numbers for this can be found in the *British National Formulary*.

Physical complications

The complications of self-injection may require treatment in a general hospital. They include accidental overdose, skin infections, abscesses, septicaemia, hepatitis, and HIV infection. Drug misusers will also need help with general health problems such as nutrition and dental care. Immunization against hepatitis B may be advisable.

Principles of withdrawal

The withdrawal of misused drugs is sometimes called *detoxification*. For many drugs, particularly opioids, withdrawal may sometimes be most effectively undertaken in hospital (see below). Withdrawal from stimulant drugs and benzodiazepines can often be an outpatient procedure, provided that the doses are not very large and that barbiturates are not taken as well. Nevertheless, the risk of depression and suicide should be borne in mind.

Drug maintenance

Some clinicians undertake to prescribe certain drugs to dependent people who are not willing to give them up. The usual procedure is to prescribe a drug which has a slower action (and is therefore less addictive) than the 'street' drug. For example, methadone is prescribed in place of heroin. When this procedure is combined with help with social problems and a continuing effort to encourage the person to accept withdrawal, it is called *maintenance therapy*.

The rationale of this approach is twofold.

1. Prolonged prescribing will remove the need for the patient to obtain 'street' drugs, and will thereby reduce the associated physical and social damage.

2. Social and psychological help, aided by the natural process of maturing, will give the patient the confidence and skills to be able to give up drugs eventually.

Maintenance drug treatment is used in particular for patients with opioid dependence. If maintenance drug therapy is used, it should be remembered that some drug-dependent people convert tablets or capsules into material for injection, which is a particularly dangerous practice. Furthermore, some attend a succession of GPs in search of supplementary supplies of drugs. They may withhold information about attendance at clinics or pose as temporary residents.

Some patients who receive maintenance drugs achieve a degree of social stability, but others continue heavy drug misuse and deteriorate both medically and socially. Patients who are on maintenance methadone are more likely to be retained in treatment than those in drug-free programmes. This may be important because the length of time spent in treatment, regardless of type, is the best predictor of favourable outcome. (The use of methadone maintenance treatment in the management of opioid dependence is considered in more detail below.)

Harm reduction

The increase in HIV and hepatitis C infection has emphasized the importance of *harm reduction programmes*, of which prescribing maintenance may be one component. The purpose of such programmes is to increase the number of substance misusers who enter and comply with treatment. The aim is to identify intermediate treatment goals which, although not involving total abstinence, nevertheless reduce the risk of drug misuse to the individual and society. For example, even if a patient continues to misuse drugs, the risk of hepatitis and HIV infection can be reduced by providing appropriate education and practical help. Such interventions may result in the drug misuser using safer routes of drug administration or sterile injection equipment. Counselling and screening for hepatitis and HIV may also be worthwhile, and hepatitis B vaccination should be offered to non-immune patients.

Psychosocial treatments

Treatment for drug misuse should always include psychosocial approaches. The usual way to deliver this is through a *key worker* who institutes measures such as *counselling, education*, and *motivational interviewing*. Practical help with benefits and information about services can also be provided. All patients should be aware of self-help and mutual aid groups such as Narcotics Anonymous, which can be of great benefit to many individuals. Some patients are helped by treatment in a therapeutic community in which there can be frank discussion of the effects of drug taking on the person's character and relationships within the supportive setting of the group (for an outline of community therapy, see Chapter 24).

More formal psychological treatments, as described for the management of alcohol misuse (see Box 20.11), can also be helpful, and have been reviewed by the National Institute for Health and Clinical Excellence (2007). The aim of such treatment is to increase recreational and personal skills so that the patient becomes less reliant on drugs and the drug culture as a source of satisfaction. Involvement of the patient's partner and family in structured couple and family therapy is often helpful.

As with alcohol dependence, cognitive behavioural techniques can be used to identify, in advance, situations that act as triggers for drug use. In this way alternative methods of coping can be planned (*relapse prevention*). It has already been mentioned that when a drug misuser is confronted with a situation that contains personal cues for drug use, they can experience acute discomfort associated with a strong desire to use the drug. The technique of cue exposure aims, through repeated exposure, to desensitize the drug misuser to these effects and thus improve their ability to remain abstinent. Although *contingency management* is not currently widely used in the UK, and is politically sensitive, there is good evidence for its effectiveness in reducing drug misuse, and it appears more effective than other psychosocial approaches such as cognitive behaviour therapy. Contingency management provides a variety of incentives in the form of vouchers, privileges, or modest financial rewards to encourage individuals to modify their drug misuse and increase health-promoting behaviours (National Institute for Health and Clinical Excellence, 2007; Luty, 2015a).

Rehabilitation

Many drug takers have difficulty in establishing themselves in normal society. The aim of rehabilitation is to enable the drug-dependent person to leave the drug sub-culture and to develop new social contacts. Unless this can be achieved, any treatment is likely to fail.

Rehabilitation may be undertaken after treatment in a therapeutic community. Patients first engage in work and social activities in sheltered surroundings, and then take greater responsibility for themselves in conditions that are increasingly similar to those of everyday life. Hostel accommodation is a useful stage in this gradual process. Continuing social support is usually required when the person makes the transition to normal work and living.

Dual-diagnosis patients

As noted above, the management of patients with both substance misuse and serious psychiatric illness, such as schizophrenia or mood disorders, poses several additional challenges. Such comorbidity is associated with an increased risk of violence and suicide, and poorer clinical and social outcomes (National Institute for Health and Clinical Excellence, 2011b). Patients with dual diagnoses are particularly difficult to retain in treatment, and frequently present in crisis with many unmet social needs. Drake *et al.* (2007) identified the following components of a successful integrated treatment service for patients with substance misuse and serious psychiatric illness:

- appropriate staff training
- use of a recovery-based approach with expectation of recovery in the longer term
- multidisciplinary case management with assertive outreach to engage and retain patients in treatment
- some form of peer-orientated group intervention led by a professional facilitator
- emphasis on motivational interviewing, harm reduction, and skills training
- long-term community support, including daycare and residential care
- pharmacotherapy (e.g. naltrexone and disulfiram), with particular consideration of clozapine for those with schizophrenia and substance misuse.

It is worth emphasizing that in many settings the co-occurrence of serious mental illness and drug and alcohol misuse is the norm rather than the exception. Recent guidance from the National Institute for Health and Clinical Excellence highlights the importance of recognizing patients with *comorbid psychosis and substance misuse*, and the development of suitably integrated services to tackle both problems (National Institute for Health and Clinical Excellence, 2011b).

Misuse of specific types of drug

Opioids

This group of drugs includes morphine, heroin, codeine, and synthetic analgesics such as pethidine and methadone. The pharmacological effects of opioids are mediated primarily through interaction with specific opioid receptors, with morphine and heroin being quite selective for the μ-opioid-receptor type. The main medical use of opioids is for their powerful analgesic actions; they are misused for their euphoriant and anxiolytic effects.

In the past morphine was misused widely in western countries, but it was largely replaced as a drug of misuse by *heroin*, which has a particularly powerful euphoriant effect, especially when taken intravenously. However. the main source of illicit opioid use currently comes from *medically prescribed analgesics;* in fact, prescription opioids such as tramadol, oxycodone, and dihydrocodeine are the second most commonly misused illicit substances after cannabis. In the USA there are now more deaths from prescription opioids than from heroin (Luty, 2014).

Epidemiology

The Psychiatric Morbidity Survey reported that in households in England the prevalence of illicit opiate use over the past year was about 0.3%, and the rate of dependence was 0.1%. The lifetime rate of illicit opiate use was almost 2% (McManus *et al.*, 2009). Higher rates would be expected in the homeless and in prisons.

Use and misuse

The epidemiological data indicate that many people use heroin without becoming dependent on it. However, there is no doubt that repeated heroin use can lead to the rapid development of dependence and marked physiological tolerance. As well as the intravenous route, opioid users may employ other methods of administration—for example, subcutaneous administration ('skin-popping') or sniffing ('snorting'). Heroin may also be heated on a metal foil and inhaled ('chasing the dragon'). Heroin users may change their customary method of drug administration from time to time. From the perspective of harm reduction, methods that avoid intravenous administration are preferable.

Clinical effects

As well as *euphoria* and *analgesia*, opioids cause *respiratory depression, constipation, reduced appetite,* and *low libido.* Tolerance develops rapidly, leading to the need for an increasing dosage. Tolerance does not develop equally to all of the effects, and constipation often continues when the other effects have diminished. When the drug is stopped, tolerance diminishes rapidly, so a dose taken after a period of abstinence has greater effects than it would have had previously. This loss of tolerance can result in dangerous—sometimes fatal—respiratory depression when a previously tolerated dose is resumed after a drug-free interval (e.g. after a stay in hospital or prison).

Withdrawal from opioids

Withdrawal symptoms from opioids may include the following:

- intense craving for the drug
- restlessness and insomnia
- pain in muscles and joints

- running nose and eyes
- abdominal cramps, vomiting, and diarrhoea
- piloerection, sweating, dilated pupils, and raised pulse rate
- disturbance of temperature control.

These features usually begin about 6 hours after the last dose, reach a peak after 36–48 hours, and then wane. Withdrawal symptoms rarely threaten the life of someone in reasonable health, although they cause great distress and so drive the person to seek further supplies of the drug.

Methadone

Methadone is approximately as potent, weight for weight, as morphine. It causes cough suppression, constipation, and depression of the central nervous system and of respiration. Pupillary constriction is less marked. The withdrawal syndrome is similar to that of heroin and morphine, and is at least as severe. Because methadone has a long half-life (1–2 days), symptoms of withdrawal may begin only after 36 hours and reach a peak after 3–5 days. For this reason, methadone is often used to replace heroin in patients who are dependent on the latter drug.

The natural course of opioid dependence

Longer-term follow-up studies of opioid misusers have revealed that in most cases the disorder appears to run a chronic relapsing and remitting course, with a significant mortality (10–20%) over 10 years. Nevertheless, up to 50% of opioid users have been found to be abstinent at 10-year follow-up, which suggests a trend towards natural remission in survivors (Robson, 2009).

Deaths are not infrequently due to accidental overdosage, often related to loss of tolerance after a period of enforced abstinence (see above). Suicide is also a common cause of death. Deaths from HIV infection and hepatitis have become more frequent in recent years. Factors associated with a good outcome include substantial periods of employment and marriage. Abstinence is often related to a change in life circumstances. This is illustrated by the report of 95% abstinence among soldiers who returned to the USA after becoming dependent on opioids during service in the Vietnam War (Robins, 1993).

Prevention

Because dependence develops rapidly and treatment of dependent opioid misusers is unsatisfactory, preventive measures (see 'Prevention' above) are particularly important with regard to this group of drugs.

Treatment of crises

Opioid misusers may present in crisis to a doctor in any of three situations. First, when their *supplies have run out*, they may seek drugs either by requesting them directly or by feigning a painful disorder. Although withdrawal symptoms are very unpleasant, so that the misuser will go to great lengths to obtain more drugs, these symptoms are not usually dangerous to an otherwise healthy person. Therefore it is best to offer drugs only as the first step of a planned maintenance or withdrawal programme. This programme is described in the following sections. The second form of crisis is *drug overdose*. This requires medical treatment, directed in particular towards any respiratory depression caused by the drug. The third form of crisis is an *acute complication of intravenous drug usage*, such as local infection, necrosis at the injection site, or infection of a distant organ, often the heart or liver.

Planned withdrawal (detoxification)

The severity of withdrawal symptoms depends on psychological as well as pharmacological factors. Therefore the psychological management of the patient during withdrawal is as important as the drug regimen. The speed of withdrawal should be discussed with the patient to establish a timetable which is neither so rapid that the patient will not collaborate nor so protracted that the state of dependence is perpetuated. During withdrawal, much personal contact is needed to reassure the patient; the relationship that is formed in this way can be important in later treatment. The duration of opioid

---

> ### Box 20.19 Pharmacological management of opioid withdrawal
>
> - If short-term, non-opiate treatment is desired, use an α_2-adrenoceptor agonist such as lofexidine
> - Buprenorphine can be used for short-term opioid withdrawal
> - Methadone treatment for withdrawal can be successful, but needs to be carried out slowly with a gradual tapering of the dose
>
> Reproduced from Journal of Psychopharmacology, 26(7), Lingford-Hughes AR *et al.,* BAP updated guidelines: evidence-based guidelines for the pharmacological management of substance abuse, harmful use, addiction and comorbidity: recommendations from BAP, pp. 899-952, Copyright (2012), with permission from SAGE Publications.

detoxification is usually about 4 weeks in a residential setting and up to 12 weeks in a community setting.

When the dose is low, opioids can be withdrawn more quickly while giving symptomatic treatment for the withdrawal effects (Box 20.19). Drugs such as *loperamide* or *metoclopramide* can be useful for gastrointestinal symptoms. *Non-steroidal analgesics* may be useful for aches and pains. Another drug that may be useful is the α$_2$-adrenoceptor agonist, *lofexidine*. Lofexidine has a similar action to clonidine, but causes less hypotension and is preferred for managing opiate withdrawal.

When the daily dose of heroin is high, it may be necessary to prescribe an opioid, reducing the dose gradually. One approach is to use *methadone*, which has a more gradual action. The difficulty lies in judging the correct dose of methadone, because patients may either overstate their use of heroin because they fear the withdrawal symptoms, or understate it in an attempt to avoid censure. In addition, as noted below, the strength of street drugs varies.

Methadone should be given in a liquid form to be taken by mouth. The initial methadone dose is normally 10–40 mg daily, depending on the patient's usual consumption. Users with evidence of opioid tolerance may require dosing at the higher end of this range. If 4 hours after an initial dose there is evidence of withdrawal symptoms, a supplementary dose may be given, but caution is needed because methadone is a long-acting drug, and accumulation and toxicity could result. Street heroin varies in potency in different places and at different times. Therefore, if possible, advice about the equivalent dose of methadone should be obtained from a doctor with experience of treating drug dependence. The rate of methadone reduction depends on the clinical circumstances and the patient's clinical responses. The most rapid regimen may take about 10 days to 3 weeks, but slower reductions over several months may sometimes be appropriate.

Buprenorphine, a partial agonist at opioid receptors, can also be used to manage opioid withdrawal. Again, tapering doses are used at a rate that has been agreed with the patient. Buprenorphine is often well tolerated, but care needs to be taken when starting treatment, especially in the case of patients who are transferring from methadone. This is because the partial agonist action of the drug may precipitate acute withdrawal in patients who are transferring from higher doses of methadone (more than 30 mg) or heroin. This can usually be avoided by beginning treatment when the patient is already in mild withdrawal.

When opioid drugs are prescribed to drug-dependent patients, there is the possibility of diversion of the medication to the illegal market. This can be avoided by supervision of consumption of each daily dose—for example, by nursing or pharmacy staff. This practice also reduces the risk of overdose, and the daily personal contact probably also has other therapeutic benefits. It is generally regarded as good practice at least while treatment is being established, although daily attendance can be difficult for patients who are in full-time employment. In general, opiate detoxification can take place in the community, but inpatient management should be considered for patients who have not benefited from previous attempts at detoxification in the community, or who need a high level of nursing and medical care because of comorbid physical or psychiatric problems or polydrug abuse, or those who have significant social problems.

During and after opiate withdrawal it is important to consider and institute a suitable plan of psychosocial intervention, as outlined above (National Institute for Health and Clinical Excellence, 2007; Luty, 2015a).

Pregnancy and opioid dependence

The babies of women who misuse opioids are more likely than other babies to be premature and of low birth weight. They may also show withdrawal symptoms after birth, including irritability, restlessness, tremor, and a high-pitched cry. These signs appear within a few days of birth if the mother was taking heroin, but are delayed if she was taking methadone, which has a longer half-life in the body. Low birth weight and prematurity are not necessarily directly related to the drug, as poor nutrition and heavy smoking are common among heroin misusers.

Later effects have been reported, with the children of opioid-dependent mothers being more likely, as toddlers, to be overactive and to show poor persistence. However, these late effects may result from the unsuitable family environment rather than from a lasting effect of the intrauterine exposure to the drug.

The pregnancies of women who are in methadone maintenance programmes have a better outcome than those of women who use opioids but are not in such programmes. Some pregnant women request detoxification, but there are significant risks to the baby if this is carried out in the first or third trimester. The main aim of treatment in the first trimester is to engage the mother in a multidisciplinary care programme that will include stabilization on a suitable dose of methadone, avoidance of illegal drug use, and a high level of antenatal care. Patients who are receiving buprenorphine can remain on this treatment. Detoxification may be carried out in the second trimester, employing small frequent reductions of methadone or buprenorphine (Lingford-Hughes *et al.*, 2012).

Maintenance treatment for opioid dependence

As described above, withdrawal from opioids is the preferred treatment option, but if this is not possible, maintenance treatment, usually with methadone, may reduce the physical and social harm associated with the intravenous use of illegal drug supplies. Instead of heroin, methadone is prescribed as a liquid preparation formulated so as to discourage attempts to inject it.

Methadone maintenance treatment. Overall, patients who are receiving methadone maintenance treatment are approximately three times more likely to stay in treatment, and are about two-thirds less likely to use illegal heroin (Lingford-Hughes *et al.*, 2012). In addition, patients in methadone maintenance programmes show less risky injecting behaviours and lower rates of HIV infection.

Methadone doses of 20–40 mg daily have been widely advocated as appropriate for maintenance treatment, but there is evidence that higher doses (60–120 mg daily) are associated with lower rates of illegal opioid use and improved retention in the therapeutic programme. The latter is associated with an improved therapeutic outcome. The best approach is probably to have a flexible dosing policy, bearing in mind the potential toxicity of methadone in patients whose tolerance is unknown or difficult to assess. Generally it is better to start treatment with lower doses initially (not more than 40 mg daily), and to increase the dose over a number of weeks, titrating against the presence of withdrawal symptoms. It should be remembered that methadone levels continue to increase for about 5 days after the last dosage adjustment.

There is also a growing evidence base for the use of *buprenorphine* as an alternative to methadone for maintenance treatment for opioid users, although there is less consensus on appropriate dosing. In general, doses of 12–16 mg are used in longer-term prescribing. The same principles of treatment apply as in methadone prescribing. In controlled trials, maintenance methadone treatment is superior to buprenorphine in retaining patients in treatment; however, buprenorphine has a greater safety margin, particularly in terms of adverse cardiac effects such as prolongation of the QT interval. In practice, either buprenorphine or methadone can be offered as maintenance treatment, the decision being guided by safety considerations and patient choice (Lingford-Hughes *et al.*, 2012).

The concerns about diversion of prescribed opioid drugs, and the risk of overdose, have been described above in the section on management of opioid withdrawal. They also apply in maintenance treatment, and daily supervised consumption is commonly continued for a proportion of patients in maintenance treatment. A UK survey showed that supervision of methadone administration produced a fourfold decrease in deaths caused by methadone overdose (Strang *et al.*, 2010).

Naltrexone is a long-acting opioid antagonist that is used to help to prevent relapse in detoxified opioid-dependent patients. Although naltrexone treatment may have a role in certain dependent individuals who are highly motivated, such as doctors recovering from opioid dependence, or patients engaged in structured programmes associated with the criminal justice system, its benefit in the wider community of opioid users is less well established (Lingford-Hughes *et al.*, 2012).

Therapeutic community methods

These forms of treatment aim to produce abstinence by effecting a substantial change in the patient's attitudes and behaviour. Drug taking is represented as a way of avoiding pre-existing personal problems, and as a source of new ones. Group therapy and communal living are combined in an attempt to produce greater personal awareness, more concern for others, and better social skills. In most therapeutic communities some of the staff have previously been dependent on drugs, and so are often better able to gain the confidence of patients in the early stages of treatment. For younger populations, the use of a multimodal approach, including family involvement and community support with psychotherapy and pharmacologic interventions is important (National Institute for Health and Care Excellence, 2007).

Anxiolytic and hypnotic drugs

The most frequently misused drugs in this group are now the *benzodiazepines*. *Barbiturates* are little prescribed and their misuse has fallen. (It is worth noting, however, that sudden cessation of longer-term barbiturate treatment can cause a particularly serious withdrawal syndrome, akin to *delirium tremens*.) Other drugs with sedative properties that are currently misused include *gabapentin* and *pregabalin*. The clinical effects of these drugs are thought to result from their ability, directly or indirectly, to facilitate brain GABA function.

Benzodiazepines

These drugs were in therapeutic use for many years before it became apparent that their prolonged use could lead to tolerance and dependence, with a characteristic withdrawal syndrome. The withdrawal syndrome includes the following:

- *Anxiety symptoms*—anxiety, irritability, sweating, tremor, and sleep disturbance.
- *Altered perception*—depersonalization, derealization, hypersensitivity to stimuli, abnormal body sensations, and abnormal sensation of movement.
- *Other features* (rare)—depression, suicidal behaviour, psychosis, seizures, and delirium tremens.

Epidemiology. Benzodiazepine use has been extremely widespread—for example, it has been estimated that about 10% of the population of Europe and the USA use benzodiazepines as anxiolytics or hypnotics. Over the last few years there has been a decline in the prescription of benzodiazepines for anxiety. Most long-term users are older women. However, there is a significant misuse problem among younger people, often associated with intravenous administration of very high doses and polysubstance misuse. A significant proportion of people who are dependent on alcohol are also dependent on benzodiazepines. The Psychiatric Morbidity Survey reported that in households in England the prevalence of illegal tranquillizer use during the previous year was 0.7%, while 0.3% of those surveyed described themselves as dependent on tranquillizers (McManus *et al.*, 2009).

Dependence. Dependence on benzodiazepines often results from prolonged medical use, but may also result from the availability of benzodiazepines as street drugs because of their euphoriant and calming effects. The withdrawal syndrome closely resembles the anxiety symptoms for which the drugs are usually prescribed. Thus if symptoms appear after the dose of benzodiazepine has been reduced, the doctor may revert to a higher dosage in the mistaken belief that these symptoms indicate a persistent anxiety disorder. It has been estimated that about one-third of patients who take a benzodiazepine at therapeutic doses for more than 6 months may become dependent (Lingford-Hughes *et al.*, 2012).

Treatment. In mild dependence, minimal interventions such as a letter from the GP providing information and advising a reduction in dose can be effective. Treatment of more established dependence usually consists of gradual withdrawal over a period of at least 8 weeks. The addition of psychological therapies such as group cognitive behavioural therapy can improve cessation rates. Withdrawal appears to be more severe from benzodiazepines that have short half-lives and high potency at the benzodiazepine receptor. For this reason it is often suggested that patients who are taking such compounds should be switched to longer-acting drugs such as diazepam before withdrawal is attempted.

Current advice is that the dose of benzodiazepine should be lowered by about one-eighth every 2 weeks. However, if a patient experiences troublesome withdrawal symptoms, the dose can be maintained or even temporarily increased until the symptoms settle.

If a patient has been misusing benzodiazepines in very high doses, often in conjunction with opioid misuse, a reduction to a therapeutic dose is a good initial aim. In general, patients should be given no more than 30 mg diazepam daily, which should be enough to prevent withdrawal seizures. Carbamazepine is an alternative to benzodiazepines to control withdrawal symptoms.

Many patients experience their most troublesome withdrawal symptoms once the benzodiazepine dose has been completely tapered off. Symptoms usually subside over the next few weeks, although the time course can be irregular and some symptoms, such as muscle spasm, may not appear until other features of withdrawal have largely disappeared. A few patients continue to experience withdrawal-like symptoms for months or even years after cessation of benzodiazepines (*prolonged withdrawal syndrome*).

Prevention. The prevention of benzodiazepine dependence lies in the restriction of prescribing. Psychological treatments are effective for anxiety disorders (see Chapter 24), and non-pharmacological approaches to insomnia are also beneficial (see Chapter 13). If benzodiazepines are prescribed, this should be for the short-term relief of symptoms that are severely disabling or distressing. In some patients, who are already long-term users at modest doses, the balance of benefit and risk will favour continued prescribing, but these patients should be regularly reviewed and advised to cut their dose of medication if they can. This can be sufficient to persuade 20–40% of long-term benzodiazepine users to reduce their daily dose or discontinue treatment.

For further information about benzodiazepine dependence and its treatment, see Lingford-Hughes *et al.* (2012).

Gabapentin and pregabalin

Pregabalin is licensed for the treatment of generalized anxiety disorder (see Chapter 25) while both *gabapentin* and *pregabalin* are used as anticonvulsants and for the treatment of neuropathic pain. Both drugs are structural analogues of GABA, but they do not affect GABAergic mechanisms directly, instead modifying neurotransmitter release through interaction with the α_2-δ subunit of voltage-gated calcium channels.

Both drugs produce prominent sedative and anxiolytic effects and there is growing evidence of their misuse and dependence, particularly in people with a history of alcohol and other substance misuse, and in prison settings. Some of the misuse arises from prescribing for licensed indications; however, sales on the internet also are an important source (Kapil *et al.*, 2014). Misuse in combination with opiates is also quite common.

Sudden cessation of gabapentin and pregabalin can produce a *withdrawal syndrome*. Agitation, confusion, and disorientation are the most frequent symptoms, while sweating, gastrointestinal symptoms, tachycardia, hypertension, and insomnia are also reported. Treatment with gabapentin or pregabalin rapidly alleviates the syndrome, but administration of benzodiazepines does not seem helpful. For a review of pregabalin and gabapentin misuse, see Mersfelder and Nichols (2016).

Cannabis

Cannabis is derived from the plant *Cannabis sativa*. It is consumed either as the dried vegetative parts in the form known as marijuana or grass, or as the resin secreted by the flowering shoots of the female plant. Cannabis contains several pharmacologically active substances, of which the most powerful psychoactive compound is δ-9-tetrahydrocannabinol *(THC)*. It seems likely that the pharmacological effects of cannabinols are mediated through interaction with specific cannabinoid receptors in the central nervous system. Endogenous ligands for these receptors include 2-arachidonoyl glycerol and arachidonoyl ethanolamide (anandamide) (for a review of the pharmacology of cannabis, see Lu and Mackie, 2016). Over the past decade more potent cannabis preparations (known as 'skunk') have become widely available; these have higher levels of THC and a greater risk of adverse effects.

Epidemiology. In some parts of North Africa and Asia, cannabis products are consumed in a similar way to alcohol in western society. In North America and Europe the intermittent use of cannabis by young people is widespread. The Psychiatric Morbidity Survey reported that in households in England the lifetime use of cannabis was about 23%, with 7.5% of those surveyed reporting use in the past year, and 2.7% meeting the criteria for cannabis dependence (McManus *et al.*, 2009).

Clinical effects. The effects of cannabis vary with the dose, the person's expectations and mood, and the social setting. Users sometimes describe themselves as 'high' but, like alcohol, cannabis seems to exaggerate the preexisting mood, whether that was exhilaration or depression. Users report an increased enjoyment of aesthetic experiences, and distortion of the perception of time and space. There may be reddening of the eyes, dry mouth, tachycardia, irritation of the respiratory tract,

and coughing. Cannabis intoxication can lead to dangerous driving.

Adverse effects. No serious adverse effects have been demonstrated among those who use cannabis intermittently in small doses. Although there is no positive evidence of teratogenicity, cannabis has not been proved safe during the first 3 months of pregnancy. Inhaled cannabis smoke irritates the respiratory tract and is potentially carcinogenic. The most common adverse psychological effect of acute cannabis consumption is *anxiety*. Mild *paranoid ideation* is also not uncommon. At higher doses, *toxic confusional states* and occasionally *psychosis* in clear consciousness may occur.

Cannabis and mental illness. It is well established that cannabis can modify the course of an established schizophrenic illness, with evidence from a systematic review that users are more likely to experience more *severe positive symptoms*, more *relapses*, and *longer hospitalizations* (Schoeler *et al.*, 2016). The question of whether cannabis use can predispose to the later *development of schizophrenia* has been more controversial. Andreasson *et al.* (1987) followed up 45,570 Swedish conscripts for 15 years. They found that the relative risk of developing schizophrenia was 2.5 times higher in individuals who used cannabis, and that the relative risk for heavy users was six times higher. Although these data suggest that cannabis could be a risk factor for the development of schizophrenia, it is also possible that those who are predisposed to develop schizophrenia are also predisposed to misuse cannabis.

However, more recent prospective cohort studies that have adjusted for various baseline confounding factors such as history of mental illness, continue to demonstrate an increased risk of new-onset psychotic symptoms in young people who use cannabis. The increase in risk of psychosis is about twofold in individuals without other risk factors for schizophrenia (rising from about 7 in 1000 to 14 in 1000 in regular users). However, in people at high risk of schizophrenia due, for example, to a strong family history, a twofold increase in risk could be important, perhaps raising the risk of psychosis from about 1 in 10 to 1 in 5 (Hall and Degenhardt, 2011).

There has also been concern that cannabis use among teenagers might increase the risk of other poor psychosocial outcomes, such as mood and anxiety disorders, cognitive impairment, poor educational performance, job instability, traffic accidents, and uptake of more harmful illegal drugs. Such associations have continued to be reported consistently; however, the direction of causation is not always clear and confounding by factors such as childhood adversity is difficult to exclude completely (Hall, 2015). It is, of course, possible that genes predisposing to cannabis misuse might also predispose to mental illnesses such as depression and schizophrenia—a possibility supported by recent GWAS studies (Walters and Owen, 2016).

Tolerance and dependence. There is evidence that tolerance to the effects of cannabis can occur in individuals who are exposed to high doses for a prolonged period of time, but it is less evident in those who use small or intermittent doses. However, some patients do report inability to control cannabis use despite personal and social harm resulting from it. The *lifetime risk* of cannabis dependence in those who have ever used it is estimated at about 9%, compared to 32% for nicotine, 23% for heroin, 17% for cocaine, and 15% for alcohol (Hall, 2015). Withdrawal from high doses of cannabis gives rise to a syndrome of *irritability, nausea, insomnia, and anorexia*. These symptoms are generally mild in nature. The best way to manage cannabis dependence is unclear, but psychosocial interventions are commonly provided. Although abstinence may be difficult to achieve, treatment does appear to lower cannabis use and the associated harms.

For a review of the adverse effects of cannabis use, see Hall (2015), and for an outline of the management of cannabis dependence, see Winstock *et al.* (2010).

Stimulant drugs

These drugs include *amphetamines*, and related substances such as methylphenidate. *Cocaine* is also a stimulant drug, but is considered separately in the next section.

Amphetamines

Amphetamines play a significant role in the pharmacological treatment of attention deficit disorder (see Chapter 16) and narcolepsy (see Chapter 13), but have very little other use in medical practice. The psychomotor stimulant effects of amphetamines are believed to result from their ability to release and block the reuptake of dopamine and noradrenaline.

Epidemiology. Amphetamines are currently used rather less than cocaine in the UK. The Psychiatric Morbidity Survey reported that in households in England the lifetime use of amphetamines was about 8.6%, with 0.7% reporting use in the past year, and 0.2% of those surveyed meeting the criteria for amphetamine dependence (McManus *et al.*, 2009).

In the past, addiction to stimulant drugs arose chiefly from injudicious prescribing. However, most amphetamines are now illegally synthesized and used as a 'street drug', known as 'speed' or 'whizz'. As well as being taken orally or intravenously, amphetamines can also be 'snorted' (taken like snuff). A pure form of amphetamine ('ice') can be smoked or injected, and is said to produce particularly powerful effects.

Clinical effects. Apart from their immediate effect on mood, amphetamines cause over-talkativeness, overactivity, insomnia, dryness of the lips, mouth, and nose, and anorexia. The pupils dilate, the pulse rate increases, and the blood pressure rises. With large doses there may be *cardiac arrhythmia, severe hypertension, cerebrovascular accident*, and, occasionally, *circulatory collapse*. At increasingly high doses, neurological symptoms such as seizures and coma may occur. Acute adverse psychological effects of amphetamines include dysphoria, irritability, insomnia, and confusion. Anxiety and panic can also be present. *Obstetric complications* include miscarriage, premature labour, and placental abruption (see Box 20.20).

Amphetamine-induced psychosis. Prolonged use of high doses of amphetamines may result in repetitive stereotyped behaviour (e.g. repeated tidying). A *paranoid psychosis* that has been likened to paranoid schizophrenia may also be induced by prolonged high doses. The features include persecutory delusions, auditory and visual hallucinations, and sometimes hostile and dangerously aggressive behaviour. Usually the condition subsides within about a week, but occasionally it persists for months. It is not certain whether these prolonged cases represent true drug-induced psychoses, schizophrenia provoked by the amphetamine, or are merely coincidental. Whatever the nature of the association, it is not uncommon for patients with a history of amphetamine misuse to present to general psychiatric

---

Box 20.20 Some complications of amphetamine and cocaine misuse

Medical

Cardiovascular—hypertension, stroke, arrhythmias, myocardial infarction
Infective—abscesses, septicaemia, hepatitis, HIV
Obstetric—reduced fetal growth, miscarriage, premature labour, placental abruption
Other—weight loss, dental problems, epilepsy, general neglect

Psychiatric

Anxiety, depression, antisocial behaviour, insomnia, paranoid psychosis services. The ability of amphetamines to provoke psychosis has been one of the observations that has supported the dopamine hypothesis of schizophrenia (see Chapter 11).

Tolerance and dependence. From the epidemiology of amphetamine use, it seems that many recreational users do not progress to misuse and dependence. In more persistent users, tolerance to amphetamines leads to higher doses of the drug being taken. A withdrawal syndrome ('*crash*') of varying severity follows cessation of amphetamine use. In mild cases it consists mainly of low mood and decreased energy. In some cases, particularly in heavy users, depression can be severe, and accompanied by anxiety, tremulousness, lethargy, fatigue, and nightmares. Craving for the drug may be intense, and suicidal ideation may be prominent. Dependence on amphetamines can develop quickly. Dependence on stimulant drugs may be recognized from a history of overactivity and high spirits alternating with inactivity and depression. Whenever amphetamine use is at all likely, a urine sample should be taken for analysis as soon as possible because these drugs are quickly eliminated.

Prevention and treatment. Prevention of amphetamine misuse depends on restriction of the drugs and careful prescribing. Doctors should be wary of newly arrived patients who purport to suffer from narcolepsy.

Treatment of acute overdoses requires sedation and management of hyperpyrexia and cardiac arrhythmias. Most toxic symptoms, including paranoid psychoses, resolve quickly when the drug is stopped. An antipsychotic drug may be needed to control florid symptoms.

The treatment of amphetamine dependence is difficult, as craving for the drug can be intense. Abstinence is the usual goal and to achieve this a full range of social and psychological interventions may be needed (see above). Benzodiazepines may be helpful for managing acute distress caused by a severe withdrawal syndrome. Antidepressants do not appear to be effective in promoting abstinence, although they may be appropriate for treatment of a persistent depressive disorder. Abstinence-based programmes are not suitable for all misusers, and in view of the considerable harm that is associated with repeated intravenous misuse, some specialist centres have undertaken maintenance treatment with oral dexamphetamine. While retrospective studies show a possible benefit, at present there are no large randomized trials supporting this practice. Psychosocial approaches such as cognitive behaviour therapy and contingency management continue to be the mainstay of treatment (Lingford-Hughes *et al.*, 2012).

Cocaine

Cocaine is a central nervous stimulant with effects similar to those of amphetamines (described above). It is a particularly powerful positive reinforcer in animals, and causes strong dependence in humans. These latter effects probably stem from the ability of cocaine to block the reuptake of dopamine into presynaptic dopamine terminals. This leads to substantial increases in extracellular levels of dopamine in the ventral striatum, and consequent activation of the physiological 'reward system' (Lingford-Hughes *et al.*, 2010).

Cocaine is administered by injection, by smoking, and by sniffing into the nostrils. The latter practice sometimes causes perforation of the nasal septum. In 'freebasing', chemically pure cocaine is extracted from the street drug to produce 'crack', which has a very rapid onset of action, particularly when inhaled.

Epidemiology. The Psychiatric Morbidity Survey reported that in households in England the lifetime use of cocaine was about 6.3%, with 2.5% of those surveyed reporting use in the past year, and 0.4% meeting the criteria for cocaine dependence.

Clinical effects. The psychological effects of cocaine include excitement, increased energy, and euphoria. This can be associated with grandiose thinking, impaired judgement, and sexual disinhibition. Higher doses can result in visual and auditory hallucinations. *Paranoid ideation* may lead to *aggressive behaviour*. More prolonged use of high doses of cocaine can result in a *paranoid psychosis* with violent behaviour. This state is usually short-lived, but may be more enduring in those with a pre-existing vulnerability to psychotic disorder. *Formication* ('cocaine bugs')—a feeling as if insects are crawling under the skin—is sometimes experienced by heavy cocaine users.

The physical effects of cocaine include increases in pulse rate and blood pressure. Dilatation of the pupils is often prominent. Severe adverse effects of cocaine use include *cardiac arrhythmias, myocardial infarction, myocarditis,* and *cardiomyopathy.* Cocaine use has also been associated with cerebrovascular disease, including cerebral infarction, subarachnoid haemorrhage, and transient ischaemic attacks. Seizures and respiratory arrest have been reported. *Obstetric complications* include miscarriage, placental abruption, and premature labour.

Tolerance and dependence. In persistent users, tolerance of the effects of cocaine develops and a withdrawal syndrome similar to that seen following withdrawal of amphetamines can occur. After acute cocaine use, the 'crash' consists of dysphoria, anhedonia, anxiety, irritability, fatigue, and hypersomnolence. If the preceding cocaine use has been relatively mild, such symptoms resolve within about 24 hours. After more prolonged use, the symptoms are more severe and extended, and are associated with intense craving, depression, and occasionally severe suicidal ideation. Craving for cocaine can re-emerge after months of abstinence, particularly if the individual is exposed to psychological or social cues previously associated with its use.

Treatment. Acute intoxication may require sedation with benzodiazepines or, in severe cases, an antipsychotic agent. Concurrent medical crises such as seizures or hypertension should be managed in the usual way.

As with amphetamines, the treatment of cocaine dependence is difficult because of the intense craving associated with abstinence from the drug. For moderate cocaine users it may be sufficient to provide psychological and social support on an outpatient basis. Heavy and chaotic users with strong dependence will need more intensive management, perhaps in a residential setting. There is little evidence to support substitute pharmacological treatments to date, although several approaches have been evaluated (Lingford-Hughes *et al.*, 2012). Various psychosocial approaches can be helpful for patients with cocaine dependence. These include cognitive behavioural therapies, contingency management, and programmes that incorporate twelve-step approaches. With regard to individual treatment programmes, it is worth noting that people who misuse cocaine often misuse other drugs, such as opioids and alcohol.

MDMA ('ecstasy')

The recreational use of *3,4 methylenedioxymethamphetamine (MDMA)*, also known as 'ecstasy', increased rapidly at the end of the twentieth century but might now be declining to some extent. In 1998, about 5% of 16–24-year-olds reported using ecstasy in the past year, and in 2002 the number had risen to about 7% (Aust *et al.*, 2002). In 2007, the Psychiatric Morbidity Survey found a corresponding figure of 3.4% (McManus *et al.*, 2009). Lifetime use of ecstasy in this survey across all ages was about 5%. Ecstasy is a synthetic drug that is classified in the DSM-IV substance list as a hallucinogen. However, it has stimulant as well as mild hallucinogenic properties. It is usually taken in tablet or capsule form in a dose of about 50–150 mg. Given in this way, its effects last for about 4–6 hours. Like amphetamines, ecstasy increases the release of dopamine, but it also releases 5-hydroxytryptamine (5-HT), which may account for its hallucinogenic properties.

Clinical effects. Ecstasy produces a positive mood state, with feelings of euphoria, sociability, and intimacy. It also produces sensations of newly discovered insights and heightened perceptions. The physical effects of ecstasy include *loss of appetite, tachycardia, bruxism, and sweating*. Tolerance of successive doses of ecstasy develops quickly. Weekend users describe a midweek 'crash' in mood, which may represent withdrawal effects.

Adverse reactions. Rarely, ecstasy can cause severe adverse reactions, and deaths due to hyperthermia and its complications have been reported in healthy young adults. Hyperthermia probably results from the effect of ecstasy in increasing brain 5-HT release, together with the social setting in which the drug is customarily taken (crowded parties with prolonged and strenuous dancing). Deaths have also been reported due to cardiac arrhythmias, although pre-existing cardiac disease may have played a role. Intracerebral haemorrhage has occurred in ecstasy users, probably as a consequence of hypertensive crises. Cases of toxic hepatitis could reflect impurities in manufacture or an idiosyncrasy in metabolism.

The use of ecstasy has been associated with acute and chronic paranoid psychoses. However, as with other drug-induced psychotic states, it is not clear how far such disorders represent idiosyncratic reactions of vulnerable individuals. There are also reports of 'flashbacks', which are the recurrence of abnormal experiences weeks or months after drug ingestion. Such effects have been reported with other hallucinogens (see below). It is possible that repeated use of ecstasy may increase the risk of adverse psychiatric outcomes such as depression, anxiety, and depersonalization.

In experimental animals, including primates, repeated treatment with ecstasy causes degeneration of 5-HT nerve terminals in the cortex and forebrain. Therefore it is possible that such effects could occur in humans, and some brain imaging studies have shown changes in serotonin transporter binding that could equate to 5-HT terminal damage; however, the findings are not consistent. Whether such a change could be associated with long-term neuropsychological or psychiatric sequelae is disputed, but there is evidence for memory impairments in former ecstasy users (Parrott, 2013).

Prevention and harm reduction. Although the risk of serious harm following acute ecstasy use appears to be low, it is important to inform potential users about the acute risks and the potential long-term hazard of *neurotoxicity, cognitive impairment*, and *adverse longer-term psychiatric sequelae*. Consumption of large doses and pre-existing psychiatric disorder are likely to be associated with increased risk of adverse reactions. Education may also help users to avoid heatstroke by encouraging them to take breaks from dancing and to consume sufficient *isotonic* replacement fluid during vigorous exercise. However, the consumption of large amounts of water has sometimes caused death due to *hyponatraemia*.

For a review of ecstasy and the complications of its use, see Winstock and Schifano (2009) and Parrott (2013).

Hallucinogens

Hallucinogens are sometimes known as psychedelics, but we do not recommend this term because it does not have a single clear meaning. The term psychotomimetic is also used, because the drugs produce changes that bear some resemblance to those of psychotic symptoms. However, the resemblance is not close, so we do not recommend this term either.

The synthetic hallucinogens include LSD, dimethyltryptamine, and methyldimethoxyamphetamine. Of these drugs, LSD is encountered most often in the UK. Hallucinogens also occur naturally in some species of mushroom ('magic mushrooms'), and varieties containing *psilocybin* are consumed for their hallucinogenic effects. The mode of action of hallucinogenic drugs is unclear, but most act as partial agonists at brain 5-HT$_{2A}$ receptors.

Epidemiology. The Psychiatric Morbidity Survey reported that in households in England the lifetime use of LSD was 3.5%, while that of magic mushrooms was 5.0%. The corresponding figures for use in the past year were 0.2% and 0.6%, respectively (McManus *et al.*, 2009).

Clinical effects. The effects of LSD have been most well studied, and will be described here. The physical actions of LSD are variable. There are initial sympathomimetic effects—heart rate and blood pressure may increase and the pupils may dilate. However, overdosage does not appear to result in severe physiological reactions.

In predisposed individuals, the hypertensive effects of hallucinogens can cause adverse myocardial and cerebrovascular effects. The psychological effects develop within a period of 2 hours after LSD consumption, and generally last from 8 to 14 hours. The most remarkable experiences are distortions or intensifications of *sensory perception*. There may be confusion between sensory modalities (*synaesthesia*), with sounds being perceived as visual, or movements being experienced as if heard. Objects may be seen to merge with one another or to move rhythmically. The passage of time appears to be slowed, and experiences seem to have a profound meaning.

A distressing experience may be *distortion of the body image*, with the person sometimes feeling that they are outside their own body. These experiences may lead to panic, with fears of insanity. The patient's mood may be one of exhilaration, distress, or acute anxiety. According to early reports, behaviour could be unpredictable and extremely dangerous, with users sometimes injuring or even killing themselves as a result of behaving as if they were invulnerable. Since then there may have been some reductions in such adverse reactions, possibly because users are more aware of the dangers and take precautions to ensure support from other people during a 'trip'.

Whenever possible, adverse reactions should be managed by 'talking down' the user, explaining that the alarming experiences are due to the drug. If there is not time for this, an anxiolytic such as diazepam should be given and is usually effective. Tolerance of the psychological effects of LSD can occur, but a withdrawal syndrome has not been described. It is uncertain whether dependence occurs, but it is likely to be rare.

It has been argued that the use of LSD can cause long-term abnormalities in thinking and behaviour, or even schizophrenia, but the evidence for this is weak. However, *flashbacks* (i.e. the recurrence of psychedelic experiences weeks or months after the drug was last taken) are a recognized event. A number of medications, including benzodiazepines and anticonvulsants, have been reported to be helpful in the management of flashbacks, but there have been no controlled trials (Abraham, 2009).

Recently, there have been calls for a clinical re-evaluation of psychedelic drugs such as LSD, with claims that their adverse effects, particularly when taken in safe and controlled conditions, have been overstated. It is also suggested that, following their use, there can be an improved sense of wellbeing and therapeutically relevant 'openness to change'. For an expression of this view, see Carhart-Harris *et al.* (2016).

Phencyclidine and ketamine

Phencyclidine and ketamine are sufficiently different from the hallucinogens in their actions to require a separate description. They can be synthesized easily, taken by mouth, smoked, or injected. Phencyclidine was developed as a *dissociative anaesthetic*, but its use was abandoned because of adverse effects such as delirium and hallucinations. It is related to the currently used anaesthetic agent ketamine. Ketamine is also misused, and has similar effects to those of phencyclidine. However, ketamine has a shorter half-life than phencyclidine and is less likely than the latter to be associated with grossly disturbed behaviour.

Both phencyclidine and ketamine antagonize neurotransmission at *N-methyl-D-aspartate (NMDA) receptors,* which may account for their hallucinogenic effects. The psychological effects of ketamine in healthy volunteers have been used to model some of the clinical symptoms and cognitive changes that are seen in patients with schizophrenia, and are discussed in Chapter 11. Ketamine has also aroused interest because of its unexpected ability to produce a striking temporary *remission of depression* in treatment-refractory patients.

Phencyclidine is widely available in the USA but is little used in the UK. Most users of phencyclidine also use other drugs, particularly alcohol and cannabis. Ingestion of phencyclidine may be inadvertent, as it is often added to other street drugs to boost their effects. Ketamine is growing in popularity and is mainly used in the 'club scene' (Winstock and Schifano, 2009). Ketamine has a good safety profile when used as an anaesthetic, for which purpose it is given intravenously. Illicit use of ketamine can involve intravenous use or 'snorting'. When taken by either of these routes the drug has short duration of action (about 1–2 hours).

Clinical effects. Small doses of phencyclidine produce drunkenness, with analgesia of the fingers and toes, and even anaesthesia. Intoxication with the drug is prolonged, the common features being agitation, depressed consciousness, aggressiveness and psychotic-like symptoms, nystagmus, and raised blood pressure. With high doses there may be ataxia, muscle rigidity, convulsions, and absence of response to the environment even though the eyes are wide open. Phencyclidine can be detected in the urine for 72 hours after it was last taken.

If serious overdoses are taken, sympathomimetic crises may occur with hypertensive heart failure, cerebrovascular accident, or malignant hyperthermia. Status epilepticus may appear. Rhabdomyolysis can lead to renal failure. Fatalities have been reported, due mainly to hypertensive crisis but also to respiratory failure or suicide. Other people may be attacked and injured. Chronic use of phencyclidine may lead to aggressive behaviour accompanied by memory loss. Tolerance of the effects of phencyclidine occurs, although withdrawal symptoms are rare in humans. Animal studies suggest that dependence could occur in heavy users (Abraham, 2009).

Low doses of ketamine produce mood elevation, while at higher doses the user experiences sensory and perceptual distortions and out-of-body experiences similar to those reported with LSD. Frightening hallucinations, thought disorder, and confusion can also occur. These usually remit after a few hours. Patients who are admitted to hospital with ketamine intoxication show evidence of sympathetic overactivity, with chest pain, tachycardia, and palpitations. They may also experience nausea and vomiting, difficulty in breathing, ataxia, mutism, and temporary paralysis. Rarely, severe agitation and rhabdomyolysis can occur.

Treatment of intoxication. Treatment of acute phencyclidine intoxication is symptomatic, according to the features listed above. Haloperidol, diazepam, or both may be given. Caution should be exercised if using benzodiazepines alone, because of the risk of further behavioural disinhibition. Chlorpromazine should be avoided, as it may increase the anticholinergic effects of phencyclidine and worsen the patient's mental state. Hypertensive crisis should be treated with antihypertensive agents such as phentolamine. Respiratory function must be carefully monitored because excessive secretions may compromise the airway in an unconscious patient. Treatment of ketamine intoxication is also supportive and symptomatic. Antipsychotic drugs have little effect on the psychiatric symptoms, but benzodiazepines are reported to be helpful.

For reviews, see Abraham (2009) and Winstock and Schifano (2009).

Volatile substances (solvents, inhalants)

The misuse of *volatile substances* (also known as solvents) is not new, but public concern about widespread misuse first became apparent in the USA in the 1950s. Similar concerns emerged in the UK in the early 1970s. Although public interest has waned since then, there is a continuing high level of volatile substance misuse, particularly among adolescents. The pharmacological actions of volatile substances in the central nervous system are unclear but, like alcohol, they may increase the fluidity of neuronal cell membranes and are active at many different kinds of ion channel. This seems to result in increases in brain GABA function and decreases in NMDA receptor activity (Beckley and Woodward, 2013).

Epidemiology. Volatile substance misuse is a worldwide problem. The Psychiatric Morbidity Survey (McManus *et al.*, 2009) reported that in households in England the lifetime use of volatile substances was about 1.4%, with 0.1% of those surveyed reporting use in the past year. However, the survey did not include teenagers under the age of 16 years, among whom current use may be highest. *Amyl nitrite ('poppers')* appears to be more commonly used (see Box 20.14), but has a different pattern of use and is not discussed here. Volatile substance misuse is highly prevalent among the very young homeless populations in South American countries.

Volatile substance use occurs mainly in young men, and is more common in individuals from lower socio-economic groups. Most of the young people who are known to use volatile substances do so as a group activity, and only about 5% are solitary users. There is some evidence that a subgroup of volatile substance users have antisocial personality disorder and are likely to use and misuse multiple substances. However, the epidemiological data suggest that most individuals who use volatile substances do so only a few times and then abandon the practice (Ives, 2009).

Substances used and methods of use. The volatile substances used are mainly solvents and adhesives (hence the name 'glue-sniffing'), but also include many other substances, such as petrol, cleaning fluid, aerosols of all kinds, agents used in fire extinguishers, and butane. Toluene and acetone are frequently used. In this chapter the term 'volatile substance' will be used to denote all of these various substances. The methods of ingestion depend on the substance, and include inhalation from the tops of bottles, beer cans, cloths held over the mouth, plastic bags, and sprays. Volatile substance use may be associated with the taking of other illicit drugs, or with tobacco or alcohol consumption, which can be heavy.

Clinical effects. The clinical effects of volatile substances are similar to those of alcohol. The central nervous system is first stimulated and then depressed. The stages of intoxication are similar to those of alcohol, namely euphoria, blurring of vision, slurring of speech, incoordination, staggering gait, nausea, vomiting, and coma. Compared with alcohol intoxication, volatile substance intoxication develops and wanes rapidly (within a few minutes, or up to 2 hours). There is early disorientation, and 40% of cases may develop hallucinations, which are mainly visual and often frightening. This combination of symptoms may lead to serious accidents.

Adverse effects. Volatile substance misuse has many severe adverse effects, of which the most serious is sudden death. These fatalities occur during acute intoxication, and about 100 such deaths occurred annually in the UK in the 1990s, although there has been a decline subsequently, with 36 deaths being recorded in 2008 (Ghodse *et al.*, 2010). Around 50% of the deaths are due to the direct toxic effects of the volatile substance, particularly cardiac arrhythmias and respiratory depression. The rest are due to trauma, asphyxia (due to plastic bag over the head), or inhalation of stomach contents.

Chronic users may show evidence of neurotoxic effects, and severe and disabling peripheral neuropathy has been described in teenager misusers. Other neurological adverse effects, particularly associated with toluene, include impaired cerebellar function, encephalitis, and dementia. Volatile substance misuse can also damage other organs, including the liver, kidney, heart, and lungs. Gastrointestinal symptoms include nausea, vomiting, and haematemesis.

Tolerance and dependence. Dependence can develop if use is regular, but physical withdrawal symptoms are unusual. When such symptoms occur they usually consist of sleep disturbance, irritability, nausea, tachycardia, and, rarely, hallucinations and delusions. With sustained use over a period of 6–12 months, tolerance can develop.

Diagnosis. The diagnosis of acute volatile substance intoxication is suggested by several features, including glue on the hands, face, or clothes, a chemical smell on the breath, rapid onset and waning of intoxication, and disorientation in time and space. Chronic misuse is diagnosed mainly on the basis of an admitted history of habitual consumption, increasing tolerance, and dependence. A suggestive feature is a facial rash ('glue-sniffer's rash') caused by repeated inhalation from a bag.

Treatment. As noted above, for many users experimentation with volatile substances is a temporary phase that does not appear to lead to persistent misuse or dependence. Advice and support may be sufficient for such individuals. However, a significant subgroup of those who misuse volatile substances also misuse other substances, such as alcohol and opioids. Such individuals are more likely to have an antisocial personality disorder and to have experienced a chaotic and abusive family life. Treatment of this group is difficult, and a full range of psychological and social treatments is likely to be needed (see above). There is no specific pharmacotherapy for volatile substance misuse, but associated psychiatric disorders such as depression may require treatment in their own right.

Prevention. Prevention of volatile substance misuse may best be directed at the large numbers of young people who experiment with volatile substances as a result of curiosity or peer pressure. Policies include the restriction of sales of volatile substances to children and adolescents. Education, particularly concerning the risk of severe injury and death (which can, of course, occur in occasional or first-time users), seems to be worthwhile. Wider social measures, such as the provision of improved recreational facilities, have also been advocated.

For a review of volatile substance misuse, see Beckley and Woodward (2013).

Table 20.6 Some examples of substances used as 'recreational' drugs

Drug	Pharmacology	Intoxication syndrome
Spice ('Genie', 'Yucatan Fire')	Herbal mixture with addition of synthetic cannabinoids	Changes in mood and perception, cognitive impairment, psychosis, scleral injection, hunger
Salvia ('Magic Mint', 'Mystic Sage')	Plant extract from *Salvia divinorum*. Active substance is salvinorin A, an opiate kappa receptor agonist	Alterations in mood and somatic sensations. Striking changes in perception of external reality, confusion, amnesia, anxiety
Mephedrone, ('Meow-Meow'), MDPV ('Vanilla Sky', 'Purple Wave')	Synthetic cathinone derivatives, related to active substance in *khat*. Cause release of monoamine neurotransmitters, including dopamine	Euphoria, increased sociability, agitation, psychosis, seizures, tachycardia chest pain, hyponatraemia

Reproduced from The Journal of Emergency Medicine, 44(6), Johnson LA, Johnson RL and Portier RB, Current "legal highs", pp. 1108–1115, Copyright (2013), with permission from Elsevier.

Legal highs

The phrase '*legal high*' refers to a substance with psychotropic properties whose sale or use is not banned (or not yet banned) by legislation. The recreational use of such substances appears to be increasing in the UK and Europe. A European survey, conducted in 2011, found that between 5% and 10% of young people admitted taking a legal high at least once in the previous year (Luty, 2014). Legal highs can be purchased on the internet and may also be sold by dealers together with more established illicit drugs.

Because the development and uptake of legal highs evolves quickly, with the aim of circumventing usual regulatory channels, their effects, particularly in terms of intoxication, may not be well recognized. Generally, legal highs are designed to mimic effects of more traditional drugs of abuse. As one substance is banned, manufacturers search for replacements with a similar pharmacology that have not yet been caught in the regulatory framework. Because of this, any description of available compounds is always likely to be dated, but a few examples are given in Table 20.6. The passage of legislation by the UK Government in 2016 (The 'Psychoactive Substances Act') is designed to lessen the use of legal highs by making it an offence to produce or supply psychoactive substances for human consumption. There are exceptions for approved medical and scientific use. How well this legislation will work in practice remains to be seen.

Further reading

Gelder MG, López-Ibor JJJr, Andreasen NC and Geddes JR (eds) (2009). Section 4.27: Substance use disorders. In: *The New Oxford Textbook of Psychiatry*. Oxford University Press, Oxford.

National Institute for Health and Clinical Excellence (2011). *Alcohol-Use Disorders: Diagnosis, assessment and management of harmful drinking and alcohol dependence*. Clinical Guideline 115. National Institute for Health and Clinical Excellence, London. (A periodically updated comprehensive review.)

Robson P. (2009). *Forbidden Drugs*. Oxford University Press, Oxford. (A very readable account of illegal drugs, the reasons for their use, and treatment of misuse.)

CHAPTER 21
Suicide and deliberate self-harm

Introduction

Suicide is among the ten leading causes of death in most countries for which information is available and the second most common cause of death in young people (Hawton, 2012). There are some indications that the overall rate is decreasing (see Figure 21.1), and the most recent figures confirm that this reduction has continued (World Health Organization, 2014): between 2000 and 2012 the age-standardized suicide rate has fallen by 26% internationally (23% in men and 32% in women). However, these changes have not been uniform and range from a decline of nearly 70% in some countries to an increase of over 250% in others. In the UK, suicide is the third most important contributor to life years lost after coronary heart disease and cancer. Over the past 50 years, several countries have reported a considerable increase in the number of young men who kill themselves, although there have been some signs that this trend may be reversing (Bridge *et al.*, 2006). The subject is important to all doctors who may at times encounter people who are at risk for suicide, and who may also at times be involved in helping family members or others after a suicide. The importance of the subject is reflected in national and international initiatives for suicide prevention (US Office of Surgeon General, 2012; World Health Organization, 2012, 2014; Department of Health, 2012; Mann *et al.*, 2005).

For every suicide it is estimated that more than 30 non-fatal episodes of self-harm occur. Depression, substance misuse, and other mental health problems are more common in people who deliberately harm themselves, and the rate of suicide in the year following an episode of deliberate self-harm (DSH) is some 60–100 times that of the general population (Hawton *et al.*, 2003a). The rate of suicide is also raised in the period following discharge from inpatient psychiatric care. For these reasons, psychiatrists need to be particularly well informed about the nature of DSH and suicidal behaviour, and about strategies aimed at their prevention. For an overview of relevant aspects of suicide and DSH, see Wasserman and Wasserman (2009).

Suicide

The act of suicide

Suicide has been defined as an act with a fatal outcome, deliberately initiated and performed in the knowledge or expectation of its fatal outcome. People who take their lives do so in a number of different ways. In England and Wales, according to the Office for National Statistics in 2008, hanging was the most commonly used method

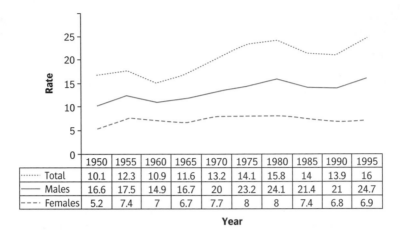

Figure 21.1 Global suicide rates (per 100,000), by gender, for the period 1950–95 (selected countries indicated in Table 21.1).

Reproduced from Figures and Facts about Suicide, pp. iv, Copyright (1999), with permission from World Health Organization http://whqlibdoc.who.int/hq/1999/WHO_MNH_MBD_99.1.pdf accessed 26/03/12 with permission.

for suicide by men (53%), followed by drug overdose (16%), self-poisoning by car exhaust fumes, drowning, and jumping. The commonest methods for women were drug overdose (36%), hanging (34%), and drowning (Wasserman and Wasserman, 2009). In the USA, gunshot and other violent methods are more frequent than in the UK.

Most completed suicides have been planned. Precautions against discovery are often taken—for example, choosing a lonely place or a time when no one is expected. However, in most cases a warning is given. In a US study, suicidal ideas have been expressed by more than two-thirds of those who die by suicide, and clear suicidal intent by more than one-third. Often the warning had been given to more than one person. Over 40% of people who committed suicide had consulted their general practitioner in the preceding weeks (Pirkis and Burgess, 1998). Data from the National Confidential Inquiry into Suicide and Homicide (2015) suggest that 25–29% of suicides have been in recent contact with mental health services.

The epidemiology of suicide

The accuracy of the statistics

Accurate statistics about suicide are difficult to obtain because information about the exact cause of a sudden death is not always available. For example, in England and Wales, official figures depend on the verdicts reached in coroners' courts. A verdict of suicide is recorded by a coroner only if there is clear evidence that the injury was self-inflicted and that the deceased intended to kill

himself. If there is any doubt about either point, a verdict of accidental death or an open verdict is recorded. Open verdicts are more often recorded when the method of self-harm is less active (e.g. drowning compared with hanging) and when the deceased is younger (Neeleman and Wessely, 1997). It is accepted that official statistics underestimate the true rates of suicide. Local culture and customs, in particular the stigma attached to suicide and the procedure and requirements for classifying a death as suicide have a marked effect (Hawton and van Heeringen, 2009). For instance, a ninefold to tenfold underestimation of reported suicides has been suggested for India (Gajalakshmi and Peto, 2007). An attempt has been made to overcome these problems by reporting 'probable suicides', which combine deaths attributed to suicide and 'open verdicts' (Schapira *et al.*, 2001).

Differences in suicide rates

For these reasons, caution should be exercised when comparing rates of suicide in different time periods and between different countries. Despite this, long-standing and fairly stable differences in rates of suicide between different countries are apparent. The finding of Sainsbury and Barraclough (1968) that, within the USA, the rank order of suicide rates among immigrants from 11 different nations reflected those within the 11 countries of origin supports these differences in national rates. The current suicide rate in the UK (10.1 per 100,000 in men and 2.8 per 100,000 in women) is in the lower range of those reported in western countries. Generally, higher rates are reported in eastern and northern European countries, and lower rates in Mediterranean countries. The suicide rates in the former

Soviet Union have increased substantially since its break-up, particularly among men (53.9 per 100,000 for the Russian Federation and for Lithuania, and 63.3 per 100,000 for Belarus (World Health Organization, 2010). Reported suicide rates are very low in Islamic countries. The gender differences are less in Asian than in western countries. Some methods of suicide reflect local culture; for example, self-immolation or ritual disembowelment (Cheng and Lee, 2000), or carbon monoxide poisoning produced by burning charcoal in Hong Kong (Leung et al., 2002).

Changes in suicide rates

Suicide rates have changed in several ways since the beginning of the last century. Recorded rates for both men and women fell during each of the two world wars. There were also two periods during which rates increased. The first, during 1932 and 1933, was a time of economic depression and high unemployment. However, the second period, between the late 1950s and the early 1960s, was not. Following this, from 1963 to 1974 the rates declined in England and Wales but not in other European countries (with the exception of Greece) or in North America. The decline in England and Wales has been attributed to a change from coal gas, which has been the most common method of suicide, to non-toxic North Sea gas.

Variations with the seasons

In England and Wales, suicide rates have been highest in spring and summer for every decade since 1921–1930. A similar pattern has been found in other countries in both hemispheres. The reason for these fluctuations is not known, although it has been suggested that they relate to changes in the incidence of mood disorders. Seasonal variations in suicide rates may be diminishing (Ajdacic-Gross et al., 2008).

Demographic characteristics

Suicide is about three times as common in men as in women. The highest rates of suicide in both men and women are in the elderly. Suicide rates are lower among the married than among those who have never been married, and increase progressively through widowers, widows, and the divorced. Rates are higher in the unemployed. Rates of suicide are high among prisoners, especially among those on remand (Fazel et al., 2005).

Rates are particularly high in certain professions, particularly those with access to lethal materials. The rate in veterinary surgeons is four times the expected rate (Bartram and Baldwin, 2010); in pharmacists and farmers it is double the expected rate (Charlton et al., 1993); and it is also higher in doctors, particularly female doctors (Meltzer et al., 2008). Suicide among doctors is discussed further on page 615.

The causes of suicide

Methods of investigation

Hawton and van Heeringen (2009) have helpfully divided risk factors into distal and proximal (see Box 21.1).

Investigations into the causes of suicide face several difficulties. Information about the health and wellbeing of the deceased at the time of suicide cannot be obtained directly. Prospective studies of suicide are difficult to arrange because of its relative rarity. Two strategies have been used to overcome these difficulties.

1. *'The psychological autopsy'.* Retrospective studies have pieced together the circumstances that surrounded the suicide by examining records and interviewing doctors, relatives, and friends who knew the deceased well.

2. Epidemiological studies have examined associations between social and demographic factors and rates of suicide in different populations at different times.

Both approaches have methodological problems. However, the psychological autopsy has helped to identify factors that precede suicide, the proximal factors. The second approach has informed our understanding

---

Box 21.1 Risk factors for suicide

Distal

- Genetic loading
- Personality characteristics (e.g. impulsivity, aggression)
- Restricted fetal growth and perinatal circumstances
- Early traumatic life events
- Neurobiological disturbances (e.g. serotonin dysfunction and hypothalamic–pituitary axis hyperactivity)

Proximal

- Psychiatric disorder
- Physical disorder
- Psychosocial crisis
- Availability of means
- Exposure to models

Reproduced from The Lancet, 373(9672), Hawton K, van Heeringen K, Suicide, pp. 1372–1381, Copyright (2009), with permission from Elsevier.

of social circumstances that may give rise to increased rates of suicide, the distal factors.

Individual psychiatric and medical factors (proximal factors)

The most consistent finding of studies of proximal factors (see Table 21.1) is that the large majority (90%) of those who die from suicide have some form of mental disorder at the time of death, and psychiatric disorders account for over 40% of the population risk (Cavanagh et al., 2003). Similar results have been reported in several countries (Cheng and Lee, 2000), although in some rural regions the association of diagnosed psychiatric disorder with suicide appears to be less strong (Manoranjitham et al., 2010; Tong and Phillips, 2010). The most frequent conditions include the following:

- *Depression*. About 4% of individuals with depression will die by suicide and those who do are more likely to have a past history of self-harm and to have had recent contact with mental health services, and have experienced a sense of hopelessness (Coryell and Young, 2005). They are also more often single, separated, or widowed, are older, and are more often male. However, suicide risk is higher in the first episode of depression, often related to alcohol use. A review of community studies found suboptimal or no treatment for their illness in the majority (Wasserman and Wasserman, 2009). Those receiving no treatment were 1.8 times more likely to commit suicide. In bipolar disorder the lifetime risk is elevated to 10–15%, more often early on in the course of the illness (Goodwin and Jamison, 2007).

- *Personality disorder*. This is diagnosed in 40–50% of people who commit suicide, according to some surveys

(Foster et al., 1997). Rates are particularly high in borderline and antisocial disorder (Lieb et al., 2004).

- *Alcohol misuse*. This is strongly associated with suicide risk, especially in the presence of dependence (Conner and Duberstein, 2004). The lifetime risk is 7% (Inskip et al., 1998; Wilcox, 2004). Among those who are alcohol-dependent, suicide is more likely when the patient is male, older, has a long history of drinking, and has a history of depression and of previous suicidal attempts. Suicide risk is also increased among those whose drinking has caused physical complications, relationship problems, difficulties at work, or arrests for drunkenness offences.

- *Drug misuse*. This is relatively common among those who die by suicide, particularly in the young (Wilcox, 2004).

- *Schizophrenia*. The suicide rate is increased among young men early in the course of the disorder, particularly when there have been relapses, when there are depressive symptoms, and when the illness has turned previous academic success into failure. The lifetime risk is estimated at about 5% (see Chapter 11).

Other factors associated with suicide are a *past history of DSH* (see page 622) and *poor physical health*, especially *epilepsy, eating disorders,* especially *anorexia nervosa* (Chapter 13) and *ADHD*. For a review, see Stenager and Stenager (2000).

Social factors

Comparisons of the rates of suicide between and within different countries have been conducted over a period of many years. None has been more influential than that undertaken by Emile Durkheim at the end of the nineteenth century (Durkheim, 1951). Durkheim examined variations in the rate of suicide within France, and between France and other European countries. He demonstrated that a range of social factors have an impact on rates of suicide. Rates were lower at times of war and revolution, and increased during periods of both marked economic prosperity and economic depression. He concluded that social integration and social regulation were central to the rate of suicide. Durkheim described four types of suicide, including *'anomic' suicide*. This refers to suicide by a person who lacks ties with other people and no longer feels part of society. (Durkheim's other types of suicide were egoistic, altruistic, and fatalistic.)

More recent studies have repeatedly demonstrated that areas with *high unemployment, poverty* (Gunnell et al., 1995), *divorce*, and *social fragmentation* (Whitley et al., 1999) have higher rates of suicide. There is

Table 21.1 Rates of mental disorders in five psychological autopsy studies on completed suicides using DSM-III or DSM-III-R criteria

Depressive disorders	36–90%
Alcohol dependence or abuse	43–54%
Drug dependence or abuse	4–45%
Schizophrenic disorders	3–10%
Organic mental disorders	2–7%
Personality disorders	5–44%

Source: data from Lonnqvist JK, Epidemiology and causes of suicide. In: Gelder MG, Andreasen NC, López-Ibor JJ Jr and Geddes JR (eds), The New Oxford Textbook of Psychiatry, 2nd edn, Copyright (2009), Oxford University Press.

evidence that the economic recession of 2008, with its following austerity and rising unemployment, has been associated with a rise in the male suicide rate even in relatively protected countries such as the UK (Barr *et al.*, 2012), with reports of even greater effects in those most affected, such as Greece. The increased rates of suicide are most marked in areas of greater unemployment (Barr *et al.*, 2012) and among men aged 45–54 (Appleby *et al.*, 2015). Such studies cannot be used as a means of examining the characteristics of individuals who kill themselves, but they do provide important information about factors within society that may affect the rate of suicide. Cross-cultural evidence indicates wide variation in the meaning of suicide and social attitudes to it, which appears to be associated with differences in suicide rates (Stack, 2000).

Another social factor that appears to affect rates of suicide is *media coverage of suicide*. Suicide and attempted suicide rates were shown to increase after television programmes and films depicting suicide (Stack, 2003). The precise nature of the media content may also be influential in increasing or decreasing the risk of imitative behaviour (Niederkrotenthaler *et al.*, 2010).

Biological factors

A family history of suicide increases the risk at least twofold (Qin *et al.*, 2003), and genetic factors account for 45% of variance in suicidal behaviour (Bondy *et al.*, 2006). The genetic mechanism may be largely independent of mechanisms giving rise to psychiatric disorders (Roy *et al.*, 2000), but related to impulsivity and aggression.

Suicidal behaviour has been linked to decreased activity of brain 5-HT pathways. Markers of 5-HT function, such as cerebrospinal fluid (CSF) 5-HIAA and the density of 5-HT transporter sites, are lowered in suicide victims. The association between underactivity of 5-HT pathways and suicidal behaviour appears to extend across diagnostic boundaries, and may be related to increased impulsivity and aggression in those with low brain 5-HT function. The link between 5-HT function and suicidality has prompted genetic association studies in people with suicidal behaviour. However, reliable associations with 5-HT-related and other genes have not yet emerged (Antypa *et al.*, 2013). For reviews of the neurobiology and genetics of suicide, see Ernst *et al.* (2009) and Niculescu *et al.* (2016).

Psychological factors

Psychological factors in suicide have been derived mainly by extrapolation from studies of non-fatal DSH, but the factors may not be the same. Research has indicated that hopelessness, impulsivity, dichotomous thinking, cognitive constriction, problem-solving deficits, and overgeneralized autobiographical memory are all associated with suicidal behaviour. All of these could act by predisposing an individual to act impulsively (Williams and Pollock, 2000).

Conclusion

The associations considered above do not, of course, establish causation, but they do suggest three sets of interacting influences:

1. Medical factors, including depressive disorder, alcohol misuse, and abnormal personality.
2. Psychological factors, of which hopelessness is the strongest.
3. Social factors, especially social isolation and poverty.

Personality traits of impulsivity and aggression could be important, and these may have a biological basis, possibly related to dysregulation of the 5HT system.

Special groups

Suicide among those in contact with psychiatric services

Given the strong association between mental disorder and suicide, it is not surprising that many people who kill themselves are in contact with psychiatric services. The National Confidential Inquiry into Suicide and Homicide, which was set up in 1997, collects information on all patients who committed suicide while in contact with the mental health services (National Confidential Inquiry into Suicide and Homicide, 2015). Between 1997 and 2007, coroners recorded a verdict of suicide or an open verdict in 54,808 deaths, of which 14,249 (26%) had been in contact with mental health services during the preceding 12 months. During this period the annual number of inpatients dying by suicide had decreased by 46% and the number dying by strangulation or hanging had decreased by 69%.

Suicide after discharge from hospital occurred within 1 month in 43% of 238 patients studied, and nearly 50% of these suicides occurred before the first follow-up appointment (Hunt *et al.*, 2009). Figures from the 2015 Inquiry indicate that the rate of suicide by patients in contact with mental health services has increased considerably. These figures are complicated by the fact that there are more patients overall so they are not rates. A striking increase has been in the number of suicides of patients under the care of Crisis Resolution/Home Treatment teams. There are now three times as many suicides under the care of these teams as inpatient suicides, and in 37% of these the patient had been under their care for less than a week. The first week after discharge is the period of highest risk.

These findings indicate that the following measures are necessary.

- *Support patients intensively* during the first few weeks after discharge from hospital. The first follow-up should take place within 7 days of discharge.
- *Plan in advance* the steps that should be taken if the patient ceases to cooperate with treatment.
- *Monitor the side effects* of drugs, and change to one with fewer side effects if these seem likely to lead to refusal to continue with the medication.
- *Ward design*. Since hanging was a common method of suicide by inpatients, wards are regularly inspected to eliminate 'ligature points'.

'Rational' suicide

Despite the findings reviewed above, suicide can be the rational act of a mentally healthy person. Several European countries (e.g. Switzerland, the Netherlands, Belgium) have recognized this and made changes in their law to allow those with a long-term illness to take their own life with help from friends, family, or even medical practitioners. An established and well-documented decision is generally required, together with confirmation that the individual does have capacity. The law has not yet changed in the UK, but interpretation of recent cases and parliamentary activity indicates that there soon may be a change. The major concern is to draft a bill with wording to protect elderly people from pressure from family who are either burdened by their care or likely to benefit financially by their death. Public opinion has certainly shifted towards a recognition that reasonable people may, in some circumstances, want to end their own lives. Lack of personal autonomy and perceived dignity due to infirmity and chronic pain are the commonest reasons advanced by those who pursue this path.

It is a good general rule to assume, until further enquiry has proved otherwise, that a person who talks of suicide has an abnormal state of mind. If the assumption is correct—and it is sometimes difficult to identify a depressive disorder when the person is first seen—the patient's urge to die is likely to diminish when their abnormal mental state recovers. Moreover, even when the decision to die was arrived at rationally, it is still reasonable to attempt to prevent the person from self-harm. This is because a decision about suicide may have been made rationally but on the basis of incomplete information or mistaken assumptions. It may change

when the person is better informed—for example, when it has been explained to them that death from cancer need not be as painful as they formerly believed.

Older people

In most countries the highest rate of suicide is among people aged over 75 years. The most frequent methods are hanging among men, and drug overdose among women (Harwood *et al.*, 2000). In addition to active self-harm, some older adults die from deliberate self-neglect (e.g. by refusing food or necessary treatment). As in younger age groups, depression is a strong predictor of suicide in the elderly. Other risk factors are social isolation, bereavement, and impaired physical health (Harwood *et al.*, 2006). Personality is also important, especially anxious and obsessional traits (Harwood *et al.*, 2001). For further information about suicide in the elderly, see Harwood and Jacoby (2000).

Children and adolescents

Children

Suicide is rare in children. In 1989, the suicide rate for children aged 5–14 years was estimated to be 0.7 per 100,000 in the USA and 0.8 per 100,000 in the UK. Little is known about the factors that lead to suicide in childhood, except that it is associated with severe personal and social problems. Children who have died by suicide have usually shown antisocial behaviour. Suicidal behaviour and depressive disorders are common among their parents and siblings (Shaffer, 1974). Shaffer distinguished two groups of children. The first group consisted of children of superior intelligence who seemed to be isolated from less educated parents. Many of their mothers were mentally ill. Before death, the children had appeared depressed and withdrawn, and some had stayed away from school. The second group consisted of children who were impetuous, prone to violence, and resentful of criticism (Shaffer *et al.*, 2000).

Adolescents

Suicide rates among adolescents have increased in recent years. In England and Wales the increase has mainly been in male adolescents aged 15–19 years (McClure, 2000), and the principal methods among males have been hanging, and poisoning with car exhaust fumes (Hawton *et al.*, 1999). The risk factors are similar to those in adults, with high rates of comorbid psychiatric disorders (Bridge *et al.*, 2006). A psychological autopsy study (Houston *et al.*, 2001) showed that about 70% of adolescents who killed themselves had had psychiatric disorders, mainly depressive and personality disorders, which were sometimes comorbid. Many of them had misused alcohol or drugs. The suicide was often the culmination of long-term difficulties with relationships and other psycho-social problems. Approximately two-thirds of these individuals had made a previous suicide attempt.

Ethnic groups

Rates among immigrants closely reflect those in their countries of origin. In the UK, there is particular concern about possible high rates of suicide among Asian women (Ahmed *et al.*, 2007).

High-risk occupational groups

Doctors. The suicide rate among doctors is higher than that in the general population, and the excess is greater among female doctors (Meltzer *et al.*, 2008). Many reasons have been suggested for the excess, including the ready availability of drugs, increased rates of addiction to alcohol and drugs, the stresses of work, reluctance to seek treatment for depressive disorders, and the selection into the medical profession of predisposed personalities. A psychological autopsy study of 38 working doctors who had died by suicide (Hawton *et al.*, 2004) found psychiatric disorder—mainly depressive disorder and/or drug or alcohol misuse—in about two-thirds of cases, and problems at work in a similar proportion. About one-third of cases had relationship problems, and about a quarter had financial problems. Self-poisoning with drugs was more common than in the general population, and 50% of the anaesthetists used anaesthetic agents. Rates have been reported to be higher in anaesthetists, community health doctors, general practitioners, and psychiatrists (Hawton *et al.*, 2001). Much of this increased risk is accounted for by female doctors. It is not known whether this relates more to factors in the individual (contributing to specialty choice and to suicide rate) or to the nature of the work. However, significant personal and mental health problems, beyond work stress, are generally identifiable in those who do commit suicide (Hawton *et al.*, 2004a).

Veterinary surgeons have the highest suicide rates of any professional group. The reasons for this are unclear, but are likely to closely parallel those identified for doctors, and include managerial issues, a high workload, and possibly the impact of regularly euthanizing sick animals (Platt *et al.*, 2010).

Farmers also have high rates of suicide. Possible causes include the ready availability of means of self-harm (e.g. poisons and firearms), together with work stress and financial difficulties (Malmberg *et al.*, 1999).

Students, contrary to popular belief, are not a high-risk group, with rates close to their age group in the general population.

Suicide pacts

In suicide pacts, two (or occasionally more) people agree that at the same time each will take his or her own life. Completed suicide pacts are uncommon. In Far Eastern countries, those involved are usually lovers aged under 30 years, and in western countries they are usually interdependent couples aged over 50 years. Suicide pacts have to be distinguished from cases where murder is followed by suicide (especially when the first person dies but the second is revived), or where one person aids another person's suicide without intending to die himself or herself.

The psychological causes of these pacts are not known with certainty. Usually the two people have a particularly close relationship but are socially isolated from others. Often a dominant partner initiates the suicide (Brown and Barraclough, 1997). *Mass* suicide is occasionally reported. For example, 913 followers of the People's Temple cult died at Jonestown, Guyana, in 1978, and 39 members of the Heaven's Gate Cult in California died in 1997. These tragic events are generally initiated by a charismatic leader who has strong convictions and is sometimes deluded. Sometimes there is evidence to suggest murder followed by suicide within the group.

There have been several cases in which the internet has been used to arrange suicide pacts (Naito, 2007).

The assessment of suicidal risk

General issues

Every doctor should be able to assess the risk of suicide. There are two requirements. The first is a willingness to make direct but tactful enquiries about the patient's intentions. There is no convincing evidence that asking a patient about suicidal inclinations makes suicidal behaviour more likely. On the contrary, someone who has already thought of suicide is likely to feel better understood when the doctor raises the issue, and this feeling may reduce the risk.

The second requirement is to be alert to factors that predict suicide. However, prediction based on these factors has a low sensitivity and specificity. Even if the risk is correctly assessed as high, it is difficult to predict when the suicide will take place. The limitations of prediction have been illustrated by a study by Goldstein *et al.* (1991). They tried to develop a statistical model to predict the suicides from among a group of high-risk hospital patients, but failed to identify a single one of the 46 patients who later committed suicide. The same conclusion was drawn by Kapur and House (1998).

Assessment of risk

The most obvious warning sign is a direct statement of intent. It cannot be repeated too often that there is no truth in the idea that people who talk of suicide do not do it. On the contrary, two-thirds of those who die by suicide have told someone of their intentions. However, a difficulty arises with people who talk repeatedly of suicide. In time their statements may no longer be taken seriously, being discounted as manipulation. However, some who repeatedly make such threats do eventually kill themselves. Just before the act, there may be a subtle change in their way of talking about dying, sometimes in the form of oblique hints instead of former more open statements.

Risk is assessed further by considering factors that have been shown to be associated with suicide (see page 611). Factors that point to greater risk include the following:

- marked hopelessness
- a history of *previous suicide attempts*: around 40–60% of those who die by suicide have made a previous attempt
- social isolation
- older age
- *depressive disorder*, especially with severe mood change with insomnia, anorexia, and weight loss
- *alcohol dependence*, especially with physical complications or severe social damage
- drug dependence
- *schizophrenia*, especially among young men with recurrent severe illness, depression, intellectual deterioration, or a history of a previous suicide attempt
- chronic painful illness
- epilepsy
- abnormal personality.

Completing the history

When these general risk factors have been assessed, the rest of the history should be evaluated. The interview should be conducted in an unhurried and sympathetic way that allows the patient to admit any despair or self-destructive intentions. It is usually appropriate to start by asking about current problems and the patient's reaction to them. Enquiries should cover losses, both personal (e.g. bereavement or divorce) and financial, as well as loss of status. Information about conflict with other people and social isolation should also be elicited. Physical illness should always be enquired after, particularly any painful condition in the elderly. (Some depressed suicides have unwarranted fears of physical illness as a feature of their psychiatric disorder.)

When assessing previous personality, it should be borne in mind that the patient's self-description may be coloured by depression. Whenever possible, another informant should be interviewed. The important points include mood swings, impulsive or aggressive tendencies, and attitudes towards religion and death.

Mental state examination

The assessment of mood should be particularly thorough, and cognitive function must not be overlooked. The interviewer should then assess suicidal intent. It is usually appropriate to begin by asking whether the patient thinks that life is too much for them, or whether they no longer want to go on. This first question can lead to more direct enquiries about thoughts of suicide, specific plans, and preparations for suicide, such as saving tablets. It is important to remember that severely depressed patients occasionally have homicidal ideas—they may believe that it would be an act of mercy to kill other people, often their partner or a child, to spare them intolerable suffering. Such homicidal ideas should always be taken extremely seriously.

Assessment of risk among inpatients

The suicide of a hospital inpatient is always of particular concern, and it is important to be able to identify those at risk. Unfortunately, the general guiding risk factors noted above are present in so many of those admitted that they differentiate poorly between degrees of risk.

The management of suicidal patients

General issues

Having assessed the suicidal risk, the clinician should make a treatment plan and try to persuade the patient to accept it. The first step is to decide whether the patient should be admitted to hospital or treated as an outpatient or day-patient. This decision depends on the intensity of the suicidal intention, the severity of any associated psychiatric illness, and the availability of social support outside hospital. If outpatient treatment is chosen, the patient should be given a telephone number so that they can obtain help at any time if they feel worse. Frustrated attempts to find help can be the last straw for a patient with suicidal inclinations.

If the immediate risk of suicide is judged to be high, inpatient care is likely to be required unless there is an effective crisis management team available, or reliable relatives who wish to care for the patient themselves, understand their responsibilities, and are able to fulfil them. Such a decision requires an exceptionally thorough knowledge of the patient and their problems, and of the relatives. It is best if in doubt to play safe. If hospital treatment is essential and the patient refuses it, admission under a compulsory order will be necessary. In most countries imminent suicide risk is sufficient for detention for observation, but the duration and conditions will vary. Readers should be aware of and follow the legal requirements of the jurisdiction in which they work.

Management in the community

The management of patients who have been identified as being at risk of suicide but do not require admission involves continuing assessment of the suicidal risk, and agreed plans for appropriate treatment and support (see Box 21.2). Where they are available and the patient consents to this, relatives or other carers should be involved. The key worker should liaise closely with other members of the community team to ensure that there will be a prompt and appropriate response if the patient or the carers ask for additional help. If medication is required—for example, to treat a depressive disorder—the drug that is least dangerous in overdose should be chosen. The choice should be discussed with the general practitioner, and small quantities should be prescribed. When appropriate, medication should be kept safely by the carer. Both patients and carers need to know how to obtain immediate help in an emergency.

Management in hospital

The obvious first requirement is to prevent patients from harming themselves. These arrangements require adequate staffing and a safe ward environment. A policy (see Box 21.3) should be agreed with all staff members when the patient is admitted.

Ward arrangements. Ward design should minimize the availability of means of self-harm. This includes preventing access to open windows and other places where jumping could lead to serious injury or death, removing ligature points from which hanging could take place (e.g. by boxing in pipework), preventing access to ward areas in which self-injury would be easier to enact, and removing potentially dangerous personal possessions such as razors and belts. If the risk is high, special nursing arrangements may be needed to ensure that the patient is never alone.

The *management policy* (see Box 21.3) should be:

- *reviewed* carefully at frequent intervals until the danger passes
- *explained to and agreed with each new shift of staff*, especially when the review has led to changes in the plan
- *explained to and, if possible, agreed with the patient.* If the patient does not agree to necessary parts of the plan, the reasons for these should be carefully explained. If the patient still refuses to collaborate, and the risk is high, compulsory treatment may be required.

If intensive supervision is needed for more than a few days, the patient may become irritated by it and try to

> ### Box 21.2 Care of the potentially suicidal patient in the community
>
> Full assessment of patient and proposed carers
> Organization of adequate social support
> Regular review of the suicide risk and the arrangements
> Safe psychiatric medications given in adequate dosage using less toxic drugs
> Small prescriptions
> Involvement of relatives in the safe storage of tablets
> Arrangements for immediate access to extra help for patient and carers

---

Box 21.3 Care of the suicidal patient in hospital

General requirements

Safe ward environment

An adequate number of well-trained staff

Good working relationships among staff, and between staff and patients

Agreed policies for the observation, assessment, and review of patients

On admission

Assess risk

Agree the level of observation

Remove any objects that might be used for suicide

Discuss and agree plans with the patient

Agree a policy for visitors (number, duration of visit, and what they need to know)

During admission

Regular review of risk and plans

Agreed plans for the level of supervision

Clear communication of assessments and plans between staff, especially when shifts change

Agree action to be taken if the patient leaves the ward without notice or permission

At discharge

Agree date and plan for aftercare in advance of discharge

Discuss and agree the plan with the patient and those involved in their care

Prescribe in adequate but non-dangerous amounts

Arrange follow-up, and agree action to be taken if the patient does not attend

---

evade it. Staff should anticipate this, ensure that treatment of any associated mental illness is not delayed, and support the patient intensively while waiting for the treatment to have an effect. However determined the patient is to die, there is usually some small remaining wish to go on living. If the staff adopt a caring and hopeful attitude, those remaining positive feelings can be encouraged, generating a more positive view of the future. The patient can then be helped to see how an apparently overwhelming accumulation of problems can be dealt with one by one.

The risk of suicide is higher during periods of home leave arranged to test readiness for discharge. It is also greater during the period immediately before discharge and in the first few weeks after discharge (see page 613). Therefore the discharge plan should include early reassessment, effective psychological and social support, and rapid response to any need for extra help. Plans for leave and for discharge should be discussed with the patient and their concerns elicited. If appropriate, the plans should be modified.

However carefully patients are cared for, suicide will happen, despite all the efforts of the staff. The doctor then has an important role in supporting others, particularly nurses who have come to know the patient particularly well. Although it is essential to review every suicide carefully to determine whether useful lessons can be learned, this process should never become a search for a scapegoat.

The relatives

When a patient has died by suicide, the relatives require not only the support that is appropriate for any bereaved person, but also help with the common responses of anger, guilt, and a feeling that they could have done more to prevent the death. Barraclough and Shepherd (1976) found that relatives usually reported that the police conducted their enquiries in a considerate way, but that the public inquest was very distressing. Subsequent newspaper publicity caused further grief, reactivating the events surrounding the death and increasing feelings of stigma. Sympathetic listening, explanation, and counselling are likely to help relatives with these difficulties. Anger is often a part of this grief, and should be met by a willingness to listen and to provide full information. Wertheimer (2001) has reviewed the consequences of suicide for relatives.

Suicide prevention

In population terms, suicide is a rare event. In Western Europe it accounts for approximately one to two deaths per 10,000 people per year. Therefore a controlled trial of an intervention to reduce suicide would require many thousands of participants. Such trials have not been conducted. However, there is some evidence from observational studies to suggest measures that could affect the rate of suicide in the population (see Box 21.4). Such possible measures will be discussed next. For further information, see Hawton (2000b).

Service changes

Educating primary care physicians. The effectiveness of interventions based in primary care is equivocal. The Gotland study evaluated the impact of teaching all the island's GPs about the diagnosis and treatment of affective disorder. The suicide rate fell significantly below both the long-term suicide trend, but 3 years after the project ended it had returned almost to baseline values (Rutz *et al.*, 1992). The researchers concluded that the programme had been effective, but that it would need to be repeated every 2 years to have long-term benefits, and that it appeared to benefit only females. A similar finding was demonstrated in Hungary (Szanto *et al.*, 2007).

Improving psychiatric services. Earlier recognition and better treatment of the psychiatric disorders might be expected to reduce suicide rates. However, it has proved difficult to demonstrate this empirically.

Targeting high-risk groups. The usual clinical approach is to provide additional help for high-risk groups, such as patients who have recently received inpatient psychiatric treatment and those who have recently deliberately harmed themselves. (Crisis services are discussed below.)

Long-term medication. Although the continued prescribing of antidepressants during the period following an episode of depression reduces the risk of a subsequent episode of depression, a reduction in suicidal behaviour has not been demonstrated. However, there is accumulating evidence that lithium prophylaxis reduces suicide rates (Cipriani *et al.*, 2013), and some evidence that clozapine may reduce suicide attempts among people with schizophrenia or schizoaffective disorder (see page 296).

Prescribing less toxic antidepressants. Selective serotonin reuptake inhibitors (SSRIs) are less toxic in overdose than tricyclic antidepressants. On the other hand, SSRIs have been reported to cause the emergence or worsening of suicidal ideas in young people, possibly because they can cause agitation and insomnia initially. Although it is not possible to reach a decisive conclusion on the basis of the available evidence, it seems that the overall risk of suicide associated with SSRIs is similar to that with tricyclic antidepressants (Cipriani *et al.*, 2005). A US study demonstrated an increased rate of suicide attempts in the month *before* antidepressant medication was prescribed (Simon *et al.*, 2006). In addition, there is some evidence from epidemiological studies that increased prescribing of less toxic antidepressants such as SSRIs is associated with a decrease in population suicide rates, although this has been contested (Isacsson *et al.*, 2010). Until the evidence is conclusive, the most appropriate drug should be decided for individual patients, and their progress monitored and support provided during the first few weeks of treatment.

Counselling services. In the UK, the best known service for people who are suicidal is the Samaritan organization, which was founded in London in 1953 by the Reverend Chad Varah. People who are in despair are encouraged to contact a widely publicized telephone number. The help that is offered ('befriending') is provided by nonprofessional volunteers, who have been trained to listen sympathetically without attempting to take on tasks that are in the province of a professional. It is often quoted that people who telephone the Samaritans have a higher suicide rate in the ensuing year than the general population (Barraclough and Shea, 1970). This finding is difficult to interpret. Undoubtedly the Samaritans attracts people at risk for suicide, and it remains unclear how far the help that is offered may be beneficial. Even if this is so, the Samaritans provide valuable support for many lonely and despairing people.

Box 21.4 Suicide prevention

Better and more accessible psychiatric services
Restriction of the means of suicide
Encouragement of responsible media reporting
Educational programmes
Improved care for high-risk groups
Crisis centres and telephone 'hotlines'

Population strategies

Reducing the availability of methods of suicide

The ease with which people can access lethal methods of self-harm may affect the rate of suicide using those methods, and may have some effect on suicide rates in general. If the available methods are less harmful, more people will be resuscitated. No matter what changes are made, however, people who are determined to kill themselves can eventually find the means to do so. Several changes have been made.

Detoxification of gas. In Britain, between 1948 and 1950, poisoning by domestic coal gas accounted for 40% of reported suicides among men and 60% of those among women. Following the introduction of less toxic North Sea gas, the number of suicides using this method decreased dramatically, and the national rate of suicide also fell. Kreitman (1976) argued that the removal of coal gas was responsible for this change, but some care is indicated as rates were falling worldwide.

Detoxification of car exhaust fumes. The fitting of catalytic converters to motor vehicles to reduce the toxicity of car exhaust fumes appears to have reduced the number of deaths using this method (Routley, 2007).

Restricting amounts of analgesics. In the UK, government legislation has limited the amount of paracetamol, salicylates, and their compounds that an individual can buy at one time. There is evidence that this legislation has reduced suicides from overdoses of these drugs (Hawton *et al.*, 2004b).

Removing and preventing access to hazards. In hospital wards and police and prison cells, ligature points from which hanging could take place should be removed or enclosed (see page 617). Physical barriers on bridges, train platforms, and other potentially dangerous places may reduce the number of suicides at these places (Bennewith *et al.*, 2007). Campaigns are currently under way to restrict access to lethal pesticides that are used in rural communities in the developing world (Mishara, 2007).

Improving access to mental health care. A review of the implementation of the national suicide strategy has demonstrated a significant reduction in suicides in those known to mental health services by the introduction of 24-hour crisis services (While *et al.*, 2012).

Other measures

More responsible media reporting. Sometimes people copy methods of suicide that have received widespread media coverage. For this and other reasons, reporters and editors have been encouraged to report suicide responsibly. In 2006, following a submission from the Samaritans, the Press Complaints Commission added a new subclause to the section 'Intrusion into Grief and Shock', which now states that 'when reporting a suicide, care should be taken to avoid excessive detail about the method used' (Press Complaints Commission, 2007).

Social policy. Given the repeatedly demonstrated association between unemployment and suicide, it has been argued that policies aimed at reducing rates of unemployment may help to reduce the rate of suicide (Lewis *et al.*, 1997). Factors such as increasing social isolation may also need to be tackled in this way. Although the means of fulfilling such strategies are far from clear, and it would be difficult to evaluate their effectiveness, such calls remind us of the relationship between social policy and health.

Public education. Campaigns to educate the public about mental illness and its treatment have included outreach to schools, which has involved teaching about solving problems and seeking help when distressed. The value of such approaches is uncertain. Some screening has been tried in schools but suffers from an excessive false-positive rate (Gould *et al.*, 2005).

Deliberate self-harm

Until the 1950s, little distinction was made between people who killed themselves and those who survived after an apparent suicidal act. In the UK, Stengel (1952) was the first to identify epidemiological differences between the two groups. He proposed the term 'attempted suicide' to describe self-injury that the person could not be sure to survive. Subsequent studies of the motivation for such episodes found that the intention of many of the survivors had not been to die. As a result, several terms—*deliberate self-poisoning, parasuicide,* and *deliberate self-harm*—were introduced to describe episodes of intentional self-harm that did not lead to death and may or may not have been motivated by a desire to die (see Box 21.5). Kreitman (1977) defined this behaviour as 'a non-fatal act in which an individual deliberately causes self-injury or ingests a substance in excess of any prescribed or generally recognized dosage.' The Royal College of Psychiatrists encourages the use of the term 'self-harm', and 'non-suicidal self-injury' (NSSI) has also been proposed. In this chapter, the term 'deliberate self-harm' (DSH) will be used to describe such incidents.

Acts that end in suicide and acts of DSH overlap one another. Some people who had no intention of dying succumb to the unintended effects of an overdose. Others who intended to die are revived. Importantly, many people were ambivalent at the time of the act, uncertain whether they wished to die or to survive. It should be remembered that, among people who have been involved in DSH, the suicide rate in the subsequent 12 months is about 100 times greater than in the general population. It remains high for many years, with over 5% committing suicide within 9 years (Owens *et al.*, 2002). Therefore DSH should not be regarded lightly.

The act of deliberate self-harm

Methods of deliberate self-poisoning

In the UK, about 90% of the cases of DSH that are referred to general hospitals involve a drug overdose, and most of them present no serious threat to life. The type of drug used varies somewhat with age, local prescription practices, and the availability of drugs. The most commonly used drugs are the non-opiate analgesics, such as paracetamol and aspirin. Paracetamol is particularly dangerous because it damages the liver and may lead to the delayed death of patients who had not intended to die. It is particularly worrying that younger patients, who are usually unaware of these serious risks,

often take this drug. Antidepressants (both tricyclics and SSRIs) are taken in about 25% of episodes. About 50% of people consume alcohol in the 6 hours before the act (Hawton *et al.*, 2007).

Methods of deliberate self-injury

Deliberate self-injury accounts for about 10% of all DSH presenting to general hospitals in the UK. The commonest method of self-injury is laceration, usually cutting of the forearms or wrists; it accounts for about 80% of the self-injuries that are referred to a general hospital. (Self-laceration is discussed further below.) Other forms of self-injury include jumping from a height or in front of a train or motor vehicle, shooting, and drowning. These violent acts occur mainly among older people who intended to die (Harwood and Jacoby, 2000).

Deliberate self-laceration

There are three forms of deliberate self-laceration:

1. Deep and dangerous wounds inflicted with serious suicidal intent, more often by men.

2. Self-mutilation by schizophrenic patients (sometimes in response to hallucinatory voices) or people with severe learning difficulties.

3. Superficial wounds that do not endanger life, more often inflicted by women.

Only the last group will be described here.

Usually, the act of laceration is preceded by increasing tension and irritability, which diminish afterwards.

Box 21.5 Terms for non-fatal self-inflicted harm

Attempted suicide

Used widely (especially in North America) for episodes where there was at least some suicidal intent, or sometimes without reference to intent. Repetitive bodily harm may be excluded.

Deliberate* self-harm

Used in UK for all episodes survived, regardless of intent. North American usage refers to episodes of bodily harm without suicidal intent, especially if repetitive. Usually excludes overdoses and methods of high lethality.

Parasuicide

Episodes survived, with or without suicidal intent (especially in Europe) or episodes without intent. Repetitive bodily harm may be excluded.

Self-poisoning or self-injury

Self-harm by these methods regardless of suicidal intent.

Self-mutilation

Serious bodily mutilation (such as enucleation of eye) without suicidal intent. Repetitive superficial bodily harm without suicidal intent (synonymous with North American term 'deliberate self-harm'). Also known as self-injurious behaviour, self-wounding.

Sometimes the term is used to describe both the above meanings and also stereotypical self-harm in intellectually disabled people.

*The adjective 'deliberate' is now not favoured by patients in the UK.

Reproduced from The Lancet, 366(9495), Skegg K, Self-harm, pp. 1471–83, Copyright (2005), with permission from Elsevier.

After the act, the patient often feels shame and disgust. Some of these individuals report that they lacerated themselves while in a state of detachment from their surroundings, and that they experienced little or no pain. The lacerations are usually multiple, made with glass or a razor blade, and inflicted on the forearms or wrists. Some also injure themselves in other ways (e.g. by burning with cigarettes, or inflicting bruises).

Self-cutters who attend hospital are more often men (Hawton *et al.*, 2004c). People who cut themselves superficially do not always seek help from the medical services, and many of these people are young females, often with problems of low self-esteem, and sometimes impulsive or aggressive behaviour, unstable moods, difficulty in interpersonal relationships, and problems with alcohol and drug misuse.

The epidemiology of deliberate self-harm

DSH is the main risk factor for completed suicide. Although there is no national DSH register, there are several local registers that track its incidence. In the early 1960s, a substantial increase in DSH began in most western countries. In the UK, the rates varied during the 1970s and 1980s and increased again through the 1990s. A national suicide prevention strategy in 2002 aimed to reduce suicide by 20% by 2010. DSH has been falling during this decade, particularly in males, and this parallels falling suicide rates (Bergen *et al.*, 2010). Current estimates of the rate of DSH in the UK suggest a figure of about 4 per 1000 per year. The rates in most European countries are lower (see Kerkhof, 2000), and there are remarkable international variations which defy a simple explanation (Skegg, 2005).

Variations according to personal characteristics

DSH is more common among younger people, with the rates declining sharply in middle age (see Figure 21.2). The Oxford Suicide Centre report for 2013 demonstrates the persistence of this distribution (Hawton *et al.*, 2013). Over recent years, the proportion of men presenting following DSH has risen. In the 1960s and 1970s the female-to-male ratio was about 2:1, whereas recent studies show much smaller differences. The peak age for men is older than that for women. For both sexes, rates are very low under the age of 12 years. DSH is more prevalent in those of lower socioeconomic status and who live in more deprived areas. Rates are higher for both men and women among the divorced, and among teenage

wives, and younger single men and women (Hawton *et al.*, 2003b).

Rates of DSH in the elderly have changed little in recent years. Their characteristics seem to be more similar to those of individuals who kill themselves than of younger people who harm themselves deliberately (Harwood and Jacoby, 2000).

Causes of deliberate self-harm

Precipitating factors

People who harm themselves deliberately report more *stressful life events*, especially quarrels with a partner, girlfriend, or boyfriend.

Predisposing factors

Familial and developmental factors may predispose to DSH. These have been studied in great detail, often drawing on large samples (Skegg, 2005). The whole range of adverse early circumstances (abuse, parental divorce, parental discord, or mental illness) is associated with an increased risk, particularly in adolescents and young patients (Beautrais, 2000; Brent *et al.*, 2002).

Economic and social environment. Rates of DSH are higher among the unemployed. However, unemployment is related to other social factors associated with DSH, such as financial difficulties, and it is difficult to determine whether unemployment is a direct cause. Rates of DSH are also higher in areas of socioeconomic deprivation (Hawton *et al.*, 2001).

Personality disorder. In the UK (Haw *et al.*, 2001) and other countries (e.g. Suominen *et al.*, 1996), personality disorder is identified in almost 50% of patients who deliberately self-harm. Borderline personality disorder has been reported to be common, but other studies have found anxious, anankastic (obsessional), and paranoid personality disorders more frequently (Haw *et al.*, 2001). Impulsiveness, and poor skills in solving interpersonal problems, may also predispose to DSH.

Ill health. A background of poor physical health is common.

Sociological and cultural factors. Rates of self-harm vary enormously between different cultures, probably reflecting societal attitudes towards such behaviour (Schmidtke *et al.*, 1996). Echoing Durkheim's groundbreaking study, a professed religious faith does appear to reduce the risk of self-harm, as it does with suicide (Statham *et al.*, 1998; Dervic *et al.*, 2004). Sexual orientation, particularly homosexuality in men, has been associated with higher rates (Skegg *et al.*, 2003), though whether this is still so is not clear.

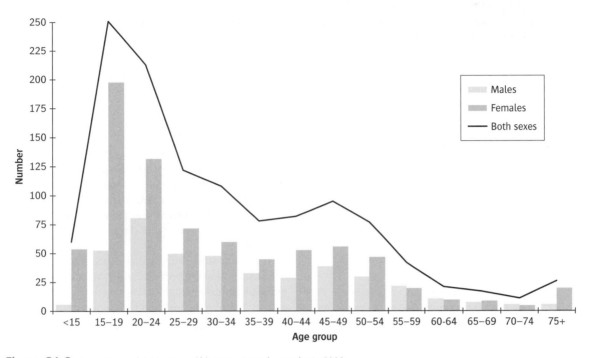

Figure 21.2 Age groups of deliberate self-harm patients by gender in 2002.

Reproduced from Self-harm in Oxford 2014, Centre for Suicide Research, Department of Psychiatry, University of Oxford, by permission of Professor KE Hawton, Oxford University, UK.

Psychiatric disorder

It used to be held that, with the exception of adjustment disorder, psychiatric disorder was uncommon among people who harmed themselves deliberately. However, if standardized assessments are used, psychiatric disorder has been detected in about 90% of patients who DSH who are seen in hospital (Suominen *et al.*, 1996; Haw *et al.*, 2001). Even allowing for the lower thresholds of standardized instruments this does indicate a need for vigilance. Depressive disorder is the most frequent diagnosis in both sexes, followed by alcohol and drug abuse in men, and anxiety disorders in women. Comorbidity is frequent, especially between psychiatric disorder and personality disorder.

Motivation and deliberate self-harm

The motives for DSH are usually mixed and often difficult to identify with certainty. Even when patients know their own motives, they may try to hide them from other people. For example, people who have taken an

overdose in response to feelings of frustration and anger may feel ashamed and say instead that they wished to die. Conversely, people who truly intended to kill themselves may deny it with the intention of repeating it. For this reason, when individuals are assessed, more emphasis should be placed on a common-sense evaluation of their actions leading up to self-harm than on their subsequent accounts of their motives.

Useful information has, however, been obtained by questioning groups of patients about their motives., A study in 13 European countries found similar reported motives in all of the study sites listed in Box 21.6 (Hjelmeland *et al.*, 2002). Only a few patients stated that the act was premeditated. About 25% said that they wished to die. Some stated that they were uncertain whether they wanted to die or not, others that they were leaving it to 'fate' to decide, and yet others that they were seeking a temporary escape. Another group admitted that they were trying to influence someone—for example, that they were seeking to make a relative feel guilty for having failed them in some way. This motive of influencing other people was first emphasized by Stengel and Cook (1958), who wrote that these people hoped to call forth 'action from the human environment'. This behaviour has since been referred to as 'a cry for help'. Although some acts of DSH result in increased help for the patient, others may arouse resentment, particularly when they are repeated, prompting 'a cry for help' to be rephrased as 'a cry of pain' (Williams and Pollock, 2000).

The outcome of deliberate self-harm

Repetition of self-harm

In the weeks after DSH, many patients report changes for the better. Those with psychiatric symptoms often report that they have become less intense. This improvement may result from help provided by professionals, or from improvements in the person's relationships, attitudes, and behaviour. Some people do not improve and harm themselves again, in some cases fatally. A systematic review of 90 studies (Owens *et al.*, 2002) concluded that, among people who have engaged in DSH:

- about one in six repeats the DSH within 1 year
- about one in four repeats the DSH within 4 years.

Factors associated with repetition of attempted suicide are listed in Box 21.7.

Suicide following deliberate self-harm

People who have intentionally harmed themselves have a much increased risk of later suicide. The same systematic review (Owens *et al.*, 2002) concluded that among these people:

- between 1 in 200 and 1 in 40 commit suicide within 1 year
- about 1 in 15 commits suicide within 9 years or more.

These risks are compiled from several countries, so they cannot be compared directly with the general population rate of about 1 in 10,000 people per annum in the UK. Nevertheless, the risk is clearly greatly increased.

Among people who deliberately harm themselves, the risk of eventual suicide is even greater among those who are older, male, depressed, or alcohol-dependent. Use of a dangerous or violent method also indicates a high risk. However, a non-dangerous method of self-harm does not necessarily indicate a low risk of subsequent suicide, partly because the patient may have incomplete knowledge of the dangerousness of the available methods (see Box 21.8).

It is more difficult to predict which patients will die by suicide following previous self-harm because the rate of suicide, although higher than that in the general population, is still quite low, and the predictive factors have low specificity.

Results of treatment after deliberate self-harm

Although randomized controlled studies have shown decreases in psychopathology and improvements in

> **Box 21.8 Risk factors for suicide after self-harm**
>
> Older age
> Male sex
> Past psychiatric care
> Psychiatric disorder
> Social isolation
> Repeated self-harm
> Avoiding discovery at time of self-harm
> Medically severe self-harm
> Strong suicidal intent
> Substance misuse (especially in young people)
> Hopelessness
> Poor physical health
>
> Reproduced from The Lancet, 366(9495), Skegg K, Self-harm, pp. 1471–83, Copyright (2005), with permission from Elsevier.

social problems after various treatments, there is less evidence that treatment prevents the repetition of DSH. One reason for this lack of evidence is that several kinds of treatment have been investigated, and the numbers in most studies have been rather low. Hawton conducted a meta-analysis of 20 randomized controlled trials (of 10 different interventions), with repetition of DSH as an outcome measure (Hawton, 2005). His conclusions were as follows.

- A trend towards greater reduction of repetition was found for problem-solving therapies, although this was only statistically significant in one out of six randomized controlled trials. One study that used a self-help manual found no benefit.
- Brief psychodynamic interpersonal therapy has been shown in one randomized controlled trial to reduce self-reported attempts at self-harm more than treatment as usual (Guthrie *et al.*, 2001).
- For patients with borderline personality disorder, rates of repetition were lower with dialectical behaviour therapy than with standard aftercare (based on a single trial).
- The provision of emergency contact cards (allowing immediate access to help) showed some benefits, but not in all studies and probably only for first-attenders. There was some suggestion that such cards may be detrimental for repeat attenders.

- The provision of increased intensity of care with outreach showed modest benefit, but only for the home visit/outreach component.

An Australian study showed some benefit, in terms of decreased repetition rates, from sending a series of postcards to patients over a 12-month period after an episode of self-harm (Carter *et al.*, 2007). However, this was not confirmed by a similar study in New Zealand (Beautrais *et al.*, 2010).

Special groups

Mothers of young children

Mothers of young children require special consideration because of the known association between DSH and child abuse. It is important to ask about the mother's feelings towards her children, and to enquire about their welfare. In the UK, information about the children can usually be obtained from the general practitioner, who may ask their health visitor to investigate the case. Caring for young children can put strains on already shaky relationships, and there is evidence of an increased risk of partner violence against vulnerable young mothers (Vaughn *et al.*, 2015).

Children and adolescents

DSH among children and adolescents increased in the 1990s in many parts of the developed world. It is difficult to obtain the exact rates because many of these acts are minor drug overdoses or self-injuries that do not reach the medical services (Hawton *et al.*, 2002). It is generally agreed that DSH is rare among preschool children, and becomes increasingly common after the age of 12 years. Except in the youngest age groups, it is more common among girls.

Methods. Drug overdose is the most common method among those attending hospital. Self-cutting is common, especially among females, although it less often results in attendance at hospital. More dangerous forms of self-injury are more frequent among males (Hawton *et al.*, 2003c).

Motivation. It is difficult to determine the motivation for self-harm in young children, especially as a clear concept of death is not usually developed until around the age of 12 years. It is probable that only a few younger children have any serious suicidal intent. Their motivation may be more often to communicate distress, to escape from stress, or to influence other people. Epidemics of DSH occasionally occur as a result of imitative behaviour among adolescents (de Wilde, 2000).

Causes. DSH in adolescents is associated with family breakdown, familial psychiatric disorder, and child abuse, or simply not feeling 'heard' or validated within the family environment (Sinclair and Green, 2005). It is often precipitated by social problems—for younger adolescents most often family problems, for older ones difficulties with boyfriends or girlfriends, and for both age groups problems with schoolwork. Among adolescents it is also associated with alcohol and drug misuse (especially among males), violence and being the victim

of violence, mood disorder, and personality disorder (Hawton *et al.*, 2003c).

Outcome. For most children and adolescents, the outcome of DSH is relatively good, but a significant minority continue to have social and psychiatric problems, and to repeat acts of DSH. A poor outcome is associated with poor psychosocial adjustment, a history of previous DSH, and severe family problems.

Management.

When children or adolescents harm themselves, it is better for them to be assessed by child and adolescent psychiatrists rather than members of the adult DSH service. Treatment usually involves the family, and is directed to the causal problems and to the coping skills of the child or adolescent.

The management of deliberate self-harm

The organization of services

The care of patients with DSH involves a variety of services, including primary care teams, ambulance services, emergency department staff, and social services. All of these staff require training to enable them to respond appropriately and to make the necessary decisions, including how to assess immediate risk, to obtain informed consent, and to assess capacity to consent and in what circumstances necessary care can be given without consent. The organization of the medical and surgical response to these patients is beyond the scope of this book; for such information, see National Institute for Clinical Excellence (2004b).

Arrangements for psychosocial assessment vary and a debate has long persisted about who should assess these patients. Whatever arrangement is made, it is important to ensure that all patients do receive a psychosocial assessment as well as an assessment of the medical effects of the self-harm (see below). Each hospital site should have a code of practice detailing the arrangements for psychosocial assessment agreed by general medical and psychiatric services and known to those who work there.

Provision should be available for the special needs of patients from ethnic minorities. Children and adolescents should, whenever possible, be assessed by staff who have been trained in the assessment and care of young people and who are familiar with the problems of confidentiality and consent that can arise in such cases. If possible, patients over the age of 65 years should be assessed by staff who are familiar with the special

problems of the elderly, and who are aware of the greater risk of completed suicide in this age group.

The assessment of patients after deliberate self-harm

General aims

Assessment is concerned with three main issues:

1. The immediate risks of suicide.
2. The subsequent risks of further DSH.
3. Current medical or social problems.

The assessment should be conducted in a way that encourages patients to undertake a constructive review of their problems and of the ways in which they could deal with them themselves. It is important to encourage self-help, because many of these people are unwilling to be seen again by a psychiatrist.

Usually the assessment has to be carried out in an accident and emergency department or a ward in a general hospital, where there may be little privacy. Whenever possible, the interview should be conducted in a side room so that it will not be overheard or interrupted. If the patient has taken an overdose, the interviewer should first make sure that they have recovered sufficiently to be able to give a satisfactory history. If consciousness is still impaired, the interview should be delayed. Information should also be obtained from relatives or friends, the family doctor, and any other person (such as a social worker) who is already attempting to help the patient. Wide enquiry is important, as sometimes information from other sources may differ substantially from the account given by the patient. For a review of general hospital assessment, see Hawton (2000b).

Specific enquiries

The interview should address five questions.

1. What were the patient's intentions when they harmed themselves?
2. Do they now intend to die?
3. What are their current problems?
4. Is there a psychiatric disorder?
5. What helpful resources are available?

Each of these questions will now be considered in turn.

What were the patient's intentions when they harmed themselves?

Patients sometimes misrepresent their intentions. For this reason the interviewer should reconstruct, as fully as possible, the events that led up to the act of self-harm to find the answers to five subsidiary questions.

- *Was the act planned or carried out on impulse?* The longer and more carefully the plans have been made, the greater is the risk of a fatal repetition.
- *Were precautions taken against being found?* The more thorough the precautions were, the greater is the risk of a further fatal overdose. Of course, events do not always take place as the patient expected—for example, a partner may arrive home earlier than usual so that the patient is discovered alive. In such circumstances it is the patient's reasonable expectations that are of importance in predicting the future risk.
- *Did the patient seek help?* Serious intent can be inferred if there were no attempts to obtain help after the act.
- *Was the method thought to be dangerous?* If drugs were used, what were they and what amount was taken? Did the patient take all of the drugs available? If self-injury was used, what form did it take? Not only should the actual dangerousness of the method be assessed, but also the dangerousness anticipated by the patient, which may be inaccurate. For example, some people wrongly believe that paracetamol overdoses are harmless, or that benzodiazepines are dangerous.
- *Was there a 'final act'* (e.g. writing a suicide note or making a will)? If so, the risk of a further fatal attempt is greater.

By reviewing the answers to these questions, the interviewer can form a judgement of the patient's intentions at the time of the act (see Box 21.9).

Do they now intend to die?

The interviewer should ask directly whether the patient is pleased to have recovered or wishes that they had died. If the act suggested serious suicidal intent and if the patient now denies such intent, the interviewer should try to find out by tactful questioning whether there has been a genuine change of resolve.

What are their current problems?

Many patients will have experienced a mounting series of difficulties in the weeks or months leading up to the act. Some of these difficulties may have been resolved by the time that they are interviewed, sometimes as a result of the act of self-harm—for example, a partner who had threatened to leave the patient may have decided to stay. The more serious the problems that remain, the greater is the risk of a fatal repetition. This risk is particularly strong if the problems include loneliness or ill health. The review of problems should be systematic and should cover the following:

- intimate relationships with the partner or another person
- relationships with children and other relatives
- employment, finances, and housing
- legal problems
- social isolation, bereavement, and other losses
- physical health.

Drug and alcohol problems can be considered either at this stage of the assessment or later when the psychiatric state is reviewed.

Is there a psychiatric disorder?

It should be possible to answer this question from the history and from a brief but systematic examination of the mental state. Particular attention should be directed to depressive disorder, alcoholism, anxiety disorder, and personality disorder. Schizophrenia and dementia should also be considered, although they will be found less often. Adjustment disorders are diagnosed in many individuals in response to major life changes and stresses (e.g. bereavement, relationship break-up, migration). The presence of an obvious precipitating event does not rule out the presence of a psychiatric disorder.

What helpful resources are available?

These include capacity to solve problems, material resources, and the help that others are likely to provide. The best guide to patients' abilities to solve future problems is their record of dealing with difficulties in the past—for example, the loss of a job or a broken relationship. The availability of help should be assessed by asking about friends and confidants, and about any support the patient is receiving or can be expected to receive from the general practitioner, social workers, or voluntary agencies.

Is there a continuing risk of suicide?

The interviewer now has the information required to answer this important question. The answers to the first five questions outlined above are reviewed:

- Did the patient originally intend to die?
- Do they intend to do so now?
- Are the problems that provoked the act still present?
- Is there a psychiatric disorder?
- Is additional support available, and is the patient likely to accept it?

Having reviewed the answers to these questions, the interviewer compares the patient's characteristics with those that are found in people who have died by suicide. These characteristics are summarized in Box 21.9.

Is there a risk of further non-fatal self-harm?

The predictive factors are summarized in Box 21.7. All of the points should be considered before deciding on the risk.

What treatment is required and will the patient agree to it?

If the risk of suicide is judged to be high, the procedures are those outlined in the first part of this chapter (see page 617). Around 5–10% of patients who DSH require admission to a psychiatric unit; most need treatment for depression or alcoholism, and a few for schizophrenia. Some need a period of respite from overwhelming stress.

If admission to hospital is not indicated, a plan of management has to be agreed with the patient and any potential carers. If the patient refuses the offer of help, their care should be discussed with the general practitioner before they are allowed to return home (see below and Box 21.10). For most patients it is useful to provide an emergency telephone number that allows immediate

> ### Box 21.9 Factors that suggest high suicidal intent
>
> Act carried out in isolation
>
> Act timed so that intervention is unlikely
>
> Precautions taken to avoid discovery
>
> Preparations made in anticipation of death (e.g. making a will, organizing insurance)
>
> Preparations made for the act (e.g. purchasing the means of suicide, saving up tablets)
>
> Communicating intent to others beforehand
>
> Extensive premeditation
>
> Leaving a note
>
> Not alerting potential helpers after the act
>
> Admission of suicidal intent
>
> Reproduced from Hawton K and Taylor T, Treatment of suicide attempters and prevention of suicide and attempted suicide. In: Gelder MG, Andreasen NC, López-Ibor JJ Jr and Geddes JR (eds), The New Oxford Textbook of Psychiatry, Copyright (2009), with permission from Oxford University Press.

access to advice or an urgent appointment should there be a further crisis.

Management after the assessment

Patients who have harmed themselves are often reluctant to accept further help, and it is important to conduct the assessment interview in a way that fosters a therapeutic relationship. Plans should be discussed with the patient, and, if they are not agreed, an alternative plan that is mutually acceptable should be negotiated. Patients' needs fall into three groups:

1. A small minority need admission to a psychiatric unit for treatment.
2. About one-third have a psychiatric disorder that requires treatment in primary care, or from a psychiatric team in the community.
3. The remainder need help with various psychosocial problems, and assistance with improving their ways of coping with stressors. This help is needed even when the risk of immediate suicide or non-fatal repetition is low, as continuing problems

> **Box 21.10 Patients who harm themselves and refuse treatment**
>
> Note that there are international differences in laws and practices.
> - The most senior experienced doctor available should see the patient and discuss the proposed treatment, the alternatives, and the patient's concerns. It is often helpful to involve the patient's relatives or close friends. Sympathetic, patient discussion of the person's concerns is often followed by consent.
> - A patient who has harmed himself or herself but is alert and conscious should be presumed to have the mental capacity to refuse medical advice unless shown otherwise. This capacity should be assessed (see page 78, Box 4.2) as soon as possible. All staff should be able to perform this assessment, but, where possible, incapacity should be confirmed by a psychiatrist. If appropriate, assessment for compulsory treatment should be arranged.
> - When a patient is assessed as mentally incapable (e.g. because of persistent intoxicating effects of overdose), staff have a responsibility under common law to act in that person's best interests. This may include taking the patient to hospital, keeping them there for assessment, and giving immediate life-saving treatment.
> - Staff should remember that mental capacity may change over time, and attempts should be made to explain each new procedure or treatment and to obtain consent before it is carried out.
> - When, after full discussion, a competent patient continues to refuse to consent and there are no grounds for compulsory treatment, a further attempt should be made to find an acceptable alternative plan. If the attempt does not succeed, the consequences of the decision should be explained clearly, and the discussions recorded fully in the notes. If the patient insists on leaving, they have to be allowed to go, but they should be encouraged to return, and given an emergency contact number and options for further treatment. The situation should be discussed as soon as possible with the patient's general practitioner.
> - It is generally appropriate to attempt to contact the patient on the following day and repeat the offer of help. The case should be discussed with the general practitioner to decide who should make the contact.
>
> For further guidance, see National Institute for Clinical Excellence (2004b).

increase the risk of later repetition. Apart from practical help, problem-solving is usually the best approach, starting with the problems identified during the assessment interview. Unfortunately, such help is often refused.

The general principles of care are summarized in Box 21.11. If the episode of self-harm is associated with problems in a specific interpersonal relationship, it is often helpful to interview the other person involved if the patient agrees, first alone and then together with the patient. This joint interview can lead to an improved dialogue between the couple, and this may help to decrease the risk of acute repetition.

Some special problems of management

Patients who refuse assessment

Patients who refuse to be interviewed, or who seek to discharge themselves, have very high rates of repetition (Crawford and Wessely, 1998). It is essential to gather as much information as possible from other sources before allowing the patient to leave. The problem should be discussed with the general practitioner and community mental health team if they are involved. If the risk of suicide is judged to be high, it may be necessary to keep the patient until an assessment is made for detention under a compulsory order.

Frequent repeaters

Some patients take overdoses repeatedly at times of stress. Often the behaviour seems intended to reduce tension or gain attention. However, when overdoses are taken repeatedly, relatives often become unsympathetic or even overtly hostile, and staff of hospital emergency departments may feel frustrated. These patients usually have a personality disorder and many insoluble social problems. Unfortunately, neither counselling nor intensive psychotherapy is usually effective. All of those involved in the patient's management should agree a care plan which should seek to reward constructive behaviour. An opportunity for continuing support by one individual should be arranged. However, whatever

> ### Box 21.11 General principles of care after self-harm
>
> - Monitor patient for further suicidal or self-harm thoughts
> - Identify support available in a crisis
> - Come to a shared understanding of the meaning of the behaviour and the patient's needs
> - Treat psychiatric illness vigorously
> - Attend to substance abuse
> - Help patient to identify and work towards solving problems
>
> - Enlist support of family and friends where possible
> - Encourage adaptive expression of emotion
> - Avoid prescribing quantities of medication that could be lethal in overdose
> - Assertive follow-up in an empathic relationship
> - Affirm the values of hope and of caring for oneself
>
> Reproduced from The Lancet, 366(9495), Skegg K, Self-harm, pp. 1471–83, Copyright (2005), with permission from Elsevier.

help is arranged, the risk of eventual death by suicide is high. Since the UK government initiative to provide better care for personality disordered patients (National Institute for Mental Health in England [NIMHE], 2003), most services have established dedicated services for those with borderline personality disorders (Chapter 15), which can often be of particular value to these patients if they will accept referral.

Repeated self-cutting

The management of self-laceration presents many problems. Patients often have difficulty in expressing their feelings in words, so formal psychotherapy may not be helpful. Simple efforts to gain the patient's confidence and increase their self-esteem are more likely to succeed. Assessment should include a behavioural analysis of the sequences of events that lead to self-cutting. This may help to formulate ways in which treatment could either interrupt the chain of events that leads to self-cutting, or replace the cutting with an alternative method of obtaining relief.

Medication appears to have a limited role, although atypical antipsychotic agents such as risperidone or olanzapine in low dose may be valuable as a short-term measure to reduce tension. Many people who cut themselves have significant personality difficulties. Treatment should be directed towards these problems, although it may be difficult and prolonged. Admission to a psychiatric unit is occasionally necessary, but carries risks, and is advised against unless absolutely necessary (National Institute for Health and Clinical Excellence, 2009b). If the patient is admitted, a clear and detailed policy is needed, as self-cutting is very often difficult to manage in an inpatient unit, and indeed may be imitated by other patients. Referral to the newly established 'complex needs' services for personality disordered patients makes more sense for such patients. Simple referral is rarely enough, but energy invested in supporting engagement with such psychotherapy services is time well spent.

Further reading

Gelder MG, Andreasen NC, López-Ibor JJJr and Geddes JR (eds) (2009). Section 4.15. Suicide. In: *The New Oxford Textbook of Psychiatry*, 2nd edn. Oxford University Press, Oxford. (The four chapters in this section comprehensively review deliberate self-harm and suicide.)

Hawton K *et al.* (2013). *Self-Harm in Oxford 2013*. Centre for Suicide Research, University of Oxford, Oxford.

Wasserman D and Wasserman C (eds.) (2009). *Oxford Textbook of Suicidology and Suicide Prevention*. Oxford University Press, New York.

CHAPTER 22
Psychiatry and medicine

Introduction

This chapter considers the relevance of psychiatry to the rest of medical practice. It covers two related, but distinct, areas. The first is the application of psychiatric knowledge and expertise in a general medical setting. The second covers the psychiatric conditions associated with specific medical disorders.

The chapter is organized as follows:

1. Psychiatry, medicine and the concept of mind–body dualism.
2. Psychiatric disorders in medical settings.
3. Medically unexplained symptoms: somatic symptoms unexplained by medical conditions.
4. Somatoform and dissociative disorders.
5. Services and consultation–liaison psychiatry.
6. Psychiatric aspects of specific medical conditions.
7. Psychiatric aspects of obstetrics and gynaecology.

This chapter should be read in conjunction with the chapters on stress-related disorders (Chapter 7) and neuropsychiatry (Chapter 14); aspects of psychiatry and medicine in children are discussed in Chapter 16.

Psychiatry, medicine, and mind–body dualism

Patients usually attend their doctors because of symptoms that are causing distress and/or dysfunction; that is, when they have an *illness*. Medical assessment is directed to making a diagnosis of the illness, and this diagnosis is used to guide the plan of management. The diagnosis is conventionally defined as either medical or psychiatric.

Medical diagnosis

Most medical diagnoses are based on symptoms and physical signs and the results of biological investigations that together indicate the presence of bodily pathology (abnormal structure and/or function), which is referred to as *disease*. Not all medical diagnoses are arrived at in this way (e.g. migraine) and ultimately a medical diagnosis is a label for a condition that is conventionally treated by medical doctors and listed in classifications of disease such as ICD-10.

Psychiatric diagnosis

Psychiatric diagnosis was discussed in Chapter 2 and the following brief account is intended to remind the reader of that discussion. A psychiatric diagnosis, like a medical one, is essentially a label for a condition that is conventionally treated by doctors, sometimes psychiatrists, but often by other practitioners too. Psychiatric diagnoses are listed in the classifications of diseases, along with medical diagnoses but, although some have associated physical pathology, many do not. Because they generally lack known pathology, they are generally referred to as disorders rather than diseases.

In the past, psychiatric diagnoses have been regarded as 'mental' in nature, in contrast to the 'physical' nature of medical diagnoses. This distinction reflects the absence of gross pathology in most psychiatric disorders, and the fact that these conditions usually present with disturbed mental states or behaviour rather than physical symptoms. Presentations with physical symptoms are considered later in this chapter.

Medicine, psychiatry, and dualism

Underlying this division of illnesses into physical and mental is the assumption that a parallel distinction can be made in healthy people—that there is 'mind–body dualism', an idea commonly attributed to the philosopher Descartes. So-called Cartesian dualism had, and continues to exert, a profound influence on western medical thinking (Miresco and Kirmayer, 2006). Whilst this division has some utility it can also be problematic.

Limitations of dualism

Dualism is at best an oversimplification. It can be convincingly argued that there are no such things as purely

physical or psychological conditions, whether in health or illness. The associated assumption that psychological symptoms indicate psychopathology and physical symptoms physical pathology leads to the categories shown in Table 22.1. Two of these, disease and disorder, have been considered; the other two—comorbidity and somatization—will be considered next.

Comorbidity means the co-occurrence of two disorders. The term has been extended in the table to describe the co-occurrence of prominent mental symptoms and bodily pathology since these patients are usually given both a psychiatric and a physical diagnosis (Kisely and Goldberg, 1996). In practice neither of these diagnoses may lead to effective treatment because a focus on either may lead to neglect of the other. An example is the widespread neglect of depression in patients with medical disease (Moussavi *et al.*, 2007; Walker *et al.*, 2013a).

Somatization. Some patients have somatic symptoms but no evidence of bodily pathology. It is unclear whether their illness should be categorized as medical (with presumed but unidentified somatic pathology) or as psychiatric (with assumed psychopathology). In the past these conditions were generally given the medical diagnosis of *functional illness* (function is abnormal but there is no pathology). In psychiatric practice these conditions would usually be called a *somatoform disorder*. This latter diagnosis implies that: (i) the somatic symptoms are caused by psychopathology; and (ii) there is a hypothetical process—somatization—by which the psychopathology has caused the bodily symptoms. Such patients can therefore receive both a medical diagnosis (functional disorder) and a psychiatric diagnosis (somatoform disorder), with the resulting confusion and controversy being well illustrated by literature about the condition called chronic fatigue syndrome (CFS) or myalgic encephalomyelitis (ME) (see below). In DSM-5, somatoform disorder has been abandoned because of significant overlap between the different disorders and the perceived lack of utility of the boundary between medically explained and medically unexplained symptoms (Sharpe, 2013). DSM-5 now refers to them as somatic symptom disorders. It has also reduced the number of these disorders and subcategories to avoid

Table 22.1 Traditional 'dualistic' categories of mental and physical illness

	Psychological symptoms	Physical symptoms
Bodily pathology	Comorbidity	Medical disease
Psychopathology	Psychiatric disorder	Somatization

the problematic overlaps. Since the term somatoform disorder is used in ICD-10, it will continue to be used in this chapter.

Practical consequences of dualism

One consequence of this way of thinking is the professional and organizational separation of medicine and psychiatry, which in turn contributes to its persistence. This makes it difficult to provide integrated care for patients with comorbidity and those with somatoform disorders. One organizational response to this problem has been the establishment of psychological medicine (also known as liaison psychiatry) services to general hospitals (see below).

An integrated approach

New scientific knowledge, such as the demonstration of a neural basis to many psychiatric disorders, has shown that crude dualistic thinking is untenable. Evidence for the effect of psychiatric disorder on the outcome of medical conditions such as myocardial infarction (Meijer *et al.*, 2011) and cancer (Walker *et al.*, 2013a)

has pointed to the same conclusion. Such integration is strengthened by evidence that the same psychological interventions can be effective in reducing fatigue in CFS (White *et al.*, 2011), where the underlying medical condition is uncertain, or in multiple sclerosis (Van Kessel *et al.*, 2008), where it is clear. Mind and brain are now increasingly regarded as two sides of the same coin. This paradigm shift implies that psychiatric disorders are no more distinct from medical conditions than the higher nervous system is from the rest of the body (Sharpe and Carson, 2001).

For the present, however, Cartesian dualism continues to shape everyday thinking and practice. Illnesses are given separate medical and psychiatric diagnoses linked to separate knowledge bases and distinct systems of care. The psychiatrist working in medical settings needs to be aware of these problems and help by ensuring that both the biological and psychological and social aspects of illness are considered in every case. This is referred to as the 'biopsychosocial' approach, proposed many years ago by Engel (1977) (and which is implicitly, if not explicitly, adopted throughout this book). The factors to consider in a biopsychosocial formulation are shown in Box 22.1. They can be divided further into *predisposing*, *precipitating*, and *perpetuating* causes. The last group of causes is the usual target for treatment, while the first two are relevant to prevention.

Psychiatric disorders in medical settings

Although common in all settings, the type and presentation of psychiatric disorders differs from one medical setting to another. The most common diagnoses in each setting are shown in Table 22.2.

Epidemiology

General practice. The most common psychiatric disorders in general practice are the somatoform disorders (somatic symptom disorder in DSM-5), depression, anxiety and stress-related disorders, and substance misuse. Patients with psychosis are uncommon (Ansseau *et al.*, 2004).

Casualty departments. Deliberate self-harm is the major psychiatric problem in casualty departments. Although only a minority of these patients have persistent psychiatric disorders, many have stress-related disorders and some have depressive disorders. Intoxication and delirium related to alcohol and drugs are also

common, particularly in inner-city hospitals and among people involved in accidents. Some patients with somatoform disorders, and a few with factitious disorders, are frequent attenders at casualty departments (Wooden *et al.*, 2009).

Medical and surgical outpatient clinics. About a third of people attending medical and surgical outpatient clinics have a psychiatric disorder (Maiden *et al.*, 2003). Half of these have depressive and anxiety disorders, and most of the remainder have somatoform disorders. In both groups, adequate recognition and treatment of the psychiatric disorder should be an integral part of management, since it has been shown to improve outcome: depression is a common cause of apparent worsening of a medical condition.

Medical and surgical wards. About 20% of medical and surgical inpatients have a depressive or anxiety disorder coexisting with their medical disease, 10% have a significant alcohol misuse problem, and at least a quarter

Table 22.2 The relative prevalence of common psychiatric disorders in medical settings other than psychiatry

	General practice	Casualty	Medical/surgical outpatients	Medical /surgical inpatients
Depression/anxiety	++	++	+++	+++
Delirium	−	+	−	+++
Alcohol misuse	++	+++	++	+++
Psychosis	+	+	−	−
Somatoform disorders	+++	+	+++	++

— rare; + uncommon; ++ common; +++ very common.

of elderly inpatients have an episode of delirium (Saxena and Lawler, 2009). Some patients with severe somatoform disorders undergo multiple investigations and even surgery before the diagnosis is made.

Presentation of psychiatric disorder in medical settings

Although psychiatric disorders commonly present in medical settings with psychological symptoms or behavioural disturbance, other less obvious presentations are common. These are as: (a) somatic symptoms; (b) a medical management problem and/or difficulties with adherence to treatment; (c) an apparent exacerbation of a medical condition.

> ### Box 22.1 The biopsychosocial formulation
>
> **Biological factors**
> Disease
> Physiology
>
> **Psychological factors**
> Cognition
> Mood
> Behaviour
>
> **Social factors**
> Interpersonal
> Social and occupational
> Relating to the health care system

Psychiatric disorder presenting with somatic symptoms

A significant minority of patients seen in general practice and in hospital outpatient clinics have somatic symptoms that cannot be explained by medical disease, and many of these have a psychiatric disorder (Steinbrecher *et al.*, 2011).

Somatic symptoms due to depressive and anxiety disorders. Depression is associated with somatic symptoms, such as fatigue, weight loss, and pain, which may lead to referral to a medical specialty. Anxiety is associated with symptoms of autonomic arousal, such as palpitations, and with breathlessness and sensory symptoms. A World Health Organization (WHO) collaborative study of patients presenting to primary care in 14 countries found a strong association between somatic symptoms and depressive and anxiety disorders in all centres, despite different cultures and health services. Also, there was a linear relationship between number of somatic symptoms and the presence of depression and anxiety disorder (Simon *et al.*, 1999). Among the anxiety disorders, panic disorder is an especially important cause of medically unexplained symptoms, such as chest pain, dizziness, and tingling.

Somatoform disorders. Medically unexplained somatic symptoms in the absence of a depressive or anxiety disorder are either diagnosed as medically unexplained symptoms or as somatoform disorders. Somatoform disorders are diagnosed when there is a strong suspicion of a psychogenic cause, not just as a diagnosis of exclusion. DSM-5 emphasizes the burden of symptoms rather than whether they are unexplainable or not on the basis of an identifiable medical condition (see above; also Sharpe, 2013). This change may begin to influence practice during the next few years; however, currently most clinicians cling to the concept of somatoform disorders.

Psychiatric disorder presenting as apparent worsening of a medical condition

An exacerbation of complaints about symptoms or disability associated with a chronic medical condition is sometimes caused by a comorbid depressive disorder.

Refusal of treatment is sometimes the first pointer to a psychiatric disorder.

Comorbidity: the co-occurrence of psychiatric and medical conditions

Comorbidity of psychiatric disorders with medical conditions is important. For example, an eating disorder may greatly complicate the treatment of diabetes, and depression is a risk factor for increased mortality and morbidity following myocardial infarction.

Epidemiology

Psychiatric disorder is present in as many as a third of patients with serious acute, recurrent, or progressive medical conditions. It is difficult to ascertain the exact proportion because standard criteria for the diagnosis of psychiatric disorder include some symptoms that can also be caused by medical illness; for example, fatigue and poor sleep. Although modifications have been suggested to make the criteria more appropriate for use with people with physical as well as psychiatric disorder, none is wholly satisfactory. It is best to start with standard criteria and then use knowledge of the medical condition to decide which of the symptoms that point to psychiatric disorder could have originated in this other way. However, this approach requires skilled interviewers and is difficult to achieve on a large scale.

Suicide is easier to identify and there is an increased risk in the medically ill as compared with the general population. There are associations with cancer, multiple sclerosis, and a number of other conditions (Webb *et al.*, 2012).

Common associations between psychiatric and physical illness are shown in Box 22.2. Epidemiological surveys consistently reveal extensive comorbidity between physical illness and mental health problems (Jacobi *et al.*, 2004).

The importance of psychiatric comorbidity in the medically ill

A comorbid psychiatric disorder can greatly affect the impact and outcome of medical conditions; for example, in patients with ischaemic heart disease (Surtees *et al.*, 2008), diabetes (Holt *et al.*, 2014), and cancer (Walker *et al.*, 2013b). Anxiety and depression are also risk factors for non-compliance with medical treatment (Rieckmann *et al.*, 2006).

The causes of psychiatric comorbidity in the medically ill

Psychiatric disorder may be present in medical patients for three main reasons:

1. By chance, as both are common.
2. The psychiatric disorder may have caused the medical condition; for example, alcohol dependence causing cirrhosis of the liver.
3. The medical condition may have caused the psychiatric disorder, either through an action of the disease or its treatment on the brain, or as a reaction to the psychological impact of the medical condition or its treatment, or as a result of the social effects of the

---

Box 22.2 Psychiatric disorders that are common in the medically ill

Adjustment disorder
Major depression
Anxiety disorders
Acute stress disorder
Post-traumatic stress disorder
Somatoform disorder
Substance misuse
Eating disorder
Sleep disorder
Factitious disorder
Sexual disorders

medical condition or its treatment (for example, loss of employment). These factors interact with the person's premorbid vulnerability.

The medical condition and its treatment

Biological mechanisms. In addition to delirium and dementia, a number of other psychiatric disorders may be caused by effects of the medical condition on the brain. Conditions that may act in this way include acute infection, endocrine disorders, and some forms of malignancy. This resulting psychiatric condition is referred to as an 'organic' mental disorder (see Chapter 2). The principal medical conditions that may act in this way are listed in Box 22.3.

Medical treatment may also cause psychiatric disorder by its effect on the brain. Table 22.3 lists some commonly used drugs that may produce psychiatric disorder as a side effect. Other treatments associated with psychiatric disorder include radiotherapy, cancer chemotherapy, and mutilating operations such as mastectomy.

Psychological and social mechanisms. The most common means by which a medical condition can cause psychiatric disorder is by its psychological impact. Certain types of medical condition are particularly likely to provoke serious psychiatric consequences. These include life-threatening acute illnesses and recurrent progressive conditions. Psychiatric disorder is more common in chronic medical illness when there are distressing symptoms such as severe pain, persistent vomiting, and breathlessness; and where there is significant disability (Katon *et al.*, 2007).

Patients at risk for both acute and persistent psychiatric disorder in the course of medical illness include those who:

- have developed psychological problems in relation to stress in the past
- have suffered other recent adverse life events
- are in difficult social circumstances.

The reactions of family, friends, employers, and doctors may affect the psychological impact of a medical condition. They may reduce the consequences by their support, reassurance, and other help, or they may increase it by their excessive caution, contradictory advice, or lack of sympathy.

> ### Box 22.3 Medical conditions that may cause psychiatric disorder directly
>
> **Depression**
> Carcinoma
> Infections
> Neurological disorders (see Chapter 14)
> Diabetes, thyroid disorder, Addison's disease
> Systemic lupus erythematosus
>
> **Anxiety**
> Hyperthyroidism
> Hyperventilation
> Phaeochromocytoma
> Hypoglycaemia
> Drug withdrawal
> Some neurological disorders (see Chapter 14)

Prevention of psychiatric disorder in the medically ill

There are three main strategies.

- Identify those at risk.
- Minimize the negative effect of illness by providing good medical and nursing care.
- Detect, and treat effectively, the early stages of any psychiatric disorder.

Prevention should focus on those suffering illnesses or undergoing treatments that are known to be associated with the development of psychiatric disorder, and on patients who are psychologically vulnerable as evidenced, for example, by a previous history of psychiatric disorder.

Effectiveness of psychiatric treatments in the medically ill

Clinical experience indicates that psychiatric treatments are generally effective in patients who are also medically ill. There was, however, limited evidence from randomized controlled trials because comorbid patients are usually excluded—but there are now more trials of antidepressants in medically ill patients

Table 22.3 **Some drugs with psychological side effects**

Drug	Side effect
Antiparkinsonian agents	
Anticholinergic drugs	Delirium, visual hallucinations
L-Dopa	Delirium, depression, psychotic symptoms
Cardiovascular drugs	
Methyldopa	Tiredness, weakness, depression
Clonidine	
Sympathetic blockers	Impotence, mild depression
Digitalis	Delirium, mood disturbance
Diuretics	Weakness, apathy, and depression (owing to electrolyte depletion)
Analgesics	
Salicylamide	Confusion, agitation, amnesia
Phenacetin	Dementia with chronic abuse
Other examples	
Isoniazid	Acute organic syndrome and mania
Steroids	Irritability, mania, depression
Mefloquine	Psychotic symptoms, abnormal dreams, insomnia, depression, anxiety

and a clearer indication of their value (Taylor *et al.*, 2011). Clinical experience also suggests that psychological treatments such as cognitive behaviour therapy are effective in medically ill patients, and again there is now some limited evidence from clinical trials (Van Kessel *et al.*, 2008). There is better evidence for the benefits of 'collaborative care', in which medical and psychiatric treatment are coordinated. This is especially in the management of chronic medical conditions (Katon, 2003) where there is evidence of considerably reduced treatment costs, primarily because of shorter inpatient stays (Koopmans *et al.*, 2005).

Management of psychiatric disorder in the medically ill

Assessment

Assessment is as for psychiatric disorder in other circumstances, but with the additional need to:

- Be well informed about the medical condition and its treatment.
- Distinguish anxiety and depressive disorders from normal emotional responses to physical illness and its treatment. Symptoms that seldom occur in normal distress (such as hopelessness, guilt, loss of interest, and severe insomnia) help to make the distinction.
- Be aware that medical conditions and their treatment may cause symptoms such as fatigue and loss of appetite that are commonly used to diagnose psychiatric disorder.
- Explore the patient's understanding and fears of the medical condition and its treatment.

General considerations

The nature of the medical condition and its treatment should be explained clearly and the opportunity provided for patients to express their worries and fears.

The treatment for the associated psychiatric disorder is conducted using the methods appropriate for the same disorder in a physically healthy person. Careful consideration should be given to possible interactions between the proposed psychiatric treatment and the medical condition and its treatment. Treatment can often usually be given by the general practitioner or medical specialist, but more complex cases require the skills of a psychiatrist.

Medication

Anxiolytic and sedative drugs can give valuable short-term relief when distress is severe. The indications for antidepressants are the same as those for patients who are not physically ill. The side effects and possible interactions of the psychotropic drugs with other medication should be considered carefully before prescribing.

Psychological treatments

Explanation and advice are part of the treatment of every patient. Cognitive behaviour therapy may be chosen to reduce distress, increase adherence to treatment, reduce disproportionate disability, and to modify lifestyle risk factors.

Somatic symptoms not explained by somatic pathology

Somatic symptoms that are not clearly associated with physical pathology are common in the general population and in patients in all medical settings (Mayou and Farmer, 2002). Although most of these symptoms are transient, a minority are persistent and disabling, and a cause of frequent medical consultations. Some conditions that may give rise to somatic symptoms are shown in Box 22.3.

As noted already, the most common association of physical symptoms with psychiatric disorder is with anxiety and depressive disorders, and some conditions meet the criteria for a somatoform disorder. A few of these patients have a factitious disorder, and a very small number indeed are malingering. However, many of those who present to doctors with unexplained somatic symptoms do not meet the diagnostic criteria for any of these conditions. Even in these undiagnosed cases, however, psychological and social factors are often important as causes of the symptoms and as reasons for seeking help, and psychological measures are often helpful.

Terminology

Many terms have been used to describe medically unexplained somatic symptoms, and none is wholly satisfactory. These terms include hysteria, hypochondriasis, somatization, somatoform symptoms, functional somatic symptoms, and functional overlay. Some of these terms will now be considered further.

- *Somatization.* The term was introduced at the beginning of the twentieth century by Stekl, a German psychoanalyst, to describe the expression of emotional distress as bodily symptoms. More recently, the term has been used to describe the disorder as well as the process producing it. Some current usage is even broader, covering the perception of bodily sensations as symptoms and the behaviour of consulting about them. Most usage accepts, explicitly or implicitly, Stekl's original idea that these physical symptoms are an expression of psychopathology; for example, 'a tendency to experience and communicate psychological distress in the form of somatic symptoms and to seek medical help for them' (Lipowski, 1988). Some definitions of somatization reject Stekl's view and use criteria that require physical symptoms to be accompanied by anxiety or mood disorder diagnosed according to standard criteria. Also, current research suggests that emotional distress and somatic symptoms are positively related rather than inversely related, as they would be if they were alternative expressions of an underlying psychopathology. Because there is no agreed definition, and because of the unsubstantiated aetiological assumptions, the term somatization is unsatisfactory.

- *Somatoform disorder* is the term used originally in DSM-III to describe a group of disorders, including traditional psychiatric diagnoses such as hysteria and hypochondriasis, and newly proposed categories, including somatization disorder. In DSM-5, somatoform disorders have been replaced with the diagnosis of *somatic symptom disorders* in an attempt to do away with the influence of mind/body dualism.

- *Functional somatic symptoms* is the term used often by physicians. It refers to a condition caused by a disturbance of bodily function without any known pathology. The term is relatively acceptable to patients, but the use of word functional (as opposed to organic) has been criticized.

- *Medically unexplained symptoms.* This term has the advantage of describing a clinical problem without implying any assumptions about its causes. However, it has been criticized as implying that understanding of the condition is not possible. Despite this limitation we use it in this chapter.

Epidemiology

Medically unexplained symptoms are common in the general population and in people attending primary care; and they are more frequent in women than in men (Guthrie, 2008). Although most of these symptoms are recognized as not serious and although most are short-lived, a sizeable minority lead to distress, functional disability, and role impairment with more time off work, consulting doctors, and taking medication (Harris *et al.*, 2009).

Aetiology

Although unexplained by any physical pathology, something is known about the causes of medically unexplained symptoms. Most arise from misinterpretation of the significance of normal bodily sensations: they are interpreted as a sign of disease. Concern leads to the focusing of attention on the sensations and this leads to even greater concern, apprehension, and anxiety, which exacerbate and maintain the symptom. For example, awareness of increased heart rate when excited or anxious may lead to worry about heart disease, restriction of daily activities, and repeated requests for investigation and reassurance. Good communication by clinical staff can help to counter the effects of such misinterpretations.

Box 22.4 lists sources of bodily sensations that may be misinterpreted as symptoms of disease.

Predisposing factors include:

- *Beliefs about illness* shape a person's response to sensations and symptoms. These beliefs may be related to personal experience of illness in earlier life, to involvement in the illness of family or friends, or to portrayals of illness in the media (see Box 22.5).
- *Adverse experiences in childhood.* Adults with medically unexplained symptoms commonly report adversities

> **Box 22.4 Physiological sources affecting bodily sensations**
>
> Sinus tachycardia and benign arrhythmias
>
> Effects of fatigue
> Hangover
> Effects of overeating
> Effects of prolonged inactivity
> Autonomic effects of anxiety
> Effects of lack of sleep

in childhood; for example, poor parenting and various forms of abuse.

- *Social circumstances.* Medically unexplained symptoms are associated with poor socioeconomic circumstances and acute or chronic adversity.
- *Personality.* Some people with medically unexplained symptoms have had concerns about bodily health going back to adolescence or earlier, and these can be viewed as part of their personality.

Perpetuating factors include:

- *Behavioural factors,* such as repeatedly seeking information about illness, and inactivity.
- *Emotional factors,* especially chronic anxiety and depression.
- *The reactions of others,* including doctors as well as family and friends. Doctors may inadvertently prolong the problem by failing to give clear, relevant information which takes account of the patient's individual fears and other concerns.

See Kanaan *et al.* (2007) for a review of the causes of unexplained symptoms.

> **Box 22.5 Experiences that may affect the interpretation of bodily sensations**
>
> Childhood illness, with encounters with medical services, and absence from school
> During childhood, illness of close family members
> Physical illness in adult life
> In adult life, illness among family and friends
> Accounts of illness in the media
> Other sources of information about illness

Medically unexplained symptoms

Classification

The classification of medically unexplained symptoms has been considered from two perspectives.

1. *The medical approach* has been to identify patterns of physical symptoms such as irritable bowel syndrome and fibromyalgia. The syndromes differ somewhat in different countries; for example, low blood pressure syndrome is accepted in Germany, and *mal de foie* in France, but neither is accepted in England. These are descriptive syndromes, not aetiological entities, and they overlap with other disorders. Diagnostic criteria have been produced for some of these syndromes and these criteria are useful in research and service planning.

2. *The psychiatric approach.* The alternative approach is to attempt to identify psychiatric syndromes that are the basis of the symptoms. These include *anxiety and depressive disorders, somatoform disorder*, and *factitious disorder*. A psychiatric and a medical diagnosis can be made in the same patients; for example, a patient with chest pain and no heart disease may receive a medical diagnosis of 'non-cardiac chest pain' and a psychiatric diagnosis of panic disorder, both describing the same symptoms.

Prevention

Until we know more of the causes of medically unexplained symptoms, there is no solid basis for prevention. While a reduction in predisposing factors in the population, such as childhood abuse and poor parenting, might have some effect, if they were achievable, it is more plausible to address factors such as poor communication by doctors (Ring *et al.*, 2004) and inadequate treatment of depression and anxiety in patients who present with somatic complaints. See Hotopf (2004) for a fuller discussion of prevention.

Assessment

An adequate medical assessment is essential. At the end of this the physician should explain:

- The purpose and results of all investigations carried out, and why it has been concluded that there is no medical cause for the symptoms.
- That the symptoms are nevertheless accepted as real and that it makes sense to seek other causes.

If the patient is then referred to a psychiatrist, the latter should be informed about the results of the investigations and of the way these have been explained to the patient.

The psychiatrist explores the nature and significance to the patient of the unexplained symptoms, and completes the usual psychiatric history and a mental state examination, with particular attention to:

- Previous concerns about illness.
- Current beliefs about illness.
- Personality.
- Social and psychological problems.
- Detection of a depressive or anxiety disorder.

Information should be sought from other informants as well as from the patient.

Management

The basic plan of management is the same for all medically unexplained symptoms, but individual treatment plans should take account of the patient's special concerns, the type of unexplained symptoms, and any associated psychiatric disorder.

The management of CFS and some other special functional medical syndromes is discussed below. The management of somatoform disorders is described later in the chapter.

After completing the basic procedures outlined in Box 22.6, many patients will be reassured. Those who

---

Box 22.6 Basic approaches to medically unexplained symptoms

- Emphasize that the symptoms are real and familiar to the clinician.
- Explain the role of psychosocial factors in all medical conditions.
- Offer and discuss a psychosocial explanation of the symptoms.
- Allow adequate time for the patient and partner/family to ask questions.
- Agree a treatment plan to include:
- Treatment of any minor medical problem contributing to the symptoms
- Treatment of any associated psychiatric disorder (commonly anxiety or depression)
- If appropriate, improve fitness by graded activity
- If appropriate, diary keeping to explore the relationship between symptoms and possible psychosocial causes.

are not reassured may seek repeated investigation and reassurance. Therefore, when all medically necessary investigations have been completed, the clinician should explain thoroughly why no further investigation is required. After these initial discussions, it is seldom helpful to engage in repeated arguments about the causes. Most patients are willing to accept at least that psychological as well as biological factors may influence their symptoms, and this acceptance can provide a basis for psychological management. Keeping a diary to explore the relationship of symptoms to psychosocial causes can be more convincing than further explanation.

Much can usually be achieved by the primary care team, and by the physicians using these basic procedures. However, chronic and recurrent problems may need to be referred to a psychiatrist or clinical psychologist for further treatment of associated psychiatric disorder, possibly involving cognitive therapy or dynamic psychotherapy. The psychiatrist can also help to coordinate any continuing medical care, especially when this involves several specialties and professions.

Further treatment should be based on the formulation of the person's individual problems. The treatment plan might include, for example, antidepressant medication, anxiety management, and cognitive therapy to change the inaccurate beliefs about the origin and significance of symptoms.

Regarding the evidence about the effectiveness of treatments for medically unexplained symptoms, there have been some trials of medication and of cognitive behaviour therapy, some of which are cited in the course of this chapter.

Antidepressant medication has been shown to benefit several kinds of medically unexplained symptoms, including fibromyalgia and irritable bowel syndrome. Facial pain may be helped by tricyclics. This benefit is especially (but not exclusively) in patients with marked depressive symptoms (Somashekar *et al.*, 2013).

Cognitive behaviour therapy is moderately effective in the treatment of non-cardiac chest pain, irritable bowel, and CFS. Treatment delivered by psychologists has greater benefit than that given by primary care physicians (Gerger *et al.*, 2015).

Prognosis

The prognosis for less complex cases of fairly recent onset is good, but for chronic, multiple, or recurrent conditions it is much less so. For such cases the realistic goal may be to limit disability and requests for unnecessary medical investigation. Doctors need to recognize that they may also contribute to this process. Bensing and Verhaak (2006) review evidence from studies in primary care, which demonstrate that doctors are as active in proposing biological explanations and tests as these patients are in asking for them.

For fuller information about the management of medically unexplained symptoms, see Isaac and Paauw (2014).

Chronic fatigue syndrome

Many terms have been used to describe this syndrome, whose most prominent feature is chronic disabling fatigue: the terms include *postviral fatigue syndrome*, *neurasthenia*, and *myalgic encephalomyelitis* (ME). The descriptive term *chronic fatigue syndrome* (CFS) is now preferred. The diagnosis requires that the illness must have lasted for at least 6 months and that other causes of fatigue have been excluded (Fukuda *et al.*, 1994).

CFS has a long history. In the nineteenth century the symptoms were diagnosed as neurasthenia, and in ICD-10 the syndrome can still be recorded in this way, an option that is chosen widely in China and some other countries. The diagnostic criteria for CFS overlap with those for a number of other psychiatric disorders, including depression, anxiety, somatoform disorders, and fibromyalgia. CFS remains a highly contested disorder with a powerful lobby against any psychiatric interpretation. The persistence of this conflict exemplifies the problems with defining these disorders.

Recently the US Institute of Medicine has proposed renaming CFS as '*systemic exertion intolerance disease*', with the aim of improving acceptance and understanding of the patient experience and stimulating research into the pathophysiology of key symptomatology (Anonymous, 2015).

Clinical features

The central features are fatigue at rest and prolonged exhaustion after minor physical or mental exertion. These features are accompanied by muscular pains, poor concentration, and other symptoms from the list in Box 22.7. People with this condition are commonly most concerned to avoid activity. Frustration, depression, and loss of physical fitness are common.

Epidemiology

Surveys of the general population indicate that persistent fatigue is reported by up to a quarter of the population at any one time. The complaint is common amongst people attending primary care and medical outpatient clinics. However, only a small proportion of people who complain of excessive fatigue meet the diagnostic criteria for CFS. Estimates of prevalence are around 0.5% of

---

Box 22.7 Case definition of chronic fatigue syndrome

Inclusion criteria

Clinically evaluated, medically unexplained, fatigue of at least 6 months' duration that is:

- of new onset (not lifelong)
- not a result of ongoing exertion
- not substantially alleviated by rest
- a substantial reduction in previous level of activities

The occurrence of four or more of the following symptoms:

- subjective memory impairment
- sore throat
- tender lymph nodes
- muscle pain
- joint pain
- headache
- unrefreshing sleep
- post-exertional malaise lasting more than 24 hours

Exclusion criteria

- Active, unresolved, or suspected disease
- Psychotic, melancholic, or bipolar depression
- Psychotic disorders
- Dementia
- Anorexia or bulimia nervosa
- Alcohol or other substance misuse
- Severe obesity

Reproduced from Annals of Internal Medicine, 121(12), Fukuda K et al, Chronic fatigue syndrome: a comprehensive approach to its definition and management, pp. 953–9, Copyright (1994), with permission from The American College of Physicians.

---

the general population with a marked (20–40-fold) predominance of females (Prins *et al.*, 2006). CFS in children is considered in Chapter 16.

Aetiology

The aetiology of CFS is controversial. Suggested factors include:

- *Biological causes.* Several biological causes have been proposed, including chronic infection, immune dysfunction, a muscle disorder, neuroendocrine dysfunction, and ill-defined neurological disorders. Despite strong claims for several specific causative agents, evidence is lacking. For example, *Lyme disease* (Lyme borreliosis) has been said to produce chronic fatigue, myalgia, and impaired concentration, but there are no reliable data to support a link (Stanek *et al.*, 2012).

- *Psychological and behavioural factors.* These appear to be important, especially concerns about the significance of symptoms, the resulting focusing of attention on symptoms, and avoidance of physical mental and social activities that worsen them. Many patients are depressed and/or anxious. However, not all are, and the intense opposition to a psychological understanding in some patients is very striking.

- *Social factors.* Stress at work is sometimes important. Belief that there must be a physical cause may be influenced by the stigma attached to a psychiatric diagnosis, and by some of the information provided by patient groups and practitioners.

An alternative approach to aetiology is to consider predisposing, precipitating, and perpetuating factors:

- *Predisposing factors* include a past history of major depressive disorder and perhaps personality characteristics such as perfectionism.

- *Precipitating factors* include viral infection and life stresses.

- *Perpetuating factors* may include neuroendocrine dysfunction, emotional disorder, attribution of the whole disorder to physical disease, coping by avoidance, chronic personal and social difficulties, and misinformation from the media and other sources.

Course and prognosis

For established cases, the long-term outcome has been considered poor. However, it must be remembered that most studies of prognosis relate to patients referred to specialist centres who may have experienced fatigue for a long time before the referral. Also, most studies refer to prognosis before modern treatments (see below) were widely used. A recent long-term study found a sixfold increase in suicide, but no overall excess mortality, in CFS (Roberts *et al.*, 2016).

Treatment

Many treatments have been suggested but very few are of proven efficacy. There have been several randomized controlled trials of cognitive behavioural therapy and of graded exercise regimes, which have shown the benefits of these procedures over standard medical care alone, and over relaxation therapy.

The PACE study (White *et al.*, 2011) and its follow up (Sharpe *et al.*, 2015) indicate a strong advantage to cognitive behavioural therapy and graded exercise rather than 'living within the dictates of the disorder' as recommended by many CFS groups.

Management

Assessment

As with all medically unexplained conditions, assessment should exclude treatable medical or psychiatric causes of chronic fatigue. It is important to enquire carefully about depressive symptoms, especially as patients may not at first reveal them. Although extensive medical investigations are unlikely to be rewarding, the psychiatrist can usefully collaborate with a physician when assessing these patients. The formulation should refer to any relevant aetiological factors (see above).

Starting treatment

The six basic steps are to:

1. Acknowledge the reality of the patient's symptoms and the disability associated with them.

2. Provide appropriate information about the nature of the syndrome to the patient and to the family.

3. Present the aetiological formulation as a working hypothesis to be tested, not argued over.

4. Treat identifiable depression and anxiety.

5. Encourage gradual return to normal functioning by overcoming avoidance and regaining the capacity for physical activity.

6. Help with any occupational and other practical problems.

Medication

When there is a definite evidence of a depressive disorder, antidepressant drugs should be prescribed in usual doses. Clinical experience suggests that selective serotonin reuptake inhibitor (SSRI) drugs are best tolerated. Antidepressant drugs are also useful in reducing anxiety, improving sleep, and reducing pain. Low-dose tricyclic antidepressants may have a role here.

Psychological treatment

On the simplest level, these include education about the condition, and the correction of misconceptions about cause and treatment. Cognitive behavioural methods include addressing misconceptions about the nature of the condition and excessive concerns about activity; and encouraging a gradual increase in activity. Associated personal or social difficulties can be addressed using a problem-solving approach.

See Harvey and Wessely (2009) for review of CFS.

Irritable bowel syndrome

Irritable bowel syndrome is characterized by abdominal pain or discomfort, with or without an alteration of bowel habits, persisting for longer than 3 months in the absence of any demonstrable disease.

Epidemiology

The condition occurs in as many as 10% of the general population (Wilson *et al.*, 2004), the majority of whom do not consult a doctor.

Aetiology

The cause of the syndrome is uncertain, although there appears to be a disturbance of bowel function and sensation. Depressive and anxiety disorders are common among people who attend gastroenterology clinic with irritable bowel syndrome, especially among those who fail to respond to treatment.

Treatment

People with mild symptoms usually respond to education, reassurance about the absence of serious pathology, change in diet and, when required, antimotility drugs. More severe and chronic symptoms may need additional treatment. Cognitive behavioural therapy has been shown to be of benefit, and so have tricyclic antidepressants, although SSRIs do not seem effective (Hookway *et al.*, 2015).

See Cashman *et al.* (2016) for a review of irritable bowel syndrome.

Fibromyalgia

The term fibromyalgia refers to a syndrome of generalized muscle aching, tenderness, stiffness, and fatigue, often accompanied by poor sleep. A physical sign of multiple specific tender points has been described, but it is probably non-specific. Women are affected more than men, and the condition is more common in middle age. The aetiology is uncertain, but there is a marked association with depression and anxiety. A network meta-analysis shows limited evidence for the efficacy of either pharmacological or psychological therapy, but a combination of antidepressant, aerobic exercise, and cognitive behavioural therapy shows some promise (Nuesch *et al.*, 2013).

See Clauw (2014) for a review of fibromyalgia.

Factitious disorder

DSM-5 defines factitious disorder as the 'Falsification of physical or psychological signs or symptoms, or induction of injury or disease, associated with identified deception'. The category is divided further into that imposed on the self and that imposed on another. It distinguishes single episodes from those that are recurring but no longer distinguishes on the basis of psychological or physical symptoms. In factitious disorder, symptoms are feigned to enable the person to adopt a sick role and obtain medical care (in malingering, symptoms are feigned to obtain other kinds of advantage—see below). The term *Munchausen's syndrome* denotes an extreme form of this disorder (described below).

Epidemiology

The prevalence of factitious disorder is not known with certainty, but it accounts for about 1% of referrals to consultation liaison services. The disorder usually begins before the age of 30 years. 'Illness deception' in physical disorder, covering both factitious disorder and malingering, is considered relatively common, albeit mild, in occupational health services, where one study (Poole, 2010) found it in 8% of consecutive attendees.

Aetiology

The cause is uncertain, in part because many affected individuals give histories that are inaccurate. There is often a history of parental abuse or neglect, of chronic illness in early life with many encounters with the medical services, sometimes long periods in hospital, and sometimes alleged medical mismanagement. Previous substance misuse, mood disorder, and personality disorder are other common features. Many patients have worked in medically related occupations.

Prognosis

This is variable but the condition is usually longlasting. Few patients accept psychological treatment, but some improve during supportive medical care. In some cases there is evidence of other disturbed behaviours, including abuse of children and (on the part of those working in health professions) harm to patients.

Management

Assessment

When factitious disorder is suspected, the available information should be reviewed carefully, including the history given by informants as well as that provided by the patient. A psychiatrist may be able to assist in this assessment, and in cases of doubt further specialist medical investigation may be needed. Additional evidence may be obtained by careful observation of the patient, but the ethical and legal aspects of any proposal to make covert observations should be considered most carefully.

Starting treatment

When the diagnosis has been made, the doctor should explain to the patient the findings and discuss their implications. This should be done in a way that conveys an understanding of the patient's distress and makes possible a discussion of potential psychosocial causes. Although some patients admit at this point that the symptoms are self-inflicted, others persistently deny this. One should not simply assume in this case that the patient is being deliberately misleading. Examining these patients often yields a sense of self-deception where the process lies somewhere between conscious (fabulist) and unconscious processes. In these cases, management should still be directed to helping the patient identify and overcome associated psychological and social difficulties, in the hope that improvement in such problems may be followed eventually by a lessening of the factitious disorder.

Staff who have been caring for the patient while the investigations were being carried out, may become angry when they discover that the patient has deceived them. Such feelings make management more difficult and the psychiatrist should play a part in resolving them through discussion, and by explaining the nature and severity of the patient's psychosocial problems. All closely involved staff should be involved in agreeing a treatment plan which defines what future medical care, and what help with the associated problems is needed, both for the patient and/or the family. Special risks and difficult ethical problems may arise when the patient is a healthcare worker—see Box 22.8.

See Bass and Halligan (2014) for a review of factitious disorder.

Munchausen's syndrome

Richard Asher (Asher, 1951) suggested the term Munchausen's syndrome for an extreme form of factitious disorder, in which patients attend hospital with a false but plausible and often dramatic history suggesting serious acute illness. Often the person is found to have attended and deceived the staff of many other hospitals, and to have given a different false name at each. Many of these people have scars from previous (negative) exploratory operations.

People with this disorder may obstruct efforts to obtain information about them, and some interfere with diagnostic investigations. When further information is

> ## Box 22.8 Health care workers with factitious disorder
>
> Highly publicized cases of serious physical harm to patients caused by a small number of health care workers with factitious disorder, or by those producing factitious disorder by proxy, have aroused great public concern. It is essential, therefore, in the management of these patients to consider the risk to others if the patient continues to work in health care.
>
> These infrequent cases can present difficult medico-legal problems. If the diagnosis is in doubt, it may be judged necessary to seek additional evidence by searching the patient's belongings for items (such as needles or medication) that could have been used to simulate symptoms. In general, it is unethical to search patients' belongings without first explaining the reason and obtaining permission. If the patient refuses to be searched, and there is a serious risk to others should the diagnosis be missed, it is usually appropriate to obtain advice from one or more experienced professionals, including a medicolegal opinion. Advice may be needed also when judging risk, when the risk is serious, and when the patient refuses to allow discussion with the employers in deciding whether to breach confidentiality.

obtained, especially that about previous hospital attendance, the patient often leaves. The aetiology and long-term outcome of this puzzling disorder are unknown.

Fabricated or induced illness

Fabricated or induced illness (FII; sometimes known as *factitious disorder by proxy* or *Munchausen disorder by proxy*) is a rare form of child abuse. A parent or carer, usually the child's mother, exaggerates or gives false accounts of symptoms in their child, and may fake or deliberately induce signs of illness and seek repeated medical investigations and needless treatment for the child. The first cases were described by Meadow in 1977 (Meadow, 1985).

The signs reported most commonly are neurological signs, bleeding, and rashes. Some children collude in the production of the symptoms and signs. The perpetrators (usually mothers) often have a severe personality disorder, including pathological lying, and many suffer from somatoform disorder themselves. Early abusive experiences are common (Bass and Jones, 2011). Hazards for the children include disruption of education and social development. The prognosis is usually poor for both children and perpetrators, and there is a significant mortality. Occasional cases of murder of children by professional carers have been described as an extreme form of this disorder.

FII is a child protection issue. Hence possible cases need to be investigated by a multiprofessional team, including social care and police, and the diagnosis should be made with great caution, and only after detailed investigation. In the UK, a number of high profile legal cases have highlighted the danger of diagnosis on insufficient positive evidence and without adequate exclusion of other causes of the child's symptoms.

Malingering

Malingering is not a medical diagnosis but a description of behaviour. The term denotes the deliberate simulation or exaggeration of symptoms for the purpose of obtaining some gain, such as financial compensation. The distinction from factitious disorder and from somatoform disorder can be difficult because it requires an accurate understanding of the person's motives (Bass and Halligan, 2014).

Malingering is infrequent and is most often encountered among prisoners, the military, and people seeking compensation for accidents. Several kinds of clinical picture have been described:

- malingered medical conditions and disability;
- malingered psychosis, seen in those wishing to obtain admission to hospital for shelter or to prolong their stay in hospital, and in criminal defendants trying to avoid standing trial or to influence sentencing;
- malingered or exaggerated post-traumatic stress disorder;
- malingered cognitive deficit.

Ganser's syndrome (see page 657) is thought by some to be a form of malingering.

Assessment

Assessment depends on careful history-taking and clinical examination, and a watch for discrepancies in the person's behaviour. Lawyers or insurers sometimes use surveillance by video or other means to detect the behaviour but, for ethical reasons, clinicians seldom do. Psychological tests have been used to aid detection, but none is of proven validity.

Management

When malingering is certain, the patient should be informed tactfully and his situation discussed non-judgementally. He should be encouraged to deal more appropriately with any problems that led to the behaviour and, in appropriate cases, offered some brief face-saving intervention as a way to give up the symptoms. See Eastwood and Bisson (2008) for review.

Somatoform and dissociative disorders

Classification in this area is problematic and confusing, with significant differences between ICD-10 and DSM, and between DSM-IV and DSM-5. Because of this, we discuss DSM-IV as well as ICD-10 and DSM-5 approaches.

Somatoform and dissociative disorders are considered together in this chapter because they were classified together in DSM-IV. Apart from this, the disorders are not closely linked. Some of the key terms used are defined in Box 22.9.

Note also that, although *somatoform disorder* has been replaced by *somatic symptom disorder* in DSM-5, this change is not yet widely accepted practice, and may lead to confusion in discussion with medical colleagues in the near future. For this reason we have retained the term somatoform disorder. See Mayou (2014) for discussion.

Classification

In DSM-IV, the overall term *somatoform disorder* was used to denote a group of conditions (listed in Table 22.4) characterized by physical symptoms occurring without an adequate physical cause. In DSM-5 the new term *somatic symptom disorder* emphasizes the burden of symptoms, rather than their unclear aetiology (Sharpe, 2013). In ICD-10, these disorders are not allocated a separate category; instead they are classified within the broader category of *neurotic, stress-related*, and *somatoform disorders*.

A further confusing difference between the classifications concerns the status of conversion disorder and its relationship to somatoform and dissociative disorders. In ICD-10, the category is *dissociative (conversion) disorders*; that is, conversion (Box 22.9) is viewed, in effect, as synonymous with dissociation. In DSM-IV, conversion disorder was classified as a specific subtype of dissociative disorder. However, in DSM-5, conversion disorder is classified as a type of somatoform disorder, and has the alternative name of *functional neurological symptom disorder*. This emphasizes the essential importance of the neurological examination and recognition that the relevant psychological factors may not be demonstrable at the time of diagnosis. Here, we follow the DSM-IV convention. See Table 22.4.

Somatoform disorder

This section is concerned only with the groups of unexplained physical symptoms classified within the somatoform disorder category. The defining feature is the presence of:

physical symptoms suggesting a physical disorder for which there are no demonstrable organic findings or known physiological mechanisms, and for which there is strong evidence, or a strong presumption, that the symptoms are linked to psychological factors or conflicts.

Many people experience such symptoms, and they are associated with significant distress and disability. However, there is doubt about the value of grouping together under this one rubric conditions which are dissimilar in many ways and which overlap (are comorbid)

> ### Box 22.9 Some definitions
>
> **Somatoform disorders.** A generic term used in DSM-IV for a group of disorders characterized by physical symptoms that are not explained by organic factors.
>
> **Somatic symptom disorders.** The DSM-5 replacement for somatoform disorders. It emphasizes the disability from symptoms, not whether they lack a physical explanation.
>
> **Dissociation.** A hypothetical mechanism whereby psychological processes relating to consciousness are split or fragmented. Dissociation is discussed further in Chapter 7 under Stress-related disorders.
>
> **Dissociative symptoms.** Symptoms that have been thought to arise through the mechanism of dissociation.
>
> **Conversion.** A term introduced by Freud for a hypothetical mechanism by which psychological stress leads to (is converted into) physical symptoms.
>
> **Conversion disorder.** A term for conditions that may result from conversion; conditions that in the past were called hysteria.

Table 22.4 Categories of somatoform disorders in disorders in ICD-10, DSM-IV, and DSM-5

ICD–10	DSM-IV	DSM-5
Somatization disorder	Somatization disorder	Somatic symptom and related disorders
Undifferentiated somatoform disorder	Undifferentiated somatoform disorder	Somatic symptom and related disorders
Hypochondriacal disorder	Hypochondriasis	Illness anxiety disorder
Somatoform autonomic dysfunction	*No category*	*No category*
Persistent pain disorder	Pain disorder associated with psychological factors (and a general medical condition)	Somatic symptom disorder with predominant pain or psychological factors affecting other medical conditions
Other somatoform disorders	Somatoform disorders not otherwise specified	Unspecified somatic symptom disorder
No category	Body dysmorphic disorder	Moved to obsessive compulsive and related disorders
No category	Conversion disorder	Functional neurological symptom disorder
Neurasthenia	*No category*	*No category*
		Factitious disorder moved to somatic symptom disorder and related disorders

Source: data from The ICD-10 classification of mental and behavioural disorders: clinical descriptions and diagnostic guidelines, Copyright (1992), World Health Organization; Diagnostic and Statistical Manual of Mental Disorders: DSM-IV, Copyright (2000), American Psychiatric Association; Diagnostic and Statistical Manual of Mental Disorders, Fifth Edition, Copyright (2013), American Psychiatric Association.

with anxiety disorders and depressive disorders (Sharpe and Mayou, 2004). Also, two of the conditions—hypochondriasis and somatization disorder—are so enduring that it has been suggested that they should be classified as personality disorders. (Hypochondriasis as a term has been abandoned in DSM-5, as it was considered to have become too pejorative. It has been replaced with 'illness anxiety disorder', although such patients may also sometimes be diagnosed as having a somatic symptom disorder.)

Classification in DSM-IV, DSM-5 and ICD-10

Although there are broad similarities, there are also two important differences between the subtypes of somatoform disorder in ICD-10, DSM-IV, and DSM-5 (see Table 22.4).

- *Neurasthenia* is not included in DSM-IV or DSM-5 because the category is seldom used in the USA (despite being first popularized there by George Beard and

being called for a time 'the American neurosis'). It is included in ICD-10 because it is an international classification and the category is used in some Far Eastern countries.

- *Conversion disorder* is a somatoform disorder in DSM-IV (and a somatic symptom disorder in DSM-5), but is not used to describe a specific disorder in ICD-10.

- *Body dysmorphic disorder* does not exist as a category in ICD-10; instead, it is listed as a type of hypochondriacal disorder.

There are also problems which both classifications share:

- Diagnostic criteria within the group are based on a mixture of principles—aetiology, symptom count, consultation, and response to medical treatment.

- Diagnostic criteria for hypochondriacal disorder were derived largely from patients attending hospitals and do not apply readily to many of the people with unexplained medical symptoms in the community.

- Many cases in the community did not meet the diagnostic criteria for any specific somatoform disorder in

DSM-IV and had to be placed in non-specific categories, leading to the change in name to somatic symptom disorder in DSM-5.

- The seemingly small differences between DSM-IV and ICD-10 criteria resulted in large differences in estimates of prevalence of somatoform disorder as a whole and of the subcategories.

Conversion disorder

Conversion disorder was a term introduced in DSM to replace the older term hysteria; as noted, in DSM-5 it is now also known as functional neurological symptom disorder. The term refers to a condition in which there are isolated neurological symptoms that cannot be explained in terms of known mechanisms of pathology and in which there has been a significant psychological stressor. The study of such symptoms has a long history. Some understanding of this history provides helpful background to understand the present status of the concept of conversion disorder (Box 22.10); more broadly, the evolution of thinking about hysteria was important for Freud's ideas which in turn greatly influenced twentieth-century psychiatry.

Clinical features

In DSM-IV, conversion disorder was divided into four subtypes (with motor symptoms, with sensory symptoms, with seizures or convulsions, and mixed). In DSM-5 the coding simply indicates the predominant symptom (e.g. speech, swallowing, seizures).

Conversion symptoms do not normally reflect the appropriate physiological or pathological mechanisms. They are also highly responsive to suggestion and may vary considerably in response to the comments of other people, especially doctors. Symptoms may be 'reinforced' by measures such as providing a wheelchair for the patient who has difficulty walking. Patients with conversion disorders may seem surprisingly unconcerned about the nature and implications of the symptoms ('belle indifference'). This belle indifference is not invariable.

The original psychoanalytical understanding focused on the concepts of primary and secondary gain. Secondary gain implies a significant external benefit or avoidance of unwanted responsibilities from the symptoms. The primary gain was the relief obtained by the conversion of the mental distress generated by a hypothesized neurotic conflict into physical symptoms, thereby allowing the conflict to remain unconscious. Secondary gains are usually prominent in conversion disorders, but are also common in other psychiatric—and physical—disorders.

Epidemiology

The prevalence of conversion disorder in the general population is difficult to determine, and estimates vary widely. A review of five studies indicated an incidence rate of 5–12 per 100,000 per annum, with the lowest rates in a study of psychiatric practice, in keeping with the view that many of these patients are not referred to psychiatrists. Estimates of prevalence vary even more, but with figures around 50 per 100,000. The few studies that examined change over time do not support the belief that the condition is disappearing (Akagi and House, 2002).

Aetiology

The aetiology is unknown, reflected in the wide range of theories with few research findings to support them. For review, see Lehn *et al.* (2016).

- *Psychodynamic theories* use the explanatory concept of conversion of emotional distress into physical symptoms, which often have a symbolic meaning.
- *Social factors* appear to be major determinants of the onset and development of conversion symptoms.
- *Neurophysiological mechanisms:* little is known of the neural basis of conversion disorder. Functional neuroimaging shows alterations in brain activation related to how adverse events are processed, and in the links between emotion, memory, and body schema (Aybek *et al.*, 2014).
- *Cognitive explanations*: Brown (2002) suggested that the symptoms are caused by the chronic activation of representations of the symptoms stored within memory, the process being driven by attention directed to these representations.
- *Cultural explanations*: some of the phenomena classified as conversion disorder in western countries may, in some other cultures, be accepted as possession states (see below).

Prognosis

Prognosis for subsequent neurological disorder

Owing to the limited numbers of studies and their high heterogeneity, there is a lack of rigorous empirical evidence to identify relevant prognostic factors in patients presenting with persistent medically unexplained symptoms. However, it seems that a more serious condition at baseline is associated with a worse outcome (Olde Hartman *et al.*, 2009).

Most of the patients seen in general practice or hospital emergency departments with conversion disorders of recent onset recover quickly. Disorders lasting longer

Box 22.10 A brief history of hysteria

There are descriptions of hysteria in ancient Greek medical texts. The disorder was thought to result from abnormalities of position or function of the uterus, hence the name. This view persisted until the seventeenth century. Gradually, the idea became accepted that hysteria is a disorder of the brain and, by the nineteenth century, the importance of predisposing constitutional and organic causes was recognized. It was accepted also that the usual provoking cause was strong emotion.

In the later years of the nineteenth century, the studies of hysteria by Charcot, a French neurologist working at the Salpêtrière Hospital in Paris, were particularly influential. Charcot believed at first that the symptoms of hysteria were caused by a functional disorder of the brain, and that this disorder also rendered patients susceptible to hypnosis. As a result of his susceptibility, new symptoms could be induced in these patients by suggestion, and existing ones could be modified. Later, Charcot became interested in the idea of his former pupil, Janet, that the basic disorder in hysteria is not suggestibility but a tendency to dissociation. By this Janet meant that the patients had lost the normal integration between various parts of mental functioning, and that it did not require a prior organic lesion—anyone could be hypnotized. Janet believed that this dissociation led to a loss of awareness of certain aspects of psychological functioning that would otherwise be within awareness. Janet's ideas were influential for a while but never had the impact of those of Freud.

Freud visited Charcot in the winter of 1895–1896 and was impressed by demonstrations of the susceptibility of patients to hypnosis, and of the power of suggestion. On his return to Vienna, Freud and his colleague Breuer studied patients with hysteria, published in the seminal monograph *Studies on Hysteria* (1893–1895). They proposed that hysteria was caused by emotionally charged ideas, usually sexual, which had become lodged in the patient's unconscious mind as a result of some past experience, and which were excluded from conscious awareness by repression. Freud adopted the word 'conversion' to refer to the hypothetical process whereby this hidden, unexpressed, emotion was transformed into physical symptoms. He summarized this idea in the phrase 'hysterics suffer mainly from reminiscences'.

In the years that followed, Freud came to believe that this original formulation was wrong and had been based on fabricated accounts ('screen memories'), and from then on he wrote no more on hysteria. Hysteria was thought to be a declining problem in developed countries and the erroneous view that many apparent cases were in fact unrecognized organic disease was put vigorously by Slater (1965). Subsequent changes of opinion are considered on page 648.

For the history of hysteria see Shorter (1992); for the history of the concept of conversion see Mace (2001).

---

than a year are likely to persist for many years. Slater's widely cited 1965 follow-up described the development of a physical and psychiatric disorder in a high proportion of patients. Slater's sample was highly atypical even for his tertiary clinic. A more recent follow-up of patients attending the same hospital found a very low incidence of physical or psychiatric diagnoses. A systematic review has demonstrated that misdiagnosis has steadily declined over the past several decades and is now only in the region of about 4% (Stone *et al.*, 2005). When the diagnosis of conversion disorder was made, it remained stable over time.

Prognosis for subsequent psychiatric disorder

Although subsequent neurological disorder is uncommon in these patients, psychiatric morbidity is high. Usually the psychiatric symptoms are present when the patients were first seen.

Predictors of prognosis

Predictors of good outcome are short history and young age; predictors of poor outcome are long history, personality disorder, and receipt of disability benefit or involvement in litigation (Gelauff *et al.*, 2014).

Treatment

For acute conversion disorders seen in primary care or hospital emergency departments, reassurance and suggestion of improvement are often sufficient, together with immediate efforts to resolve any stressful circumstances that provoked the reaction (Box 22.11). The doctor should be sympathetic and positive, and provide a socially acceptable opportunity for rapid return to normal physical functioning; for example, by arranging a brief course of physiotherapy. The patient should feel that the problem is accepted as deserving assessment, that it is common, and that a good outcome can be

> ### Box 22.11 Treatment of acute conversion disorder
>
> - Obtain medical and psychiatric history from patient and informants
> - Carry out appropriate medical and psychiatric examination and arrange investigations for physical causes
> - Reassure that the condition is temporary, well recognized and, for motor disorders, due to a problem of converting intention into action
> - Avoid reinforcing symptoms or disability
> - Offer continuing help with any related psychiatric or social problems

expected. The therapist should discuss any personal difficulties that have been identified, and suggest that they deserve attention in their own right.

Where symptoms have persisted for more than a few weeks more elaborate treatment is required. The general approach is to focus on removing any factors that are reinforcing the symptoms and disability and on encouraging normal behaviour. It should be explained that the symptoms and disability (as in remembering, or moving his arm) are not caused by physical disease but by an inability to convert willed intention into action; and that sensory problems are caused by an inability to become aware of sensory information, and not by a lesion interfering with sensory pathways. This problem is provoked by psychological factors. Patients should be told also that they can regain control of the disturbed function and, if necessary, offered help to do so—usually through physiotherapy. Psychotherapists often call this providing a 'licence for change'.

Attention is then directed away from the symptoms and towards problems that have provoked the disorder. Staff should show concern for the patient, but at the same time should encourage self-help. They should not make undue concessions to patients' disabilities; for example, a patient who cannot walk should be encouraged to walk again, not be provided with a wheelchair. The approach should be supportive and sympathetic: it should not appear in any way uncaring or punitive. To achieve this end, there must be a clear plan so that all members of staff adopt a consistent approach to the patient.

Medication can play a role in the treatment of these disorders if there are prominent and significant depressive or anxiety symptoms. Cognitive behaviour therapy

appears to be of little specific value, although it may act as a non-specific aid to recovery.

It is essential that measures to reduce symptoms are accompanied by help with any associated personal and social difficulties. Brief and focused psychological treatments are helpful, but more intensive therapy risks complex transference reactions.

Those who do not improve should be reviewed thoroughly for undiscovered physical illness. All patients, whether improved or not, should be followed carefully for long enough to exclude any organic disease that might have been missed at the original assessment.

For review of treatment of conversion disorder, see Lehn *et al.* (2016).

'Epidemic hysteria'

Occasionally, dissociative (or conversion) disorder spreads within a group of people as an 'epidemic'. This spread happens most often in closed groups of young women; for example, in a girls' school, a nurses' home, or a convent. Often anxiety has been heightened by some fear of an epidemic of disease present in the neighbourhood. Typically, the epidemic starts in one person who is highly suggestible, histrionic, and a focus of attention in the group. Gradually, other cases appear, first in the most suggestible, before spreading. The symptoms are variable, but fainting and dizziness are common. Outbreaks among schoolchildren have been documented.

Somatization disorder

In 1962, psychiatrists in St Louis (Perley and Guze, 1962) described a syndrome of chronic multiple somatic complaints without any identified organic cause, which they regarded as a form of hysteria. They named it *Briquet's syndrome* after a nineteenth-century French physician who wrote a monograph on hysteria. A similar syndrome, called *somatization disorder*, was introduced in DSM-III. The core feature was multiple somatic complaints of long duration, beginning before the age of 30 years. A similar category is found in ICD-10. In DSM-5 the disorder has been abandoned and is absorbed into the broader somatic symptom disorder category.

Hypochondriasis

The term hypochondriasis is one of the oldest medical terms, originally used to describe disorders believed to be due to disease of the organs situated in the hypochondrium. It was defined in DSM-IV (and ICD-10, under the heading of *hypochondriacal disorder*) in terms of conviction and/or fear of disease unsupported by the results of appropriate medical investigation. As noted earlier, it has been abandoned in DSM-5 and replaced by 'illness anxiety disorder', but hypochondriasis as a diagnostic entity has been under sustained attack for decades without disappearing and is likely to be encountered often in discussion with colleagues.

DSM-IV described the condition as a:

preoccupation with a fear or belief of having a serious disease based on the individual's interpretation of physical signs of sensations as evidence of physical illness. Appropriate physical evaluation does not support the diagnosis of any physical disorder that can account for the physical signs or sensations or for the individual's unrealistic interpretation of them. The fear of having, or belief that one has a disease, persists despite medical reassurance.

The criteria exclude patients with panic disorder or delusions, and require that symptoms have been present for at least 6 months.

Epidemiology

Attempts to estimate prevalence have been hindered by the absence of standardized assessment. Whilst some primary care surveys have estimated a prevalence of around 5%, the WHO multicentre primary care survey (Gureje et al., 1997) found a prevalence of 0.8%, or 2.2%, despite using a less restrictive definition. This later definition omitted the criterion 'persistent refusal to accept medical reassurance' but retained the triad of illness worry, associated distress, and medical help-seeking. Comorbidity with depression and anxiety disorders is frequent.

Prognosis

Evidence about course and prognosis is limited. A review of medically unexplained symptoms, somatization, and hypochondriasis (Olde Hartman et al., 2009) failed to find prognostic factors other than severity of disorder at baseline associated with a worse outcome. One study found that personality predicted the time to remission in hypochondriasis (Greeven et al., 2014).

Aetiology

The cause is unknown. Cognitive formulations suggest that there is faulty appraisal of normal bodily sensations, which are interpreted as evidence of disease. Misinterpretation is maintained by continually seeking reassurance and examining or rubbing the supposedly affected part.

Treatment

Since the disorder is chronic or recurrent, management is difficult (Starcevic, 2015). Care should be exercised to ensure that a hypochondriacal presentation of depression is not missed and left untreated. Repeated reassurance is unhelpful and may prolong the patient's concerns. Investigations should be limited to those indicated by the medical priorities and not extended to satisfy the patient's demands. Misinterpretations of the significance of bodily sensations should be corrected, and encouragement given to constructive ways of coping with symptoms. Trials have shown more benefit for hypochondriacal symptoms from cognitive behavioural treatment than from short-term dynamic psychotherapy or routine medical care (Sørensen et al., 2011).

See Noyes (2009) for a review of hypochondriasis.

Body dysmorphic disorder

Body dysmorphic disorder is the DSM term for a subgroup of the broader but ill-defined syndrome of *dysmorphophobia*, which was first described by Morselli in 1886 as 'a subjective description of ugliness and physical defect which the patient feels is noticeable to others'. In DSM-5, the term body dysmorphic disorder denotes dysmorphophobia that is not better accounted for by another psychiatric disorder. The preoccupation with the imagined defect in appearance is usually an overvalued idea, but individuals 'can receive an additional diagnosis of delusional disorder, somatic type' (Chapter 12); there is also overlap with hypochondriasis and obsessive–compulsive disorder. In DSM-5, body dysmorphic disorder is classified with 'obsessive compulsive and related disorders' while in ICD-10 it is subsumed within the category of hypochondriacal disorder.

Patients with dysmorphophobia are convinced that some part of their body is too large, too small, or is misshapen. To other people the appearance is normal, or there is a trivial abnormality. In the latter case, it may be difficult to decide whether the preoccupation is disproportionate. The common concerns are about the nose, ears, mouth, breasts, buttocks, or penis, but any part of the body may be involved. Patients may be constantly preoccupied with and tormented by their mistaken beliefs. It seems to them that other people notice and talk about the supposed deformity. They may blame all their other difficulties on it: if only their nose/breasts were a better shape, they would be more successful in their work, social life, or sexual relationships. Time-consuming behaviours which aim to re-examine, improve, or hide the perceived defect are frequent. Social impairment is considerable. There is substantial comorbidity, especially with major depression and social phobia.

The condition usually begins in adolescence. It is chronic, though it often fluctuates over time. It is probable that there is some improvement over many years but there have been no long-term prospective studies.

The severe cases described in the psychiatric literature are infrequent, but less severe forms of dysmorphophobia are more common, especially among those seeking plastic surgery or consulting dermatologists. As with the more severe cases, many meet diagnostic criteria for other disorders.

Assessment

Assessment should include questions about the nature of the preoccupations with appearance and of the ways in which this has interfered with personal and social life. Diagnosis can be difficult because some sufferers fail to reveal the precise nature of their symptoms because of embarrassment. This failure may result in misdiagnosis as social phobia, panic disorder, or obsessive–compulsive disorder.

Treatment

When body dysmorphic disorder is secondary to a psychiatric disorder such as major depression, the latter should be treated in the usual way. The treatment of primary body dysmorphic disorder is often difficult. It is essential to establish a working relationship in which the patient feels that the psychiatrist is sympathetic, understands the severity of the problems, and is willing to help. Since many patients will be requesting surgery, it is important to explain the lack of success of this approach and suggest that there are other effective treatments. There is some modest support with SSRIs (Phillips, 2008), and for cognitive behaviour therapy (Wilhelm *et al.*, 2014). Counselling and practical help should be provided for any occupational, social, or sexual difficulties that accompany the condition. Although some patients are helped by this approach coupled with continued support, many are not.

Cosmetic surgery is often successful for patients with conditions other than dysmorphophobia. Surgery is usually contraindicated, however, for people who have body dysmorphic disorder, many of whom are very dissatisfied after the operation. Selection for surgery therefore requires careful assessment of the patient's expectations. Those with the most unrealistic hopes generally have poorer prognoses. Assessment is difficult, and collaboration between plastic surgeons, psychiatrists, and psychologists is valuable. Unintended rebuffs by surgeons or psychiatrists can increase the difficulties of management.

Somatoform pain disorder

This term was used to denote patients with chronic pain that did not appear to be caused by any physical or specific psychiatric disorder. DSM-IV emphasized that the essential feature of this disorder is pain that is the predominant focus of the clinical presentation and is of sufficient severity to cause distress or impairment of functioning. It also proposed that neither organic pathology nor pathophysiological mechanism has been found to account for it or that it was grossly disproportionate to any identified causes. DSM-5 takes a radically different approach, not dichotomizing the origins of pain but accepting that physical and psychological factors are essential aspects of all chronic pain. The diagnosis is based on the need for intervention rather than the purported aetiology.

In DSM-5 some individuals with chronic pain can still be diagnosed as having somatic symptom disorder with predominant pain. Others, however, may be diagnosed within the new category of 'psychological factors affecting other medical conditions'. This diagnosis prioritizes the intervention needed to manage the very special experience of an identified medical disorder that is present.

Epidemiology

Pain is widely reported in surveys of the general population. Most people report pain that is transient, but a minority describe persistent or recurrent pain leading to disability (Gureje *et al.*, 1998). Pain is the most common symptom among people who consult doctors. Acute pain usually has an organic cause, but psychological factors can affect the subjective response to pain whatever the main cause.

In general practice, pain is a common presenting symptom of emotional problems. In psychiatric practice, it has been reported that pain is experienced by about one-fifth of inpatients and over half of outpatients. Pain is particularly associated with depression, anxiety, panic, and somatoform disorders. Patients with multiple pains are especially likely to have associated psychiatric disorder (Gureje *et al.*, 1998).

Aetiology

Chronic pain occurs in many conditions, including neurological or musculoskeletal disorders. It often has both physical and psychological causes (Bushnell *et al.*, 2013). A 'pain-prone disorder' has been suggested as a variant of depressive disorder, but there is little evidence for this. It is more likely that in these cases the pain arises from personal and social factors, and that beliefs about pain are important in maintaining it (Linton, 2000). Chronic pain may impose great burdens on the patient's family; also, the attitude of family members and other caregivers can influence the perception of pain, its course, and the response to treatment.

Assessment

The assessment of a patient complaining of pain of unknown cause should include:

- Thorough investigation of possible physical causes. When the results of this investigation are negative, it should be remembered that pain may be the first symptoms of a physical illness that cannot be detected at an early stage.
- Full description of the pain and the circumstances in which it occurs.
- Search for symptoms of a depressive or other psychiatric disorder.
- Description of pain behaviours—for example, the presentation of symptoms, requests for medication, and responses to pain.
- Exploration of the patient's beliefs about the causes and implications of the pain.

Treatment

The management of chronic pain should be individually planned, comprehensive, and involve the patient's family. Skill is required to maintain a working relationship with patients unwilling to accept an approach that uses psychological treatments as part of the treatment of pain. Any associated physical disorder should be treated and adequate analgesics provided. The treatment of pain associated with a psychiatric disorder is the treatment of the primary condition.

Psychological care is directed to assessing:

- The presence of any associated mental disorder. This assessment should be made on positive findings and not solely because no specific organic cause has been identified. If depressive illness is present it should be treated vigorously. Tricyclic antidepressant medication is effective in some patients with chronic pain even without evidence of a depressive disorder. Duloxetine, gabapentin, and pregabalin may also be helpful (Finnerup *et al.*, 2015).
- Whether psychological techniques are indicated to modify the pain or any associated behaviours. Cognitive behavioural treatment aims to encourage the use of distraction, relaxation, and other ways of coping with the pain, and to reduce social reinforcement of pain-related behaviour. In a meta-analysis these treatments had a significant though modest effect (Morley *et al.*, 2013).

Multidisciplinary pain clinics bring together expertise in somatic and psychological treatments for pain. See Grandhe *et al.* (2016) for a review of treatment approaches to chronic pain.

Specific pain syndromes

Many kinds of pain are common in the population. This section is concerned with headache, facial pain, back pain, and pelvic pain.

Headache

Patients with chronic or recurrent headache are sometimes referred to psychiatrists. There are many physical causes of headache, notably migraine, which affects about one in ten of the population at some time of their life. Many patients attending neurological clinics have headaches for which no physical cause can be found. The commonest of these is 'tension' headache, which is usually described as a dull generalized feeling of pressure or tightness extending around the head. It is frequently of short duration and is relieved by analgesia or a good night's sleep, but may occasionally be constant and unremitting. Some patients describe depressive symptoms and others describe anxiety in relation to obvious life stresses. Psychological factors seem to contribute to aetiology, but there is no evidence that the headaches result from increased muscle tension, and vascular mechanisms are more likely.

Most patients with headaches for which no physical cause can be found are reassured by an explanation of the negative results of investigations. Antidepressants and stress management both produce modest improvement (Bendtsen, 2015).

Facial pain

Facial pain has many physical causes; there are at least two forms in which psychological variables appear to be important. The more common is temporomandibular dysfunction (*Costen's syndrome* or facial arthralgia). There is a dull ache around the temporomandibular joint, and the condition usually presents to dentists. 'Atypical' facial pain is a deeper aching or throbbing pain, which is more likely to present to neurologists. Patients with either of these symptoms are often reluctant to see a psychiatrist, but several trials suggest that some antidepressants can relieve symptoms even when there is no evidence of a depressive disorder. Cognitive behaviour therapy has been found to enhance the effect of the usual dental care for temporomandibular disorders (Litt *et al.*, 2009).

See Shepherd *et al.* (2014) for a review of psychological aspects of facial pain.

Back pain

Back pain is the second leading cause for visits to primary care doctors and a major cause of disability. Most acute pain is transient, but in about a fifth of patients it persists for more than 6 months. Psychological and behavioural problems at the onset predict a poor outcome (Linton, 2000). Treatment includes the provision of accurate information about the cause and outcome of the condition, limited use of analgesics, and a graded increase in activity. Patients who fail to improve with these measures should be offered a combined programme of psychological and physical treatment. Cognitive and behavioural approaches may have some effects in chronic low back pain (Fersum *et al.*, 2013); the evidence for antidepressants is inconclusive but, as with other pain syndromes, low-dose tricyclic antidepressants can also be helpful (Williamson *et al.*, 2014).

Chronic pelvic pain

Pelvic pain is one of the most common symptoms reported by women attending gynaecology clinics. It is a feature of several gynaecological disorders, notably endometriosis. However, in other cases pain often persists despite negative investigations, and psychological factors appear to be significant causes of the pain and the disability, which often includes sexual dysfunction. Multimodal treatment approaches, often including behavioural modification and stress management, have been developed (Shah *et al.*, 2015).

Dissociative disorders

The essential feature of dissociative disorders is a disruption of the usually integrated functions of consciousness, memory, identity, or perception. This disturbance may be sudden or gradual, transient or chronic. Dissociation is a crucial concept in the development of psychiatry and a history of the term is reviewed briefly in Box 22.12.

Types of dissociative disorder

The types of dissociative disorders recognized in ICD-10 and DSM-5 (Spiegel *et al.*, 2013) are shown in Table 22.5. The inclusion in ICD-10 of the bracketed term '*conversion*' in the title of the group, reflects the previous convention of classifying these conditions with the conversion disorders (see above).

Some authors consider that these disorders are well established and common (Carota and Calabrese, 2014), while some doubt the evidence base for the category (Merskey, 2000).

Dissociative amnesia

The essential feature is an inability to recall important personal memories, usually of a stressful nature, that is too extensive for normal forgetfulness. Dissociative

---

> **Box 22.12 A brief history of dissociation**
>
> The term dissociation is associated particularly with the French philosopher and psychiatrist, Janet (1859–1947), who worked for a time with Charcot at the Salpêtrière in Paris (see Box 22.10). Janet studied aspects of sensory perception and mental integration in hysteria and other neuroses, and used the term 'désagrégation psychologique' (translated as dissociation) to describe the breakdown of this integration. For a while Janet's ideas were influential; however, his theories were overshadowed by those of Freud.
>
> In the 1970s interest in dissociation revived as a result of studies of the effects of psychological trauma, especially among Vietnam war veterans. These studies documented symptoms occurring in response to traumatic events, and suggested a common origin in the mechanism of dissociation, a new name of dissociative symptoms (see Table 22.5), and a new diagnostic category of dissociative disorders.

---

amnesia occurs alone and during the course of other dissociative disorders and of post-traumatic stress disorder, acute stress disorder, and somatization disorder. The diagnosis is made only when these other conditions are not present.

Dissociative amnesia must be distinguished from amnesia having a medical cause. It has been described in two forms:

1. Circumscribed amnesia for a single recent traumatic event.

2. Inability to recall long periods of childhood. Amongst patients who present in this way, some have concurrent organic disease.

See Staniloiu and Markowitsch (2014) for review.

Dissociative fugue

Dissociative fugue is no longer a separate diagnosis in DSM-5 but a specifier for dissociative amnesia. It is extremely rare, with a loss of memory coupled with wandering away from the person's usual surroundings. These people usually deny all memory of their whereabouts during the period of wandering, and some deny knowledge of personal identity. Many dramatic case histories have been published. The disorder must be distinguished from organic disorder, including epilepsy and substance intoxication.

Table 22.5 **DSM-5 and ICD-10 classification of dissociative disorder**

DSM-5	ICD–10
Dissociative disorders	**F44 Dissociative (conversion) disorders**
Dissociative amnesia	Dissociative amnesia
Dissociative amnesia with fugue	Dissociative fugue
Dissociative identity disorder	Multiple personality disorder
Depersonalization/derealization disorder	(classified in F48.1)
Other specified dissociative disorders	Dissociative (conversion) disorder not otherwise specified
	Dissociative stupor
	Trance and possession disorders
	Ganser's syndrome

Source: data from Diagnostic and Statistical Manual of Mental Disorders, Fifth Edition, Copyright (2013), American Psychiatric Association; The ICD-10 classification of mental and behavioural disorders: clinical descriptions and diagnostic guidelines, Copyright (1992), World Health Organization.

Dissociative identity disorder

In this disorder (widely known by the ICD-10 term 'multiple personality disorder') there are sudden alternations between two patterns of behaviour, each of which is forgotten by the patient when the other is present. One pattern is the person's normal personality, while the other 'personality' is an integrated array of emotional responses, attitudes, memories, and social behaviour, which contrasts, often strikingly, with the normal. Sometimes there is more than one additional 'personality'. The criteria for the DSM-5 diagnosis are shown in Box 22.13. The condition is probably rare, but it has been reported more frequently in certain periods, notably around the end of the nineteenth century. These variations over time probably reflect the changing interests of doctors rather than true changes in prevalence. In the course of past 40 years there has been another increase in the number of reported cases, especially in the USA. It is not certain whether this change is real, and epidemiological studies do not provide the answer because they report such widely varying prevalence rates. The disorder has been highly controversial and, along with the associated 'recovered memory syndrome', generates fierce debate and legal challenges.

Patients who meet the criteria in Box 22.13 often meet the criteria for other diagnoses, including schizophrenia, personality disorder, and substance abuse. Many also have symptoms of anxiety and depression. The relationship between dissociative identity disorder and these other conditions would be clarified by long-term follow-up studies, but no systematic studies of this kind have been reported.

Two issues have dominated the discussion of *aetiology*:

1. *The role of severe trauma*. Clinical experience and research find that many of those with the disorder describe severe physical or sexual abuse taking place in childhood. It has been suggested that dissociation began as a psychological defence mechanism that

---

Box 22.13 DSM-5 diagnostic criteria for dissociative identity disorder

A Disruption of identity by two or more distinct personality states. Involves a marked discontinuity in sense of self and agency, plus alterations in behaviour affect, cognition, which may be observed by others or reported by the individual.

B Recurrent gaps in recall of everyday events, personal information, or traumatic events.

C Symptoms cause clinically significant distress or impairment.

D Not a normal part of a broadly accepted religious or cultural practice.

E Not attributable to intoxication or other medical condition (e.g. complex partial seizures).

Note: in children, the symptoms are not attributable to imaginary playmates or other fantasy play.

Source: data from Diagnostic and Statistical Manual of Mental Disorders, Fifth Edition, Copyright (2013), American Psychiatric Association.

reduced distress at the time of the original trauma but had unfortunate lasting consequences.

2. *Iatrogenic factors*. It has been argued that the widespread publicity given to some people with multiple personality, the credulity of some therapists, and the use of hypnosis, have been responsible for at least some instances of the disorder.

For review, see Dorahy *et al.* (2014).

Depersonalization disorder

Depersonalization disorder is characterized by an unpleasant state in which external objects or parts of the body are experienced as changed in their quality, and feel unreal or remote. In DSM-5 derealization has been incorporated into depersonalization, and the condition is termed *depersonalization/derealization disorder*. Transient symptoms of depersonalization are quite common as a minor feature of other syndromes (see Chapter 1), and the symptoms of depersonalization disorder occur occasionally in association with other psychiatric disorders (see differential diagnosis, below). However, primary depersonalization disorder is rare. How rare is uncertain because estimates of the prevalence vary so widely that no useful conclusion can be reached (Reutens *et al.*, 2010).

Although classified as a dissociative disorder in DSM-5, it is not certain whether dissociation is indeed the causal mechanism (see aetiology, below). In ICD-10 this uncertainty is recognized by giving depersonalization disorder its own place in the classification, separate from the dissociative disorders.

Clinical picture

The central features are a feeling of being unreal and an unreal quality to perceptions. Emotions seem dulled and actions feel mechanical. Paradoxically, this lack of feeling is experienced as extremely unpleasant. Insight is retained into the subjective nature of their experiences. These symptoms may be intense, and accompanied by *déjà vu* and by changes in the experience of passage of time. Some patients complain also of sensory distortions affecting a single part of the body (usually the head, the nose, or a limb), a feeling which some describe as if made of cotton wool.

Two-thirds of the patients are women. The onset is often sudden, in adolescence or early adult life, with the condition starting before the age of 30 years in about half the cases. Once established, symptoms may persist for years, though with periods of partial or complete remission.

Differential diagnosis

Before diagnosing depersonalization disorder, any primary disorder must be excluded, especially temporal lobe epilepsy, schizophrenia, depressive disorder, another dissociative disorder, and anxiety disorders (Sierra *et al.*, 2012). Most patients who present with depersonalization will be found to have one of these other conditions.

Aetiology

The causes of a primary depersonalization disorder are not known. Apart from the possible association with schizoid personality disorder, no definite constitutional factors have been identified. Jay *et al.* (2014) suggest that depersonalization is due to excessive inhibition of the insula by ventrolateral prefrontal cortex. At the same time, autonomic responses to unpleasant stimuli are reduced, suggesting inhibition of emotional processing, which could lead to a subjective sense of emotional numbing.

Prognosis

The rare primary depersonalization disorder has not been followed systematically; clinical experience indicates that cases lasting longer than a year have a poor long-term outcome.

Treatment

When depersonalization is secondary to another disorder, treatment should be directed to the primary condition. Supportive interviews can help the patient to function more normally despite the symptoms, and any stressors should be addressed. No specific pharmacological or psychological treatments are well established. In this, as in other conditions that are difficult to treat, it is important to resist the temptation to give ineffective treatments to appear to be doing something for the patient. It is better to give adequate time for supportive care. For review, see Reutens *et al.* (2010).

Other dissociative syndromes in ICD-10

ICD-10 contains three further dissociative syndromes which are absent from DSM-5; in the latter they would be coded as 'dissociative disorder NOS' (Table 22.5).

Dissociative stupor

In dissociative stupor, patients show the characteristic features of stupor. They are motionless and mute, and they do not respond to stimulation, but they are aware of their surroundings. Dissociative stupor is rare. It is essential to exclude other possible conditions, namely schizophrenia, depressive disorder, mania, and organic brain diseases.

Ganser's syndrome

Ganser's syndrome is a very rare condition with four features:

- giving 'approximate answers' (see below) to questions designed to test intellectual functions
- psychogenic physical symptoms
- hallucinations
- apparent clouding of consciousness.

The syndrome was described in 1898 by Ganser in prisoners, but it is not confined to them. The term 'approximate answers' denotes answers (to simple questions) that are plainly wrong but are clearly related to the correct answer in a way that suggests that the latter is known. For example, when asked to add two and two a patient might answer five. The obvious advantage to be gained from the condition, coupled with the approximate answers, suggests malingering. However, the condition is often maintained so consistently that unconscious mental mechanisms have been thought to play a part. For some naïve individuals this may represent their only way of communicating effectively their distress. It is important to exclude an organic brain disease or schizophrenia; the former should be considered particularly carefully when muddled thinking and visual hallucinations are part of the clinical picture.

For a review, see Dwyer and Reid (2004).

Trance and possession disorder

Trance and possession states are characterized by a temporary loss of the sense of personal identity and of full awareness of the surroundings. Such states are induced temporarily in willing participants in religious or other ceremonies, and also recreationally in 'raves', often aided by drug use. When they arise in this way, the states are not recorded as disorders. According to DSM-5, a dissociative trance involves:

… acute narrowing or complete loss of awareness of immediate surroundings that manifests as profound unresponsiveness or insensitivity to environmental stimuli. …. accompanied by minor stereotyped behaviours of which the individual is unaware or cannot control … is not a normal part of a broadly accepted cultural or religious practice.

Some cases resemble multiple personality disorder, in that the person behaves as if taken over by another personality for a brief period. When the condition is induced by religious ritual, the person may feel taken over by a deity or spirit. The focus of attention is narrowed to a few aspects of the immediate environment; for example, to the priest carrying out a religious ceremony. The affected person may repeatedly perform the same movements, or adopt postures, or repeat utterances.

Miscellaneous other syndromes associated with dissociation

Cultural syndromes

Certain patterns of unusual behaviour, restricted to certain cultures, have been thought to reflect psychological mechanisms of dissociation. Some of these behaviours can be classified as 'cultural-bound syndromes'. This term has been criticized because of its 'ethnocentric' implications—that all mental disorders are best, or only, understood from a European perspective. It is applied to syndromes in non-western cultures but not to syndromes which are found particularly in western cultures—for example, eating disorders and CFS. Many of the early descriptions were associated with explicit or implicit racist ideas, and these terms should be used with circumspection. Examples of cultural syndromes include the following:

- *Latah*, which is found among women in Malaya, is characterized by echolalia, echopraxia, and other kinds of abnormally compliant behaviour. The condition usually follows a frightening experience.
- *Amok* has been described among men in Indonesia and Malaya. It begins with a period of brooding, which is followed by violent behaviour and sometimes dangerous use of weapons. Amnesia is usually reported afterwards. It is unlikely that all patients with this pattern of behaviour are suffering from a dissociative disorder; the others may be suffering from mania, schizophrenia, or a postepileptic state.
- *Arctic hysteria (Piblokto)* is seen among the Inuit, more often in the women. The affected person tears off her clothing, screams and cries, runs about in distress, and may endanger her life by exposure to cold. Sometimes the behaviour is violent. The relationship of this syndrome to dissociative disorder is not firmly established, and there may be more than one cause.

It has been suggested that these cultural syndromes are becoming less common or altering in presentation as a result of globalization (Ventriglio *et al.*, 2016).

Recovered memories and false-memory syndrome

These conditions are described on page 158.

Factitious dissociative identity disorder

There is wide agreement, even among those who believe that dissociative identity disorder is common, that both factitious and malingered presentations are also common (Dorahy *et al.*, 2014).

Psychiatric services in medical settings

Psychiatric services for general hospitals are named and organized in several ways.

Consultation–liaison psychiatry (sometimes known as C–L psychiatry or as *liaison psychiatry*) is the traditional term. In consultation work, the psychiatrist gives opinions on patients referred by physicians and surgeons; in liaison work the psychiatrist is a member of a medical or surgical team, and offers advice about any patient to whose care he feels able to contribute. However, in contemporary psychiatry, the term *psychological medicine* is often preferred, reflecting an increasing integration of psychiatry into general medicine rather than just consulting or liaising with it (Sharpe, 2014).

Behavioural medicine is the term for similar arrangements provided by clinical psychologists rather than psychiatrists.

Psychosomatic medicine is a term used widely in the past in some countries, and which is still current in Germany. It has been revived in the USA as the name for consultation–liaison psychiatry as a recognized subspecialty (Gitlin *et al.*, 2004).

The make-up of services

Consultation and liaison units vary in their size and organization. Some are staffed entirely by psychiatrists, and others by a multidisciplinary team of psychiatrists, nurses, social workers, and clinical psychologists. A few services have inpatient beds for patients who are both medically and psychiatrically ill. In some North American hospitals with large consultation–liaison services, up to 5% of all admissions are referred to psychiatrists. In the UK and many other countries, a smaller proportion of inpatients are referred, most being emergencies, especially those with deliberate self-harm (see Chapter 21). Most of the literature on consultation–liaison psychiatry has focused on inpatients, but most of the patients referred are from outpatient clinics and emergency departments.

Consultation–liaison psychiatry is increasingly concerned with the provision of psychiatric and psychological assessment, and the collaborative management of patients with either medically unexplained symptoms or psychiatric disorders comorbid with chronic medical illness. A major challenge is to find ways of extending these overstretched services to similar patients treated in primary care.

For further information about consultation and liaison psychiatry and psychosomatic medicine, see Leentjens *et al.* (2011).

Psychiatric consultation in a medical setting

The consultation has two parts: the *assessment* of the patient, and *communication* with the patient and with the doctor who is making the referral. Assessment is similar to that of any other patients referred for a psychiatric opinion with the addition that it is necessary to take into account their medical condition and treatment, and their willingness to see a psychiatrist.

First steps

Having received the request for a consultation, the psychiatrist should make sure that the referring doctor has adequately discussed the psychiatric referral with the patient and that the latter has agreed to see the psychiatrist. Before interviewing the patient, the psychiatrist should read the relevant medical notes and ask the nursing staff about the patient's mental state and behaviour. The psychiatrist should find out what treatment the patient is receiving, and if necessary consult a work of reference about the side effects of any drugs.

The assessment interview

In most respects, the assessment is as described in Chapter 3, but it is modified to reflect the circumstances (see also Chapter 3, page 55). Thus, at the start of the interview the psychiatrist should make clear to the patient the purpose of the consultation. It may be necessary to discuss the patient's concerns about seeing a psychiatrist (for example, it does not imply that they are 'mad' or that the referring doctor disbelieves them) and to explain how the interview may contribute to the treatment plan (by adding another kind of expertise to their medical care).

Clinical notes

In the past, the psychiatrist would usually keep a separate, detailed, record of the assessment and conclusions, with a much briefer entry being made in the medical notes, which contained only the essential information and conclusions. However, it is now usual for each patient to have only one medical record, and thus no separate psychiatric notes. Nevertheless, it is important that the psychiatrist includes a concise, clear summary that will be understandable to the medical team, within the full record of the assessment.

Writing the response to the referral

It is often appropriate to discuss the proposed plan of management with the medical and nursing team managing the patient before writing a final opinion. In this way the psychiatrist can make sure that recommendations are feasible and acceptable, and that answers have been given to the questions asked about the patient.

The entry in the medical notes should be along the lines of a letter to a general practitioner (see page 65). It is important to make clear the nature of any immediate treatment that is recommended, and who is to carry it out. If the assessment is provisional until other informants have been interviewed, the psychiatrist should state when the final opinion will be given. The note should be signed legibly, and should tell the ward staff where the psychiatrist or a deputy can be found should further help be required.

Management

Treatment is similar to that of a similar psychiatric disorder in a medically well patient. However, when psychiatric drugs are prescribed, special attention should be paid to the possible effects of the patient's medical condition on their metabolism and excretion, and to any possible interactions with other drugs that the patient is taking. The plan should be based on a realistic assessment of the amount of supervision available on a medical or surgical ward, for example, for a depressed patient with suicidal ideas. With support from a psychiatrist the nursing staff can manage most brief psychiatric disorders that arise in a general hospital, although some support may be needed from a psychiatric nurse (who may be a member of the consultation–liaison team).

Continuing care

The psychiatrist may need to review the patient's progress whilst in hospital. After discharge it is important to attempt to ensure continuity of care by speaking or writing to the general practitioner. According to the needs of the case, care may be continued by the general practitioner, or the liaison psychiatrist may continue to see the patient, or care may be transferred to the community psychiatric team.

Some common emergency problems

General approach

The successful management of any psychiatric emergency depends importantly on the initial clinical interview. The aims are those of any assessment interview: to establish a good relationship with the patient, elicit information from the patient and other informants, and observe the patient's behaviour and mental state. A relaxed, sympathetic, and firm approach helps to calm the situation enough for the doctor to reach an understanding of the patient's concerns and suggest a plan that the patient will agree. In an emergency, it may not be possible to conduct a full assessment interview, but the assessment should be as systematic and as complete as the circumstances permit.

The anxious patient

Panic attacks. The somatic symptoms of a panic attack are frequent reasons for an emergency presentation. Common features include non-cardiac chest pain, tingling in the extremities, and the effects of hyperventilation (see page 162). Most patients can be talked through an episode of panic, and hyperventilation responds to rebreathing into a paper bag. Occasionally a small dose of a benzodiazepine is needed to control the anxiety. Follow-up with treatment for panic disorder may be required.

Severe generalized anxiety may complicate any medical presentation. Attendance at an emergency department can be a frightening experience and the consequent anxiety may be made worse by the response of unaware staff. It is usually possible to reduce the anxiety by explaining what is happening in a sympathetic manner. Occasionally a small dosage of a benzodiazepine may be necessary to control the anxiety.

See also Chapter 3 for assessment of anxious patients.

The angry or aggressive patient

It can be very upsetting to clinicians and other carers when the person they are trying to help responds with anger. When this happens, it is essential to keep calm and avoid doing or saying anything that may increase the person's anger, and to be careful about physical safety (see below). The clinician should try to find out and understand why the person is angry. Sometimes it is helpful to comment on the anger and to ask directly why the person is so upset. It is always unwise either to show anger in return or to be unduly submissive. It may be necessary to apologize for the problem that has caused the anger, for example, if the patient has been kept waiting for a long time.

If the patient is potentially violent, it is essential to arrange for adequate but unobtrusive help to be available. Physical contact (including physical examination) should not be attempted unless the purpose has been clearly understood by and agreed with the patient. If restraint cannot be avoided, it should be accomplished quickly by an adequate number of people using the minimum of force. Staff should not attempt single-handed restraint. Extreme caution is, of course, required if the patient could be in possession of an offensive weapon.

See also Chapter 18 for discussion of prevention and management of violence in psychiatric settings.

Emergency drug treatment of disturbed or violent patients

Diazepam (5–10 mg) may be useful for a patient who is frightened. For more severely disturbed patients intramuscular lorazepam can be used; intramuscular haloperidol (2–5 mg) can also be used for those who are psychotic and who have previously been exposed to antipsychotics. For further details, see Chapter 25. For treatment of delirium, see Chapter 14.

When the patient has become calm, medication may be continued in smaller doses, usually three to four times a day and preferably by mouth, using syrup if the patient will not swallow tablets. The dosage depends on the patient's weight and on the initial response to the drug. Careful observations by nurses of the physical state and behaviour are necessary during this treatment.

Problems in consent to treatment

General principles relating to consent to treatment are discussed in Chapter 4. Psychiatrists can often be asked to advise on issues around the competency of patients, and are sometimes asked to advise about patients who are refusing to accept medical or surgical treatment. There are several reasons why patients may be unwilling to accept treatment that is recommended to them. They may not have understood the information they have been given, they may be frightened or angry, or, occasionally, they may have a mental illness that interferes with their ability to make an informed decision.

It has to be accepted that a conscious mentally competent adult has the right to refuse treatment even after a full and rational discussion of the reasons for carrying it out. When the patient's condition is such that he cannot give consent, then, in the UK and many other countries, the doctor in charge of the patient has the right to give immediate treatment in life-threatening emergencies. The medicolegal issues are summarized in Box 22.14.

See Boland *et al.* (2000) for a review of the management of psychiatric syndromes in intensive care units.

Psychiatric aspects of medical procedures and conditions

Genetic counselling

Genetic counselling about the reproductive risks of hereditary disease is mainly given to couples contemplating marriage, or planning or expecting a child. Psychiatrists used to be involved in this but it is now the responsibility of medical geneticists, not least because of rapid developments in the range and methods of testing available. However, psychiatrists do need to keep up to date with the increasing number of clinical situations in which genetic counselling may be indicated (see Chapter 5).

Counselling includes:

- providing information about risks
- helping people to cope with concerns about the diagnosis

- enabling patients to take informed decisions about family planning.

Occasionally medical geneticists may request the collaboration or advice of psychiatrists, particularly when potential parents appear to be significantly distressed by the advice and unable to concentrate on making decisions.

Psychiatric aspects of surgical treatment

Preoperative problems

Patients about to undergo surgery are often anxious, and those who are most anxious before operation are likely

> ### Box 22.14 Medicolegal and ethical issues: patients who refuse to accept advice about emergency treatment
>
> - *In life-threatening emergencies* where it is not possible to obtain the patient's consent (consciousness is impaired, or there is evidence of psychiatric disorder which cannot be immediately assessed), opinions should be obtained from medical and nursing colleagues, and, if possible, from the patient's relatives. Detailed records should be kept of the reasons for the decision. It is essential for all doctors to know the law about these matters in the country in which they are practising.
>
> - If a patient has a *mental disorder that impairs the ability to give informed consent,* it may be appropriate to use legal powers of compulsory assessment and treatment of the mental disorder. In the UK, the powers for compulsory treatment of a mental disorder do *not* give the doctor a right to treat concurrent physical illness against the patient's wishes. However, after successful treatment of the psychiatric disorder, the patient may decide to give informed consent for the treatment of the physical illness. See also Chapter 4.

to be anxious afterwards. Most studies of psychological preparation for surgery have shown that it can reduce postoperative distress, especially when the preparation includes measures to improve coping.

Psychiatrists may be asked to assess patients before surgery. Common reasons for such a request include:

- clarification of the role of emotional factors in the patient's physical complaints
- uncertainty about the patient's cognitive state and capacity to provide informed consent
- help in the management of current psychiatric problems
- help in predicting the patients' response to surgery and their capacity to cooperate with postoperative treatment and rehabilitation.

Psychiatric problems in the postoperative period

Delirium

Delirium is common after major surgery, especially in the elderly. Whether delirium develops depends on the type of surgery, the type of anaesthetic, the presence of postoperative physical complications, and the type of medication. Delirium is associated with increased mortality and longer stay in hospital (see Chapter 14).

Pain

Psychiatrists are sometimes asked to advise on the management of patients with unusually severe postoperative pain. Patients who are given greater control over the timing of analgesia usually experience less pain and make less use of analgesia. Some are helped by anxiety management, and others by help in resolving anger

arising, for example, from disagreements with the staff who are caring for them.

Long-term psychological problems after surgery

Adjustment problems are particularly common after mastectomy and laryngectomy, and after surgery that has not led to the expected benefit. Psychiatrists can sometimes contribute to the management of such problems, especially when the surgery is part of the treatment of a relapsing, chronic, or progressive disorder. The psychiatrist may help to discover psychosocial factors that are impeding adjustment, and to help the patient resolve or come to terms with the problems. Some patients require antidepressant medication.

See Hales *et al.* (2009) for review.

Plastic surgery

People with physical deformities often suffer embarrassment and distress, and this may markedly restrict their lives as children and as adults. When such patients are psychiatrically healthy, plastic surgery usually gives good results. Even when there is no major objective defect to match the concerns about appearance, cosmetic surgery to the nose, face, and breasts is usually successful. Nevertheless, psychological assessment can contribute to assessment before plastic surgery: the outcome is likely to be poor in patients who have delusions about their appearance, dysmorphophobia, or greatly unrealistic expectations, or have been dissatisfied with previous surgery. See Van Soest *et al.* (2009) for a review.

Bariatric surgery

There is a high prevalence of psychiatric disorders amongst candidates for bariatric surgery. There is also evidence that psychiatric symptoms decrease post-surgery, although these improvements may not persist. See Muller *et al.* (2013) for review.

Limb amputation

Limb amputation has different psychological consequences for young and for elderly people. Young adult amputees, such as those losing a leg in a road accident or in military action, characteristically show denial at first, and may later experience depression and phantom limb pains which resolve slowly. Children and adolescents seem to have a similar outcome. Older people usually undergo amputation after prolonged problems associated with vascular disease. Such patients do not commonly report severe distress immediately after the operation, but they often develop phantom limb pain. Some have difficulty with the prosthesis and show a degree of functional incapacity disproportionate to their physical state.

Organ transplantation

These operations have considerable associated psychiatric consequences related to the nature of the surgery, and the need for continuing intensive medical care.

Selection for transplantation. The selection process can be stressful, and so can the wait for a suitable organ, though the latter tends to be less so for kidney transplants because there is the alternative of continuing dialysis during the waiting period. There are few psychological contraindications for these operations, mostly relating to inability to cope with the demands of the necessary long-term postoperative care. After operation, transplantation is associated with the same psychiatric and emotional problems that occur after other major surgery, especially anxiety, delirium, and depression. There are also some problems specific to a particular type of transplant; for example, liver transplantation has the highest rate of preoperative and postoperative neuropsychiatric complications.

These problems are sufficiently frequent and serious to justify psychiatric liaison with transplant units to support staff and train them to recognize and respond appropriately to patients who have such problems (Heinrich and Marcangelo, 2009).

Diabetes mellitus

Diabetes is a chronic condition requiring prolonged medical supervision and informed self-care, and many physicians emphasize the psychological aspect of treatment. It is associated with an increased prevalence of psychiatric disorder. Moreover, type 2 diabetes is two to three times more common in patients with severe mental disorder, related both to shared disease mechanisms and the effects of antipsychotic drugs (Holt and Mitchell, 2015), highlighting the need for psychiatrists to be aware of the features and management of diabetes.

For review of the psychiatric aspects of diabetes, see Ducat *et al.* (2014).

Psychological factors and diabetic control

Psychological factors are important in established diabetes because they influence its control, and it is now generally accepted that good control of blood glucose is the most important single factor preventing long-term complications. Psychological factors can impair control in two ways. First, stressful experiences can lead to endocrine changes. Second, many diabetics do not adhere well to their treatment regime, especially at times of stress, and this is an important cause of 'brittle' diabetes.

Problems of being diabetic

Psychological and social problems may be caused by restrictions of diet and activity, the need for self-care, and the possibility of serious physical complications such as vascular disease and impaired vision. Although most diabetic people overcome or adapt to such problems, an important minority have difficulties. Adherence to regimes for testing, diet, and insulin is often unsatisfactory so that glycaemia control is less than optimal. Problems of this kind are particularly likely in adolescents with type 1 diabetes.

Other problems

Associated eating disorder. Control of diabetes is more difficult when the diabetic person has an eating disorder, in particular when insulin is part of the treatment regimen, since it can be misused to lose weight.

Associated medical complications. Psychosocial problems are more than usually common in diabetics who have severe medical complications such as loss of sight, renal failure, and vascular disease. Diabetic neuropathy is often very painful and can restrict activities.

Sexual problems are common among diabetics. Two kinds of impotence occur in diabetic men. The first is psychogenic impotence of the kind found in other chronic debilitating diseases. The second kind is more common in diabetes, and may pre-date other features of the disease. It is thought to be associated with pelvic autonomic neuropathy and vascularity, while endocrine factors may play a part.

Pregnancy is a difficult time for diabetic women, with problems in the control of diabetes and increased risks of miscarriage and fetal malformations.

Organic psychiatric syndromes in diabetic patients

Delirium. The first evidence of developing diabetic coma is sometimes an episode of disturbed behaviour, starting either abruptly or insidiously. The cause of the behaviour becomes clearer as other prodromal symptoms develop, including thirst, headaches, abdominal pain, nausea, and vomiting. The pulse is rapid and blood pressure is low. Dehydration is marked and acetone may be smelt on the breath.

Dementia. Diabetes is a risk factor for dementia (see Chapter 14).

Psychiatric aspects of diabetes management

Diabetes has been the object of considerable psychiatric research, involving a range of psychological treatments and particularly in adolescent and brittle diabetics. Possible measures include: treatment for depressive disorder; blood glucose awareness training to improve the ability to recognize and act on fluctuations in blood glucose concentrations; weight management programmes; cognitive behavioural approaches to improve self-care; help with psychosocial problems; and treatment of sexual dysfunction. Tricyclic antidepressants may be helpful in relieving the pain of neuropathy. See Plack *et al.* (2010) for a review of psychological care of patients with insulin-dependent diabetes.

Other endocrine disorders

Many endocrine disorders, most conspicuously thyroid and adrenal dysfunction, have been associated with psychiatric complications. Box 22.15 summarizes some of the more common associations, together with aspects of steroid therapy.

See Harrison and Kopelman (2009) for a review of the psychiatric aspects of endocrine disorder.

Other metabolic and autoimmune disorders

Psychiatric aspects of systemic lupus erythematosus and autoimmune encephalitis are covered in Chapter 14. For other metabolic and medical disorders, such as the porphyrias, sarcoidosis, and myasthenia gravis, see Harrison and Kopelman (2009).

Cardiac disorders

It has long been suggested that emotional disorder predisposes to ischaemic heart disease. Dunbar (1954) described a 'coronary personality'. Recent research has concentrated on several possible risk factors, including chronic emotional disturbance, social and economic disadvantage, overwork and other chronic stress, and the so-called 'type A personality'. The latter consists of hostility, excessive competitive drive, ambitiousness, a chronic sense of urgency, and a preoccupation with deadlines (Friedman and Rosenman, 1959). Although type A behaviour has been widely accepted as an independent risk factor for ischaemic heart disease, recent evidence has cast doubt on this conclusion. However, there is evidence that cardiac patients with 'type D' personality (high levels of distress and negative affect) have a poorer outcome (Denollet *et al.*, 2010).

Angina

Angina is often precipitated by emotions such as anxiety, anger, and excitement. It is a frightening symptom, and some patients become overcautious despite reassurance and encouragement to resume normal activities. Angina is sometimes accompanied by atypical chest pain and breathlessness caused by anxiety or hyperventilation, and it is important to identify this rather than increasing medical anti-angina therapy.

Myocardial infarction

Patients often respond to the early symptoms of myocardial infarction with denial, and consequently delay seeking treatment. In the first few days in hospital, acute organic mental disorders and anxiety symptoms are common.

Recent research has concentrated on the replicated finding that depression, anxiety, and social isolation are important risk factors for both a lower quality of life (Dickens *et al.*, 2006) and for a 22% increased risk of death after myocardial infarction (Meijer *et al.*, 2013).

Some survivors of cardiac arrest suffer cognitive impairment. When such impairment is mild, it may show up later as apparent personality change or as behavioural symptoms, which may be attributed wrongly to an emotional reaction to the illness.

When patients return home from hospital, they commonly report non-specific symptoms such as fatigue, insomnia, and poor concentration, as well as excessive concern about somatic symptoms and an unnecessarily cautious attitude to exertion. Most patients overcome

> ## Box 22.15 **Psychiatric aspects of other endocrine disorders and steroid therapy**
>
> **Hyperthyroidism (thyrotoxicosis).** May present with psychiatric symptoms such as anxiety, irritability, emotional lability, and difficulty in concentrating. These, together with hyperactivity, fatigue, and tremor, may make differential diagnosis from anxiety disorder difficult. Treatment of thyroid dysfunction usually results in improvement of the psychiatric symptoms.
>
> **Hypothyroidism (myxoedema).** Cognitive impairment and other psychiatric disorders are common. Mood disorder may take a rapid-cycling form. Replacement therapy may reverse the mood symptoms but neuropsychiatric problems may persist. See Dugbartey (1998) for a review.
>
> **Hyperadrenalism (Cushing's syndrome).** Depressive symptoms are common. Their severity is not closely related to plasma cortisol concentrations, and personality and stressful circumstances may play a part. Psychological symptoms usually improve quickly when
>
> the medical condition is controlled. Paranoid symptoms also occur, especially in those with the most severe illness. See Pivonello *et al.* (2015).
>
> **Steroid therapy.** Affective symptoms, especially euphoria or mild mania, are frequent. Paranoid symptoms are less common. The severity of the mental disorder is not closely associated with dosage. Symptoms usually improve when the dosage is reduced but, when severe, lithium prophylaxis should be considered for patients who need to continue steroid treatment after a mood disorder has been controlled. Withdrawal of corticosteroids may cause lethargy, weakness, and joint pain.
>
> **Anabolic steroids.** Anabolic–androgenic steroids are widely used by athletes. Significant mood disturbances and increased aggression have been reported (Oberlander and Henderson, 2012).

these problems and return to a fully active life. A few continue with emotional distress and social disability out of proportion to their physical state, often accompanied by atypical somatic symptoms. Such problems are more common in patients with longstanding psychiatric or social problems, overprotective families, and myocardial infarction with a complicated course.

The finding that depression and social isolation are associated with increased mortality after myocardial infarction has led to research to evaluate interventions to treat them. In the large trials so far completed, nursing support to combat social isolation was ineffective. Cognitive behaviour therapy, medication, and exercise all show some efficacy in treating depression after myocardial infarction, but antidepressants must be used with caution, and tricyclic antidepressants are best avoided. Reductions in cardiac events and mortality have not been demonstrated reliably (Shapiro, 2015).

Non-cardiac chest pain

During the American Civil War, Da Costa described a condition which he called 'irritable heart'. This syndrome consisted of a conviction that the heart was diseased, together with palpitations, breathlessness, fatigue, and inframammary pain. This combination has also been named 'disorderly action of the heart', 'effort syndrome', and 'neurocirculatory asthenia'. The symptoms were originally thought to indicate a disorder of the functioning of the heart.

Non-cardiac chest pain is very common among patients in primary care and in cardiac outpatient clinics. Most patients are reassured by a thorough assessment, but a significant minority continue to complain of physical and psychological symptoms and to limit their everyday activities. Follow-up studies of patients with chest pain and normal coronary angiograms have consistently found subsequent mortality and cardiac morbidity to be little greater than those without cardiac disease, but persistent disability to be common.

Many causes have been suggested for atypical cardiac symptoms, including pain originating in the chest wall, oesophageal reflux and spasm, microvascular angina, mitral valve prolapse, and psychiatric disorder. In most patients chest pain appears to be due to minor non-cardiac physical causes or to hyperventilation, which are misconstrued as heart disease and associated with anxiety. The aetiology is as for other medically unexplained symptoms. The most common psychiatric concomitant is panic disorder; less common are depressive disorder and hypochondriasis.

Management should follow the principles described in Chapter 8, with a particular emphasis on the treatment of hyperventilation, graded increase in activity, and discussion of beliefs about the cause of the pain. Cognitive behaviour therapy may be effective in the management of anxiety with hyperventilation. Depressive disorder should be treated with antidepressant medication.

See George *et al.* (2016) for a review.

Sensory disorders

Deafness

Deafness may develop before speech is learned (prelingual deafness) or afterwards. Profound early deafness interferes with speech and language development, and with emotional development. Prelingually deaf adults often maintain their own social groups and communicate by sign language. When they have problems, it appears that these are more often diagnosed as behaviour problems and social maladjustment than emotional disorder. These problems are managed best by those with special knowledge of the effects of deafness.

Deafness of later onset has less severe effects than those just described. However, the acute onset of profound deafness can be extremely distressing, whilst milder restriction of hearing may cause depression and considerable social disability.

Kraepelin was the first to suggest that deafness is an important factor in the development of persecutory delusions. Subsequent evidence supports an association between deafness and paranoid disorders in the elderly (see Chapter 12). See Landsberger *et al.* (2013) for a review.

Tinnitus

Tinnitus is very common, but few patients seek treatment and most are able to live a normal life. Persistent tinnitus may be associated with low mood. Some patients are helped by devices that mask tinnitus with a more acceptable sound. Antidepressant medication may improve mood and reduce the intensity of the tinnitus. Cognitive and behavioural methods may enable people to accept their tinnitus and to minimize their social handicaps and perhaps protect against the increased risk of suicide in this disorder. For review, see Langguth *et al.* (2013).

Blindness

Although it imposes many difficulties, blindness in early life need not lead to abnormal psychological development in childhood or to unsuccessful later development. In previously sighted people, the later onset of blindness often causes considerable distress. Initial denial and subsequent depression are common, as are prolonged difficulties in adjustment. See Berman and Brodaty (2006).

Infections

Psychological factors may affect the course of recovery from an acute infection (Hotopf *et al.*, 1996). In a classic early study, psychological tests were completed by 600 people who subsequently developed Asian influenza. Delayed recovery from the influenza was no more common among people whose initial illness had been severe, but it was more frequent among those who had obtained more abnormal scores on the psychological tests before the illness (Imboden *et al.*, 1961). More recent findings of research on viral illness in general practice and infectious mononucleosis have reported similar conclusions.

In addition, some infectious diseases (for example, hepatitis A, influenza, and brucellosis) are frequently followed by periods of depression and fatigue. The possible role of infections, such as Lyme disease, as a cause of chronic fatigue was discussed on page 642. *Viral encephalitis* is discussed in Chapter 14.

HIV infection

HIV infection affects the brain at an early stage and the disease has a chronic progressive course associated with a wide range of psychiatric consequences. With modern combined antiretroviral therapy, most patients with AIDS lead relatively healthy lives for substantial periods; indeed, their life expectancy is no longer significantly reduced. The nature of the physical symptoms, their progressive course, and the reactions of other people all explain why emotional distress is common in people with HIV infection. A further reason is that some of those at high risk for HIV (for example, drug abusers) may have other psychological problems. Effects on the family may be considerable, especially where the partner and or one or more of the children are infected. Women might first find out about their diagnosis when pregnant, and so will have to navigate the difficult adjustment of having a potentially life-limiting condition at the same time as preparing to become a parent and their concerns about how the infection might affect their parenting as well as the physical and psychological health of their child. Psychiatrists can contribute to the care of AIDS patients by providing counselling and specialist treatment for neuropsychiatric and other psychiatric complications.

Reactions to testing. Although HIV antibody testing is worrying for most of those who undergo it, the distress is usually short-lived whatever the outcome of the test. People who have persistent and unjustified worries about having AIDS require psychiatric help of the kind appropriate for other illness fears.

Psychiatric problems, including adjustment disorder, depressive disorder, and anxiety disorder, are frequent at the time of diagnosis, although they may occur at any stage of the disease. People with previous psychological problems, longstanding social difficulties, or lack of social support are especially vulnerable.

Suicide and *deliberate self-harm* may occur in people who are concerned about the possibility of HIV infection as well as in people with proven disease. Among the latter, the risk is greater in those with advanced symptoms. However, it is not certain how much greater is the risk of suicide and deliberate self-harm in AIDS patients than in the general population.

Neuropsychiatric disorders occur secondary to the complications of immune suppression and as a result of the direct effects of HIV on the brain (Saylor *et al.*, 2016). Minor cognitive disorders are frequent. HIV-associated dementia (AIDS–dementia complex), HIV encephalopathy, and subacute encephalitis occur late in the illness in around a third of patients. There is usually an insidious onset with progression to profound dementia. HIV infection can also result in neurological symptoms and dementia in those who do not have AIDS. Delirium may occur when there is an opportunistic infection or cerebral malignancy (Dilley and Fleminger, 2009).

Social consequences are considerable because of the public fears of the condition and stigma. Cultural differences in acceptance or rejection, and in the availability of family and other support, are major determinants of quality of life.

Problems in relation to illicit drug use are considered in Chapter 20. The disorganized lives of some HIV-positive drug users and their personal and social problems can make treatment of HIV difficult.

Ethical problems are related to confidentiality. They include the importance of maintaining confidentiality, disclosure to third parties who are at risk of infection, disclosure to insurers and to employers, and protection of the public from risk of transmission from HIV-infected health care workers.

Cancer

The psychological consequences of cancer are similar to those of any other serious physical illness:

- *Delay in seeking medical help* because of fear or denial.
- *Response to the diagnosis*, which may be anxiety, shock, anger, disbelief, or depression. Sometimes the response is severe enough to meet the criteria for a psychiatric disorder, usually an adjustment disorder or sometimes a depressive disorder. The risk of suicide is increased, particularly in the year after diagnosis (Hem *et al.*, 2004).
- *Later consequences*. Major depression occurs throughout the course of cancer and appears to be more frequent in those suffering pain. Prevalence estimates for depression in cancer range from 5% to 15%, with higher rates in palliative care settings (Walker *et al.*, 2013a).
- *The progression and recurrence* of cancer are often associated with increased psychiatric disturbance, which may result from a worsening of physical symptoms such as pain and nausea, from fear of dying, or from the development of an organic psychiatric syndrome.
- *Delirium and dementia* may arise from brain metastases, which originate most often from carcinoma of the lung, but also from tumours of the breast and alimentary tract, and from melanomas. Occasionally, brain metastases produce psychiatric symptoms before the primary lesion is discovered (see also Chapter 14).
- *Neuropsychiatric problems (paraneoplastic syndromes)* are sometimes induced by certain kinds of cancer in the absence of metastases, notably by ovarian teratomas, lung tumours, and Hodgkin's lymphoma. The mechanism is thought to be an autoimmune response or secretion of psychoactive substances by cancer cells (see Chapter 14).

Treatment for cancer may cause psychological disorder. Emotional distress is particularly common after mastectomy and other mutilating surgery. *Radiotherapy* causes nausea, fatigue, and emotional distress. *Chemotherapy* often causes malaise and nausea, and anxiety about chemotherapy may cause anticipatory nausea before the treatment. The latter may be helped by behavioural treatments in addition to antiemetic medication.

Family and other close relatives of cancer patients may experience psychological problems, which may persist even if the cancer is cured. Nevertheless, many patients and relatives make a good adjustment to cancer. The extent of their adjustment depends partly on the information they receive.

Treatment for psychological consequences of cancer

In the past doctors were reluctant to tell patients that the diagnosis was cancer, but most patients prefer to know the diagnosis and how it will affect their lives. However, the information must be communicated well; otherwise there may be problems in achieving a psychological adjustment. Depression and anxiety disorders are often missed in these patients, and systematic screening has been recommended (Andersen *et al.*, 2014), but is often not carried out in practice (Shaw *et al.*, 2016).

Depression in cancer patients can be effectively treated (Walker *et al.*, 2013b). A significant improvement in depressive symptoms, and an improved quality of life, was reported using an integrated collaborative care model that includes psychological therapy and antidepressants (Sharpe *et al.*, 2014).

Earlier findings suggesting specific reaction types (e.g. 'fighting spirit') or targeted psychotherapy have not been confirmed by later work.

Childhood cancer

Childhood cancer presents special problems. Communication of the diagnosis is particularly difficult but it is generally better to explain the diagnosis in terms appropriate to the child's stage of development. The child often reacts to the illness and its treatment with behaviour problems. Many parents react at first with shock and denial, and may take months to accept the full implications of the diagnosis. Some mothers develop an anxiety or depressive disorder, and other family members may be affected. In the early stages of the illness parents are usually helped by advice about practical matters, and later by discussions of their feelings, which often include guilt. Adult survivors of cancer in childhood or adolescence appear to be at risk of social difficulties.

Accidents

Psychiatric associations

Psychiatric disorder predisposing to accidents. This is often through cognitive impairment occurring, for example, in alcohol or drug intoxication, delirium, or dementia, and less so in depression and some personality disorders.

Psychiatric disorder caused by accidents includes adjustment disorder, anxiety and depressive disorders, and post-traumatic stress disorder. Avoidance of situations associated with the accident is common and may be severe enough to meet diagnostic criteria for phobic anxiety disorder. *Head injury* may cause specific cognitive disorders and personality change (see page 378).

Associations with particular kinds of accident

Criminal assault can have especially severe and persistent consequences for victims (Kilpatrick and Acierno, 2003). Victims' problems are discussed further on page 527.

Road traffic accidents are the leading cause of death in people aged under 40 years and a major cause of physical morbidity. Psychiatric factors contributing to road accidents include the misuse of alcohol and drugs, psychiatric illness, suicidal and risk-taking behaviour, and the side effects of some prescribed psychotropic drugs. Psychiatric consequences include acute stress disorder, anxiety and depressive disorders, post-traumatic stress disorder, phobias of travel, and disorders caused by brain injury. Some of these conditions are transient, but others persist and may cause considerable disability. Most of those affected do not seem to have been psychologically vulnerable before the accident (Chossegros *et al.*, 2011).

Occupational injury. The psychiatric consequences of occupational injury resemble those of other accidents. It is sometimes alleged that hopes of compensation or other benefits help to maintain the symptoms and disability—see 'Compensation neurosis', below.

Spinal cord injury. Around a quarter of patients admitted to a spinal injury unit suffer from psychiatric problems requiring treatment. Depression is common in the period immediately after a spinal cord injury, but usually improves with time. Nevertheless, suicide appears to be more common among these patients than in the general population.

Burns. In children, burns are associated with overactivity, learning disability, child abuse, and child neglect. In adults, burns are associated with alcohol and drug misuse, deliberate self-harm, and dementia. Severe burns and their protracted treatment may cause severe psychological problems. Hamburg *et al.* (1953) described three stages:

- *Stage 1* lasts days or weeks; denial is common. The most frequent psychiatric disorders are organic syndromes. At this stage the relatives often need considerable help.
- *Stage 2* is prolonged and painful; here denial recedes and emotional disorders are more common. Patients need to be helped to withstand pain, to express their feelings, and gradually accept disfigurement.
- *Stage 3*: the patient leaves hospital and has to make further adjustments to deformity or physical disability and the reaction of other people to their appearance.

Post-traumatic stress disorder is common among those with severe burns, and persistent anxiety and depression occur in more than a third (Palmu *et al.*, 2011). The outcome is worse for patients with burns affecting the face. Such patients are likely to withdraw from social activities. These patients need considerable support from the staff of the burns unit, but only a minority also require referral to a psychiatrist.

'Compensation neurosis'

The term compensation neurosis (or accident neurosis) refers to psychologically determined physical or mental symptoms occurring when there is an unsettled claim for compensation. It was believed that such psychological factors were important in claims for persistent physical disability after occupational injuries and road accidents. Compensation claims were thought to prolong symptoms and that settlement was followed by recovery, although evidence has failed to substantiate this extreme view (Margoshes and Webster, 2000).

In fact, many accident victims do not claim compensation, and few become involved in prolonged litigation. However, it does appear that time off work and disability are affected by the type of accident, social factors, and the prospect of compensation, social security, or other benefits.

See Malt (2009) for a review of the psychiatric aspects of accidents, burns, and other trauma.

Psychiatric aspects of obstetrics and gynaecology

Pregnancy

Psychiatric disorder is more common in the first and third trimesters of pregnancy than in the second. In the *first trimester* unwanted pregnancies are associated with anxiety and depression. In the *third trimester* there may be fears about the impending delivery or doubts about the normality of the fetus. Psychiatric symptoms in pregnancy are more common in women with a history of previous psychiatric disorder and probably also in those with serious medical problems affecting the course of pregnancy, such as diabetes. It is sometimes said that psychiatric disorders are less common in pregnant than non-pregnant women, but this is not borne out by systematic reviews of depression (Gavin *et al.*, 2005) and anxiety (Goodman *et al.*, 2014) disorders. Maternal depression during pregnancy is associated with an increased rate of premature delivery and some other adverse perinatal outcomes (Jarde *et al.*, 2016), highlighting the need for effective screening to improve detection and thence treatment (O'Connor *et al.*, 2016).

Management of depression in pregnancy involves careful assessment, consideration of treatment options, and providing the woman with accurate information about risks and benefits (Box 22.16). In particular, care must be taken when using antidepressants, as with all psychotropic drugs, during pregnancy (Chisolm and Payne, 2016). Nevertheless, if the woman has a history of recurrent moderate to severe depression and has been effectively maintained on antidepressant medication, it is generally better to continue this treatment during pregnancy because the risk of relapse is high if medication is withdrawn, and because of the risks to the fetus of untreated maternal depression (Jarde *et al.*, 2016).

Women with a history of less severe depression can often withdraw antidepressant medication successfully (Yonkers *et al.*, 2011).

Women not taking antidepressant medication who become depressed during pregnancy should be provided with psychoeducation and psychological treatment in a stepped care manner, depending on the severity of their condition. If the depression is severe, or if a moderate depressive episode fails to respond to psychological

---

Box 22.16 Depression in pregnancy

- Offer all pregnant women information about depression, its significance for her and her baby, and the recommended treatment options
- Women with a history of recurrent depression of moderate to severe intensity who are successfully maintained on antidepressant treatment may be advised to continue treatment
- Women who experience the onset of a mild–moderate depressive episode should be offered education and psychological treatment using a stepped care approach
- Women with severe depression or those with moderate depression not responding to psychological treatment should be offered antidepressant medication, usually an SSRI other than paroxetine
- The absolute risks of harms to the fetus from antidepressants in pregnancy are low and need to be placed in the context of the risks of untreated depression in the mother

management, antidepressant medication should be offered, usually an SSRI (Vigod *et al.*, 2016). Indeed, generally the risks of SSRI treatment in pregnancy are low and are outweighed by those of untreated depression. However, self-limiting neonatal withdrawal syndromes have been described, although the incidence across studies varies widely. SSRI use in later pregnancy may also be associated with a small increase (1–2 per 1000 live births) in the risk of pulmonary hypertension of the newborn, a potentially fatal condition (Huybrechts *et al.*, 2015). Paroxetine has been associated with cardiac defects and should therefore be avoided in pregnancy; other antidepressants appear to be safe in this respect (Huybrechts *et al.*, 2014).

For review of depression in pregnancy, see Vigod *et al.* (2016).

Hyperemesis gravidarum

About half of all pregnant women experience nausea and vomiting in the first trimester. In the past it was sometimes suggested that these symptoms, as well as the severe condition of hyperemesis gravidarum, have a psychological basis, but there is no evidence for this.

Pseudocyesis

Pseudocyesis is a rare condition in which a woman believes that she is pregnant when she is not, and develops amenorrhoea, abdominal distension, and other changes similar to those of early pregnancy. The condition is more common in younger women. Pseudocyesis usually resolves quickly once diagnosed, but some patients persist in believing that they are pregnant. Recurrence is common. Only rarely is the condition associated with a psychiatric disorder.

Couvade syndrome

In this syndrome, the partner of the pregnant woman reports that he is experiencing some of the symptoms of pregnancy, complaining of nausea, morning sickness, and often of toothache. These complaints generally resolve after a few weeks.

Termination of unwanted pregnancy

In the past, psychiatrists in the UK were often asked to see pregnant women who were seeking a therapeutic abortion on the grounds of mental illness. The provisions of current legislation in the UK and many other countries now make it generally more appropriate for decisions to be made by the family doctor and the gynaecologist, without involving a psychiatrist. Nevertheless, psychiatric opinions are still sought at times, not only about the grounds for termination of pregnancy but also for an assessment of the likely psychological effects of termination in a particular patient (Morris *et al.*, 2012). Most of the evidence suggests that the psychological consequences of termination are usually mild and transient (Fergusson *et al.*, 2009).

In vitro fertilization

The process of *in vitro* fertilization (IVF) is often protracted and, not surprisingly, associated with emotional distress (Rockliff *et al.*, 2014). However, postpartum depression is no more common than in women following spontaneous pregnancy (Gressier *et al.*, 2015).

Spontaneous abortion

Approximately a fifth of diagnosed pregnancies do not progress beyond 20 weeks, mainly because of fetal defects. Distress is common after miscarriage, although most women improve rapidly (Broen *et al.*, 2005).

Antenatal death

Antenatal death (stillbirth) causes an acute bereavement reaction and, for some women, long-term psychiatric problems, as well as concern about future pregnancy. It is believed by many midwives that parents should be helped to mourn by encouraging them to hold the baby, to name it, and to have a proper funeral. However, the evidence regarding this issue is weak (Hennegan *et al.*, 2015). Parents may need some continuing support and the next pregnancy may be a particularly worrying time.

The risk of stillbirth is higher in women with a psychiatric history, but this may reflect factors such as antenatal care attendance rather than the psychiatric disorder itself (King-Hele *et al.*, 2009).

Caesarian section

Caesarian section has been said to have adverse psychological consequences for parents and infants. Most of the research has failed to test this association because it has not separated the effects of surgery from other adverse factors. However, it would seem sensible to pay particular attention to parental support and to initial bonding.

See Brockington (2009) for a review of the psychiatric aspects of pregnancy.

Postpartum mental disorders

These disorders can be divided into minor mood disturbance (maternity blues), puerperal psychosis, and chronic depressive disorders of moderate severity.

Minor mood disturbance—'maternity blues'

Amongst women giving birth to a normal child, between half and two-thirds experience brief episodes of irritability, lability of mood, and episodes of crying. Lability of mood is particularly characteristic, taking the form of rapid alternations between euphoria and misery. The symptoms reach their peak on the third or fourth day postpartum. Patients often speak of being 'confused', but tests of cognitive function are normal. Although frequently tearful, patients may not be feeling depressed at the time but tense and irritable.

'Maternity blues' is more frequent among primigravida. The condition is not related to complications at delivery or to the use of anaesthesia. 'Blues' patients have often experienced anxiety and depressive symptoms in the last trimester of pregnancy; they are also more likely to give a history of premenstrual tension, fears of labour, and poor social adjustment.

Both the frequency of the emotional changes and their timing suggest that maternity blues may be related to readjustment in hormones after delivery, although this has not been established. No treatment is required because the condition resolves spontaneously in a few days.

Postpartum psychosis (puerperal psychosis)

In the nineteenth century, puerperal and lactational psychoses were thought to be specific entities distinct from other mental illnesses. Later psychiatrists such as Bleuler and Kraepelin regarded the puerperal psychoses as no different from other psychoses, and neither ICD-10 nor DSM-5 have a specific diagnostic category for puerperal psychosis. Nevertheless, the term continues to be used widely by clinicians and patients.

For a review, see Jones *et al.* (2014).

Epidemiology

The incidence of postpartum psychoses has been estimated at 1–2 per 1000 births. This incidence is substantially above the expected rate for psychoses in non-puerperal women of the same age. Puerperal psychoses are more frequent in primiparous women and in those who have suffered previous major psychiatric illness. In particular, women with a history of bipolar disorder have a 20% risk of puerperal relapse. However, about half of women who develop puerperal psychosis do not have any form of 'high-risk' history (Jones *et al.*, 2014). Puerperal illnesses are reported to be more common in developing than in developed countries; the excess may reflect cases with an organic aetiology.

Aetiology

There is a genetic predisposition, which overlaps with that of bipolar disorder, but apart from a possible susceptibility locus on chromosome 16, no specific genes or genetic pathways have been identified. The early onset of puerperal psychoses has led to speculation that they might be caused by the dramatic hormonal changes that follow delivery. There is, however, no evidence that hormonal changes in women with puerperal psychoses differ from those in other women in the early puerperium. Hence if endocrine factors do play a part, they would seem to act only as precipitating factors in predisposed women. Immunological factors have also been implicated. The sleep deprivation associated with childbirth may play a role since disrupted sleep can precipitate mania in vulnerable individuals.

Clinical features

The onset of puerperal psychosis is often within 2–3 days of delivery, and usually within the first 1–2 weeks. A sudden onset and rapid deterioration is typical. Three types of clinical picture are observed: delirium, mood disorder, and schizophreniform disorder. Delirium was common in the past, but is now much less frequent since the incidence of puerperal sepsis was reduced by antibiotics. Nowadays affective psychoses predominate, either bipolar disorder with mania or mixed features, or depressive psychosis. Schizophreniform disorders presenting for the first time occur, but are rare. The clinical features of these syndromes are similar to those of the corresponding non-puerperal syndrome. Insomnia and overactivity are often early features. Perplexity and confusion are common.

Management

Assessment should be prompt and pay attention to the potential risks to mother and baby (Spinelli, 2009). As well as the usual psychiatric assessment it is essential to ascertain the mother's ideas concerning the baby. Severely depressed or psychotic patients may have delusional ideas that the child is malformed, imperfect in some way, or evil. These false ideas may lead to attempts to kill the child to spare it from future suffering, or to protect others. Infanticide is extremely rare, but suicide, though also uncommon, is a leading cause of maternal death.

Treatment usually requires inpatient care, often under the Mental Health Act. If available, admission is often best to a mother and baby unit, where the child can remain with the mother to minimize adverse effects on maternal bonding. Once the admission is arranged, all contacts between mother and baby should be supervised, at first, by nursing staff and thereafter reviewed in the light of clinical progress. Child protection considerations should always be an integral part of management.

As with other psychoses, antipsychotics are a mainstay of treatment, with antidepressants also used if depressive symptoms are prominent. Adjunctive benzodiazepines are helpful for insomnia and sleep disturbance. Lithium may also be worth considering if there is a clear bipolar component, though it is advised that women taking lithium should not breastfeed. Where pharmacological treatment and psychological support do not resolve symptomatology, the early use of ECT, which can be rapidly effective in puerperal psychosis, should be considered. For review, see Bergink *et al.* (2015).

Prognosis

Over 75% of women have a good outcome after puerperal psychosis. Recovery usually occurs within a few months. After a puerperal psychosis there is a high (at least 35%) risk of relapse after the next delivery (Wesseloo *et al.*, 2016), and almost 70% of women will have a non-puerperal recurrence, usually of bipolar disorder (Blackmore *et al.*, 2013). Given these risks, women with a history of puerperal psychosis should be offered preconception care and regular psychiatric support during and immediately after each pregnancy. In this instance, the benefits of maintenance medication (antipsychotics and mood stabilizers) often outweigh the risks. However, sodium valproate should be avoided, as in all women of childbearing age, unless no other treatment is effective or tolerable. For review, see Jones *et al.* (2014).

Postnatal depression

Less severe depressive disorders are much more common than the puerperal psychoses. Systematic reviews suggest a point prevalence of 5% in the first 3 months after delivery, rising to 19% if minor depression is included (Gavin *et al.*, 2005). It is estimated that about a third of these cases start during pregnancy. Higher figures have been reported in low- and middle-income countries. Tiredness, irritability, and anxiety are often more prominent than depressive mood change, and there are often phobic and obsessional symptoms concerning fears about harming the baby. It is important to distinguish such obsessional thinking from delusional beliefs related to puerperal psychosis, as discussed above.

Most patients recover after 2–6 months, but up to 30% still have some depressive symptoms in the year following childbirth. There is a high risk (about 40%) of depressive relapse subsequently, either postnatally or at other times.

For review, see Howard *et al.* (2014a).

Aetiology

Clinical observation suggests that postnatal disorders are often precipitated in vulnerable mothers by the psychological adjustment required after childbirth, as well as by the loss of sleep and the hard work involved in the care of the baby. There is little evidence of a specific biological basis different from depression in other situations. The main risk factors are a previous history of depression (especially when accompanied by obstetric complications) and indications of social adversity. Low levels of partner or other support, relationship difficulties, and domestic violence are also risk factors. Unintended pregnancy is associated with a twofold increase in postnatal depression (Abajobir *et al.*, 2016).

Management

Despite the medical and other care given to women after childbirth, many postpartum depressions are undetected or, if detected, untreated. Therefore those providing care to mother and baby need to be alert to the possibility of depression. Screening appears to decrease the prevalence of postnatal depression (O'Connor *et al.*, 2016), and the Edinburgh Postnatal Depression Scale performs reasonably well as a screening tool.

Many women can be treated effectively in primary care, with non-directive counselling and help with solving practical problems (Clarke *et al.*, 2013). A small proportion need specific psychological interventions or antidepressant medication, and a few with severe or complex problems require referral to psychiatric services. Evidence shows efficacy of psychological and pharmacological therapies comparable to depressive episodes in other situations. Exposure of the infant to drug via breast milk needs to be considered but is generally low with SSRIs such as sertraline. For review, see Larsen *et al.* (2015).

Other psychiatric disorders in the postnatal period

There has been much less emphasis on other disorders in the postnatal period, but research indicates that anxiety disorders, eating disorders, and post-traumatic stress disorder can all present at this time and require treatment. For review, see Howard *et al.* (2014a,b).

Effects of maternal mental health on the child

Maternal psychiatric disorders, especially depression, during pregnancy and in the postnatal period have significant effects on the development of the child (Goodman *et al.*, 2011). For example, both antenatal and postnatal depression in the mother are associated with an increased risk in the child for emotional problems, behavioural difficulties, disorganized attachment, and depression. Postnatal depression also impacts on intellectual development in the child, although the long-term effects on cognitive functioning are uncertain. Although most studies have focused on mothers, there is increasing evidence that paternal depression shows similar associations with child development.

The mechanisms linking parental mental health with child health and development are complex. They likely include an interplay of genetic, epigenetic, biological, and social factors, acting both as mediators and moderators of risk.

A number of interventions to reduce the adverse effects of parental psychiatric disorder on the health of children have been tested. Treatment of maternal perinatal disorders has yielded a mixed pattern of results, with not all studies showing benefits for the child even when the mother has been treated successfully. Greater effects on the child have emerged from specific parenting interventions, including home-visiting programmes to improve the quality of interactions and the attachment between mother and infant. There are no data regarding effects of interventions in fathers.

For further discussion, see Chapter 16. For review, see Stein *et al.* (2014).

Psychiatric aspects of gynaecology

Premenstrual syndrome and premenstrual dysphoric disorder

These categories denote a group of psychological and physical symptoms starting a few days before and ending shortly after the onset of a menstrual period. The psychological symptoms include anxiety, irritability, mood lability, food cravings, and depression; the physical symptoms include breast tenderness, abdominal discomfort, and a feeling of distension. Premenstrual syndrome (PMS) is not included in current classifications of psychiatric disorder, but premenstrual dysphoric disorder (PMDD) is included in DSM-5 within the 'Depressive disorders' chapter. For a diagnosis of PMDD,

there must be a minimum of five symptoms, including affective ones, which are clearly related to menstruation. Both PMS and PMDD should be distinguished from the much more frequent occurrence of similar symptoms that are not strictly premenstrual in timing.

For review, see Ryu and Kim (2015).

Epidemiology

The frequency of PMS in women of reproductive age is estimated at 30–40%, and 3–8% for PMDD. Such estimates should be interpreted with caution. First, there is a problem of definition. Mild and brief symptoms are frequent premenstrually, and it is difficult to decide when they should be classified as PMS. Second, information about symptoms is often collected retrospectively by asking women to recall earlier menstrual periods, and this is an unreliable way of establishing the time relationships. Prospective ratings are more likely to be accurate. Third, the description of premenstrual symptoms is subjective and may be influenced by knowledge that the enquiry is concerned specifically with the premenstrual syndrome.

Aetiology

The aetiology is uncertain. Biological explanations have been based on ovarian hormones (excess oestrogen, lack of progesterone), pituitary hormones, and disturbed fluid and electrolyte balance. None of these theories has been proved. Various unproven psychological explanations have been based on possible associations of the syndrome with neuroticism or with attitudes towards menstruation.

Treatment

PMS has been treated with progesterone, and also with oral contraceptives, bromocriptine, diuretics, and psychotropic drugs. There is no convincing evidence that any of these is effective, and treatment trials suggest a high placebo response (up to 65%). Psychological support and encouragement may be as helpful as medication.

For PMDD, SSRIs and oral contraceptives are considered the treatment of choice, with the latter primarily improving the physical symptoms. Cognitive behaviour therapy and lifestyle modifications also have a role (Lustyk *et al.*, 2009).

See O'Brien *et al.* (2011) for a review of premenstrual syndromes and their treatment.

The menopause

In addition to the physical symptoms of flushing, sweating, and vaginal dryness, menopausal women often complain of headache, dizziness, and depression. It is not certain whether depressive symptoms are more common in menopausal women than in non-menopausal women (Rössler *et al.*, 2016). Nevertheless, amongst patients who consult general practitioners because of emotional symptoms, a disproportionately large number of women are in the middle-age group that spans the menopausal years.

Depressive and anxiety symptoms at the time of the menopause could have several causes. Hormonal changes have often been suggested, notably deficiency of oestrogen, but a causal role has not been established. Psychiatric symptoms at this time of life could equally well reflect changes in the woman's role as her children leave home, her relationship with her husband alters, and her own parents become ill or die.

There are no specific treatments for depression associated with the menopause, and it should be treated in the usual fashion. For review, see Llaneza *et al.* (2012).

Hysterectomy

The alleged relationship between hysterectomy and psychiatric disorder has been controversial. A systematic review concluded that hysterectomy is associated with an improvement in depressive symptoms and no effect on anxiety symptoms (Darwish *et al.*, 2014). Moreover, patients who are free from psychiatric symptoms before hysterectomy seldom develop them afterwards (Gath *et al.*, 1982).

Sterilization

Considerations similar to those for hysterectomy apply to these procedures. Although retrospective studies suggested that sterilization leads to psychiatric disorder and sexual dysfunction, prospective enquiry has contradicted this. Indeed, sexual relationships are more likely to improve than worsen, and definite regrets are unusual.

For review of psychiatric aspects of obstetrics and gynaecology, see Brockington (2009).

Further reading

Gelder MG, Andreasen NC, López-Ibor JJ Jr and Geddes JR (eds.) (2009). *New Oxford Textbook of Psychiatry*. Oxford University Press, Oxford. (See Sections 4.6.3, 4.9, and 5.)

Global psychiatry

In this chapter the basic concerns of the global mental health movement are described:

- The prevalence of psychiatric illness across the globe, with an emphasis on low- and middle-income countries (LMICs).
- The influence of increased psychosocial adversity in LMICs on the prevalence and treatment of mental illness.
- The question of resources, and the challenge of how to make treatments available to the large proportion of the global population who have limited access to services despite their high need.

The term *neurological, mental health, developmental, and substance use (NMDS) disorders* is often used in the context of global health. NMDS disorders constitute a large proportion of the global burden of disease, and increasing recognition of this fact provides important momentum to the emerging field of global mental health (Patel and Prince, 2010).

Other aspects of psychiatry that differ between countries and cultures are discussed elsewhere in the book, as summarized in Box 23.1.

The global burden of mental illness

With the use of Disability Adjusted Life Years (DALY), the importance of neurological and psychiatric disorders as a global contributor of disease has become undeniable; by 2010, NMDS disorders were estimated to account collectively for more than 29% of the global burden of disease in LMICs (Table 23.1) (Silberberg *et al.*, 2015). In tandem with increased global life expectancy, non-communicable diseases have become the major cause of death and disability, with the burden of NMDS increasing by around 40% in the past two decades (Whiteford *et al.*, 2013).

There are many challenges to the improvement of mental health care across the globe (Collins *et al.*, 2011). They include:

- Lack of knowledge and evidence on:
  - the positive and negative influences on the development of mental illness in LMICs, including the impact of poverty, violence, war, migration, and disaster;
  - the most effective and cost-effective forms of management in low-resource settings. For example, how to better integrate with primary care treatment approaches; developing interventions that can be delivered by non-mental health professionals, and appropriate use of medication.
- Systemic difficulties in:
  - work force capacity. There are fewer opportunities in LMICs to train, practice, and conduct research in psychiatry. This is often referred to as the *mental health gap (mhGAP)* between what is needed for mental health services and what is available (World Health Organization, 2010);
  - health system and policy responses. Care for those with mental illness often falls well below those with physical illness, with legislation needed to protect

---

Box 23.1 Areas relevant to global psychiatry discussed in other chapters

Classification (Chapter 2)
Diagnosis in different cultural contexts (page 32)

Assessment (Chapter 3)
Patients from another culture (page 57)

Aetiology (Chapter 5)
Social sciences: transcultural studies (page 98)

Reactions to stressful experiences (Chapter 7)
Refugees and victims of torture (page 148)

Anxiety and obsessive–compulsive disorders (Chapter 8)
Transcultural variations in anxiety disorders (page 184)

Depression (Chapter 9)
Transcultural factors (page 198)

Schizophrenia (Chapter 11)
Migration and ethnicity (page 277)

Misuse of alcohol and drugs (Chapter 20)
Religion, tolerance, and ethnicity (page 570)
Epidemiology of substance misuse disorders (page 586)

Suicide and deliberate self-harm (Chapter 21)
Differences in suicide rates (page 610)

Psychiatry and medicine (Chapter 22)
Trance and possession disorders (page 657)
Cultural syndromes (page 657)

Psychiatric services (Chapter 26)
Members of ethnic minorities and migrants (page 797)
Refugees (page 798)

---

their rights and to ensure that there are facilities equipped to manage their care.

Compared to a number of other major contributors to the global burden of disease, many NMDS disorders manifest in early life and so interventions should incorporate a life-course approach to ensure that children and families are considered, and that their educational and occupational needs are also prioritized (Patton *et al.*, 2016). Furthermore, the impact of NMDS extends beyond the patient to other family members and communities, requiring health system-wide changes to offer improved treatment together with attention to the widespread social exclusion, discrimination, and stigma those with mental illness can experience in LMICs.

Socioeconomic deprivation and chronic adversity

There is growing international evidence that mental ill health and poverty interact, such that those who live in poverty have increased risk of mental illness, and those living with a mental illness will drift into or remain in poverty (Lund *et al.*, 2011). An important element to breaking this cycle is to address both the social causes of mental illness and the disabilities and economic deprivation that are a consequence of mental illness.

There are marked demographic and urban shifts taking place in a number of LMICs. These shifts place increasing stress on systems of governance and care, and can have important impacts on the development of mental illness and the provision of psychiatric services, given the poor availability of specialist services. The increasing proportion of older adults living in high-income countries (Chapter 19) is markedly different to the large proportions of children in many LMICs. Indeed, over 80%

of children and adolescents live in LMICs (Fazel *et al.*, 2014). Global urbanization will be most prominent in LMICs in the next decades, with 90% of the projected population growth and urbanization concentrated in Asia and Africa (UN Population Division, 2015). As areas transition economically to higher income brackets, associated socioeconomic deprivation can also occur, with income inequality becoming more prominent, further impacting on potential risk factors for mental illness. These include changing community structures, more fractured families with reductions in support for young families, changing gender roles, changing diets (with increasing non-communicable diseases such as type 2 diabetes), and the leap into technology with marked social media use, especially by young adult populations. The psychological impacts of all of these factors and their interactions are poorly studied (Patton *et al.*, 2016).

Table 23.1 **Proportions of age-standardized estimated disability adjusted life years (>0.5%) attributable to mental health, substance-use and non-communicable neurological disorders by high-income and low- and middle-income countries**

Disorder	Absolute DALYs* as global per thousand people (Rank**)	Percentage in high-income countries (developed)	Percentage in LMICs (developing)
Mental health and behavioural disorders			
Mental health (all)	185,200	11.1	6.73
Major depressive disorder	63,200 (2)	3.42	2.39
Anxiety disorders	26,830 (9)	1.60	0.98
Schizophrenia	15,000 (11)	0.85	0.49
Bipolar disorders	12,870 (17)	0.63	0.50
Dysthymia	11,100 (16)	0.6	0.42
Substance-use disorders			
Drug-use disorders	20,000 (19)	1.53	0.67
Alcohol-use disorders	17,640 (22)	1.52	0.56
Neurological disorders: non-communicable			
Cerebrovascular disease and strokes	102,200	5.97	3.79
Neurological disorders (all)	73,800	4.42	2.71
Migraine	22,360 (6)	1.21	0.84
Epilepsy	17,400 (23)	0.44	0.75
Alzheimer's disease and other dementias	11,350 (21)	1.75	0.22
Other neurological disorders	17,870	0.53	0.76

* DALY is defined as a measure of overall disease burden and expressed as the sum of years of potential life lost due to ill health, disability, or premature mortality.
** Number in brackets specifies where the disorder comes in the DALY ranking of all neurological, psychiatric and substance abuse disorders. For further details of categories and estimates, see Silberberg et al. (2015).

Adapted from Nature, 527(7578), Silberberg D et al., Brain and other nervous system disorders across the lifespan—global challenges and opportunities, pp. S151–4, Copyright (2015), with permission from Nature Publishing Group, reproduced under the Creative Commons License 4.0.

Finally, people with serious mental disorders and disabilities bear a disproportionate burden of human rights abuses, with limited basic entitlements, such as freedom and the denial of the right to care. The need to address them has been equated to a global emergency on a par with the worst human rights scandals in the history of global health (Patel et al., 2011).

Resources and service development considerations

The barriers to providing better mental health care to large swathes of the global population, which include poorly resourced services and the lack of the most basic human rights for the mentally unwell, have been referred to as a 'failure of humanity' (Kleinman, 2009).

Health systems in LMICs need increased resources to scale up care. Budgetary allocations for mental health care are still significantly out of proportion to the burden posed by mental health problems (Eaton et al., 2011). Furthermore, there is a need to ensure that the increasing resources for developing services account for the unique needs of people who are particularly vulnerable, notably children and those affected by serious mental disorders and disabilities.

The challenges facing the implementation of packages of care in LMICs include:

- the lack of priority for mental health over the other health needs of countries;
- high levels of poverty and social deprivation;
- diverse cultural settings;
- broader health system challenges such as weak coordination between national and local authorities, inadequate medication supply, and weak health management information systems;
- burden on the front-line health care workers;
- shortages of human resources;
- inflexible bureaucracy;
- lack of accountability among the implementing agencies;
- demand-side constraints, including limited community awareness, high levels of stigma and discrimination against people living with mental illness, and diverse explanatory models, which may influence the acceptability and uptake of services (Lund *et al.*, 2016).

Integration of mental health into existing systems of primary and physical health care must be viewed as a priority given the significant resource limits of current mental health provision. An analysis of data from the WHO Atlas projects identified widespread, systematic, and long-term neglect of resources for mental health care in LMICs (Saxena *et al.*, 2006, 2007). In 2007, it was estimated that one-third of all countries have no national policy or plan to improve mental health and reduce the burden of mental disorders. And, of those countries with a policy, almost 40% had not revised them for two decades; there were similar figures regarding legislation to protect the rights of those requiring involuntary treatment for serious mental illnesses.

The mhGAP guidelines mentioned earlier (World Health Organization, 2010) highlight how important it is to ensure that treatments used are based on evidence of efficacy. Unfortunately, the use of scarce resources for ineffective treatments and inefficient models of care is not uncommon and needs to be reduced. Delivery of effective treatments depends crucially on the development of human resources, especially among the front-line health workforce. This often requires innovative solutions, and methods should be developed to share these practices (Kakuma *et al.*, 2011).

Lay mental health workers

The mhGAP has focused attention on *task shifting*: the delegation of responsibilities to lower level cadres who are supported and supervised by more senior professionals; for example, using lay health workers to deliver psychological interventions in LMICs (Chibanda *et al.*, 2015). In South Africa, a study using trained community lay health workers improved the quality of mother–infant engagement (Cooper *et al.*, 2002). Similarly, in Pakistan, it was possible to integrate a cognitive behaviour therapy intervention in the routine work of community health workers, resulting in better outcomes than usual care in reducing depression (Rahman *et al.*, 2008). In India, a trained lay counsellor-led collaborative stepped care intervention improved recovery from depressive and anxiety disorders among patients attending primary health care facilities (Patel *et al.*, 2010). In Chile, a multicomponent stepped-care intervention was more effective than usual care for depression at a public health care level (Araya *et al.*, 2006). Finally, Murray *et al.* (2014) have developed a 'common elements' approach to treatment of mood, post-traumatic stress, or anxiety problems, where lay workers were trained to deliver a treatment intervention using a transdiagnostic approach for which early data showed a decrease in clinical symptoms with good retention in treatment, suggesting acceptability. It has been piloted in the USA, Iraq, and on the Thai–Burma border.

Integration into primary health care

The challenge of scaling up mental health services in LMICs is less one of what to implement than one of how to implement. There is already robust evidence for a range of cost-effective interventions, but little evidence on how these may be delivered in diverse low-resource settings. A key element is to increase the capacity to treat common mental disorders within primary health care settings. The Programme for Improving Mental health carE (PRIME) (Lund *et al.*, 2016) was a large multisite study in five LMICs to develop district mental health care plans. They highlighted some key components, including having shared objectives; the need for participation and engagement with local stakeholders; focusing on community, health facility, and health organization levels; challenges of overburdened primary health care systems; and the limited impact of training without systemic changes in the form of new mental health resources (usually in the form of an experienced mental health professional to provide support), referral pathways, improved medication supply, and reorientation of health facility managers (Hanlon *et al.*, 2015).

Specific populations of concern

HIV/AIDS pandemic

People living with HIV/AIDS have a prevalence of over 30% of mental disorders (depression, anxiety, and related conditions) in LMICs. The rates are higher than for non-HIV-infected individuals (Brandt, 2009; see also Chapter 22), and these disorders contribute significantly to poor HIV disease outcomes, such as increased HIV treatment failure and increased risk of HIV acquisition (Chibanda *et al.*, 2015). The identification of highly active antiretroviral treatments and the welcome expansion in access to them has resulted in a new global health challenge resulting from these chronic mental disorder comorbidities of HIV. A large treatment gap, in particular for depression, exists in sub-Saharan Africa, where the ratio of mental health professionals to the population in sub-Saharan Africa is 1 per 2.5 million for psychologists, 1 per 1 million for mental health nurses and 1 per 2 million for psychiatrists. There are some promising results for the effectiveness of cognitive behaviour therapy for common mental disorders in HIV/AIDS-affected populations, but the evidence is limited.

In considering the needs of mothers, 90% of the global number of pregnant women with HIV live in sub-Saharan Africa (Stein *et al.*, 2014). Being diagnosed with HIV during pregnancy, which is when many African women learn of their diagnosis, increases the risk of depression. It is a cause for concern that women who are depressed are less likely to adhere to antiretroviral therapy, which is critical for the mother's survival and to prevent transmission of HIV to the child.

Perinatal mental illness

Evidence is emerging that poor perinatal maternal mental health, especially depression in women at socioeconomic disadvantage, is linked to poor infant growth and stunted development (Stein *et al.*, 2014; Howard *et al.*, 2014; see Chapter 16). Postnatal depression in LMICs is associated with high rates of diarrhoeal diseases in children, which could contribute to their poor growth. Furthermore, comorbidity is more common in LMICs, likely increasing the adverse consequences of perinatal mental illness. There is evidence that perinatal depression raises the risks for children even into late adolescence in terms of increased rates of depression. Of particular concern is the extent to which outcomes for children are moderated by persistent maternal disorder and socioeconomic disadvantage. Perinatal mental illness might also account for a substantial proportion of maternal deaths in low-income countries if suicide were properly classified and reported. There is evidence that trained non-specialist health workers can provide effective interventions for postnatal depression in LMICs.

Several randomized controlled trials in LMICs showed that psychological interventions delivered by local community health workers can have a positive effect on parenting and child development. A study in Pakistan used a form of cognitive behavioural therapy together with parenting support that began during pregnancy (Rahman *et al.*, 2008). No effect was noted on child growth, the principal outcome, but rates of postnatal depression were reduced, and parents reported decreased rates of children's diarrhoea, increased rates of immunization, and increased play with children. In Jamaica, an intervention targeting child rearing and parenting self-esteem led to improvements in both maternal depressive symptoms and infant global development compared with standard care (Baker-Henningham *et al.*, 2008). As a final example, in a socioeconomically disadvantaged South African community, an intervention focused on helping mothers to attend to the details of the infant's communication and to respond to sensitively led improvements in the quality of mother–child interaction and increased rates of secure attachment (Cooper *et al.*, 2009).

Children and adolescents

Children and adolescents comprise more than a third of the global population. Addressing their mental health needs more effectively than is currently the case might alleviate suffering, improve educational attainment in childhood, and potentially reduce the burden of mental disorders in adulthood (Kieling *et al.*, 2011; Patton *et al.*, 2016). Schools provide a potentially valuable location for mental health support services given the scarcity of dedicated mental health services for children in LMICs, since schools exist in almost all urban and rural contexts (Fazel *et al.*, 2014). For example, the School HeAlth Promotion and Empowerment programme (SHAPE) intervention in India successfully trained lay school health counsellors to conduct physical health screening (visual and hearing) as well as mental health interventions. The programme included skilled supervision of the counsellors, the provision of which diminished over time as the counsellor's skills improved, and also incorporated whole school interventions around violence and bullying (Rajaraman *et al.*, 2012). The intervention had a number of impacts noted from qualitative interviews, including parent-reported improved behaviour and success noted following individual counselling sessions, which were accessed by about 6% of students.

The Lancet Commission on adolescent health and wellbeing (Patton *et al.*, 2016) highlighted how the current lack of mental health provision leaves adolescents vulnerable to the harmful consequences of the current societal economic and cultural changes taking place, as well as noting the equally positive opportunities to improve their health and wellbeing if their health needs are better addressed. Better childhood health and nutrition, extensions to education, delays in family formation, and new technologies offer positive possibilities, but global trends of concern include those promoting unhealthy lifestyles and commodities, youth unemployment, less family stability, environmental degradation, armed conflict, and mass migration, all of which pose major threats to adolescent wellbeing. Of note, just over half of adolescents grow up in multi-burden countries, characterized by high levels of all types of health problems, including diseases of poverty (HIV and other infectious diseases, undernutrition, and poor sexual and reproductive health), injury and violence, and non-communicable diseases. The Commission argued that the most powerful actions are intersectoral, multi-level, and multicomponent, involving young people themselves.

For more information on the background and issues relevant to child and adolescent psychiatry across the globe, see Rahman *et al.* (2015) and Patton *et al.* (2016).

Humanitarian emergencies

Natural disasters, conflicts, and other humanitarian disasters provide not only a high need but also a unique opportunity to scale up care to the affected population. The prevalence of mental health and psychosocial problems in these situations is high. Most frequently, mental health researchers in humanitarian settings have focused on identifying rates of post-traumatic stress disorder and other common mental disorders. However, severe mental disorders (e.g. psychotic disorders), non-specific forms of psychological distress, and psychosocial problems specific to young people are also important (Reed *et al.*, 2012). Evidence also exists of the effect of deteriorated environmental conditions on mental health and wellbeing in humanitarian settings, including undermined social support networks, loss of opportunities for generating income, and lack of respect for human rights.

Interventions in these settings have been reported in a systematic review (Tol *et al.*, 2011). In 160 reports, the five most commonly reported activities were basic counselling for individuals (39%); facilitation of community support of vulnerable individuals (23%); provision of child-friendly spaces (21%); support of community-initiated social support (21%); and basic counselling for groups and families (20%). Most interventions took place and were funded outside national mental health and protection systems. Two studies showed promising effects of strengthening community and family supports. Studies on refugee children have shown that interventions delivered within the school setting can be successful in helping children overcome difficulties associated with forced migration (Tyrer and Fazel, 2014), as well as specific trauma-focused interventions (Fazel *et al.*, 2015).

With increasing appreciation of the importance of *mental health and psychosocial support* (MHPSS), international guidelines have been agreed integrating key components of mental health interventions into humanitarian assistance programmes (Inter-Agency Standing Committee, 2007). The key factors include preparedness steps to be taken before emergencies occur, minimum responses to be implemented during the acute phase of the emergency, and comprehensive responses to be implemented once the minimum responses have been applied.

Further reading

Patel V and Minas H (2013) *Global Mental Health: Principles and Practice*. Oxford University Press, Oxford.

CHAPTER 24

Psychological treatments

Introduction

This chapter is concerned with various kinds of coun-selling, psychotherapy, behavioural and cognitive therapies, and some related techniques. The UK is almost unique in having a separate faculty and spe-cialist training in psychotherapy for psychiatrists. In most countries, psychotherapy is considered a core aspect of a psychiatrist's role, fundamental to their professional identity. It is no longer routine for trainee psychiatrists to be trained fully in one or other form of psychotherapy, but rather they gain an overview. It will be obvious, however, that much of what fol-lows below is inevitably woven into the daily prac-tice of psychiatry. Expectations of this competence are likely to vary in the near future, but it is unlikely to disappear.

The subject is large, and some basic principles underly this chapter.

- Psychological treatment is not given in isolation, and this chapter complements the chapters on physical treatment and services.

- This chapter focuses on the general nature of the treatments; their use in specific disorders is covered in the relevant chapters.

- Psychological treatments are often combined with medication, considered in more detail with the rele-vant disorders.

- Many different techniques are considered here, so one will be described in detail.

- Supervised experience is essential before any of these treatments can be used with patients.

Terminology. The word psychotherapy is used in two ways. It can denote all forms of psychological treatment, including counselling and cognitive behaviour ther-apy (CBT). More traditionally it indicates established psychotherapies (usually broadly psychodynamic) that require a specific and elaborate training. These usually involve personal therapy, and exclude counselling and CBT. Psychological treatment is used for the broader sense and psychotherapy is used more precisely; for example, 'brief dynamic psychotherapy'.

How psychological treatments developed

The use of psychological healing is as old as the practice of medicine—parallels have been drawn with the ceremonial healing in temples in ancient Greece. In psychiatry, psychological treatment evolved towards the end of the eighteenth century with developments in hypnosis. Anton Mesmer (1734–1815), physician, challenged the prevailing practice of 'casting out devils' in 1775. He proposed that the body could be influenced by magnetism, initially actual magnets, but more importantly the therapist's force of personality or 'animal magnetism' (Burns, 2013). 'Mesmerism' was renamed hypnosis by a Manchester doctor, James Braid, who believed it was related to sleep (Braid, 1843).

Treatment with hypnosis was revived in France by the eminent neurologist Jean-Martin Charcot (1825–1893). He treated many patients suffering from hysteria and recognized that it worked by suggestion. Freud visited Charcot to study hypnosis, and used it with his patients back in Vienna. He used hypnosis not to modify symptoms directly, but to release the emotions associated with repressed conflicts that he believed to be their cause. Freud's revolutionary advance was his recognition that patients could recall forgotten events and conflicts without hypnosis. Recall was achieved by the patient lying on a couch and being encouraged to let their mind wander with the therapist out of sight—'free association'. In time he attended to the intensity of the relationship with his patients—'transference'. These discoveries formed the basic technique of psychoanalysis and subsequently of the larger group of dynamic psychotherapies.

Freud published vivid accounts of his new treatment and elaborated his increasingly complex theories, collecting a group of followers. Some of these later broke away, forming their own 'schools' of dynamic psychotherapy. These developments will be described briefly. More detailed descriptions are widely available, and for a brief overview see Burns (2006) and Burns and Lundgren (2015).

Early departures from Freud's original group

Alfred Adler left Freud's group in 1910; he stressed social factors in personal development and rejected the libido theory. He also stressed social factors in personal development, introducing the term 'inferiority complex'. His 'individual analysis' focused on current problems and solutions, and was highly influential with American analysts. Carl Jung emphasized the inner world of fantasy, and the interpretation of unconscious material, deduced from dreams, paintings, and other artistic productions. Jung believed that part of the content of the unconscious mind was common to all people (the 'collective unconscious') and was expressed in universal images which he called *archetypes*. The Jungian relationship between therapist and patient is more equal, and the therapist is more active and reveals more about himself (Storr, 2000).

The neo-Freudians formed in the USA in the 1930s from predominantly Jewish refugees from Nazi Germany. While they accepted that the origins of neurosis were in childhood, they rejected Freud's emphasis on early infantile sexuality and considered family and social factors more important.

Melanie Klein in London adapted psychoanalytical techniques for use with very young children. She interpreted their play and originated the 'object relations' school of psychoanalysis. 'Object' is a confusing term here as it refers both to people (e.g. the mother), to parts of that person (e.g. the mother's breast), and, most importantly, to their internal psychological representation. Klein's language is excessively dramatic, emphasizing strong instinctual feelings of love and hate. She described emotional development, moving through a 'paranoid-schizoid position' to the 'depressive position'. Klein has been widely influential, particularly for therapists working with severely ill patients (see Segal, 1963).

Attachment theory originated in the work of John Bowlby, a British analyst. The theory is that infants need a secure relationship with their parents in reality—not just in fantasy. Insecure attachments can lead to difficulty in establishing relationships, and emotional problems later. Bowlby's ideas had a considerable effect on the care of children, such as the need to maintain contact with the parents when a child is admitted to hospital. For a review of the historical development of attachment theory, see Holmes (2000).

Brief psychodynamic psychotherapy. Ferenczi saw the need to develop treatments shorter than psychoanalysis. He did this by setting time limits, making the role of the therapist less passive, and planning the main themes of treatment. These innovations have found their way into the brief dynamic psychotherapy that is used today.

The trend has continued towards briefer treatment that attends more to the patient's current problems than to those in the past. *Interpersonal therapy* (see page 687), directed to current interpersonal problems in depressed patients, and *cognitive analytic therapy* (see page 698), using cognitive therapy techniques within a framework of psychodynamic understanding, are two current forms.

The development of cognitive behaviour therapy

Behaviour therapy. Interest in a treatment based on scientific psychology arose in the early twentieth century. Watson and Rayner (1920) in the USA used learning principles in the treatment of children's fears, and aversion therapy for alcoholism. Maudsley psychologists in the 1930s used learning principles in treatments for phobic disorders. Joseph Wolpe in South Africa published *Psychotherapy by Reciprocal Inhibition* (Wolpe, 1958), describing a treatment for neurotic disorders, based on learning theory and making use of relaxation. In the USA, Skinner (1953) proposed operant conditioning in the treatment of psychiatric disorders. Wolpe's ideas were adopted in the UK, and Skinner's ideas were initially more influential in the USA. These approaches converged, and practice in the two countries is now similar.

There has always been an emphasis on evaluation for these new methods. The first clinical trial was reported in 1978 (Gelder *et al.*, 1978), followed by several trials establishing a strong evidence base for behavioural methods.

Cognitive therapy began with the work of A. T. Beck, a US psychiatrist who was dissatisfied with psychoanalytical psychotherapy for depressive disorders. Beck noted recurring themes in the thinking of depressed patients, and he concluded that these themes were an essential part of the disorder and had to be changed by challenging them in specific ways (see Box 24.8.). US psychologists were also dissatisfied with operant conditioning and its 'black-box' approach. They proposed that the recurrent thoughts played a part in maintaining distress, with suggestions of how these thoughts might be controlled (Meichenbaum, 1977).

Cognitive behaviour therapy. These cognitive approaches were integrated with behaviour therapy to produce CBT. The strong evidence base, clearly described procedures, and relatively brief treatment time of CBTs have made them the preferred psychological treatment for many disorders.

Classification of psychological treatments

Several simple classifications of psychological treatments have been proposed. Two are given here, with a further classification given below, with hints to identify their use in most healthcare systems.

1. Classification by *technique*:
   - *Eclectic*
   - *Psychodynamic*
   - *Cognitive behavioural*
   - *Other* (e.g. systems theory).

2. Classification by *number* of patients taking part:
   - *Individual therapy*
   - *Couple therapy*
   - *Family therapy*
   - *Small and large group therapy*

These two classifications can be combined—for example, *individual cognitive behavioural* or *psychodynamic group* therapy.

Psychotherapy in public services

Psychological treatment is the principal treatment for some psychiatric disorders, alone or with medication. Counselling, crisis intervention, and CBTs are used in this way when they have been shown to be effective in clinical trials. Dynamic psychotherapy, because there is limited evidence of its efficacy and because training is long and expensive, is less available. This is especially so of long-term psychodynamic therapy. 'Subthreshold' conditions are now generally offered counselling, and psychodynamic treatment for them now occurs mainly in private practice.

Planning their uses within a public health service has generated a third classification:

A *Simple psychological aspects of all health care.* This refers to skills and techniques to help individuals to adjust to stressful situations or confront difficult decisions. These are often considered aspects of a good doctor–patient relationship.

B *Moderately complex and provided by most mental health professionals.* This includes simpler CBT and brief dynamic psychotherapies. These treatments are usually an identified part of the management plan that includes medication and social measures.

C *Highly complex and provided by formally trained therapists.* This group includes the more complex psychodynamic and CBTs. These are used to treat more severe or complex disorders, alone or as part of a wider plan of management.

Common factors in psychological treatment

Different psychological treatment methods achieve results that are broadly equal and are greater than placebo. The features that psychotherapies share may be more important than their differences. Jerome Frank (1967) identified them and they are listed in Box 24.1.

Transference and countertransference

Therapeutic relationships are inevitably emotional but they can sometimes become very intense. These powerful emotions were labelled 'transference' and 'countertransference' by Freud because he believed their force derived from earlier, key relationships that had been 'transferred' to them. Transference and countertransference features mark all psychological treatments, and therapists overlook them at their peril.

Transference often becomes increasingly intense as treatment progresses, and is especially strong when patients reveal intimate personal problems. Transference can be positive, with warm feelings, or negative, with critical or hostile feelings. What is characteristic of them is their excess. Initially considered an impediment, transference, and its resolution, is now seen as an essential part of successful treatment.

Countertransference refers to intense feelings in the therapist towards the patient. Analysts debate whether the term countertransference should be restricted to 'neurotic' or distorted responses, or whether it can include all emotional responses. *Transference problems* may arise from excessive dependency on or idealization of the therapist and make it difficult to end treatment, with a resurgence of symptoms. However, dependency is a normal feature of much therapy and does not necessarily cause difficulties.

Box 24.1 Common factors in psychotherapy

The therapeutic relationship. The most important of the common factors in psychotherapy but can become too intense.

Listening. Listening attentively shows concern for the patient's problems and develops the helping relationship in which the patient feels understood.

Release of emotion. Helpful early in treatment, but repeated release is seldom useful. Intense and rapid emotional release is called *abreaction*.

Restoration of morale. Many patients have suffered repeated failures, and may feel helpless. Improved morale enables the patient to begin to help himself or herself.

Providing information. Patients may remember little of what they have been told about their condition because of poor concentration. Information should be as simple as possible, expressed clearly, repeated, and perhaps written down.

Providing a rationale. All psychotherapies provide some explanation for the current problem, which improves the patient's confidence. It may be by direct explanation (as in short-term psychotherapy), or fostered indirectly (as in much long-term psychotherapy).

Advice and guidance. These are part of all psychotherapy, whether direct as in brief therapies or indirect as in long-term therapies.

Suggestion. All psychological treatment contains an element of suggestion, which is powerful during the early stages.

Counselling and crisis intervention

Counselling

There is no distinct boundary between psychotherapy and counselling. Broadly speaking, counselling is less formal and less extensive (fewer sessions) than psychotherapy. Counsellors have shorter training than psychotherapists and are more open and equal in their relationships. Often counselling is focused on a specific problem (bereavement, drug abuse) rather than an attempt to permanently alter personality or uncover obscure conflicts.

Counselling is more widespread than formal psychotherapy, and counselling skills are a valued part of the professional identity of nurses and social workers. It is widely provided by voluntary bodies, often by unpaid staff. These voluntary bodies, such as the Samaritans, Cruise, and Relate in the UK, maintain a high profile and are easily accessible.

Counselling incorporates the non-specific factors shared by psychotherapies (see Box 24.1). The relationship between the counsellor and the person who is being counselled is believed to be the primary therapeutic agent in all counselling, but the relative importance of giving information, allowing the release of emotion, and exploring the situation, vary. Counselling developed from Carl Rogers' *client-centred approach*. In this the counsellor largely restricts his interventions to helping the client understand their feelings better by reflections back to the emotional content of the client's utterances, often simply repeating the last statement with an interrogative tone. They rarely seek clarification of facts nor offer explanations. The approach is optimistic in tone and actively encouraging but focused on increasing self-awareness, 'That seems to make you angry' (*reflection of feelings*) or 'You were disappointed' (*repeating for clarification the last statement*). Rogerian, or client-centred, counselling is widely available in primary care and voluntary agencies but has been largely replaced in secondary mental health care by the more structured and focused procedures.

Approaches to counselling

Problem-solving counselling is highly structured, particularly suitable for problems related to stressful circumstances or when life problems are exacerbating or maintaining other disorders. Basic counselling is combined with a systematic approach to the resolution of problems. The patient is helped to:

- *identify and list* problems causing distress
- *consider courses of action* to solve or reduce problems
- *select a problem and course of action* that appear feasible and likely to succeed
- *review the results* and select another problem if successful, or another course of action if not.

Interpersonal counselling was developed by Klerman *et al.* (1987) from interpersonal therapy (described on page 687), and has many similarities to the problem-solving approach. Attention is focused on current problems in personal relationships within the family, at work, and elsewhere. These problems are considered under four headings—*loss, interpersonal disputes, role transitions*, and *interpersonal deficits*. Using a problem-solving approach, the therapist encourages patients to consider alternative ways of coping with these difficulties, and to try these out between sessions. For a review see Blanco *et al.* (2009).

Psychodynamic counselling places more emphasis on unconscious processes by which previous relationships influence current feelings and relationships. The patient's emotional reactions (transference) are used to understand problems in other relationships. Its developmental approach fits well in student health centres.

Counselling for specific purposes

Debriefing

Debriefing for survivors of disasters has become a worldwide phenomenon. Survivors are encouraged to recall the distressing events, with emphasis on emotional release, and responses to the immediate problems. Evidence from clinical trials is discouraging, suggesting that this approach may prolong ruminations (Mayou *et al.*, 2000) and distract from essential social supports and the traditional advice to 'get back on the horse as soon as possible'. NICE guidance (National Institute for Health and Clinical Excellence, 2013a) specifically advises against its routine use.

Counselling for relationship problems

Couples are encouraged to talk constructively about problems in their relationship. The focus is on the need for each partner to understand the point of view, needs, and feelings of the other, and also to identify positive aspects of the relationship and potential strategies to move forward. A 'safe space' to explore can prevent a spiral down into mutual recrimination.

Bereavement counselling

Bereavement counselling draws heavily on following the identified stages of normal grief (see page 155, Box 7.9.). It combines an opportunity for emotional release (including anger), information about the normal course of grieving, and sensitive encouragement about viewing the body and disposing of clothing. It also involves advice on practical problems of living without the deceased person.

Counselling about health risks

Genetic counselling and counselling about the risks of sexually transmitted disease are probably not counselling as we generally understand it. These focus on giving information and providing an opportunity for reflection. However, to be effective counselling skills such as sensitivity and respect are essential.

Counselling in primary care

In primary care, many patients are referred to practice counsellors and IAPT (Improving Access to Psychological Therapies) workers who have received a relatively limited training but often have no background in health or social care professions. GP counsellors use various methods of brief treatment, although most often they employ non-directive Rogerian approaches, usually 4–6 sessions. Although very popular, the effectiveness of counselling in primary care is modest (Bower *et al.*, 2003). IAPT workers are trained in basic CBT.

Crisis intervention

Crisis intervention was originally conceived to use the crisis as an entry to longer-term problems but now is used mainly to cope with current crises. It originated in dealing with disasters (Lindemann, 1944); Caplan, 1961), and draws on Caplan's four stages of coping:

1. Emotional arousal with efforts to solve the problem.
2. Increasing arousal leading to a disorganization of behaviour.
3. Trials of alternative ways of coping.
4. Exhaustion and decompensation.

Crisis intervention seeks to limit the reaction to the first stage, or to avoid the fourth stage.

Problems leading to crisis

Common problems include:

- *Loss and separation*, such as bereavement or divorce, but also during severe illness.
- *Role changes*, such as marriage, parenthood, or even a new job.
- *Relationship problems*, such as those between sexual partners, or between parent and child.
- *Conflicts*, arising from pressing but impossible choices.

Crisis intervention methods

The methods used in crisis intervention (see Box 24.2) resemble interpersonal counselling and problem-solving counselling, but with a greater emphasis on reducing arousal. Treatment starts as soon as possible after the crisis and consists of a few sessions over a period of days or, at most, a few weeks. The focus is on current problems, although relevant past events can be considered. High levels of emotional arousal interfere with problem-solving, and the first aim of treatment is to reduce arousal. Reassurance and ventilation of emotions are usually effective, but anxiolytic medication is often used.

Supportive psychotherapy

Supportive psychotherapy is one of the most difficult but also one of the most important skills that any psychiatrist must acquire. It is used to help a person to cope with enduring difficulties such as chronic mental or physical illness, and in the care of the dying (page 152). Supportive therapy is based on the common factors of psychological treatment (see Box 24.1). Its basic elements, listed in Box 24.3, are:

- *The therapeutic relationship*. A trusting and supportive relationship is central in sustaining patients with long-term difficulties. The most common anxiety voiced by staff is the risk of excessive dependence. An effective relationship is most often achieved by an acceptance of the realistic need for dependence. After all, the patient is seeing you because they 'need' you. We, after all, have achieved our independence through the successful resolution of our own dependence.
- *Listening*. As in all forms of psychological treatment, the patient must feel that they have their doctor's full attention and sympathy while he is with them, and that their concerns are being taken seriously.

during the first session. Indeed, the patient may need to receive information gradually, giving time to absorb it. Most patients indicate, directly or indirectly, how much detail they wish.

- *Emotional release* and its acceptance can be helpful.
- *Encouraging hope* is important, but unrealistic reassurance can destroy trust. Reassurance should always be specific, offered only when the patient's concerns have been fully understood. A positive approach builds on encouraging the patient to exploit their assets and opportunities.
- *Persuasion.* Doctors can use their powers of persuasion to help patients to take difficult but necessary decisions and actions.

Self-help groups can give valuable support to some patients and to relatives, more effective because it comes from others who have struggled with the same problems. Support groups vary enormously, and it is important have some familiarity with a particular group before recommending it. For an account of supportive treatment, see Bloch (2006).

Box 24.2 Crisis intervention

Treatment is immediate, brief, and collaborative

Stage 1

Reduce arousal
Focus on current problems
Encourage self-help

Stage 2

Assess problems
Consider solutions
Test solutions

Stage 3

Consider future coping methods

- *Information and advice* are important, but their timing should be considered carefully. Information should be accurate, but it is not necessary to explain everything

---

Interpersonal psychotherapy

Interpersonal psychotherapy (IPT) was developed as a structured psychological treatment for the interpersonal problems of depressed patients (Klerman *et al.*, 1984). IPT fully embraces the medical model, encouraging the patient to recognize that depression is an illness and that they are suffering from it. The treatment is highly structured. The number and content of treatment sessions are planned carefully. The initial

assessment period lasts from one to three sessions. Interpersonal problems are considered under the following four headings:

1. bereavement and other loss
2. role disputes
3. role transitions
4. 'interpersonal deficits' such as loneliness.

Each problem is considered using specific situations, and alternative ways of coping are evaluated. Clear goals are set and progress towards them is monitored, with new coping strategies tried out in homework assignments. In the middle phase of treatment, specific methods are used for each of the four kinds of problem listed above. For grief and loss, the methods resemble grief counselling (page 156). For interpersonal disputes and role transitions, patients are helped to identify clearly the issues in the dispute, as well as any differences between their own values and those of the relevant others. They are helped to recognize their own contributions to problems that they ascribe

---

Box 24.3 Basic procedures of supportive treatment

Develop a therapeutic relationship
Listen to the patient's concerns
Inform, explain, and advise
Allow the expression of emotion
Encourage hope
Review and develop assets
Encourage self-help

to that person. Interpersonal deficits are addressed by analysing present relationship problems and previous attempts to overcome them, and then discussing alternatives. In the final two or three sessions, future problems are anticipated and considered.

Several clinical trials have shown that IPT is effective for depressive disorders in adults and adolescents (Mufson *et al.*, 2004), dysthymia (Markowitz, 2003), and bulimia nervosa. For an account of IPT, see Blanco *et al.* (2009).

Cognitive behaviour therapy

All psychiatric disorders have cognitive and behavioural components, and both have to change if the patient is to recover. With other treatments, change comes about indirectly—for example, as mood improves with antidepressant therapy, or as conflicts become resolved with psychotherapy. CBT aims to change cognitions and behaviour directly. Unlike dynamic psychotherapy, it is not concerned with the origins of the disorder, but what is maintaining it now.

Behaviour therapy focuses on what provokes symptoms or abnormal behaviour. *Avoidance* is particularly important in phobic and anxiety disorders, as it prevents the normal extinction of the anxiety response. Many behaviours are *maintained by their consequences*. For example, the reduction in anxiety following escape from stressful situations reinforces the phobic avoidance. *Reinforcement* also entrenches symptoms, such as when parents pay more attention to a child's noisy and unruly behaviour.

Cognitive therapy generally focuses on two kinds of abnormal thinking—*automatic thoughts* and *dysfunctional beliefs and attitudes*. Automatic thoughts are often stereotyped and exaggerated responses to stressors such as 'everybody despises me' after mild criticism. They provoke an immediate emotional reaction, usually of anxiety or depression, and undermine self-esteem. Dysfunctional beliefs and attitudes determine the way in which situations are perceived and interpreted.

Three factors are thought to maintain dysfunctional beliefs and attitudes.

1. *Attending selectively* to evidence that confirms them, and ignoring or discounting evidence that contradicts them. For example, patients with social phobias attend more to the critical behaviour of others than to signs of approval.
2. *Thinking illogically* in stereotyped ways (Box 24.4).
3. *Safety-seeking behaviour*, believed to reduce an immediate threat, but perpetuates the fear.

General features of cognitive behaviour therapy

Core features of CBT.

- *The patient is an active partner*. The patient takes an active part in treatment, with the therapist acting as an expert adviser who asks questions, and offers information and guidance.
- *Socratic questioning*. Automatic thoughts are challenged by questioning them—are there other ways of understanding what is happening? What are the implications of thinking this way?
- *Attention to provoking and maintaining factors*. The patient keeps daily records to identify factors that precede or follow the disorder and which may be provoking or maintaining it. This kind of assessment is sometimes called the *ABC approach*, the initials referring to **A**ntecedents, **B**ehaviour, and **C**onsequences.
- *Attention to ways of thinking*, revealed by recording thoughts associated with the behavioural or emotional disturbances.

Box 24.4 Examples of illogical thinking

Overgeneralization. Drawing general conclusions from single instances (e.g. 'He does not love me, so no one will ever love me').

Selective abstraction. Focusing on a single unfavourable aspect of a situation and ignoring favourable aspects.

Personalization. Blaming themselves for the actions of other people.

All-or-nothing thinking. Viewing people or situations as 'black-and-white'.

- *Treatment as investigation ('collaborative empiricism').* Therapeutic procedures are usually presented as experiments which, even if they fail, help reveal more about the condition.
- *Homework assignments and behavioural experiments.* Patients practise new behaviours between sessions with the therapist, or carry out experiments to test explanations suggested by the therapist (Box 24.5).
- *Highly structured sessions.* At each session, an agenda is agreed, and progress since the last session is reviewed, including any homework. New topics are considered, the following week's homework is planned, and the main points of the session are summarized.
- *Monitoring.* Assessment includes checking daily records kept by the patient, and often includes rating scales.
- *Treatment manuals* describe procedures and how they are applied. Manuals ensure that therapists stick to effective procedures.

Assessment for cognitive behaviour therapy

Topics to be covered

As well as a full psychiatric history, certain additional topics are addressed (see Box 24.6). For each of the

---

> **Box 24.6 Topics to be considered during assessment for cognitive behaviour therapy**
>
> 1. **A description of each problem, including behaviour, thoughts, and emotions associated with it**
>   - Where it occurs most often
>   - Common prior events
>   - Response to these events
>   - What follows the problem
> 2. **Factors that alleviate or worsen the problem**
> 3. **Maintaining factors**
>   - Avoidance
>   - Safety behaviours
>   - Selective attention
>   - Ways of thinking
>   - The responses of others

> **Box 24.5 An agoraphobic patient's record of a behavioural experiment**
>
> **Situation:** Shopping in a crowded supermarket.
>
> **My predictions:** I shall panic and feel dizzy. Unless I tense my stomach muscles and breathe deeply, I shall faint.
>
> **Experiment:** When anxious, do not tense stomach muscles or breathe deeply.
>
> **Outcome:** I did panic quite badly. I felt dizzy, but less so than usual. I did not faint.
>
> **What I learned:** I did not faint despite a severe panic, and without actions to prevent fainting. I may be wrong thinking I shall faint whenever I panic; tensing and deep breathing may not help. My therapist could be right in thinking that deep breathing makes me feel more dizzy.
>
> **What I should do next:** Repeat the experiment next time I go shopping.

---

presenting problems, the therapist enquires about antecedents, behaviour, and consequences (the ABC approach). *The term 'behaviour' is used to include thinking and emotion, as well as actions.* By considering the sequence ABC on several occasions, regular patterns of thinking and responding are identified. The therapist focuses on the patient's reasons for their beliefs, which is essential for planning experiences that will change them.

Sources of information

Self-monitoring: records of thoughts, behaviours, and experiences over days or weeks, made in real time. The record sheet usually has columns for symptoms, thoughts, emotions, and actions, plus the day and time at which they occurred. Events immediately preceding the problem are noted, as well as those occurring at the time and afterwards.

Observations during treatment sessions: the patient may be asked to imagine situations in which problems arise, and to report accompanying thoughts and emotions. Symptoms resembling the disorder may be induced (e.g. panic-like symptoms produced by hyperventilation), and accompanying thoughts and emotions noted.

Special interviewing: some patients need help to become aware of their maladaptive beliefs. *Laddering* involves a series of questions, each about the answer to the previous question. For example, a patient with an eating disorder might be asked what would happen if she were to gain weight, and she answers that she would lose her friends. To the question 'Why?' she might reply that she would be unlikeable. To a further question 'Why?' she might say that only thin people are attractive and popular.

The formulation

The information obtained in these various ways is combined with the usual psychiatric history in a formulation consisting of:

- the type of *events that provoke symptoms*
- any *special features of these events*
- *background factors*
- *maintaining factors*, including avoidance, safety behaviours, and ways of thinking.

The formulation is guided by a cognitive model of the disorder. The therapist discusses the formulation with the patient and may build it up, step by step, perhaps using a diagram on paper or whiteboard. The formulation is modified in light of the discussion.

Behavioural techniques

There are many behavioural techniques, some for a single disorder (such as the enuresis alarm; see page 692), and others such as exposure that can be used for a variety of disorders. Here we describe the more commonly used methods. Evidence for them is considered in the relevant chapters for the particular disorders.

Relaxation training

This is the simplest behavioural technique, and is mainly useful for subthreshold states of anxiety, for stress-related disorders such as initial insomnia (Viens *et al.*, 2003), and for mild hypertension (Yung and Keltner, 1996). In 'progressive relaxation', patients are trained to relax individual muscle groups one by one, and to regulate their breathing (Jacobson, 1938). Relaxation is used in anxiety disorders with good effects (Öst and Breitholtz, 2000) and can be learned in part from pre-recorded instructions or in a group. However, it has to be practised regularly, and many patients lack the motivation to do this.

Exposure

Exposure is used to reduce avoidance behaviour, especially in the treatment of phobic disorders. For simple phobias it is often sufficient to use exposure alone, but for complex phobic disorders exposure is usually combined with cognitive procedures. Exposure can be carried out *in practice* by confronting the actual situations that provoke anxiety or *in imagination* by imagining the phobic situations vividly enough to induce anxiety. Exposure can be gradual, progressing through a series of increasingly difficult situations (*desensitization*), or abrupt and intensive (*flooding*). In practice, exposure is usually paced between these two extremes, preferably in practice rather than in imagination.

Desensitization

In desensitization the patient is helped to:

1. *Construct a hierarchy* of situations that provoke increasing degrees of anxiety. About 10 items are chosen with an equal increment of anxiety between them. Sometimes two or more hierarchies can be constructed if no obvious theme links the stressful situations.
2. *Enter or imagine entering the situations* on each step of the hierarchy until achieved without anxiety.
3. *Use relaxation* while entering or imagining the situation to reduce the anxiety response, and enhance the imagery.

Flooding

In flooding, the patient enters the most feared situation from the start, and remains there until the anxiety has diminished. The process is repeated with other near-maximal stimuli. The experience is distressing and the results are no better than those obtained with desensitization, so flooding is seldom used.

Exposure in routine practice

Sessions last for about 45 minutes of entering a feared situation every day, either alone or with a relative or friend. Usually anxiety diminishes with each exposure. Sometimes, if the anxiety becomes overwhelming, the treatment has to restart from a less stressful situation. Disengagement from anxiety-provoking situations by thinking of other things is a commonly encountered defence.

Exposure with response prevention

This is a treatment for obsessional rituals. The pressure for rituals decreases if they can be resisted for periods of about an hour.

1. The therapist *explains the rationale for treatment and agrees targets* for exposure, such as to touch a 'contaminated' object such as a door handle and not to wash their hands for the next hour. A more advanced target might be to do all the household cleaning without washing their hands until the task is completed. Patients need to feel confident that every task will be agreed in advance and that they will never be faced with the unexpected.

2. The therapist may demonstrate the necessary exposure, a procedure known as *modelling*.

3. Initially the therapist accompanies and supports the patient during prevention, but later the patient does this on their own.

4. With progress the patient practises entering previously avoided situations that normally provoke rituals. This is called *exposure*.

The obsessional thoughts that accompany rituals usually improve as the rituals are brought under control. Obsessional thoughts that occur without rituals are more difficult to treat. *Habituation training* is a form of mental exposure treatment in which patients dwell on the obsessional thoughts for long periods or listen repeatedly to a recording of the thoughts spoken aloud for an hour or more. Alternatively, *thought stopping*, is used (see distraction techniques on page 692).

Social skills training

Some aspects of social behaviour include skills that can be learned—for example, making eye contact, or starting a conversation. These skills can be improved through modelling, guided practice, role-play and video feedback. The training is mainly useful for socially anxious people to improve self-confidence and in the management of adolescents with autism and Asperger's syndrome. It was also, for a time in the 1970s and 1980s, intensively pursued within rehabilitation for people with psychoses (Leff *et al.*, 1982). Although it failed to deliver the expected reductions in relapse, the techniques were adapted successfully with families to reduce high expressed emotion.

Assertiveness training

Assertiveness training is a form of social skills training in which patients practise appropriate self-assertion. By a combination of coaching, modelling, and role reversal, patients are encouraged to practise appropriate verbal and non-verbal behaviour, and to judge the level of self-assertion that is appropriate to various situations. Assertiveness training has, surprisingly, been found helpful not just with timid people but also with aggressive individuals, as it teaches a more appropriate way of channelling anger.

Anger management

In this form of social skills training, patients are helped to:

- identify situations that lead to anger
- identify attitudes that lead to anger that is out of proportion

- identify factors that reduce restraints on anger, especially the use of alcohol
- discover and practise alternative ways of dealing with situations that provoke anger—for example, delaying their response until anger can be brought under control ('count to 10').

Self-control techniques

All behavioural treatments aim to increase patients' control over their own behaviour. Self-control techniques attempt to do this directly without the intermediate step of changing thoughts or emotions as in cognitive therapy. Self-control techniques are based on operant conditioning principles, and on the studies by Bandura (1969) of the role of self-reward in social behaviour. Overeating and excessive smoking are examples of target behaviours. Self-control training is usually part of a wider cognitive behaviour programme.

Self-control treatment has three stages:

1. *Self-monitoring.* Daily records are kept of the problem behaviour and the circumstances in which it arises. Keeping a record enhances motivation by demonstrating the severity of the problem. These records are subsequently used to assess progress.

2. *Self-evaluation.* Achievements to be rewarded are agreed with the patient, and progress is monitored by the patient.

3. *Self-reward.* A system of reward points that can be accumulated to earn a material reward such as a week without smoking may be rewarded by going out for dinner.

Contingency management

Contingency management, like self-control techniques, provides rewards for desired behaviour and removes reinforcement from undesired behaviour. However, instead of relying on self-monitoring and self-reinforcement, in contingency management another person monitors the behaviour and provides the reinforcers. The latter are usually social reinforcers, such as indications of approval or disapproval, or enjoyable activities earned by accumulating points. Contingency management in the form of *token economies* was used mainly in the treatment of children and people with learning disability in residential settings, but is now seldom used because of its limited effect and generalizability. More recently, direct financial rewards have been given for changes in behaviour in various public health initiatives (Marteau *et al.*, 2009), including in mental health (Burton *et al.*, 2010). Direct payments have been shown to increase adherence to antipsychotic maintenance management (Priebe *et al.*, 2013), but this approach meets stern resistance.

Contingency management involves four stages.

1. *Define and record the behaviour*. The behaviour to be changed is defined and another person (usually a nurse or a parent) is trained to record it.

2. *Identify the stimuli and reinforcements*. The events that regularly precede the behaviour are identified. Similarly, the events that immediately follow the behaviour, *reinforcers*. Those involved may be quite unaware of their role in stimulating or reinforcing such behaviours.

3. *Change the reinforcement*. Reinforcement is directed away from the problem behaviours and towards desired behaviours. For example, parents are helped to attend less when their child shouts and more when he is quiet—always a difficult thing to keep up.

4. *Monitor progress*. Records are kept of the frequency of the problem and desired behaviours.

Enuresis alarms

This behavioural treatment is based on classical conditioning and was developed specifically for nocturnal enuresis (page 469). The original 'pad and bell' comprised two metal plates under the sheets attached to a battery and a buzzer, activated if the child passed urine. Nowadays a small sensor is attached to the pyjamas. The noise of the alarm wakes the child, who must then rise to empty his bladder and, if necessary, change the bed sheet. With repetitions the child begins to wake before his bladder empties involuntarily.

Complex behavioural techniques

Habit reversal

Habit reversal is a complex procedure that is generally used to treat tics, Tourette's syndrome, and stuttering. The classical treatment has five components—training in becoming aware of the onset of the behaviour, monitoring the behaviour, training in initiating competing responses that are incompatible with the behaviour, relaxation, and social support.

Eye movement desensitization and reprocessing

This treatment was developed for post-traumatic stress disorder (PTSD). It has three components:

- *exposure* using imagined scenes of the traumatic events
- *a cognitive component* in which the patient attempts to replace negative thoughts associated with the images with positive ones

- *saccadic eye movements* induced by asking the patient to follow rapid side-to-side movements of the therapist's finger.

Eye movement desensitization and reprocessing (EMDR) remains controversial, particularly with regard to whether the eye movements contribute to its efficacy (Russell, 2008). A review (Silver *et al.*, 2008) suggests that it is effective, although the quality of the evidence is relatively poor.

Behavioural techniques that are no longer in general use

Biofeedback has not been proved to add to the effects of relaxation alone. *Aversion therapy*, one of the earliest behavioural techniques, was developed in the 1930s as a treatment for alcohol dependence. Negative reinforcement was used to suppress unwanted behaviour. Its effects are temporary, and it was criticized as being more of a punishment than a treatment.

Cognitive techniques

Four methods are commonly used to bring about cognitive restructuring (i.e. change in cognitions).

1. *Distraction*, or focusing attention away from distressing thoughts. This is done by attending to something in the immediate environment (e.g. the objects in a shop window), by engaging in a demanding mental activity (e.g. mental arithmetic), or by producing a sudden sensory stimulus (e.g. snapping a rubber band on the wrist), called 'thought stopping.'

2. *Neutralizing*. The emotional impact of anxiety-provoking thoughts can be reduced by rehearsing a reassuring response (e.g. 'My heart is beating fast because I feel anxious, not because I have heart disease'). Patients may carry a 'prompt card' on which the reassuring thoughts are written.

3. *Challenging beliefs*. The therapist produces evidence that contradicts the patient's beliefs. However, such beliefs persist and, for these, if they are severe, CBT is indicated. CBT therapists do this by asking questions, as in Box 24.7, and arranging behavioural experiments, as in Box 24.5.

4. *Reassessing the patient's responsibility*. We all overestimate our responsibility for events that have many determinants. Constructing a *pie chart* that shows all of the determinants can help reassess such responsibility. Allocating appropriately sized sectors to other identified factors before entering their own contribution demonstrates that there is less room for the patient's contribution than had been supposed.

Cognitive behavioural treatments

CBT is now the most widely used psychological treatment internationally. It dominates UK provision for a range of disorders—mainly anxiety and depression, but also eating disorders, and it has even been used in psychosis. It has a coherent theory and a set of practices based on a collaborative approach between patient and therapist over a limited (often predetermined) number of sessions. The approaches are succinctly explained by Westbrook *et al.* (2011).

Treatments for anxiety disorders

In anxiety disorders, cognitive techniques are combined with exposure. The importance of exposure relates to avoidance behaviour, more in the phobic disorders and less in generalized anxiety disorders.

Three kinds of cognition are considered in treatment:

1. *Fear of fear*: general concerns about the effects of being anxious (e.g. losing control).

2. *Fear of symptoms*: concerns about specific symptoms (e.g. fears that palpitations are a sign of heart disease).

3. *Fear of negative evaluation*: concerns that other people will react unfavourably to the patient.

The balance of these cognitions varies in different anxiety disorders. In generalized anxiety disorder, fear of fear and general worry predominate (page 167). In social phobia, fears of negative evaluation are particularly important, as are concerns about blushing and trembling. In agoraphobia, fear of fear (especially thoughts that the person will faint, die, or lose control) and fears about the symptoms of a panic attack are central. Treatment involves the techniques outlined above—giving information, questioning the logical basis of the fears, and arranging behavioural experiments.

Information about the physiology of anxiety helps patients to attribute symptoms such as dizziness and palpitations correctly, instead of to physical illness, often heart disease. The *illogical basis of the fears* is discovered by questioning the patient's own evidence for the beliefs. *Behavioural experiments* are devised to test the patient's beliefs and the alternative explanation suggested by the therapist.

Anxiety management is a general treatment for anxiety disorders. It has six stages:

1. *Assessment*. The patient keeps a diary record of:
   - the frequency and severity of symptoms
   - the situations in which they occur
   - avoidance behaviour.

2. *Information* about the physiology of anxiety and any other matters that will correct misconceptions.

3. *Explanation* of the various vicious circles of anxiety.

4. *Relaxation* training as a means of controlling anxiety.

5. *Exposure* to situations that provoke anxiety.

6. *Distraction* to reduce the impact of anxiety-provoking thoughts.

Treatment for panic disorder is focused on the belief that physical symptoms of anxiety are evidence of a serious physical condition, usually heart disease. These beliefs create a vicious circle in which anxiety symptoms such as tachycardia generate additional anxiety, and this further increases the physical symptoms. Treatment consists of:

1. *Explanation* of how physical symptoms are part of the normal response to stress, and how fear of these symptoms sets up a vicious circle of anxiety.

2. *Record keeping*. Patients record the anxious cognitions that precede and accompany their panic attacks.

3. *Demonstration*. The therapist demonstrates that:

- physical symptoms can provoke anxious thoughts (e.g. by asking the patient to induce such symptoms by over-breathing or strenuous exercise and noting the accompanying thoughts and fears)

- these thoughts can induce anxiety (e.g. by asking the patient to focus their mind on the cognitions and observe the effect).

This demonstration that physical symptoms lead to anxious thoughts, which in turn lead to anxiety, helps to *validate the vicious circle account* of the aetiology of panic attacks.

4. *Safety-seeking behaviours*. Attention is given to safety behaviours, and to any dysfunctional beliefs that make ordinary situations stressful.

5. *Behavioural experiments* to test the patient's ideas against those proposed by the therapist.

6. *Cognitive restructuring* follows the observation that symptom changes affect the severity of the panic attacks. Repeating the sequence gradually leads to control of the panic attacks.

Treatment for PTSD includes attention to the characteristic intrusive visual images in the condition. Patients repeatedly imagine the situations depicted in these images, as they would do in systematic desensitization. They try to change the content in small steps to images that are less distressing. Research into the use of imagery in CBT and in desensitization has become a focus for several treatment initiatives in PTSD and beyond (Hackmann *et al.*, 2011). Patients are also helped to integrate and process the fragmentary and distressing recollections of the traumatic events. (Treatment for PTSD is considered further on page 147.)

Overall, CBT is the psychological treatment of choice for anxiety disorders (Olatunji *et al.*, 2010). For a review of the current status and practice, see Clark and Beck (2011).

Cognitive behaviour therapy for depressive disorders

Cognitive therapy for depressive disorders was developed by A. T. Beck (1976). It is a complex procedure intended to alter three aspects of the thinking of depressed patients—negative intrusive thoughts, beliefs and assumptions that render ordinary situations stressful, and errors of logic that allow these beliefs and assumptions to persist despite evidence to the contrary.

Monitoring is of three kinds.

1. Patients identify intrusive thoughts (e.g. 'I am a failure') by writing down their thoughts when their mood is low.

2. Therapists uncover dysfunctional beliefs and assumptions by asking questions such as those shown in Box 24.7. A typical belief of a depressed patient is 'Unless I always try to please other people, they will not like me.'

3. Patients record their activities and identify if it was pleasurable and if it was accompanied by a sense of mastery and achievement.

If the patient is severely depressed, the monitoring of thoughts is deferred and attention is focused on activities. The resulting 'activity schedule' is used to encourage activities that have been identified as leading to pleasure and mastery. The schedule also helps to bring a sense of order and purpose. At this stage the therapist helps the patient to reduce the need to make decisions, which are difficult for someone who is severely depressed.

If the patient is less severely depressed, treatment begins with an explanation of the cognitive model of depression, and an attempt is made to reduce intrusive thoughts. This is done through distraction and by rehearsing reassuring alternatives (e.g. 'Even though I think my work is bad, my boss praised me yesterday'). To help the patient to concentrate on the positive statement, the alternative can be written on a prompt card. As treatment proceeds, more time is spent in challenging depressive cognitions using the techniques outlined in Box 24.8 combined with behavioural experiments.

The following points are important in relation to cognitive therapy for depression.

- *Reviewing evidence*. Depressed patients are particularly prone to focus on evidence that supports their negative ideas, and to overlook evidence that contradicts them. The therapist should help the patient to give appropriate weight to the positive evidence.

- *Considering alternatives*. Depressed patients often reject positive alternatives to their thoughts and beliefs. The therapist can help the patient to consider alternatives by asking questions such as 'What do you think that another person would think about this situation?' or 'What would you think if another person had done what you have done?' (For additional questions, see Box 24.8.) Behavioural experiments are used to challenge beliefs and assumptions.

- *Considering consequences*. Patients should be helped to see the consequences of thinking negative thoughts. For example, the thought that everything

Box 24.8 Logical errors in depressive disorders

Box 24.8 Logical errors in depressive disorders

Exaggeration: magnifying small mistakes and thinking of them as major failures.

Catastrophizing: expecting serious consequences from minor problems (e.g. thinking that a relative who is late home has been involved in an accident).

Overgeneralizing: thinking that the bad outcome of one event will be repeated in every similar event in future (e.g. that having lost one partner, the person will never find a lasting relationship).

Ignoring the positive: dwelling on personal shortcomings or on the unfavourable aspects of a situation while overlooking the favourable aspects.

is hopeless may prevent them from attempting even small changes that could accumulate beneficially.

- *Considering errors of logic* (Box 24.8). The patient should be helped to ask questions such as 'Am I thinking in black-and-white terms?', 'Am I drawing too wide conclusions from this single event?', 'Am I blaming myself for something for which I am not responsible?', or 'Am I exaggerating the importance of events?' These questions are asked in relation to specific ideas, beliefs, and situations.

- *Considering beliefs.* As depression improves, more attention is given to the patient's beliefs, as abnormal beliefs can lead to relapse. Laddering (page 689) can uncover such beliefs. Useful questions include 'In what ways is this idea helpful?', 'In what ways is it unhelpful?' and 'What alternatives are there?'

- *'Mindfulness.'* People who are prone to depression may have a cognitive set in which thoughts and feelings are experienced as events rather than as aspects of the self. Modifying this set reduces the risk of relapse. Mindfulness-based cognitive therapy (MBCT) is an 8-week programme conducted in groups of 8–15 patients (Segal *et al.*, 2012), designed to modify these cognitive routines and reduce the risk of relapse. MBCT in addition to standard care significantly reduces the relapse rate in patients suffering from recurrent major depression (Chiesa and Serretti, 2010), and is recommended by the National Institute for Health and Clinical Excellence (2009a). The contribution of the specific 'mindfulness' component of treatment is unclear.

Cognitive behaviour therapy for bulimia nervosa

Currently CBT therapists emphasize the applicability of their approach for all eating disorders and believe the strict distinction between bulimia nervosa and anorexia nervosa is unhelpful and the same approach (CBT-E) should be applied. Evidence for effectiveness is strong for bulimia nervosa but weaker for anorexia nervosa. See Chapter 13 for review of the evidence for, and contemporary approaches to, psychological treatment for eating disorders.

The treatment of bulimia nervosa with CBT is based on the idea that the central problems are excessive concern about shape and weight, and low self-esteem. This leads to extreme dieting, followed by binge eating and often by self-induced vomiting and abuse of laxatives and diuretics. This vicious circle can be interrupted by:

- restoring a regular pattern of eating three meals a day
- increasing restraint on binge eating
- discussing ideas about shape, weight, and self-esteem.

The therapist attends first to the disordered pattern of eating before attempting to modify cognitions. He *explains the cognitive model* and relates it to the patient's experience. He emphasizes the importance of regular meals, the causal role of long periods of fasting, and the adverse effects of repeated vomiting, and of repeatedly taking laxatives and diuretics. The patient *keeps a record* of what they eat, when they eat, and when they induce vomiting or take laxatives and diuretics. The situations that provoke binge eating are recorded. With this information, the patient is better able to control the urge to overeat and, subsequently, the bouts of vomiting. The patient takes a number of precautions to help them to control their eating:

- Meals are eaten in a place separate from that in which food is prepared or stored.

- A limited amount of food is available at each meal—for example, two slices of bread are put on the table, rather than a whole loaf.

- A small amount of food is left on the plate and then thrown away, to mark the end of the meal.

- When shopping for food, a list is made in advance and purchases are strictly limited to the items and quantities on the list.

The therapist strongly discourages frequent checking of weight and of appearance, as both habits maintain the disorder.

Because patients often binge when they are unhappy, lonely, or bored, they are helped to *find other ways of dealing with unpleasant emotions*. For example, they might seek out friends, listen to music, or simply go out for a walk. Vomiting usually stops when the binges are under control. The dangers of abuse of laxatives and diuretics are emphasized once more, and the patient is strongly encouraged to dispose of all such drugs safely.

When eating is under better control, *attention turns to cognitions*. The patient records these together with the eating behaviour. Relevant cognitions are concerned not only with body shape and weight, but also with self-esteem. Examples of these cognitions include the following:

- to be fat is to be a failure
- dieting is a sign of strong will and self-control
- it is necessary to be thin if one is to be happy and successful.

Such beliefs persist because of the *illogical ways of thinking* (see Box 24.4). Identifying these illogical ways of thinking is not to deny that many of them receive strong social endorsement. The fact that many people agree with such cognitions does not mean that the thinking is not wrong. The questioning used to identify cognitions and illogical thinking resembles that described in Box 24.7.

Treatment also exists in a self-help format that can be effective with well-motivated patients (Box 24.9).

Cognitive behaviour therapy for hypochondriasis

The approach is twofold—first, to identify behaviours that maintain the disorder and, second, to change hypochondriacal ideas directly. The relevant behaviours include:

- repeatedly seeking reassurance, which relieves anxiety briefly but reinforces the concerns in the longer term
- checking bodily functions (e.g. measuring the pulse rate)
- checking bodily structure (e.g. palpating for lumps).

Hypochondriacal ideas are treated in the same way as anxiety and depressive disorders, using questioning and behavioural experiments. CBT has been found to be moderately helpful and MBCT has also been tested (Williams *et al.*, 2011).

Cognitive behaviour therapy for schizophrenia

Two approaches are used. The first aims to help the patient to *reduce and cope better with stressors* that may be exacerbating the disorder, and to *cope better with hallucinations*. The techniques for dealing with stressors are similar to those described above—namely, identifying and finding ways

> ### Box 24.9 Self-help for bulimia nervosa
>
> **Monitoring**
> - A daily record of eating, binges, and vomiting
> - Weighing no more than once a week
>
> **Regular planned meals**
> - Three normal-sized meals a day
> - Three small between-meal snacks
>
> **Stop binges**
> - Eat only the planned amount
> - Keep other food out of sight
> - Keep limited stocks of food
> - Take just enough money when buying food
>
> **Control vomiting**
> - Urge to vomit declines as binges stop
>
> **Control purging**
> - Reduce laxatives/diuretics, if necessary, in stages
>
> **Find alternatives to binge eating**
> - List distracting activities
> - Try them
>
> **Reduce life problems**
> - Problem-solving counselling
>
> For further information, see Fairburn (2013).

of dealing with stressful situations. Patients are helped to cope with hallucinations by distancing themselves and repeating statements that neutralize their effects.

The aim of the second approach is to *challenge delusions*. This approach is directed to secondary delusions, especially those that seem to have developed to explain hallucinations. The therapist encourages the patient to regard the delusions as beliefs rather than facts, and to discuss alternatives. To do this effectively requires a detailed formulation of each patient's delusions and other beliefs. When questioning the basis of the delusions, the therapist should avoid challenging them directly. Instead, he should try to persuade the patient to consider the consequences of holding the delusion and what would be the consequences of thinking in another way. The therapist then tries to reformulate the delusion as a way of making sense of certain experiences, which can be understood in terms of the knowledge the patient had at the time, but should now be reconsidered.

Turkington *et al.* (2005) have taught the approach to nurses with considerable success, and it is a module in several postgraduate mental health nursing courses (www.thorn-initiative.org.uk).

CBT is included as an integral component of treatment in current schizophrenia treatment guidelines. For details, see Chapter 11.

Cognitive therapy for personality disorder

Beck suggested that the techniques he had developed for the treatment of depressive disorders could be adapted for personality disorders. He described beliefs and ways of thinking that characterize each type of personality disorder in terms of self-view, the views of others, general beliefs, perceived threats, main strategies for coping, and primary affective responses. Beck also suggested a 'schema' characteristic of each type of personality disorder and consisting of statements that can be challenged in treatment. For example, the schema for histrionic personality disorder includes the following statements:

- 'Unless I captivate people, I am nothing'
- 'To be happy, I need other people to admire me'
- 'I must show people that they have hurt me.'

Schemas are challenged using the general techniques of cognitive therapy (see Box 24.7). There is some weak evidence for the value of schema-based CBT in borderline personality disorder (Blum *et al.*, 2008) and they are widely used in forensic settings.

Dialectic behaviour therapy for borderline personality disorder

Marsha Linehan (Linehan *et al.*, 1994) developed this treatment for patients with borderline personality disorder who repeatedly harmed themselves. Despite the name, it uses cognitive as well as behavioural techniques. The treatment is highly structured and described in a manual. Therapy is intensive, with individual sessions, skills training in a group, and access by telephone to the therapist between sessions. It is delivered by a small team of therapists and lasts for up to a year.

Individual sessions have four elements:

1. *Cognitive behavioural techniques*, including self-monitoring, and a collaborative style of working with the patient.
2. *Dialectical ways of thinking about problems*, such as seeing causality in terms of 'both/and' rather than 'either/or', and the possibility of reconciling opposites. This approach is particularly valuable to avoid unhelpful confrontations.
3. *'Mindfulness'*—the practice of detachment from experience.
4. *Aphorisms*—that is, phrases that encapsulate the approach (e.g. 'Although I may not have caused all my problems, I still have to solve them').

During the sessions, treatment goals are prioritized, dealing first with life-threatening situations, then with matters that could reduce collaboration with treatment, and after that with behaviours that impair quality of life.

Skills training sessions are usually provided in weekly groups lasting for 2 hours or more. Patients learn how to control anger and other strong emotions, how to tolerate distress, how to develop interpersonal skills, and mindfulness. The procedures for teaching these skills are described in a manual.

Telephone contact is designed to help patients get through crises by using the skills that have been learned in the sessions. The hours at which contact will be available are agreed in advance between patient and therapist.

Dialectic behaviour therapy has been claimed to give good results with borderline personality disorder, and has become widely available, although providing the full programme can be difficult. The beneficial effects are primarily on behaviour (i.e. reducing self-harming and suicide attempts) rather than on mood and self-esteem, and the degree of prescription in its provision may be a barrier to better understanding of what is effective within it.

Individual dynamic psychotherapies

Brief insight-oriented psychotherapy

This kind of psychotherapy seeks to uncover the origins of a psychiatric disorder in early life experience, identifying unconscious factors that account for abnormal thinking, emotions, and behaviour. In its usual form, it aims to produce change, with weekly sessions over 6–9 months. The treatment is focused upon specific problems—hence an alternative term *focal psychotherapy*. The procedures can be summarized as follows.

Starting treatment

The initial assessment is considered very important and is not hurried. It assesses suitability for brief treatment and selects the problems that will be the focus of treatment. This focus and the length of treatment are agreed with the patient, and that not all problems will be resolved is acknowledged. The therapist explains the general aim of linking past and present behaviour patterns, and that the therapist's role is to help the patient to find their own solutions. An atmosphere is created in which the patient feels involved and listened to, and one that is safe to explore ideas and fantasies that were previously hidden.

Subsequent sessions

In subsequent sessions the patient is encouraged to:

- give specific examples of the selected problems, and consider how they thought, felt, and acted at the time
- talk freely about these emotionally painful subjects
- express ideas and feelings even if they seem illogical or shameful
- review their own part in difficulties they usually ascribe to other people
- look for common themes in their problems and their responses
- consider how their present patterns of behaviour began, their original function, and why they persist
- consider alternative ways of thinking and behaving in distressing situations
- try out new responses to their emotions.

The therapist's role is to respond to the emotional as well as the intellectual content of the patient's descriptions (e.g. 'It sounds as though you felt angry when this happened'). He helps the patient to examine feelings previously denied, and to consider past situations in which similar feelings were experienced. Non-verbal behaviour can point to problems that are not being expressed directly. He maintains the agreed focus—avoiding problem areas too complex to address.

Interpretations are key features of dynamic therapy. These are essentially hypotheses linking present to past events and behaviours. They can include observations of defence mechanisms, such as blocks in recall during the sessions.

Transference and countertransference. The therapist has to be alert to intense emotions arising in sessions—transference and countertransference. *Transference* feelings about the therapist are a key to how the patient responded to key figures in childhood. In brief therapy, *countertransference* is usually taken to include all the therapist's emotional responses to the patient. Insight into countertransference can be difficult so therapists have their own regular supervision.

Ending treatment. The difficulty, and inevitability, of termination is discussed from an early stage. As it approaches, the patient should have a better understanding of their problems and be more confident about dealing with them. Endings often involve a 'flare up' of symptoms, allowing their understanding to be refreshed. It is common to arrange a couple of follow-up appointments spaced over 2 or 3 months.

Indications

The indications for short-term dynamic psychotherapy are based predominantly on clinical experience. It is chosen when the problem:

- can be conceptualized in psychodynamic terms
- is emotional or interpersonal (rather than a specific psychiatric disorder)
- involves low self-esteem, and recurrent problems in forming intimate relationships.

In addition, treatment is more effective when the patient:

- has adequate social support while treatment continues
- is willing to attempt change through their own efforts
- can look honestly at their own motives
- is capable of ceasing self-exploration when the sessions end.

Contraindications include obsessional or hypochondriacal disorders, severe mood disorder, psychoses, and some personality disorders, especially those characterized by acting out. For a review of the theories and methods of brief individual dynamic psychotherapy, see Hobbs (2005).

Cognitive analytic therapy

Cognitive analytic therapy is a brief therapy developed by a GP, Tony Ryle. Treatment is based on a 'procedural sequence model'. This proposes that behaviour follows a set sequence. Procedural sequences can be faulty in three ways.

- *Traps* are repetitive cycles of behaviour in which the consequences of behaviour perpetuate it. For example, depressed people think in ways that lead to failure, making further depression more likely.

- *Dilemmas* are false choices or unduly narrowed options. For example, people who fear angry feelings may think that the only alternative to aggression is excessive submission. This allows others to take advantage of them, making them even more angry.

- *Snags* are the anticipation of highly negative consequences of actions such that the action is never carried out and therefore never subjected to a reality check.

The *theory of reciprocal roles* was developed when cognitive analytic therapy was used with borderline personality disorder patients. Ryle proposed that people develop internalized 'templates' of social roles which consist of a role for the self, a role for the other person, and a paradigm of the relationship. Such roles include teacher/pupil, bully/victim, and abuser/abused. When one person adopts one of the roles, the other person feels under pressure to adopt the reciprocal role. These 'templates' can become narrow and inflexible.

Outline of the treatment

Following assessment and an explanation of the treatment, the patient is helped to construct a list of problems, moods, and behaviours, and records them in a diary. Recurrent maladaptive behaviours, role problems, and faulty procedural sequences are identified and formulated, often using diagrams to explain the procedural sequences. Specific examples of general procedures are sought in the diaries, and homework is arranged to try out alternative procedures—for example, asserting oneself appropriately. The origins of maladaptive procedures are also considered from a psychodynamic perspective—present maladaptive behaviour may have arisen from behaviour that was adaptive when the person was younger.

The formulation is summarized in the form of a letter to the patient. The therapist helps the patient become aware of and change their behaviours, procedural sequences, and role problems. Transference and countertransference problems are anticipated, identified, and discussed. Treatment usually lasts either 16 or 24 sessions. When it ends, the therapist writes another letter to the patient summarizing their progress, prognosis, and future action, and the patient is asked to write to the therapist summarizing their experience. Patients often need help to become aware of their problems ('develop an observing I'). This is achieved by modelling the evaluation and analysis of problems using diagrams. There is some early evidence of its value in young patients and those with borderline personality disorder (Chanen *et al.*, 2008). For further information about cognitive analytic therapy, see Ryle and Kerr (2016).

Long-term individual dynamic psychotherapy

Long-term dynamic psychotherapy is a general term for most individual psychotherapy that lasts for longer than 9 months. The best known is psychoanalysis, and most methods are derived from it. Long-term dynamic psychotherapy is costly, and because it has not been shown to be superior to shorter forms, it is rarely available in public health services. It is reserved for patients judged too difficult for short-term psychotherapy and is still used in training for psychotherapists.

Long-term dynamic psychotherapy aims to increase insight—that is 'the conscious recognition of the role of unconscious factors on current experience and behaviour' (Fonagy and Kächele, 2009). It also involves integrating these insights into current functioning, called 'working through'. Insight is achieved by bringing feelings and ideas previously outside consciousness into conscious awareness, and then interpreting their significance and linking past experiences to present ones.

The basic tools are free association, and examining the content of fantasies and dreams. Analysis of transference provides further information about unconscious processes, as does analysis of the countertransference. Recognizing countertransference is a key goal of personal psychotherapy during training.

Resistance to accessing unconscious material takes three forms:

1. *Repression:* active blocking access to unconscious material.
2. *Transference resistance:* restricting the intensity of the therapeutic relationship.
3. *Negative therapeutic reactions:* such as new symptoms that retard progress.

Analysis of resistance, as with analysis of transference, can often markedly increase insight.

Interpretations are considered the hallmark of this treatment. Interpretations link together seemingly unrelated mental phenomena and involve defences, unconscious processes, transference, or the links between past experience and present patterns. Transference interpretations are particularly emphasized in long-term therapy.

Long-term psychodynamic psychotherapy also differs from brief dynamic psychotherapy in that:

- *It is less structured*—the patient is encouraged to talk and associate ideas freely without a specific focus.
- *The therapist is less active* and guides the patient less.
- *Patients may be seen twice a week* (up to five times a week in vanishingly rare classical analysis).

Treatment in groups

Small-group psychotherapy

This is psychotherapy carried out with a group of usually about eight patients. Small-group psychotherapy is used most often to modify interpersonal problems, as a form of supportive treatment, or to encourage adjustment to the effects of physical or mental illness.

The origins of group psychotherapy

Group therapy's early origins were in American physician Joseph Pratt's supportive and educational groups for patients with pulmonary tuberculosis (Pratt, 1908). Modern group therapy originated in the treatment of war neuroses in the UK. Group analysis (Foulkes and Lewis, 1944) was based on psychoanalysis with a rather passive group leader using analytical interpretations. Bion, a Kleinian analyst, focused specifically on the unconscious defences of the group as a whole rather than on the problems of individual members (Bion, 1961). In the USA, so-called 'action groups' in the 1960s and early 1970s provided a more intense experience. Group techniques are legion, but what they have in common seems more important than the differences.

Classification of small-group therapies

One classification of groups is by their goals (specific versus non-specific) and the activity of the leader (high versus low) (Schlapobersky and Pines, 2009):

1. *Specific goals—high leader activity*: such as structured alcohol and drug programmes and CBT in groups.
2. *Specific goals—low leader activity*: includes problem-solving groups.
3. *Non-specific goals—high leader activity*: includes the many short-term group therapies, including psychodrama.
4. *Non-specific goals—low leader activity*: includes various psychodynamic groups.

Terminology

Groups can be described in terms of their structure, process, and content.

- *Structure* describes the enduring reciprocal relationships between each member of the group and the therapist, and between the members.

- *Process* describes the short-term changes in emotions, behaviours, relationships, and other experiences of the group.
- *Content* refers to the observable events in the group meetings—the themes, responses, discussions, and silences.

Therapeutic factors in group therapy

Group treatments share the therapeutic factors common to all kinds of psychological treatment, including restoring hope, releasing emotion, giving information, providing a rationale, and suggestion (see Box 24.1). Group treatment also shares additional factors, such as shared experience, support for and from group members, socialization, imitation, and interpersonal learning (Yalom and Leszcz, 2005), summarized in Box 24.10.

General indications for group therapy

Group or individual therapy?

There is no strong evidence that the results of group therapy differ from those of equivalent individual psychotherapy. Nor is there evidence of differing results for forms of group therapy. Clinical experience suggests that they are somewhat less effective than individual therapies unless they build on shared clinical features.

What problems are suitable?

Group therapy appears most appropriate for patients whose problems are mainly in relationships. Contraindications are similar to those for individual psychotherapy.

Types of small-group psychotherapy

Supportive groups

Many of the therapeutic factors in a group (Box 24.10) work in supportive treatment. In supportive groups, the therapist encourages self-help and ensures that the experiences are used positively. He should also ensure that relationships do not become too intense, protect vulnerable patients when necessary, and ensure that each member is supported by and gives support to other members.

Self-help ('mutual-help') groups

Self-help groups are organized and led by patients or former patients who have learned ways of overcoming

Box 24.10 Therapeutic factors in group therapy

Universality (shared experience). This helps the patient to realize that they are not alone and that others have similar experiences and problems. Hearing about others' experiences is often more convincing and helpful than reassurance from a therapist.

Altruism. Supporting others increases self-esteem of the giver, as well as helping the receiver. Mutual support leads to a sense of belonging to the group.

Group cohesion. Belonging to a group is especially valuable for those who have previously felt isolated. Group cohesion sustains the group through difficult patches.

Socialization. Social skills are acquired in the group from the comments and reactions of members in response to one another's behaviour. Members can try out new behaviours within the safety of the group.

Imitation. This involves learning from observing and adopting the behaviours of other group members. Patients imitate adaptive behaviours, although there is a risk that maladaptive behaviours can also be learnt.

Interpersonal learning. This involves learning from the interactions within the group and from practising new ways of interacting. Interpersonal learning is an important component of group therapy.

Recapitulation of the family group. Interactions can become over time increasingly based on past relationships between patients and their parents and siblings. This group transference is encouraged and used in analytical groups.

---

or adjusting to their difficulties. Group members benefit from the opportunity to talk about their own problems and express their feelings, and from mutual support. Group processes develop very strongly in these groups. Some such groups, such as Alcoholics Anonymous, have strict rules of procedure.

There are countless self-help groups for people who suffer from a wide range of different problems. These include Alcoholics Anonymous (page 584), Weight Watchers, groups for patients with chronic physical conditions, and groups for the bereaved (CRUSE Clubs). Few self-help groups (now often referred to as 'mutual-help groups') have been evaluated.

Therapeutic groups

Interpersonal group therapy

Interpersonal group therapy developed in particular from the work of Yalom and Leszcz (2005), and characterizes most group therapy. Treatment is focused on problems in current relationships, and examines the ways in which these problems are reflected in the group. The past is discussed only in so far as it helps to make sense of present problems.

Patients are prepared for their experience in a group by emphasizing:

- *Confidentiality*: the proceedings of the group are confidential.

- *Reliability*: members must attend regularly and on time, and not leave early.
- *Disclosure*: members are required to disclose their problems.
- *Concern*: members must show concern for the problems of others.
- *Disappointment*: at first members may be disappointed by the lack of rapid change, or frustrated by the need to share the time available for speaking.
- *Keeping apart*: The group members should not meet outside the group, and if they do so this should be reported at the next meeting.
- *Duration*: the length of the group is explained (e.g. '10 weeks' or '2 years'), together with the need to remain until the end.

Setting up the group

General considerations. About eight members are chosen. They should have some problems in common, and no member should have exclusive problems that set them apart from the rest. Meetings need a room of adequate size, with the chairs in a circle so that all members can see one another.

Meetings usually last for 60–90 minutes to allow adequate time for every member to take part; they are usually held once a week, and generally continue for 12–18 months. Most groups are 'slow open', with new members joining only to replace those who leave. Totally *closed* groups are very difficult to maintain, and rare outside residential settings. Groups that accept new members frequently, known as *open* groups, are usually supportive or psychoeducational.

One or two therapists? Most groups are run by one therapist, but many have cotherapists. The advantage of having two therapists is both practical and theoretical. It ensures continuity if one of the therapists has to be away, and it also provides an excellent training opportunity. Theoretically it can also help with countertransference problems. A risk is that cotherapists may compete with or behave defensively towards one another. However, in general if differences are discussed as they arise, they can provide further insight into the group process and offer healthy modelling of problem exploration and resolution.

Some problems in group therapy

However skilful the therapist, certain problems commonly arise.

- *Formation of subgroups.* Some members may form a coalition based on age, social class, shared values, or other characteristics. The therapist should discourage such groupings, encouraging the group to discuss the reasons for their formation.
- *Members who talk too much.* The therapist needs to address this at an early stage, before the group rejects the talkative member. He may ask the group why they allow one person to absolve the rest from the need to speak about themselves.
- *Members who talk too little.* The therapist should assist silent members to speak and should therefore understand the reasons for silence.
- *Conflict between members.* The therapist should not take sides in conflicts but should encourage the whole group to discuss the issue in ways that lead to understanding of its arising, perhaps a hostile transference.
- *Avoidance of the present.* Members may talk excessively about the past to avoid present conflicts. The therapist can ask questions or use interpretations to bring the discussion back to the present, or actively relate it to current group process.
- *Potentially embarrassing revelations.* Common sense and judgement have to be used to protect vulnerable patients from blurting out potentially devastating information (e.g. about sexual or even criminal activity) early in the group.

Group analysis

This technique has been widely used within the UK health service. It differs from the interpersonal method described above in the greater use of interpretations about transference and unconscious mechanisms and in encouraging 'free-floating discussion' rather than a specific focus. Particular attention is given to transferences to the therapist and between members generating hypotheses about previous relationships to understand current problems.

Encounter groups and psychodrama (action techniques)

In *encounter groups* the interaction between members is actively intensified to provoke change. The encounter can be verbal, using challenging language, but it can also include touching or hugging between the participants. Sessions can last several hours. These groups are attractive to volatile individuals and undoubtedly carry some risks of things getting worse. *Psychodrama* groups enact events from the life of one member, in scenes reflecting either current relationships or those of their family of origin. Such enactments often provoke strong feelings reflecting the problems of other group members. Members often swap roles to understand the other person's perspective. The drama is followed by a group discussion. Psychodrama is found useful with less educated and verbal patients, and is favoured in some prison settings.

Ward groups

Group meetings, often called 'community meetings', are part of the daily programme of many psychiatric wards. The approach originated in therapeutic communities. These are large groups, usually including all of the patients in a treatment unit together with some or all of the staff. At the simplest level, large groups allow patients to examine and deal with the problems of living together. They can confront individual patients about disordered or disruptive behaviour, and provide opportunities for social learning. Care needs to be exercised to avoid bullying, and a predominantly supportive atmosphere is needed for these groups to work. The group is sometimes used as a kind of governing body that formulates rules and seeks to enforce them.

Therapeutic communities

In a therapeutic community, every shared activity is viewed as a potential source of learning and change. Members live, work, and play together, and learn about themselves through the reactions of other members in the course of these activities. Within the safe environment of the community, they are encouraged to experiment with new behaviours and appreciate points of view other than their own. Members take part in frequent group meetings. Maxwell Jones, its founder, called it a *living-learning*

> ### Box 24.11 Principal features of a therapeutic community
>
> **Informality.** There are few rules, and staff dress and behave informally.
>
> **Mutual help.** Members support each other and help others to change.
>
> **Permissiveness.** Members tolerate behaviour that they might not accept elsewhere.
>
> **Directness and honesty.** Members respond directly to distortions of reality and other kinds of self-deception.
>
> **Shared decisions.** Members and staff join in the day-to-day decisions about the running of the unit, the behaviour of its members, and often about the admission of new members.
>
> **Shared activities.** Members provide some of the 'hotel' services in the community, so that each has a job involving responsibilities to other people.

situation (Jones, 1968), others a culture of enquiry. The underlying principles of the regimen have been summarized as *democracy, reality confrontation, permissiveness*, and *communality* (Rapoport, 1960). These translate into the features shown in Box 24.11. Residential therapeutic communities are no longer available in the NHS but the approach is still predominant in day units and in drug rehabilitation and some offender institutions.

Therapeutic day hospitals

Therapeutic day units are increasingly widespread for the treatment of personality disorder (Bateman and Fonagy, 2008). They have a similar structure to therapeutic communities, with a culture of enquiry, but emphasize 'mentalization'. They are informed by psychoanalytical theory, but emphasize group work and a supportive environment. Using nurse therapists, the aim is to help patients to become aware of their strong emotions and reflect and learn to tolerate them, rather than act them out impulsively. There is no emphasis on understanding past experiences as long as the patient can begin to manage their intense emotions.

Psychotherapy with couples and families

Couple therapy

Couple therapy is usually proposed either because conflict in a relationship appears to be the cause of emotional disorder in one of the partners or to save a threatened relationship. The problem is conceived in terms of how the couple interact, and treatment is directed to this interaction. Couples are required themselves to identify the difficulties that they would like to put right.

Several techniques of therapy have developed, based on psychodynamic, behavioural, and systems theory approaches, and on a combination of techniques drawn from these latter two.

Family therapy

Several, sometimes all, members of a family take part in this treatment. Usually both parents are involved, often together with the child whose problems have led the family to seek help. They may be joined by other members of the extended family. The aim of treatment is to improve family communication and functioning,

and consequently to help the identified patient. Since success depends on the collaboration of several people, dropout rates are high. Whatever their method, family therapists have the following goals for the family:

- improved communication
- improved autonomy for each member
- improved agreement about roles
- reduced conflict
- reduced distress in the member who is the patient.

The systems approach is very influential, and was developed in the USA by Salvador Minuchin, who in his structural family therapy, advocated a practical approach to resolving problems. In Italy, the Milan school used hypotheses about the family system to suggest ways of promoting change. These approaches are described briefly below, together with an eclectic approach. The reader will find more detailed accounts in the chapter by Bloch and Harari (2009). Family therapy is used in the treatment of some young people with anorexia nervosa after weight has been restored by other means. Special kinds of family treatment have been developed to reduce relapses in schizophrenia (page 290).

Systemic family therapy

Systemic family therapy is concerned with the present functioning of the family, rather than with members' past experiences. The therapist's task is to identify the family's unspoken rules, their disagreements about who makes these rules, and their distorted ways of communicating. The therapist helps the family to understand and modify the rules, and to improve communication.

The *Milan approach* (Palazzoli *et al.*, 1978) usually consists of 5–10 sessions, spaced at intervals of 1 month or more ('long brief therapy'). *Circular questioning* is often used to assess the family. In this technique, one person is asked to comment on the relationships of others—for example, the mother may be asked how her husband relates to their son, and others are asked to comment on her response. The purpose is to discover and clarify confused or conflicting views. A hypothesis is then constructed about the family functioning and presented to the family, who are asked to consider the hypothesis during and between sessions. The family may be asked to try to behave in new ways. Sometimes the therapist provokes change with *paradoxical injunctions* designed to provoke the family into making changes that they cannot make in other ways. Paradoxical injunctions are impossible or counterintuitive suggestions that force the family to confront their hidden or unacceptable motives. A review of 10 outcome studies of Milan therapy found symptomatic improvement in about two-thirds of patients, and improved functioning in about 50% of the families (Carr, 1991).

Eclectic family therapy

In everyday clinical work, especially with adolescents, it is almost impossible to do without simple short-term interventions to bring about limited changes in the family. The present situation of the family and how the members communicate with one another is usually the focus.

Assessment

Constructing a genogram using conventional symbols (Figure 24.1) is a particularly useful step in family therapy, leading to questions on current and past family life, and the roles of the members. The therapist tries to answer two questions: namely how the family functions and whether family factors are involved in the patient's problems. Bloch and Harari (2009) have proposed a helpful framework in which to consider these questions.

1. How does the family function?
   - *structure* recorded in the genogram (e.g. single parent, a step-parent, size and age spread of the sibship)
   - *changes and events* (e.g. births, deaths, departures, and financial problems)
   - *relationships* (e.g. close, distant, loving, conflictual, etc.)
   - *patterns of interaction* involving two or more people (e.g. a child who sides with one parent against the other).

2. Are family factors involved in the patient's problems? The family may be:

   - *reacting* to the patient's problems (note that there may be other, unrelated, problems)
   - *supporting* the patient
   - *contributing* to the patient's problems (e.g. the problems of a daughter who cannot leave her lonely mother).

Intervention

Specific goals for change are agreed with the members of the family, who are asked to consider how any changes will affect themselves and others, and what has prevented the family from making the changes. Paradoxical injunctions may be included, but should be made only after the most careful consideration of the range of possible responses. The therapist should remember that interchanges in the sessions are likely to continue when the family return home, and should try to ensure that this does not lead to further problems.

Psychotherapy for children

The kinds of psychotherapy discussed so far do not lend themselves to the treatment of young children, who lack the necessary verbal skills. In practice many emotional problems of younger children are secondary to those of

their parents, and it is often appropriate to direct psychotherapy mainly to them.

Melanie Klein believed it was possible to use the child's play as equivalent to the words of the adult in

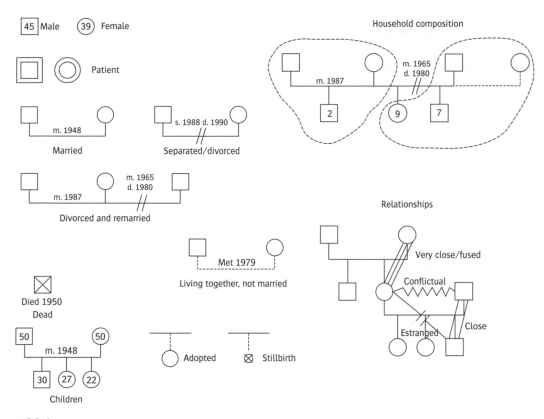

Figure 24.1 Symbols used in the construction of a genogram.

Reproduced from Bloch and Harari, Family Therapy in the Adult Psychiatric Setting. In: MG Gelder, Andreasen NC, López-Ibor JJ Jr, Geddes JR (eds), The New Oxford Textbook of Psychiatry, Copyright (2009), with permission from Oxford University Press.

psychotherapy. Anna Freud developed child psychotherapy by a less extreme adaptation of her father's techniques to the needs of the child. She accepted that non-analytical techniques could be helpful, including reassurance, suggestion, the giving of advice, and acting as a role model (an 'auxiliary ego'). For many neurotic disorders, she advocated analytical techniques to identify the unconscious content and to interpret it to strengthen ego function.

In the UK, most psychotherapy for children is eclectic; the therapist tries to establish a good relationship with the child and to learn about their feelings and thoughts, partly through talking and listening, and partly through play. Older children can communicate verbally with adults, but younger children can communicate better through play. The therapist can help children to find words that express their thoughts and feelings, and can thus make it easier for them to control and modify them. Child psychotherapy is discussed further in Chapter 16. For a more detailed account, see Pearce (2009).

Psychotherapy for older people

Increasing emphasis is being placed on the provision of psychological treatments as part of the care plan for elderly patients. Provided that they do not have cognitive impairment, elderly patients can take part in any of the treatments described for younger adults. When using cognitive therapy, it is important to be aware of minor cognitive impairment that, while insufficient to affect general functioning, may impair the patient's engagement in therapy. For a more detailed account see Cook et al. (2005).

Treatments of mainly historical and cultural interest

In our evidence-based era it may seem inappropriate to list treatments that have fallen into disuse because of lack of effect. However, many of these treatments have entered our culture and have a strong hold on the public imagination. Psychiatrists are likely to be approached by patients who are keen to receive such treatments, and we need to be familiar with them in the same way as we are with outdated but influential concepts such as the 'schizophrenogenic' mother.

Hypnosis is a state in which the person is relaxed and drowsy, and more suggestible than usual. Hypnosis can be induced in many ways. The main requirements are that the subject should be willing to be hypnotized and convinced that hypnosis will occur. Most hypnotic procedures contain some combination of a task to focus attention (e.g. watching a moving object), rhythmic monotonous instructions, and the use of a graduated series of suggestions (e.g. that the person's arm will rise). The therapist uses the suggestible state either to implant direct suggestions of improvement, or to encourage recall of previously repressed memories.

Hypnosis is used infrequently in psychiatry but is used widely for stopping smoking, dieting, etc. A light trance is used occasionally as a form of relaxation. For this purpose hypnosis has not been shown to be generally superior to relaxation. A deeper trance is used occasionally to enhance suggestion to relieve symptoms, especially those of conversion disorder. Although sometimes effective in the short term, this method has not been shown to be superior to suggestion without hypnosis. The authors do not recommend the use of hypnosis in clinical psychiatry.

Autogenic training was described by Schultz in 1905 and was in use mainly in continental Europe as a treatment for physical symptoms caused by emotional disorder. Patients practise exercises to induce feelings of heaviness, warmth, or cooling in various parts of the body, and to slow their respiration. Repeated use of these exercises is supposed to induce changes in autonomic nervous activity, thereby alleviating physical symptoms in stress-related and anxiety disorders, including hypertension. Its results do not differ substantially from those achieved with simple relaxation, nor is there any good evidence that it has a specific therapeutic effect.

Abreaction (the unrestrained expression of emotion) has long been used to relieve mental distress and some psychiatric symptoms. Abreaction is part of many forms of religious healing (see below). It was used to great acclaim during the Second World War, using rapid-acting barbiturates to bring prompt relief from acute war neuroses (predominantly acute stress disorders), notably by Sargant and Slater. In civilian practice, abreaction is less effective, perhaps because fewer disorders are the result of discrete overwhelming stresses. For more information about the procedure, see Sargant and Slater (1963).

Meditation and yoga are increasingly used by people with minor psychiatric problems as an alternative or adjunct to psychiatric treatment. There are many approaches, each associated with different systems of belief, but sharing common features. They involve relaxation and the regulation of breathing, and directing attention away from the external world and from the stream of thoughts that would otherwise occupy the mind, often by repeating a word or phrase (a mantra). An important feature is setting time aside when calm can be restored. In addition, the espousal of a value system and association with similar-minded individuals (the activities are commonly group-based) may explain some of the reported successes of the methods. Aspects of meditation have been incorporated into MBCT.

Traditional healing still plays an important part in many individuals' lives, and is often a precursor to seeking professional help. It is not restricted, as is often assumed, to ethnic minority groups. Alternative medicines and treatments are ubiquitous in all strata of society. However, the use of traditional healers is generally restricted to minority groups. Traditional healers can be broadly divided into four groups (Jilek, 2000).

- *Herbalists* are concerned mainly with plant remedies, some of which are known to contain active ingredients, while others appear to be placebos.
- *Medicine men and women* use ritual methods of healing, sometimes combined with plant remedies. They are believed to have special powers, often of supernatural origin.
- *Shamans* use methods like those of medicine men and women, but also enter into altered states of consciousness in which they are believed to communicate with spirits or ancestors, and to recover the abducted souls of people made ill by this supposed loss.
- *Diviners* discover and name the cause of illness by interpreting oracles (in either clear or altered consciousness) from the content of dreams, or through some form of communication with ancestors or spirits.

Traditional healers use methods that incorporate the non-specific processes in western psychological treatment (Box 24.1). In addition, they are aware of the value of naming a condition and answering the questions 'Why am I (or my son) afflicted?' This ends uncertainty and relieves blame and guilt. Some traditional healers use therapeutic suggestion, and many involve the family both in the diagnostic process and in the rituals of treatment. Some employ cleansing or purification rituals to eliminate supposed polluting agents. A few healers use sacrificial rites to appease supernatural beings, sometimes combining these with confession and a promise of changed behaviour. They may involve the wider community to reinforce their message. Traditional healing is not necessarily incompatible with modern medicine, and may be running parallel with it more often than we think.

Ethical problems in psychological treatment

Autonomy

The need for informed consent is as great in psychological treatments as in any other medical procedure. To give such consent the patient must understand the nature of the treatment and its likely consequences. Such preparation is not only ethically desirable but also likely to improve the therapeutic alliance.

Confidentiality

Group psychotherapy presents special problems of confidentiality. Patients should understand fully the requirement to talk of personal matters in the group, but they need to understand equally clearly the requirement to treat as confidential all they hear in the group. Family therapy presents similar problems, especially if the therapist agrees to see one member outside the family session, and is told of a family secret (e.g. an extramarital affair). Wherever possible the therapist should avoid such individual meetings and arrange for a colleague to see the family member if this is necessary (e.g. if one member is seriously depressed). Similar problems arise in couple therapy.

The answer to the question of when a therapist should reveal confidential material to a third party is the same as in other treatment situations, namely that it is justified when there is a substantial risk to a third party. Confidentiality is often confused with secrecy in psychotherapy (both by patients and by some therapists). Modern mental healthcare utilizes a model of shared responsibility, and often information must be shared. Only in exceptional cases should patients be promised that 'absolutely no one else will ever know of this'.

Exploitation

Patients who are receiving psychological treatment are particularly vulnerable to exploitation. This arises from the experiences that cause them to seek psychotherapy, but also because of the intense and often dependent relationship with the therapist. As in other branches of medicine, exploitation may be financial or sexual. Financial exploitation is a potential problem in private practice, in which treatment may be prolonged for longer than is necessary. Occasionally the exploitation is sexual. In the medical and other caring professions, such exploitation is prohibited in professional codes of conduct. Several rogue therapists have defended inappropriate sexual contact as 'therapeutic' and, remarkably, in some cases have succeeded in this defence. However, it is never acceptable to form a sexual relationship with a current or previous patient. In some jurisdictions (e.g. some US states) there are evolving guidelines about the time that must elapse before such relationships can be considered acceptable.

Another form of exploitation is the imposition of the therapist's values on the patient. This may be open and direct (e.g. when a therapist imposes his view that termination of pregnancy is morally wrong) or it may be concealed and indirect (e.g. when a therapist expresses no opinion, but nevertheless gives more attention to the arguments against termination than to those for it). Similar problems may arise, for example, in couple therapy when the therapist's values may affect his approach to the question of whether the couple should separate. A controversial issue is that of 'implanting' erroneous explanations. This has been very contested in relation to 'recovered memory' syndrome, where the recall, after many years, of early familial sexual abuse has been attributed to therapists exploiting suggestibility. Although there has been no suggestion that this is deliberate, there is considerable professional doubt about its status, and the consequences are so potentially catastrophic that it requires very careful monitoring.

In group psychotherapy, one patient may be exploited by another. This is one of the reasons for proscribing contact outside the group. One patient may bully or scapegoat another within the sessions, or may seek a sexual relationship outside. The therapist should try to protect vulnerable patients within the sessions. Clearly it is not possible to be as strict in this matter as in a professional relationship, but strongly emphasizing the purpose of the therapy rules is key to minimizing the problem.

Further reading

Bateman A, Brown D and Pedder J (2000). *Introduction to Psychotherapy: An outline of psycho-dynamic principles and practice*, 3rd edn. Tavistock/Routledge, London. (An account of dynamic theory, and practice in individual, couple, family, and group formats.)

Bloch S (2013). *An Introduction to the Psychotherapies*, 4th edn. Oxford University Press, Oxford. (An introduction to the commonly used psychological treatments, with a chapter on ethics.)

Frank JD and Frank JB (1993). *Persuasion and Healing*, 3rd edn. Johns Hopkins Press, Baltimore, MD. (A revised version of a landmark account of the non-specific factors in psychotherapy.)

Gabbard G, Beck JS and Holmes J (2005). *Oxford Textbook of Psychotherapy*. Oxford University Press, Oxford. (A comprehensive set of reviews of the major forms of psychotherapy and their use in clinical practice.)

Gurman AS (ed.) (2003). *Family Therapy: Theory, practice and research*. Brunner-Routledge, London. (A comprehensive work of reference.)

Hawton K *et al.* (2000). *Cognitive Behavioural Approaches for Adult Psychiatric Disorders: A practical guide*, 2nd edn. Oxford University Press, Oxford. (An introduction with many valuable practical examples.)

CHAPTER 25

Drugs and other physical treatments

Introduction

This chapter is concerned with the use of drugs and other physical treatments, such as electroconvulsive therapy (ECT) and neurosurgical procedures. Psychological treatments are the subject of Chapter 24. This separation, although convenient when treatments are described, does not imply that the two kinds of therapy are to be thought of as exclusive alternatives when an individual patient is considered; on the contrary, many patients require both. In this book, the ways of combining treatments are considered in other chapters, where the treatment of individual syndromes is discussed. It is important to keep this point in mind when reading this chapter.

Our concern is with clinical therapeutics rather than basic psychopharmacology, which the reader is assumed to have studied already. An adequate knowledge of the mechanisms of drug action is essential if drugs are to be used in a rational way, but a word of caution is appropriate. The clinician should not assume that the therapeutic effects of psychotropic drugs are necessarily explained by the pharmacological actions that have been discovered so far. In addition, there is relatively little knowledge about the neuropsychological mechanisms through which pharmacological manipulation can ameliorate psychological symptomatology.

This caution does not imply that a knowledge of pharmacological mechanisms has no bearing on psychiatric therapeutics. On the contrary, there have been substantial advances in pharmacological knowledge since the first specific psychotropic drugs were introduced in the 1950s, and it is increasingly important for the clinician to relate this knowledge to their use of drugs. As noted in Chapter 6, evidence-based clinical guidelines are increasingly used to assist practitioners in their use of medication, and it is important to be aware of these. However, in specialist psychiatric practice there is often rather less high-quality evidence to guide prescribing, and a knowledge of pharmacology will help to ensure that safe and reasonable prescribing practices are followed.

History of physical treatments

Physical treatments have been applied to patients with psychiatric disorders since antiquity, although, in retrospect, the most that could be claimed for the best of these interventions is that they were relatively harmless. Of course, the same holds for the management of patients with general medical disorders, for which similar treatments, such as bleeding and purging, were often used regardless of diagnosis. It is wise not to be too censorious about the treatment of disorders of which the aetiology is still largely unknown, but to bear in mind that 'it may well be that in a hundred years current therapies, psychotherapies as well as physical therapies, will be looked upon as similarly uncouth and improbable' (Kiloh *et al.*, 1988).

Historically, physical treatments can be divided into two main classes:

- Those that were aimed at producing a direct change in a pathophysiological process, usually by some alteration in brain function.
- Those that were aimed at producing symptomatic improvement through a dramatic psychological impact.

The latter interventions were often based on philosophical theories about the moral basis of madness. For example, many physicians appear to have followed the proposal of Heinroth (1773–1843) that insanity was the product of evil and personal wrongdoing. Accordingly, restraint with chains and corporal punishment were seen as appropriate remedies. Other physical treatments, such as the spinning chair introduced by Erasmus Darwin (1731–1802), seemed to be designed to produce a general 'shock to the system', and perhaps thereby to interrupt the morbid preoccupations of the patient. A less arduous regimen was the use of continuous warm baths, often given in combination with cold packs. This treatment was recommended by clinicians as distinguished as John Conolly (1794–1866) and Emil Kraepelin (1856–1926), and was still in use at the Bethlem Hospital in the 1950s.

Drugs that produce changes in the function of the central nervous system, such as opiates and anticholinergic agents, have been used in the treatment of mental disorders for hundreds of years. Although some of these drugs may have had calming effects, they were of no specific value in the treatment of psychiatric disorders. Often a physical treatment was used not because of its proven efficacy, but because it was recommended by an eminent and vigorous physician. Also, the assessment of efficacy depended almost entirely on uncontrolled clinical observation.

In 1933, about 10 years after the isolation of insulin by Frederick Banting and Charles Best, Manfred Sakel introduced *insulin coma treatment* for psychosis. A suitable dose of insulin was used to produce a coma, which was terminated by either tube feeding or intravenous glucose. A course of treatment could include up to 60 comas. Not surprisingly, serious side effects were common, and a mortality of at least 1% could be expected, depending on the standard of the clinic and the physical state of the patient. Insulin coma treatment was rapidly taken up throughout Europe, and many specialized treatment units were built. There was a great improvement in the morale of patients and staff because of the belief that this dramatic treatment could cure symptoms of some of the most serious psychiatric disorders.

There were always some practitioners who doubted the efficacy of insulin coma treatment. Their doubts were reinforced by a controlled trial by Ackner and Oldham (1962), who found that, in patients with schizophrenia, insulin coma was no more effective than a similar period of unconsciousness induced by barbiturates. This study was published about the time when chlorpromazine was introduced, and both factors led to a rapid decline in the use of insulin coma treatment. It should be noted that the controlled studies did not exclude the efficacy of insulin treatment in some circumstances, and a number of workers continued to maintain that it was effective. Therefore it is interesting that recent experimental studies have shown that insulin administration causes striking changes in the release of monoamine neurotransmitters, as well as other brain changes; for example, in inflammatory processes and cytokine production (Kleinridders *et al.*, 2014). Perhaps the main lesson to be learned from insulin coma treatment is that the introduction of a new medical treatment should be preceded by adequate controlled trials to determine whether it is therapeutically more effective or safer than current therapies (see Chapter 6). This lesson is particularly important in psychiatry, because the aetiology of most disorders is obscure and outcome may vary widely, even among patients with the same clinical syndrome.

ECT was introduced about the same time as insulin coma treatment. Unlike the latter, ECT has retained a place in current clinical practice. The rationale for convulsive therapy was a postulated antagonism between schizophrenia and epilepsy such that the one would exclude the other. This view is erroneous in so far as schizophrenia-like illnesses are actually more common in patients with temporal lobe epilepsy than would be expected by chance (see Chapter 11). Astute clinical observation, in combination with controlled trials, has shown that ECT is effective in the acute treatment of severe mood disorders. Thus, even though the rationale for the introduction of ECT was incorrect and its mode of action remains unclear, controlled trials have confirmed that, in carefully defined clinical situations, ECT is a safe and effective treatment.

The action of *lithium* in reducing mania was a chance finding by Cade (1949), who had been investigating the effects of urates in animals and had decided to use the lithium salt because of its solubility. Lithium is a toxic agent, so Cade's important observations did not have a significant impact on clinical practice until the following decade, when controlled trials showed that lithium was effective in both the acute treatment of mania and the prophylaxis of recurrent mood disorders.

Other agents that revolutionized psychopharmacology were introduced about this time (see Box 25.1). Their efficacy and their indications were first recognized through clinical observation, and were subsequently confirmed by controlled clinical trials. None of these agents was introduced on the basis of an aetiological hypothesis. Indeed, such aetiological hypotheses as there are in biological psychiatry have been largely derived from knowledge of the mode of action of effective drugs. Thus the dopamine-receptor-antagonist properties of antipsychotic drugs have given rise to the dopamine hypothesis of schizophrenia, while the action of tricyclic antidepressants and monoamine oxidase inhibitors (MAOIs) in facilitating the effects of noradrenaline and 5-hydroxytryptamine (5-HT) has led to the various monoamine hypotheses of mood disorders.

The past few decades have brought a period of consolidation in psychopharmacology. Clinical trials have been widely used to refine the indications of particular drug treatments and to maximize their risk/benefit ratios. New compounds have become available, but because most of them have been derived from previously described agents, their range of activity is not strikingly different from that of their predecessors. In general, however, the newer agents are better tolerated and sometimes safer—developments that are important for clinical practice.

There may now be grounds for more optimism about the prospects for advances in psychopharmacology. For example, there is rapidly increasing knowledge about chemical signalling in the brain. Numerous neurotransmitters and neuromodulators interact with specific families of receptors, many of which exist in a number of different subtypes. Most of these receptors have been cloned, and selective ligands for them are becoming available. There is increasing knowledge as to how these chemical messengers may modify behaviour through their interactions with specific brain regions and distributed neuronal circuits.

Future compounds that are developed as a consequence of these scientific advances are likely to differ from current drugs in their range of behavioural effects, and could lead to important new developments in psychopharmacology. Given the complex causes of psychiatric disorders, it seems likely that detailed knowledge of aetiology and pathophysiology may lag behind advances in therapeutics. Of course, this disparity is not uncommon in general medicine. It serves to reinforce the importance of *randomized clinical trials* in the assessment of new psychopharmacological treatments.

Box 25.1 Introduction of some physical treatments in psychiatry

1934 Insulin coma treatment (Sakel)

1936 Frontal leucotomy (Moniz)

1936 Metrazole convulsive therapy (Meduna)

1938 Electroconvulsive therapy (Cerletti and Bini)

1941 Amphetamine for hyperactivity in children (Bradley)

1949 Lithium (Cade)

1952 Chlorpromazine (Delay and Deniker)

1954 Benzodiazepines (Sternbach)

1957 Iproniazid (Crane and Kline)

1957 Imipramine (Kuhn)

1966 Valpromide (valproate) in bipolar disorder (Lambert *et al.*)

1967 Clomipramine in obsessive–compulsive disorder (Fernandez and Lopez-Ibor)

1971 Carbamazepine in bipolar disorder (Takezaki and Hanaoka)

1988 Clozapine in treatment-resistant schizophrenia (Kane *et al.*)

1999 Lamotrigine in bipolar depression (Calabrese *et al.*)

2001 Atypical antipsychotic augmentation in depression (Shelton *et al.*)

2005 Quetiapine in bipolar depression (Calabrese *et al.*)

General considerations

The pharmacokinetics of psychotropic drugs

Before psychotropic drugs can produce their therapeutic effects, they must reach the brain in adequate amounts. The extent to which they do so depends on their absorption, distribution, passage across the blood–brain barrier, metabolism, and excretion. A short review of these processes is given here. The reader who has not studied them before is referred to the chapters on pharmacokinetics in *Rang and Dale's Pharmacology* (Rang *et al.*, 2015). The following processes are important:

- absorption
- distribution
- metabolism
- excretion.

Absorption

In general, psychotropic drugs are easily absorbed from the gut because most of them are *lipophilic* and are not highly ionized at physiological pH values. Like other drugs, they are absorbed faster from an empty stomach, and in reduced amounts by patients suffering from intestinal hurry or malabsorption syndrome.

Distribution

Psychotropic drugs are distributed in the plasma, where most of them are largely bound to proteins—for example, diazepam and amitriptyline are about 95% bound. They pass easily from the plasma to the brain, across the blood–brain barrier, because they are highly lipophilic. For the same reason, they enter fat stores, from which they are released slowly long after the patient has ceased to take the drug. This means that psychotropic drugs tend to have *large volumes of distribution*.

Metabolism

Most psychotropic drugs are *metabolized in the liver*. This process begins as the drugs pass through the liver in the portal circulation on their way from the gut. This 'first-pass' metabolism reduces the amount of available drug, and is one of the reasons why larger doses are needed when a drug such as chlorpromazine is given by mouth than when it is given intramuscularly. The extent of this liver metabolism differs from one person to another. It is altered by certain other drugs which, if taken at the same time, induce liver enzymes (e.g. carbamazepine) or inhibit them (e.g. selective serotonin reuptake inhibitors [SSRIs]).

Some drugs, such as carbamazepine, induce their own metabolism, especially after being taken for a long time. Not all drug metabolites are inactive—for example, fluoxetine is metabolized to a hydroxy derivative, norfluoxetine, which is also a potent 5-HT reuptake inhibitor. Where drugs give rise to active metabolites, measurements of plasma concentrations of the parent drug alone are a poor guide to therapeutic activity.

Excretion

Psychotropic drugs and their metabolites are excreted mainly through the *kidney*. When kidney function is impaired, excretion is reduced and a lower dose of drug should be given. Lithium is filtered passively and then partly reabsorbed by the same mechanism that absorbs sodium. The two ions compete for this mechanism; hence reabsorption of lithium increases when that of sodium is reduced (e.g. by thiazide diuretics). Certain fractions of lipophilic drugs such as chlorpromazine are partly excreted in the bile, enter the intestine for the second time, and are then partly reabsorbed (i.e. a proportion of the drug is recycled between intestine and liver).

Plasma half-life

Plasma concentrations of drugs vary throughout the day, rising immediately after the dose and falling at a rate that differs between individual drugs. The rate at which a drug level declines after a single dose ranges from hours for lithium carbonate to weeks for slow-release preparations of injectable antipsychotic agents. Knowledge of these differences allows more rational decisions to be made about appropriate intervals between doses.

The concept of *plasma half-life* is useful here. The half-life of a drug in plasma is the time taken for its concentration to fall by a half, once dosing has ceased. For most psychotropic drugs, the amount eliminated over time is proportional to the plasma concentration, and in this case it will take approximately five times the half-life for the drug to be eliminated from plasma. Equally, when dosing with a drug begins, it will take five times the half-life for the concentration in plasma to reach steady state. This can be important when planning treatment. For example, MAOIs should not be given with SSRIs. Therefore if a patient is taking sertraline, which has an elimination half-life of about 26 hours, it will be important to leave at least five times the half-life (a week is recommended) before starting MAOI treatment. When sertraline treatment begins, the plasma concentrations will continue to rise for about a week before reaching a steady state.

Measurement of circulating drug concentrations

As a result of individual variations in the mechanisms described above, plasma concentrations after standard doses of psychotropic drugs can vary substantially from one patient to another. For example, tenfold differences have been observed with the antidepressant drug nortriptyline. Therefore it might be expected that measurements of the plasma concentration of circulating drugs would help the clinician. However, with a few exceptions (e.g. lithium and clozapine), this practice is rarely helpful because the plasma drug levels that predict therapeutic response or toxicity within individuals vary so much. Clearly, for any drug to work it must be present in plasma above a certain minimum concentration, and for some medications 'target' levels have been suggested. However, it is still not unusual for some individuals to show a therapeutic response when plasma levels are lower than recommended.

Pharmacodynamic measures

As an alternative to these assays, it may be possible to measure the pharmacological property that is thought to be responsible for the therapeutic effect of a particular drug. For example, positron emission tomography (PET) can be used to measure directly the degree of brain dopamine-receptor blockade produced by antipsychotic drugs during treatment. Such information has proved valuable in designing appropriate dosage regimens of antipsychotic drugs (see Table 25.4). However, these pharmacodynamic measures have not yet been able to identify why some patients do not respond to medication. For example, the degree of dopamine-receptor blockade is the same in patients who respond to antipsychotic drugs as in those who do not. Pharmacogenetic approaches to prediction of treatment response (see Box 25.2) are a topic of current interest, although most of the findings remain controversial and are yet to have an impact on routine clinical practice. For a review, see Harrison (2015b).

Drug interactions

When two psychotropic drugs are given together, one may interfere with or enhance the actions of the other. Interference may arise through alterations in absorption, binding, metabolism, or excretion (*pharmacokinetic interactions*), or by interaction between the pharmacological mechanisms of action (*pharmacodynamic interactions*).

Pharmacokinetic interactions

Interactions that affect *drug absorption* are seldom important for psychotropic drugs, although it is worth noting that absorption of chlorpromazine is reduced by antacids. Interactions due to *protein binding* are also uncommon, even though many psychotropic drugs are highly protein-bound. Interactions that affect *drug metabolism* are of considerable importance. Examples include the inhibition of the metabolism of antipsychotic drugs by some SSRIs, and the stimulation of the metabolism of many psychotropic drugs by carbamazepine, which induces the relevant *cytochrome P450 enzymes* (see below). Interactions that affect *renal excretion* are mainly important for lithium, the elimination of which is decreased by thiazide diuretics.

Cytochrome P450 enzymes. There have been significant developments in the understanding of the microsomal cytochrome P450 enzyme system. These enzymes are located mainly in the liver but also in other tissues, including the gut wall and brain. Their role is to detoxify exogenous substances such as drugs, and their activity can be increased or decreased by concomitant drug administration. This can give rise to clinically important drug interactions. Importantly, several antidepressants, particularly SSRIs, potently inhibit P450 enzymes (see Table 25.9).

Pharmacodynamic interactions

Pharmacodynamic interactions are exemplified by the serotonin syndrome, in which drugs that potentiate brain 5-HT function by different mechanisms (e.g. SSRIs and MAOIs) can combine to produce dangerous 5-HT toxicity (see below).

As a rule, a single drug can be used to produce all of the effects required of a combination—for example, many antidepressant drugs have useful antianxiety effects. It is desirable to avoid combinations of psychotropic drugs whenever possible, and, if a combination is to be used, it is essential to know about possible interactions. The *British National Formulary* provides a useful guide.

Drug withdrawal

Many psychotropic drugs do not achieve useful therapeutic effects for several days or even weeks. After the drugs have been stopped, there is often a comparable delay before their effects are lost. Psychotropic and, indeed, many other classes of drugs produce neuroadaptive changes during repeated administration. Tissues therefore have to readjust when drug treatment is stopped; this readjustment may appear clinically as a *withdrawal or abstinence syndrome*. Characteristic abstinence syndromes have been described for antidepressants,

---

Box 25.2 **Pharmacogenetics in psychiatry**

Polymorphic (allelic) variation in DNA may affect the expression (and therefore the function) of genes involved in the actions, or metabolism, of psychotropic drugs. That is, they may modify the likelihood of therapeutic response or the development of adverse effects. Examples are listed below.

- Genetic variation in CYP-metabolizing enzymes can affect blood levels of drugs and thereby brain exposure. Mutations in the gene for CYP2D6 may be associated with antipsychotic drug-induced tardive dyskinesia.
- Alleles associated with decreased expression of 5-HT transporter may be associated with poorer response to SSRIs.
- Therapeutic response to clozapine may be associated with specific alleles of the 5-HT$_{2A}$ receptor.
- Weight gain with antipsychotic drugs is associated with an allele of the 5-HT$_{2C}$ receptor.

---

antipsychotics, and anxiolytics, while sudden discontinuation of lithium can provoke a 'rebound' mania in patients with bipolar disorder. It is important to be able to distinguish withdrawal syndromes from relapse of the disorder that is being treated. In addition, the risk of abstinence symptoms makes it prudent to withdraw psychotropic drugs slowly wherever possible.

General advice about prescribing

Use well-tried drugs

It is good practice to use well-tried drugs with therapeutic actions and side effects that are thoroughly understood. Clinicians should become familiar with a small number of drugs from each of the main classes. In this way they can become used to adjusting the dosage and recognizing side effects. Well-tried drugs are usually less expensive than new preparations.

Give an adequate dose

Having chosen a suitable drug, the doctor should prescribe it in *adequate doses*. They should not change the drug or add others without a good reason. In general, if there is no therapeutic response to one established drug, there is no likelihood of a better response to another that has very similar pharmacological properties (provided that the first drug has been taken in adequate amounts). However, since the main obstacle to adequate dosage is usually side effects, it may be appropriate to change to a drug with a different pattern of side effects—for example, from a tricyclic antidepressant to an SSRI, or vice versa.

Use drug combinations cautiously

Occasionally, combinations of psychotropic drugs are given deliberately in the hope of producing interactions that will be more potent than the effects of either drug taken alone in full dosage (e.g. an SSRI with an atypical antipsychotic agent). This practice, if it is to be used, is best carried out by experienced psychiatrists (or under their guidance) because the adverse effects of combinations are less easy to predict than those of single drugs.

Dosing and treatment duration

When a drug is prescribed, it is necessary to determine the dose, the interval between doses, and the likely duration of treatment. The dose ranges for commonly used drugs are indicated later in this chapter. Ranges for others can be found in the manufacturers' literature, the *British National Formulary*, or a comparable work of reference. Within the therapeutic range, the correct dose for an individual patient should be decided after considering the severity of symptoms, the patient's age and weight, and any factors that may affect drug metabolism (e.g. other drugs that are being taken, or liver disease).

Next, the interval between doses must be decided. Psychotropic drugs have often been given three times a day, even though their duration of action is such that most can be taken once or twice a day without any undesirable fall in plasma concentrations between doses. Less frequent administration has the advantage that outpatients are more likely to be reliable in taking drugs. In hospital, less frequent drug rounds mean that nurses have more time for psychological aspects of treatment. Some drugs, such as anxiolytics, are required for immediate effect rather than continuous action; they should not be given at regular intervals, but shortly before occasions on which symptoms are expected to be at their worst or 'as needed' with an individually defined daily limit. The duration of treatment depends on the disorder under treatment; it is considered in the chapters that deal with the relevant clinical syndromes.

What patients want to know

Psychotropic drugs have the aim of changing what people think and feel; not surprisingly, many patients have misgivings about taking them. It is therefore important to make it clear what the drug is being used for, what therapeutic effects are expected, and when they should start to appear. Other key questions that must be dealt with include the following:

- What effects will I experience on first taking the drug?
- What side effects can I expect?
- What serious side effects should I report immediately?
- For how long should I take the drug?
- Is the drug addictive?
- What will I notice when I stop the drug?

Compliance, concordance, and collaboration

Many patients do not take the drugs that are prescribed for them. Of course this problem is not restricted to psychiatric practice, but the use of psychotropic drugs raises additional issues in terms of societal stigma and the nature of the adverse effects. Problems with compliance are mainly manifested when treating outpatients, but also occur in hospital, where some patients find ways of avoiding taking the drugs administered by nurses.

If patients are to take medication reliably, they must be convinced of the need to take it, be free from unfounded fears about its dangers, and be aware of how to take it. Each of these requirements presents particular problems when the patient has a psychiatric disorder. Thus patients with schizophrenia or seriously depressed patients may not be convinced that they are ill, or they may not wish to recover. Deluded patients may distrust clinical staff, and hypochondriacal patients may fear dangerous side effects. Anxious patients often forget the prescribed dosage and frequency of their drugs. Therefore it is not surprising that many psychiatric patients do not take their drugs in the prescribed way. It is important for the clinician to pay attention to this problem. Time spent discussing the patient's concerns is time well spent, for it often increases compliance with treatment. Written instructions and information can be a valuable adjunct, and are now included with drug packaging.

The successful and safe use of medication requires a *collaborative* relationship between patient and doctor. Some have proposed that the terms *concordance* or *adherence* should therefore be preferred to *compliance*, which carries the implicit assumption that the patient's job is to obey instructions. Whatever the term used, it is

clearly important to recognize that the use of drug treatment, particularly in psychiatry, requires a thorough understanding of the *patient's attitude* to both their illness and its treatment (Britten *et al.*, 2010).

Ethical aspects of drug prescription

The ethical issues in this complex area have been reviewed by Kader and Pantelis (2009).

1. The basis of ethical prescribing is the practitioner's comprehensive knowledge of the risks and benefits of drug therapies. This will be derived from evidence-based approaches where possible.

2. The doctor–patient relationship is the appropriate framework through which this knowledge is communicated to the patient.

3. The therapeutic partnership between patient and doctor must lead to true informed consent, which includes the right of competent patients to refuse treatment.

Difficulties arise when the evidence base for treatment is lacking and when there is uncertainty about what approach to pursue. Here the clinician has the responsibility to advise treatments that would be supported by peer opinion and to use clinical guidelines. The clinician should also support the right of patients to genuinely effective treatment where this is being hindered by cost constraint and other economic factors. Another difficult problem concerns refusal of treatment when capacity is impaired and the health and safety of the patient or others are at risk. In fact, empirical research suggests that refusal of treatment in these circumstances is often transient and due to current clinical factors. Indeed, most patients whose refusal of treatment is clinically overridden apparently conclude eventually that the decision to treat them was justified (Kader and Pantelis, 2009). It is, of course, important to elucidate and document the reasons for treatment refusal, and to respect the right of competent patients to refuse treatment.

Prescribing for special groups

Children and the elderly

Psychotropic drugs usually lack specific licences for use in young people, and relevant controlled trials are sparse. However, in the case of antidepressants, for example, only fluoxetine has a licence for the treatment of depression in young people, with accompanying advice from NICE that it should be used in combination with a specific psychological treatment in this age group (see Chapter 16). Practitioners need to make themselves aware of local guidelines concerning the use of psychotropic medication in young people, and should seek specialist advice when in doubt.

Clinical trials of most psychotropic medications often exclude older patients, even though conditions such as depression are more common in the elderly. Elderly patients are often sensitive to side effects of medication, and may have impaired renal or hepatic function; for these reasons it is important to start treatment with low doses.

Pregnant women

There are special problems with regard to prescribing psychotropic drugs in pregnancy, because of the risk of *teratogenesis*. Information about the teratogenic risk of individual drugs can be obtained from the relevant manufacturer and from the *British National Formulary*, although the available evidence is often sparse or difficult to interpret. In addition, illnesses such as depression are known to have adverse effects on pregnancy outcomes (Grote *et al.*, 2010). The practitioner and patient therefore have the difficult task of weighing available information against the risk of managing the illness without medication. In addition, a substantial number of pregnancies are unplanned. For this reason, it is prudent, where possible, to advise women of childbearing age who require psychotropic drugs specifically to avoid pregnancy until the need for the drug treatment is over. For reviews of the use of psychotropic drugs in pregnancy, see National Institute for Health and Care Excellence (2014) and Chisolm and Payne (2016).

Anxiolytics and antidepressants

Anxiolytic drugs are seldom essential in early pregnancy, and psychological treatments can usually be used. If short-term medication is needed, *benzodiazepines* have in general not been shown to be teratogenic, although one meta-analysis has shown an increased risk of oral clefts after first-trimester exposure. If an *antidepressant drug* is required, it is probably better to use long-established preparations such as *imipramine* or *amitriptyline*, for which there is no consistent evidence of a teratogenic effect after many years of use. There is also reasonable experience with *fluoxetine* and *sertraline*, which do not appear to be associated with an increased risk of major malformations. However, *paroxetine* treatment in the first trimester may result in increased cardiac defects, and SSRIs taken after 20 weeks' gestation may result in an increased risk of pulmonary hypertension in the newborn.

Antipsychotic drugs and mood stabilizers

It is seldom necessary to start *antipsychotic drugs* in early pregnancy. There is little evidence that high-potency agents such as *haloperidol* carry an increased teratogenic risk. However, there may be a higher rate of congenital malformations in babies who are exposed to lower-potency agents such as *chlorpromazine*. There is less information on the teratogenic risk of newer ('atypical') antipsychotic agents, but a recent epidemiological study in over 1000 women found, after careful controlling, no evidence of an increase in adverse outcomes for either mother or baby (Vigod *et al.*, 2015).

Lithium treatment early in pregnancy has been associated with cardiac abnormalities in the fetus, particularly *Ebstein's anomaly*. Therefore women who are considering pregnancy have been recommended to discontinue lithium before conceiving. Similarly, women who become pregnant while taking lithium have usually been advised to stop the treatment. However, recent epidemiological studies have suggested that, although the relative risk of Ebstein's anomaly is increased at least tenfold in infants who are exposed to lithium in the first trimester, the absolute risk is still fairly low, at 0.05–0.1%. Withdrawal of lithium carries a high risk of relapse in patients with bipolar illness, and the balance of risk to mother and baby may therefore suggest continuation of lithium treatment during pregnancy in some cases.

Anticonvulsant drugs such as *carbamazepine* and *valproate* are increasingly used as mood stabilizers. However, both of these agents are clearly associated with an increased risk of neural-tube defects as well as other fetal abnormalities. The neural-tube defects associated with anticonvulsant use may be associated with changes in folate metabolism. However, a role for folate treatment in their prevention has not been established. Because many pregnancies are unplanned, current guidelines suggest that valproate should not be prescribed to women of childbearing age unless no alternative treatment is found effective or sufficiently well tolerated (National Institute for Health and Care Excellence, 2014).

Neonatal toxicity

Exposure to psychotropic drugs in the later stages of pregnancy can give rise to *neonatal toxicity*, either through the presence of the drug or through a withdrawal syndrome. For example, it has been reported that among babies born to mothers who have been receiving *tricyclic antidepressants* there may be withdrawal reactions that include tremulousness, vomiting, poor feeding, and seizures. Direct anticholinergic effects, such as gastrointestinal stasis and bladder distension, have also been reported. These reactions, although clearly problematic, appear to settle quickly without causing lasting sequelae.

There are also reports that late exposure to SSRIs may be associated with an increased risk of neonatal complications, including jitteriness, hypoglycaemia, poor muscle tone, and respiratory difficulties. The perinatal toxicity associated with *lithium* use includes 'floppy baby syndrome', with cyanosis and hypotonicity, whereas *benzodiazepine* treatment can result in impaired temperature regulation together with breathing and feeding difficulties.

Animal studies suggest that fetal exposure to psychotropic medication can cause *longer-term abnormalities in brain development and behaviour*, and it is possible that similar effects might occur in humans (see, for example, Pederson *et al.*, 2010). However, disentangling such effects from those associated with illness in the mother is difficult (Grote *et al.*, 2010).

Breastfeeding

Psychotropic drugs should be prescribed cautiously to women who are breastfeeding. *Diazepam* and other *benzodiazepines* pass readily into breast milk, and may cause sedation and hypotonicity in the infant. Antipsychotic drugs and antidepressants also enter breast milk, although rather less readily than diazepam. However, *sulpiride* is excreted in significant amounts and should be avoided. *Fluoxetine* and *citalopram* could also accumulate, but imipramine, nortriptyline, and sertraline are present in small amounts and breastfeeding can be permitted while the baby is observed for sedation or feeding difficulties. It is usually advised that mothers should express and discard breast milk that has been exposed to peak plasma levels of the drug concerned.

Lithium salts enter the milk freely, and serum concentrations in the infant can approach those of the mother, so breastfeeding is best avoided. However, the amounts of *carbamazepine* and *valproate* in breast milk are considered too low to be harmful. A general problem is that, even when the concentration of a particular drug in breast milk is low and no detectable clinical effect on the infant can be discerned, it is nevertheless possible that subtle longer-term effects on brain development and behaviour could occur. For this reason, some authorities recommend that women who are receiving psychotropic medication should not breastfeed at all. A more pragmatic view is provided by the *British National Formulary* (see also National Institute for Health and Care Excellence, 2014 and Taylor *et al.*, 2015).

What to do if there is no therapeutic response

1. Is the drug being taken as recommended? The first step is to find out whether the patient has been taking the drug in the correct dose. They may not have understood the original instructions, or may be worried that a full dose will produce unpleasant side effects. Some patients fear that they will become dependent if they take the drug regularly. Other patients may have little wish to take drugs for the reasons discussed above.

2. Is the patient taking any other drug that could affect the metabolism or pharmacological action of the psychotropic agent? Misuse of legal or illegal substances might interfere with the therapeutic actions of psychotropic drugs.

3. Is the diagnosis correct? Review the diagnosis to make sure that the treatment is appropriate before deciding whether to increase the dose.

Failure to respond adequately to psychotropic medication is a common reason for psychiatric referral. Specific pharmacological approaches for individual disorders are discussed in the relevant chapters.

The classification of drugs used in psychiatry

Drugs that have effects mainly on mental symptoms are referred to as *psychotropic*. Psychiatrists also use the term *antiparkinsonian agents*, which refers to drugs that are employed to control the side effects of some psychotropic drugs. Anticonvulsant drugs have a growing role in the treatment of mood disorders.

Psychotropic drugs are conventionally divided into different classes, as shown in Table 25.1, but the therapeutic actions of particular compounds are not confined to one diagnostic category. For example, SSRIs are classified as antidepressants and are effective in the treatment of major depression, but they also produce useful therapeutic effects in anxiety states, obsessive–compulsive disorders, and some eating disorders. Of course, this breadth of effect does not mean that the latter syndromes are forms of depression. It merely highlights the fact that the neuropsychological consequences of facilitating brain 5-HT function may provide beneficial effects in a variety of psychiatric disorders.

Although there is considerable understanding of the pharmacological actions of psychotropic drugs, little is known about the neuropsychological consequences of these pharmacological actions and about the ways in which neuropsychological changes are translated into clinical benefit in different diagnostic syndromes.

At present, therefore, the best plan is to classify drugs according to their major therapeutic use, but to bear in mind that the therapeutic effects of different classes of drugs *may overlap considerably*.

Each of the main groups of drugs will now be reviewed in turn. For each group, an account will be given of therapeutic effects, pharmacology, the principal compounds available, pharmacokinetics, unwanted effects, and contraindications. General advice will also be given about the use of each group in everyday clinical practice, but specific applications to the treatment of individual disorders will be found in the chapters that deal with those conditions. Drugs that have a limited use in the treatment of a single disorder—for example, *disulfiram* for alcohol problems, or *cholinesterase inhibitors* for dementia—are discussed in the chapters that deal with the relevant clinical syndromes.

Anxiolytic drugs

Anxiolytic drugs, such as *benzodiazepines*, have been prescribed widely and often inappropriately. Before prescribing anxiolytic drugs it is always important to seek the causes of anxiety and to try to modify them. It is also essential to recognize that a degree of anxiety can motivate patients to take steps to reduce the problems that are causing it. Therefore removing all anxiety in the short term is not always beneficial to the patient in the long run. Anxiolytics such as benzodiazepines are most useful when given for a short time, either to tide the patient over a crisis or to help them to tackle a specific problem.

Tolerance is a particular problem with benzodiazepine-like anxiolytic drugs, and drug dependence can develop. Because the benzodiazepines are still widely used anxiolytics, they will be considered first. *Antidepressants* are increasingly used to treat specific anxiety syndromes, but their therapeutic actions differ in important ways from benzodiazepine-like drugs. Their indications in the treatment of anxiety disorders will be considered here, but their detailed pharmacology is discussed in the section on antidepressant drugs. When reading this section, it is important to bear in mind that psychological treatments are effective in the management of anxiety disorders and have certain advantages over drug treatment, including more sustained efficacy after treatment cessation, as well as fewer adverse effects.

Benzodiazepines

Pharmacology

Benzodiazepines have several actions:

- anxiolytic
- sedative and hypnotic
- muscle relaxant
- anticonvulsant.

Their pharmacological actions are mediated through specific receptor sites located in a supramolecular complex with gamma-aminobutyric acid ($GABA_A$) receptors. Benzodiazepines enhance GABA neurotransmission, thereby indirectly altering the activity of other neurotransmitter systems, such as those involving noradrenaline and 5-HT.

Compounds available

Many different benzodiazepines are available. They differ both in the potency with which they interact with benzodiazepine receptors and in their plasma half-life (see Box 25.3). In general, *high-potency benzodiazepines* and those with *short half-lives* are more likely to be associated with dependence and withdrawal. Benzodiazepines with short half-lives (less than 12 hours) include lorazepam, temazepam, and lormetazepam.

Because of problems with dependence, long-acting benzodiazepines are preferable for the management of

Table 25.1 Classification of clinical psychotropic drugs

Class of drug	Examples of classes	Class indications (examples)
Antipsychotic	Phenothiazines	Acute treatment of schizophrenia and mania; prevention of relapse in schizophrenia
	Butyrophenones	
	Substituted benzamides	
Antidepressant	Tricyclic antidepressants	Major depression (acute treatment and prophylaxis), anxiety disorders
	MAOIs	
	SSRIs	
Mood stabilizer	Lithium	Prophylaxis of bipolar disorder and recurrent mood disorder
	Anticonvulsants	
Anxiolytic	Benzodiazepines	Anxiety disorders (short-term use)
	Azapirones (buspirone)	
Hypnotic	Benzodiazepines	Insomnia
	Cyclopyrrolones ('Z drugs')	
Psychostimulant	Methylphenidate	Hyperkinetic syndrome of childhood
	Modafinil	Narcolepsy

anxiety, even if such treatment is to be given intermittently on an 'as-required' basis. Long-acting benzodiazepines include drugs such as diazepam, chlordiazepoxide, alprazolam, and clonazepam. *Diazepam* is rapidly absorbed and can be used both for the continuous treatment of anxiety and for treatment 'as required'. *Alprazolam*, a high-potency benzodiazepine, is effective in the treatment of panic disorder. This therapeutic efficacy is not confined to alprazolam, because equivalent doses of other high-potency agents such as *clonazepam* are also effective.

Flumazenil is a benzodiazepine-receptor antagonist that produces little pharmacological effect by itself, but blocks the actions of other benzodiazepines. Therefore it may be useful in reversing acute toxicity produced by benzodiazepines, but carries a risk of provoking acute benzodiazepine withdrawal. Flumazenil is available only for intravenous use.

Pharmacokinetics

Benzodiazepines are rapidly absorbed. They are strongly bound to plasma proteins but, because they are lipophilic, pass readily into the brain. They are metabolized to a large number of compounds, many of which have therapeutic effects of their own; temazepam and oxazepam are among the metabolic products of diazepam. Excretion is mainly as conjugates in the urine.

Benzodiazepines with short half-lives, such as temazepam and lorazepam, have a 3-hydroxyl grouping, which allows a one-step metabolism to inactive glucuronides. Other benzodiazepines, such as diazepam and clorazepate, are metabolized to long-acting derivatives, such as desmethyldiazepam, which are themselves therapeutically active.

It is now common practice to give benzodiazepines (often in combination with low-dose antipsychotic drugs) to produce a rapid calming effect in psychosis. In this situation, benzodiazepines may be given parenterally, and it is worth noting that the absorption of diazepam following intramuscular injection is poor, and lorazepam should be preferred if this route of administration is used.

Unwanted effects

Benzodiazepines are well tolerated. When they are given as anxiolytics, their main side effects are due to the sedative properties of large doses, which can lead to *ataxia* and *drowsiness* and *falls* (especially in the elderly), and occasionally to *confused thinking* and *amnesia*. Minor

---

Box 25.3 Half-lives of some drugs that act at the GABA–benzodiazepine-receptor complex

Diazepam	20–100 h*
Chlordiazepoxide	5–30 h*
Lorazepam	8–24 h
Temazepam	5–11 h
Zopiclone	4–6 h
Zolpidem	1.5–2 h
Chlormethiazole	4–6 h
	(4–12 h in the elderly)
Chloral	6–8 h

* Active metabolite increases half-life further.

---

degrees of drowsiness and of impaired coordination and judgement can *affect driving skills* and the operation of potentially dangerous machinery; moreover, people who are affected in this way are not always aware of it. For this reason, when benzodiazepines are prescribed, especially those with a longer action, patients should be advised about these dangers and about the potentiating effects of alcohol. The prescriber should remember that these effects are more common among elderly patients and those with impaired renal or liver function. Use of benzodiazepines for more than 3 months has been linked to an *increased risk of dementia* but residual confounding cannot be excluded (National Institute for Health and Care Excellence, 2015)

Although in some circumstances benzodiazepines reduce tension and aggression, they can also rarely lead to a *release of aggression* by reducing inhibitions in people with a tendency to aggressive behaviour. In this they resemble alcohol. This possible effect should be remembered when prescribing for those judged to be at risk of child abuse, or for any person with a previous history of impulsive aggressive behaviour.

Toxic effects

Benzodiazepines have few toxic effects. Patients usually recover from large overdoses because these drugs do not depress respiration and blood pressure as barbiturates

do. Even so, fatal overdoses of benzodiazepines have occasionally been reported.

Drug interactions

Benzodiazepines, like other sedative anxiolytics, potentiate the effects of alcohol and of drugs that depress the central nervous system. Significant respiratory depression has been reported in some patients receiving combined treatment with benzodiazepines and clozapine.

Dependence and withdrawal

It is now generally agreed that *dependence* develops after prolonged use of benzodiazepines. The frequency depends on the drug and the dosage, and has been estimated to be up to 50% of patients who are long-term users. Benzodiazepines are associated with a withdrawal syndrome and tolerance. Although drug-seeking behaviour is less common, it certainly can occur, and benzodiazepines are not uncommonly involved in polydrug misuse and dependence.

The *withdrawal syndrome* associated with benzodiazepines is characterized by several different kinds of symptoms:

- apprehension, anxiety, and insomnia
- tremor
- nausea
- heightened sensitivity to perceptual stimuli and perceptual disturbances
- depression and suicidal thinking
- epileptic seizures (rarely).

Since many of these symptoms resemble those of anxiety disorder, it can sometimes be difficult to decide whether the patient is experiencing a benzodiazepine withdrawal syndrome or a recrudescence of the anxiety disorder for which the drug was originally prescribed. Perceptual disturbances are more likely to indicate benzodiazepine withdrawal.

Withdrawal symptoms generally begin within 2–3 days of stopping a short-acting benzodiazepine, and within 7 days of stopping a long-acting one. The symptoms generally last for 3–10 days. Withdrawal symptoms seem to be more frequent after taking drugs with a short half-life than after taking those with a long one. If benzodiazepines have been taken for a long time, it is best to withdraw them gradually over a period of several weeks. If this is done, withdrawal symptoms can be minimized or avoided (see Chapter 20). Benzodiazepines do have the advantage of becoming quickly effective. Therefore current advice is that they should be administered on a short-term basis only (not more than 4 weeks) to help a patient to cope with functionally disabling anxiety while other treatment measures are instituted.

Azapirones (buspirone)

Indications and pharmacology

The only drug in the azapirone class that is currently marketed for the treatment of anxiety is *buspirone*. It is effective in the treatment of generalized anxiety disorder but is not helpful in the treatment of panic disorder. Unlike the benzodiazepines, the anxiolytic effects of buspirone take several days to develop and require dose-titration. It is also important to note that buspirone cannot be used to treat benzodiazepine withdrawal. Perhaps for these reasons it has relatively little use.

Pharmacologically, buspirone has no affinity for benzodiazepine receptors, but stimulates a subtype of 5-HT receptor called the *5-HT$_{1A}$ receptor*. This receptor is found in high concentration in the raphe nuclei in the brainstem, where it regulates the firing of 5-HT cell bodies. Administration of buspirone lowers the firing rate of 5-HT neurons and thereby decreases 5-HT neurotransmission in certain brain regions. This action may be the basis of its anxiolytic effect.

Pharmacokinetics and adverse effect

Buspirone has poor systemic availability because it has an extensive first-pass metabolism. The side effect profile differs from that of benzodiazepines. For example, buspirone treatment does not cause sedation, but instead is often associated with *lightheadedness, nervousness*, and *headache* early in treatment. There is little evidence that tolerance and dependence occur during buspirone use, although such a judgement must always be made with circumspection.

Drug interactions

Buspirone is relatively free from significant drug interactions, but combination with MAOIs has been reported to cause raised blood pressure.

Antidepressant drugs used for anxiety

Antidepressant drugs usually ameliorate the anxiety that accompanies depressive disorders. Tricyclic antidepressants have also been shown to be effective in the management of *generalized anxiety disorder, panic disorder*, and *post-traumatic stress disorder*, whether or not significant depressive symptoms are present. Similarly, SSRIs are effective in a broad range of anxiety disorders, including *obsessive–compulsive disorder* (Baldwin *et al.*, 2014). Both venlafaxine and duloxetine, which are classified

as *selective serotonin and noradrenaline reuptake inhibitors (SNRIs)*, are licensed for the treatment of generalised anxiety disorder as well as depression.

The therapeutic profile of antidepressant drugs in the treatment of anxiety differs significantly from that of benzodiazepines. The time of onset of effect is much slower with antidepressants and, particularly in panic disorder, there may be an *exacerbation of symptoms* early in treatment. However, the ultimate therapeutic effect of antidepressants is as least as great as that of benzodiazepines, and they are less likely to produce cognitive impairment (Baldwin *et al.*, 2014). In addition, the use of antidepressants is not associated with tolerance and dependence although, as noted above, sudden cessation of treatment can cause abstinence symptoms.

Antipsychotic drugs used for anxiety

Conventional antipsychotic drugs have sometimes been prescribed in low doses for their anxiolytic effects, particularly in patients with persistent anxiety who have become dependent on other drugs, and those with aggressive personalities who respond badly to the disinhibiting effects of benzodiazepines. However, even low-dose antipsychotic treatment, if maintained, is not free from the risk of *tardive dyskinesia*. Newer antipsychotic drugs, such as quetiapine, may also possess anxiolytic effects when given either as a sole treatment or as augmentation treatment in patients who are non-responsive to more standard drug therapies (Baldwin, 2014). However, the adverse-effect profile of antipsychotic drugs, together with the lack of well-controlled studies, suggests that such an indication should be restricted to specialist use in patients with anxiety disorders that have not responded to other pharmacological and psychological approaches (Baldwin *et al.*, 2014).

Beta-adrenoceptor antagonists that are used for anxiety

These drugs relieve some of the autonomic symptoms of anxiety, such as tachycardia, almost certainly by a peripheral effect. They are best reserved for anxious patients whose main symptom is palpitation or tremor, particularly in social situations. An appropriate drug is *propranolol* in a dose of 20–40 mg three times a day. Contraindications are heart block, systolic blood pressure below 90 mmHg, or a pulse rate of less than 60 beats/minute, and a history of bronchospasm. Beta-adrenoceptor antagonists precipitate heart failure in a few patients, and should not be given to those with atrioventricular node block, as they decrease conduction in the atrioventricular node and bundle of His. They can exacerbate Raynaud's phenomenon and hypoglycaemia in diabetics.

Pregabalin

Indications and pharmacology

Pregabalin is a derivative of the anticonvulsant drug, *gabapentin*. Like gabapentin, pregabalin has anticonvulsant and analgesic properties. It is licensed for the treatment of *generalized anxiety disorder* but not other anxiety disorders. Both gabapentin and pregabalin are analogues of GABA; however, neither compound is active at GABA or benzodiazepine receptors. It is believed that their therapeutic effects are mediated through interaction with the α2-δ subunit of voltage-gated calcium channels with a consequent modification of neurotransmitter release.

Controlled trials have shown that, in doses of 150–600 mg, pregabalin is effective in the treatment of generalized anxiety disorder, and is at least as efficacious as other agents used to treat generalized anxiety disorders, including the SSRIs (Baldwin *et al.*, 2014).

Pharmacokinetics and adverse effect

Pregabalin is rapidly absorbed, with peak plasma concentrations occurring within about 1 hour. Its half-life is about 6 hours, and it is eliminated unchanged primarily through renal excretion. Dose adjustment is therefore required in patients with impaired renal function. Because of its pattern of elimination, pregabalin treatment is not expected to cause pharmacokinetic interactions with other drugs, but the effects of central sedatives (e.g. benzodiazepines and alcohol) may be potentiated.

In clinical trials of patients with generalized anxiety disorder, discontinuation owing to adverse events with pregabalin was about 12%, compared with 5% with placebo. The most common adverse effects are somnolence and dizziness. Other common unwanted effects of pregabalin include increased appetite, mood changes, confusion, ataxia, tremor, and memory impairment. The most potentially serious reactions are visual disturbances, including vision loss, blurred vision, and other changes of visual acuity. These symptoms mostly improve when pregabalin is discontinued. It also seems likely that withdrawal of pregabalin is associated with discontinuation

symptoms, such as insomnia, headache, nausea, diarrhoea, anxiety, sweating, and dizziness.

Advice on management

Before an anxiolytic drug is prescribed, the cause of the anxiety should always be sought. In addition, it is helpful to classify the nature of the anxiety disorder, as this can have implications for drug treatment. It is worth remembering that, although medication is undoubtedly helpful in the treatment of anxiety syndromes, *psychological treatments* are as effective and are often preferred by patients. In practice, medication tends to be used when psychological treatments are not readily available or have not been successful.

For most patients with *anxiety symptoms*, attention to life problems, an opportunity to talk about their feelings, and reassurance from the doctor are enough to reduce anxiety to tolerable levels. If an anxiolytic is needed, a benzodiazepine should be given for a short time—not more than 3 weeks—and withdrawn gradually. It is important to remember that dependency is particularly likely to develop among people with alcohol-related problems. If the drug has been taken for several weeks, the patient should be warned that they may feel tense for a few days when it is stopped.

A compound such as *diazepam* is suitable for both the intermittent treatment of anxiety and continuous treatment throughout the day. The use of diazepam on an 'as-needed' basis usually means that lower total doses are consumed and the risk of tolerance and dependence is diminished. For longer-term treatment of severe generalized anxiety disorder, *antidepressant medication* is more appropriate (see Chapter 8).

Antidepressants are often helpful in the treatment of *panic disorder*, although the risk of early symptomatic worsening must be remembered and explained to the patient. The use of small doses early in treatment (e.g. 10 mg imipramine, 5 mg citalopram) can be helpful. High-potency benzodiazepines such as *alprazolam* and *clonazepam* are effective in panic disorder, but can cause cognitive impairment and withdrawal problems. However, they may be helpful in patients who do not respond to other treatments. *MAOI treatment* can also be used in treatment-resistant patients (Baldwin *et al.*, 2014).

Hypnotics

Hypnotics are drugs that are used to improve sleep. Many anxiolytic drugs also act as hypnotics, and these

have been reviewed in the previous section. Hypnotic drugs are prescribed widely and are often continued for too long. This reflects the frequency of insomnia as a symptom. Effective psychological treatments are available for the management of insomnia, and they appear to have a more sustained duration of action than hypnotics (Espie and Kyle, 2009).

Pharmacology

The ideal hypnotic would increase the length and quality of sleep without residual effects the next morning. It would do so without altering the pattern of sleep and without any withdrawal effects when the patient ceased to take it. Unfortunately, no drug meets these exacting criteria. It is not easy to produce drugs that affect the whole night's sleep and yet are sufficiently eliminated by morning for there to be no residual sedative effects (Wilson *et al.*, 2010).

Most prescribed hypnotics *enhance the action of GABA* through interaction with either the benzodiazepine receptor or other adjacent sites located on the GABA macromolecular complex. Antihistamines and low doses of sedating antidepressants such as amitriptyline and trazodone are also used to facilitate sleep. The pineal hormone, melatonin, is involved in organizing circadian rhythms and is sometimes used for the treatment of primary insomnia.

Compounds available

The most commonly used hypnotics are *benzodiazepines* or non-benzodiazepine ligands, which act at or close to the benzodiazepine-receptor site. The latter include *zopiclone* and *zolpidem* (*'the Z drugs'*). The actions of these drugs can be reversed by the benzodiazepine-receptor antagonist, flumazenil. Other available hypnotic agents include *chloral hydrate* (or its derivatives), *chlormethiazole*, and *sedating antihistamines* (the latter are often present in 'over-the-counter' preparations). A sustained-release form of melatonin is also licensed for the short-term treatment of insomnia in the middle-aged and elderly (Lemoine and Zisapel, 2012).

Of the benzodiazepines, the shorter-acting compounds such as temazepam and lormetazepam are appropriate as hypnotics because of their relative lack of hangover effects (see Box 25.3). Other benzodiazepines that were previously marketed as hypnotics, such as flurazepam and nitrazepam, have a long duration of action and produce significant impairments in tests of cognitive function on the day following treatment.

Zopiclone is a cyclopyrrolone. It produces fewer changes in sleep architecture than benzodiazepine hypnotics. The most common side effect is a *bitter aftertaste* following ingestion, but behavioural disturbances,

including *confusion, amnesia*, and *depressed mood*, have been reported. *Zolpidem* is a similar agent, with a shorter half-life. Like benzodiazepines, an epidemiological study has linked prolonged use of Z drugs with an increased risk of dementia (National Institute for Health and Care Excellence, 2015).

Clomethiazole edisylate is a hypnotic drug with anticonvulsant properties. It has often been used to prevent withdrawal symptoms in patients who are dependent on alcohol. For this reason, it is sometimes mistakenly believed to be a suitable hypnotic for alcoholic patients. This belief is erroneous because the drug is as likely as any other hypnotic drug to cause dependency, and can cause *respiratory depression* when combined with alcohol. It retains a place in the treatment of insomnia in the elderly because of its short duration of action. Unwanted effects *include sneezing, conjunctival irritation*, and *nausea*.

Unwanted effects

As well as the specific side effects of individual compounds noted above, there are a number of general problems associated with the use of all hypnotics. One of the most important is the presence of *residual effects*, which are experienced by the patient on the next day as feelings of being *slow* and *drowsy*. These are accompanied by deficits in daytime performance and an increased risk of falls and other accidents. Such effects are less apparent with the shorter-acting compounds noted above but can still be detected even with drugs such as zolpidem. Other problems include the *development of tolerance*, whereby the original dose of the drug has progressively less efficacy, and *'rebound' insomnia* on withdrawal, which makes preparations difficult to stop. *Tolerance* is less of a problem with sedating antidepressants, but such drugs have long half-lives accompanied by residual psychomotor effects the next day.

Interactions

The most important interaction of hypnotic drugs is with *alcohol*, where a potentiated effect can be seen. The *interaction between clomethiazole and alcohol* is particularly dangerous, and can result in death from respiratory failure. It should not be prescribed for alcoholics who continue to drink. Hypnotics will also potentiate the effect of other drugs with sedating actions, such as some antidepressant and antipsychotic agents.

Advice on management

Before prescribing hypnotic drugs, it is important to find out whether the patient is really sleeping badly and, if so, why. Many people have unrealistic ideas about the number of hours for which they should sleep. For example, they may not know that duration of sleep often becomes shorter in middle and late life. Others take 'cat naps' in the daytime, perhaps through boredom, and still expect to sleep as long at night. Some people ask for sleeping tablets in anticipation of poor sleep for one or two nights (e.g. when travelling). Such temporary loss of sleep is soon compensated for by increased sleep on subsequent nights, and any supposed advantage in terms of alertness after a full night's sleep is likely to be offset by the residual effects of the drugs.

The common causes of disturbed sleep include excessive caffeine or alcohol, pain, cough, pruritus, dyspnoea, and anxiety and depression. When any primary cause is present, this should be treated, not the insomnia. Often simple 'sleep hygiene' measures may be helpful (see Chapter 13). If, after careful enquiry, a hypnotic appears to be essential, it should be prescribed for a few days only. The clinician should explain this to the patient, and should warn them that a few nights of restless sleep may occur when the drugs are stopped,

but that this restlessness will not be a reason for prolonging the prescription.

The prescription of standard hypnotics for children is not justified, except for the occasional treatment of night terrors and somnambulism. However, *melatonin* has been regarded as helpful in improving sleep in children with neurodevelopmental disorders or sleep disorders such as sleep-onset insomnia and delayed-phase sleep syndrome (see Chpater 13; Wilson *et al.*, 2010). Hypnotics should also be prescribed with particular care for the elderly, who may become confused and get out of bed in the night, and perhaps injure themselves. Many patients are started on long periods of dependency on hypnotics by the prescribing of 'routine night sedation' in hospital. Prescription of these drugs should not be routine, but should only be a response to a real need, and should be stopped before the patient goes home. Guidance from the National Institute for Health and Care Excellence (2015) reinforces advice to use hypnotic medicines only for *short periods in disabling insomnia.*

Antipsychotic drugs

This term is applied to drugs that reduce psychomotor excitement and control symptoms of psychosis. Alternative terms for these agents are *neuroleptics* and *major tranquillizers*. None of these names is wholly satisfactory. 'Neuroleptic' refers to the side effects rather than to the therapeutic effects of the drugs, and 'major tranquillizer' does not refer to the most important clinical action. The term 'antipsychotic' is used here because it appears in the *British National Formulary*.

The main therapeutic uses of antipsychotic drugs are to reduce *hallucinations, delusions, agitation*, and *psychomotor excitement* in schizophrenia, mania, or psychosis secondary to a medical condition. The drugs are also used prophylactically to *prevent relapses* of schizophrenia and other psychoses. The introduction of chlorpromazine in 1952 led to substantial improvements in the treatment of schizophrenia, and paved the way to the discovery of the many psychotropic drugs that are now available.

Pharmacology

Antipsychotic drugs (see Box 25.4) share the property of *blocking dopamine receptors*. This may account for their therapeutic action, a suggestion that is supported by the close relationship between their potency in blocking dopaminergic receptors *in vitro*, and their

therapeutic strength. Imaging studies show that acute psychosis is associated with increased dopamine release in striatal regions, and that the extent of this increase correlates with the subsequent therapeutic effect of antipsychotic drugs (see Chapter 11). A persuasive formulation of antipsychotic drug action suggests that these agents block the ability of increased dopamine release to attribute *abnormal salience* to irrelevant stimuli (Kapur, 2003).

Dopamine receptors are of several subtypes. It is the D_2 receptor that is critical for antipsychotic action, and all licensed drugs in the category are antagonists at this receptor, with varying affinities for the D_2 subtype. PET studies suggest that an antipsychotic effect is obtained when D_2-receptor occupancy lies in the range 60–70%. Higher levels are associated with extrapyramidal movement disorders and hyperprolactinaemia, but not with greater efficacy (Kapur *et al.*, 1999). Other side effects are attributable to binding to a variety of other receptors (see below).

Distinction between typical and atypical antipsychotic drugs

The term *atypical* antipsychotic agent was introduced to distinguish the newer antipsychotic drugs from

> ### Box 25.4 A list of antipsychotic drugs
>
> **Phenothiazines**
> Chlorpromazine
> Trifluoperazine
>
> **Thioxanthenes**
> Flupenthixol
> Clopenthixol
>
> **Butyrophenones**
> Haloperidol
>
> **Dibenzodiazepines**
> Clozapine
> Olanzapine
>
> **Dibenzothiazepine**
> Quetiapine
>
> **Substituted benzamides**
> Sulpiride
> Amisulpride
>
> **Benzisoxazole**
> Risperidone
>
> **Quinolinone**
> Aripiprazole

In addition, the risk of tardive dyskinesia appears to be lower with the newer antipsychotic drugs (Correll *et al.*, 2014).

Another property that is sometimes attributed to atypical antipsychotic drugs is improved efficacy relative to typical agents. Although this is true in terms of positive psychotic symptoms for the prototypic atypical antipsychotic, clozapine, it is not clear how far more recently developed compounds meet this exacting criterion. A multiple treatments meta-analysis of placebo-controlled trials showed that evidence in this respect is strongest for amisulpride, olanzapine, and risperidone (Leucht *et al.*, 2013). However, pragmatic trials have so far failed to demonstrate important therapeutic differences between conventional and newer antipsychotic drugs, and even clozapine does not have proven efficacy against negative or cognitive symptoms. For these and other reasons, most authorities now believe that the terms 'atypical' and 'typical' antipsychotic are not useful, and that attention is better directed towards the pharmacological properties of individual drugs and their associated therapeutic profile (Leucht *et al.*, 2013) (see Table 25.2). See Chapter 11 for further discussion.

Pharmacology of typical (conventional) antipsychotics

All of these drugs are effective dopamine-receptor antagonists, but many possess additional pharmacological properties that influence their *adverse-effect profile*.

Phenothiazines

Chlorpromazine is the prototypic phenothiazine. It antagonizes α_1-adrenoceptors, histamine H_1-receptors, and muscarinic cholinergic receptors. Blockade of α_1-adrenoceptors and histamine H_1-receptors gives chlorpromazine a sedating profile, while α_1-adrenoceptor blockade also causes hypotension. The anticholinergic activity may cause dry mouth, urinary difficulties, and constipation, while on the other hand offsetting the liability to cause extrapyramidal side effects. In contrast to chlorpromazine, piperazine compounds such as *trifluoperazine* and *fluphenazine* are more selective dopamine-receptor antagonists, and are therefore less sedating but more likely to cause extrapyramidal effects.

Thioxanthenes and butyrophenones

Thioxanthenes such as *flupenthixol* and *clopenthixol* are similar in structure to the phenothiazines. The therapeutic effects are similar to those of the piperazine group. Butyrophenones such as *haloperidol* have a different structure but are clinically similar to the thioxanthenes.

conventional *typical* agents, such as chlorpromazine and haloperidol. An alternative term is *second generation*. Although the definition of the term 'atypical' varies in the literature, a fundamental property of an atypical antipsychotic is its ability to produce an antipsychotic effect *without causing extrapyramidal side effects*. This definition is problematic, not least because antipsychotics do not fall clearly into two classes in this respect, but lie along a spectrum. For example, low-potency conventional antipsychotic drugs such as chlorpromazine have a relatively low risk of producing extrapyramidal symptoms when prescribed at modest dosages; conversely, extrapyramidal side effects can also occur with the atypical antipsychotic risperidone. However, it is true to say that atypical antipsychotic agents have a lower likelihood of causing extrapyramidal side effects within their usual therapeutic range.

Table 25.2 **Atypical antipsychotics**

Drug	EPS*	Prolactin elevation	Weight gain	Adverse effects
Amisulpride	+	+++	+	Insomnia, agitation, nausea, constipation, QT prolongation
Sulpiride	+	+++	+	Insomnia, agitation, abnormal liver function tests
Clozapine	0	0	+++	Agranulocytosis—white cell monitoring mandatory, myocarditis and myopathy (rare), fatigue, drowsiness, dry mouth, sweating, tachycardia, postural hypotension, nausea, constipation, ileus, urinary retention, seizures, diabetes
Olanzapine	+/0	+	+++	Somnolence, dizziness, oedema, hypotension, dry mouth, constipation, diabetes, QT prolongation
Quetiapine	0	0	++	Somnolence, dizziness, postural hypotension, dry mouth, abnormal liver function tests, QT prolongation, diabetes
Risperidone	++	+++	++	Insomnia, agitation, anxiety, headache, impaired concentration, nausea, abdominal pain, diabetes, QT prolongation
Aripiprazole	+	0	0	Agitation, insomnia, nausea, vomiting
Lurasidone	+	+	0	Somnolence, insomnia, anxiety, agitation, nausea, dyspepsia, abdominal pain

* EPS, extrapyramidal symptoms; 0, not present; +, sometimes; ++, often; +++, can be excessive.

They are potent dopamine-receptor antagonists, with few effects at other neurotransmitter receptors. They are not sedating, but have a high propensity to cause extrapyramidal side effects.

Pharmacology of atypical antipsychotic drugs

Selective D2-receptor antagonists.

Atypical antipsychotic drugs have a diverse pharmacology, but currently two main groupings can be discerned. On the one hand are substituted benzamides such as *sulpiride* and *amisulpride*. These drugs are highly selective D_2-receptor antagonists which, for reasons that are not well understood, seem less likely to produce extrapyramidal movement disorders. They also lack sedative and anticholinergic properties. However, they do cause a substantial increase in plasma prolactin.

5-HT2-D2-receptor antagonists

The other major group of atypical antipsychotic drugs possess *5-HT$_2$-receptor-antagonist properties*. In other aspects—for example, potency of dopamine D_2-receptor blockade, these drugs differ significantly from one another (Meltzer, 2004; Citrome, 2013). *Risperidone* is a potent antagonist at both 5-HT$_2$ receptors and dopamine D_2 receptors. It also possesses α_1-adrenoceptor-blocking properties, which can cause mild sedation and hypotension. *Paliperidone* is an active metabolite of risperidone

and has very similar pharmacological properties when given orally.

Olanzapine is a slightly weaker D_2-receptor antagonist than risperidone, but has anticholinergic and powerful histamine H_1-receptor-blocking activity. This gives it strong sedating effects. *Quetiapine* is also a histamine H_1-receptor antagonist; it has modest 5-HT$_2$-receptor-antagonist effects, and rather weaker D_2-receptor-antagonist properties. It has a low propensity to cause movement disorders and, like olanzapine, is highly sedating. *Lurasidone* is a potent 5-HT$_2$ and D_2 receptor antagonist. It binds only weakly to histamine H_1 receptors, which makes it less likely to cause weight gain and sedation than olanzapine or quetiapine. *Asenapine* binds potently to 5-HT$_2$ receptors. It also binds significantly to D_2 receptors, as well as to a range of other 5-HT receptors and the alpha-2-adrenoreceptor, but the contribution of these latter properties to its therapeutic effect is unclear. In the UK and Europe, asenapine is licensed for the treatment of mania but not schizophrenia. It requires sublingual administration.

Sertindole is a potent 5-HT$_2$-receptor antagonist with weak D_2-receptor-antagonist effects. It causes clinically significant effects on the QT interval in the electrocardiogram, and its use is currently suspended. *Ziprasidone* is another 5-HT$_2$ and D_2-receptor antagonist, which differs from the other 5-HT$_2$/D$_2$-receptor antagonists described here, because it also binds to 5-HT$_{1A}$ receptors and is a noradrenaline reuptake inhibitor. Somnolence and dizziness are common side effects of ziprasidone, and it causes relatively little weight gain. It has a tendency to increase the QT interval, and has not been licensed in the UK. *Aripiprazole* is a partial dopamine agonist that also has 5-HT$_2$-receptor-blocking and 5-HT$_{1A}$-agonist properties. It has an activating profile and pro-dopaminergic side effects such as insomnia, nausea, and vomiting. It is less likely to cause weight gain than quetiapine or olanzapine.

To some extent these latter drugs were designed to reproduce the pharmacological profile of *clozapine*, which was the first antipsychotic agent to show definite benefit in the treatment of patients whose psychotic symptoms had failed to respond to conventional agents. In addition, clozapine has a low liability to cause movement disorders, and is therefore usually regarded as the prototypic atypical antipsychotic drug (Kane *et al.*, 1988). Clozapine is a *weak dopamine D$_2$-receptor antagonist but has a high affinity for 5-HT$_2$ receptors*. It also binds to a variety of other neurotransmitter receptors, including histamine H$_1$, α$_1$-adrenergic and muscarinic cholinergic receptors (Meltzer, 2004). Various studies have attempted to define a therapeutic plasma range for clozapine, with inconsistent results. A reasonable compromise between efficacy and safety is 350–500 µg/l. Above 600 µg/l the risk of seizures increases significantly.

The pharmacological basis for the increased efficacy of clozapine is not well understood. However, it is clear that the use of clozapine is associated with a significant risk of *leucopenia*, which restricts its use to patients who do not respond to or who are intolerant of other antipsychotic drugs. The adverse effects and haematological monitoring of clozapine treatment is discussed below.

Depot antipsychotic drugs

Slow-release preparations are used for patients who need to take antipsychotic medication to prevent relapse but cannot be relied upon to take it regularly. These 'depot' preparations include the esters of conventional antipsychotic drugs such as *fluphenazine decanoate, flupenthixol decanoate, zuclopenthixol decanoate, haloperidol decanoate*, and *pipotiazine palmitate*. All are given intramuscularly in an oily medium. *Zuclopenthixol acetate* reaches peak plasma levels within 1–2 days and has a shorter duration of action than other depots. It is used for the immediate control of acute psychosis, but its superiority to ordinary intramuscular injections is not established. Slow-release injections of atypical antipsychotic drugs such as *risperidone, paliperidone* (an active metabolite of risperidone), *aripiprazole*, and *olanzapine* are also available.

Pharmacokinetics

Antipsychotic drugs are well absorbed, mainly from the jejunum. When they are taken by mouth, part of their hepatic metabolism is completed as they pass through the portal system on their way to the systemic circulation (first-pass metabolism). Antipsychotic drugs are *highly protein-bound.*

With the exception of *sulpiride and amisulpride*, which are excreted unchanged by the kidney, antipsychotic drugs are extensively metabolized by the liver to produce a range of active and inactive metabolites. For example, following administration of chlorpromazine, about 75 metabolites have been detected in the blood or urine. This complex metabolism has made it difficult to interpret the clinical significance of plasma concentrations of most antipsychotics; for this reason the plasma measures are seldom used in everyday clinical work. The half-life of most antipsychotic drugs (around 20 hours) is sufficient to allow once-daily dosing. However, *quetiapine* has a half-life of about 3 hours, and twice-daily dosing in the treatment of schizophrenia is recommended, although modified-release preparations are available.

The pharmacokinetic profile of *depot preparations* differs substantially from that of standard preparations. For all compounds except zuclopenthixol acetate, it takes several weeks for steady-state drug levels to be reached in the plasma (see Table 25.3). This means that relapse after treatment discontinuation is likely to be similarly delayed.

Drug interactions

Antipsychotic drugs potentiate the effects of other *central sedatives*. They may delay the hepatic metabolism of tricyclic antidepressants and antiepileptic drugs, leading to increased plasma levels of the latter agents. The *hypotensive* properties of chlorpromazine may enhance the effects of *antihypertensive drugs*, including ACE inhibitors.

Some antipsychotic drugs, and particularly *pimozide*, can increase *the QT interval* (QTc is often cited, which is the QT interval corrected for heart rate) and should not be given with other drugs that are likely to potentiate this effect, such as antiarrhythmics, astemizole and terfenadine, cisapride, and tricyclic antidepressants. There are also reports of an increased risk of cardiac arrhythmias when pimozide has been combined with clarithromycin and erythromycin.

Table 25.3 Some pharmacokinetic properties of depot antipsychotic drugs

Depot	Time to peak plasma level (days)	Time to steady state (weeks)	Licensed dosing interval (weeks)	Typical clinical dose (mg)
Flupenthixol decanoate	3–7	8	2–4	60
Fluphenazine decanoate	1–2	8	2–5	50
Haloperidol decanoate	7	8–12	4	100
Pipotiazine palmitate	7–14	8	4	50
Zuclopenthixol decanoate	7	8	2–4	300
Risperidone microspheres	28	8	2	37.5
Olanzapine pamoate	2–4	12	2-4	300
Paliperidone palmitate	13	20	Monthly	100
Aripiprazole	7	20	Monthly	300

Adapted from Taylor D, Paton C and Kapur S, The Maudsley Prescribing Guidelines, 12th edition, Copyright (2015), with permission from John Wiley & Sons.

Clozapine should not be given with any agent that is likely to *potentiate its depressant effect on white cell count*, such as carbamazepine, co-trimoxazole, and penicillamine. Some *SSRIs* (notably fluoxetine and paroxetine) slow the hepatic metabolism and increase blood levels of several antipsychotic drugs, including haloperidol, risperidone, aripiprazole, and clozapine.

Unwanted effects

The many different antipsychotic drugs share a broad pattern of unwanted effects that are mainly related to their *antidopaminergic, antiadrenergic*, and *anticholinergic* properties (see Box 25.5). Details of the effects of individual drugs can be found in the *British National Formulary* or a similar work of reference. Here we give an account of the general pattern, with examples of the side effects associated with a few commonly used drugs.

Extrapyramidal effects

These are related to the antidopaminergic action of the drugs on the *basal ganglia*. As already noted, the therapeutic effects may also derive from the antidopaminergic action, although at mesolimbic and mesocortical sites. The effects on the extrapyramidal system fall into four groups, which are summarized below.

Acute dystonia

This occurs soon after treatment begins, especially in young men. It is most often observed with butyrophenones and with the piperazine group of phenothiazines. The main features are torticollis, tongue protrusion, grimacing, and opisthotonos, an odd clinical picture that can easily be mistaken for histrionic behaviour. It can be controlled by an anticholinergic agent given carefully by intramuscular injection.

Akathisia

This is an unpleasant feeling of physical restlessness and a need to move, leading to an inability to keep still. Agitation with suicidal ideation can also occur. Akathisia may wrongly be mistaken for a worsening of psychosis, and more antipsychotic medication may then be inappropriately prescribed. It usually occurs during the first 2 weeks of treatment with antipsychotic drugs, but may begin only after several months. Akathisia is not reliably controlled by antiparkinsonian drugs. Beta-adrenoceptor antagonists and short-term treatment with benzodiazepines may be helpful. The best strategy is to reduce the dose of antipsychotic drug, if possible.

Parkinsonian syndrome

Antipsychotic-induced parkinsonism is characterized by akinesia, an expressionless face, and lack of associated movements when walking, together with rigidity, coarse tremor, stooped posture, and, in severe cases, a festinant gait. This syndrome often does not appear until a few months after the drug has been taken, and then sometimes diminishes even though the dose has not been reduced. The symptoms can be controlled with

Box 25.5 Some unwanted effects of antipsychotic drugs

Antidopaminergic movement effects

Acute dystonia
Akathisia
Parkinsonism
Tardive dyskinesia

Antiadrenergic effects

Sedation
Postural hypotension
Inhibition of ejaculation

Anticholinergic effects

Dry mouth
Reduced sweating
Urinary hesitancy and retention
Constipation
Blurred vision
Precipitation of glaucoma

Antihistaminic effects

Sedation
Weight gain

Other effects

Cardiac arrhythmias
Metabolic syndrome and diabetes
Amenorrhoea
Galactorrhoea
Hypothermia
Pulmonary embolus

antiparkinsonian drugs. However, it is not good practice to prescribe antiparkinsonian drugs prophylactically as a routine, because not all patients will need them. Moreover, these drugs themselves have undesirable effects in some patients; for example, they occasionally cause an acute organic syndrome, and may worsen or unmask concomitant tardive dyskinesia.

Tardive dyskinesia

This is particularly serious because, unlike the other extrapyramidal effects, it does not always recover when the drugs are stopped. It is characterized by chewing and sucking movements, grimacing, choreoathetoid movements, and possibly akathisia. The movements usually affect the face, but the limbs and the muscles of respiration may also be involved. Although the syndrome is seen occasionally among patients who have not taken antipsychotic drugs, it is more common among those who have taken antipsychotic drugs for a number of years. It is also sometimes seen in patients who are taking dopamine-receptor blockers for other indications (e.g. metoclopramide for chronic gastro-intestinal problems).

Epidemiology. Tardive dyskinesia is more common among *women, the elderly*, and patients who have *diffuse brain pathology*. A diagnosis of *mood disorder* is also a risk factor. In about 50% of cases, tardive dyskinesia disappears when the antipsychotic drug is stopped. Estimates of the frequency of the syndrome vary in different series, but it seems to develop in about 20% of patients with schizophrenia who have been treated with long-term conventional antipsychotic medication. Current evidence suggests that the incidence of tardive dyskinesia is lower with *atypical antipsychotic agents* such as clozapine, olanzapine, and risperidone than with haloperidol (Correll *et al.*, 2014). However, cases still occur, albeit at a lower level.

Pathophysiology. The cause of tardive dyskinesia is uncertain, but it could be due to supersensitivity to dopamine as a result of prolonged dopaminergic blockade. This explanation is consistent with the observations that tardive dyskinesia may be aggravated by stopping antipsychotic drugs or by the administration of anticholinergic antiparkinsonian drugs (presumably by upsetting further the balance between cholinergic and dopaminergic systems in the basal ganglia).

Treatment. Many treatments for tardive dyskinesia have been tried, but none of them is universally effective. Therefore it is important to reduce its incidence as far as possible by limiting long-term antipsychotic drug treatment to patients who really need it. At the same time, a careful watch should be kept for abnormal movements in all patients who have taken antipsychotic drugs for a long time. If dyskinesia is observed, the antipsychotic drug should be stopped if the state of the mental illness allows this.

Although tardive dyskinesia may first worsen after stopping the drug, in many cases it will improve over several months. If the dyskinesia persists after this time or if the continuation of antipsychotic medication is essential, a trial can be made of an atypical agent such as quetiapine. This can sometimes lead to remission of the disorder. Olanzapine and aripiprazole are also possibilities. Clozapine may be the most effective atypical agent in treating tardive dyskinesia but because of its side effect profile is best reserved for patients who do not respond to other atypicals (unless the patient also has a con-comitant treatment-resistant psychotic illness). Other agents that have been tried include vitamin E, although the evidence for its efficacy is conflicting. A dopamine-depleting agent called tetrabenazine is licensed for the treatment of tardive dyskinesia but tends not to be well tolerated (see Taylor *et al.*, 2015).

Tardive dystonia

Although the two conditions can coexist, tardive dys-kinesia needs to be distinguished from *tardive dystonia*, which is the long-term persistence of a dystonic move-ment disorder. Clinically the condition is indistin-guishable from the various idiopathic dystonias which present, for example, with blepharospasm or torticol-lis. The diagnosis of drug-induced tardive dystonia is made on the basis of exposure to dopamine-receptor-blocking agents and a negative family history of dys-tonia. Treatment is unsatisfactory. Anticholinergic drugs are ineffective, and the condition often persists after withdrawal of the antipsychotic agent. However, clozapine has been reported to be useful, as has local injection of botulinum toxin into the affected muscle group.

Antiadrenergic effects

These include sedation, postural hypotension with reflex tachycardia, nasal congestion, and inhibition of ejaculation. The effects on blood pressure are particu-larly likely to appear after intramuscular administration, and may appear in the elderly whatever the route of administration.

Anticholinergic effects

These include dry mouth, urinary hesitancy and reten-tion, constipation, reduced sweating, blurred vision, and, rarely, the precipitation of glaucoma.

Antihistaminic effects

H_1-histamine receptor antagonism causes sedation and also increased appetite. The latter can result in excessive weight gain, which contributes towards the develop-ment of the metabolic syndrome and type 2 diabetes.

Other effects
Cardiac conduction defects

Cardiac arrhythmias are sometimes reported. ECG changes are more common in the form of *prolongation of the QT interval* and T-wave changes. It was noted above that the use of *pimozide* has been associated with ser-ious cardiac arrhythmias. Cautious dose adjustment with ECG monitoring is recommended. A similar effect

led to the withdrawal of the phenothiazine, *thiorida-zine*. Other antipsychotic drugs with moderate effects to lengthen the QT interval are amisulpride, quetiapine, chlorpromazine, and haloperidol. Antipsychotic drugs are also associated with an increased risk of venous thrombosis and pulmonary embolus, which appears to be greater with the newer agents and in those who have started treatment more recently (Parker *et al.*, 2010). For a review of the cardiac effects of antipsychotic drugs and the role of ECG monitoring, see Abdelmawla and Mitchell (2006a, b).

Depression

Depression of mood has been said to occur, but this is difficult to evaluate because untreated patients with schizophrenia may have periods of depression. It is certainly possible that excessive dopamine-receptor-blockade in the mesolimbic forebrain could be asso-ciated with anhedonia and loss of drive, which could then resemble depression or negative symptoms of schizophrenia.

Diabetes and metabolic syndrome

We have already seen that, probably due to histamine H_1 receptor antagonism, patients may *gain weight* when tak-ing antipsychotic drugs, especially chlorpromazine and atypical agents such as olanzapine, quetiapine, and clo-zapine (see Table 25.2). Weight gain can result in obesity, which increases the risk of type 2 diabetes. Schizophrenia itself has been associated with an increased risk of diabe-tes, and this risk is probably increased by antipsychotic drugs, partly but not completely through the associated weight gain. Weight gain is probably least likely to be a problem with haloperidol, amisulpride, aripiprazole, and lurasidone.

Other pharmacological properties of antipsychotic drugs may increase the risk of diabetes, independently of weight gain—for example, via blockade of peripheral M_3 muscarinic receptors. Similarly, newer antipsychotic drugs such as olanzapine, clozapine, and quetiapine are associated with increased lipid levels. These adverse effects are of great clinical importance because they increase the risk of *cardiovascular disease* and may there-fore contribute to the increase in overall mortality seen in patients with schizophrenia. A meta-analysis reported that just over a third of patients taking antipsychotic drugs have the '*metabolic syndrome*' (a combination of central obesity with two out of four of: hypertension, raised fasting glucose, low HDL cholesterol, and raised triglycerides). The presence of this syndrome signifi-cantly increases the risk of cardiovascular disease such as myocardial infarction and stroke.

Patients who are receiving treatment with antipsychotic drugs require careful monitoring of metabolic aspects of their general health (Box 25.6). For a review, see Cooper *et al.* (2016). For a review of the pharmacological mechanisms involved in the adverse metabolic effects of antipsychotic drugs, see Reynolds and Kirk (2010).

Endocrine changes

Galactorrhoea and *amenorrhoea* are induced in some women by *high prolactin levels*, and it is possible that low libido and sexual dysfunction may also result. There may also be an increased risk of osteoporosis. Some atypical agents do not increase prolactin levels significantly (see Table 25.2). For a review of the adverse effects of hyperprolactinaemia, see Wieck and Haddad (2004).

Other unwanted effects

In the elderly, *hypothermia* is an important unwanted effect. Some antipsychotic drugs, particularly lower-potency agents, such as chlorpromazine and clozapine, *lower the seizure threshold* and can increase the frequency of seizures in epileptic patients. Prolonged *chlorpromazine* treatment can lead to *photosensitivity* and to accumulation of pigment in the skin, cornea, and lens.

Sensitivity reactions. Phenothiazines, particularly *chlorpromazine*, have been associated with cholestatic jaundice, but the incidence is low (about 0.1%). Blood cell dyscrasias also occur rarely with antipsychotic drugs, but are most common with clozapine. Skin rashes can also occur.

Adverse effects of clozapine

The use of clozapine is associated with a significant risk of *leucopenia* (about 2–3%), which can progress to agranulocytosis. Weekly blood counts for the first 18 weeks of treatment and at 2-weekly intervals thereafter are mandatory. After 1 year, the frequency of blood sampling may be reduced to monthly intervals. With this intensive monitoring, the early detection of leucopenia can be followed by immediate withdrawal of clozapine and by reversal of the low white cell count. This procedure greatly reduces, but does not eliminate, the risk of progression to agranulocytosis. It is usually recommended that clozapine be used as the sole antipsychotic agent in a treatment regimen. Clearly, it is wise to avoid concomitant use of drugs such as *carbamazepine*, which may also lower the white cell count.

Because of its relatively weak blockade of dopamine D_2 receptors, clozapine is unlikely to cause extrapyramidal movement disorders, including tardive dyskinesia. It does not increase plasma prolactin, so galactorrhoea does not occur. However, its use is associated with

---

> ### Box 25.6 Metabolic monitoring and interventions for patients taking antipsychotic drugs
>
> *Monitoring* (if possible, should start before treatment or as soon as possible afterwards)
> 1. Body mass index (once every 4 weeks for 12 weeks, then at least biannually)
> 2. Blood glucose (fasting or random: 12 weeks, 6 months, and then annually—switch to HbA_{1c})
> 3. Lipid profile (fasting or random: 12 weeks, 6 months, and then annually)
> 4. Blood pressure (12 weeks, 6 months, and annually)
> 5. Enquire about tobacco smoking and alcohol use at each visit
>
> #### Possible interventions
>
> 1. 'Lifestyle' interventions: diet and exercise, advice about smoking and alcohol intake
> 2. Switch to antipsychotic drug less likely to cause weight gain (Table 25.2)
> 3. Adjunctive metformin for weight gain (requires monitoring of renal function and B_{12} levels)
> 4. Medical management of diabetes, dyslipidaemia, and hypertension according to NICE guidelines
>
> Reproduced from Journal of Psychopharmacology, 30(8), Cooper SJ et al, BAP guidelines on the management of weight gain, metabolic disturbances and cardiovascular risk associated with psychosis and antipsychotic drug treatment, pp. 717-48, Copyright (2016), with permission from SAGE Publications.

---

hypersalivation, drowsiness, postural hypotension, weight gain, and *hyperthermia. Seizures* may occur at higher doses. Clozapine is a sedating compound, and cases of respiratory and circulatory embarrassment have been reported during combined treatment with clozapine and benzodiazepines. *Constipation i*s common and should be treated or a dangerous *ileus* may result. Rarely, fatal *myocarditis* and *myopathy* have been reported. The weight gain is at least partly responsible for an increased risk of *diabetes mellitus.*

The neuroleptic malignant syndrome

This rare but serious disorder occurs in a small minority of patients who are taking antipsychotic drugs, especially high-potency compounds. Most reported cases have followed the use of antipsychotic agents for schizophrenia, but in some cases the drugs were used for mania, depressive disorder, or psychosis secondary to a medical condition. *Combined lithium and antipsychotic* drug treatment may be a predisposing factor. The overall incidence is probably about 0.2% of patients who are treated with antipsychotic drugs.

The onset is often, but not invariably, during the first 10 days of treatment. The clinical picture includes the rapid onset (usually over 24–72 hours) of severe motor, mental, and autonomic disorders, together with *hyperpyrexia*.

- The prominent motor symptom is generalized muscular hypertonicity. Stiffness of the muscles in the throat and chest may cause dysphagia and dyspnoea.
- The mental symptoms include akinetic mutism, stupor, or impaired consciousness.
- Hyperpyrexia develops, with evidence of autonomic disturbances in the form of unstable blood pressure, tachycardia, excessive sweating, salivation, and urinary incontinence.
- In the blood, *creatinine phosphokinase (CPK)* levels may be greatly elevated, and the white cell count may be increased.
- Secondary complications may include pneumonia, thromboembolism, cardiovascular collapse, and renal failure.

The mortality rate of neuroleptic syndrome appears to have been declining over recent years, but can still be of the order of 10%. The syndrome lasts for 1–2 weeks after stopping an oral neuroleptic, but may last two to three times longer after stopping long-acting preparations. Patients who survive are usually, but not invariably, without residual disability.

The differential diagnosis includes encephalitis, and in some countries heat stroke. Before the introduction of antipsychotic drugs, a similar disorder was reported as a form of catatonia sometimes called acute lethal catatonia. The condition can probably occur with any antipsychotic agent, but in many reported cases the drugs used have been haloperidol or fluphenazine. Cases have also been reported with atypical antipsychotic drugs, including clozapine. The cause could be related to excessive dopaminergic blockade, although why this should affect only a minority of patients cannot be explained.

Treatment is symptomatic. The main priorities are to stop the drug, cool the patient, maintain fluid balance, and treat intercurrent infection. No drug treatment is certainly effective. *Diazepam* can be used for muscle stiffness. *Dantrolene*, a drug used to treat malignant hyperthermia, has also been tried. *Bromocriptine*, a dopamine agonist, is also recommended. Very ill patients require support in an intensive care unit, with intubation and paralysis to maintain respiration and deal with renal failure.

Some patients who developed the syndrome on one occasion have been given the same drug again safely after the acute episode has resolved. Nevertheless, if an antipsychotic has to be used again, it is prudent to restart treatment cautiously with an atypical agent with weaker dopamine-receptor-blocking properties, used at first in low doses. At least 2 weeks should elapse before antipsychotic drug treatment is reinstated.

Contraindications to antipsychotic drugs

There are few absolute contraindications to antipsychotic medication, and they vary with individual drugs. Before any of these drugs are used, it is important to consult the *British National Formulary* or a comparable work of reference. Contraindications include myasthenia gravis, Addison's disease, glaucoma (where compounds have significant anticholinergic activity), and, in the case of clozapine, any evidence of bone marrow depression. For patients with liver disease, chlorpromazine should be avoided and other drugs used with caution. Caution is also required when there is renal disease, cardiovascular disorder, epilepsy, or serious infection. Patients with Parkinson's disease sometimes require antipsychotic medication to deal with psychotic states induced by dopaminergic agents; quetiapine or clozapine is advised in these circumstances.

Antipsychotic drugs can produce severe movement disorders and changes in consciousness in some patients with dementia, particularly *Lewy body dementia*. In the elderly, especially those with pre-existing cerebrovascular disease, they are also associated with an increased risk of stroke. Current recommendations are to use antipsychotic drugs with great caution, and to avoid their use if possible, in these clinical situations. For discussion, see Chapter 14.

Dosage

Doses of antipsychotic drugs need to be adjusted for the individual patient, and changes should be made gradually. Doses should be lower for the elderly, for patients with brain damage or epilepsy, and for the physically ill. The dosage of individual drugs can be found in the *British National Formulary* or a comparable work of reference, or in the manufacturer's literature.

PET imaging studies

There has been an important trend towards the recommendation of lower doses of typical antipsychotic drugs such as haloperidol. This is based in part on studies with PET, which have demonstrated that adequate dopamine D_2-receptor blockade (in the basal ganglia at least) can be obtained with what were previously considered *low doses* of conventional antipsychotic drugs (e.g. about 5 mg of haloperidol) (see Table 25.4) (Nord and Farde, 2011). For newer antipsychotic drugs, sufficient PET data are usually available to allow clear dosage recommendations.

Low recommended doses produce an adequate antipsychotic effect in the majority of patients. Higher doses may cause further calming, but are likely to be associated with significant adverse effects, some of which may be serious (e.g. cardiac arrhythmias). A prevailing view is that the combination of modest doses of antipsychotic drugs with a benzodiazepine is a safer and more effective means of producing rapid sedation than high doses of antipsychotic drugs.

Antipsychotic drugs and the risk of sudden death

The association of *sudden unexplained death* with antipsychotic drug treatment is a matter of continuing debate. Patients with schizophrenia treated with antipsychotic drugs appear to have higher rates of cardiac arrest and ventricular arrhythmias than controls. They are also more likely to die through choking (Ruschena *et al.*, 2003). This could be due to the illness or to treatment. However, antipsychotic drugs are known to alter *cardiac conduction*, and drugs such as chlorpromazine also have hypotensive effects. Epidemiological studies show that the increased risk of sudden death (about

twofold) in patients who are taking antipsychotic drugs is similar for the older and newer agents, and is related to increasing dose (Ray *et al.*, 2009). Although this association may not be causal, it is clearly prudent to use as low a dose of an antipsychotic drug as the clinical circumstances permit. Particular caution is needed in patients with pre-existing cardiac disease and those taking other medications that might increase the QT interval (Abdelmawla and Mitchell, 2006a, b).

An indication of the relative dosage of some commonly used antipsychotic drugs taken by mouth is given in Table 25.4. Some practical guidance on the most frequently used drugs is given in the next section.

Pharmacological treatment of acute behavioural disturbance

The role of antipsychotic drugs in the treatment and management of schizophrenia and related disorders is covered in Chapter 11. Here we cover the appropriate use of antipsychotic agents in control of acute behavioural disturbance—sometimes called rapid tranquillization.

Antipsychotic drugs and benzodiazepines are used to control psychomotor excitement, hostility, and other abnormal behaviour resulting from schizophrenia, mania, or organic psychosis. If the patient is very excited and is displaying abnormally aggressive behaviour, the aim should be to bring the behaviour under control as quickly and safely as possible. Drug treatment in this situation should only be used if psychological or

Table 25.4 Dosage and D_2 receptor blockade of some antipsychotic drugs

Drug	Relative dose (oral)	Maximum *BNF* dose (mg)	D_2-receptor occupancy *in vivo* (%) [daily dose (mg)][*]
Chlorpromazine	100	1000	80 [200]
Trifluoperazine	5	NA	80 [10]
Haloperidol	2	20	80 [4]
Flupenthixol	1	18	74 [10]
Sulpiride	200	2400	74 [800]
Clozapine	60	900	47 [600]
Risperidone	2	16	75 [4]
Olanzapine	8	20	75 [15]
Aripiprazole	5	30	80 [15]

NA, not available.
[*]Source: Nord and Farde, 2011; Yokoi *et al.*, 2002.

behavioural approaches cannot be employed or have failed to calm the situation.

If the patient is already taking an antipsychotic drug, the addition of *lorazepam* (1–2 mg) or *promethazine* (25–50 mg) can be helpful. If the patient is not taking regular antipsychotic medication, the use of *olanzapine* (10 mg), *quetiapine* (100–200 mg), *risperidone* (1–2 mg), or *haloperidol* (5 mg) (the latter combined with *promethazine* 25 mg) can be considered, although the product licence for haloperidol recommends pre-treatment ECG monitoring, which might be difficult to arrange in an emergency situation.

If parenteral treatment is needed, lorazepam (2 mg), promethazine (50 mg), and olanzapine (10 mg) are available as intramuscular preparations, as is haloperidol (5 mg), which, as with oral treatment, is best combined with promethazine. An intramuscular preparation of aripiprazole (9.75 mg) is licensed for emergency use; it may be somewhat less effective than olanzapine, but is less likely to cause hypotension. When using olanzapine intramuscularly it is important to be aware of the contraindications to its use, particularly with regard to patients with cardiovascular disease. *Intramuscular olanzapine should not be given with parenteral benzodiazepines.* Whatever treatment is used, it is important to check for possible respiratory depression, particularly in the elderly and in patients with concomitant physical illness. The benzodiazepine antagonist *flumazenil* should be available. For a summary of the emergency pharmacological management of disturbed behaviour, see Taylor *et al.* (2015).

There are several other practical points concerning the management of the acutely disturbed patient that can be dealt with conveniently here. Although it may not be easy in the early stages to differentiate between mania and schizophrenia as causes of the disturbed behaviour, it is necessary to try to distinguish them from psychosis secondary to medical conditions and from outbursts of aggression in abnormal personalities. Among medical conditions it is important to consider postepileptic states, the effects of head injury, transient global amnesia, and hypoglycaemia. If the patient has been drinking alcohol, the danger of potentiating the sedative effects of antipsychotic drugs and benzodiazepines should be remembered. Similarly, antipsychotic drugs that may be more likely to provoke seizures should be used with caution in postepileptic states.

For further information about the management of violence in health care settings, and clinical guidelines, see Chapter 18.

Anticholinergic drugs

Although these drugs have no direct therapeutic use in psychiatry, they are sometimes required to control the *extrapyramidal side effects* of typical antipsychotic drugs.

Pharmacology

Of the drugs that are used to treat idiopathic parkinsonism, currently only the *anticholinergic compounds* are used for drug-induced extrapyramidal syndromes. These drugs are antagonists of *muscarinic cholinergic receptors* both centrally and in the periphery. Some also possess *antihistaminic* properties.

Preparations available

Many anticholinergic drugs are available, and there is little to choose between the various compounds. However, some authorities suggest that the use of agents that are more selective for the M_1 subtype of the muscarinic receptor—for example, *biperiden*—may be associated with fewer peripheral anticholinergic effects. Other preparations that are employed include *procyclidine* and *benzhexol*. *Orphenadrine* and *benztropine* have combined antihistaminic and anticholinergic properties.

Pharmacokinetics

Limited data are available. Anticholinergic drugs appear to be well absorbed and are extensively metabolized in the liver. They are highly protein-bound. Their half-lives are generally in the range of 15–20 hours.

Unwanted effects

In large doses these drugs may cause delirium (*acute organic syndrome*), especially in the elderly. Their anticholinergic activity can summate with those of antipsychotic drugs so that glaucoma or retention of urine in men with enlarged prostates may be precipitated. Drowsiness, dry mouth, and constipation also occur. These effects tend to diminish as the drug is continued.

Orphenadrine may be more toxic than other anticholinergic drugs in overdose, whereas *benztropine* has been associated with heat stroke. All anticholinergic drugs can exacerbate tardive dyskinesia, but are probably not a predisposing factor in its development. Anticholinergic drugs can worsen cognitive function and should be avoided in patients with dementia. It is also possible that long-term use of drugs with anticholinergic properties (this will include drugs such as tricyclic antidepressants and some antipsychotics) can increase the risk of dementia (Gray *et al.*, 2015).

Drug interactions

Antiparkinsonian drugs can induce *drug-metabolizing enzymes* in the liver, so that plasma concentrations of antipsychotic drugs are sometimes reduced. As noted above, anticholinergic agents can potentiate the effects of other drugs with anticholinergic activity, such as chlorpromazine and amitriptyline.

Advice on management

As noted previously, anticholinergic drugs should not be given routinely because they may increase the manifestation of tardive dyskinesia. Also, the presence of persistent extrapyramidal side effects is a sign that the dose of medication is excessive for that patient, in terms of D_2-receptor occupancy. Patients who are receiving injectable long-acting antipsychotic preparations may require anticholinergic drugs for only a few days after injection, if at all. There have been reports of misuse of and dependence on anticholinergic drugs, possibly resulting from a mood-elevating effect.

If anticholinergic drugs are required, *biperiden* (2–12 mg daily) or *procyclidine* (5–30 mg daily) are appropriate for routine use. These drugs are usually given three times daily, although their half-lives would suggest that less frequent dosing should be possible. It is best not to give anticholinergic drugs in the evening because of the possibility of excitement and *sleep disruption*.

Antidepressant drugs

Currently used antidepressant drugs can be divided into three main classes, depending on their acute pharmacological properties.

1. *Monoamine reuptake inhibitors.* These are compounds that inhibit the reuptake of noradrenaline and/or 5-HT. They include tricyclic antidepressants, selective serotonin reuptake inhibitors (SSRIs), selective noradrenaline and serotonin reuptake inhibitors (SNRIs), and selective noradrenaline reuptake inhibitors (NARIs).

2. *Monoamine oxidase inhibitors (MAOIs).* These are compounds that deactivate monoamine oxidase irreversibly (phenelzine and tranylcypromine) or reversibly (moclobemide).

3. *5-HT$_2$ receptor antagonists.* These drugs (mirtazapine and trazodone) have complex effects on monoamine mechanisms but share the ability to block 5-HT$_2$ receptors.

In the broad range of major depression, these drugs are of equivalent efficacy. The main differences between them are in their *adverse effects and safety* (see Table 25.5). Each of these three classes of drugs will be considered in turn after some comments on the possible mechanism of action of antidepressants.

Mechanism of action

The acute effect of reuptake inhibitors and of MAOIs is to enhance the functional activity of noradrenaline and/or 5-HT. These actions can be detected within hours of the start of treatment, yet the full antidepressant effects of drug treatment can be delayed for several weeks. For example, it has been suggested that at least 6 weeks should elapse before an assessment of the effects of an antidepressant drug can be made in an individual patient.

To some extent, this delay in the onset of therapeutic activity may be due to pharmacokinetic factors. For example, the half-life of most antidepressant drugs is around 24 hours, which means that steady-state plasma drug levels will be reached only after 5–7 days. However, it seems unlikely that this can completely account for the lag in antidepressant activity.

The delay in onset of obvious therapeutic effect with antidepressant medication led to suggestions that the antidepressant effect of current treatments is a consequence of slowly evolving neuroadaptive changes in the brain, which are triggered by acute potentiation of monoamine function. Studies in experimental animals have implicated various mechanisms that might underlie this effect, including desensitization of inhibitory autoreceptors on 5-HT and noradrenaline cell bodies, increased production of neurotrophins, such as brain-derived neurotrophic factor (BDNF), and increased synaptogenesis and neurogenesis.

Recently, however, attention has focused on the effects of antidepressant drugs on the neuropsychological

Table 25.5 Groups of antidepressant drugs

Drug	Advantages	Disadvantages
Tricyclic antidepressants	Well studied Efficacy never surpassed	Cardiotoxic*, dangerous in overdose
		Anticholinergic side effects**
	Useful sedative effect in selected patients	Cognitive impairment
		Weight gain during longer-term treatment
SSRIs/SNRIs	Lack cardiotoxicity***: relatively safe in overdose[†]	Long-term toxicity not fully evaluated
	Not anticholinergic	Gastrointestinal disturbance, sexual dysfunction
	No cognitive impairment	May worsen sleep and anxiety symptoms initially
	Relatively easy to give effective dose	Greater risk of drug interaction
Trazodone	Lacks cardiotoxicity[††], relatively safe in overdose	Daytime drowsiness
Mirtazapine	Useful sedative effect in selected patients	Weight gain common Less well-established efficacy in severe depression

*Lofepramine is relatively safe in overdose.

**Long-term use of anticholinergic drug may increase risk of dementia

***Citalopram and escitalopram increase QT interval

[†]Venlafaxine is more dangerous than SSRIs in overdose

[††]Cardiac arrhythmias have rarely been reported with trazodone.

mechanisms involved in the processing of emotional information. Emotional processing is known to be negatively biased in depressed patients, and it is therefore of great interest that *single doses* of antidepressant drugs produce positive biases in emotional processing in healthy volunteers and reverse the negative biases present in depressed patients, in the absence of any changes in subjective mood. These findings suggest that relevant *neuropsychological* effects of antidepressants can be detected from the beginning of treatment, and the delay in the appearance of obvious therapeutic effects of antidepressant medication may stem from the time taken for changes in emotional processing to be experienced as subjective changes in mood as an individual with this new emotional 'set' interacts with their environment. The latter process could well involve the 'relearning' of emotional associations, which makes the changes in synaptic plasticity and neurogenesis that have been reported in animal studies of antidepressants of great interest. For a review, see Sharp and Cowen (2011).

Selective serotonin reuptake inhibitors

In general, SSRIs are now preferred to tricyclic antidepressants in the first-line treatment of depression because they are moderately better tolerated and markedly less toxic in overdose (National Institute for Health and Clinical Excellence, 2009a).

Pharmacological properties

Six SSRIs—citalopram, escitalopram, fluoxetine, fluvoxamine, paroxetine, and sertraline—are available at present for clinical use in the UK. SSRIs are a structurally diverse group, but they all *inhibit the reuptake of 5-HT* with high potency and selectivity. None of them has an appreciable affinity for the noradrenaline uptake site, and the present data suggest that they have a low affinity for other monoamine neurotransmitter receptors.

Pharmacokinetics

In general, SSRIs are absorbed slowly and reach peak plasma levels after about 4–8 hours, although citalopram and escitalopram are absorbed more quickly. The half-lives of citalopram, escitalopram, fluvoxamine, paroxetine, and sertraline are between 20 and 30 hours, whereas the half-life of fluoxetine is 48–72 hours. The SSRIs are primarily eliminated by hepatic metabolism. Fluoxetine is metabolized to norfluoxetine, which is also a potent 5-HT uptake blocker and has a half-life of

7–9 days. Sertraline is converted to desmethylsertraline, which has a half-life of 2–3 days and is 5–10 times less potent than the parent compound in inhibiting the reuptake of 5-HT. The contribution of desmethylsertraline to the antidepressant effect of sertraline during treatment is unclear.

Efficacy of SSRIs in depression

SSRIs have been extensively compared with placebo and with reference tricyclic antidepressants. The SSRIs are all *superior to placebo* and are *generally as effective as tricyclics* in the treatment of major depression. Most comparative studies have been of moderately depressed outpatients, and there has been concern that SSRIs may be less effective than conventional tricyclic antidepressants for more severely depressed patients, particularly inpatients (Anderson, 2003).

Unwanted effects of SSRIs

Side effects can be grouped as follows (see Table 25.6):

- *Gastrointestinal effects.* Nausea occurs in about 20% of patients, although it often resolves with continued administration. Other side effects include dyspepsia, bloating, flatulence, and diarrhoea. Over longer-term treatment weight gain can occur—most significantly with paroxetine.
- *Neuropsychiatric effects.* These include insomnia, daytime somnolence, agitation, tremor, restlessness, irritability, and headache. SSRIs have also been associated with seizures and mania, although they are less likely than tricyclics to cause the latter effects. Extrapyramidal side effects such as parkinsonism and akathisia have been reported, but are uncommon.
- *Other effects.* Sexual dysfunction, including ejaculatory delay and anorgasmia, is common during SSRI treatment. Sweating and dry mouth are also reported. Cardiovascular side effects are rare with SSRIs, but some reduction in pulse rate may occur, and postural hypotension has been reported. SSRIs have been associated with skin rashes and, rarely, a more generalized

allergic reaction with arthritis. SSRIs can cause low sodium states secondary to inappropriate antidiuretic hormone secretion, especially in the elderly. Elevation of liver enzymes can occur but is generally reversible on treatment withdrawal. *SSRIs may increase the risk of upper gastrointestinal bleeding,* particularly when combined with non-steroidal anti-inflammatory drugs or aspirin. Long-term use of SSRIs has been associated with an increased risk of osteoporotic fracture. Part of this risk probably stems from depression itself, but 5-HT mechanisms play a role in bone physiology, and SSRIs are associated with a greater risk of fracture than antidepressants with a low affinity for the 5-HT transporter (Verdel *et al.*, 2010).

SSRIs and suicidal behaviour

There have been anecdotal reports that SSRI treatment may be associated with hostile and suicidal behaviour. Meta-analyses of placebo and comparator controlled trials of SSRIs in adults have found no significant increase in *completed suicide* in SSRI-treated patients, and no difference in rates of *non-fatal suicidal behaviour* between patients taking SSRIs and those taking tricyclics.

Relative to placebo there may be a small risk that SSRIs can increase rates of *self-harm*, but in the largest meta-analysis, involving over 700 studies, the number needed to harm with SSRIs (759) was much greater than the number needed to treat (estimated to be between 4 and 7) (Gunnell *et al.*, 2005). Ecological studies, although difficult to control, show fairly consistently that SSRI prescription at a population level is associated with a decline in completed suicide (Isacsson *et al.*, 2010).

In adolescents and children the risk of self-harm with SSRIs might be greater. In a meta-analysis of 27 placebo-controlled trials in children and adolescents with a variety of diagnoses, including depression, Bridge *et al.* (2007) found no completed suicides but a small, significant increase in suicidal ideation and self-harm attempts with SSRIs compared with placebo (number needed to harm = 143). Again there are hints that, in adolescents, rates of SSRI prescribing at a population level may be

Table 25.6 **Side effects of SSRIs**

Gastrointestinal	*Common:* nausea, appetite loss, dry mouth, diarrhoea, constipation, dyspepsia *Uncommon:* vomiting, weight loss
Central nervous system	*Common:* headache, insomnia, dizziness, anxiety, fatigue, tremor, somnolence *Uncommon:* extrapyramidal reaction, seizures, mania
Other	*Common:* sweating, delayed orgasm, anorgasmia *Uncommon:* rash, bleeding, pharyngitis, dyspnoea, serum sickness, hyponatraemia, alopecia

inversely related to completed suicide, but this has been disputed (Gibbons *et al.*, 2007).

As noted above, SSRIs can cause agitation and restlessness early in treatment, and it is possible that in predisposed individuals this might trigger dangerous behaviour. An epidemiological study of depressed patients in primary care who received a first prescription for an antidepressant found no significant difference in rates of suicidal behaviour or completed suicide in patients taking SSRIs compared with those taking tricyclic antidepressants (Jick *et al.*, 2004). Noteworthy, however, was the fourfold increase in risk of attempted suicide seen with all antidepressants in the first 9 days of treatment, relative to the risk with longer-term treatment (greater than 90 days). In the small number of completed suicides, the relative risk in the first 9 days of treatment was increased almost 40-fold (Jick *et al.*, 2004).

There are a number of possible reasons for this important phenomenon. For example, depressed people may visit their doctor and start treatment when they are at a particularly low ebb. Thus it is possible that suicidal feelings and behaviour are important factors in bringing people into treatment in the first place. Alternatively, the observation may be a reflection of the traditional view that the greatest risk of suicidal behaviour occurs during the early stages of antidepressant treatment, because improvement in motor retardation precedes resolution of depressed mood. Whatever the explanation, it reinforces advice that patients should be closely monitored when starting antidepressant medication. Interestingly, a similar phenomenon of increased rates of self-harm has been reported in patients with depression in the early stages of psychological treatment (Simon and Savarino, 2007).

Interactions with other drugs

Pharmacodynamic interactions

The most serious interaction reported is where simultaneous administration of SSRIs and MAOIs has provoked a *5-HT toxicity syndrome* (the 'serotonin syndrome'), with agitation, hyperpyrexia, rigidity, myoclonus, coma, and death (for further details, see the section below on MAOIs). Other drugs that increase brain 5-HT function and that must therefore be used with caution in combination with SSRIs include lithium and tryptophan, which have been reported to be associated with mental state changes, myoclonus, and seizures.

Other medical drugs that have been implicated in the serotonin syndrome when combined with SSRIs include tramadol and linezolid. Serotonin toxicity can also occur if SSRIs are combined with 5-HT receptor agonists such as sumatriptan.

SSRIs may potentiate the induction of *extrapyramidal movement disorders* by antipsychotic drugs, although this effect could be partly due to a pharmacokinetic interaction whereby SSRIs increase plasma levels of certain antipsychotic drugs (see below). The risk of *gastrointestinal bleeding* is increased when SSRIs are combined with aspirin or non-steroidal anti-inflammatory drugs. The risk of clinically significant bleeding is also elevated with combined administration of SSRIs and anticoagulants such as warfarin.

Pharmacokinetic interactions

Some SSRIs, particularly fluvoxamine, fluoxetine, and paroxetine, can produce substantial inhibition of hepatic cytochrome P450 enzymes, and can decrease the metabolism of several other drugs, thereby elevating their plasma levels (see Table 25.7). Examples where clinically important reactions have been reported include tricyclic antidepressants, antipsychotic agents (including clozapine and risperidone), anticonvulsants, and warfarin. *Citalopram, escitalopram*, and *sertraline* cause fewer reactions of this nature.

The clinical use of SSRIs in depression

Whether meta-analyses reveal clinically important differences in efficacy between SSRIs has been disputed (Gartlehner *et al.*, 2008; Cipriani *et al.*, 2009). However, there are significant differences in pharmacokinetic profile, which have a bearing on the likelihood of a withdrawal syndrome and the potential for drug interactions (see Table 25.8).

Fluvoxamine appears to have *higher dropout rates* from trials, and may be somewhat less well tolerated. *Fluoxetine* has the *most activating effect*, and also has a distinctive pharmacokinetic profile in relation to its *long-acting metabolite*, which has a half-life of about 1 week. On the one hand, this results in potential for troublesome *drug interactions* several weeks after fluoxetine has been stopped. For example, at least 5 weeks should elapse between stopping fluoxetine and starting an MAOI. On the other hand, this slow tapering of plasma concentration results in fluoxetine being the least likely of the SSRIs to cause a *withdrawal syndrome*.

Escitalopram is the active isomer of citalopram, and is marketed as being more effective than the parent compound, although whether any difference between the two drugs is of clinical significance is disputed. Both citalopram and escitalopram have been associated with prolongation of the QT interval and their maximum allowable doses lowered accordingly. *Paroxetine* appears to have the most troublesome withdrawal syndrome of the SSRIs (Table 25.8).

Table 25.7 Inhibition of P450 enzyme by SSRIs

	CYP 1A2	CYP 2D6	CYP 2C9	CYP 2C19	CYP 3A/4
Inhibitors	Fluvoxamine (+++)	Fluoxetine (+++)	Fluoxetine (+++)	Fluvoxamine (+++)	Fluvoxamine (++)
	Duloxetine (+)	Paroxetine (+++)	Fluvoxamine (+++)	Fluoxetine (++)	Fluoxetine (+)
		Duloxetine (++)			
		Sertraline (+)		Venlafaxine (+)	
		Citalopram (+)			
		Escitalopram (+)			
Some substrates (plasma level increased)	Olanzapine	Tricyclic antidepressants	Warfarin	Tricyclic antidepressants	Benzodiazepines
	Clozapine		Tolbutamide		Carbamazepine
	Haloperidol	Venlafaxine	Phenytoin	Diazepam	Quetiapine
	Tricyclic antidepressants	Haloperidol		Propranolol	Clozapine
		Thioridazine		Omeprazole	
	Theophylline	Risperidone			
		Clozapine			
		Olanzapine			

Inhibition: +, mild; ++, modest; +++, strong.

When treating depressive disorder, dosing with SSRIs is straightforward because the recommended starting dose is often sufficient to produce significant therapeutic benefit. Higher doses may be a little more effective but this is offset by a greater rate of treatment discontinuation due to side effects (Jakubovski *et al.*, 2015).

Patients who are starting SSRIs should be warned about the likely side effects, including nausea and some restlessness during sleep—a forewarned patient is more

Table 25.8 Differences between SSRIs

Drug	Risk of pharmacokinetic interaction[*]	Discontinuation syndrome	Other
Citalopram	+	+	Increases QT interval
Escitalopram	+	+	Increases QT interval
Fluoxetine	+++	0	Increased risk of agitation, slower onset of action
Fluvoxamine	+++	+++	Less well tolerated
Paroxetine	+++	+++	Weight gain
Sertraline	++	++	May have dopaminergic effects

[*] Based on inhibition of cytochrome P450 enzymes. See Table 25.7.
+, present; ++, common; +++, marked.

likely to continue with medication. A number of patients become more anxious and agitated early during SSRI treatment; therefore it is important to explain that such effects are sometimes experienced during treatment but do not mean that the underlying depression is worsening. If the patient persists with treatment, such anxiety and agitation usually diminish, but *short-term treatment with a benzodiazepine* may be helpful, particularly if sleep disturbance is a problem. Small doses of *trazodone* (50–150 mg) may also help sleep, although there are occasional reports of serotonin toxicity with this combination.

Patients should be *reviewed frequently* during the first few weeks of treatment, when support and advice are helpful both to maintain morale and to ensure compliance with medication. Often the clinician can detect improvements in rapport and initiative early in treatment. It can then be useful to discuss these changes with the patient.

When patients respond to SSRIs there is good evidence that *continuing treatment for at least 6 months* lowers the rate of relapse. In addition, placebo-controlled studies have shown that SSRIs are effective in the prophylaxis of recurrent depressive episodes. SSRIs should not be stopped suddenly, as there have been reports of *withdrawal reactions* (insomnia, nausea, agitation, and dizziness) after the cessation of treatment, particularly with paroxetine (for a review of antidepressant discontinuation syndromes, see Haddad and Anderson, 2007). Liquid preparations of SSRIs can facilitate a slow withdrawal, as can a switch to fluoxetine.

Tricyclic antidepressants

Tricyclic antidepressants continue to be useful agents because of their efficacy in severely ill depressed patients and those with treatment-refractory illness (Cowen and Anderson, 2015). At low doses tricyclics are still used widely for the treatment of neuropathic pain syndromes.

Pharmacology

Tricyclic antidepressants have a three-ringed structure with an attached side chain. A useful distinction is between compounds that have a terminal methyl group on the side chain (*tertiary amines*) and those that do not (*secondary amines*). In general, compared with the secondary amines, tertiary amines (e.g. amitriptyline, clomipramine, and imipramine) have a higher affinity for the 5-HT uptake site and are more potent antagonists of α_1-adrenoceptors and muscarinic cholinergic receptors. Therefore, in clinical use, tertiary amines are more sedating and cause more anticholinergic effects than secondary amines (e.g. desipramine and nortriptyline).

Tricyclic antidepressants inhibit the reuptake of both 5-HT and noradrenaline. They also have *antagonist*

activities at a variety of neurotransmitter receptors. In general, these receptor-blocking actions have been thought to cause adverse effects (see Table 25.9), although some investigators have argued that the ability of some tricyclic antidepressants to antagonize brain 5-HT_2 receptors may also mediate some of their therapeutic effects. Tricyclics have quinidine-like *membrane-stabilizing effects*, and this may explain why they impair cardiac conduction and cause high toxicity in overdose.

Pharmacokinetics

Tricyclic antidepressants are well absorbed from the gastrointestinal tract, and peak plasma levels occur 2–4 hours after ingestion. Tricyclics are subject to significant first-pass metabolism in the liver and are highly protein-bound. The free fraction is widely distributed in body tissues. In general, the elimination half-life of tricyclics is such that it is unnecessary to give them more than once daily.

Tricyclics are metabolized in the liver by hydroxylation and demethylation. It is noteworthy that demethylation of tricyclics with a tertiary amine structure gives rise to significant plasma concentrations of the corresponding secondary amine. There can be substantial (10- to 40-fold) differences in plasma tricyclic antidepressant levels between individual subjects when fixed-dose regimens are employed. Despite this, plasma level monitoring does not have a clearly established role in the use of tricyclics. Plasma measures have been suggested to be helpful for safety reasons when high doses of tricyclics are employed, but ECG monitoring is probably more useful (Taylor *et al.*, 2015).

Compounds available

These include amitriptyline, clomipramine, desipramine dosulepin, doxepin, imipramine, lofepramine, nortriptyline, and trimipramine. Clomipramine and lofepramine are sufficiently distinct from amitriptyline and imipramine to warrant separate mention.

Clomipramine is the most potent of the tricyclic antidepressants in inhibiting the reuptake of 5-HT. However, its secondary amine metabolite, desmethylclomipramine, is an effective noradrenaline reuptake inhibitor. In studies of depressed inpatients, the antidepressant effect of clomipramine was found to be superior to that of the SSRIs citalopram and paroxetine (Clear *et al.*, 2015). Unlike other tricyclic antidepressants, clomipramine is also useful in ameliorating the symptoms of *obsessive–compulsive disorder* (whether or not there is a coexisting major depressive disorder).

Lofepramine is a tertiary amine which is metabolized to desipramine. However, during lofepramine treatment, desipramine levels are probably too low to contribute

Table 25.9 **Some adverse effects of tricyclic antidepressants**

Pharmacological action	Adverse effect
Muscarinic-receptor blockade (anticholinergic)	Dry mouth, tachycardia, blurred vision, glaucoma, constipation, urinary retention, sexual dysfunction, cognitive impairment
α_1-Adrenoceptor blockade	Drowsiness, postural hypotension, sexual dysfunction, cognitive impairment
Histamine H_1 receptor blockade	Drowsiness, weight gain
Membrane-stabilizing properties	Cardiac conduction defects, cardiac arrhythmias, epileptic seizures

significantly to the therapeutic effect. Lofepramine is a fairly selective inhibitor of noradrenaline reuptake, and has fewer anticholinergic and antihistaminic properties than amitriptyline. Lofepramine has been widely compared with other tricyclic antidepressants, and in general its antidepressant efficacy appears to be equivalent (Anderson, 2003).

The most important feature of lofepramine is that, unlike conventional tricyclic antidepressants, *it is not cardiotoxic in overdose.* This means that it is likely to be safer than other tricyclics for patients with cardiovascular disease, although caution is still recommended. There have been reports of *hepatitis* in association with lofepramine, but it is not clear whether the incidence is higher than with other tricyclic antidepressants.

Unwanted effects of tricyclic antidepressants

These are numerous and important (see Tables 25.5 and 25.9).

- *Anticholinergic effects.* These include dry mouth, disturbance of accommodation, difficulty in micturition, leading to retention, constipation, leading rarely to ileus, postural hypotension, tachycardia, and increased sweating. Retention of urine, especially in elderly men with enlarged prostates, and worsening of glaucoma are the most serious of these effects; dry mouth and accommodation difficulties are the most common.

- *Psychiatric effects.* These include tiredness and drowsiness with amitriptyline and other sedative compounds, insomnia with desipramine and lofepramine, and acute organic syndromes. Mania may be provoked

in patients with bipolar disorders and generally tricyclics are not recommended for patients with bipolar illness (see Chapter 10).

- *Cardiovascular effects.* Tachycardia and postural hypotension occur commonly. The electrocardiogram frequently shows prolongation of PR and QT intervals, depressed ST segments, and flattened T-waves. Ventricular arrhythmias and heart block develop occasionally, more often in patients with pre-existing heart disease.

- *Neurological effects.* These include fine tremor (commonly), incoordination, headache, muscle twitching, epileptic seizures in predisposed patients, and, rarely, peripheral neuropathy.

- *Other effects.* Allergic skin rashes, cholestatic jaundice, and, rarely, agranulocytosis; weight gain and sexual dysfunction are also common.

- *Withdrawal effects.* Tricyclic antidepressants should be withdrawn slowly if at all possible. Sudden cessation may be followed by nausea, anxiety, sweating, gastrointestinal symptoms, and insomnia with vivid dreaming.

Toxic effects

In overdosage, tricyclic antidepressants produce a large number of effects, some of which are extremely serious. Therefore urgent expert treatment in a general hospital is required, but the psychiatrist should know the main signs of overdosage. These can be listed as follows. The cardiovascular effects include *ventricular fibrillation, conduction disturbances*, and *low blood pressure.* Heart rate may be increased or decreased depending partly on the degree of conduction disturbance. Sedation and coma lead to *respiratory depression.* The resulting hypoxia increases the likelihood of cardiac complications. Aspiration pneumonia may develop. In practice most patients need only supportive care, but cardiac monitoring is important, and arrhythmias require urgent treatment by a physician in an intensive care unit.

Interactions with other drugs

- Tricyclic antidepressants antagonize the hypotensive effects of α_2-adrenoceptor agonists such as clonidine, but can be safely combined with thiazides and angiotensin-converting enzyme (ACE) inhibitors.

- The ability of tricyclics to block noradrenaline reuptake can lead to hypertension with systemically administered noradrenaline and adrenaline.

- Tricyclics should not be used in conjunction with antiarrhythmic drugs, particularly amiodarone. Tricyclics increase the QT interval and should not be given with other psychotropic or general medical drugs that can produce a similar effect, for example, pimozide, astemizole, erythromycin, clarithromycin, diphenhydramine, and tamoxifen.

- Plasma levels of tricyclics can be increased by numerous other drugs, including cimetidine, sodium valproate, calcium-channel blockers, and SSRIs. Tricyclics may increase the action of warfarin. Interactions of tricyclic drugs with MAOIs are considered later.

Contraindications

Contraindications include agranulocytosis, severe liver damage, glaucoma, prostatic hypertrophy, uncontrolled epilepsy, and significant cardiovascular disease. Tricyclics must be used cautiously in epileptic patients and in the elderly.

Clinical use of tricyclic antidepressants

It is probably sufficient to be familiar with one sedating compound (e.g. amitriptyline) and one less sedating drug (e.g. nortriptyline). Other tricyclics can then be reserved for special purposes. For example, lofepramine can be used for patients who present a risk of overdose, while clomipramine can be reserved for patients in whom a depressive disorder is related to obsessive–compulsive disorder.

The prescribing of amitriptyline can be taken as an example. At the outset it is important to explain to the patient that, although side effects may be noticed early in treatment, any significant improvement in mood may be delayed for a week or more, and therefore it is important to persist. Early signs of improvement may include better sleep and a lessening of tension.

The usual practice of starting with a *low dose* of amitriptyline and building up is probably wise, because side effects are generally milder and the patient is more likely to develop tolerance to them. The starting dose will depend to some extent on the patient's age, weight, physical condition, and history of previous exposure to tricyclics; daily doses of 25–50 mg for an outpatient and 50–75 mg for an inpatient would be reasonable. The whole dose can be given at night about 1–2 hours before bedtime, because the sedative effects of the drug will aid sleep.

The dose of amitriptyline to be aimed for is about 125 mg daily or above. With careful monitoring and encouragement, this dose can usually be reached over a period of 2–4 weeks. Whether lower doses of tricyclics are effective in less severe depressive states in primary care is still debated.

In some patients, *side effects* limit the rate of dosage increase, but if there is clinical improvement it is reasonable to settle for lower doses. In general, side effects should not be greater than the patient can comfortably tolerate. For patients who show little or no improvement, it is usually advisable to continue amitriptyline for 4 weeks at the maximum tolerated dose before deciding that the drug is ineffective.

Some patients respond only to *higher doses* (up to 300 mg daily), and cautious increases towards this level are warranted in patients with resistant depression provided that the side effects are tolerable. In doses above 225 mg daily, it is wise to *monitor* the *ECG* before each further dosage increase.

In the ECG it is important to note any evidence of impaired cardiac conduction—for example, *lengthening of the QT interval* and the appearance of bundle branch block or arrhythmias. Because of the half-life of amitriptyline, each dose increase will take about a week to reach steady state. If the patient has not improved, and if they cannot tolerate an increase in dose or fail to respond to higher doses, other treatments should be considered. Some possible strategies are outlined in Chapter 9 (see page 228).

Maintenance and prophylaxis

If patients respond to amitriptyline, they should be maintained on treatment for *at least 6 months*, as continuation therapy greatly reduces the risk of early relapse. The same dose of amitriptyline should be maintained if possible, but if side effects become a problem the dose can be lowered until tolerance is again satisfactory.

It is often not clear when antidepressant drug treatment should be withdrawn, because in some patients depression is a recurrent disorder. Long-term prophylactic treatment may then be justified. Obviously the risk of recurrence increases with the number of episodes that the patient suffers, but other clinical and biochemical predictors of relapse are not well established (see Chapter 9).

Monoamine oxidase inhibitors

MAOIs were introduced just before the tricyclic antidepressants, but their use has been less widespread because of both troublesome *interactions with foods and drugs* and uncertainty about their *therapeutic efficacy*. However, in adequate doses MAOIs are useful antidepressants, often producing clinical benefit in depressed patients who have not responded to other medication or ECT. In addition, MAOIs can be useful in *refractory anxiety states* (Baldwin *et al.*, 2014; Cowen and Anderson, 2015).

These beneficial effects have to be weighed against the need to adhere to *strict dietary and drug restrictions* to avoid reactions with tyramine and other sympathomimetic agents. In practice this means that conventional MAOIs are used only in patients who failed to respond to multiple other treatments.

Pharmacological properties

MAOIs inactivate enzymes that oxidize noradrenaline, 5-HT, dopamine, and tyramine, and other amines that are widely distributed in the body as transmitters, or are taken in food and drink or as drugs. Monoamine oxidase (MAO) exists in a number of forms that differ in their substrate and inhibitor specificities. From the point of view of psychotropic drug treatment, it is important to recognize that there are two forms of MAO—type A and type B—which are encoded by separate genes. In general, *MAO-A* metabolizes intraneuronal noradrenaline and 5-HT, whereas both MAO-A and MAO-B metabolize dopamine and tyramine.

Compounds available

Phenelzine is the most widely used and widely studied compound. *Isocarboxazid* is reported to have fewer side effects than phenelzine, and can be useful for patients who respond to the latter drug but suffer from its side effects of hypotension or sleep disorder. *Tranylcypromine* differs from the other compounds in combining the ability to inhibit MAO with an *amphetamine-like stimulating effect*, which may be helpful in patients with anergia and retardation. However, some patients have become dependent on the stimulant effect of tranylcypromine. Moreover, compared with phenelzine, tranylcypromine is more likely to give rise to hypertensive crises, although it is less likely to damage the liver. For these reasons, tranylcypromine should be prescribed with particular caution.

Moclobemide differs from the other compounds in *selectively binding* to MAO-A, which it inhibits in a *reversible* way. This results in a lack of significant interactions with foodstuffs, and a quick offset of action (see below).

Pharmacokinetics

Phenelzine, isocarboxazid, and tranylcypromine are rapidly absorbed and widely distributed. They have short half-lives (about 2–4 hours), as they are quickly metabolized in the liver by acetylation, oxidation, and deamination. People differ in their capacity to acetylate drugs. For example, in the UK, approximately 60% of the population are 'fast acetylators', who would be expected to metabolize hydrazine MAOIs more quickly than 'slow acetylators'. Some studies have shown a better clinical response to phenelzine in 'slow acetylators', but this finding has not been consistently replicated. However, it may underlie the observation that the best response rate with MAOIs occurs in studies that have used *higher dose ranges*, presumably because even patients who metabolize MAOIs quickly will receive an adequate dose.

Phenelzine, isocarboxazid, and tranylcypromine bind irreversibly to MAO-A and MAO-B by means of a covalent linkage. This means that the enzyme is permanently deactivated and MAO activity can be restored only when new enzyme is synthesized. Thus, despite their short half-lives, irreversible MAOIs cause a *long-lasting inhibition of MAO*.

In contrast to these compounds, moclobemide binds reversibly to MAO-A. This compound has a short half-life (about 2 hours), and therefore its inhibition of MAO-A is brief, declining to some extent even during the latter periods of a three times daily dosing regimen. Full MAO activity is restored within 24 hours of stopping moclobemide, whereas with the irreversible MAOIs, a period of 2 weeks or more may be needed for synthesis of new MAO.

Efficacy of MAOIs in depression

For many years MAOIs were in relative disuse because several studies, in particular a large controlled trial by the Medical Research Council (Clinical Psychiatry Committee, 1965), found phenelzine to be no more effective than placebo in the treatment of depressive disorders. It seems likely that the doses of MAOIs were too low in these early investigations; in the Medical Research Council study the maximum dose of phenelzine was 45 mg daily, in contrast to the current practice of using doses of up to 90 mg daily if side effects permit. Subsequent studies have shown that in this wider dose range MAOIs are *superior to placebo* and are *generally equivalent to tricyclic antidepressants* in their therapeutic activity (Cleare *et al.*, 2015).

Unwanted effects

These include dry mouth, difficulty in micturition, postural hypotension, confusion, mania, headache, dizziness, tremor, paraesthesia of the hands and feet, constipation, and oedema of the ankles. Hydrazine compounds can give rise to hepatocellular jaundice (see Box 25.7).

Interactions with foodstuffs

Some foods contain *tyramine*, a substance that is normally inactivated by MAO in the liver and the gut wall. When MAO is inhibited, tyramine is not broken down and is free to exert its *hypertensive effects*. These effects are due to release of noradrenaline from sympathetic nerve terminals with a consequent elevation in blood pressure. This may reach dangerous levels and may occasionally result in *subarachnoid haemorrhage*. Important early symptoms of such a crisis include a severe and usually throbbing headache.

Box 25.7 Adverse effects of MAOIs

Central nervous system

Insomnia, drowsiness, agitation, headache, fatigue, weakness, tremor, mania, confusion

Autonomic nervous system

Blurred vision, difficulty in micturition, sweating, dry mouth, postural hypotension, constipation

Other

Sexual dysfunction, weight gain, peripheral neuropathy (pyridoxine deficiency), oedema, rashes, hepatocellular toxicity (rare), leucopenia (rare)

The incidence of hypertensive reactions is about 10% in patients who are taking MAOIs, even in those who have received dietary counselling. Therefore regular reminders about dietary restrictions may be helpful, particularly in patients on longer-term treatment (see Box 25.8). There have been reports of a wide range of foods being implicated in hypertensive reactions with MAOIs, but many of these have cited single cases and therefore are of uncertain validity. Another complication is that the tyramine content of a particular food item may vary, as may the susceptibility of an individual patient to a hypertensive reaction. If a forbidden food has been consumed on one occasion without adverse effects, this does not preclude a future reaction.

Box 25.8 Foods to be avoided during MAOI use

- All cheeses except cream, cottage, and ricotta cheeses
- Red wine, sherry, beer, and liquors
- Pickled or smoked fish
- Brewer's yeast products (e.g. Marmite, Bovril, and some packet soups)
- Broad bean pods (e.g. Italian green beans)
- Beef or chicken liver
- Fermented sausage (e.g. bologna, pepperoni, salami)
- Unfresh, overripe, or aged food (e.g. pheasant, venison, unfresh dairy products)

It is notable that about 80% of all reported reactions between foodstuffs and MAOIs, and nearly all of the deaths, have followed the *consumption of cheese*. Hypertensive reactions should be treated with parenteral administration of an α_1-adrenoceptor antagonist, such as *phentolamine*. If this drug is not available, *chlorpromazine* can be used. The use of oral *nifedipine* has also been advocated. Whatever treatment is given, blood pressure must be monitored carefully.

Moclobemide and tyramine reactions

Tyramine is metabolized by both MAO-A and MAO-B. Experimental studies have shown that the hypertensive effect of oral tyramine is potentiated *much less by moclobemide* than by non-selective MAOIs. In patients who are taking moclobemide in doses of up to 900 mg daily, the dose of tyramine required to produce a significant pressor response is above 100 mg. Even a five-course meal with red wine would be unlikely to result in a tyramine intake of more than 40 mg.

Tyramine has relatively little effect in patients who are receiving moclobemide because MAO-B (present in the gut wall and the liver) is still available to metabolize much of the tyramine ingested. Another factor may be that the interaction between moclobemide and MAO-A is reversible, thus allowing displacement of moclobemide from MAO when tyramine is present in excess.

Interactions with drugs

Patients who are taking MAOIs must not be given drugs whose metabolism depends on enzymes that are affected by the MAOI. These drugs include *sympathomimetic amines* such as *adrenaline, noradrenaline,* and *amphetamine*, as well as *phenylpropanolamine* and *ephedrine* (which may be present in proprietary cold cures). *L-Dopa* and *dopamine* may also cause hypertensive reactions. Local anaesthetics often contain a sympathomimetic amine, which should also be avoided. Some *opiates* (particularly *pethidine, tramadol,* and *fentanyl*), as well as *cocaine*, and *insulin* can be involved in dangerous interactions. Sensitivity to *oral antidiabetic* drugs is increased, with a consequent risk of hypoglycaemia. The ability of MAOIs to cause postural hypotension can increase the hypotensive effects of other agents. Finally, the metabolism of carbamazepine, phenytoin, and other drugs that are broken down in the liver may be slowed.

The serotonin syndrome. A number of drugs that potentiate brain 5-HT function can produce a severe *neurotoxicity syndrome* when combined with MAOIs. The main features of this syndrome are listed in Box 25.9. It is worth noting that some of these

> ## Box 25.9 Clinical features of the serotonin syndrome
>
> ### Neurological
>
> Myoclonus, nystagmus, headache, tremor, rigidity, seizures
>
> ### Mental state
>
> Irritability, confusion, agitation, hypomania, coma
>
> ### Other
>
> Hyperpyrexia, sweating, diarrhoea, cardiac arrhythmias, death

symptoms resemble the neuroleptic malignant syndrome with which 5-HT neurotoxicity is occasionally confused. In view of the interactions between dopamine and 5-HT pathways, it is possible that similar mechanisms may be involved.

Current clinical data indicate that combination of *MAOIs* with *SSRIs, venlafaxine,* and *clomipramine* is contraindicated. The combination of MAOIs with *L-tryptophan* has also been reported to cause 5-HT toxicity. Adverse reactions have been reported between the 5-HT$_{1A}$ receptor agonist, *buspirone,* and MAOIs. In addition, the use of 5-HT$_1$ receptor agonists, such as *sumatriptan,* should be avoided. If used with caution, the combination of *lithium* with MAOIs appears to be safe, and it can be effective in patients with resistant depression.

If a 5-HT syndrome develops, all medication should be stopped and supportive measures instituted. In theory, drugs with 5-HT-receptor-antagonist properties such as cyproheptadine or propranolol may be helpful, but controlled studies have not been carried out. For a review of the serotonin syndrome, see Gillman and Whyte (2004).

Combination of MAOIs with tricyclic antidepressants. The combined use of MAOIs and tricyclic antidepressants fell into disuse because of the severe reactions associated with the 5-HT syndrome. Current views are that combination therapy is safe provided that the following rules are observed:

- Clomipramine and imipramine are not used. The most favoured tricyclics in combination with MAOIs are amitriptyline and trimipramine.
- The MAOI and tricyclic are started together at low dosage, or the MAOI is added to the tricyclic (adding tricyclics to MAOIs is more likely to provoke dizziness and postural hypotension).

The advantages and disadvantages of combined tricyclic and MAOI therapy have not been fully established. On the one hand, patients who are taking tricyclics with MAOIs are less likely to suffer from *MAOI-induced insomnia*, but on the other hand, they are more likely to experience *postural hypotension* and troublesome *weight gain*. The combination is said to be useful in patients with *resistant depression*. Although formal studies have not been carried out in this patient group, there are case reports of patients for whom combined MAOI and tricyclic treatment was successful when either treatment alone had not been helpful. Low doses of *trazodone* (50–150 mg) are also used to ameliorate MAOI-induced insomnia; present experience suggests that this combination is generally well tolerated, although there are occasional reports of adverse effects that could represent serotonin toxicity.

Contraindications

These include liver disease, phaeochromocytoma, congestive cardiac failure, and conditions that require the patient to take any of the drugs that react with MAOIs.

Clinical use of MAOIs in depression

The clinical use of phenelzine can be taken as an example. Treatment should start with 15 mg daily, increasing to 30 mg daily in divided doses (with the final dose taken not later than 3.00 pm) in the first week. Patients should be given *clear written instructions about foods to be avoided* (see below), and should be warned to take no other medication unless it has been specifically checked with a pharmacist or doctor who knows that the patient is taking MAOIs. As always, patients should be warned about the delay in therapeutic response (up to 6 weeks) and about common side effects (sleep disturbance and dizziness).

In the second week, the dose of phenelzine can be increased to 45 mg daily. At this stage a greater increase to 60 mg may produce a quicker response, but is also associated with more adverse effects. Accordingly, if feasible, it is better to find out whether an individual patient will respond to lower doses (about 45 mg) before increments are made (up to 90 mg daily). If the patient does not respond to 45 mg, the dose can be increased by 15 mg weekly if side effects permit.

The response to MAOIs can often be sudden; over the course of a day or two the patient suddenly feels better. If there are signs of *overactivity* or *excessive buoyancy* in mood, the dose can be reduced and the patient monitored for signs of developing hypomania. Side effects that are likely to be particularly troublesome are insomnia and postural hypotension. Insomnia is best managed by lowering the dose of MAOI, if feasible. Otherwise, the addition of a benzodiazepine or trazodone (50–150 mg at night) can be helpful, although the latter drug can sometimes increase problems of dizziness and postural hypotension.

Postural hypotension can be a disabling problem with MAOIs. Again, dose reduction is worth considering. Various measures have been suggested—for example, the use of support stockings, an increase in salt intake, or even the use of a mineralocorticoid. Of course, the latter two measures have their own adverse effects.

Withdrawal from MAOIs

Patients who respond to MAOIs have often suffered from disabling depression for many months or even years. For such patients the usual practice is to continue therapy for at least 6 months to a year. With MAOIs, it is wise to lower the dose if the patient can tolerate the reduction without relapsing. Sudden cessation of MAOIs can lead to *anxiety* and *dysphoria*. Even gradual withdrawal can be associated with increasing anxiety and depression.

Clinical experience indicates that it is more difficult to stop MAOI than tricyclic antidepressant treatment. An explanation for this difference may be that MAOIs produce a more severe discontinuation syndrome than other antidepressants; another possible explanation is that MAOIs are given to patients with chronic disabling disorders who frequently relapse. It is emphasized that, because of the time taken to synthesize new MAO, *2 weeks should elapse* between the cessation of irreversible MAOI treatment and the easing of dietary and drug restrictions.

Moclobemide

In their freedom from tyramine reactions and their quick offset of activity, reversible type A MAOIs, such as *moclobemide*, have clear advantages over conventional MAOIs. However, the therapeutic efficacy of moclobemide, particularly in more severely depressed patients, is not as well established. Also, it is not clear that moclobemide is effective for patients with the various forms of atypical depression and drug-resistant depression for which conventional MAOIs can be useful (Cleare *et al.*, 2015).

The starting dose of moclobemide is 150–300 mg daily, which can be increased to 600 mg over a number of weeks. Treatment-resistant patients may require higher doses, but above levels of 900 mg daily it is prudent to institute the usual MAOI dietary restrictions. Moclobemide is better tolerated than tricyclic antidepressants or irreversible MAOIs, but side effects such as

nausea, insomnia, and agitation occur in about 20–30% of patients.

Drug interactions of moclobemide

Moclobemide should not be combined with *SSRIs, venlafaxine*, or *clomipramine* because a serotonin syndrome may result. Caution is needed with *sumatriptan*. Like the irreversible MAOIs, moclobemide may react adversely with some *opiates*. Similarly, moclobemide may potentiate the pressor effects of *sympathomimetic amines*; therefore combined use should be avoided. Moclobemide should not be combined with *L-dopa* because of the risk of hypertensive crisis. *Cimetidine* delays the metabolism of moclobemide.

Other antidepressant drugs

Other antidepressant drugs are available for use in the UK and other countries. Their mechanism of action is such that they cannot easily be grouped with SSRIs, tricyclic antidepressants, or MAOIs. These drugs also have differing adverse-event profiles. Therefore they are discussed individually below.

Agomelatine

Agomelatine is a more recently licensed antidepressant which is a melatonin receptor agonist and a somewhat weaker antagonist at 5-HT$_{2C}$ receptors. The mechanism of antidepressant action of agomelatine is not established, but could be mediated through a melatonin-like action on circadian rhythms. It is also possible that 5-HT$_{2C}$-receptor blockade might lead to increased dopamine release in the prefrontal cortex, though whether agomelatine blocks 5-HT$_{2C}$ receptors at clinically used doses is unclear (Whiting and Cowen, 2013).

Pharmacokinetics

Agomelatine is rapidly absorbed, reaching maximum levels within 1–2 hours of ingestion. However, it has a high first-pass metabolism, with a bioavailability of only 5–10%. It has a short half-life of about 2 hours and no metabolites likely to contribute to its therapeutic action.

Efficacy

Controlled trials indicate that agomelatine appears comparable in efficacy to venlafaxine and paroxetine, although the doses of the latter agents were relatively modest. However, efficacy relative to placebo is somewhat equivocal and long-term efficacy in terms of relapse prevention is not well established (Koesters *et al.*, 2013). In clinical trials, agomelatine was dosed once-daily at 9.00 pm, which is sufficiently in advance of the endogenous night-time melatonin peak to produce effects on circadian rhythm. Therefore it seems sensible when prescribing agomelatine to use the same treatment schedule.

Unwanted effects

The most common adverse effects of agomelatine are *nausea* and *dizziness*. Agomelatine is not sedating, but some patients experience *somnolence*, and *insomnia* has also been reported. Other possible side effects include *anxiety and fatigue, diarrhoea*, and *constipation*. *Sexual dysfunction* is less frequent than with SSRIs. The most serious potential adverse effect of agomelatine is an increase in liver enzymes (ALT and AST), with a rate of 1.4% and 2.5% in agomelatine-treated patients (25 mg and 50 mg, respectively) compared with 0.6% in patients taking placebo. For this reason, treatment with agomelatine should be preceded by measurement of liver function tests, which should be repeated after approximately at 3, 6, 12, and 24 weeks. Any clinical suspicion of impaired hepatic function should be followed by urgent liver function tests, and treatment with agomelatine should be stopped if the results are abnormal.

Drug interactions

The main interaction of agomelatine is with drugs that inhibit the hepatic microsomal enzymes, CYP1A2 and CYP2C9/19. This is because these enzymes metabolize agomelatine, and higher blood levels of agomelatine are likely to increase the risk of hepatic dysfunction. Therefore agomelatine should not be given with potent CYP1A2 inhibitors such as fluvoxamine and ciprofloxacin. Coadministration of agomelatine with more moderate inhibitors (oestrogens, propranolol, and grepafloxacin) should be employed with caution.

Mirtazapine

Mirtazapine is a quadricyclic compound with complex pharmacological actions. It is a fairly potent antagonist at several 5-HT-receptor subtypes, particularly 5-HT$_2$ and 5-HT$_3$ receptors. Mirtazapine is also a competitive antagonist at histamine H$_1$ receptors and α_1- and α_2-adrenoceptors. The latter action leads to an increase in noradrenaline cell firing and release. Mirtazapine is not a muscarinic cholinergic antagonist and is not cardiotoxic. Because of these various actions, mirtazapine has a *sedating profile*, but it is not anticholinergic and is relatively *safe in overdose*.

Pharmacokinetics

Mirtazapine is well absorbed, with peak plasma levels being reached between 1 and 2 hours. The half-life is about 16 hours, and the daily dose can be given at night. Mirtazapine is extensively metabolized by the liver, and has only minor inhibitory effects on cytochrome P450 isoenzymes.

Efficacy

Mirtazapine has demonstrated clinical efficacy in both *placebo-controlled and comparator trials* with SSRIs and tricyclic antidepressants in moderate to severely depressed patients. The effective dose is usually between 10 mg and 45 mg daily.

Unwanted effects

The common adverse effects of mirtazapine are attributable to its potent antihistaminic actions, and include *drowsiness* and *dry mouth*. *Increased appetite* and *body weight* are also common. Thus far leucopenia does not appear to be more common with mirtazapine than with other antidepressants. However, the data sheet recommends that physicians be vigilant for possible signs that might reflect low white cell count.

Drug interactions

Mirtazapine may potentiate other centrally acting sedatives. There is a theoretical risk that mirtazapine could reverse the therapeutic effect of α_2-adrenoceptor agonists such as clonidine.

Trazodone

Trazodone is a triazolopyridine derivative with complex actions on 5-HT pathways. Studies *in vitro* suggest that trazodone has some weak 5-HT-reuptake-inhibiting properties, which are probably not manifested during clinical use; for example, repeated administration of trazodone does not lower platelet 5-HT content.

Trazodone has antagonist actions at 5-HT$_2$ receptors, but its active metabolite, *m*-chlorophenylpiperazine (*m*-CPP), is a 5-HT receptor agonist. Therefore the precise balance of effects on 5-HT receptors during trazodone treatment is difficult to determine, and may depend on relative blood levels of the parent compound and metabolite. Trazodone also blocks postsynaptic α_1-adrenoceptors. Overall it has a distinct *sedating profile*.

Pharmacokinetics

Trazodone has a short half-life (about 4–14 hours). It is metabolized by hydroxylation and oxidation, with the formation of a number of metabolites, including *m*-CPP. During treatment, plasma levels of *m*-CPP may exceed those of trazodone itself.

Efficacy

Several controlled studies have shown that trazodone in doses of 150–600 mg is *superior to placebo* in the treatment of depressed patients. Trazodone also appears to have equivalent antidepressant activity to reference compounds such as imipramine. Many of these studies were carried out in moderately depressed outpatients, and the efficacy of trazodone relative to other antidepressants in more severely ill patients is not well established (Anderson, 2003).

Some have maintained that the efficacy of trazodone is improved if treatment is started at low doses (50 mg) and increased slowly to 300 mg over 2–3 weeks. Despite the short half-life of trazodone, once-daily adminstration of the drug is often sufficient. The drug is usually given in the evening to take advantage of its sedative properties. Doses above 300 mg daily are usually better given in divided amounts. Lower doses (50–150 mg) are sometimes used in combination with SSRIs and MAOIs to ameliorate the sleep-disrupting effects of the latter agents.

Unwanted effects

The major unwanted effect of trazodone is *excessive sedation*, which can result in significant cognitive impairment. *Nausea* and *dizziness* are also reported, particularly if the drug is taken on an empty stomach. The α_1-adrenoceptor-antagonist properties of trazodone may *lower blood pressure* to some extent, and postural hypotension has been reported. Trazodone is less cardiotoxic than conventional tricyclics, but there are reports that *cardiac arrhythmias* may be worsened in patients with cardiac disease. Nevertheless, trazodone is less toxic in overdose than tricyclic antidepressants.

The most serious side effect of trazodone is *priapism*. This reaction is seen rarely (about 1 in 6000 male patients). It can cause considerable problems, requiring the local injection of noradrenaline agonists such as adrenaline, or even surgical decompression. Long-term sexual dysfunction has sometimes resulted. It is recommended that male patients be warned of this potential side effect and advised to seek medical help urgently if persistent erection occurs.

Drug interactions

As with all sedative antidepressants, trazodone may potentiate the sedating effects of alcohol and other central tranquillizing drugs. Studies in animals have raised the possibility that trazodone could attenuate the hypotensive effect of clonidine, but it is not known whether such an interaction occurs in humans.

Venlafaxine

Venlafaxine is a phenylethylamine derivative which produces a *potent blockade of 5-HT reuptake*, with lesser effects on noradrenaline reuptake, which probably only become apparent at higher doses. In this respect the pharmacological properties of venlafaxine resemble those of clomipramine to some extent. However, unlike clomipramine and other tricyclic antidepressants, venlafaxine has a negligible affinity for other neurotransmitter receptor sites, and so lacks sedative and anticholinergic effects. Because of these pharmacological properties, venlafaxine has been classified as a *selective serotonin and noradrenaline reuptake inhibitor (SNRI)*.

Pharmacokinetics

Venlafaxine is well absorbed, achieving peak plasma levels about 1.5–2 hours after oral administration. The half-life of venlafaxine is 3–7 hours, but it is metabolized to desmethylvenlafaxine, which has essentially the same pharmacodynamic properties as the parent compound and a half-life of 8–13 hours. The extended-release formulation of venlafaxine (venlafaxine XL) reaches a peak plasma level after about 6 hours. This gives a longer apparent half-life (about 15 hours), but the drug is still quickly eliminated. Once-daily dosing is possible with this preparation.

Efficacy

Venlafaxine has been studied in both inpatients and outpatients with major depression and compared with placebo and active comparators. Current studies suggest that it is more effective than placebo and of at least equal efficacy to other available antidepressant drugs, including tricyclic antidepressants. Some meta-analyses suggest that venlafaxine is more effective than SSRIs, particularly for more severely depressed patients, but the data are inconsistent (Cleare *et al.*, 2015).

Venlafaxine has a wider dosage range than SSRIs, from 75 to 375 mg daily in two divided doses, or up to 225 mg of the extended-release preparation given as a single dose. The usual starting dose of venlafaxine is 75 mg daily, which may be sufficient for many patients. Upward titration can be considered in cases where there is insufficient response.

Unwanted effects

The adverse-effect profile of venlafaxine resembles that of SSRIs, with the most common adverse effects being *nausea, headache, somnolence, dry mouth, dizziness*, and *insomnia. Anxiety* and *sexual dysfunction* may also occur. Venlafaxine occasionally causes *postural hypotension* but, in addition, dose-related *increases in blood pressure* can occur. Blood pressure monitoring is advisable in patients who are receiving more than 150 mg venlafaxine daily.

Overdoses of venlafaxine have been associated with cardiac arrhythmias, so it is probably prudent to avoid using venlafaxine in patients with significant cardiac disease. Like SSRIs, venlafaxine can lower plasma sodium levels. Venlafaxine may be somewhat less well tolerated than SSRIs (Cleare *et al.*, 2015).

Venlafaxine appears to be *more toxic than SSRIs* in acute overdose (Cheeta *et al.*, 2004), with a toxicity intermediate between that of conventional tricyclic antidepressants and SSRIs. Similarly to some SSRIs, sudden discontinuation of venlafaxine has been associated with troublesome symptoms of *fatigue, nausea, abdominal pain,* and *dizziness*. It is recommended that patients who have received venlafaxine for 6 weeks or more should have the dose reduced gradually over at least a 1-week period, and longer if possible.

Drug interactions

Unlike the SSRIs, venlafaxine appears to produce relatively modest effects on hepatic drug-metabolizing enzymes, and therefore should be less likely to inhibit the metabolism of coadministered drugs. Venlafaxine is metabolized partly by CYP34A4, and caution is recommended where venlafaxine is coprescribed with CYP3A4 inhibitors such as ketoconazole and clarithromycin. Like other drugs that potently inhibit the uptake of 5-HT, venlafaxine should not be given concomitantly with MAOIs because of the danger of a toxic serotonin syndrome. It is also recommended that 14 days should elapse after the end of MAOI treatment before venlafaxine is started, and that at least 7 days should elapse after venlafaxine cessation before MAOIs are given. As with SSRIs, venlafaxine should be used with caution in combination with other 5-HT promoting drugs (for example, lithium, triptans, and tramadol).

Duloxetine

Like venlafaxine, duloxetine is also classified as an SNRI. It is about five times more potent in inhibiting the reuptake of 5-HT than in inhibiting that of noradrenaline. It has little effect on other neurotransmitter receptors (Cowen *et al.*, 2005).

Pharmacokinetics

Duloxetine is well absorbed, with maximum blood levels occurring about 6 hours post ingestion. It has a half-life of about 12 hours. It is extensively metabolized to therapeutically inactive compounds.

Efficacy

Duloxetine given in a single dose of 60 mg daily has greater antidepressant efficacy than placebo, and is equivalent in therapeutic activity to SSRIs. Currently there is no consistent evidence that the efficacy of duloxetine is greater than that of SSRIs, or that it has a role in SSRI-resistant depression (Cipriani *et al.*, 2009).

Unwanted effects

The adverse-effect profile of duloxetine is similar to that seen with other 5-HT-promoting antidepressants, and includes *nausea, dry mouth, dizziness, gastrointestinal disturbances, insomnia, somnolence,* and *sexual dysfunction*. Like venlafaxine, duloxetine can increase blood pressure; there are few data on toxicity in overdose. As would be expected from its pharmacology and half-life, abrupt cessation of duloxetine is associated with troublesome dizziness, insomnia, anxiety, and headache (Cowen *et al.*, 2005).

Drug interactions

Duloxetine produces a moderate inhibition of CYP2D6 and, to a lesser extent, of CYP1A2. It is therefore likely to increase blood levels of other drugs that are metabolized by these enzymes (see Table 25.7). On the basis of its pharmacology, duloxetine should not be given concomitantly with MAOIs because of the danger of a toxic serotonin syndrome. For the same reason it seems advisable that 14 days should elapse after the end of MAOI treatment before duloxetine is started, and that at least 7 days should elapse after duloxetine cessation before MAOIs are given. Combination with drugs such as lithium, triptans, and tramadol should be approached with caution.

Vortioxetine

Vortioxetine is a recently licensed antidepressant which blocks the reuptake of 5-HT and also antagonizes a variety of 5-HT receptors, including the 5-HT_{1D}, 5-HT_3, and 5-HT_7 receptors, while acting as an agonist at 5-HT_{1A} receptors. Hence vortioxetine produces complex effects on 5-HT neurotransmission but probably overall leads to an increase in brain 5-HT function, particularly at postsynaptic 5-HT_{1A} receptors. At higher doses (20 mg) vortioxetine produces a similar occupancy of brain 5-HT transporter sites as standard therapeutic doses of SSRIs.

Pharmacokinetics

Vortioxetine is slowly absorbed, with peak plasma concentrations being reached between 7 and 11 hours. Vortioxetine is metabolized principally through CYP2D6 to an inactive metabolite. The half-life is about 65 hours. Poor CYP2D6 metabolizers (about 5–7% of the Caucasian population) have about a twofold increase in plasma vortioxetine levels.

Efficacy

Short-term studies show superior efficacy of vortioxetine relative to placebo at doses of 10–20 mg (Citrome, 2014), with a number needed to treat for clinical response of 7 and remission of 11. In one randomized study of patients who had failed to respond to first-line SSRI treatment, a switch to vortioxetine was superior to agomelatine (Montgomery *et al.*, 2014). A relapse prevention study over 1 year showed superiority of vortioxetine relative to placebo. It is claimed that vortioxetine has a particularly beneficial effect on depression-associated cognitive impairment, but systematic studies in comparison to SSRIs have yet to be carried out.

Unwanted effects

The main adverse effects of vortioxetine are *nausea, vomiting, diarrhea*, and *constipation. Dizziness, abnormal dreaming*, and *pruritis* are also reportedly common. At lower doses (10–15 mg) the incidence of sexual dysfunction appears less than that of other 5-HT reuptake blockers, but at 20 mg the advantage for vortioxetine is lost.

Drug interactions

Data are currently rather limited, but similar precautions as those taken with SSRIs are recommended. Accordingly, concomitant treatment with vortioxetine and MAOIs or within 2 weeks of stopping a conventional MAOI is contraindicated. As with other 5-HT reuptake blockers, caution is needed when vortioxetine is given to patients at increased risk of bleeding, through, for example, anticoagulant treatment or therapy with non-steroidal anti-inflammatory agents. Similarly, caution should be exercised when coadministering vortioxetine with other 5-HT potentiating agents such as tryptophan, lithium, triptans, and tramadol. Vortioxetine levels are likely to be increased by strong inhibitors of CYP2D6, such as ritonavir, bupropion, and quinidine.

Reboxetine

Reboxetine is a morpholine and is structurally related to fluoxetine. It is a *selective noradrenaline reuptake inhibitor (NARI)*, with no clinically significant effects on other neurotransmitter receptors.

Pharmacokinetics

After oral administration, reboxetine reaches peak plasma levels after about 2 hours. Its half-life is around 13 hours, and twice-daily administration is recommended. Reboxetine is metabolized by the liver, where it is a substrate for cytochrome P450 CYP3A.

Efficacy

Reboxetine reportedly shows efficacy in both *placebo-controlled trials* and against active comparators such as SSRIs. However, different meta-analyses have come to differing conclusions, and overall in moderately depressed outpatients reboxetine may be less effective than some other classes of antidepressants, including SSRIs (Cipriani *et al.*, 2009). It is claimed that reboxetine produces better improvement in social function in depressed patients than SSRIs, but this possibility has not been confirmed. The usual dose of reboxetine is 4 mg twice daily, with a maximum dose of 12 mg daily.

Unwanted effects

Despite its low affinity for muscarinic receptors, reboxetine produces adverse effects characteristic of cholinergic-receptor blockade, presumably through interactions of noradrenergic and cholinergic pathways. The most common side effects are *dry mouth, constipation, sweating*, and *insomnia. Urinary hesitancy, impotence, tachycardia*, and *vertigo* are also occasionally described.

Drug interactions

Limited information is available. It is recommended that reboxetine should not be given with other agents that might *potentiate noradrenaline function*, such as MAOIs, or that might increase blood pressure, such as ergot derivatives. Plasma reboxetine levels might be increased by drugs that inhibit cytochrome P450 3A4, such as some antifungal agents, fluvoxamine, and macrolide antibiotics.

L-Tryptophan

L-Tryptophan is a naturally occurring amino acid which is present in the normal diet; about 500 mg of tryptophan are consumed daily in the typical western diet. Most ingested tryptophan is used for protein synthesis and the formation of nicotinamide nucleotides, and only a small proportion (about 1%) is used to synthesize 5-HT via 5-hydroxtryptophan (5-HTP). Tryptophan hydroxylase, the enzyme that catalyses the formation of 5-HTP from L-tryptophan, is normally unsaturated with tryptophan. Accordingly, increasing tryptophan availability to the brain increases 5-HT synthesis.

Pharmacokinetics

L-Tryptophan is rapidly absorbed, with plasma levels peaking about 1–2 hours after ingestion. It is extensively bound to plasma albumin. The amount of L-tryptophan available for brain 5-HT synthesis depends on several factors, including the proportion of L-tryptophan free in plasma, the activity of the tryptophan-metabolizing enzyme, tryptophan pyrrolase, and the concentration of other plasma amino acids that compete with L-tryptophan for entry into the brain.

Efficacy

There is only weak evidence that L-tryptophan has anti-depressant activity when given alone, though it may be superior to placebo in moderately depressed outpatients. There is rather better evidence that L-tryptophan combined with MAOI treatment can enhance the antidepressant effects of MAOIs. Similar synergistic effects have been reported in some studies of L-tryptophan combined with tricyclic antidepressants, although overall the therapeutic benefit of this combination is inconsistent.

Unwanted effects

L-Tryptophan is generally well tolerated, although *nausea* and *drowsiness* soon after dosing are not unusual. However, the prescription of L-tryptophan has been associated with the development of a severe scleroderma-like illness, the *eosinophilia–myalgia syndrome (EMS)*, in which there is a very high circulating eosinophil count (about 20% of peripheral leucocytes), with severe muscle pain, oedema, skin sclerosis, and peripheral neuropathy. Fatalities have been reported.

It is now reasonably well established that EMS is not caused by L-tryptophan itself but rather by a *contaminant* formed in the manufacturing process used by a particular manufacturer (Kilbourne *et al.*, 1996). L-Tryptophan may be used for the treatment of *refractory depression*, when it can be used as an *adjunct* to other antidepressant medication. Patients who are receiving L-tryptophan should be monitored for possible symptoms of EMS. L-Tryptophan should be withdrawn if there is any evidence that EMS may be developing, and an urgent blood eosinophil count should be obtained.

Drug interactions

The only significant drug interactions of L-tryptophan are with drugs that also increase brain 5-HT function. Thus, although administration of L-tryptophan with MAOIs may produce clinical benefit, there are also reports that this combination may lead to 5-HT neurotoxicity as described above. Similarly, the combination of L-tryptophan with SSRIs has been reported to cause myoclonus, shivering, and mental state changes (Gillman and Whyte, 2004).

St John's wort

St John's wort is an extract from the plant, *Hypericum perforatum*. It has been used in medicine for centuries for numerous indications, including burns, arthritis, snakebite, and depression. The active principles are probably derived from six major product groups, including *hypericins* and *hyperforins*. The pharmacology of St John's wort is complex, but animal experimental and some human studies indicate that it potentiates aspects of monoamine neurotransmission (Linde, 2009).

Efficacy

There have been numerous trials of St John's wort, although these are difficult to interpret because the preparations and dosages have been difficult to standardize. In addition, the trials have been conducted in mild to moderately depressed subjects. More recent meta-analyses suggest that standardized extracts of hypericum (in doses of 600–1800 mg) are more effective than placebo, and about equal in efficacy to other antidepressants, in patients with clearly diagnosed major depression (Linde *et al.*, 2005; Cleare *et al.*, 2015). However, there is a lack of longer-term efficacy data, and the available hypericum preparations are not standardized.

Adverse effects and drug interactions

St John's wort is well tolerated, with the most common side effects being *gastrointestinal disturbance, dizziness*, and *tiredness*. Cases of mania during treatment have been described. Photosensitivity is also rarely reported. Hypericum extracts may *induce hepatic enzymes*, and there are reports that treatment with St John's wort was associated with lowered levels of theophylline, cyclosporin, digoxin, and ethinyloestradiol. Finally, St John's wort may cause *serotonin neurotoxicity* when combined with SSRIs and other 5-HT-potentiating drugs (Linde, 2009).

Bupropion

Bupropion has significant use as an antidepressant in the USA. In the UK it is licensed as an adjunct to smoking withdrawal but not as an antidepressant. It is structurally and pharmacologically distinct from other antidepressants, being a unicyclic aminoketone derivative. Bupropion modestly enhances both dopamine and noradrenaline function in the brain, probably via reuptake blockade.

Efficacy and adverse effects

Numerous controlled trials have shown that the antidepressant effect of bupropion is superior to that of placebo and equivalent to that of SSRIs. In some respects the adverse-effect profile of bupropion is similar to that of the SSRIs, with insomnia, agitation, tremor, and nausea being most frequently reported. However, mania and psychosis can also occur, as can raised blood pressure. Bupropion is less likely than SSRIs to cause sexual dysfunction and weight gain, which gives it an important advantage in some patients.

The main concern with the use of bupropion has been the increased risk of seizures. In its original formulation the risk of seizures at higher doses (0.4%) was about four times greater than that associated with SSRIs (about 0.1%). The risk appears to be less with the slow-release formulation (bupropion SR), which has been marketed for smoking cessation. At doses of 300 mg or less, the risk of seizures with bupropion SR appears to be about the same as that seen with SSRIs. This is the maximum dose recommended for smoking cessation, and is the standard dose used when treating depression. Bupropion should not be used in patients with a history of seizures or eating disorder.

Drug interactions

Bupropion should not be given with other drugs that might lower the seizure threshold, such as tricyclic antidepressants, antipsychotic drugs, and antimalarial drugs. Administration with MAOIs is also contraindicated. Bupropion has been combined safely with lithium, and in the USA is used by specialists to augment ineffective SSRI treatment. Bupropion inhibits CYP2D6, and drugs metabolized by this pathway (including some other antidepressants and antipsychotics) should be coprescribed only with caution.

Mood-stabilizing drugs

Several agents are grouped under this heading, such as *lithium* and a number of anticonvulsant drugs, including *carbamazepine* and *sodium valproate*. These three drugs are effective in the *prevention of recurrent affective illness* and also in the *acute treatment of mania*. In addition, lithium has useful antidepressant effects in some circumstances, but the antidepressant activity of carbamazepine and sodium valproate is less well established. Another anticonvulsant, *lamotrigine*, shows promise in the acute treatment and prevention of bipolar depression, but does not appear to be effective against manic states.

Lithium

Placebo-controlled trials have shown that lithium is effective in a number of conditions, including the following:

- the acute treatment of mania
- the prophylaxis of unipolar and bipolar mood disorder
- augmentation therapy in resistant depression
- the prevention of aggressive behaviour in patients with learning disabilities.

Mechanism of action

Animal studies have shown that lithium has important effects on the intracellular signalling molecules or 'second messengers' that are activated when a neurotransmitter or agonist binds to a specific receptor. At clinically relevant doses, lithium inhibits the formation of *cyclic adenosine monophosphate (cAMP)* and also attenuates the formation of various *inositol lipid-derived mediators*. Through these actions lithium could exert profound effects on a wide range of neurotransmitter pathways, many of which use the above messenger systems. More recent interest has focused on the ability of lithium to promote cell survival and increase synaptic plasticity, perhaps through inhibition of the activity of the enzyme glycogen synthase kinase-3 (GSK-3).

Pharmacokinetics

Lithium is rapidly absorbed from the gut and diffuses quickly throughout the body fluids and cells. Lithium moves out of cells more slowly than sodium. It is removed from the plasma by renal excretion and by entering cells and other body compartments. Therefore there is rapid excretion of lithium from the plasma, and a slower phase reflecting its removal from the whole-body pool.

Like sodium, lithium is filtered and partly reabsorbed in the kidney. When the proximal tubule absorbs more water, lithium absorption increases. Therefore *dehydration* causes the plasma lithium concentration to rise. Because lithium is transported in competition with sodium, more is reabsorbed by the kidney when sodium concentrations fall. This is the mechanism whereby *thiazide diuretics* can lead to toxic concentrations of lithium in the blood.

Dosage and plasma concentrations

Because the therapeutic and toxic doses are close together, it is essential to measure plasma concentrations of lithium during treatment. Measurements should first be made after about 7 days, then about every 2 weeks, and then, provided that a satisfactory steady state has been achieved, once every 6 weeks. Subsequently, lithium levels are often very stable, and serum measures can be carried out at intervals of approximately 3 months unless there are clinical indications for more frequent monitoring.

After an oral dose, serum lithium levels rise by a factor of two or three within about 4 hours. For this reason, concentrations are normally measured approximately *12 hours after the last dose*, usually that given at night. It is important to follow this routine, as published information about lithium levels refers to the concentration 12 hours after the last dose, and not to the 'peak' reached in the 4 hours after that dose. If an unexpectedly high concentration is found, it is important to establish whether the patient has inadvertently taken a morning dose before the blood sample was taken.

Previously, the accepted range for prophylaxis was 0.7–1.2 mmol/l measured 12 hours after the last dose. However, current trends are to maintain lithium at *lower serum levels* because this decreases the burden of side effects. Severus *et al.* (2008) concluded that, in the prophylaxis of bipolar disorder, the minimum efficacious serum level of lithium was 0.4 mmol/l, but in most patients the best therapeutic response was obtained with levels in the range 0.6–0.75 mmol/l. Higher levels benefited some patients with more persistent manic symptomatology. In the treatment of acute mania, serum concentrations below 0.8 mmol/l appear to be ineffective, and a range of 0.8–1.0 mmol/l is probably required. Serious toxic effects appear with concentrations above 2.0 mmol/l, although early symptoms may appear at concentrations above 1.2 mmol/l (Macritchie and Young, 2004).

A number of delayed-release preparations of lithium are now available, but their pharmacokinetics *in vivo* do not differ significantly from those of standard lithium carbonate preparations. Liquid formulations of lithium citrate are available for patients who have difficulty in taking tablets. Lithium may be administered once- or twice-daily. Frequency of administration does not appear to affect urine volume. In general, it is more convenient to take lithium as a single dose at night, but patients who experience gastric irritation on this regimen may be helped by divided daily doses.

Unwanted effects

A mild *diuresis* due to sodium excretion occurs soon after the drug is started. Other common effects include *tremor of the hands, dry mouth*, a *metallic taste, feelings of muscular weakness*, and *fatigue* (Table 25.10).

Some degree of *mild thirst* and *polyuria* is common in patients taking lithium, probably because lithium blocks the effect of antidiuretic hormone on the renal tubule. This may not be of clinical significance, but up to one-third of patients can show progression to a *diabetes insipidus-like syndrome* with pronounced polyuria and polydipsia. This may necessitate withdrawal of lithium

treatment, although the use of lower serum lithium levels may cause the syndrome to remit.

Some patients, especially women, *gain weight* when taking the drug. Persistent fine tremor, mainly affecting the hands, is common, but coarse tremor suggests that the serum concentration of lithium has reached toxic levels. Most patients adapt to the fine tremor; for those who do not, propranolol up to 40 mg three times daily may reduce the symptom. Both *hair loss* and *coarsening of hair texture* can occur.

Thyroid gland enlargement occurs in about 5% of patients who are taking lithium. The thyroid shrinks again if thyroxine is given while lithium is continued, and it generally returns to normal a month or two after lithium has been stopped. Lithium interferes with thyroid production, and *hypothyroidism* occurs in up to 20% of women patients, with a compensatory rise in thyroid-stimulating hormone.

Tests of thyroid function should be performed every 6 months to help to detect these changes, but these intermittent tests are no substitute for a continuous watch for suggestive clinical signs, particularly *lethargy* and substantial *weight gain*. If hypothyroidism develops and the reasons for lithium treatment are still strong, thyroxine treatment should be added. Lithium has also been associated with elevated serum calcium levels in the context of *hyperparathyroidism*. This is occasionally associated with severe depression, making distinction from the underlying mood disorder difficult.

Reversible ECG changes also occur. These may be due to displacement of potassium in the myocardium by lithium, as they resemble those of hypokalaemia, with T-wave flattening and inversion or widening of the QRS. They are rarely of clinical significance. Other changes include a reversible *leucocytosis* and occasional papular or maculopapular *rashes*.

Effects on *memory* are sometimes reported by patients, who complain in particular of everyday lapses of memory, such as forgetting well-known names. It is possible that this impairment of memory is caused by the mood disorder rather than by the drug itself, but there is also evidence that lithium can be associated with impaired performance on certain cognitive tests.

Long-term effects on the kidney. As noted above, lithium treatment decreases *tubular concentrating ability* and can occasionally cause a nephrogenic diabetes inspidus. In addition, there have been reports that over many years of treatment, lithium can sometimes cause an increasing and in some cases *irreversible decline* in tubular function. This may be more likely in patients with higher serum concentrations of lithium, and

Table 25.10 **Some adverse effects of lithium, carbamazepine, and valproate**

	Lithium	Carbamazepine	Valproate
Neurological	Tremor, weakness, dysarthria, ataxia, impaired memory, seizures (rare)	Dizziness, weakness, drowsiness, ataxia, headache, visual disturbance	Tremor, sedation
Renal/fluid balance	Increased urine output with decreased urine-concentrating ability. Thirst, diabetes insipidus, oedema	Acts to increase urine-concentrating ability, low sodium states, oedema	Increased plasma ammonia
Gastrointestinal	Altered taste, anorexia, nausea, vomiting, diarrhoea, weight gain	Anorexia, nausea, constipation, hepatitis	Anorexia, nausea, vomiting, diarrhoea, weight gain, hepatitis (rare), pancreatitis (rare)
Endocrine	Decreased thyroxine with increased TSH. Goitre, hyperparathyroidism (rare)	Decreased thyroxine with normal TSH	Menstrual disturbances
Haematological	Leucocytosis	Leucopenia, agranulocytosis (rare)	Low platelet count, abnormal platelet aggregation
Dermatological	Acne, exacerbation of psoriasis	Erythematous rash	Hair loss
Cardiovascular	ECG changes (usually clinically benign)	Cardiac conduction disturbances	

where concomitant psychotropic medication has been employed (Macritchie and Young, 2004).

Several follow-up studies have examined the effect of longer-term lithium maintenance treatment on *glomerular function*. In general, it has been thought that any decline in glomerular function is usually mild and related to lithium intoxication. However, more recent epidemiological studies suggest that lithium treatment is associated with an increased risk of chronic kidney disease, particularly in patients with a greater number of prescriptions for lithium (Kessing *et al.*, 2015). Whether lithium is associated with an increased risk of *end-stage renal failure* is unclear (Close *et al.*, 2014; Kessing *et al.*, 2015). Clarifying this possibility is difficult because patients with bipolar disorder (the group most likely to receive lithium) may have an increased risk of renal disease anyway through associated medical morbidities; for example, hypertension and diabetes (see Chapter 10).

With the current trends towards long-term prophylaxis of mood disorders, it is clearly wise to monitor plasma creatinine levels regularly and to supplement this with estimated glomerular filtration rate (e-GFR; see Box 25.10). It seems likely that the risk of nephrotoxicity will be minimized by maintaining plasma lithium levels at the lower end of the therapeutic range, provided that they are therapeutically effective for the individual

patient. Also, careful attention to medical comorbidity in bipolar patients is important.

Toxic effects

These are related to dose. They include *ataxia, poor coordination of limb movements, muscle twitching, slurred speech*, and *confusion*. They constitute a serious medical emergency, as they can progress through *coma* and *fits* to *death*.

If these symptoms appear, lithium must be stopped at once and a high intake of fluid provided, with extra sodium chloride to stimulate an osmotic diuresis. In severe cases, renal dialysis may be needed. Lithium is rapidly cleared if renal function is normal, so that most cases either recover completely or die. However, cases of permanent neurological and renal damage despite haemodialysis have been reported.

As noted earlier, lithium can increase *fetal abnormalities*, particularly of the heart, although the magnitude of the individual risk is low. The decision as to whether or not to continue with lithium treatment during pregnancy must therefore be carefully considered. Important factors include the likelihood of affective relapse if lithium is withheld, and the difficulty that could be experienced in managing an episode of affective illness in the particular individual.

Box 25.10 Lithium, renal function, and estimated glomerular filtration rate

The *estimated glomerular filtration rate (e-GFR)* in a healthy young adult is about 100 ml/min, and it falls by about 1 ml/min per year as people get older, so many healthy 75-year-olds will have an e-GFR of 50–60 ml/min.

Chronic kidney disease (CKD)

CKD stage 1: e-GFR >90 ml/min, normal kidney function, but urine findings or structural abnormalities or genetic trait indicate kidney disease

CKD stage 2: e-GFR 60–90 ml/min, mildly reduced kidney function, and other findings (as for stage 1) indicate kidney disease

CKD stage 3: e-GFR 30–59 ml/min, a moderate reduction in kidney function

CKD stage 4: e-GFR 15–29 ml/min, a severe reduction in kidney function

CKD stage 5: e-GFR <15 ml/min, established kidney failure, when dialysis or a kidney transplant may be needed.

Stage 3 CKD is asymptomatic, but is associated with a greater subsequent risk of cardiovascular disease. People with stage 3 CKD require regular cardiovascular monitoring and tests of renal function, including urinalysis every 3 months.

Indications for referral to a specialist renal physician in a patient taking lithium

Referral is required if any of the following are present:

- e-GFR is decreasing by >4 ml/min annually
- progressive rise in blood creatinine concentration in three or more serial tests
- proteinuria
- haematuria
- symptoms suggestive of chronic renal failure (e.g. tiredness, anaemia)
- e-GFR <30 ml/min.

Source: data from British Journal of Psychiatry, 193(2), Morriss R and Benjamin B, Lithium and eGFR: a new routinely available tool for the prevention of chronic kidney disease, pp. 93–95, Copyright (2008), The Royal College of Psychiatrists.

If pregnant patients continue with lithium, serum levels should be monitored closely. Ultrasound examination and fetal echocardiography are valuable screening tests as the pregnancy progresses. Patients with a history of *bipolar disorder* have a substantially *increased risk* of relapse in the postpartum period. In such patients it may be worth considering the introduction of lithium shortly after delivery to provide a prophylactic effect. However, significant concentrations of lithium can be measured in the serum of breastfed infants, which may make bottle-feeding advisable.

Drug interactions

Because of the narrow therapeutic index of lithium, *pharmacokinetic* drug interactions are of major clinical importance (Box 25.11). *Pharmacodynamic* interactions may involve potentiation of *5-HT-promoting agents*, leading to a serotonin syndrome. In addition, therapeutic serum levels of lithium can be associated with *neurotoxicity* in the presence of certain other centrally acting agents; for example, calcium channel blockers and carbamazepine.

ECT and surgery. It is possible that the continuation of lithium during *ECT* may lead to neurotoxicity. If feasible, lithium treatment should be suspended or serum levels reduced during ECT, because the customary overnight fast beforehand may leave patients relatively dehydrated the following morning. If possible, lithium treatment should be discontinued before *major surgery*, because the effects of *muscle relaxants* may be potentiated. However, the risk of acute withdrawal and 'rebound' mania must be considered.

Lithium withdrawal

In some studies, abrupt *lithium withdrawal* has been associated with the rapid onset of mania. Undoubtedly there is an increased risk of recurrent mood disorder after lithium discontinuation, probably because lithium is an effective prophylactic agent and because it is used for disorders that have a high risk of recurrence. However, there is probably also a lithium withdrawal syndrome with 'rebound' mania, although this may be restricted to patients with bipolar disorder.

The risk of rapid relapse is reduced if lithium is *discontinued slowly* over a period of several weeks. Even patients who have remained entirely well for many years may experience a further episode of affective disorder after lithium discontinuation. Most of these individuals

> ### Box 25.11 Some drug interactions of lithium
>
> #### Pharmacokinetic
>
> **Increased lithium levels**
>
> - Diuretics (furosemide is safest)
> - Non-steroidal anti-inflammatory drugs (aspirin/sulindac is safest)
> - ACE inhibitors
> - Angiotensin-II-receptor antagonists
> - Antibiotics (metronidazole)
>
> **Decreased lithium levels**
>
> - Theophylline
> - Sodium bicarbonate
>
> #### Pharmacodynamic
>
> - *5-HT neurotoxicity*
>   SSRIs (can be used safely with care)
> - *Extrapyramidal side effects enhanced*
>   Antipsychotic agents, metoclopramide, domperidone
> - *Enhanced neurotoxicity*
>   Carbamazepine, phenytoin, calcium-channel blockers, methyldopa

will respond to the reintroduction of lithium (Tondo *et al.*, 1997).

Contraindications

These include renal failure or recent renal disease, current cardiac failure or recent myocardial infarction, and chronic diarrhoea sufficient to alter electrolytes. Lithium should not be prescribed if the patient is judged to be unlikely to observe the precautions required for its safe use. This includes a propensity to discontinue it suddenly against advice.

The management of patients on lithium

Preparation. A careful routine of management is essential because of the effects of therapeutic doses of lithium on the thyroid and kidney, and the toxic effects of excessive dosage. The following routine is one of several that have been proposed, and can be adopted safely. Successful treatment requires attention to detail, so the steps are described below at some length.

Before starting lithium, a *physical examination* should be performed, including the measurement of blood pressure. It is also useful to weigh the patient and calculate the BMI.

Blood should be taken for estimation of *electrolytes, calcium, creatinine, e-GFR*, and a *full blood count. Thyroid function tests* are also necessary. If indicated, an ECG and pregnancy tests should be performed as well.

If these tests show no contraindication to lithium treatment, the doctor should check that the patient is not taking any drugs that might interact with lithium. A careful explanation should then be given to the patient. They should understand the possible early toxic effects of an unduly high blood concentration, and also the circumstances in which this can arise—for example, during intercurrent gastroenteritis, renal infection, or the dehydration secondary to fever. They should be advised that if any of these arise, they should stop the drug and seek medical advice.

It is usually appropriate to include another member of the family in these discussions. Providing *printed guidelines* on these points is often helpful (either written by the doctor, or in one of the forms provided by pharmaceutical firms). In these discussions a sensible balance must be struck between alarming the patient by overemphasizing the risks, and failing to give them the information that they need to take a collaborative part in the treatment.

Starting treatment. Lithium should normally be prescribed as the carbonate, and treatment should begin and continue with a *single daily dose* unless there is gastric intolerance, in which case divided doses can be given. If the drug is being used for prophylaxis, it is appropriate to begin with 200–400 mg daily in a single dose. The lower end of the range is appropriate when patients are taking concomitant medication such as SSRIs that might interact with lithium.

Blood should be taken for lithium estimations every week or two, adjusting the dose until an appropriate concentration is achieved. A lithium level of 0.4–0.7 mmol/l (in a sample taken 12 hours after the last dose) may be adequate for prophylaxis, as explained above. If this is not effective, the previously accepted higher range of 0.8–0.9 mmol/l can be tried if side effects permit and the predominant symptomatology is manic. When judging the response, it should be remembered that several months may elapse before lithium achieves its full effect.

Continuation treatment. As treatment continues, lithium estimations should be carried out about *every 12 weeks*. It is important to have some means of reminding patients and doctors about the times at which repeat investigations are required. Computerized databases may be helpful in this respect. *Every 6 months*, blood samples should be taken for electrolytes, urea, creatinine, e-GFR, calcium, and thyroid function tests. If two consecutive thyroid function tests 1 month apart show evidence of *hypothyroidism*, lithium should be stopped or L-thyroxine prescribed. Troublesome *polyuria* is a reason for attempting a reduction in dose, whereas severe persistent polyuria is an indication for specialist renal investigation, including tests of concentrating ability. A persistent *leucocytosis* is not uncommon and is apparently harmless. It reverses soon after the drug is stopped.

When lithium is given, the doctor must keep in mind the interactions that have been reported with psychotropic and other drugs (see above). It is also prudent to be extra vigilant for toxic effects if ECT is being given. If the patient requires an anaesthetic for any reason, the anaesthetist should be told that they are taking lithium; this is because, as noted above, there is some evidence that the effects of muscle relaxants may be potentiated.

Lithium is usually continued for at least a year, and often for much longer. The need for the drug should be reviewed once a year, taking into account any persistence of mild mood fluctuations, which suggest the possibility of relapse if treatment is stopped. Continuing medication is more likely to be needed if the patient has previously had several episodes of mood disorder within a short time, or if previous episodes were so severe that even a small risk of recurrence should be avoided.

Some patients have taken lithium continuously for 15 years or more, but there should always be compelling reasons for continuing treatment for more than 5 years. As noted above, lithium should be withdrawn slowly, over a number of months if possible. The patient should be advised not to discontinue lithium suddenly on their own initiative.

Carbamazepine

Carbamazepine was originally introduced as an *anticonvulsant*, and was found to have useful effects on mood in certain patients. Subsequently it was found to be beneficial in some bipolar patients, including those who had proved *refractory to lithium*. There is reasonable evidence that carbamazepine is effective in the management of *acute mania* and also in the *prophylaxis of bipolar disorder*, although overall its efficacy is probably less than that of lithium (Goodwin et al, 2016).

Mode of action. Like certain other anticonvulsants, carbamazepine blocks *neuronal sodium channels*. It is unclear whether this action plays a role in the mood-stabilizing effects. In both humans and animals, carbamazepine facilitates 5-HT neurotransmission, an action that it shares with lithium.

Pharmacokinetics

Carbamazepine is slowly but completely absorbed and widely distributed. It is extensively metabolized, and at least one metabolite, carbamazepine epoxide, is therapeutically active. The half-life during long-term treatment is about 20 hours. Carbamazepine is a strong *inducer of hepatic microsomal enzymes*, and can lower the plasma concentrations of numerous other drugs.

Dosage and plasma concentrations

The dosage of carbamazepine in the treatment of mood disorders is similar to that used in the treatment of epilepsy, within the range 400–1600 mg daily. Treatment is usually given in divided doses twice-daily, because this practice may improve tolerance. No clear relationship has been established between plasma carbamazepine concentrations and therapeutic response, but it seems prudent to monitor levels (about 12 hours after the last dose) and to maintain them in the usual anticonvulsant range as a precaution against toxicity.

Unwanted effects

Side effects are common at the beginning of treatment. They include *drowsiness, dizziness, ataxia, diplopia*, and *nausea*. Tolerance to these effects usually develops quickly. A potentially serious side effect of carbamazepine is *agranulocytosis*, although this complication is very rare (variously estimated to be from 1 in 10,000 to 1 in 125,000 patients).

A *relative leucopenia* is more common, with the white cell count often falling during the first few weeks of treatment, although it usually remains within normal levels. Rashes occur in about 5% of patients, and, rarely, severe exfoliative dermatitis develops. Elevations in liver enzymes may also occur, and, rarely, *hepatitis* has been reported. Carbamazepine can cause disturbances of *cardiac conduction*, and is therefore contraindicated in patients with pre-existing abnormalities of cardiac conduction. Carbamazepine is an established *human teratogen*.

Carbamazepine lowers plasma *thyroxine levels*, but thyroid-stimulating hormone levels are not elevated and clinical hypothyroidism is unusual. Carbamazepine has also been associated with *low sodium states*. The unwanted effects of carbamazepine are compared with those of lithium and valproate in Table 25.10.

Drug interactions

Carbamazepine increases the metabolism of many other drugs, including tricyclic antidepressants, benzodiazepines, antipsychotic drugs, oral contraceptive agents, thyroxine, warfarin, other anticonvulsants, and some antibiotics. A similar mechanism may underlie the decline in plasma carbamazepine levels that occurs after the first few weeks of treatment.

Carbamazepine levels may be increased by SSRIs and erythromycin. The pharmacodynamic effects and plasma levels of carbamazepine may be increased by some calcium-channel blockers, such as diltiazem and verapamil. Conversely, carbamazepine may decrease the effect of certain other calcium-channel antagonists, such as felodipine and nicardipine. Neurotoxicity has been reported when carbamazepine and lithium have been combined even in the presence of normal lithium levels. The manufacturers of carbamazepine recommend that combination of carbamazepine with MAOIs should be avoided. However, there are case reports of these drugs being used safely together. It is possible that some MAOIs may increase plasma carbamazepine levels.

Clinical use of carbamazepine

Current clinical guidelines (see, for example, Goodwin *et al.*, 2016) place carbamazepine rather low down the list of therapeutic options, after drugs such as lithium, valproate, and lamotrigine. To some extent this reflects the liability of carbamazepine to cause significant drug interactions, as well as its perceived poorer tolerability. Also, there is less recent controlled evidence concerning its use. With this is mind, the usual indications for carbamazepine are as follows:

- The prophylactic management of bipolar illness in patients for whom lithium and valproate treatment is ineffective or poorly tolerated.
- The treatment of patients with frequent mood swings and mixed affective states for which carbamazepine may be more effective than lithium.
- Added to lithium treatment in patients who have shown a partial response to the latter drug; in these circumstances it is important to remember that this combination can cause neurotoxicity.
- In the acute treatment of mania, again usually as an alternative or addition to lithium and valproate.

If clinical circumstances permit, it is preferable to start treatment with carbamazepine slowly at a dose of 100–200 mg daily, increasing in steps of 100–200 mg twice-weekly. Patients show wide variability in the blood levels at which they experience adverse effects; accordingly, it is best to titrate the dose against the side effects and the clinical response.

Because of the risk of a *lowered white cell count*, it is prudent to monitor the blood count before treatment and after 3 and 6 months of treatment. Some guidelines also recommend monitoring liver function tests and plasma electrolytes; however, clinical vigilance is probably the best safeguard. Patients should be instructed to seek help urgently if they develop a fever or other sign of infection. When patients have responded to the addition of carbamazepine to lithium, it is possible subsequently to attempt a cautious withdrawal of lithium. However, the current clinical impression is that, for many patients, the maintenance of mood stability requires continuing treatment with both drugs.

Sodium valproate

Like carbamazepine, sodium valproate was first introduced as an anticonvulsant. In recent years there has been increasing interest in using the drug in the management of mood disorders.

There have been several controlled studies indicating that valproate is effective in the *acute management of mania*. As yet there is less clear evidence that it is effective in *longer-term prophylaxis* of bipolar disorder. In a randomized trial, Bowden *et al.* (2000) showed a marginal benefit for valproate over lithium and placebo in bipolar patients over a 1-year follow-up. However, in the large pragmatic BALANCE trial, valproate was less effective than lithium (BALANCE Study Group, 2010). There have been numerous case studies and open series that have reported useful prophylactic effects of valproate in patients who were *unresponsive to lithium* and *carbamazepine*, including those with rapid-cycling mood disorders.

Mode of action. Valproate is a simple branch-chain fatty acid with a mode of action that is unclear. However, there is some evidence that it can slow down the breakdown of the *inhibitory neurotransmitter GABA*. This action could account for the anticonvulsant properties of valproate, but whether it also underlies the psychotropic effects is unclear.

Pharmacokinetics

Valproate is rapidly absorbed, with the peak plasma concentrations occurring about 2 hours after ingestion. It is widely and rapidly distributed and has a half-life of 8–18 hours. Valproate is metabolized in the liver to produce a wide variety of metabolites, some of which have anticonvulsant activity. Unlike carbamazepine, valproate does not induce hepatic microsomal enzymes and, if anything, it tends to delay the metabolism of other drugs.

Dosing and plasma concentrations

Valproate can be started at a dose of 200–400 mg daily, which may be increased once- or twice-weekly to a range of 1–2 g daily. Plasma levels of valproate do not correlate well with either the anticonvulsant or the mood-stabilizing effects, but it has been suggested that efficacy in the treatment of acute mania is usually apparent when plasma levels are *greater than 50 µg/ml*.

Unwanted effects

Common side effects of valproate include *gastrointestinal disturbances, tremor, sedation*, and *tiredness*. Other troublesome side effects include *weight gain* and *transient hair loss*, with changes in hair texture on regrowth.

Patients who are taking valproate may show some elevation in *hepatic transaminase enzymes*. Provided that this increase is not associated with hepatic dysfunction, the drug can be continued while enzyme levels and liver function are carefully monitored. However, there have been several reports of fatal *hepatic toxicity* associated with the use of valproate; most of these cases have occurred in children taking multiple anticonvulsant drugs. Valproate must be withdrawn immediately if vomiting, anorexia, jaundice, or sudden drowsiness occur.

Valproate may also cause *thrombocytopenia*, and may inhibit platelet aggregation. *Acute pancreatitis* is another rare but serious side effect, and *increases in plasma ammonia levels* have also been reported. Other possible side effects include *oedema, amenorrhoea*, and *rashes*. Valproate has been associated with *polycystic ovary disease*, and is an important human teratogen. The National Institute for Health and Clinical Excellence (2014) has recommended that valproate should not be used for the treatment of bipolar disorder in women of childbearing age unless no alternative treatment is effective or can be tolerated.

Drug interactions

Valproate potentiates the effects of central sedatives. It has been reported to increase the side effects of other anticonvulsants (without necessarily improving anticonvulsant control). It may increase plasma levels of lamotrigine, phenytoin, and tricyclic antidepressants. The interaction with lamotrigine necessitates careful adjustment of lamotrigine dosage (see below). Valproate can increase the adverse effects of *olanzapine*.

Clinical use

The efficacy of valproate in the acute and continuation treatment of mania has been established by several controlled trials (Goodwin *et al.*, 2016), and it is licensed for this indication in the UK in the form of the semi-sodium preparation. In the treatment of acute mania it has a quicker onset of action than lithium and carbamazepine because it can be dosed at high levels initially. For example, a therapeutic effect can be apparent within 1 or 2 days of employing a loading dose of valproate of 20 mg/kg. Valproate may also be more effective than lithium in the management of patients with *mixed affective states*.

In terms of prophylaxis, valproate appears to be effective in the prevention of both manic and depressive episodes (Miura *et al.*, 2014). It has often been used in combination with lithium in bipolar patients who have shown a partial response to lithium, and this combination appears to be safe. Valproate has also been used in combination with carbamazepine. For patients who continue to show episodes of mood disturbance, valproate can also be combined with atypical antipsychotic drugs (Goodwin *et al.*, 2016). Guidelines recommend that body weight, blood count, and liver function tests are assessed prior to treatment and thereafter at 6-monthly intervals.

Lamotrigine

Lamotrigine is a triazine derivative that blocks voltage-dependent *sodium channels* and reduces excitatory neurotransmitter release, particularly that of *glutamate*. It is licensed in the UK as a monotherapy and adjunctive treatment for epilepsy.

Lamotrigine is not licensed for the treatment of mood disorders in the UK, but there are open studies showing therapeutic benefit when it has been added to the medication of patients with *bipolar illness that is refractory to standard treatments*. In addition, placebo-controlled trials have shown that lamotrigine has efficacy as monotherapy in the *acute treatment of bipolar depression* (Geddes *et al.*, 2009), and also in the *longer-term prevention of bipolar depression* (Benyon *et al.*, 2009). Lamotrigine was also effective in patients with bipolar depression when added to quetiapine (Geddes *et al.*, 2016). Used alone, lamotrigine does not seem to have significant acute or prophylactic antimanic actions.

Pharmacokinetics

Following oral administration, lamotrigine is rapidly absorbed, with peak plasma levels occurring after about 1.5 hours. The drug is extensively metabolized by the liver but does not induce cytochrome P450 enzymes. Its half-life is about 30 hours. A plasma therapeutic range has not been identified.

Adverse effects

Skin eruptions, usually maculopapular in nature, occur in about 3% of patients and may be associated with fever. They are most common in the first few weeks of treatment, and their incidence can be reduced by careful initial dosing (see below). Other side effects include *nausea, headache, diplopia, blurred vision, dizziness, ataxia*, and *tremor*. Rarely, very serious adverse effects, such as *angioedema, Stevens–Johnson syndrome*, and *toxic epidermal necrolysis*, have been reported.

Drug interactions

Plasma levels of lamotrigine can be lowered by drugs that induce hepatic-metabolizing enzymes, such as *carbamazepine*. Combination of carbamazepine and lamotrigine can also cause neurotoxicity. Lamotrigine levels are increased by concomitant administration of *valproate*.

Clinical use

Lamotrigine has a useful role to play in the acute and prophylactic management of the depressive pole of bipolar disorder. Because lamotrigine appears to be ineffective in the treatment or prevention of mania, it is often used in combination with other drugs such as lithium. However, in bipolar patients where the burden of illness is almost exclusively depressive, it can be used as a monotherapy (Goodwin *et al.*, 2016).

When initiating lamotrigine treatment, to minimize the risk of rash it is important to follow the dosage recommendations in the *British National Formulary* (25 mg daily for the first 2 weeks, followed by 50 mg daily for the next 2 weeks). The usual therapeutic dose in bipolar disorder is in the range 50–300 mg daily. If the patient is also taking valproate, dosage initiation must be even more cautious (for guidance, see the *British National Formulary*).

Gabapentin

Gabapentin was developed as a structural analogue of GABA. Despite its structural relationship to GABA, its anticonvulsant mechanism of action is thought to be mediated through inhibition of the α_2-δ subunit of voltage-gated calcium channels.

Gabapentin is licensed as an adjunctive treatment for seizure disorders, and is not licensed for the treatment of mood disorders. There are published case series that show benefit when gabapentin has been used as an adjunctive therapy in patients with bipolar disorder resistant to standard medication regimens. However, controlled trials in mania and refractory bipolar depression have yielded disappointing results (Goodwin *et al.*, 2016). Gabapentin has a *sedating* profile and may also have *anxiolytic* properties. Its analogue, *pregabalin*, has not been studied in bipolar disorder, but is licensed for the treatment of *generalized anxiety disorder* and *neuropathic pain*.

Pharmacokinetics

After oral absorption, peak plasma levels of gabapentin are reached after 2–3 hours. Gabapentin is not metabolized by the liver and is excreted entirely by the kidney. Its half-life is about 5–7 hours, and three times daily dosing is recommended.

Unwanted effects

The most common side effects of gabapentin are *somnolence, dizziness, fatigue*, and *nystagmus*. No serious adverse effects have been reported.

Drug interactions

Probably because of its lack of hepatic metabolism, to date no significant pharmacokinetic interactions of gabapentin with other medications have been described. It may potentiate the effects of other central sedatives.

Clinical use

Gabapentin has a wide dosage range, but the usual dose in bipolar illness is between 600 mg and 2400 mg daily. Sedative and anxiolytic effects are often apparent at lower doses. Although effects of this nature might be useful in patients with refractory bipolar illness, there is currently *no evidence from controlled trials* that gabapentin has a place in the treatment of bipolar disorder.

Psychostimulants

This class of drugs includes mild stimulants, of which the best known is *caffeine*, and more powerful stimulants, such as *amfetamine* and *methylphenidate*. *Cocaine* is a powerful psychostimulant, with a particularly high potential for inducing dependence (see Chapter 20). It is useful as a local anaesthetic, but has no other clinical indications. All potent psychostimulants *increase the release* and *block the reuptake* of dopamine and noradrenaline. A newer compound, *modafinil*, produces increases in alertness and decreases sleepiness, and, although its mechanism of action is uncertain, it may also involve dopaminergic mechanisms (Young and Geyer, 2010).

Indications

The main current indication for psychostimulant treatment with methylphenidate and amfetamine is attention-deficit hyperactivity disorder (ADHD) in children, and in adults where ADHD symptomatology has persisted from childhood. Various preparations are available and *slow-release forms of methylphenidate* are often preferred to diminish the need to take additional doses in the school day and to lessen rapid-onset stimulant effects which are believed to increase the risk of dependence. A recently licensed form of amfetamine, *lisdexamfetamine*, consists of an inactive complex of dexamfetamine and the amino acid, lysine; this prodrug is then taken up by red cells from which the active dexamfetamine is slowly released.

Another indication for stimulants is the treatment of *narcolepsy*. In the past, amfetamines were widely prescribed for the treatment of depression, but have now been superseded by the antidepressant drugs. Some specialists, mainly in the USA, believe that psychostimulants may have a role in combination with other antidepressant drugs for patients with *refractory depressive* *disorder*, but this indication is not clearly supported by evidence from controlled trials.

Modafinil is licensed for the treatment of sleepiness associated with narcolepsy, obstructive sleep apnoea, and sleep disorders associated with shift work. Modafinil has also been used with apparent benefit to treat sleepiness and fatigue in depressed patients receiving SSRIs (Cowen and Anderson, 2015).

Unwanted effects

These include restlessness, insomnia, poor appetite, dizziness, tremor, palpitations, and cardiac arrhythmias. Toxic effects from large doses include disorientation and aggressive behaviour, hallucinations, convulsions, and coma. Persistent abuse can lead to a paranoid state similar to paranoid schizophrenia. *Amfetamines* can cause severe hypertension in combination with MAOIs and, to a lesser extent, with tricyclic antidepressants. They are contraindicated in cardiovascular disease and thyrotoxicosis. *Modafinil* has been associated with dry mouth, nausea, abdominal pain, headache, tachycardia, palpitations, anxiety, and insomnia. It should not be used in patients with significant cardiovascular disease.

Other physical treatments

Electroconvulsive therapy

History

Convulsive therapy was introduced in the 1930s on the basis of the mistaken idea that epilepsy and schizophrenia do not occur together. It seemed to follow that induced fits should lead to improvement in schizophrenia. However, when the treatment was tried it became apparent that the most striking changes occurred not in schizophrenia but in *severe depressive disorders*, in which it brought about a substantial reduction in chronicity and mortality.

The first psychiatrist to employ seizures as therapy was Ladislas von Meduna who, in 1934, used medications such as camphor and pentylenetetrazole to produce grand mal fits. However, in 1938 Cerletti and Bini found that electrical stimulation, applied through bitemporal electrodes, produced fits more efficiently and quickly than drugs, and, as time went by, electrical stimulation became the rule. The subsequent addition of brief anaesthesia and muscle relaxants made the treatment safer and more acceptable.

Indications

This section summarizes the indications for ECT. Further information about the efficiency of the procedure will be found in the chapters that deal with the individual psychiatric syndromes.

ECT is a rapid and effective treatment for *severe depressive disorders*. In the Medical Research Council trial (Clinical Psychiatry Committee, 1965) it acted faster than imipramine or phenelzine, and was more effective than imipramine in women and more effective than phenelzine in both sexes. The indications for ECT have been reviewed by the National Institute for Clinical Excellence (2003) (see Box 25.12). Indications suggested by the Royal College of Psychiatrists (2005) are shown in Box 25.13.

Both sets of guidelines are in agreement with the impression of many clinicians, and with the recommendations of this book, that ECT should be used mainly when it is essential to bring about improvement quickly. Therefore the strongest indications are an immediate *high risk of suicide, depressive stupor,* or *danger to physical health* because the patient is not drinking enough to maintain adequate renal function.

Box 25.12 Indications for ECT (National Institute for Clinical Excellence, 2003)

It is recommended that electroconvulsive therapy is used only to achieve rapid and short-term improvement of severe symptoms after an adequate trial of other treatment options has proven ineffective and/or when the condition is considered to be potentially life-threatening in individuals with:

1. Severe depressive illness.
2. Catatonia.
3. A prolonged or severe manic episode.

The NICE guidelines for the use of ECT *in depression* were modified slightly in 2009 to the following:

- Consider ECT for acute treatment of severe depression that is life-threatening and when a rapid response is required, or when other treatments have failed.
- Do not use ECT routinely for people with moderate depression but consider it if their depression has not responded to multiple drug treatments and psychological treatment.

ECT can lead to a rapid resolution of *mania*, but is generally reserved for patients who do not respond to drug treatment, or for those whose manic illness is particularly severe, requiring high doses of antipsychotic drugs (Goodwin *et al.*, 2016).

On the basis of clinical case studies, it has long been held that ECT is useful for the treatment of *acute catatonic states*. Controlled studies have also shown that ECT is effective in patients with acute schizophrenia with predominantly positive symptoms. In these studies ECT is effective not only for affective symptoms but also for positive symptoms such as *delusions* and *thought disorder* (Brandon *et al.*, 1985). In general, however, ECT adds little to the effects of adequate doses of antipsychotic drugs, although it probably produces a greater rate of symptomatic improvement in the short term. It is unclear whether ECT has a role in the treatment of patients with schizophrenia whose positive symptoms do not respond to antipsychotic medication. There is more evidence for the use of clozapine in this situation, and ECT is not generally recommended (National Institute for Clinical Excellence, 2003), although the Royal College of Psychiatrists suggests that it can be considered as a fourth-line option. A randomized controlled trial indicated that ECT may be beneficial in patients with schizophrenia who do not respond to clozapine (Petrides *et al.*, 2015).

Mode of action

Role of the seizure

Presumably the specific therapeutic effects of ECT must be brought about through physiological and biochemical changes in the brain. The first step in identifying the mode of action must be to find out whether the therapeutic effect depends on the seizure, or whether other features of the treatment are sufficient, such as the passage of the current through the brain, and the use of anaesthesia and muscle relaxants.

Box 25.13 Indications for ECT (Royal College of Psychiatrists, 2005)

In severe depressive illness, ECT may be the treatment of choice when the illness is associated with:
- life-threatening illness because of refusal of foods and fluids
- a high suicide risk.

ECT may be considered for the treatment of severe depressive illness associated with:
- stupor
- marked psychomotor retardation
- depressive delusions and hallucinations.

ECT may be considered as second- or third-line treatment of depressive illness that is not responsive to antidepressant drugs.

ECT may be considered for the treatment of mania:

- that is associated with life-threatening physical exhaustion
- that has not responded to appropriate drug treatment.

ECT may be considered for the treatment of acute schizophrenia as a fourth-line option for treatment-resistant schizophrenia after treatment with two antipsychotic drugs and then clozapine has proved ineffective.

ECT may be indicated in patients with catatonia where treatment with a benzodiazepine (usually lorazepam) has proved ineffective.

Reproduced from Advances in Psychiatric Treatment, 11(2), Scott A, College Guidelines on electroconvulsive therapy: an update for prescribers, pp. 150–6, Copyright (2005), with permission from The Royal College of Psychiatrists.

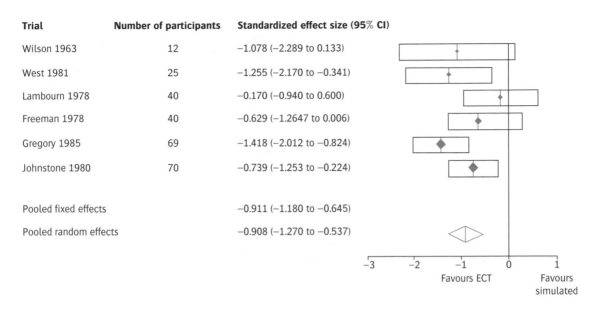

Trial	Number of participants	Standardized effect size (95% CI)
Wilson 1963	12	−1.078 (−2.289 to 0.133)
West 1981	25	−1.255 (−2.170 to −0.341)
Lambourn 1978	40	−0.170 (−0.940 to 0.600)
Freeman 1978	40	−0.629 (−1.2647 to 0.006)
Gregory 1985	69	−1.418 (−2.012 to −0.824)
Johnstone 1980	70	−0.739 (−1.253 to −0.224)
Pooled fixed effects		−0.911 (−1.180 to −0.645)
Pooled random effects		−0.908 (−1.270 to −0.537)

Figure 25.1 Meta-analysis of randomized, placebo-controlled studies of ECT in depression.

Reproduced from The Lancet, 361(9360), The UK ECT Review Group, Efficacy and safety of electroconvulsive therapy in depressive disorders: a systematic review and meta-analysis, pp. 799–808, Copyright (2003), with permission from Elsevier.

Clinicians have generally been convinced that the patient does not improve unless a convulsion is produced during the ECT procedure. This impression has been confirmed by several double-blind trials which, taken together, show that ECT is strikingly more effective than a full placebo procedure that includes anaesthetic and muscle relaxant (UK ECT Review Group, 2003) (see Figure 25.1).

This evidence does not necessarily support the view that a full seizure is the sufficient and necessary therapeutic component of ECT, and recent studies have shown that this notion is incorrect. Modern ECT machines deliver brief pulses of electrical current that enable a seizure to be induced by administration of relatively low doses of electrical energy. With this mode of administration, both *electrode placement* and *electrical dosage* can have profound effects on the therapeutic efficacy of ECT. In particular, it appears that the *amount by which the applied electrical dose exceeds the seizure threshold of the individual patient* is an important determinant of both efficacy and cognitive side effects of ECT. Furthermore, the seizure threshold varies greatly (about 15-fold) between individuals.

This situation has important implications for the practical management of ECT when the clinician's aim is to find the best balance between *therapeutic efficacy* and *cognitive side effects* (see below). From a theoretical viewpoint, however, it can be concluded that an important determinant of ECT efficacy is how far the applied electrical energy *exceeds the seizure threshold* of the individual patient.

Neurobiological effects of ECT

Electrical seizures in animals produce many biochemical and electrophysiological changes, and therefore it is difficult to identify the processes that are important in the antidepressant effect of ECT. It is of interest that some of the changes in brain monoamine pathways found in rodents after ECT (e.g. *downregulation of noradrenaline β-adrenoceptors*) resemble those found after antidepressant drug treatment. In addition, both ECT and antidepressants increase the expression of *dopamine D_2 receptors* in the nucleus accumbens, which could be associated with improvements in motivational behaviour. In the case of ECT, this may involve interaction with *glutamatergic pathways*. Like antidepressant medication, electrical seizures in animals result in changes in neurotropins such as *BDNF*, and increases in *neurogenesis* in the hippocampus. The hippocampus is likely to play an important role in the pathophysiology of depression, and changes in hippocampal activity could therefore underpin some of the therapeutic effects of ECT. Of course, altered hippocampal function could also play a role in the amnestic side effects of ECT. Finally, in terms of network theories of depression (see Chapter 9), ECT appears to decrease the hyperconnectivity of the default mode network that is characteristic of depressive states (Perrin *et al.*, 2012). For a review, see Anderson and Fergusson (2013).

Physiological changes during ECT

If ECT is given without anticholinergic premedication, the pulse first slows and then rises quickly to 130–190 beats/minute, falling to the original resting rate or beyond towards the end of the seizure, before a final less marked tachycardia that lasts for several minutes. Marked increases in blood pressure are also common, and the systolic pressure can rise to 200 mmHg. Cerebral blood flow also increases by up to 200%.

Unilateral or bilateral ECT

Overall, bilateral ECT has a superior efficacy to unilateral ECT. However, bilateral treatment is associated with more cognitive impairment (UK ECT Review Group, 2003). When right unilateral ECT is dosed to about six times the seizure threshold, its efficacy approaches that of bilateral ECT, but the associated cognitive impairment is also similar (Kellner *et al.*, 2010).

These data suggest that the appropriate electrode placement for ECT should balance efficacy against cognitive disturbance according to the needs of the individual patient. If the need for improvement is particularly urgent, bilateral ECT should be considered, dosed to about two and a half times the seizure threshold.

For a meta-analytical review of treatment factors that affect the efficacy of ECT, see UK ECT Review Group (2003) (see also Box 25.14).

Unwanted effects after ECT

Subconvulsive shock may be followed by anxiety and headache. ECT can cause a brief *retrograde amnesia* as well as loss of memory for up to 30 minutes after the fit. *Brief disorientation* can occur, particularly with bilateral electrode placement. *Headache* can also occur. Some patients complain of confusion, nausea, and vertigo for a few hours after the treatment, but with modern methods these unwanted effects are mild and brief.

A few patients complain of *muscle pain*, especially in the jaws, which is probably attributable to the relaxant. There have been a few reports of sporadic major seizures in the months after ECT, but these may have had other causes. Occasional damage to the teeth, tongue, or lips can occur if there have been problems in positioning the gag or airway. Poor application of the electrodes can lead to *small electrical burns*. *Fractures*, including crush fractures of the vertebrae, have occurred occasionally when ECT was given without muscle relaxants.

All of these physical consequences are rare if a good technique of anaesthesia is used and the fit is modified

adequately. Other complications of ECT are rare and mainly occur in people suffering from physical illness. They include *cardiac arrhythmia, pulmonary embolism, aspiration pneumonia,* and *cerebrovascular accident.* Prolonged apnoea is a rare complication of the use of muscle relaxants. Rarely, *status epilepticus* may occur in predisposed individuals or in those taking medication that prolongs seizure duration.

Since the introduction of ECT, there has always been concern as to whether it may cause *brain damage.* When ECT is given to animals in the usual clinical regimen, there is no evidence that brain damage occurs. Also, structural imaging studies in patients have been reassuring on this point (UK ECT Review Group, 2003).

Memory disorder after ECT

Short-term effects. As already mentioned, the immediate effects of ECT include loss of memory for events shortly before the treatment (*retrograde amnesia*), and impaired retention of information acquired soon after the treatment (*anterograde amnesia*). These effects depend on both electrode placement (unilateral versus bilateral) and electrical dose, but electrode placement appears to be the more important factor.

> ### Box 25.14 Efficacy of ECT in depression in relation to antidepressant treatment and different stimulus parameters
>
> | Treatment comparison | HAM-D difference (with 95% CI) | Effect size* |
> | --- | --- | --- |
> | ECT superior to antidepressant medication | 5.2 (1.4–8.9) | 0.46 |
> | Bilateral ECT superior to unilateral ECT | 3.6 (2.2–5.2) | 0.32 |
> | Higher ECT dose superior | 4.1 (2.4–5.9) | 0.57 |
>
> Source: UK ECT Review Group (2003).
>
> HAM-D, Hamilton Rating Scale for Depression.
>
> * For explanation of effect sizes, see Chapter 6

Controlled studies indicate that the *anterograde amnesia* produced by ECT is *temporary*. Depressive disorders substantially impair cognitive function, and many patients report their memory as subjectively improved after ECT. ECT-induced cognitive impairment can be detected for the first days after the end of the course of treatment. However, this usually remits within about 2 weeks. A meta-analysis showed improvements in various objective measures of cognitive function, including, for example, processing speed, working memory, and executive function 2 weeks after the end of ECT treatment (Semkovska and McLoughlin, 2010).

Long-term effects. The major concern regarding long-term effects of ECT on memory is the loss of *memories for personal remote events* (retrograde amnesia for remote events) or autobiographical memory loss. In a systematic review, Fraser and colleagues (2008) concluded that ECT can produce a definite loss of autobiographical memory. While objective measures suggested that this loss largely resolved within 6 months, subjective reports by patients indicated that the loss could extend for longer and, in some cases, could be permanent. Autobiographical memory loss was less when treatment employed right unilateral electrode placement and when dose of electricity was titrated to the level of the individual patient's seizure threshold.

It seems reasonable to conclude that, when used in the usual way, *ECT is not normally followed by persisting anterograde memory disorder*, or problems with *working memory* and *executive function*, and that where these do occur they are mild and may be accounted for by concurrent depressive symptomatology. However, ECT, particularly when applied bilaterally, may cause a persisting retrograde amnesia for personal memories. Although this is not a significant problem for most patients, some, for reasons that are unclear, have much greater autobiographical memory loss, to the extent that their lives and sense of self are adversely affected. For a review of the cognitive effects of ECT, see Freeman (2013).

The mortality of ECT

The death rate attributable to ECT has been estimated to be less than 1 per 70,000 treatments. This is similar to that seen with general anaesthesia for minor surgical conditions. The risks are related to the anaesthetic procedure, and are greatest in patients with cardiovascular disease. When death occurs it is usually due to *ventricular fibrillation* or *myocardial infarction* (see Benbow and Waite, 2013).

Contraindications

The contraindications to ECT are any medical illnesses that increase the risk of anaesthetic procedure by an unacceptable amount—for example, respiratory infections, serious heart disease, and serious pyrexial illness. Other contraindications are diseases that are likely to be made worse by the *changes in blood pressure and cardiac rhythm* that occur even in a well-modified fit. These include serious heart diseases, recent myocardial infarction, cardiac failure, cerebral or aortic aneurysm, deep vein thrombosis, and raised intracranial pressure.

In Mediterranean and Afro-Caribbean patients who might have *sickle-cell trait*, additional care is needed to ensure that oxygen tension does not fall. Extra care is also required with diabetic patients who take insulin. Although risks rise somewhat in old age, so do the risks of untreated depression and drug treatment.

Technique of administration

In this section we outline the technical procedures used at the time of treatment. Although the information in this account should be known, it is important to remember that ECT is a *practical procedure* that must be learned by apprenticeship as well as by reading. For a review of the medical evaluation of patients for ECT, see Tess and Smetana (2009).

ECT clinic. ECT should be given in pleasant safe surroundings. Patients should not have to wait where they can see or hear treatment being given to others. There should be waiting and recovery areas separate from the room in which treatment is given, and adequate emergency equipment should be available, including a sucker, endotracheal tubes, adequate supplies of oxygen, and facilities to carry out full resuscitation. The nursing and medical staff who give ECT should receive *special training and accreditation*.

Arrival of the patient. The first step in giving ECT is to put the patient at ease and to check their identity. The case notes should then be seen to make sure that there is a *valid consent form* and that *the patient continues to consent to treatment*. The drug sheet should be checked to ensure that the patient is not receiving any drugs that might complicate the anaesthetic procedures. It is also important to check for evidence of drug allergy or adverse effects of previous general anaesthetics. The drug sheet should be available for the anaesthetist to see. A full physical evaluation should have been carried out by the patient's treating doctor. Specialist advice should be sought if there may be medical contraindications to ECT.

Electrode placement. A decision about electrode placement should have been made by the treating doctor prior to treatment. When using unilateral treatment, it is important to apply the electrodes to the *non-dominant hemisphere.* In right-handed people, the left hemisphere is nearly always dominant; in left-handed people, either hemisphere may be dominant. Therefore, if there is evidence that the patient is not right-handed, it is usually better to use bilateral electrode placements.

Anaesthetic procedures. Prior to administering the anaesthetic it is necessary to make sure that the patient has taken nothing by mouth for at least 5 hours, and then, with the anaesthetist, to remove any dentures and check for loose or broken teeth. Finally, the record of any previous ECTs should be examined for evidence of delayed recovery from the relaxant (due to deficiency in pseudocholinesterase) or other complications.

The anaesthetic should be given by a trained anaesthetist (although this cannot always be achieved in developing countries). Suction apparatus, a positive-pressure oxygen supply, and emergency drugs should always be available. A tilting trolley is also valuable. As well as the psychiatrist and the anaesthetist, at least one nurse should be present.

Anaesthesia for ECT was previously induced with *methohexitone,* a short-acting barbiturate. However, this agent became increasingly difficult to obtain, and *propofol* is the most widely used alternative. The injection of propofol can be painful, and it can also *decrease seizure length* and *delay or abolish convulsions. Etomidate* may be preferred in patients in whom it is difficult to induce a seizure.

The induction agent is followed immediately by a *muscle relaxant* (often suxamethonium chloride) from a separate syringe, although the same needle can be used. The anticholinergic agent *glycopyrrolate* can be used to prevent ECT-induced increases in parasympathetic tone and bradycardia. The anaesthetist is responsible for the choice of drugs, and should also ensure that the lungs are well oxygenated before a mouth gag is inserted.

Application of ECT. While the anaesthetic is being given, the psychiatrist checks both the *dose of electricity* and the *electrode placement* that has been prescribed for the patient. The skin is cleaned in the appropriate areas and moistened electrodes are applied. (If good electrical contact is to be obtained, it is also important that grease and hair lacquer are removed by ward staff before the patient is sent for ECT.) Although dry electrodes can cause skin burns, it is also important to remember that excessive moisture causes shorting and may prevent a seizure response.

Although enough muscle relaxant should have been given to ensure that convulsive movements are minimal, a nurse or other assistant should be ready to restrain the patient gently if necessary. The electrodes are then secured firmly. For unilateral ECT, the first electrode is placed on the non-dominant side, 3 cm above the midpoint between the external angle of the orbit and the external auditory meatus. The second electrode is placed *at least 10 cm away from the first one,* vertically above the meatus of the same side (see Figure 25.2). A wide separation of the electrodes is thought to maximize the efficacy of unilateral ECT. The stimulus is then given.

For *fixed-dose right unilateral ECT* the initial dose should be set at 400 millicoulombs and subsequently adjusted according to clinical efficacy and cognitive side effects. However, dose titration offers advantages in terms of individualizing the dose for each patient. In dose titration the seizure threshold for the individual patient is determined during the first ECT session by starting with a very low dose and increasing it until a fit occurs (Scott, 2005).

For *bilateral ECT,* electrodes are placed on opposite sides of the head, each 3 cm above the midpoint of the line joining the external angle of the orbit to the external auditory meatus—usually just above the hairline (see Figure 25.2). When using bilateral electrode placement, the present practice is to administer a dose of electricity that is only modestly (about 1.5 to 2.5 times) above the seizure threshold for the individual. The seizure threshold for ECT is best determined by dose titration as described above. Otherwise an appropriate dose can be estimated from the fact that two-thirds of the population have seizure thresholds in the range 100–200 millicoulombs. In addition, seizure thresholds are higher in men than in women, and increase with age. For example, a reasonable starting dose for a male

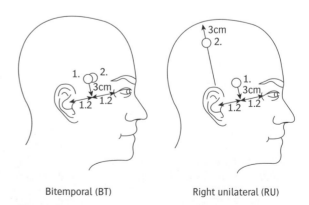

Bitemporal (BT)   Right unilateral (RU)

Figure 25.2 Electrode placements for ECT.

patient under 40 years of age who is to receive bilateral ECT would be 150 millicoulombs.

Subsequently this dose could be adjusted, depending on the length of the seizure, the cognitive side effects, and the clinical response. The dose might be increased if the seizure was short or absent, or if there was no improvement after several treatments. Conversely, troublesome post-ECT cognitive disturbance would indicate that the dose of electricity should be reduced or that unilateral placement of the electrodes should be used.

It is important to note that seizure duration may *decrease* during a course of ECT, because repeated treatment tends to increase the seizure threshold. Thus if a dose of electricity initially produced a seizure of satisfactory duration, it may subsequently need to be increased.

The seizure. It is essential to observe carefully for evidence of seizure. If satisfactory muscle relaxation has been achieved, the seizure takes the following form. First, the muscles of the face begin to twitch and the mouth drops open. Then the upper eyelids, thumbs, and big toes jerk rhythmically for about half a minute. It is important not to confuse these convulsive movements with muscle twitches due to the depolarization produced by suxamethonium.

EEG monitoring is now often used to check whether a seizure has been induced, but the records can be difficult to interpret because of the muscle artefact produced by direct stimulation of the frontalis muscle. A seizure can be detected by the appearance in the EEG of high frequency spike waves followed by slower spike and wave complexes with a frequency of around 3 Hz (Scott and Waite, 2013). An alternative is to *isolate one forearm from the effects of the muscle relaxant.* This can be done by blowing up a blood pressure cuff to above systolic pressure before the relaxant is injected; this pressure is maintained during the period in which the seizure should occur and then released. Seizure activity can then be observed in the muscles of the isolated part of the arm. When determining the appropriate cuff pressure, it is important to remember that systolic pressure rises during the seizure, so if the cuff is not at sufficient pressure the relaxant will pass into the forearm at this stage.

There is no direct correlation between treatment outcome and duration of seizure activity, but it is recommended that the dose of electricity is adjusted so as to achieve a seizure duration of *between 20 and 50 seconds*. This duration is recommended because short seizures are likely to be therapeutically ineffective, whereas long seizures are more likely to be associated with cognitive disturbance.

Psychotropic drugs may alter the seizure threshold and seizure duration. For example, most antidepressant and antipsychotic drugs lower the seizure threshold, whereas benzodiazepines, valproate, and lamotrigine have the opposite effect. Adverse effects, including increased cognitive impairment, have been reported when ECT has been given with *lithium*, and it may be prudent to suspend lithium treatment or omit the lithium dose the evening before treament. *SSRIs* have been associated with prolonged seizures during ECT. Some anaesthetists prefer not to anaesthetize patients who are taking *MAOIs*, but ECT can in fact be given safely to patients who are receiving MAOI treatment. The usual practice in the UK has been to continue antidepressant medication during a course of ECT. Sackheim *et al.* (2009) found that the introduction of nortriptyline to unmedicated patients during a course of ECT improved efficacy and lessened cognitive adverse effects. On the other hand, venlafaxine had a weaker effect in improving efficacy, and tended to worsen cognitive adverse effects.

Recovery phase. After the seizure, the lungs are oxygenated thoroughly with an airway in place. The patient remains in the care of the anaesthetist and under close nursing observation until breathing resumes and consciousness is restored. During recovery, the patient should be turned on to their side and cared for in the usual way for any patient recovering from an anaesthetic after a minor surgical procedure. A qualified nurse should be in attendance to supervise the patient and reassure them. Meanwhile, the psychiatrist makes a note of the date, type of electrode placement, drugs used, and amount of current, together with a brief description of the fit and any problems that have arisen. When the patient is awake and orientated, they should rest for an hour or so on their bed or in a chair.

If ECT is given to a day-patient, it is especially important to make certain that no food or drink has been taken before they arrive at the hospital. They should rest for several hours and should not leave until it is certain that their recovery is complete; they should leave in the company of a responsible adult, and certainly not riding a bicycle or driving a car.

Failed stimulations. The most important problem, apart from those relating to the anaesthetic procedure, is failure to produce a clonic convulsion (a tonic jerk produced by the current must not be mistaken for a seizure). If it is certain that no seizure has appeared, checks should be made of the machine, the electrodes, and contact with the skin. The possibility of shorting due to excess moisture on the scalp should also be considered. If all of these are excluded, the patient may have either an unusually high resistance to the passage of current through the extracranial tissues and skull, or a high convulsive threshold. The charge can then be increased by 50% and a further stimulus given.

Frequency and number of treatments

ECT is usually given twice a week. In general, ECT given three times weekly has *little therapeutic advantage* over a twice-weekly regimen, and may produce more cognitive impairment (UK ECT Review Group, 2003).

Decisions about the length of a course of ECT must depend on clinical experience, as relevant information is not available from clinical trials. *A course of ECT usually consists of between six and a maximum of twelve treatments.* Progress should be reviewed after each treatment. There is usually little response until two or three treatments have been given, after which increasing improvement occurs. If the response is more rapid than this, fewer treatments may be given. If there has been no response after six to eight treatments, the course should usually be abandoned, as it is unlikely that more ECT will produce a useful change.

Clinical change and memory should also be assessed after each treatment. It is better to use reliable, validated scales for this purpose. For clinical change, the Clinical Global Impression of Improvement is suitable and the patient's subjective report should also be noted. Measurement of the various aspects of memory in a routine clinical setting is more difficult. NICE (2003) has recommended the Mini Mental State Examination, which will capture confusion and short-term memory impairment but not, for example, autobiographical memory loss. Significant cognitive impairment should lead to a reappraisal of the electrical dose and electrode placement.

Prevention of relapse

It is important that, whereas ECT may produce striking benefit in depressed patients, there is *a high relapse rate* unless continuation therapy with antidepressant medication is undertaken. Sometimes the choice of antidepressant drug can be difficult because, if a patient does not respond to an adequate dose of an antidepressant drug prior to ECT, continuing the same drug after the course of ECT is completed *may not provide a useful prophylactic effect.* Thus, if a patient has required ECT because of nonresponse to antidepressant medication, it is good practice to consider a different class of antidepressant drug or lithium carbonate in the continuation and prophylactic phases of drug treatment. A randomized study of 200 patients found post-ECT prophylaxis with a combination of lithium and nortriptyline as effective as maintenance ECT in sustaining remission in the 6 months following a successful course of treatment. Despite this, just over 50% of the patients in each group relapsed (Kellner *et al.*, 2006).

A few patients respond well to ECT but continually relapse even when maintained on multiple drug therapy. In these circumstances, some practitioners have given *maintenance ECT* at a reduced frequency (e.g. fortnightly or monthly). However, this practice was not recommended by the National Institute for Clinical Excellence (2003).

Consent to ECT

Before a patient is asked to agree to ECT, it is essential to provide a full *explanation of the procedure* and indicate its *expected benefits and possible risks,* especially the effects on memory. Appropriately written information sheets should be a standard part of the consent procedure (National Institute for Clinical Excellence, 2003).

Many patients expect severe and permanent memory impairment after treatment, and some even expect to experience unmodified fits. Once the doctor is sure that the patient understands what they have been told, the patient is asked to sign a standard form of consent. It should be made clear to them that consent is being sought for the whole course of ECT, and not just for one treatment, although it is also essential to make sure that they understand that consent can be withdrawn at any time. It is also good practice to ensure that patients continue to give consent prior to each treatment throughout the course. Part of the consent process should involve the assessment of *capacity* (see Chapter 4). Patients cannot give informed consent if they lack capacity, and advance directives declining ECT should be respected unless treatment is considered life-saving and can be administered under the Mental Health Act.

In the UK, if a patient refuses consent, or is unable to give it because they are in a stupor or for some other reason, and if the procedure is essential, further steps must be considered. The first is to decide whether there are grounds for involving the appropriate section of the Mental Health Act (see Chapter 4). The section does not allow anyone to give consent on behalf of the patient, but it does establish formally that they are mentally ill and in need of treatment. In England and Wales, the opinion of a second independent consultant is required by the Mental Health Act 1983. Readers working outside the UK should familiarize themselves with the relevant legal requirements.

Patient attitude to treatment

Surveys carried out by clinicians have generally reported positive experiences of ECT, with the majority of patients reporting that the procedure was tolerable and helpful. The presence of friendly and helpful clinic staff was regarded as important in reducing anxiety about treatment. The major complaint about ECT concerned autobiographical memory loss, which in some patients was persistent and severe. Service user-led research on ECT generally elicits less positive responses about treatment, with about half the patients reporting that they would not have ECT again. Again, the presence of persistent memory loss is usually the main complaint, but some patients also reported a lack of information about ECT and its adverse effects and also experiences of coercion. Not surprisingly, patients who believe that ECT has helped them are more positive about treatment (Waite, 2013).

These experiences underline the need for careful selection of patients for ECT, as well as adequate time being taken to explain the procedure and its possible adverse effects as fully and carefully as possible.

Ethical aspects of ECT

As with drug treatment, the key issue for a competent patient is the concept of *full informed consent*. In general, ECT is widely regarded as a safe and effective treatment—a view that is supported by randomized controlled trials. However, it is important that patients are warned about the possibility of loss of remote memories outlined above. In addition, in the case of medication-resistant patients, the issue of relapse should be discussed.

ECT in the case of non-competent patients raises particularly difficult issues. Usually, in these circumstances, ECT is needed to treat a patient whose life is placed at risk as a result of their illness. The legal safeguards for patients are outlined above, but the clinician has a duty to explain to the patient and their family the reasons for the action taken, and to follow carefully the ethical principles outlined in Chapter 4.

Bright light treatment

The use of *phototherapy*, or *artificial bright light*, as a psychiatric treatment was first studied systematically by Rosenthal *et al.* (1984). These workers used bright light to treat patients with the newly identified syndrome of *seasonal affective disorder*. Since then, phototherapy has become the mainstay of treatment of *winter depression*, particularly in patients with *atypical depressive features* such as hyperphagia and hypersomnia.

Mechanism of action

The light–dark cycle is believed to be one of the most important 'zeitgebers' regulating circadian and seasonal rhythmicity in mammals. Initially, phototherapy was believed to ameliorate the symptoms of winter depression by extending the photoperiod. This was based on the view that patients with winter depression were particularly sensitive to the effects of short winter days, and that bright light treatment produced a day length equivalent to that of summer.

More recent formulations have suggested that the antidepressant effect of bright light may be attributable to a *phase advance in circadian rhythm*. This is supported by the fact that controlled trials show that, in most patients, morning phototherapy is more effective than evening phototherapy. However, other studies have shown that bright light given at midday is also therapeutically effective. It is difficult to devise a truly plausible placebo condition for bright light treatment, and some have argued that the antidepressant effects of bright light may be mediated in large measure by placebo effects, particularly patient expectation. Mårtensson and colleagues (2015) found in a meta-analysis of eight randomized studies that bright light was significantly superior to a dim light control in reducing depressive symptomatology in patients with seasonal affective disorder, with an effect size of 0.54 (95% CI: –0.95, –0.13) at study endpoint. In winter depression the therapeutic effects of bright light treatment, fluoxetine, and cognitive behaviour therapy appear generally equivalent, although cognitive therapy had a better long-term outcome (Cleare *et al.*, 2015).

Equipment

A conventional light box contains fluorescent tubes mounted behind a translucent plastic diffusing screen. The tubes provide an output that can vary between 2500 and 10,000 lux. Light sources that produce 10,000 lux are more expensive, but may allow a *reduced duration of exposure* (30 minutes, compared with 120 minutes) to secure a therapeutic effect.

Phototherapy has also been administered using *head-mounted units* or *light visors*. These instruments are attached to the head and project light into the eyes, allowing the subject to remain mobile while receiving treatment. Although light visors are more convenient to use than light boxes, results from placebo-controlled trials of light visors have proved disappointing and their use is not currently recommended.

Therapeutic efficacy and indications

The major indication for light therapy is seasonal affective disorder in which patients experience winter depressions. Bright light treatment is more effective than placebo in patients with winter depression, particularly if patients experience:

- increased sleep
- carbohydrate cravings
- an afternoon slump in energy.

Patients with more typical melancholic symptoms—for example, weight loss and insomnia—do less well with phototherapy as a sole treatment, even where the disorder is seasonal in nature. Although there are studies to suggest that morning light treatment may augment the therapeutic effect of antidepressant medication in *non-seasonal depression*, the effect may not be well sustained. However, bright light given as *a sole treatment* in non-seasonal depression may be helpful (Mårtensson *et al.*, 2015). Phototherapy may also be of benefit in other disorders characterized by depressed mood and appetite changes—for example, premenstrual syndrome and bulimia nervosa. The literature contains a number of controlled trials in such disorders where light treatment has improved ratings of depression. However, the difficulty of distinguishing specific and placebo effects of bright light makes the current data difficult to interpret.

Adverse effects

In general, phototherapy is well tolerated, although mild side effects occur in up to 45% of patients early in treatment. These include *headache, eye-strain, blurred vision, eye irritation,* and *increased tension.* Insomnia can also occur, particularly with late evening treatment. Rare adverse events that have been reported include *manic mood swings* and *suicide* attempts, the latter putatively through light-induced alerting and energizing effects prior to mood improvement. Whether these rare events are actually adverse reactions to light is uncertain. There is no evidence that phototherapy employed in recommended treatment schedules causes ocular or retinal damage.

Clinical use of phototherapy

Since the best-established indication for phototherapy is winter depression, the following account will describe the use of bright light treatment in winter depression. One of the major practical difficulties in phototherapy is the time needed to administer the treatment. For this reason, a 10,000 lux light box may be preferred because the daily duration of therapy can be reduced to 30 minutes. It seems likely that cool-white light and full-spectrum light have equivalent clinical efficacy, but because cool-white light is free of ultraviolet light it is theoretically safer.

The evidence suggests that bright light treatment of winter depression is most effective when administered in the early morning. However, treatments given at other times of day may prove beneficial and can be more convenient for individual patients. In an initial trial, therefore, it is best to recommend early morning treatment but to advise the patient that the exact timing of therapy can eventually represent a balance of therapeutic efficacy and practical convenience. Treatment should not be given late in the evening because of the possibility of *sleep disruption*.

Early morning phototherapy should start within a few minutes of awakening. Patients should allow an initial duration of treatment of 30 minutes with a 10,000 lux light box or 2 hours with 2500 lux equipment. They should seat themselves about 30–40 cm away from the light box screen. They should not gaze at the screen directly, but face it at an angle of about 45° and glance across it once or twice each minute.

The antidepressant effect of light treatment can appear within a few days, but in controlled trials longer periods (up to 3 weeks) can be necessary before the therapeutic effects of bright light exceed those of placebo treatment. As noted above, mild side effects are common in the early stages of treatment, but usually settle without specific intervention. If they are persistent and troublesome, the patient can sit a little further away from the light source or reduce the duration of exposure. Exposure should also be reduced if elevated mood occurs.

Once a therapeutic response has occurred, it is necessary to continue phototherapy up to the point of natural remission, otherwise relapse will occur. However, it may be possible to lower the daily duration of treatment. Phototherapy may also be started in advance of the anticipated episode of depression, as this appears to have a *prophylactic effect*, although doubts about the robustness of this effect have been expressed.

Neurosurgery for psychiatric disorders (psychosurgery)

History of procedure

Psychosurgery refers to the use of *neurosurgical procedures* to modify the symptoms of psychiatric illness by operating on either the nuclei of the brain or the white matter. Psychosurgery began in 1936 with the work of Egas Moniz, whose operation consisted of an extensive cut in the white matter of the frontal lobes (*frontal leucotomy*). This extensive operation was modified by Freeman and

Watts (1942), who made smaller coronal incisions in the frontal lobes through lateral burr holes.

Although their so-called 'standard leucotomy' was far from standardized anatomically, and although it produced unacceptable side effects (see below), the procedure was widely used in the UK and other countries. There was enthusiasm for the initial improvements observed in patients, but this was followed by growing evidence of adverse effects, including *intellectual impairment, emotional lability, disinhibition, apathy, incontinence, obesity,* and *epilepsy.*

These problems led to a search for more restricted lesions capable of producing the same therapeutic benefits without these adverse consequences. Some progress was made, particularly with the incorporation of *stereotactic techniques* (see Christmas *et al.*, 2004), but at the same time advances in pharmacology made it possible to use drugs to treat the disorders for which surgery was intended.

Current approaches

The term *psychosurgery* is now often replaced by the phrase *neurosurgery for mental disorders*. This change in terminology is intended to emphasize that:

- The techniques involved now involve placement of localized lesions in specific cerebral sites.
- The treatment is for specific psychiatric conditions (treatment-resistant major depression and obsessive–compulsive disorder), not for primary behavioural disturbance.

Indications

In the UK the indications for neurosurgery for mental disorders are restricted to major depression and obsessive–compulsive disorder that is chronic, treatment-refractory, and disabling. Neurosurgery is not indicated where these conditions arise as a consequence of organic brain disease or a pervasive developmental disorder.

Types of operation

Nowadays the older 'blind' operations have been replaced by stereotactic procedures that allow the lesions to be placed more accurately (see Box 25.15). In the UK, current procedures are limited to anterior capsulotomy and anterior cingulotomy. The lesions are produced either by radiofrequency thermocoagulation or by gamma radiation (the 'gamma knife'). Lesions are made bilaterally.

Effectiveness

In the absence of controlled trials, assessment has been in the form of long-term *follow-up studies*. A report by the

---

> ### Box 25.15 Stereotactic procedures used in psychosurgery
>
> **Subcaudate tractotomy**
>
> Lesion made beneath the head of each caudate nucleus, in the rostral part of the orbital cortex
>
> **Anterior cingulotomy**
>
> Bilateral lesions within the cingulate bundles
>
> **Limbic leucotomy**
>
> Subcaudate tractotomy combined with cingulotomy
>
> **Anterior capsulotomy**
>
> Bilateral lesions in the anterior limb of the internal capsule

Royal College of Psychiatrists (2000) found a 'marked improvement' rate in 63% of patients with major depression and in 58% of patients with obsessive–compulsive disorder (see Box 25.16). A recent literature review reported a slightly but significantly greater improvement in symptomatology in intractable obsessive–compulsive disorder following anterior capsulotomy in comparison to deep brain stimulation of ventral striatum and nucleus accumbens (51% reduction versus 40%) (Pepper *et al.*, 2015).

> ### Box 25.16 Outcome of psychosurgery in the UK, 1961–1997
>
> | | Depression (*n* = **727**) | Obsessive–compulsive disorder (*n* = **478**) |
> | --- | --- | --- |
> | Marked improvement | 63% | 58% |
> | Lesser improvement | 22% | 27% |
> | No response | 14% | 14% |
> | Worse | 1% | 1% |
>
> Source: data from Royal College of Psychiatrists, Copyright (2000).

Adverse effects

With modern procedures, severe adverse effects are rare. After the operation, headache and nausea are common, and confusion occurs in about 10% of patients. These adverse effects typically last for a few days, but can persist for up to a month. Long-term cognitive impairment does not seem to occur (see Box 25.17).

Clinical use

Neurosurgical procedures for mental disorders should not be performed until the effects of several years of vigorous multimodal treatment have been observed. If this rule is followed, the operation will hardly ever be used. In fact, less than 20 psychosurgical operations a year are currently performed in the UK, about 25% of the annual rate in the early 1980s. If the surgery is to be considered at all, it should only be for chronic intractable obsessional disorder and severe chronic depressive disorders in older patients. There is no clear justification for neurosurgery for anxiety disorders or schizophrenia. For a review, see Christmas *et al.* (2004).

Ethical issues

The brain is the organ of judgement and decision-making, but it is regarded as ethically permissible to operate, for example, on a brain tumour, if a patient gives their consent. The situation with regard to psychosurgery is different because the tissue that is lesioned is not overtly diseased. However, surgeons do sometimes operate on tissue that is not diseased. The practical problems with regard to psychosurgery (which distinguish it from ECT) are as follows:

- the lack of randomized studies to demonstrate that it is effective
- the irreversibility of the procedure
- the potentially serious nature of some of the adverse effects.

For these reasons it seems ethically appropriate that psychosurgery should be offered only to competent patients who are able to give their full informed consent. Determining competence may, of course, be difficult in a patient with chronic severe mood disorder. In the UK, this has led to the development of safeguards under Section 57 of the 1983 Mental Health Act, which require that:

1. The patient gives their full informed consent.
2. A multidisciplinary panel appointed by the Mental Health Act Commission confirms that the patient's consent is valid.
3. The doctor on the multidisciplinary panel certifies that the treatment should be given. Before doing so, the doctor must consult two people, one a nurse and the other neither a nurse nor a doctor, who have been concerned with the patient's treatment.

Brain stimulation techniques

Transcranial magnetic stimulation

The use of transcranial magnetic stimulation (TMS) is based on the principle that, if a conducting medium such as the brain is adjacent to a magnetic field, a current will be induced in the conducting medium. In TMS, an electromagnetic coil is placed on the scalp. The passage of high-intensity pulses of current in the coil produces a powerful magnetic field—typically about 2 Tesla—which results in current flow in neural tissue and neuronal depolarization. Neuropsychological effects of TMS are particularly likely when pulses of current are delivered rapidly, so-called *repetitive TMS (rTMS)*. If the stimulation occurs more quickly than once per second (1 Hz), it is called *fast rTMS*. The use of appropriately shaped coils allows reasonably localized stimulation of the main specific cortical areas.

Uses of TMS

TMS has been used for many years in clinical neurophysiology to explore, for example, the integrity of the motor cortex after stroke. In research settings, TMS is used to localize the cortical substrates of specific neuropsychological functions. For example, short-term verbal recall can be disrupted by rTMS administered over the left temporal cortex.

Box 25.17 Adverse effects of stereotactic psychosurgery

Acute effects

Operative mortality (less than 0.1%)
Haemorrhage, hemiplegia (less than 0.3%)
Transient confusion, lethargy (common)

Long-term effects

Epilepsy (1–2%)
Weight gain (10%)
Frontal lobe syndrome (very rare)
Personality changes (usually mild)

Clinically, rTMS has been used to relieve *depressive states*. Initially, studies used fast rTMS applied to the left prefrontal cortex. However, other investigations have employed different kinds of electromagnetic coil, stimulation parameters, and sites of coil application, making comparison between studies difficult. Typically in the treatment of depression, 40 pulses of stimulation are delivered over 4 seconds followed by a gap of 26 seconds before the next 40 pulses. Around 2400–3000 pulses are delivered over a single session, which may last for about 30 minutes. To achieve a clinical antidepressant effect, TMS is usually repeated daily for 2–3 weeks (Tracy and David, 2015).

Meta-analyses suggest that, overall, TMS is more effective in the treatment of depression than sham treatment, but it is significantly less effective than ECT (Cowen and Anderson, 2015). TMS has also been employed in treatment studies of other disorders, such as obsessive–compulsive disorder, schizophrenia, eating disorders, and depersonalization syndrome (Tracy and David, 2015). Findings in these conditions are still preliminary and the difficulty of providing a convincing sham control makes assessment difficult.

Adverse effects of TMS

The use of single-pulse TMS in neurophysiological studies has not raised significant safety concerns. The major hazard with rTMS is the risk of inducing *seizures*. This is greater with fast rTMS than with slow rTMS. Current safety protocols, which adjust the amount of magnetic stimulation in relation to the motor threshold of the individual, appear to have greatly reduced the likelihood of fits, although patients with risk factors (e.g. a family history of epilepsy) are generally excluded from TMS studies of healthy volunteers.

Minor side effects are more common, and include *muscle tension headaches*, and sufficient noise is generated by the equipment to cause short-term changes in *hearing threshold*. This can be prevented by the use of earplugs (by both patients and investigators). rTMS appropriately localized also has the potential to disrupt cognitive function, but so far such changes have been temporary, and have not persisted after the stimulation was terminated. There are insufficient data to establish whether there might be any long-term sequelae to the brain or other organs from the high-intensity magnetic field generated during TMS. No specific hazard has been revealed by current follow-up studies.

Vagal nerve stimulation

Vagal nerve stimulation (VNS) is an established treatment for patients with refractory epilepsy, in whom it was noted to improve mood. It has therefore subsequently been applied to the treatment of patients with resistant depression.

As well as providing an efferent parasympathetic outflow from the brain, the vagus nerve conveys afferent sensory fibres that synapse in the nucleus tractus solitarius and subsequently project to the forebrain. Stimulating the vagus nerve therapeutically involves an operative procedure during which a pulse generator is implanted subcutaneously in the left anterior chest wall. Bipolar electrodes, connected to the generator, are placed around the left vagus nerve in the cervical region. These electrodes are intermittently stimulated by the generator, with the stimulation parameters being regulated by a telemetric 'wand', which is connected to a personal computer. Modification of the stimulus parameters is used to balance adverse effects (see below) with therapeutic effects. Typically stimulation occurs for about 30 seconds followed by a 5-minute 'off' period (Tracy and David, 2015).

VNS in depression

Open studies have suggested that over 12 months of treatment about 50% of patients show a good clinical response to VNS. Currently the best antidepressant effects have occurred in patients who have a moderate degree of treatment resistance but who have not proved totally refractory to multiple trials of antidepressant and augmentation therapies. Berry and colleagues (2013) carried out a patient-level meta-analysis of six outpatient trials involving patients with resistant depression, which allowed comparison of VNS and treatment as usual (TAU) for up to 96 weeks postimplantation. Response rates in the VNS group at 48 and 96 weeks were 28% and 32%, whereas the corresponding figures for the TAU participants were 12% and 14%, respectively. However, in only one of these studies was there a randomized comparison of VNS and TAU, and this did not show a significant difference between the two conditions (Cowen and Anderson, 2015).

Adverse effects of VNS

During periods of VNS, hoarseness is common and throat pain, cough, and dyspnoea can occur. These adverse effects decline with time, and withdrawal from treatment is uncommon. Hypomania has rarely been reported, but its relationship to VNS treatment is uncertain (Christmas *et al.*, 2004; Tracy and David, 2015).

Deep brain stimulation

Deep brain stimulation (DBS) is established in the treatment of Parkinson's disease, where implantation of electrodes in the subthalamic nucleus significantly alleviates the motor symptoms of advanced disease. DBS was also noted sometimes to improve mood and obsessive symptomatology in patients with Parkinson's disease and this, together with increasing knowledge of the neural circuitry underlying psychiatric disorders, has led to studies of its effects in patients with refractory depression and obsessive–compulsive disorder (Tracy and David, 2015).

DBS involves bilateral implantation of electrodes into designated target locations using stereotactic guidance. The location of the electrodes is confirmed with MRI scanning. The electrodes are connected to a generator implanted into the abdomen, and the stimulation settings are adjusted according to clinical response and adverse effects. The fact that the settings can be modified and the generator switched on or off makes DBS more susceptible to controlled trial than neurosurgical treatment.

It seems likely that stimulation frequency is a key factor in determining the clinical efficacy of DBS. In Parkinson's disease, for example, stimulation starts to reduce tremor at a frequency of approximately 50 Hz and reaches a plateau at about 200 Hz. Low-frequency stimulation is believed to activate neurons, whilst high-frequency stimulation probably causes inhibition. Whereas improvement in rigidity and tremor in Parkinson's disease can be seen within minutes of DBS commencing, amelioration in depression and obsessive–compulsive symptomatology develops gradually over a period of weeks. This might be a consequence of neuroplastic changes induced by DBS, or might perhaps be due to changes in the oscillatory properties of the relevant neural networks.

DBS in obsessive–compulsive disorder

In studies of patients with intractable obsessive–compulsive disorder, electrodes have been implanted in the anterior limb of the internal capsule, with the aim of influencing the brain regions targeted by neurosurgery for obsessive–compulsive disorder (see above). Subsequent studies have also examined the effect of DBS in the ventral striatum and nucleus accumbens.

Alonso and colleagues (2015) conducted a meta-analysis of 31 studies (116 participants) of DBS in patients with refractory obsessive–compulsive disorder. Clinical response was seen in 60% of the sample, with older age of onset, religious obsessions, and compulsions being positive predictors of outcome. The different DBS studies targeted a variety of brain regions, and no particular location emerged as being the most effective site. It will be important to confirm these results with suitably powered randomized studies using sham stimulation.

DBS in depression

DBS in treatment-refractory depressed patients has also involved a number of different brain regions, based on abnormalities revealed by functional neuroimaging as well as theoretical considerations of the neural underpinnings of symptoms such as anhedonia. Studies have involved mainly the subgenual cingulate cortex and the ventral striatum. A meta-analysis of four observational studies (66 participants) of stimulation to the subgenual cortex in patients with resistant depression showed a 12-month remission rate of 26% (Berlim *et al.*, 2014). However, benefit has yet to be shown in sham controlled studies (Tracy and David, 2015).

Adverse effects of DBS

Typical adverse effects associated with DBS include throbbing or buzzing sensations, nausea, and jaw tingling. Orofacial muscle contractions, dyskinesias, dysarthria, and dysphagia are also reported. Mood changes may occur but are difficult to relate specifically to DBS. However, some patients with no history of bipolarity have experienced hypomania. More profound mood swings, including severe depression and suicidal ideation, may occur if the stimulator fails suddenly. Some patients have reported a feeling of being cognitively 'clouded', which has responded to changes in stimulus parameters. To date there is no evidence that DBS causes enduring cognitive impairment. As with any neurosurgical procedure, implantation of electrodes for DBS carries risks of haemorrhage and infection. Such complications appear to be rare; in one series of 141 patients undergoing DBS for Parkinson's disease, the overall mortality attributable to the procedure was 0.7% (Vergani *et al.*, 2010).

Ethical aspects of DBS

DBS is considered to be less invasive than neurosurgery in that the stimulation can be stopped and there is no lesioning of tissue. However, the procedure does carry risks, and there is a lack of long-term efficacy and safety data. The situation is further complicated by involvement of commercial factors, because the stimulator equipment is expensive and manufactured by industry.

This highlights once again the need for a scrupulous fiduciary relationship between the patient and the treating clinical team, as well as full informed consent to the procedure by a competent patient. It also suggests that some DBS trials should be sponsored by non-commercial organizations, and that all clinical data should be made publicly available so that there is no risk of publication bias. In view of the troubled history of direct neurosurgical interventions for psychiatric disorders, it has been proposed that DBS should only be used to treat psychiatric disorders in the context of an approved research protocol with full independent ethical review.

Transcranial direct current stimulation

A more recent stimulatory technique for treating psychiatric disorders is provided by transcranial direct current stimulation (TDCS). TDCS involves an application to the scalp of a small current of 1 or 2 milliamperes via two electrodes which function as anode and cathode. Current is typically applied for around 30 minutes. The weak electrical field thus generated is capable of altering neuronal excitability and plasticity (Tracy and David, 2015).

TDCS has been applied mainly to the treatment of depression, although even for this single indication a variety of electrode placements have been used. In patients with resistant depression, the effects of TDCS versus sham controls are inconsistent (Tracy and David, 2015). However, in a randomized, sham-controlled study of first-line treatment of 120 depressed patients, TDCS applied to prefrontal cortex was effective as a monotherapy and produced a large potentiation of the antidepressant effect of a modest dose of sertraline (Brunoni et al., 2013). TDCS may also have the ability to enhance aspects of cognitive function, which potentially could give it a role in the augmentation of psychological treatments for depression.

Further reading

Anderson IM and McAllister-Williams RH (2015). *Fundamentals of Clinical Psychopharmacology*. CRC Press, Boca Raton. (Concise evidence-based guide to mode of action of psychopharmacological agents and their clinical effects.)

Stahl SM (2013). *Stahl's Essential Psychopharmacology*. Cambridge University Press, Cambridge. (A well-illustrated account of basic and clinical use of psychotropic drugs.)

Taylor D, Paton C and Kapur S (2015). *The Maudsley Prescribing Guidelines*, 12th edn. John Wiley, Chichester. (An excellent handbook of good prescribing practice.)

Waite J and Eaton A (eds.) (2013). *The ECT Handbook*, 3rd edn. RCPsych Publications, London. (A clear, thorough, and practical guide to high-quality administration of ECT.)

CHAPTER 26

Psychiatric services

Introduction

The last two chapters dealt with the treatment of individual patients. This chapter is concerned with the provision of psychiatric care for populations. It deals mainly with the needs of and provisions for people aged 18–65 years ('adults of working age').

Services for children are described in Chapter 16, services for the elderly in Chapter 19, and services for patients with intellectual disability in Chapter 17. The organization of psychiatric services in any country inevitably depends on the organization of general medical

services in that country. This chapter will refer specifically to services in the UK, but the principles embodied apply widely.

The chapter begins with an account of the historical development of psychiatric services. This is followed by descriptions of the commonly available psychiatric services and of the problems encountered with these provisions. The chapter ends with a consideration of some innovations designed to overcome these problems.

The history of psychiatric services

What we now recognize as psychiatry dates from the end of the eighteenth century. Before that there were hardly any special provisions for the mentally ill in Europe, other than in Spain, where some hospitals were present from the Islamic Middle Ages (Chamberlain, 1966). Although mental disturbances were often considered as illnesses in antiquity, during the Middle Ages they became regarded as spiritual problems. Other than forms of exorcism and containment, little was provided.

In Britain until the middle of the eighteenth century, most mentally ill people lived with their families or, if very disturbed, were in prison. Private 'madhouses' (later to be called private asylums) were developed mainly for those who could pay, but accepted some paupers supported by their parishes (Parry-Jones, 1972). At about the same time, a few hospitals or wards were established through private benefaction and public subscription. The Bethel Hospital in Norwich was founded in 1713. In London, the lunatic ward at Guy's Hospital was established in 1728. In 1751, St Luke's Hospital was founded as an alternative to the overcrowded Bethlem Hospital, which had existed as an institution since 1247, but only latterly had become exclusively a 'madhouse.'

Moral management

At the end of the eighteenth century the Enlightenment led to a more empirical, less theological, understanding of madness. This rational approach led to increased public concern in many countries about the poor standards of private and public institutions, including efforts to improve the care of the mentally ill. In Paris in 1793, Philippe Pinel iconically released patients from their chains and introduced other changes to make the care of patients more humane. In England, similar reforming ideas were proposed by William Tuke, a Quaker philanthropist who founded the Retreat in York in 1792. The Retreat provided pleasant surroundings and adequate facilities for occupation and recreation. Treatment was based on 'moral' (i.e. social) management, consisting of kindness, calm, and activity. Tuke and Pinel both acknowledged that, although mad, patients still could respond to kindness and consideration, in contrast to the previous authoritarian approach aimed at simply controlling patients. Medical treatments such as bleeding and purging were peripheral to the routine care of the insane. Tuke's grandson, Samuel, described their system in *A Description of the Retreat* (1813), and the Retreat was replicated internationally. It became clear that many mentally ill patients could exert self-control and did not require physical restraint and punishment.

The asylum movement

Until the early nineteenth century most mentally ill people received no care and lived as vagrants or as inmates of workhouses and gaols. Public concern about the welfare of the insane in workhouses and gaols and some private madhouses led to the County Asylum Act of 1808. This provided for the building of mental hospitals in English counties. However, it was the Lunatics Act 1845 that required the building of one in every county. At first the new asylums were small and provided good treatment in spacious surroundings. Moral management was championed. The 'non-restraint movement', which had started with the work of Gardiner Hill at the Lincoln Asylum in 1837, was established by John Conolly at the Middlesex County Asylum, Hanwell, in 1845. This removed the use of all physical restraints, a practice that has characterized mental healthcare in the UK ever since.

Unfortunately, these early attitudes yielded to a more restrictive approach as the asylums expanded and became overcrowded. Initial optimism about the curability of psychiatric disorder faded with the accumulation of chronic cases and an increased focus on organic and hereditary causes. The original York Retreat housed 30 patients, and the first 16 British asylums about 100 patients each. By 1840 they averaged 300 patients, 540 patients by 1870, and 960 patients by 1900. Some patients with chronic illness were housed in detached annexes or houses in the grounds of the asylum. Other hospitals returned chronic patients to the community either by boarding them out with a family (a form of care that had long been practised successfully at Gheel in Belgium), or by returning them to workhouses. The Lunacy Commissioners, whose role was to oversee the care of the mentally ill, were concerned that these arrangements could lead to abuse, and were opposed to them. Nevertheless, nineteenth-century asylums, even when overcrowded, provided a standard of care for the mentally ill that was lacking elsewhere. They were protected from exploitation, and provided with shelter, food, and general health care, all without cost.

A change to a stricter custodial regime was endorsed by the Lunacy Act 1890, which imposed restrictions on admission and discharge from hospital. The bureaucratic and rigid 1890 Lunacy Act had resulted from years of unwarranted committal, but it handicapped British psychiatric development for nearly half a century. For accounts of psychiatric hospitals in the UK and the USA in the nineteenth century, see Jones (1992) and Rothman (1971).

Arrangements for early treatment

The opening of the Maudsley Hospital in 1923 provided an outpatient service and voluntary inpatient treatment in surroundings in which teaching and research were carried out. In the years between the wars the impetus for change increased. The Mental Treatment Act 1930 repealed many of the restrictions on discharge of patients that had been imposed by the Lunacy Act 1890. It allowed county asylums to accept voluntary patients, and changed the term 'asylum' to 'mental hospital' and the term 'lunatic' to voluntary 'mental patient'. The 1930 Act also encouraged local authorities to set up outpatient clinics and to establish facilities for aftercare. Therapeutic optimism, revived by von Jauregg's successful malaria treatment for cerebral syphilis, increased further with the introduction of insulin coma treatment (later abandoned) and electroconvulsive therapy. Efforts were made to improve conditions in hospitals, to unlock previously locked wards, and to encourage occupational activities. Similar changes took place in other countries.

In most countries, these reforms were halted by the Second World War. Psychiatric hospitals became understaffed as doctors and nurses were recruited to the war effort, and became overcrowded as some had to be evacuated for the care of the war injured (Crammer, 1990). In Germany, many psychiatric patients died in a eugenics programme—a particularly shameful episode in the history of a country that dominated psychiatric progress in the nineteenth and early twentieth centuries (Burleigh, 2000).

Social psychiatry and the beginning of community care

Several forces led to further changes in psychiatric hospitals directly after the Second World War. Social attitudes had become more liberal and sympathetic towards the disadvantaged. Wartime experience of 'battle neuroses' had encouraged interest in the early treatments, and in the use of groups and social rehabilitation. In the UK, the establishment of the National Health Service led to a general reorganization of medical services, including psychiatry. The introduction of chlorpromazine in 1952 made it easier to manage the disturbed behaviour of patients with psychosis. It became possible to open wards that had been locked (although some hospitals had done so before such drugs became available), to engage patients in social activities, and to discharge more of them into the community.

Despite these changes, services continued to be concentrated at single sites, often remote from centres of population. In the USA, Goffman (1961) vividly exposed the detrimental effects of such 'total institutions'. He described how their impersonal, inflexible, and authoritarian regimes eroded identity and, through this 'institutionalization', generated chronicity. In the UK, Wing and Brown (1970) demonstrated how large mental hospital environments characterized by 'social poverty' led to 'clinical poverty'. Vigorous social rehabilitation was introduced to improve conditions in hospital and to counteract the effects of years of institutional living. Occupational and industrial therapies were used to prepare chronically disabled patients for the move from hospital to sheltered accommodation or to ordinary housing (Bennett, 1983). Many long-stay patients were very responsive to these vigorous new methods, and optimism grew that newly admitted patients could be similarly helped.

Away from the hospitals, day units were established to provide continuing treatment and rehabilitation, and

hostels were opened to provide sheltered accommodation. The numbers of patients in psychiatric hospitals fell substantially in the UK and in other countries. The changes started later in the USA, with the introduction of Medicaid in 1965, but then progressed very rapidly. Despite these changes, services were still based in large mental hospitals that were often far from patients' homes, and the provision of community facilities remained inadequate.

Hospital closure

Early successes in discharging institutionalized patients led to expectations that asylums would soon be replaced by small psychiatric units in general hospitals, supported by community facilities. In most countries, the programme of hospital closure took place, albeit very gradually. A notable exception was Italy. In 1978, the Italian Parliament passed Law 180, which prohibited admissions to mental hospitals forthwith. It aimed to abolish Italy's neglected mental hospitals altogether over a period of 3 years and replace them with a comprehensive system of community care. Psychiatric 'diagnostic' units limited to admissions of 7 days were to be set up in general hospitals, and community services developed for each catchment area. This Italian revolution was led by Franco Basaglia in hospitals in north-east Italy, through the movement he founded. This movement—*Psichiatria Democratica*—combined a left-wing political view that patients in psychiatric hospitals were the victims of oppression by the capitalist system with the conviction that severe mental illness was induced more by social conditions than by biological causes.

Basaglia's charismatic personality and qualities of leadership (and a wife who became an Italian Senator) helped him to succeed with his reforms. Others found them more difficult, and their impact varied. Where the reforms were financed adequately and were implemented by enthusiastic staff (particularly in the wealthy north), the new provisions were successful. However, in Rome and the south facilities were often inadequate and problems encountered (Fioritti *et al.*, 1997). The state mental hospital system, however, came to a complete end in 1989 (Burti, 2001).

In the UK and elsewhere the pace of change was slower, but similar problems arose. Many patients needed ongoing intensive support, and many required repeated readmissions to hospital—so-called 'revolving-door patients'. Rehabilitation services had to adjust their expectations and provide continuing care. The early expectations of *deinstitutionalization* had clearly been overoptimistic. The policy of 'community care' was introduced to develop more adequate community provision.

The rise of community care

The development of community care falls quite neatly into two phases—before 1980 and from 1980 onwards (Burns, 2014). In the first phase, as hospitals closed, community psychiatric services acquired three responsibilities. The first was to provide treatment for those individuals with severe mental illness who would previously have remained in hospital for many years. The second was to treat severe acute psychiatric disorder as far as possible without lengthy admission to hospital, and as near as possible to the patient's home. The third was to assist primary care services in the detection, prevention, and early treatment of the less severe psychiatric disorders. Services were to be comprehensive, to deliver continuity of care, and to be provided by multidisciplinary teams.

The framework for this 'sectorized' service was laid by the 1959 Mental Health Act in the UK and a similar approach was initiated in France. The UK Act required hospitals to provide outpatient follow-up for their own discharged patients, and also required social services involvement in both compulsory admissions and community support. A highly localized service was therefore a practical necessity for effective joint working.

These general principles were applied rather differently in the UK and in the USA. In the UK, emphasis was placed initially on provision for patients discharged from long-term hospital care. In the USA, community mental health centres (CMHCs) were established, with more emphasis on prevention and early treatment to avoid admission. These CMHCs emphasized crisis intervention and the treatment of acute, often relatively minor, psychiatric disorders. Unlike the UK teams they had no outreach facility, so patients with chronic and severe mental illness (who seldom actively seek care) became neglected. A rather 'antimedical' approach in CMHCs led to difficulties in recruiting and retaining psychiatrists (Talbott *et al.*, 1987). Dissatisfaction with the centres grew as people discharged from long-term

hospital care found their way into private hospitals or prisons, or joined the homeless population of large cities (Goldman and Morrissey, 1985).

In the UK and parts of Europe, some commonly agreed principles evolved in sectorized care:

- *Minimizing inpatient care.* Hospital admissions were to be brief, and as far as possible patients were to be admitted to psychiatric units in general hospitals rather than to psychiatric hospitals. Whenever practicable, people were to be treated as outpatients or day patients.
- *Providing rehabilitation early on.* The aim of this was to protect and possibly improve residual functioning and prevent further deterioration.
- *Multidisciplinary teams.* Care was to be provided by teams, usually consisting of psychiatrists, community nurses, clinical psychologists, and social workers, often working in collaboration with members of voluntary groups.
- *Legal reform.* New laws were introduced (e.g. the 1983 Mental Health Act and its 2007 amendment in England and Wales) to limit the uses of compulsory treatment, to encourage alternatives to inpatient care, and to strengthen the rights of the individual.

As experience increased after the reforms had begun, the following additional features were introduced:

- *Care packages* based on an assessment of each patient's needs.
- *Case management* by a named, clinically trained, care worker who led and coordinated the work of others involved in care.
- Outreach to take services to vulnerable people who might otherwise find it difficult to engage with the care that is offered, and to arrange follow-up.
- *User involvement.* Service users were increasingly involved in planning both their own treatment and the services for the population.
- *Risk assessment* carried out regularly, and more formally as part of the care plan.

The components of a mental health service

From the 1960s to the mid-1980s, mental health services in the UK and, indeed, most parts of the world evolved slowly, based on professional consensus. In

the 1980s, interest in evidence-based medicine spread to mental health services research. This approach was international and increased the pace of change dramatically. The fundamental components of most care, namely inpatient wards, day hospitals, and community mental health teams (CMHTs), had not been subject to research, but were well established and have proved durable.

The publication of Stein and Test's (1980) ground-breaking trial of an Assertive Community Treatment team ushered in the second phase of development—the era of evidence-based mental health services. The more recent highly specialized teams (assertive outreach teams, crisis resolution/home treatment teams, and early-onset (psychosis) services) have been driven more by policy and this research. Since the last edition of this book we have witnessed a dramatic change in fortunes for some of these new teams as the evidence has accumulated. What follows is a description of the UK services, which addresses research and international evidence where this is relevant or helpful. The NHS has entered a phase of profound change, and the predictability and uniformity of services are likely to change markedly during the lifetime of this book. As noted earlier, issues specifically related to psychiatric services for children, those with learning disabilities, and the elderly, are discussed in Chapters 16, 17, and 19, respectively.

Inpatient wards

No comprehensive service can survive without access to 24-hour nursing supervision for acute episodes of severe illness (Thornicroft and Tansella, 2013). Surprisingly, inpatient wards are often overlooked in descriptions of comprehensive services. They serve patients at risk from neglect or suicide and those lacking insight. Wards usually accommodate 10–20 patients. It is rarely possible to staff and run stand-alone units of less than three to four such wards effectively (30–60 beds). The famed Italian Law 180 restricted wards to 15 patients, and this is a common international goal (Burns, 1998). Ward size is a trade-off between privacy and domesticity on the one hand and effective supervision on the other. Single rooms are preferable and are now the norm in new-build units. They afford maximum privacy and, although initially expensive, they improve flexibility and have been shown to reduce conflict significantly.

Single-sex accommodation

Concern for the safety and privacy of female patients has led to government requirements for single-sex wards. This reversal of the development that occurred in the 1960s and 1970s is non-negotiable, even if it may have been overtaken by the increasing availability of single ensuite accommodation in new units.

Smaller, more flexible, units such as 'crisis houses' offering 24-hour care have been a useful complement to inpatient wards. However, they are not a replacement for them, and where this has been attempted it has usually resulted in an unacceptably high rate of transfer to the psychiatric intensive care units (PICUs). Ward design and management are increasingly crucial as improved community care concentrates involuntary and disturbed inpatients in them.

Continuity of responsibility

Responsibility by the same clinical team for both community and inpatient care is unusual except in the UK and Italy, where it has delivered strikingly shorter stays and improved bed management. Continuity is difficult in dispersed populations, and increasingly even in cities as each team has fewer inpatients. A separate inpatient team ensures better inpatient standards, but with the risk of diverging approaches (e.g. a 'medical model' inpatient team and a 'psychotherapeutic' community team). It has recently become common practice in the UK at the same time that many European services are trying to overcome it, for reasons that are unclear but which may include the problems of wards having to cope with several admitting teams. Both the move to single-sex accommodation and specialized teams result in each team often having only one or two patients on a ward. Diffused responsibility and organizing multiple ward rounds have promoted the change, but not without cost (Burns, 2010). It appears to be in conflict with the expectation of continuity of clinical responsibility in the 1983 Mental Health Act, and particularly in the 2007 amendment permitting compulsory treatment in the community through the new provision of Supervised Community Treatment Orders (SCTOs, which are invariably referred to as Community Treatment Orders, or CTOs; see Chapter 4). It is unclear whether the inpatient consultant or the community consultant should make the decision.

Longer inpatient care

Acute inpatient wards admit patients for weeks or a couple of months, with rapid discharge anticipated. Across Europe the rate of compulsory admission has been rising for the past decade (Priebe et al., 2005). The reasons are unclear but bed shortages are certainly one factor (Keown et al., 2011), as is an increasing focus on risk assessment. Some patients require longer, more secure, care service because of illness severity or for legal reasons. Modern rehabilitation wards are thus generally restricted to patients with persistently unacceptable behaviour.

Diagnosis-specific wards

Diagnosis- or disorder-specific wards are relatively rare in the UK. In Scandinavia and Central Europe, separate wards for alcohol and substance abuse are long established. Wards for specific, specialized problems such as anorexia nervosa or resistant schizophrenia offer highly specific regimes. These are generally regional, and are a complement to acute admission wards, not an alternative. The current focus on organizing services along 'care pathways' may result in more specialized inpatient services.

Daycare

Daycare is provided in day hospitals and day centres, and there is no clear distinction between them. Day hospitals are generally provided by health services, include medical and nursing staff, and can offer treatments (e.g. the prescription and monitoring of medication, psychotherapies). Day centres are provided by social services or voluntary organizations. They only rarely provide specific treatments or employ clinically trained staff. However, services vary according to local context. A drop-in day centre may provide psychiatric assessment and treatment in areas of high social mobility and homelessness. Broadly speaking, day centres provide long-term social support and day hospitals provide focused interventions and treatments (Catty *et al.*, 2005).

Acute day hospitals in Europe and partial hospitalization services in the USA have been energetically proposed as acceptable and economical alternatives to inpatient care (Marshall, 2003), but have had little penetration. Day hospitals never achieved their anticipated prominence in the UK, having perhaps been overtaken as CMHTs have become more comprehensive. They serve specific groups well (e.g. mothers with small children, those with eating disorders, or personality problems). Daycare can be difficult to organize in rural settings.

Supported accommodation and residential care

The extent of inpatient care needed depends on access to other supervised accommodation. Patients remain well outside hospital only with adequate support and stable, affordable accommodation. Supervision may be needed to ensure self-care, continued medication, and to anticipate and defuse crises. This can be provided by voluntary agencies, social services, or health services. Voluntary agencies tend to be more efficient at providing long-term residential care (Knapp *et al.*, 1999), but are reluctant to accept risky patients. A mixed economy works best.

Outpatient clinics

Psychiatrists assess patients, advise them and their referrers, and provide treatments. In state-funded systems 'office-based' pure practice is rare, as most professionals work in outpatient clinics or mental health teams. Psychiatrists and psychologists may still operate independently within outpatient clinics, but with easy access to enhanced resources and second opinions. Outpatient clinics may operate either alongside CMHTs or as part of them. They work better for severe illness when fully integrated with CMHTs (Wright *et al.*, 2004). Clinics provide an efficient format for assessments and monitoring of treatment progress.

Multidisciplinary community mental health teams

Most community mental health services are made up of multidisciplinary professional groups working together to care for an identified number of patients. These are referred to generically as CMHTs. Nurses have long worked outside hospitals (e.g. midwives, health visitors), and have made psychiatric home visits since the 1950s. Social workers, psychologists, and occupational therapists are increasingly based in CMHTs rather than in their own separate departments. The staffing of these teams varies internationally, but they all hold regular review meetings. These reviews incorporate their varied professional perspectives and allocate tasks according to staff skills and patient needs. They were developed in France and the UK in the delivery of sectorized psychiatry, refined in Italy, and further elaborated in North America and Australia.

The generic sector CMHT ('the CMHT')

Who it is for

The CMHT is the fundamental building block of modern community mental health services. It originated as mental hospital catchment areas (which often covered a whole city or county) were divided into sectors of 50,000–100,000 inhabitants to facilitate ongoing care. It provides assessment and care for patients who have been discharged from psychiatric units and for outpatients who require more support than can be provided in primary care. Current sector size in Western Europe ranges from 20,000 to 50,000 members of the population, determined both by resources (the size shrinking as investment increases) and by the local configuration.

As more specialized teams are established, the CMHT's remit may be narrowed and its sector size increased.

CMHTs prioritize individuals with severe mental illnesses (SMIs), such as psychoses and severe affective disorders. Many inner-city CMHTs only see such patients. However, diagnosis is not all—complications due to social adversity, personality difficulties, or substance abuse can make secondary mental health care necessary even for apparently 'minor' disorders. Several tools have been developed for clarifying a threshold for acceptance (Slade *et al.*, 2000), but these are of limited use and most teams rely on clinical assessments. In countries with limited private care, such as the UK, CMHTs also treat mild and transient disorders.

Staffing and management

CMHTs range from 7 or 8 to over 20 full-time staff. They emphasize skill sharing and a degree of generic working, and have evolved an informal, democratic style (Burns, 2004). Senior psychiatrists initially provided clinical leadership but, with increased staff numbers and treatment complexity, 'team managers' now coordinate the workload. There is little consensus on their role, which can range from the purely administrative to determining clinical priorities and supervising staff. Clinically active team managers usually have reduced caseloads. If clinical leadership and team management are separated (which is common if there is a strong medical presence), the roles need to be well defined and relationships clarified.

Assessments

The key to good care is accurate assessment, and CMHTs vary in how they provide this. In general, psychiatrists are responsible for an initial assessment (often in an outpatient clinic) and involve the team members in treatment. Increasingly, other team members have taken a role in assessments, either individually or jointly with the psychiatrist. This issue generates strong opinions, but there has been surprisingly little research into it. With highly developed primary care, non-medical assessments may be effective, but otherwise medical time should prioritize assessments. For the most severely ill patients, home-based assessments pay considerable dividends (Stein and Test, 1980; Burns *et al.*, 2007b).

Case management

Most CMHT staff act as clinical case managers (Holloway *et al.*, 1995), taking lead responsibility for the delivery, coordination, and review of care for an agreed number of patients. Currently, clinical case managers provide direct care to build a trusting relationship and provide treatment and continuity for patients with complex needs.

They also utilize the full range of team resources. The caseloads of staff members are explicitly limited (usually 15–25), and reviews are recorded and systematic. In the UK this has been formalized as the Care Programme Approach (Department of Health, 1990), which requires a named case manager (called a *care coordinator*) and a document called a *care plan*, which records the patient's needs or problems, the proposed interventions for them, and who is responsible for each of them, plus an agreed date for *review*.

Care plans are often supplemented with a risk assessment and a contingency (crisis) plan. Optimally this should not need more than two pages, but it is often weighed down with administrative details that obscure its clinical purpose. Such simple structured paperwork can be adapted to any service. It fulfils a vital coordinating role in complex care, and serves as a natural focus for clinical reviews. The value of this document (as with the risk assessment and contingency plan) lies in its brevity. Too much information is as risky as too little, and the level of detail needs to be clinically (not managerially) determined.

Team meetings

CMHTs always have one, and often two, regular meetings per week for both clinical and administrative business. They last between 1 and 2 hours, and the level of structure varies.

Allocation of referrals. Deciding who will assess new patients need occupy only 10 minutes at the beginning of the routine meeting, or can simply be delegated to a senior member to decide. Referrals can be allocated according to who is first available, or by matching the clinical problem against available skill and training. It is remarkable how many CMHTs fail to have an agreed timetable for new assessments (as is routine in outpatient clinics). Much time is saved if each member has agreed regular assessment 'slots'. There is then no need to 'coordinate diaries' for joint assessments, and patients can be directly booked into available slots if the member is absent at allocation. Time spent discussing allocations (and particularly having a 'referral meeting') before assessment is unprofitable, and most well-functioning teams delegate the task.

Patient reviews. Reviews are needed for *new patients, routine monitoring, crises,* and *discharge.* They can range from simply reporting the problem and proposed treatment in uncomplicated cases, through to detailed, structured, multidisciplinary case conferences. These may include other services (e.g. general practitioner, housing, child protection). *New patient reviews* are particularly important for providing a broad, experienced overview, particularly if assessments are distributed across the team. They also ensure rational and fair allocation to caseloads. *Routine monitoring* is often overlooked, yet is probably the most important review for team efficiency. It shapes and redirects treatment and identifies patients who are ready for discharge. The burden on individual staff members is regularly monitored. Routine monitoring is a statutory requirement of the Care Programme Approach, and is good practice in all case management. *Crisis reviews* are unscheduled but allow case managers to seek advice when they are unsure. *Discharge reviews* provide an excellent opportunity for audit and learning within the team.

Managing waiting lists and caseloads. Effective CMHTs need to guarantee prompt access. *Routine assessments* should take place within 2–4 weeks. Striving for a shorter waiting time is rarely productive, and waiting times of much over 4 weeks have a rapidly rising rate of failed appointments. *Urgent assessments* (which include most psychotic episodes) need to be seen within a week, and usually within a couple of days. *Emergency assessments* are for those associated with immediate risk (e.g. hostile behaviour or suicidal intent) and ideally need to be seen the same day.

A practical approach to managing waiting times is to count the number of referrals in the preceding year and timetable routine assessment slots for about 120% of that rate. So, if a team that had 300 referrals in the previous year allocates seven slots a week, there will be one extra available each week for urgent assessments and emergencies. Easy access to routine assessments reduces pressure for urgent and emergency referrals, and is much more efficient than emergency rotas.

Communication and liaison

Team meetings ensure internal communication, but CMHTs also need good links with the wider network of professional colleagues. Most routine communication takes place by letter, phone, or during clinical encounters. More structured liaison is advisable with primary care and general hospitals. General hospital links may be between specific CMHTs and wards, or CMHTs may provide input to patients from their sectors. Dedicated liaison psychiatry and psychosomatic services are routine in well-resourced services.

General practice liaison. GP liaison systems originated in Balint groups but are now more likely to involve shared care or co-location of CMHTs in GP health centres (Burns and Bale, 1997). An effective and sustainable system involves regular (usually monthly) timetabled meetings between the two teams, or a 'link' CMHT member attending the GP health centre. It is important always to be clear about responsibilities; blurring of boundaries is risky.

Liaison with other agencies. The same principles apply to liaison with other agencies (social services, housing, and charitable and voluntary sector providers). Whether regular meetings are cost-effective will depend on the volume of shared work. Professional confidentiality and information sharing are more sensitive.

Mental health services research

The past 30 years have witnessed a change in how mental health services are planned and evaluated. A new academic activity, *mental health services research (MHSR)*, has come into existence, which has attempted to subject services and systems to the same evidence-based medicine approach of rigorous testing (e.g. controlled studies, randomized controlled trials, meta-analyses) widely accepted with specific treatments. This has had two profound effects. First, it has internationalized thinking about optimal services. The language of science means that findings from other parts of the world can be applied locally. Second, it has shifted the locus of control in service development away from clinicians and towards academics and policy-makers.

There are undoubted benefits to MHSR. For example, thinking and communication are markedly clearer, and some ineffective practices (e.g. traditional 'brokerage' case management) have been identified and abandoned. However, there are also drawbacks, particularly the risk of overinterpretation of results and their application without recognition of the modifying effects of the local context. This is briefly outlined in the cases of Assertive Community Treatment (ACT) teams. Three fundamental conceptual problems have dogged MHSR:

- A tendency to equate a service with a treatment, rather than with the *platform* for delivering treatments.
- The assumption that the 'control' services in randomized controlled trials are inert and consistent, when in fact they are active and very variable 'comparator' services.
- A tendency to ignore the 'pioneer' effect—shiny new demonstration services with charismatic leaders have an inherent advantage.

MHSR methodology is improving, but these pitfalls in interpreting studies always need to be considered.

Mental Health National Service Framework 1999

Mental health services in England and Wales were radically reformed following the publication of the National Service Framework (NSF) in 1999 (Department of Health, 1999) and the NHS Plan in 2000 (Department of Health, 2000). These drew heavily on MHSR and pioneering services in North Birmingham and Australia. They initially recommended the complete replacement of the UK's sectorized generic CMHTs with four separate 'functional' teams—*assertive outreach, crisis resolution and home treatment, early intervention*, and *primary care liaison* teams. The sheer impracticality of such a massive reorganization (for which there simply were not adequate trained staff) and challenges to the strength of the evidence modified the proposal, and CMHTs were retained and primary care liaison teams abandoned.

An ambitious programme to establish the first three types of functional teams was put in place, starting with the creation of 300 assertive outreach teams (AOTs). These three teams are described below. The research evidence will be briefly addressed but, as demonstrated by that on AOTs, this can change radically over time.

Assertive outreach teams

The most extensively replicated and researched specialist CMHT is the AOT. This is based on the *ACT model*, whose landmark study by Stein and Test (published in 1980 and mentioned earlier) ushered in evidence-based mental health service planning. ACT delivered improved clinical and social outcomes with substantially reduced hospitalization at slightly lower overall costs. Two Cochrane reviews with meta-analyses, one of case management showing an increase in hospitalization and one of ACT showing a reduction (Marshall and Lockwood, 1998; Marshall *et al.*, 2001), were instrumental in the adoption of ACT in the UK. AOTs (see Box 26.1) are costly, requiring one full-time case manager for about 10 patients. Consequently they are reserved for the most difficult ('hard to engage' or 'revolving-door') psychotic patients, who have frequent, often dangerous, relapses.

The AOT approach is based on proactive outreach—visiting patients at home and persisting with visits even when patients are reluctant. It exploits team-working, with daily meetings and several members working with most patients, rather than exclusive individual

> ### Box 26.1 **Core components of assertive community treatment**
>
> - Assertive follow-up
> - Small caseloads (1:10–1:15)
> - Regular (daily) team meetings
> - Frequent contact (weekly to daily)
> - *In vivo* practice (treatment in home and neighbourhood)
> - Emphasis on engagement and medication
> - Support for family and carers
> - Provision of services using all team members
> - Crisis stabilization 24 hours a day, 7 days a week

relationships. This is needed for reasons of safety (it may not be safe to visit some patients alone) and also because of the complexity of patients' needs. The approach is very practical. Staff take patients shopping, sort out their accommodation, even deliver their medicines daily if necessary. These activities go well beyond traditional professional boundaries. Advocates of AOT insisted that good outcomes depended on a strict replication of Stein and Test's approach and even developed scales to measure this ('model fidelity').

Who and what are assertive outreach teams for

Assertive outreach research has been conducted exclusively with psychotic patients, generally those with poor medication compliance and often with comorbid alcohol or drug abuse and offending behaviour. AOTs generally take only patients who cannot be stabilized despite CMHT support.

Enthusiasm for AOTs led to a preoccupation with their structure and process rather than with what they do. Despite the extensive early evidence of a reduction in hospitalization (Marshall and Lockwood, 1998), this has never been achieved against a CMHT control (Burns *et al.*, 2002), and never in the UK. Careful examination of AOT studies (Burns *et al.*, 2007b) demonstrated that this was because its practice was almost identical to standard UK CMHTs apart from the very small caseload and 24-hour availability, and these appeared to have no significant effect. In the UK, AOT teams are being abandoned and their caseloads resorbed into CMHTs. Internationally, however, ACT has become the accepted term for any multidisciplinary CMHT that offers flexible outreach.

Functional assertive community treatment teams

Functional assertive community treatment (FACT) teams are a response developed in the Netherlands to the shifting evidence base for AOT (Firn *et al.*, 2012). FACT is a hybrid between an ACT team and a generic CMHT, and uses 'zoning' to specify high-risk patients who need intensive monitoring and input. Zoning involves using a 'traffic light' classification of patients. Those in the red zone need weekly to daily contact and are considered at high risk.

Those in amber are routine patients needing weekly to monthly contact, often by a single case manager and not at great immediate risk of relapse. Those in the green zone are not in need of regular contact but only occasional assessment and are usually allowed direct self-referral. Zoning is a welcome structuring of relatively longstanding CMHT practice. Only time and research will tell whether FACT teams are significantly different from CMHTs.

Crisis teams

Crisis intervention therapy in the early 1970s built on Caplan's belief that crises (when psychological defences were breached) presented fertile opportunities for psychotherapy breakthroughs (Caplan, 1964). More recently this psychodynamic focus has faded. Crisis teams have been promoted most where local services are poorly developed (they may be the *only* community services) or social mobility is high (e.g. centres of major cities), with many transient and homeless patients for whom continuity of care cannot be established.

Crisis teams are characterized by rapid response and accessibility. Defining the duration of a crisis (and hence the window for intervention) has generated endless unprofitable debate. Most teams will see patients immediately, certainly on the same day. Their clinical aims (i.e. the assessment and management of acute episodes of mental illness) and staffing (mainly nurses and social workers) are similar to those of CMHTs. Given the acuteness of the problems, medical input is probably essential, despite attempts in some services to dispense with it. Crisis teams may be based in mental health services alongside CMHTs, or in the emergency rooms of general hospitals with 24-hour availability. Important functions include distinguishing acute mental illness from severe personal crises (especially those involving self-harm), and accessing beds for both voluntary and involuntary admissions. Hospital-based crisis teams are often run in conjunction with liaison services (see Chapter 22).

Crisis resolution/home treatment teams

Crisis resolution/home treatment (CR/HT) teams, which were introduced by the NSF, were developed in Australia (Hoult, 1986). Their primary purpose is to avoid unnecessary admissions and to reduce the duration of inpatient care. They also are, in part, a response to increased consumer demand for access out of hours. They draw heavily on assertive outreach practice, with limited, shared caseloads, flexible working, extended access, and an emphasis on outreach. Reduction in hospitalization was proposed to offset much of their cost (Smyth and Hoult, 2000). They aim to treat patients who would otherwise be in hospital, and to focus on the severely mentally ill. They offer intensive visiting (usually daily for a limited period) and considerable practical support, and they work with patients' social networks. Most aim to limit themselves to 6 weeks of involvement. Such intensive teamworking requires highly effective communication, and the teams meet daily (in some cases twice daily). Information transfer is burdensome, and liaison with CMHTs is complex, requiring absolute clarity about local arrangements for clinical responsibility.

Variations in practice and sustainability

Crisis teams are particularly difficult to research rigorously, as the informed consent required for randomized controlled trials is almost impossible to obtain. However, there is some evidence that CR/HT teams may reduce the need for hospital care (Johnson *et al.*, 2005), although this is not clear-cut (Glover *et al.*, 2006). As with AOTs, the potential for impact will depend on local provision. Although the UK model is well specified (including who it should and should not care for; see Box 26.2), in reality practice varies considerably. Unless local services are particularly undeveloped, a full 24-hour service is very wasteful, and an on-call facility to the emergency room and police station at night usually suffices. In practice, contact frequencies are generally lower, patients stay with the service longer than anticipated, and restricting the service to patients who would otherwise be in hospital is rarely achieved. CR/HT teams are inevitably referred individuals who are recurrently in crisis (often with alcohol and relationship problems), who cannot be refused care but would not 'otherwise be in hospital'.

Medical input and the team's independence from CMHTs both vary markedly. Some teams operate completely parallel to CMHTs, some share extensively (often acting as an adjunct to CMHT care—for example, making evening medication drops), and some insist on CMHT involvement. Local circumstances (and staff availability) will ultimately determine the configuration. Most CR/HT teams are now routinely involved at the threshold for admission and discharge. At its most extreme some Trusts insist that no patient can be either admitted or discharged except through the CR/HT team. Other Trusts take a more pragmatic approach—particularly when patients are well known to CMHTs.

Clarity about responsibility and leadership is crucial. Patient evaluation of CR/HT teams varies. Many appreciate the promptness of response and the level of support. Others complain about intrusiveness and having to explain themselves to a series of different staff who are often insufficiently trained to make the necessary decisions.

Traditional crisis services may have a relatively limited lifespan. A World Health Organization review found that many early crisis services had ceased to exist within a decade (Cooper, 1979). Many had successfully improved local access and consolidated as a more general service (including, but not restricted to, crisis work). Others had become overwhelmed with inappropriate referrals or patients who could not be referred on, and eventually closed. A similar pattern has been observed (but not documented) in crisis houses. Whether CR/HT teams will persist in the era of clinical commissioning is an open question.

Crisis houses and respite care

The excessive formality involved in hospital admission may prolong stays and dissuade patients from seeking help. 'Crisis houses' allow admission with a minimum of fuss, and often with reduced supervision. They are usually small (four to eight beds), in a domestic setting, and take patients for a period of days, or occasionally a week or two. They are favoured for vulnerable women and early intervention services (EIS). They do not replace inpatient care, but are generally very welcome for a minority of patients. However, without careful targeting and integration into local services they can become chaotic (and potentially dangerous) or blocked, and few survive without an active local champion.

Early intervention services

EIS are the third functional team introduced by the NSF. As discussed in Chapter 11, a long duration of untreated psychosis in schizophrenia is associated with poorer outcomes. EIS teams were developed mainly from Australian and UK models (Birchwood et al., 1998; Edwards et al., 2000). They aim to shorten DUP, protect current social functioning and networks, and improve outcome by providing prompt effective treatment. Despite a detailed prescription, UK teams vary considerably and prioritize different features of the approach. Some minimize the importance of diagnosis in favour of ease of access, while others restrict themselves to schizophrenia to maximize skills. The duration of involvement ranges from 18 to 36 months, with proposals of up to 60 months. Some have a narrow age band (a 'youth service'), while others take all first-episode patients irrespective of age (Burns, 2004). Three quite different activities are reported in the EIS literature, which may have varying emphasis in different teams (see Box 26.3).

Case management

The core of EIS is a specialized CMHT that case-manages first-episode psychosis patients. Teams prioritize the protection of social networks and functioning (by keeping the patient at college or work, and emphasizing family interventions, etc.). They assume that there will be a return to premorbid functioning, and hospitalization is avoided (crisis and respite houses are preferred) and obtaining welfare benefits is minimized. An assertive outreach approach with practical and shared case management is used during the acute phase, with less intensive follow-up thereafter. 'Zoning' is commonly used, as in FACT teams, with 'acute' patients seen at least weekly, recovering patients seen weekly to monthly, and a third category for those who are still open to the team but who are not in active treatment. Teams differ in terms of whether they insist on keeping patients registered when they have recovered and do not want contact. They also may or may not provide inpatient care.

EIS case managers aim to prevent patients and their families from lowering their expectations prematurely. As mentioned above, many avoid obtaining benefits for patients, encouraging as rapid a return to work or college as possible. Self-management of illness is strongly endorsed, with an emphasis on learning relapse signatures and devising individually appropriate responses.

Early recognition and high-risk intervention

Some EIS teams are actively involved in psychosis public awareness campaigns and lecturing in schools and colleges. A minority attempt to identify 'ultra-high-risk' patients with prodromal symptoms of schizophrenia and offer them treatment (both psychological and pharmacological) to prevent 'transition' to psychosis. This approach remains highly controversial and is generally restricted to research teams. The evidence for the efficacy of EIS interventions is outlined in Chapter 11.

Experience with EIS teams was much less than with AOTs when they were introduced in the NSF, and they included confusing and contradictory prescriptions. Even more than with AOTs, the difficulties of making them work in dispersed rural and semirural settings have posed real challenges.

A settled single model has not yet evolved for EIS teams. However, they are now well established nationally and look set to endure—probably outliving both AOT and CR/HT teams.

Forensic and rehabilitation teams

Community-focused services face particular difficulties with treatment-resistant patients, especially those with socially unacceptable or offending behaviour. Such patients do not fit well into open wards. Specialized forensic teams provide care where offending behaviour and danger to others predominate. They provide secure inpatient care (in addition to their traditional roles with prisons and the courts), which is increasing internationally (Priebe *et al.*, 2005). Some forensic teams provide community services (intensive case management of dangerous patients), but integrating them with general services can be controversial. The focus on risk assessment and extensive joint visiting are the main ways in which they differ from AOTs.

Rehabilitation services have reached out from long-stay wards to more community placements. A significant number of patients remain profoundly disabled despite receiving optimum treatments. Rehabilitation teams focus on the long-term management of disability rather than on symptoms and episode-based care. The threshold from general services to rehabilitation services varies enormously. Rehabilitation teams generally serve patients who cannot survive without some form of supervised accommodation even between relapses. These include a shrinking handful of long-stay patients, but, increasingly, a very disturbed 'new long-stay' population with comorbid substance abuse and behavioural disturbances. Inpatient provision is needed for this group, and a range of hostel care can promote stability, but is difficult to sustain. 'Hospital hostels', where patients can live in hostel-type domestic accommodation, yet be subject to the Mental Health Act, have been successfully established by some rehabilitation services.

Diagnosis-specific teams

Highly specialized teams for specific disorders (e.g. eating disorders, personality disorders, bipolar disorder) focus on developing specific skills. They provide specialized treatments, usually at regional level. They are strongly supported both by their professionals and by the families of sufferers. However, the opportunity costs of establishing such teams in a health service with finite resources require careful consideration.

Other components of a mental health service

The main components (teams and facilities) of specialized mental health services have been outlined above. It will be clear from that description that some of these components (e.g. inpatient wards, generic-sector CMHTs) are fairly ubiquitous and durable, while others (e.g. most of the specialized teams) are more variable in their availability and practice. The way in which the functions and obligations of mental health services are distributed between these different teams will vary. The most important of these components will now be outlined and described. They can be summarized as follows:

1. *Primary mental health care teams*, which support primary care and conduct initial assessments.

2. *Outpatient care.*

3. *Specialist psychological treatments*, which are often integrated into the specialist or primary mental health care teams.

4. *Crisis/home-based treatment teams*, which treat acute mental disorder in the patient's home.

5. *Accident and emergency liaison services*, which are often part of the crisis service, that assess and treat people who present to accident and emergency departments.

6. *General hospital liaison services* for medically ill people who have mental health problems.

7. *Assertive outreach teams* for severely mentally ill people who are difficult to engage or high users of services.

8. *Early intervention services* for people during their first episode of psychosis and the following 3 years.

9. *Employment services*, including supported employment to help find paid employment, training, and education.

10. *Vocational rehabilitation*, which includes sheltered workshops and transitional employment.

11. *Day hospitals and daycare services*, including drop-in centres.

12. *Self-help and service user groups and advocacy services.*

13. *Inpatient wards.*

14. *Forensic services*, with wards for high, medium, and low levels of security, and court-diversion schemes.

15. *Residential services*, providing hostels and supported accommodation, including that for acutely ill people or crises.

16. *Services for specific groups*, such as people with eating disorders, and mother and baby units.

17. *Social and welfare services*, for help with obtaining benefits, advocacy, community support workers, and home help/meals.

18. *Services for special groups*, with outreach to marginalized groups, such as the homeless and refugees.

Services for psychiatric disorder in primary care

Classification of psychiatric disorders in primary care

ICD-10 and DSM-5 were developed for use in psychiatry. They are too detailed for routine use in primary care, and their fine distinctions are seldom helpful when selecting treatment in this setting. The World Health Organization has therefore developed a simpler classification for use in primary care. Each diagnosis is linked to a plan of management.

Identification of psychiatric disorders in primary care

The most important psychiatric service in primary care is to detect disorders. This is not a simple matter, as many patients present with both physical and psychological problems, and many of the latter go undetected (see Figure 26.1). Many people with a psychiatric disorder complain only of physical symptoms, whether of a coincidental minor physical illness or a consequence of

the psychiatric disorder (e.g. palpitations in anxiety, or tiredness in depression). Some describe physical symptoms because they fear the doctor may not take emotional problems seriously. It is not just the patient who

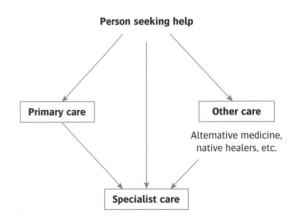

Figure 26.1 Pathways to care in the UK.

is responsible for this, as doctors often do focus on the physical symptoms. *Conspicuous morbidity* is the term for cases that are detected, and *hidden morbidity* for the rest. Hidden morbidity is generally less severe than conspicuous morbidity.

How effectively general practitioners identify undeclared psychiatric disorder depends on:

• their ability to gain the patient's confidence, thus enabling them to disclose the psychiatric problems of which they are aware

• their skill in assessing whether physical symptoms are caused by psychiatric illness; this requires a good knowledge of physical medicine as well as psychiatry.

Disorders that are treated in primary care

Most psychiatric disorders in primary care attenders can be treated successfully there. Examples include most adjustment disorders, the less severe anxiety and depressive disorders, somatization, and some cases of alcohol misuse. For a more detailed account, see Goldberg *et al.* (2009).

Patients presenting with physical symptoms. In primary care, many patients with psychiatric disorder present with physical symptoms. Such patients were called *somatizers*, but the terminology has moved to 'medically unexplained symptoms'. Many of them will reveal associated psychiatric symptoms and accept a psychiatric diagnosis when interviewed appropriately. Others deny any psychiatric symptoms and reject a psychiatric diagnosis, however skilfully they are examined, and can prove very difficult to treat. Where the concern about physical illness is unshakeable and no other psychiatric disorder is detected, the diagnosis of hypochondriasis is made. Repeated investigations fail to reassure but can be impossible to resist. Most frequent attenders are female and middle-aged (Koch *et al.*, 2007). Around 80% have a present or past psychiatric disorder, usually depression, somatization, or generalized anxiety, and around 60% have a concurrent physical illness (Katon *et al.*, 1990). Since most refuse to be referred to a psychiatric team, the general practitioner has to manage them. One approach is to help to make links between symptoms and stressful life events, leaving out psychological processes, and explore how these stresses might be reduced.

Disorders that are referred from primary care to the psychiatric services

Table 26.1 shows that on average about one in four of the patients with psychiatric disorder who are identified by

Table 26.1 Pathways to care with rates of psychiatric disorder among adults at each level of care

	Cases per 1000 per annum
In the community	260–315
Attending primary care	230
Detected in primary care[†]	102
Attending psychiatric services	24
Inpatient	6

Adapted from Goldberg D and Huxley P, Common Mental Disorders: a biosocial model, Copyright (1992), with permission from Routledge.

[†] Conspicuous psychiatric morbidity.

general practitioners are treated by the psychiatric services. This referred group includes patients with severe depressive disorders, bipolar disorders, schizophrenia, and dementia. General practitioners are more likely to refer patients with other disorders when:

• the diagnosis is uncertain
• the condition is severe
• there is a significant suicide risk
• the condition is chronic
• the necessary treatment cannot be provided by a member of the primary care team
• previous treatment in primary care has been unsuccessful
• psychiatric services are accessible and responsive
• the patient is willing to attend.

Treatments provided by the primary care team for acute disorders

Acute problems are often treated with counselling, used alone or combined with medication. Some practices also provide simple behavioural treatments. Many primary care teams include a counsellor. The availability of a counsellor has not been shown to reduce the prescribing of psychotropic drugs in the practice (Mynors-Wallis *et al.*, 1995; Sibbald *et al.*, 1996).

Improving access to psychological therapies

Psychotherapy has traditionally been a less prominent aspect of health care in the UK compared to the US or continental Europe. Psychotherapists there are either accessed directly or via GPs and paid by insurance or privately. Improving access to psychological therapies (IAPT; Clark, 2011) is an initiative to reverse this by providing easy access to basic psychotherapy (almost exclusively cognitive behavioural therapy). IAPT is a highly prescribed process, but local flexibility has been encouraged with regard to who provides it and where. IAPT has two components—a stepped-care treatment of anxiety and depressive disorders, and a supported employment service (see below). The supported employment service aims to help patients to return to work when their anxiety and depression symptoms have receded (reducing unemployment owing to psychiatric disorders was the other political stimulus for IAPT).

The first step in IAPT is self-help using telephone and internet programmes. A form of brief cognitive behaviour therapy is offered to those with residual symptoms, and referral on to specialized services only takes place after both self-help attempts and cognitive behaviour therapy. A striking feature of IAPT is the level of structure—therapists use detailed manuals, and symptomatic status is recorded after every session using the Patient Health Questionnaire (PHQ-9) (Kroenke *et al.*, 2001) for depressive symptoms and the Generalized Anxiety Disorder Assessment (GAD-7) (Spitzer *et al.*, 2006) for anxiety symptoms.

The format of IAPT is highly variable and is as yet unevaluated. The ease of access and clear commitment to psychological treatments have won widespread approval. Those who provide the service are positive about its outcome, but to date there has been little evidence of diversion from psychiatric services nor independent research evidence of its impact.

Treatments provided by the primary care team for chronic disorders

The respective roles of the general practitioner and the community team should be clearly defined in relation to any patient with chronic mental disorder, and reviewed regularly. For example, with some patients with chronic schizophrenia, the general practitioner might be responsible for their physical health, assess their general progress, administer and encourage compliance with medication, and support the family. Kendrick *et al.* (1995) found that, even with additional training, general practitioners are not very reliable at making comprehensive assessments of patients with long-term psychiatric illness. However, subsequent research demonstrated that this was possible, and financial incentives were introduced to primary care, which has improved

performance in this area. Physical monitoring of psychosis patients has become high priority, with the recognition of their dramatically reduced life expectancy (about 20 years) and the high rates of metabolic syndrome associated with the atypical antipsychotics. It has become more routine that the psychiatric team assesses these patients and agrees a plan with the general practitioner.

Work in primary care by the psychiatric team

There are several ways in which a psychiatric team can work with the primary care team, and these have changed over time (Burns and Bale, 1997).

Advising and training general practitioners and their staff (Balint groups)

Balint Groups are valued by a small group of highly motivated GPs; while some do persist they are mainly of historical interest. The psychiatrist does not see patients, but gives advice based on the general practitioner's assessment and is psychoanalytically inspired (Balint, 1964; www.balint.co.uk).

Assessing and referring

The psychiatrist assesses patients when the GP is uncertain about diagnosis or treatment. He may do this on his own or jointly with the GP, after which referral can proceed in the usual way. This approach is now very rarely used, as liaison with GPs has improved.

Assessing and treating ('shifted out patients')

There are intermittent initiatives to encourage psychiatrists to work mainly in primary care, seeing most patients there or at home, rather than in the hospital outpatient clinic. The approach rarely catches on although it often has vocal local champions. Clinical psychologists and psychiatric nurses can also work in primary care, providing assessment, counselling, or behavioural treatment. Patients no longer need to visit a psychiatric clinic, but there may be little learning between the psychiatric and primary care teams. This approach was popular in the 1980s but was shown to be generally ineffective (Wooff and Goldberg, 1988), as clinical focus shifted and skills were lost. There is more positive evidence for social workers located in primary care.

Shared care

This approach aims for 'seamless care', with enthusiastic advocates (Essex *et al.*, 1990) and several well-publicized demonstration services. However, these demonstration services rarely survived the departure of their advocates, and shared care has not caught on generally. The term is ambiguous, covering everything from GPs monitoring lithium levels to completely shared responsibility. In the care of severely mentally ill patients, absolute clarity of responsibility has repeatedly been shown to be crucial (hence the Care Programme Approach), and the risk of confusion does not seem to be worth taking.

Liaison meetings

Probably the most useful and time-efficient method is to arrange regular (usually monthly) face-to-face meetings between members of the psychiatric team and the primary care team (Burns and Bale, 1997). This can range from meetings of the entire teams to relying on identified 'link' members. The important point is that it is face to face and takes place routinely—not just over crises. Joint patients are discussed, together with possible referrals. Trust is established, along with a more realistic appraisal of what each team can do. Such liaison meetings are increasingly required by commissioners.

Specialist services for acute psychiatric disorder

Patients who are referred to specialist care

Patients who are treated by psychiatric services are a subgroup of people with mental disorders. In some countries patients can go directly to a specialist, so that those treated by the psychiatric services may not be very different from those treated in primary care. Where the general practitioner acts as the 'gatekeeper' to specialist services, as in the UK, the number and types of patient reaching the psychiatric services depend on:

- the willingness of general practitioners to treat psychiatric disorders
- the treatment skills and resources of the primary care team
- patients' willingness to attend for specialist psychiatric advice
- the general practitioner's criteria for referral to the psychiatric services
- the psychiatric services' criteria for accepting referrals.

In the UK, most patients in contact with the psychiatric services have severe and chronic anxiety disorders, severe mood disorder, schizophrenia and other psychoses, or dementia. Patients who are particularly likely to be cared for by specialists are those who are suicidal, those who are potentially dangerous to others, and those with dual diagnoses of mental disorder and substance misuse or personality disorder.

Provisions for acute specialist care

Specialist care of acute psychiatric disorder requires community teams, supported by outpatient, day patient, and inpatient provisions.

Generic versus specialized services

Community teams have traditionally been generic, dealing with all kinds of adult psychiatric problems. More recent specialized separate teams for crisis management and continuing care are described above. The potential advantages of each of these arrangements are summarized in Table 26.2.

Day hospitals

Day care is used in four main ways:

1. *Acute day hospital care* for patients with acute illness who would otherwise be admitted to hospital. Such care is generally more appropriate for those who can be with their families in the evening and at weekends. Early trials of acute day hospital treatment (involving 1568 people) found it feasible for 25% of those currently admitted to inpatient care, with comparable rates of improvement and readmission, and some found it cheaper than inpatient care (Marshall, 2003; Marshall *et al.*, 2003). However, such acute day hospitals were very different from routine day hospitals, and failed to generalize, needing either a charismatic leader or a research programme to sustain them. They are currently experiencing a resurgence as the base for CR/HT teams but have not been researched individually.

2. *Transitional daycare* to allow earlier discharge from hospital.

3. *Day treatment programmes* that provide more intensive treatment for people who are not responding to outpatient care. There is evidence for the value of this approach in personality disorder (Bateman and Fonagy, 2001), and it is increasingly being used for severe eating disorders.

Table 26.2 Generic versus specialist services

Advantages of generic services	Drawbacks of specialist services
Simple model, easy to implement	Complex model, difficult to implement
Traditional, tried and tested	New, relatively untried in clinical practice
Comprehensive	Problem of transitions between teams or falling between different team criteria
Less expensive	More expensive
Continuity of care is easier	Continuity is more difficult to achieve
Drawbacks of generic services	**Advantages of specialist services**
Evidence base is weak	Evidence base better developed
Less efficient—too many different tasks	More efficient with a smaller range of tasks
Less staff satisfaction	More staff satisfaction
Difficult to deliver complex treatments	Easier to deliver complex treatments
Heterogeneous patients, outcomes difficult to evaluate	Homogeneous patients, outcomes easier to assess

4. *Daycare centres* for the support of long-term service users. Such care needs to be planned carefully with an active treatment programme that is specific to each patient's needs, otherwise attenders easily become dependent and 'stuck'.

Day hospitals and day centres vary considerably and their clientele and activities overlap (Catty *et al.*, 2005). CR/HT teams are often integrated with day hospitals.

Inpatient units

The number of beds required for acute psychiatric disorder is difficult to determine exactly. However, it is generally accepted that bed numbers in the US, the UK, and parts of Europe are now inadequate (Priebe *et al.*, 2005). Severe bed shortage appears to be a contributor to the recent increase in compulsion (Keown, 2008) as it depends on:

- The level of morbidity, including substance misuse, in the population served by the unit.
- The willingness and ability of families to care for acutely ill relatives, which in turn depends on the quality of accommodation and the availability of other family members.
- The extent and availability of crisis services.
- Facilities for treatment of acute psychiatric disorder outside hospital, such as well-staffed hostels.
- Facilities for early discharge of patients from hospital after the acute phase of the disorder; it is

generally easier to discharge early than to avoid admission.

The design of inpatient units for acutely ill patients should strike a balance between the patients' needs for privacy and the staff's requirement to observe them, although single, ensuite accommodation is increasingly the norm. They need to be sufficiently large to ensure adequate staffing for emergencies, yet avoid an anonymous or 'institutional' feel. Three 15- to 20-bedded wards is considered to be the minimum necessary for safe effective care, and units of over 100 patients are considered probably too large. Ward design should minimize the possibility of suicide by hanging or jumping. There is a need for secure areas for the most disturbed patients, areas where patients can be alone, and areas where they can interact with others. There should be provision for occupational therapy, the practice of domestic skills, and recreation. Outdoor space is desirable. Single-sex accommodation is now mandatory.

The siting of acute inpatient units. Inpatient care for acute psychiatric disorders is generally provided as part of a general hospital complex. This siting reduces stigma and provides easy access to general medical services when required. The disadvantages of such siting include a low threshold for disruptive behaviour and inadequate space for occupational and recreational activities suitable for psychiatric care. Many of these problems can be overcome if the psychiatric unit occupies a separate building within the general hospital complex.

Collaboration with community teams. Patients are at increased risk, particularly for suicide, when they move from inpatient to community care. About 25%

of suicides among psychiatric patients in England and Wales occur within 3 months of discharge from inpatient psychiatric care, with a peak in the first 1–2 weeks, and contact in the week following discharge is essential.

Psychiatric services that provide long-term care

Characteristics of patients who require long-term care

Diagnosis

With the exception of the elderly (who are considered in Chapter 19), most psychiatric patients who require long-term care have schizophrenia, chronic affective disorders, or personality disorders associated with aggressive behaviour or substance misuse. Patients who need care in hospital for longer than 1 year, other than forensic patients, are referred to as 'new long-stay'. This distinguishes them from the 'old long-stay', who had been residents in hospital closure programmes.

Problems

There are several ways of classifying the problems of patients who need long-term psychiatric care. They can be divided into seven groups, three of which are contained in the World Health Organization's classification of disablement (page 23), on the basis of the following problems:

- *Symptoms* such as persistent hallucinations or suicidal ideas.
- *Unacceptable behaviours*, such as shouting obscenities, and threatening or carrying out violent acts.
- *Impairments* that interfere with the functioning of a psychological or physical system—for example, poor memory or lack of drive.
- *Disabilities* that interfere with the activities of the whole person, such as inability to dress.
- *Handicaps*, which are social disadvantages directly resulting from disability—for example, inability to work, or to care for children.
- *Other social disadvantages* that are not directly related to disability, but which are a consequence of the *stigmatizing attitudes* of other people—for example, unemployment, poverty, and homelessness.

- *Adverse personal reactions* to illness and social disadvantage—for example, low self-esteem, hopelessness, denial of illness, or the misuse of drugs.

Wing and Furlong (1986) proposed a list of patient characteristics that make it difficult to treat the individual in the community, which, despite its age, is still useful (see Box 26.4). Patients with severe and persistent problems of this kind may need care in a well-staffed hostel, or in a hospital that can provide appropriate rehabilitation and security.

Requirements of a community service providing long-term care

To treat patients in the community, they need all the elements of care previously provided in hospital. The following provisions are required:

1. Suitable and well-supported carers.
2. Appropriate accommodation.
3. Suitable occupation.
4. Arrangements that enlist the patient's collaboration with treatment.
5. Regular reassessment, including physical health.
6. Effective collaboration among carers (formal and informal).
7. Continuity of care and rapid response to crises.

Complicated and expensive arrangements are required to make these seven elements available as readily in the community as they would be in hospital. Lack of such arrangements may leave patients homeless, without constructive occupation, inadequately treated, and without a carer. Failure of community care may also leave carers unsupported and family life disrupted. When community care began, it was concerned mainly with patients who had become institutionalized and compliant after many years in hospital. These patients could often be managed in the community without much difficulty. Younger patients who have spent less time in hospital are often less compliant and more difficult to manage.

Carers

When people with severe mental illness live at home, *family and friends* are the main carers. They provide much of the help that would have been given by nurses had the patient remained in hospital. For example, they may have to encourage the patient to get up in the morning, maintain personal hygiene, eat regular meals, and occupy himself or herself constructively. Carers also encourage collaboration with treatment. If patients have many problem behaviours, prolonged involvement in their care is stressful. Carers may then need support and advice, and sometimes periods of respite.

Volunteers play an important part in many systems of community care. Trained volunteers can help to support patients and their families, and some charitable organizations employ professional carers, such as hostel staff.

Community psychiatric nurses are the backbone of community care by supporting patients and carers, evaluating patients, supervising drug therapy, and encouraging social interaction. Monitoring is particularly important for patients whose mental state is unstable.

Accommodation

Patients who have been discharged from hospital need food and shelter. Many live with their families, and some care for themselves in rented accommodation. Others require more extensive help, which can be provided in three ways.

In lodgings. Some families take in patients as lodgers and to provide them with extra care. This practice works well in several countries, but has not been widely adopted in the UK.

In group homes. Many patients live in group homes of four or five patients together. The houses may be owned by social or health services or by a charity. This model works well for people with schizophrenia and social handicaps but few positive symptoms. People in group homes receive regular support and supervision, usually from a community nurse or social worker. They ensure the arrangements are working well and encourage residents to take on as much responsibility as possible.

In hostels. For some people, hostels are half-way houses from which they move on to more independent living. Others need to remain in hostels for a period of years. Although most hostel residents live fairly independent lives, a few of the most disabled require additional care. Hostels have permanent staffing. Levels of supervision vary and overnight staff may sleep in, or do night shifts as in a hospital ward.

Occupation

Most patients would like to work, although rates of unemployment are higher in mental illness than any other disabled group. There are several approaches to increasing work and employment:

- *Vocational rehabilitation* is the longest established approach. Extensive training based on a detailed assessment of disabilities and following a structured programme is provided to develop the skills and confidence needed for competitive employment. Training may take place in sheltered workshops, with transitional jobs in paid posts 'owned' by the rehabilitation scheme. Progress to open employment is disappointing.

- *The Clubhouse model* is a specialized form of vocational rehabilitation that is based around a building which is jointly administered and maintained by people with mental illness (Beard *et al.*, 1987). Originating in the USA, it has established itself internationally but is not widespread and may be fading out.

- *Supported employment* was originally developed for people with learning disabilities. Individuals are placed in competitive work without any extended preparation, but with support on the job (Bond *et al.*, 1997). It has been shown in several randomized controlled trials (Bond *et al.*, 2008) to be the most effective way of obtaining open employment. Most of the studies have been conducted in the USA, but a European replication (Burns *et al.*, 2007a) confirmed equal efficacy (over 50% of psychotic patients became employed). It is government policy in the UK and several European countries and is part of the IAPT programme, but provision remains patchy.

- *Sheltered work* allows people to work productively but more slowly than would be acceptable elsewhere. Schemes include horticulture projects and craft workshops.
- *Voluntary activities*. Some patients who cannot meet the requirements for sheltered work benefit from undertaking voluntary activities.
- *Occupational therapy*. Those unable to contemplate work can benefit from occupational therapy to reduce boredom, understimulation, and lack of social contacts. Occupational activities are often provided in a day hospital or a day centre.

Reassessment

Patients living outside hospital require the same regular reassessments. The patient's mental state and of collaboration with treatment is assessed by the key worker, often a community nurse, with less frequent reassessment by a psychiatrist. Patients can forget appointments, and a recall system prompts re-establishing contact. Physical health reviews are essential because such patients often neglect physical illness, or may not accept offered help.

Risk assessment. It is more difficult to anticipate threatening or dangerous behaviour in community care than in hospital. An important part of assessment is a regular evaluation of the patient's risk to himself or herself, and to other people. Such assessment involves *static factors*, such as the patient's past behaviours, and *dynamic risk factors,* such as the current level of substance misuse or of psychosocial stressors. A risk management plan is an important component of the overall care plan. The scientific value of structured risk assessment has been disputed (Fazel *et al.*, 2014). However, they demonstrate that due consideration has been given of possible adverse consequences.

Continuity of care

Community care staff need to gain the confidence of their patients and to know them well. Neither can be achieved if there are frequent changes in staff. Continuity of care is important, and staff should be extra vigilant when care passes between workers.

Response to crisis

Staff need to respond quickly to crises. Families and the staff of voluntary organizations accept patients more readily if they know that help will be available quickly in an emergency. Furthermore, readmission to hospital may be avoided by prompt action. A crisis plan agreed in advance with the patient and carers is particularly helpful. Staffing levels need to be adequate to allow a quick response, preferably by staff who know the patient.

Working with the family and volunteers

Community care is costly, and in most countries public funds are limited, so arrangements often depend on input from families and voluntary groups. It is important that families and voluntary groups are involved in the planning of services, and that there is agreement about their responsibilities. Without such an agreement, family may feel responsible for over-demanding tasks, and professionals concerned that volunteers are taking on tasks beyond their capabilities. Similarly, it is best practice to involve families and voluntary groups in the evaluation of services.

Other components of a community service

Rehabilitation and recovery

Rehabilitation denotes procedures for helping patients to reach and maintain their best level of functioning. It is based on a careful assessment of disabilities and deficits and relies on a structured, gradual training. It may be provided in an inpatient unit, a day hospital, or a specialized rehabilitation centre. Rehabilitation procedures include medical, psychological, occupational, social, and residential. Most patients require medication to control symptoms of schizophrenia or chronic affective disorders. Psychological methods include supportive therapy, behavioural programmes, and social skills training (see Chapter 24). Work helps to structure the day and provides an opportunity for interaction with other people. It can improve self-esteem, and payment is an added incentive. For many the aim is to return to ordinary work, but those who cannot achieve this are trained for activities such as gardening, crafts, and cooking. These provide a sense of achievement and a shape to the day. Whenever practicable, patients should be encouraged to join the same social groups attended by healthy people.

The recovery movement

'Recovery' has taken on a quite specific meaning in recent years beyond the absence of symptoms. The 'recovery movement' (Slade *et al.*, 2014) emphasizes the primacy of patient determination in treatment planning and goals. What matters is the quality of life, not the absence of symptoms. Clearly it is eminently sensible to recognize that the goal of treatment is to enable patients to live the life they wish and to make the best adaptation to their residual problems. The approach does, however, raise some problems for practitioners. Firstly, much of the rhetoric unnecessarily caricatures psychiatric practice as narrow and mechanical.

A tenet of the recovery movement is that psychiatrists are overly pessimistic about outcomes, and it calls on us to be more hopeful and 'upbeat'. Most professionals believe they owe their patients honesty. Lastly, some recovery enthusiasts insist that mental health professionals should support the patient's treatment choices even if they believe them wrong. The recovery movement is a good reminder that social and personal outcomes are what matter to patients and families. Hopefully this will persist when the excesses have faded.

Inpatient care

People with long-term mental illness require inpatient care for acute treatment at times of relapse, for intensive rehabilitation, and in some instances for long stay. The basic requirements for such an inpatient unit are broadly similar to those for patients with acute illness, except that accommodation can be more domestic. Because the pace and intensity of treatment is usually slower for this group, it is advisable to have a separate facility. Patients with severely disturbed behaviour need secure areas, with outdoor space and occupational and social activities in the same building.

Services for people with particular needs

Clinical work and research have identified several groups of patients whose needs may require special attention.

Members of ethnic minorities and migrants

Members of ethnic minorities are less likely to use routine services. They are less likely to consult general practitioners when they have a psychiatric disorder or to accept referral to psychiatric services. Professionals are less likely to identify psychiatric disorder, and may be less able to explain the illness and treatment in terms that accommodate their cultural beliefs. These problems are not primarily due to a limited command of English.

The problems of minorities in the UK have been studied, in particular among those of Asian and Afro-Caribbean origin. People of Asian origin consult their general practitioners more frequently about most conditions than do members of the general population, but consult them less about psychiatric symptoms (Murray and Williams, 1986; Gillam *et al.*, 1989), and often present with physical symptoms. African-Caribbean patients with psychoses lack family support and often bypass GP referral and come to services via the police (Morgan *et al.*, 2005). In some ethnic minorities, referral to a psychiatrist is avoided because it can affect marriage prospects.

Underrecognition and overadmission of psychiatric disorder

In the 1980s and 1990s much was made of professionals' overdiagnosis of psychosis in African and African-Caribbean patients based on a lack of cultural sensitivity (Littlewood and Lipsedge, 1997). The AESOP study has dispelled this myth, confirming that the rates are indeed higher and the outcomes, if anything, marginally worse rather than better as they would be as the consequence of misdiagnosis (Fearon *et al.*, 2006).

The debate on whether the needs of ethnic minority patients are best served by separate teams has now faded out. Increased vigilance and flexible services are what is needed rather than altered diagnostic procedures or separate services (Singh and Burns, 2006).

Homeless mentally ill people

When hospitals were closed, it was feared that many discharged patients would become homeless, but when closures were planned carefully, few of them became so (Leff, 1993; Harrison *et al.*, 1994). Nevertheless, surveys have found high rates of chronic psychiatric disorder among the residents of hostels for the homeless (Geddes *et al.*, 2014). The most common disorders were alcohol and drug dependence. Psychotic illness and major depression each ranged from 3% to 42%. Alcohol dependence has increased over recent decades. Services for the homeless mentally ill vary enormously, and there is neither agreement on their need nor on their characteristics (Hwang and Burns, 2014).

Doctors with psychiatric problems

Although doctors have tried to reduce the stigma associated with psychiatric disorder, many of them do not seek help if they develop such disorders themselves. Most national medical associations provide accessible and confidential services for doctors with mental health problems. It is still important to provide arrangements to enable psychiatrically ill doctors (and other mental health staff) to obtain treatment away from their place of work. A greater acceptance of psychiatric disorder is required within the medical profession, with appropriate arrangements for aftercare and a gradual (and in some cases supervised) return to work. The issue needs greater discussion during medical education and training. When disorders are chronic or recurrent, fitness to practice has to be considered.

Refugees

Refugees have the general problems of members of ethnic minority groups (described above), together with specific problems secondary to the experiences that led them to seek refuge in another country. These experiences include persecution, physical injury, torture, rape, or the witnessing of these. The consequences include general medical as well as psychiatric conditions. The latter are mainly post-traumatic stress disorder and depressive disorder.

The specifics of care needed by refugees should be set in the context of many of the principles of global mental health, dealt with further in Chapter 23. At the very least they need integrated medical and psychiatric care from a team that is sensitive to cultural factors. Integrated care is important because general and psychiatric disorders occur together, and because refugees often come from cultures in which distress and psychiatric disorder are generally manifested by physical symptoms. In addition, aid workers are sometimes reluctant to refer refugees to a solely psychiatric service, which they think inappropriate for what appears to be a normal response to overwhelmingly stressful circumstances. As with the homeless mentally ill, acceptability is much greater with integrated services.

Staff who provide services for refugees should be experienced in the treatment of post-traumatic conditions, and should be aided by interpreters. Female members of staff are needed to help female refugees, especially those who have experienced rape. Other staff should have experience in treating children and adolescents. For a review of the psychiatric problems of refugees, see Mollica *et al.* (2009), and for a review of such problems among child and adolescent refugees, see Fazel *et al.* (2012a). See also Chapter 23.

Some difficulties with community care

The burden on relatives

If members of the family are to take responsibility for patients, by housing them, encouraging adaptive behaviour, supervising their medication, and reporting signs of relapse, they need to be well informed, adequately supported, and able to obtain help in an emergency. Such support is time-consuming and is rarely available unless community care is well resourced and the needs of the family are given high priority. In the UK a carer assessment is obligatory with long-term disorders, yet many carers report poor communication from psychiatric services. Staff experience continuing conflict over their duty of confidentiality to the patient and their wish to support and inform relatives. There is no easy answer to this dilemma. Carers report the greatest difficulties in coping with negative symptoms and socially embarrassing or aggressive behaviour, and anticipatory anxiety about such behaviour and long-term prognosis are regularly reported as more burdensome than practical help.

Care plans should always consider the possible effects of the patient's illness on any children in the home.

Problems with the distribution of resources

When resources are limited, there is a conflict between the needs of patients with acute disorders and those with chronic disorders. The conflict is most evident in primary care, where the former group of patients is generally more demanding of care and more responsive to it.

Problems with the coordination of services

In most countries, long-stay hospital care for patients with chronic psychiatric disorder is provided by a single agency (a hospital authority). Community care requires coordinated action by several agencies, each of which usually has other responsibilities—for example, social services departments have responsibilities for mentally healthy children and frail elderly people as well as for psychiatric patients. This broad responsibility generates endless problems with regard to the allocation of resources. Regular negotiation is the only possible response.

International service principles

In countries that have few specialist psychiatric resources, it is essential to decide on priorities. The World Health Organization (1984) has identified four priorities:

1. Rapid response to psychiatric emergencies.
2. Provisions for chronic severe psychiatric disorder.
3. Care for psychiatric disorders associated with general medical illness.
4. Care for any high-risk groups that are found in the country (e.g. drug misusers).

The World Health Organization advocates the training of *auxiliary workers* who can supplement the efforts of fully trained staff. Thus in countries with few trained psychiatrists, resources may be used most effectively by improving the skills of nurses who can perform the first-line management of psychiatric disorders, supported by general practitioners. See also Chapter 23.

Further reading

Goldberg D and Huxley P (1992). *Common Mental Disorders: A biosocial model*. Routledge, London. (This book is still valuable for its account of the development and utility of the 'filter' model, which relates epidemiology to the provision of services.)

Thornicroft G and Szmukler G (2001). *Textbook of Community Psychiatry*. Oxford University Press, Oxford. (A comprehensive work of reference.)

References

Abajobir AA *et al.* (2016). A systematic review and meta-analysis of the association between unintended pregnancy and perinatal depression. *Journal of Affective Disorders*, **192**, 56–63.

Abbass AA *et al.* (2013). Psychodynamic psychotherapy for children and adolescents: A meta-analysis of short-term psychodynamic models. *Journal of the American Academy of Child & Adolescent Psychiatry*, **52**, 863–75.

Abdelmawla N and Mitchell AJ (2006a). Sudden cardiac death and antipsychotics. Part 1: Risk factors and mechanisms. *Advances in Psychiatric Treatment*, **12**, 35–44.

Abdelmawla N and Mitchell AJ (2006b). Sudden cardiac death and antipsychotics. Part 2: Monitoring and prevention. *Advances in Psychiatric Treatment*, **12**, 100–9.

Abderhalden C *et al.* (2008). Structured risk assessment and violence in acute psychiatric wards: randomized controlled trial. *British Journal of Psychiatry*, **193**, 44–50.

Abel KM, Drake R and Goldstein JM (2010). Sex differences in schizophrenia. *International Review of Psychiatry*, **22**, 417–28.

Abraham HD (2009). Disorders relating to use of PCP and hallucinogens. In: Gelder MG, Andreason NC, Lopez-Ibor JJJr and Geddes JR (eds.) *New Oxford Textbook of Psychiatry*. Oxford University Press, Oxford. pp. 486–90.

Abraham A and Luty J (2010). Testing for illicit drug use in mental health services. *Advances in Psychiatric Treatment*, **16**(5), 369–79

Abrams RC and Horowitz SV (1996). Personality disorders after age 50: a meta-analysis. *Journal of Personality Disorders*, **10**, 271–81.

Academy of Medical Sciences (2004). *Calling Time. The Nation's drinking as a major health issue*. Academy of Medical Sciences, London.

Ackner B and Oldham AJ (1962). Insulin treatment of schizophrenia. A three-year follow-up of a controlled study. *Lancet*, **i**, 504–6.

Adams K and Grant I (2009). *Neuropsychological Assessment of Neuropsychiatric and Neuromedical Disorders*. 3rd edn. Oxford University Press, New York.

Adams RD *et al.* (1965). Symptomatic occult hydrocephalus with 'normal' cerebrospinal fluid pressure: a treatable syndrome. *New England Journal of Medicine*, **273**, 117–26.

Addington J, Heinssen R (2012). Prediction and prevention of psychosis in youth at clinical high risk. *Annual Review of Clinical Psychology*, **8**, 269–89.

Adshead G and Ferris S (2007). Treatment of victims of trauma. *Advances in Psychiatric Treatment*, **13**, 358–68.

Agid O *et al.* (2003). Delayed-onset hypothesis of antipsychotic action: a hypothesis tested and rejected. *Archives of General Psychiatry*, **60**, 1228–35.

Agnew-Blais JC *et al.* (2016). Evaluation of the persistence, remission, and emergence of attention-deficit/hyperactivity disorder in young adulthood. *JAMA Psychiatry*, **73**, 713–20.

Agorastos A, Haasen C, Huber CG (2012). Anxiety disorders through a transcultural perspective: implications for migrants. *Psychopathology*, **45**(2), 67–77.

Agrawal N and Govender S (2011). Epilepsy and neuropsychiatric comorbidities. *Advances in Psychiatric Treatment*, **17**, 44–53.

Ahmari SE and Simpson B (2013). Neurobiology and treatment of OCD. In: Charney DS, Sklar O, Buxbaum JD, Nestler EJ (eds.) *Neurobiology of Mental Illness*, OUP, New York, Ch. 48.

Ahmed AS (2007). Post-traumatic stress disorder, resilience and vulnerability. *Advances in Psychiatric Treatment*, **13**, 369–75.

Ahmed K, Mohan RA and Bhugra D (2007). Self-harm in South Asian women: a literature review informed approach to assessment and formulation. *American Journal of Psychotherapy*, **61**, 71–81.

Ainsworth MDS *et al.* (1978). *Patterns of Attachment: A psychological study of the strange situation*. Erlbaum, Hillsdale, NJ.

Aizenstein HJ *et al.* (2011). fMRI correlates of white matter hyperintensities in late-life depression. *American Journal of Psychiatry*, **168**, 1075–82.

Ajdacic-Gross V *et al.* (2008). Reduction in the suicide rate during Advent—a time series analysis. *Psychiatry Research*, **157**, 139–46.

Akagi H and House A (2002). The clinical epidemiology of hysteria: vanishingly rare or just vanishing? *Psychological Medicine*, **32**, 191–4.

Albanese A *et al.* (2013). Phenomenology and classification of dystonia: a consensus update. *Movement Disorders*, **28**, 863–73.

Albert FW and Kruglyak L (2015). The role of regulatory variation in complex traits and disease. *Nature Reviews Genetics*, **16**, 197–212.

Alcohol Concern (2016). Statistics on alcohol. https://www.alcoholconcern.org.uk/help-and-advice/statistics-on-alcohol/

Alexander DA (2005). Early mental health intervention after disasters. *Advances in Psychiatric Treatment*, **11**, 12–18.

Alexander GE and Crutcher MD (1990). Functional architecture of basal ganglia circuits: neural substrates of parallel processing. *Trends in Neuroscience*, **13**, 266–71.

Alexander M *et al.* (2015). Age-stratified prevalence of mild cognitive impairment and dementia in European populations: a systematic review. *Journal of Alzheimer's Disease*, **48**, 355–69.

Alexopoulos GS *et al.* (1997). 'Vascular depression' hypothesis. *Archives of General Psychiatry*, **54**, 915–22.

Alisic E *et al.* (2014). Rates of post-traumatic stress disorder in trauma-exposed children and adolescents: meta-analysis. *British Journal of Psychiatry*, **204**, 335–40.

Alloy LB *et al.* (2005). The psychosocial context of bipolar disorder: Environmental, cognitive and developmental risk factors. *Clinical Psychology Review*, **25**, 1043–75.

Alonso J *et al.* (2004). Prevalence of mental disorders in Europe: results from the European Study of the Mental Disorders (ESEMeD) project. *Acta Psychiatrica Scandinavica*, **109**, 21–7.

Alonso P *et al.* (2015). Deep brain stimulation for obsessive-compulsive disorder: a meta-analysis of treatment outcome and predictors of response. *PloS One*, **10**, e0133591.

Althof S (2010). Sex therapy: advances in paradigms, nomenclature, and treatment. *Academic Psychiatry*, **34**, 390–6.

Altman EG *et al.* (1997). The Altman Self-Rating Mania Scale. *Biological Psychiatry*, **42**, 948–55.

Altshuler D, Daly MJ and Lander ES (2008). Genetic mapping in human disease. *Science*, 322, 881–8.

Amato PR and Anthony CJ (2014). Estimating the effects of parental divorce and death with fixed effects models. *Journal of Marriage and Family*, 76(2), 370–86.

American Psychiatric Association (1998). Guidelines for assessing the decision-making capacities of potential research subjects with cognitive impairment. *American Journal of Psychiatry*, **155**, 1649–50.

American Psychiatric Association (2013). *Diagnostic and Statistical Manual of Mental Disorders, Fifth Edition (DSM-5)*. American Psychiatric Association, Washington, DC.

American Psychiatric Association (2013). *The Principles of Medical Ethics 2013 Edition*. American Psychiatric Association, Washington, DC.

American Psychiatric Association Practice Guidelines (2001). Practice guideline for the treatment of patients with borderline personality disorder. *American Journal of Psychiatry*, **158**, 1–52.

Amir N, Leiner A and Bomyea J (2010). Implicit memory and posttraumatic stress symptoms. *Cognitive Therapy and Research*, **34**, 49–58.

Amminger GP *et al.* (2015). Longer-term outcome in the prevention of psychotic disorders by the Vienna omega-3 study. *Nature Communications*, **6**, 7934.

Anand A and Charney DS (2000). Norepinephrine dysfunction in depression. *Journal of Clinical Psychiatry*, **61**, 16–24.

Anand R *et al.* (2014). Therapeutics of Alzheimer's disease: Past, present and future. *Neuropharmacology, 76*, 27–50.

an der Heiden W and Häfner (2011). Course and outcome. In: Weinberger D and Harrison PJ (eds.) *Schizophrenia*, 3rd edn. Wiley-Blackwell, Oxford. pp. 104–41.

Andersen BL *et al.* (2014). Screening, assessment, and care of anxiety and depressive symptoms in adults with cancer. *Journal of Clinical Oncology*, **32**, 1605–19.

Anderson E (2008). Cognitive change in old age. In: R Jacoby, C Oppenheimer, T Dening and A Thomas (eds.) *The Oxford Textbook of Old Age Psychiatry*, Oxford University Press, Oxford. pp. 33–50.

Anderson IM (2003). Drug treatment of depression: reflections on the evidence. *Advances in Psychiatric Treatment*, **9**, 11–20.

Anderson IM and Fergusson GM (2013). Mechanism of action of ECT. In: J Waite, A Eaton (eds.) *The ECT Handbook*. RCPsych Publications, London. pp. 1–7.

Andrade C, Kumar C and Surya S (2013). Cardiovascular mechanisms of SSRI drugs and their benefits and risks in ischemic heart disease and heart failure. *International Clinical Psychopharmacology*, **28**, 145–55.

Andreasen NC (2009). Schizophrenia: a conceptual history. In: MG Gelder, NC Andreasen, JJ Lopez-IborJr and JR Geddes (eds.) *The New Oxford Textbook of Psychiatry*, 2nd edn. Oxford University Press, Oxford. pp. 521–6.

Andreasson S *et al.* (1987). Cannabis and schizophrenia. A longitudinal study of Swedish conscripts. *Lancet*, **ii**, 1483–6.

Angel K (2010). The history of 'female sexual dysfunction' as a mental disorder in the 20th century. *Current Opinion in Psychiatry*, **23**, 536–41.

Angermeyer MC *et al.* (2011). Biogenetic explanations and public acceptance of mental illness: systematic review of population studies. *The British Journal of Psychiatry*, **199**, 367–72.

Angst J (2009). Course and prognosis of mood disorders. In: MG Gelder, NC Andreasen, JJ Lopez-Ibor and JR Geddes (eds.) *New Oxford Textbook of Psychiatry*. Oxford University Press, Oxford. pp. 665–9.

Angst J *et al.* (2013). Mortality of 403 patients with mood disorders 48 to 52 years after their psychiatric hospitalization. *European Archives of Psychiatry and Clinical Neuroscience*, **263**, 425–34.

Angst J *et al.* (2015). A Swiss longitudinal study of the prevalence of, and overlap between, sexual problems in men and women aged 20 to 50 years old. *Journal of Sex Research*, **52**, 949–59.

Anonymous (1994). Molecules and minds. *Lancet*, **343**, 681–2.

Anonymous (2015). What's in a name? Systemic exertion intolerance disease. *Lancet*, **385**, 663.

Ansseau M *et al.* (2004). High prevalence of mental disorders in primary care. *Journal of Affective Disorders*, **78**, 49–55.

Anthenelli RM (2010). Focus on: comorbid mental health disorders. *Alcohol Research and Health*, **33**, 109–17.

Anton RF *et al.* (2006). Combined pharmacotherapies and behavioural interventions for alcohol dependence: the COMBINE Study: a randomized controlled trial. *Journal of the American Medical Association*, **295**, 2003–17.

Antypa N *et al.* (2013) Serotonergic genes and suicide: A systematic review. *European Neuropsychopharmacology*, **23**, 1125–1142.

Anwar S *et al.* (2009). Is arson the crime most strongly associated with psychosis?—A national case-control study of arson risk in schizophrenia and other psychoses. *Schizophrenia Bulletin*. doi:10.1093/schbul/sbp098.

Appleby L *et al.* (2015). *The National Confidential Inquiry into Suicide and Homicide by People with Mental Illness Annual Report 2015: England, Northern Ireland, Scotland and Wales*. University of Manchester.

Arango C and Carpenter WT (2011). The schizophrenia construct: symptomatic presentation. In: D Weinberger and PJ Harrison (eds.) *Schizophrenia*, 3rd edn. Wiley-Blackwell, Oxford. pp. 9–23.

Arango C, Fraguas D (2016). Should psychiatry deal only with mental disorders without an identified medical aetiology? *World Psychiatry*, **15**, 22–3.

Araya R *et al.* (2006). Cost-effectiveness of a primary care treatment program for depression in low-income women in Santiago, Chile. *American Journal of Psychiatry*, **163**, 1379–87.

Arcelus J *et al.* (2011). Mortality rates in patients with anorexia nervosa and other eating disorders. A meta-analysis of 36 studies. *Archives of General Psychiatry*, **68**, 724–31.

Arena JE and Rabinstein AA (2015). Transient global amnesia. *Mayo Clinic Proceedings*, **90**, 264–72.

Arnold SE *et al.* (2013). Comparative survey of the topographical distribution of signature molecular lesions in major neurodegenerative diseases. *Journal of Comparative Neurology*, **521**, 4339–55.

Arnone D *et al.* (2012). Magnetic resonance imaging studies in unipolar depression: Systematic review and meta-regression analyses. *European Neuropsychopharmacology,* **22**, 1–16.

Arnone D *et al.* (2015). Indirect evidence of selective glial involvement in glutamate-based mechanisms of mood regulation in depression: Meta-analysis of absolute prefrontal neurometabolic concentrations. *European Neuropsychopharmacology,* **25**, 1109–17.

Arnow BA *et al.* (2015). Depression subtypes in predicting antidepressant response: A report from the iSPOT-D Trial. *American Journal of Psychiatry,* **172**, 743–50.

Aronson R *et al.* (1996). Triiodothyronine augmentation in the treatment of refractory depression. A meta-analysis. *Archives of General Psychiatry,* **53**, 842–8.

Arscott K, Dagnan D and Kroese B (1998). Consent to psychological research by people with an intellectual disability. *Journal of Applied Research in Intellectual Disability,* **11**, 77–83.

Arseneault L *et al.* (2006). Bullying victimization uniquely contributes to adjustment problems in young children: a nationally representative cohort study. *Paediatrics,* **118**, 130–8.

Arseneault L, Bowes L and Shakoor S (2010). Bullying victimization in youths and mental health problems: 'Much ado about nothing'? *Psychological Medicine,* **40**, 717–29.

Asher R (1951). Munchausen's syndrome. *Lancet,* **i**, 339–41.

Asperger H (1944). Die 'Autistischen Psychopathien' Kindesalter. *Archiv für Psychiatrie und Nervenkrankheiten,* **117**, 76–136.

Assum T and Sørensen M (2010). Safety performance indicator for alcohol in road accidents—international comparison, validity and data quality. *Accident Analysis and Prevention,* **42**, 595–603.

Auer RN (2004). Hypoglycemic brain damage. *Metabolic Brain Disease,* **19**, 169–75.

Aust R, Sharp C and Goulden C (2002). *Prevalence of Drug Use: key findings from the 2001/2002 British Crime Survey.* Home Office, London.

Ayala ES, Meuret AE and Ritz T (2009). Treatments for blood-injury-injection phobia: a critical review of current evidence. *Journal of Psychiatric Research,* **43**, 1235–42.

Aybek S *et al.* (2014). Neural correlates of recall of life events in conversion disorder. *JAMA Psychiatry,* **71**, 52–60.

Ayerbe L *et al.* (2012). Natural history, predictors and outcomes of depression after stroke: systematic review and meta-analysis. *British Journal of Psychiatry,* **202**, 14–21.

Bagayogo IP *et al.* (2013). Transcultural aspects of somatic disorders in the context of depressive disorders. In: RD Alarcon (ed.). *Cultural Psychiatry.* Karger, Rochester, pp. 64–74.

Bagni C *et al.* (2012). Fragile X syndrome: causes, diagnosis, mechanisms, and therapeutics. *Journal of Clinical Investigation,* **122**, 4314–22.

Baigent C *et al.* (2010). Large-scale randomized evidence: trials and meta-analyses of trials. In: Warrell DA, Cox TM and Firth JD (eds.) *Oxford Textbook of Medicine.* Oxford University Press, Oxford. pp. 31–47.

Baio J (2012). Prevalence of Autism Spectrum Disorders: Autism and Developmental Disabilities Monitoring Network, 14 Sites, United States, 2008. Morbidity and Mortality Weekly Report. Surveillance Summaries. *Centers for Disease Control and Prevention,* **61**, 1–19.

Baizabal-Carvallo J and Jankovic J (2016). Parkinsonism, movement disorders and genetics in frontotemporal dementia. *Nature Reviews Neurology,* **12**, 175–85.

Baker-Henningham H *et al.* (2005). The effect of early stimulation on maternal depression: a cluster randomised controlled trial. *Archives of Disease in Childhood,* **90**, 1230–4.

BALANCE Study Group (2010). Lithium plus valproate combination therapy versus monotherapy for relapse prevention in bipolar 1 disorder (BALANCE): a randomised open label trial. *Lancet,* **375**, 385–95.

Baldwin DS and Sinclair JM (2015). Recurrent brief depression: This too shall pass? In: D Bhugra, GS Malhi (eds). *Troublesome Disguises: Managing challenging disorders in psychiatry,* Wiley-Blackwell, Chichester, pp. 100–13.

Baldwin DS, Huusom AKT and Maehlum E (2006). Escitalopram and paroxetine in the treatment of generalised anxiety disorder: randomised, placebo-controlled, double-blind study. *British Journal of Psychiatry,* **189**, 264–72.

Baldwin DS *et al.* (2014). Evidence-based pharmacological treatment of anxiety disorders, post-traumatic stress disorder and obsessive-compulsive disorder: a revision of the 2005 guidelines from the British Association for Psychopharmacology. *Journal of Psychopharmacology,* **28**, 403–39.

Baldwin RC *et al.* (2003). Guideline for the management of late-life depression in primary care. *International Journal of Geriatric Psychiatry,* **18**, 829–38.

Balestri M *et al.* (2014). Genetic modulation of personality traits: a systematic review of the literature. *International Clinical Psychopharmacology,* **29**, 1–15.

Balint M (1964). *The Doctor, the Patient and his Illness,* 2nd edn. Pitman, London.

Ballard C and Corbett A (2013). Agitation and aggression in people with Alzheimer's disease. *Current Opinion in Psychiatry,* **26**, 252–9.

Ballard C *et al.* (2005). Quetiapine and rivastigmine and cognitive decline in Alzheimer's disease: randomised double-blind placebo-controlled trial. *British Medical Journal,* **330**, 874–7.

Ballard C *et al.* (2015). Dextromethorphan and quinidine for treating agitation in patients with Alzheimer disease dementia. *JAMA,* **314**, 1233–5.

Ballard C *et al.* (2016). Dementia in Down's syndrome. *Lancet Neurology,* **15**, 622–36.

Ballenger JC (2009). Panic disorder and agoraphobia. In: MG Gelder, NC Andreasen, JJ Lopez-IborJr and JR Geddes (eds.) *New Oxford Textbook of Psychiatry.* Oxford University Press, Oxford. pp. 750–64.

Balodis IM *et al.* (2015). Neurobiological features of binge eating disorder. *CNS Spectrums,* **20**, 557–65.

Bandura A (1969). *Principles of Behaviour Modification.* Holt, Rinehart and Winston, New York.

Bang J *et al.* (2015). Frontotemporal dementia. *Lancet,* **386**, 1672–82.

Banks R *et al.* (2007). *Challenging Behaviour: A unified approach* (Clinical and service guidelines for supporting people with learning disabilities who are at risk of receiving abusive or restrictive practices). London: The Royal College of Psychiatrists, The British Psychological Society and The Royal College of Speech and Language Therapists. College Report CR, 144.

Barahona-Corrêa J and Filipe CN (2015). A concise history of Asperger syndrome: The short reign of a troublesome diagnosis. *Frontiers in Psychology*, 6, 2024.

Barbee JG *et al.* (2011). A double-blind placebo-controlled trial of lamotrigine as an antidepressant augmentation agent in treatment-refractory unipolar depression. *Journal of Clinical Psychiatry*, 72, 1405–12.

Barbui C and Cipriani A (2011). Efficacy of antidepressants and benzodiazepines in minor depression: systematic review and meta-analysis. *British Journal of Psychiatry*, 198, 11–16.

Barnes TR (1989). A rating scale for drug-induced akathisia. *British Journal of Psychiatry*, 154, 672–6.

Barnes TRE *et al.* (2009). Antipsychotic long-acting injections: Prescribing practice in the UK. *British Journal of Psychiatry*, 195, s37–42.

Barr B *et al.* (2012). Suicides associated with the 2008–10 economic recession in England: time trend analysis. *British Medical Journal*, 345, e5142.

Barraclough B and Harris EC (2002). Suicide preceded by murder: the epidemiology of homicide–suicide in England and Wales 1988–92. *Psychological Medicine*, 32, 577–84.

Barraclough BM and Shea M (1970). Suicide and Samaritan clients. *Lancet*, ii, 868–70.

Barraclough BM and Shepherd DM (1976). Public interest: private grief. *British Journal of Psychiatry*, 126, 109–13.

Barry G (2014). Integrating the roles of long and small noncoding RNAs in brain function and disease. *Molecular Psychiatry*, 19, 410–16.

Barry H *et al.* (2015). Anti-N-methyl-D-aspartate receptor encephalitis: review of clinical presentation, diagnosis and treatment. *BJPsych Bulletin*, 39, 19–23.

Barth J *et al.* (2013). The current prevalence of child sexual abuse worldwide: a systematic review and meta-analysis. *International Journal of Public Health*, 58, 469–83.

Bartram DJ and Baldwin DS (2010). Veterinary surgeons and suicide: a structured review of possible influences on increased risk. *Veterinary Record*, 166, 388–97.

Baruk H (1959). Delusions of passion. In: SR Hirsch and M Shepherd (eds.) *Themes and Variations in European Psychiatry*. Wright, Bristol. pp. 375–84.

Bass C and Halligan P (2014). Factitious disorders and malingering: challenges for clinical assessment and management. *Lancet*, 383, 1422–32.

Bass C and Jones D (2011). Psychopathology of perpetrators of fabricated or induced illness in children: case series. *British Journal of Psychiatry*, 199, 113–18.

Basson R and Schultz WW (2007). Sexual dysfunction 1: Sexual sequelae of general medical disorders. *Lancet*, 369, 409–24.

Bateman A and Fonagy P (2008). Eight-year follow-up of patients treated for borderline personality disorder: mentalization-based treatment versus treatment as usual. *American Journal of Psychiatry*, 165, 631–8.

Bateman A and Fonagy P (2009). Randomized controlled trial of outpatient mentalization-based treatment versus structured clinical management for borderline personality disorder. *American Journal of Psychiatry*, 166, 1355–64.

Bateman A and Krawitz R (2013). *Borderline Personality Disorder: An evidence-based guide for generalist mental health professionals*. Oxford University Press, Oxford.

Bateman AW *et al.* (2015). Treatment of personality disorder. *Lancet*, 385, 735–43.

Bateson G *et al.* (1956). Towards a theory of schizophrenia. *Behavioural Science*, 1, 251–64.

Bayley N (2006). Bayley scales of infant and toddler development–third edition. San Antonio, TX: Harcourt assessment. *Journal of Psychoeducational Assessment*, 25(2), 180–90.

Beard JH, Propst RN and Malamud TJ (1987). The Fountain House model of rehabilitation. *Psychosocial Rehabilitation Journal*, 5, 47–53.

Beards S *et al.* (2013). Life events and psychosis: a review and meta-analysis. *Schizophrenia Bulletin*, 39, 740–7.

Beauchamp TL and Childress JF (2013). *Principles of Medical Ethics*. 7th edn. Oxford University Press, Oxford.

Beautler LE and Moos RH (2003). Coping and coping styles in personality and treatment planning: introduction to the special series. *Journal of Clinical Psychology*, 59, 1045–7.

Beautrais AL (2000). Risk factors for suicide and attempted suicide among young people. *Australian and New Zealand Journal of Psychiatry*, 34, 420–36.

Beautrais AL *et al.* (2010). Postcard intervention for repeat self-harm: randomised controlled trial. *British Journal of Psychiatry*, 197, 55–60.

Bebbington PE and Kuipers E (2011). Schizophrenia and psychosocial stresses. In: D Weinberger and PJ Harrison (eds.) *Schizophrenia*, 3rd edn. Wiley-Blackwell, Oxford. pp. 601–24.

Beck AT (1967). *Depression: Clinical, experimental, and theoretical aspects*. Harper and Row, New York.

Beck AT (1976). *Cognitive Therapy and the Emotional Disorders*. International Universities Press, New York.

Beck AT *et al.* (1961). An inventory for measuring depression. *Archives of General Psychiatry*, 4, 561–85.

Beck AT. (2010). Cognitive theory and therapy of anxiety and depression: Convergence with neurobiological findings. *Trends in Cognitive Sciences*, 14, 418–24.

Beck K *et al.* (2014). The practical management of refractory schizophrenia—the Maudsley Treatment Review and Assessment Team service approach. *Acta Psychiatrica Scandinavica*, 130, 427–38.

Beckley JT and Woodward JJ (2013). Volatile solvents as drugs of abuse: focus on the cortico-mesolimbic circuitry. *Neuropsychopharmacology*, 38, 2555–67.

Beckwith H *et al.* (2014). Personality disorder prevalence in psychiatric outpatients: A systematic literature review. *Personality and Mental Health*, 8, 91–101.

Beech AR *et al.* (2016). Paraphilias in the DSM-5. *Annual Review of Clinical Psychology*, 12, 383–406.

Beekman AT *et al.* (2002). The natural history of late-life depression: a 6-year prospective study in the community. *Archives of General Psychiatry*, 59, 605–11.

Beekman ATFC, Copeland JRM and Prince M (1999). Review of community prevalence of depression in later life. *British Journal of Psychiatry*, 174, 307–11.

Bell V, Halligan PW and Ellis HD (2006). Diagnosing delusions: a review of inter-rater reliability. *Schizophrenia Research*, 86, 76–9.

Belsky J *et al.* (2007). Are there long-term effects of early child care? *Child Development*, 78, 681–701.

Benbow SM and Waite J (2013). Non-cognitive adverse effects of ECT. In: J Waite, A Eaton (eds.) *The ECT Handbook*. RCPsych Publications, London. pp. 71–5.

Bendtsen L (2015). Treatment guidelines: implications for community-based headache treatment. *International Journal of Clinical Practice*, **69**, 13–16.

Bennett DH (1983). The historical development of rehabilitation services. In: FN Watts and DH Bennett (eds.) *The Theory and Practice of Rehabilitation*. John Wiley & Sons, Chichester.

Bennett S *et al.* (2015). Psychological interventions for mental health disorders in children with chronic physical illness: A systematic review. *Archives of Disease in Childhood*, **100**, 308–16.

Bennewith O *et al.* (2007). Effect of barriers on the Clifton suspension bridge, England, on local patterns of suicide: implications for prevention. *British Journal of Psychiatry*, **190**, 266–7.

Bensing JM and Verhaak PFM (2006). Somatisation: a joint responsibility of doctor and patient. *Lancet*, **367**, 452–4.

Benyon S *et al.* (2009). Pharmacological interventions for the prevention of relapse in bipolar disorder: a systematic review of controlled trials. *Journal of Psychopharmacology*, **23**, 574–91.

Berelowicz M and Tarnopolsky A (1993). Borderline personality disorder. In: P Tyrer and G Stein (eds.) *Personality Disorder Reviewed*. Gaskell, London. pp. 90–112.

Bergen H *et al.* (2010). Epidemiology and trends in non-fatal self-harm in three centres in England: 2000–2007. *British Journal of Psychiatry*, **197**, 493–8.

Bergink V *et al.* (2015). Treatment of psychosis and mania in the postpartum period. *American Journal of Psychiatry*, **172**, 115–23.

Berlim MT *et al.* (2014). Effectiveness and acceptability of deep brain stimulation (DBS) of the subgenual cingulate cortex for treatment resistant depression: a systematic review and meta-analysis of randomized trials. *Journal of Affective Disorders*, **159**, 31–8.

Berlin I (1958). *Two Concepts of Liberty*. Clarendon Press, Oxford.

Berman K and Brodaty H (2006). Psychosocial effects of age-related macular degeneration. *International Psychogeriatrics*, 18, 415–28.

Bernard S and Turk J (2009). *Developing Mental Health Services for Children and Adolescents with Learning Disabilities: a toolkit for clinicians*. Royal College of Psychiatrists, London.

Berrios GE (1992). Phenomenology, psychopathology and Jaspers: a conceptual history. *History of Psychiatry*, **3**, 303–27.

Berrios GE and Kennedy N (2002). Erotomania: a conceptual history. *History of Psychiatry*, **13**, 381–400.

Berry SM *et al.* (2013). A patient-level meta-analysis of studies evaluating vagus nerve stimulation therapy for treatment-resistant depression. *Medical Devices* (Auckland, NZ), **6**, 17.

Berson RJ (1983). Capgras' syndrome. *American Journal of Psychiatry*, **140**, 969–78.

Bienvenu OJ, Davydow DS and Kendler KS (2011). Psychiatric 'diseases' versus behavioral disorders and degree of genetic influence. *Psychological Medicine*, **41**, 33–40.

Biesecker LG and Green RC (2014). Diagnostic clinical genome and exome sequencing. *New England Journal of Medicine*, **370**, 2418–25.

Billiard M (2009). Excessive sleepiness. In: Gelder MG, Andreasen NC, Lopez-Ibor JJJr and Geddes JR (eds.), *New Oxford Textbook of Psychiatry*, 2nd edn. Oxford University Press, Oxford. pp. 938–43.

Binet A (1877). Le fétichisme dans l'amour. *Revue Philosophique*, **24**, 143.

Bion WR (1961). *Experiences in Groups*. Tavistock Publications, London.

Birchwood M, Todd P and Jackson C (1998). Early intervention in psychosis. The critical period hypothesis. *British Journal of Psychiatry Supplement*, **172**, 53–9.

Bittles A (2009). The biology of ageing. In: Gelder MG, Andreasen NC, Lopez-Ibor JJJr and Geddes JR (eds.) *New Oxford Textbook of Psychiatry*, Oxford University Press, Oxford. pp. 1507–11.

Black D and Trickey D (2009). The effects of bereavement in childhood. In: MG Gelder, NC Andreasen, JJ Lopez-IborJr and JR Geddes (eds.) *New Oxford Textbook of Psychiatry*. Oxford University Press, Oxford. pp. 1758–60.

Blackmore ER *et al.* (2013). Reproductive outcomes and risk of subsequent illness in women diagnosed with postpartum psychosis. *Bipolar Disorders*, **15**, 394–404.

Blackmore MA *et al.* (2009). Social anxiety disorder and specific phobias. In: MG Gelder, NC Andreasen, JJ Lopez-IborJr and JR Geddes (eds.) *New Oxford Textbook of Psychiatry*. Oxford University Press, Oxford. pp. 739–50.

Blair RJR (2003). Neurobiological basis of psychopathy. *British Journal of Psychiatry*, **182**, 5–7.

Blair RJR *et al.* (2014). Conduct disorder and callous–unemotional traits in youth. *New England Journal of Medicine*, **371**, 2207–16.

Blanco C *et al.* (2009). Interpersonal psychotherapy for depression and other disorders. In: Gelder MG, López-Ibor JJJr and Andreasen NC (eds.) *New Oxford Textbook of Psychiatry*. Oxford University Press, Oxford. pp. 1318–26.

Blashfield RK *et al.* (2014). The cycle of classification: DSM-I through DSM-5. *Annual Review of Clinical Psychology*, **10**, 25–51.

Blennow K *et al.* (2012). The neuropathology and neurobiology of traumatic brain injury. *Neuron*, **76**, 886–99.

Blessed G, Tomlinson BE and Roth M (1968). The association between quantitative measures of dementia and of senile change in the cerebral grey matter of elderly subjects. *British Journal of Psychiatry*, **114**, 797–811.

Bleuler E (1906). *Affektivität, Suggestibilität, und Paranoia*. Halle, Marhold.

Bleuler E (1911). *Dementia Praecox or the Group of Schizophrenias*. International University, New York (English edition published in 1950).

Bleuler M (1974). The long-term course of the schizophrenic psychoses. *Psychological Medicine*, **4**, 244–54.

Bloch MH *et al.* (2010). Meta-analysis of the dose–response relationship of SSRI in obsessive-compulsive disorder. *Molecular Psychiatry*, **15**, 850–5.

Bloch S (2006). *An Introduction to the Psychotherapies*, 4th edn. Oxford University Press, Oxford.

Bloch S and Harari E (2009). Family therapy in the adult psychiatric setting. From Psychotherapy with couples. In: MG Gelder, Andreasen NC, López-Ibor JJJr, and Geddes JR (eds.) *The New Oxford Textbook of Psychiatry*. Oxford University Press, Oxford. pp. 1380–91.

Blomstrom A *et al.* (2016). Associations between maternal infection during pregnancy, childhood infections, and the risk of subsequent psychotic disorder. A Swedish cohort study of nearly 2 million individuals. *Schizophrenia Bulletin*, **42**, 125–33.

Bloomfield PS et al. (2016). Microglial activity in people at ultra high risk of psychosis and in schizophrenia: an [11C] PBR28 PET brain imaging study. *American Journal of Psychiatry*, **173**, 44–52.

Blum N et al. (2008). Systems Training for Emotional Predictability and Problem Solving (STEPPS) for outpatients with borderline personality disorder: a randomized controlled trial and 1-year follow-up. *American Journal of Psychiatry*, **165**, 468–78.

Bockting CL et al. (2015). A lifetime approach to major depressive disorder: The contributions of psychological interventions in preventing relapse and recurrence. *Clinical Psychological Review*, **41**, 16–26.

Boeve BF et al. (2013). Clinicopathologic correlations in 172 cases of rapid eye movement sleep behavior disorder with or without a coexisting neurologic disorder. *Sleep Medicine*, **14**, 754–62.

Boland RJ, Goldstein MG and Haltzman SD (2000). Psychiatric management of behavioural syndromes in intensive care units. In: A Stoudemier, BS Fogel and DB Greenberg (eds.). *Psychiatric Care of the Medical Patient*. Oxford University Press, New York. pp. 299–314.

Bolea-Alamañac B et al. (2014). Evidence-based guidelines for the pharmacological management of attention deficit hyperactivity disorder: Update on recommendations from the British Association for Psychopharmacology. *Journal of Psychopharmacology*, **28**, 179–203.

Bond GR et al. (1997). An update on supported on the job employment for people with severe mental illness. *Psychiatric Services*, **48**, 335–46.

Bond GR, Drake RE and Becker DR (2008). An update on randomized controlled trials of evidence-based supported employment. *Psychiatry Rehabilitation Journal*, **31**, 280–90.

Bondy B et al. (2006). Genetics of suicide. *Molecular Psychiatry*, **11**, 336–51.

Bonsack C and Borgeat F (2005). Perceived coercion and need for hospitalization related to psychiatric admission. *International Journal of Law and Psychiatry*, **28**, 342–7.

Boorsma M et al. (2012). The prevalence, incidence and risk factors for delirium in Dutch nursing homes and residential care homes. *International Journal of Geriatric Psychiatry*, **27**, 709–15.

Bora E, Pantelis C (2013). Theory of mind impairments in first-episode psychosis, individuals at ultra-high risk for psychosis and in first-degree relatives of schizophrenia: systematic review and meta-analysis. *Schizophrenia Research*, **144**, 31–6.

Bornovalova MA et al. (2014). Understanding the relative contributions of direct environmental effects and passive genotype-environment correlations in the association between familial risk factors and child disruptive behavior disorders. *Psychological Medicine*, **44**, 831–44.

Borum R et al. (2005). Structured assessment of violence risk in youth. In T Grisso, G Vincent, D Seagrave (eds.), *Mental Health Screening and Assessment in Juvenile Justice*, 311–23. Guilford Press, New York,

Bosanac P, Patton GC and Castle DJ (2009). Early intervention in psychotic disorders: faith before facts? *Psychological Medicine*, **40**, 353–8.

Bostic J and Martin A (2009). Assessment in child and adolescent psychiatry. In MG Gelder, NC Andreasen, JJ Lopez-Ibor, JR Geddes (eds.) *The New Oxford Textbook of Psychiatry*, 2nd edn. Oxford University Press, Oxford. pp. 1600–6.

Bouras N and Holt G (2009). The planning and provision of psychiatric services for adults with learning disability. In: MG Gelder, NC Andreasen, JJ López-IborJr and JR Geddes (eds.) *The New Oxford Textbook of Psychiatry*, 2nd edn. Oxford University Press, Oxford. pp. 1887–92.

Bourque F et al. (2011). A meta-analysis of the risk for psychotic disorders among first- and second-generation immigrants. *Psychological Medicine*, **41**, 897–910.

Bowden CL et al. (1994). Efficacy of divalproex vs lithium and placebo in the treatment of mania. *Journal of the American Medical Association*, **271**, 918–24.

Bowden CL, Calabrese JR and McElroy SL (2000). A randomized, placebo-controlled 12-month trial of divalproex and lithium in treatment of outpatients with bipolar I disorder. *Archives of General Psychiatry*, **57**, 481–9.

Bowden CL et al. (2003). A placebo controlled 18-month trial of lamotrigine and lithium maintenance treatment in recently manic or hypomanic patients with bipolar 1 disorder. *Archives of General Psychiatry*, **60**, 392–400.

Bower P, Rowland N and Hardy R (2003). The clinical effectiveness of counselling in primary care: a systematic review and meta-analysis. *Psychological Medicine*, **33**, 203–15.

Bowlby J (1944). Forty-Four Juvenile Thieves: Their characters and home-life. International Journal of Psychoanalysis, **25**, 19–53.

Bowlby J (1951). *Maternal Care and Maternal Health*. World Health Organization, Geneva.

Bowlby J (1980). *Attachment and Loss*. Basic Books, New York.

Braak H and Braak E (1991). Neuropathological stageing of Alzheimer-related changes. *Acta Neuropathologica*, **82**, 239–59.

Braak H and Del Tredici K (2015). The preclinical phase of the pathological process underlying sporadic Alzheimer's disease. *Brain*, **138**, 2814–33.

Braam W et al. (2009). Exogenous melatonin for sleep problems in individuals with intellectual disability: a meta-analysis. *Developmental Medicine and Child Neurology*, **51**, 340–9.

Bracken P et al. (2012). Psychiatry beyond the current paradigm. *The British Journal of Psychiatry*, **201**, 430–4.

Bradford JM. (2014). Sexual Deviation: Assessment and Treatment. An Issue of *Psychiatric Clinics of North America* (Vol. 37). Elsevier Health Sciences, Amsterdam.

Braid J (1843). *Neurohypnology: or the rationale of nervous sleep, considered in relation with animal magnetism*. Churchill, London.

Brakoulias V et al. (2015). A meta-analysis of the response of pathological hoarding to pharmacotherapy. *Psychiatry Research*, **229**, 272–6.

Bramble D (2011). Psychopharmacology in children with intellectual disability. *Advances in Psychiatric Treatment*, **17**, 32–40.

Bramon E et al. (2004). Meta-analysis of the P.300 and P.50 waveforms in schizophrenia. *Schizophrenia Research*, **70**, 315–29.

Bramon E et al. (2005). Is the P300 wave an endophenotype for schizophrenia? A meta-analysis and a family study. *Neuroimage*, **27**, 960–8.

Brandon S et al. (1985). Leicester ECT trial: results in schizophrenia. *British Journal of Psychiatry*, **146**, 177–83.

Brandt R (2009). The mental health of people living with HIV/AIDS in Africa: a systematic review. *African Journal of AIDS Research*, **8**, 123–33.

Branney P and White A (2008). Big boys don't cry: depression and men. *Advances in Psychiatric Treatment, 14*, 256–62.

Bras J, Guerreiro R and Hardy J (2012). Use of next-generation sequencing and other whole-genome strategies to dissect neurological disease. *Nature Reviews Neuroscience, 13*, 453–64.

Brazier J (2010). Is the EQ-5D fit for purpose in mental health? *British Journal of Psychiatry, 197*, 348–9.

Brent D and Maalouf F (2015). Depressive disorders in childhood and adolescence. In: A. Thapar *et al.* (eds). *Rutter's Child and Adolescent Psychiatry*, John Wiley & Sons, Chichester, pp. 874–92.

Brent DA *et al.* (2002). Familial pathways to early-onset suicide attempt: risk for suicidal behavior in offspring of mood-disordered suicide attempters. *Archives of General Psychiatry, 59*, 801–7.

Breslin R and Evans H (2004). *Key Child Protection Statistics. Child homicides and deaths*. www.nspcc.org.uk/inform/Statistics/KeyCPstats/4.asp

Brewin CR (2009). Recovered memories and false memories. In: MG Gelder, NC Andreasen, JJ Lopez-Ibor and JR Geddes (eds.) *New Oxford Textbook of Psychiatry*. Oxford University Press, Oxford. pp. 713–16.

Brickell C and Munir K (2008). Grief and its complications in individuals with intellectual disability. *Harvard Review of Psychiatry, 16*, 1–12.

Bridge JA *et al.* (2006). Adolescent suicide and suicidal behavior. *Journal of Child Psychology and Psychiatry, 47*, 372–94.

Bridge JA *et al.* (2007). Clinical response and risk for reported suicidal ideation and suicide attempts in paediatric antidepressant treatment: a meta-analysis of randomized controlled trials. *Journal of the American Medical Association, 297*, 1683–96.

British Medical Association (2013). *Drugs of Dependence: The role of medical professionals*. BMA Board of Science.

Britten N, Riley R and Morgan M (2010). Resisting psychotropic medicines: a synthesis of qualitative studies of medicine-taking. *Advances in PsychiatricTreatment, 16*, 207–18.

Broadhead J and Jacoby RJ (1990). Mania in old age: a first prospective study. *International Journal of Geriatric Psychiatry, 5*, 215–22.

Brockington I (2009). Obstetric and gynaecological conditions associated with psychiatric disorder. In: MG Gelder, NC Andreasen, JJ López-IborJr and JR Geddes (eds.). *The New Oxford Textbook of Psychiatry*. Oxford University Press, Oxford. pp. 1114–27.

Broen A *et al.* (2005). The course of mental health after miscarriage and induced abortion: a longitudinal, five-year follow-up study. *BMC Medicine, 3*, 18.

Brown AS and Derkits EJ (2010). Prenatal infection and schizophrenia. A review of epidemiologic and translational studies. *American Journal of Psychiatry, 167*, 261–80.

Brown AS and Susser ES (2008). Prenatal nutritional deficiency and risk of adult schizophrenia. *Schizophrenia Bulletin, 34*, 1054–63.

Brown C and Lloyd K (2001). Qualitative methods in psychiatric research. *Advances in Psychiatric Treatment, 7*, 350–6.

Brown GW (2009). Medical sociology and issues of aetiology. In: MG Gelder, NC Andreasen, JJ Lopez-Ibor, JR Geddes (eds). *New Oxford Textbook of Psychiatry*, OUP, Oxford, pp. 268–75.

Brown GW and Birley JL (1968). Crises and life changes and the onset of schizophrenia. *Journal of Health and Social Behavior, 9*, 203–14.

Brown GW and Harris TO (1978). *Social Origins of Depression*. Tavistock, London.

Brown GW and Harris TO (1993). Aetiology of anxiety and depressive disorders in an inner-city population. 1. Early adversity. *Psychological Medicine, 23*, 143–54.

Brown GW *et al.* (1962). Influence of family life on the cause of schizophrenic illness. *British Journal of Preventive and Social Medicine, 16*, 55–68.

Brown J (2015). The use and misuse of short cognitive tests in the diagnosis of dementia. *Journal of Neurology, Neurosurgery and Psychiatry, 86*, 680–5.

Brown M and Barraclough B (1997). Epidemiology of suicide pacts in England and Wales, 1988–92. *British Medical Journal, 315*, 286–7.

Brown RJ (2002). The cognitive psychology of dissociative states. *Neuropsychiatry, 7*, 221–35.

Bruch H (1974). *Eating Disorders: Anorexia nervosa and the person within*. Routledge & Kegan Paul, London.

Brunelle S *et al.* (2013). Late-onset schizophrenia. In: T Dening, A Thomas (eds). *Oxford Textbook of Old Age Psychiatry*, 2nd edn. Oxford University Press, Oxford.

Brunoni AR *et al.* (2013). The sertraline vs electrical current therapy for treating depression clinical study: results from a factorial, randomized, controlled trial. *JAMA Psychiatry, 70*, 383–91.

Bryant-Waugh R, Markham L, Kreipe RE and Walsh BT (2010). Feeding and eating disorders in childhood. *International Journal of Eating Disorders, 43*(2), 98–111.

Bryant-Waugh R, Watkins B, Thapar A, Pine DS, Leckman JF, Scott S, Snowling MJ and Taylor E (2015). Feeding and eating disorders. *Rutter's Child and Adolescent Psychiatry*, 1016–34.

Bryant RA *et al.* (2010). The psychiatric sequelae of traumatic injury. *American Journal of Psychiatry, 167*, 312–20.

Buchanan A (2008). Risk of violence by psychiatric patients: beyond the 'actuarial versus clinical' assessment debate. *Psychiatric Services, 59*, 184–90.

Buckley PF *et al.* (2009). Psychiatric comorbidities and schizophrenia. *Schizophrenia Bulletin, 35*, 383–402.

Bulik-Sullivan C *et al.* (2015). An atlas of genetic correlations across human diseases and traits. *Nature Genetics, 47*, 1236–41.

Bundy H, Stahl D and MacCabe JH (2011). A systematic review and meta-analysis of the fertility of patients with schizophrenia and their unaffected relatives. *Acta Psychiatrica Scandinavica, 123*, 98–106.

Bunevicius R and Prange AJ (2010). Thyroid disease and mental disorders: cause and effect or comorbidity. *Current Opinion in Psychiatry, 23*, 363–8.

Burleigh M (2000). Extinguishing the ideas of yesterday: eugenics and euthanasia. In *The Third Reich. A new history*. Macmillan, London, pp. 343–81.

Burmeister M, McInnis MG and Zollner S (2008) Psychiatric genetics: progress amid controversy. *Nature Reviews Genetics* 9: 527–40.

Burns A and Illiffe S (2009). Dementia. *British Medical Journal, 338*, b75.

Burns A, Gallagley A and Byrne J (2004). Delirium. *Journal of Neurology, Neurosurgery and Psychiatry, 75*, 362–7.

Burns T (1998). Not just bricks and mortar: Report of the Royal College of Psychiatrists Working Party on the size, staffing, structure, sitting, and security of new acute adult psychiatric in-patient units. *Psychiatric Bulletin*, **22**, 465–6.

Burns T (2006). *Psychiatry: A Very Short Introduction*. Oxford University Press, Oxford.

Burns T (2009). Part 7: Planning and providing mental health services for a community. In: Gelder MG, Andreason NC, Lopez-Ibor JJJr and Geddes JR (eds.) *New Oxford Textbook of Psychiatry*. Oxford University Press, Oxford.

Burns T (2010). The dog that failed to bark. *The Psychiatrist*, **34**, 361–3.

Burns T (2013). *Our Necessary Shadow*. Allen Lane, London.

Burns T (2014). Community psychiatry's achievements. *Epidemiology and Psychiatric Sciences*, **23**, 337–44.

Burns T and Bale R (1997). Establishing a mental health liaison attachment with primary care. *Advances in Psychiatric Treatment*, **3**, 219–24.

Burns T and Burns-Lundgren E (2015). *Very Short Introduction to Psychotherapy*. Oxford University Press, Oxford.

Burns T and Firn M (due 2016). *Assertive Outreach in Community Mental Health*, 2nd edn. retitled.

Burns T, Rugkåsa J, Molodynski A, Dawson J, Yeeles K, Vazquez-Montes M, Voysey M, Sinclair J and Priebe S (2013) Community treatment orders for patients with psychosis (OCTET): a randomised controlled trial. *The Lancet*, **381**, 1627–33.

Burns T *et al.* (2002). International differences in home treatment for mental health problems. Results of a systematic review. *British Journal of Psychiatry*, **181**, 375–82.

Burns T *et al.* (2007a). The effectiveness of supported employment for people with severe mental illness: a randomised controlled trial. *The Lancet*, **370**, 1146–52.

Burns T *et al.* (2007b). Use of intensive case management to reduce time in hospital in people with severe mental illness: systematic review and meta-regression. *British Medical Journal*, **335**, 336.

Burns T *et al.* (2011). Pressures to adhere to treatment ('leverage') in English mental healthcare. *British Journal of Psychiatry*, **199**, 145–50.

Burti L (2001). Italian psychiatric reform 20 plus years after. *Acta Psychiatrica Scandinavica*, **104**, 41–6.

Burton A *et al.* (2010). Do financial incentives increase treatment adherence in people with severe mental illness? A systematic review. *Epidemiology and Psychiatric Sciences*, **19**, 233–42.

Bushnell M *et al.* (2013). Cognitive and emotional control of pain and its disruption in chronic pain. *Nature Reviews Neuroscience*, **14**, 502–11

Butler RJ (2008). Wetting and soiling. In: M Rutter *et al.* (eds.) *Child and Adolescent Psychiatry*, 5th edn, Blackwell, Oxford. pp. 916–29.

Butler RW and Braff DL (1991). Delusions: a review and integration. *Schizophrenia Bulletin*, **17**, 633–47.

Byrd AL and Manuck SB (2014). MAOA, childhood maltreatment, and antisocial behavior: meta-analysis of a gene–environment interaction. *Biological Psychiatry*, **75**, 9–17.

Cade JF (1949). Lithium salts in the treatment of psychotic excitement. *Medical Journal of Australia*, **2**, 349–52.

Cadoret RJ (1978). Psychopathology in adopted-away offspring of biologic parents with antisocial behaviour. *Archives of General Psychiatry*, **35**, 176–84.

Cain CK *et al.* (2013). Neurobiology of fear and anxiety: Contributions of animal models to current understanding. In: DS Charney, JD Buxbaum, P Sklaar, EJ Nestler (eds). *Neurobiology of Mental Illness*. Oxford University Press, Oxford, pp. 549–66.

Callicott JH *et al.* (2003). Complexity of prefrontal cortical dysfunction in schizophrenia: more than up or down. *American Journal of Psychiatry*, **160**, 2209–15.

Campbell EJ, Scadding JG and Roberts RS (1979). The concept of disease. *British Medical Journal*, **ii**, 757–62.

Canetta S *et al.* (2014). Elevated maternal C-reactive protein and increased risk of schizophrenia in a national birth cohort. *American Journal of Psychiatry*, **171**, 960–8.

Cannon M, Jones PB and Murray RM (2002). Obstetric complications and schizophrenia. Historical and meta-analytic review. *American Journal of Psychiatry*, **159**, 1080–92.

Cannon M *et al.* (2014). Priming the brain for psychosis: maternal inflammation during fetal development and the risk of later psychiatric disorder. *American Journal of Psychiatry*, **171**, 901–5.

Cannon TD (2015). How schizophrenia develops: cognitive and brain mechanisms underlying onset of psychosis. *Trends in Cognitive Sciences*, **19**, 744–56.

Cape J *et al.* (2010). Brief psychological therapies for anxiety and depression in primary care: meta-analysis and meta-regression. *BMC Medicine*, **8**, 1–11.

Caplan G (1961). *An Approach to Community Mental Health*. Tavistock Publications, London.

Caplan G (1964). *Principles of Preventive Psychiatry*. Basic Books, New York.

Cardno A, Owen MJ (2014). Genetic relationships between schizophrenia, bipolar disorder, and schizoaffective disorder. *Schizophrenia Bulletin*, **40**, 504–15.

Cardno AG and Gottesman II (2000). Twin studies of schizophrenia: from bow-and-arrow concordances to Star Wars Mx and functional genomics. *American Journal of Medical Genetics (Seminars in Medical Genetics)*, **97**, 12–17.

Carhart-Harris RL *et al.* (2016). The paradoxical psychological effects of lysergic acid diethylamide (LSD). *Psychological Medicine*, **46**, 1379–90.

Carota A and Calabrese P (2014). Hysteria around the world. *Frontiers of Neurology and Neuroscience*, **35**, 169–80.

Carr A (1991). Milan systemic family therapy: a review of ten empirical investigations. *Journal of Family Therapy*, **13**, 237–63.

Carr A *et al.* (2016). *The Handbook of Intellectual Disability and Clinical Psychology Practice*. Second Edition Routledge, Abingdon.

Carroll A (2009). Are you looking at me? Understanding and managing paranoid personality disorder. *Advances in Psychiatric Treatment*, **15**, 40–8.

Carter GL *et al.* (2007). Postcards from the edge: 24-month outcomes of a randomised controlled trial for hospital-treated self-poisoning. *British Journal of Psychiatry*, **191**, 548–53.

Caserta MT *et al.* (2009). Normal brain aging: clinical, immunological, neuropsychological, and neuroimaging features. *International Review of Neurobiology*, **84**, 1–19.

Casey P (2009). Adjustment disorder: epidemiology, diagnosis and treatment. *CNS Drugs*, (11) **23**, 927–38.

Cashman MD *et al.* (2016). Irritable bowel syndrome: a clinical review. *Current Rheumatology Reviews*, **12**, 13–26.

Caspi A and Shiner R (2008). Temperament and personality. In: M Rutter *et al.* (eds.) *Child and Adolescent Psychiatry*, 5th edn. Blackwell, Oxford. pp. 182–98.

Caspi A *et al.* (2003). Influence of life stress on depression: moderation by a polymorphism in the 5-HTT gene. *Science*, **301**, 386–9.

Caspi A *et al.* (2010). Genetic sensitivity to the environment: the case of the serotonin transporter gene and its implications for studying complex diseases and traits. *Focus*, **8**, 398–416.

Castle D (2012). The truth, and nothing but the truth, about early intervention in psychosis. *Australian and New Zealand Journal of Psychiatry*, **46**, 10–13.

Castle D and Bosanac P (2012). Depression and schizophrenia. *Advances in Psychiatric Treatment*, **18**, 280–8.

Castle D *et al.* (1991). The incidence of operationally defined schizophrenia in Camberwell, 1965–84. *British Journal of Psychiatry*, **159**, 790–4.

Castle DJ *et al.* (1993). Does social deprivation during gestation and early life predispose to later schizophrenia? *Social Psychiatry and Psychiatric Epidemiology*, **28**, 1–4.

Cattell RB (1963). *The Sixteen Personality Factor Questionnaire.* Institute for Personality and Ability Testing, Chicago, IL.

Catts VS *et al.* (2008). Cancer incidence in patients with schizophrenia and their first-degree relatives—a meta-analysis. *Acta Psychiatrica Scandinavica*, **117**, 323–36.

Catty J, Goddard K and Burns T (2005). Social services day care and health services day care in mental health: do they differ? *International Journal of Psychoanalysis*, **51**, 151–61.

Cavanagh JTO *et al.* (2003). Psychological autopsy studies of suicide: a systematic review. *Psychological Medicine*, **33**, 395–405.

Cermolacce M, Sass L and Parnas J (2010). What is bizarre in bizarre delusions? A critical review. *Schizophrenia Bulletin*, **36**, 667–79.

Chamberlain AS (1966). Early mental hospitals in Spain. *American Journal of Psychiatry*, **123**, 143–9.

Chan RCK *et al.* (2010). Neurological soft signs in schizophrenia. A meta-analysis. *Schizophrenia Bulletin*, **36**, 1089–104.

Chanen AM *et al.* (2008). Early intervention for adolescents with borderline personality disorder using cognitive analytic therapy: randomised controlled trial. *British Journal of Psychiatry*, **193**, 477–84.

Charlton J *et al.* (1993). Suicide deaths in England and Wales: trends in factors associated with suicide deaths. *Population Trends*, **71**, 34–42.

Charman T, Hood J and Howlin P (2008). Psychological assessment in the clinical context. In: M Rutter *et al.* (eds.) *Child and Adolescent Psychiatry*, 5th edn. Blackwell, Oxford. pp. 299–316.

Charman T *et al.* (2010). Defining the cognitive phenotype of autism. *Brain Research*, **1380**, 10–21.

Chaste P and Leboyer M (2012). Autism risk factors: Genes, environment, and gene–environment interactions. *Dialogues in Clinical Neuroscience*, **14**, 281–92.

Cheeta S *et al.* (2004). Antidepressant-related deaths and antidepressant prescriptions in England and Wales. *British Journal of Psychiatry*, **184**, 41–7.

Chen J *et al.* (2014). Childhood sexual abuse and the development of recurrent major depression in Chinese women. *PloS One*, **9**, e87569.

Cheng ATA and Lee CS (2000). Suicide in Asia and the Far East. In: K Hawton and K van Heeringen (eds.) *The International Handbook of Suicide and Attempted Suicide*. John Wiley & Sons, Chichester. pp. 29–48.

Chibanda D *et al.* (2015). Psychological interventions for common mental disorders for people living with HIV in low-and middle-income countries: systematic review. *Tropical Medicine and International Health*, **20**, 830–9.

Chick J *et al.* (1988). Advice versus extended treatment for alcoholism: a controlled study. *British Journal of Addiction*, **83**, 159–70.

Chisolm MS and Payne JL (2016). Management of psychotropic drugs during pregnancy. *British Medical Journal*, **352**, h5918.

Chossegros L *et al.* (2011). Predictive factors of chronic post-traumatic stress disorder 6 months after a road traffic accident. *Accident Analysis and Prevention*, **43**, 471–7.

Chouinard G *et al.* (1980). Extrapyramidal symptom rating scale. *Canadian Journal of Neurological Science*, **7**, 233.

Christensen J *et al.* (2013). Prenatal valproate exposure and risk of autism spectrum disorders and childhood autism. *JAMA*, **309**, 1696–703.

Christmas D *et al.* (2004). Neurosurgery for mental disorder. *Advances in Psychiatric Treatment*, **10**, 189–99.

Christodoulou GN (1991). The delusional misidentification syndromes. *British Journal of Psychiatry*, **14**, 65–9.

Ciompi L (1980). The natural history of schizophrenia in the long term. *British Journal of Psychiatry*, **136**, 413–20.

Cipriani A *et al.* (2009) Comparative efficacy and acceptability of 12 new-generation antidepressants: a multiple-treatments meta-analysis. *The Lancet*, **373**, 746–58.

Cipriani A, Rendell J and Geddes JR (2010). Olanzapine in the long-term treatment of bipolar disorder: a systematic review and meta-analysis. *Journal of Psychopharmacology*, **24**, 1729–38.

Cipriani A *et al.* (2011). Comparative efficacy and acceptability of antimanic drugs in acute mania: A multiple-treatments meta-analysis. *The Lancet*, **378**, 1306–15.

Cipriani A *et al.* (2013). Lithium in the prevention of suicide in mood disorders: updated systematic review and meta-analysis. *British Medical Journal*, **346**, f3646.

Cipriani A *et al.* (2016). Comparative efficacy and tolerability of antidepressants for major depressive disorder in children and adolescents: a network meta-analysis. *Lancet,* S0140-6736, 30385-3.

Citrome L (2013). A review of the pharmacology, efficacy and tolerability of recently approved and upcoming oral antipsychotics: an evidence-based medicine approach. *CNS Drugs*, **27**, 879–911.

Citrome L (2014). Vortioxetine for major depressive disorder: a systematic review of the efficacy and safety profile for this newly approved antidepressant—what is the number needed to treat, number needed to harm and likelihood to be helped or harmed? *International Journal of Clinical Practice*, **68**, 60–82.

Clancy MJ *et al.* (2014). The prevalence of psychosis in epilepsy: a systematic review and meta-analysis. *BMC Psychiatry*, **14**, 75.

Clark A (2004). Working with grieving adults. *Advances in Psychiatric Treatment*, **10**, 164–70.

Clark D (2011). Implementing NICE guidelines for the psychological treatment of depression and anxiety disorders: the IAPT experience. *International Review of Psychiatry*, **23**, 318–27.

Clark DA, Beck AT (2010). Cognitive theory and therapy of anxiety and depression: convergence with neurobiological findings. *Trends in Cognitive Sciences*, **14**, 418–24.

Clark DA and Beck AT (2011). *Cognitive Therapy of Anxiety Disorders: Science and practice*. Guilford Press, New York, NY.

Clark L and Harrison J (2001). Assessment instruments. In: W Livesley (ed.) *Handbook of Personality Disorders: theory, research, and treatment*. Guilford Press, New York. pp. 277–306.

Clark L, Chamberlain SR and Sahakian BJ (2009). Neurocognitive mechanisms in depression: implications for treatment. *Annual Review of Neuroscience*, **32**, 57–74.

Clarke A and Seymour J (2010). 'At the foot of a very long ladder.' Discussing the end of life with older people and informal care givers. *Journal of Pain and Symptom Management*, **40**, 857–69.

Clarke K *et al.* (2013). Psychosocial interventions for perinatal common mental disorders delivered by providers who are not mental health specialists in low- and middle-income countries: a systematic review and meta-analysis. *PLoS Medicine*, **10**, e1001541.

Clarke S *et al.* (2013). Cognitive analytic therapy for personality disorder: randomised controlled trial. *British Journal of Psychiatry*, **202**, 129–34.

Clarkin JF *et al.* (1999). *Transference-Focused Psychotherapy for Borderline Personality Disorder Patients*. Guilford Press, New York, NY.

Clauw DJ (2014). Fibromyalgia: a clinical review. *Journal of the American Medical Association*, **311**, 1547–55.

Clayton AH *et al.* (2016). Sexual dysfunction due to psychotropic medications. *Psychiatric Clinics of North America*, **39**, 427–63.

Cleare AJ *et al.* (2015). Evidence-based guidelines for treating depressive disorders with antidepressants: A revision of the 2008 British Association for Psychopharmacology guidelines. *Journal of Psychopharmacology*, **29**, 459–525.

Cleckley HM (1964). *The Mask of Sanity: an attempt to clarify issues about the so-called psychopathic personality*, 4th edn. Mosby, St Louis, MO.

Clinical Psychiatry Committee (1965). Clinical trial of the treatment of depression. *British Medical Journal*, i, 881–6.

Clomipramine Collaborative Study Group (1991). Clomipramine and the treatment of patients with obsessive-compulsive disorder. *Archives of General Psychiatry*, **48**, 730–8.

Cloninger CR (2009). Assessment of personality. In: MG Gelder, NC Andreasen, JJ Lopez-Ibor and JR Geddes (eds.) *The New Oxford Textbook of Psychiatry*, 2nd edn. Oxford University Press, Oxford, pp. 78-84.

Cloninger CR *et al.* (1988). Genetic heterogeneity and the classification of alcoholism. *Advances in Alcohol and Substance Abuse*, 7, 3–16.

Cloninger CR *et al.* (1993). A psychobiological model of temperament and character. *Archives of General Psychiatry*, **50**, 975–90.

Close H *et al.* (2014). Renal failure in lithium-treated bipolar disorder: a retrospective cohort study. *PloS One*, **9**, e90169.

Coccaro F, Lee R and Kavoussi RJ (2010). Aggression, suicidality, and intermittent explosive disorder: serotonergic correlates in personality disorder and healthy control subjects. *Neuropsychopharmacology* **35**, 435–44.

Cochrane AL (1972). *Effectiveness and Efficiency: random reflections on health services*. Nuffield Provincial Hospitals Trust, London.

Cochrane AL (1979). 1931–1971: a critical review with particular reference to the medical profession. In: *Medicines for the Year 2000*. Office of Health Economics, London. pp. 1–11.

Cohen CI *et al.* (2015). New perspectives on schizophrenia in later life: implications for treatment, policy, and research. *Lancet Psychiatry*, **2**, 340–50.

Cohen NJ *et al.* (2015). Adoption. In: A. Thapar *et al.* (eds). *Rutter's Child and Adolescent Psychiatry*. John Wiley & Sons, Chichester, pp. 273–84.

Cohen P *et al.* (2005). The children in the community study of developmental course of personality disorder. *Journal of Personality Disorders* **19**, 466–86.

Cohen SC *et al.* (2013). Clinical assessment of Tourette syndrome and tic disorders. *Neuroscience and Biobehavioral Reviews*, **37**, 997–1007.

Cohen-Woods S *et al.* (2013). The current state of play of the molecular genetics of depression. *Psychological Medicine*, **43**, 673–87.

Coid J and Ullrich S (2010). Antisocial personality disorder is on a continuum with psychopathy. *Comprehensive Psychiatry*, **51**, 426–33.

Coid J *et al.* (2002). Ethnic differences in prisoners. 1: Criminality and psychiatric morbidity. *British Journal of Psychiatry*, **181**, 473–80.

Coid J *et al.* (2006). Prevalence and correlates of personality disorder in Great Britain. *British Journal of Psychiatry*, **188**, 423–31.

Coid J *et al.* (2013). The relationship between delusions and violence: findings from the East London First Episode Psychosis Study. *JAMA Psychiatry*, **70**, 465–71.

Coleman E *et al.* (2012). Standards of care for the health of transsexual, transgender, and gender-nonconforming people, version 7. *International Journal of Transgenderism*, **13**, 165–232.

Collacott R *et al.* (1998). Behaviour phenotype for Down's syndrome. *British Journal of Psychiatry*, **172**, 85–9.

Collin G *et al.* (2016). Connectomics in schizophrenia: from early pioneers to recent brain network findings. *Biological Psychiatry: Cognitive Neuroscience and Neuroimaging*, **1**, 199–208.

Collinge J (2009). Prion disease. In: MG Gelder, NC Andreasen, JJ Lopez-Ibor, JR Geddes (eds.) *New Oxford Textbook of Psychiatry*, 2nd edn. Oxford University Press, Oxford. pp. 351–61.

Collings S and Llewellyn G. (2012). Children of parents with intellectual disability: Facing poor outcomes or faring okay? *Journal of Intellectual and Developmental Disability*, **37**, 65–82.

Collins PY *et al.* (2011). Grand challenges in global mental health. *Nature*, **475**, 27–30.

Collishaw S. (2015). Annual research review: Secular trends in child and adolescent mental health. *Journal of Child Psychology and Psychiatry and Allied Disciplines*, **56**, 370–93.

Collishaw S *et al.* (2004). Time trends in adolescent mental health. *Journal of Child Psychology and Psychiatry*, **45**, 1350–62.

Collishaw S *et al.* (2007). Resilience to adult psychopathology following childhood maltreatment: Evidence from a community sample. *Child Abuse & Neglect*, **31**, 211–29.

Collishaw S *et al.* (2010). Trends in adolescent emotional problems in England: a comparison of two national cohorts twenty years apart. *Journal of Child Psychology and Psychiatry and Allied Disciplines*, **51**, 885–94.

Colom F *et al.* (2009). Group psychoeducation for stabilised bipolar disorders: 5-year outcome of a randomised clinical trial. *British Journal of Psychiatry*, **194**, 260–5.

Conner KR and Duberstein PR (2004). Predisposing and precipitating factors for suicide among alcoholics: empirical review and conceptual integration. *Alcoholism: Clinical and Experimental Research*, **28**, 6S–17S.

Conron KJ *et al.* (2012). Transgender health in Massachusetts: results from a household probability sample of adults. *American Journal of Public Health*, **102**, 118–22.

CONVERGE consortium (2015). Sparse whole-genome sequencing identifies two loci for major depressive disorder. *Nature*, **523**, 588–91.

Cook JM, Gallagher-Thompson D and Hepple J (2005). Psychotherapy with older adults. In: GO Gabbard, JS Beck and J Holmes (eds.) *Oxford Textbook of Psychotherapy*. Oxford University Press, Oxford. pp. 381–92.

Cooper C *et al.* (2011). A systematic review of treatments for refractory depression in older people. *American Journal of Psychiatry*, **168**, 681–8.

Cooper C *et al.* (2013). Treatment for mild cognitive impairment: systematic review. *British Journal of Psychiatry*, **203**, 255–64.

Cooper JE (1979). *Crisis Admission Units and Emergency Psychiatric Services. Public Health in Europe, No. 2*. World Health Organization, Copenhagen.

Cooper JE, Kendell RE and Gurland BJ (1972). *Psychiatric Diagnosis in New York and London*. Oxford University Press, London.

Cooper PJ *et al.* (2002). Impact of a mother—infant intervention in an indigent peri-urban South African context. *British Journal of Psychiatry*, **180**, 76–81.

Cooper PJ *et al.* (2009). Improving quality of mother–infant relationship and infant attachment in socioeconomically deprived community in South Africa: randomised controlled trial. *British Medical Journal*, **338**, b974.

Cooper S and Greene JDW (2005). The clinical assessment of the patient with early dementia. *Journal of Neurology, Neurosurgery and Psychiatry*, **76**, 15–24.

Cooper SA and Smiley E (2009). Prevalence of intellectual disabilities and epidemiology of mental ill-health in adults with intellectual disabilities. In: MG Gelder, NC Andreasen, JJ López-IborJr, and JR Geddes (eds.) *The New Oxford Textbook of Psychiatry*, 2nd edn. Oxford University Press, Oxford. pp. 1825–9.

Cooper SJ *et al.* (2016). BAP guidelines on the management of weight gain, metabolic disturbances and cardiovascular risk associated with psychosis and antipsychotic drug treatment. *Journal of Psychopharmacology*, **30**, 717–48.

Copeland J *et al.* (1999). Depression in Europe. Geographic distribution among older people. *British Journal of Psychiatry*, **174**, 312–21.

Copeland WE *et al.* (2013). Adult psychiatric outcomes of bullying and being bullied by peers in childhood and adolescence. *JAMA Psychiatry*, **70**, 419–26.

Copeland WE *et al.* (2015). Adult functional outcomes of common childhood psychiatric problems: a prospective, longitudinal study. *JAMA Psychiatry*, **72**, 892–9.

Copen CE *et al.* (2016). Sexual behavior, sexual attraction, and sexual orientation among adults aged 18–44 in the United States: Data from the 2011–2013 National Survey of Family Growth. *National Health Statistics Reports*, **88**, 1–14.

Coppus A. (2013). People with intellectual disability: What do we know about adulthood and life expectancy? *Developmental Disabilities Research Reviews*, **18**, 6–16.

Corbett A *et al.* (2012). Assessment and treatment of pain in people with dementia. *Nature Reviews Neurology*, **8**, 264–72.

Cordeiro L *et al.* (2010). Clinical assessment of DSM-IV anxiety disorders in fragile X syndrome: prevalence and characterization. *Journal of Neurodevelopmental Disorders*, **3**, 57.

Correll CU, Leucht S and Kane JM (2014). Lower risk for tardive dyskinesia associated with second-generation antipsychotics: a systematic review of 1-year studies. *American Journal of Psychiatry*, **161**, 414–25.

Coryell W and Young EA (2005). Clinical predictors of suicide in primary major depressive disorder. *Journal of Clinical Psychiatry*, **66**, 412–17.

Costello E *et al.* (1996). The Great Smoky Mountains Study of Youth: functional impairment and serious emotional disturbance. *Archives of General Psychiatry*, **53**, 1137–43.

Costello EJ and Angold A (2009). Epidemiology of psychiatric disorder in childhood In: M Gelder *et al.* (eds.) *New Oxford Textbook of Psychiatry*. Oxford University Press, Oxford. pp. 1594–9.

Costello EJ and Maughan B (2015). Annual research review: Optimal outcomes of child and adolescent mental illness. *Journal of Child Psychology and Psychiatry and Allied Disciplines*, **56**, 324–41.

Couldwell A and Stickley T (2007). The Thorn course: rhetoric and reality. *Journal of Psychiatric and Mental Health Nursing*, **14**, 625–34.

Cousins DA, Butts K and Young A (2009). The role of dopamine in bipolar disorder. *Bipolar Disorders*, **11**, 787–806.

Cousins L and Goodyer IM (2015). Antidepressants and the adolescent brain. *Journal of Psychopharmacology*, **29**, 545–55.

Cowen PJ (2015). Neuroendocrine and neurochemical processes in depression. In: RJ DeRubies, DR Strunk (eds). *The Oxford Handbook of Mood Disorders*. OUP, Oxford.

Cowen PJ and Anderson IM (2015). New approaches to treating resistant depression. *Advances in Psychiatric Treatment*, **21**, 315–23.

Cowen PJ, Ogilvie AD, Gama J (2005). Efficacy, safety and tolerability of duloxetine 60 mg once daily in major depression. *Current Medical Research and Opinion*, **21**(3), 345.

Craddock N (2013). Genome-wide association studies: What a psychiatrist needs to know. *Advances in Psychiatric Treatment*, **19**, 82–8.

Craddock N and Mynors-Wallis L (2014). Psychiatric diagnosis: impersonal, imperfect and important. *British Journal of Psychiatry*, **2**, 93–5.

Craddock N and Sklar P (2013). Genetics of bipolar disorder. *The Lancet*, **381**, 1654–62.

Crammer J (1990). *Asylum History: Buckinghamshire County Pauper Lunatic Asylum—St Johns*. Gaskell, London.

Crawford M and Wessely S (1998). The changing epidemiology of deliberate self-harm—implications for service provision. *Health Trends*, **30**, 66–8.

Crawford MJ et al. (2012). Group art therapy as an adjunctive treatment for people with schizophrenia: multicentre pragmatic randomised trial. *British Medical Journal,* **344,** e846.

Crawford MJ et al. (2012). The prevalence of personality disorder among ethnic minorities: findings from a national household survey. *Personal Mental Health,* **6,** 175–82.

Crow TJ (1985). The two-syndrome concept: origins and current status. *Schizophrenia Bulletin,* **11,** 471–86.

Crow TJ (2002). Handedness, language lateralisation and anatomical asymmetry: relevance of protocadherin XY to hominid speciation and the aetiology of psychosis. Point of view. *British Journal of Psychiatry,* **181,** 295–7.

Crowe RR (1974). An adoption study of antisocial personality. *Archives of General Psychiatry,* **31,** 785–91.

Crowley TJ et al. (2015). Substance-related and addictive disorders. In: A. Thapar et al. (eds). *Rutter's Child and Adolescent Psychiatry.* John Wiley & Sons, Chichester, pp. 931–49.

Cuijpers P et al. (2013). The efficacy of psychotherapy and pharmacotherapy in treating depressive and anxiety disorders: A meta-analysis of direct comparisons. *World Psychiatry,* **12,** 137–48.

Cuijpers P et al. (2014a). Adding psychotherapy to antidepressant medication in depression and anxiety disorders: A meta-analysis. *World Psychiatry,* **13,** 56–67.

Cuijpers P et al. (2014b). Psychological treatment of generalized anxiety disorder: A meta-analysis. *Clinical Psychology Review,* **34,** 130–40.

Cullum S (2013). Management of dementia. In: T Dening, A Thomas (eds). *Oxford Textbook of Old Age Psychiatry,* 2nd edn. Oxford University Press, Oxford.

Cutajar MC et al. (2010). Suicide and fatal drug overdose in child sexual abuse victims: a historical cohort study. *Medical Journal of Australia,* **192,** 184–7.

Cutajar MC et al. (2010). Psychopathology in a large cohort of sexually abused children followed up to 43 years. *Child Abuse & Neglect,* **34,** 813–22.

Cuthbert BN and Insel TR (2013). Toward the future of psychiatric diagnosis: the seven pillars of RDoC. *BMC Medicine,* **11,** 126.

Czajkowski N et al. (2011). The structure of genetic and environmental risk factors for phobias in women. *Psychological Medicine,* **41,** 1987–95.

Da Costa RT, Sardinha A and Nardi AE (2008). Virtual reality exposure in the treatment of fear of flying. *Aviation Space and Environmental Medicine,* **79,** 899–903.

Dager SR et al. (2008). Research applications of magnetic resonance spectroscopy to investigate psychiatric disorders. *Topics in Magnetic Resonance Imaging,* **19,** 81–96.

Danese A et al (2015) Child maltreatment. In: A. Thapar et al. (eds). *Rutter's Child and Adolescent Psychiatry.* John Wiley & Sons, Chichester, pp. 364–75.

Daniels AM et al. (2014). Approaches to enhancing the early detection of autism spectrum disorders: A systematic review of the literature. *Journal of the American Academy of Child & Adolescent Psychiatry,* **53,** 141–52.

Danysz W and Parsons C (2012). Alzheimer's disease, beta-amyloid, glutamate, NMDA receptors and memantine—searching for the connections. *British Journal of Pharmacology,* **167,** 324–52.

Darwish M, Atlantis E, Mohamed-Taysir T (2014). Psychological outcomes after hysterectomy for benign conditions: a systematic review and meta-analysis. *European Journal of Obstetrics & Gynaecology and Reproductive Biology,* **174,** 5–19.

da Silva J et al. (2013). Affective disorders and risk of developing dementia: systematic review. *British Journal of Psychiatry,* **202,** 177–86.

Datta V and Cleare AJ (2009). Recent advances in bipolar disorder pharmacotherapy: focus on bipolar depression and rapid cycling. *Expert Review of Clinical Pharmacology,* **2,** 423–34.

Dauwan M et al. (2016). Exercise improves clinical symptoms, quality of life, global functioning, and depression in schizophrenia: a systematic review and meta-analysis. *Schizophrenia Bulletin,* **42,** 588–99.

David A et al. (1995). Are there neurological and sensory risk factors for schizophrenia? *Schizophrenia Research,* **14,** 247–51.

David AS (2009a). Basic concepts in neuropsychiatry. In: David AS, Fleminger S, Kopelman M et al. (eds.) *Lishman's Organic Psychiatry,* 4th edn. Wiley Blackwell, Oxford. pp. 3–27.

David AS (2009b). Clinical assessment. In: David AS, Fleminger S, Kopelman M et al. (eds.) *Lishman's Organic Psychiatry,* 4th edn. Wiley Blackwell, Oxford. pp. 103–63.

David AS and Kopelman MD (2009). Neuropsychology in relation to psychiatry. In: David AS, Fleminger S, Kopelman M, et al. (eds.) *Lishman's Organic Psychiatry,* 4th edn. Wiley Blackwell, Oxford. pp. 29–102.

David AS et al. (2009) *Lishman's Organic Psychiatry,* 4th edn. Wiley-Blackwell, Oxford.

David AS and Prince M (2005). Psychosis following head injury: a critical review. *Journal of Neurology, Neurosurgery and Psychiatry,* **76**(Suppl.1), 153–60.

Davidson K (2000). *Cognitive Therapy for Personality Disorders. A guide for clinicians.* Butterworth Heinemann, Oxford.

Davies G et al. (2003). A systematic review and meta-analysis of Northern Hemisphere season of birth studies in schizophrenia. *Schizophrenia Bulletin,* **29,** 587–93.

Davies LE and Oliver C. (2014). The purported association between depression, aggression, and self-injury in people with intellectual disability: A critical review of the literature. *American Journal on Intellectual and Developmental Disabilities,* **119,** 452–71.

Davies SJC, Esler M and Nutt DJ (2010). Anxiety—bridging the heart/mind divide. *Journal of Psychopharmacology,* **24,** 633–8.

Davis DHJ et al. (2012). Delirium is a strong risk factor for dementia in the oldest-old: a population-based cohort study. *Brain,* **135,** 2809–16.

Davis DHJ et al. (2017). Association of delirium with cognitive decline in late life: a neuropathologic study of 3 population-based cohort studies. *JAMA Psychiatry,* **74,** 244–51.

Davison K and Bagley CR (1969). Schizophrenia-like psychoses associated with organic disorders of the central nervous system: a review of the literature. In: RN Herrington, (ed). *British Journal of Psychiatry Special Publication No.4, Current Problems in Neuropsychiatry.* Headley, Ashford.

Dawson J (2005). *Community Treatment Orders: International comparisons.* Otago University, Dunedin.

Dawson J and Burns T (2016). Reducing legal barriers to smooth transition between forensic and general mental health care.

In: L Wooton and A Buchanan (eds.) *Care of the Mentally Disordered Offender in the Community*. Oxford University Press, Oxford.

de la Torre-Ubieta L *et al*. (2016). Advancing the understanding of autism disease mechanisms through genetics. *Nature Medicine*, **22**, 345–61.

De la Tourette G (1885). Etude sur une affection nerveuse valuation par l'incoordination motrice accompagnée d'écholalie et de coprolalie. *Archives de Neurologie*, **9**, 19–42.

DeMaso DR *et al*. (2009). Practice parameter for the psychiatric assessment and management of physically ill children and adolescents. *Journal of the American Academy of Child & Adolescent Psychiatry*, **48**, 213–33.

Department of Health (2012). *Suicide Prevention Strategy for England*. Policy Paper, Department of Health, London.

de Wilde EJ (2000). Adolescent suicidal behaviour: a general population perspective. In: K Hawton and K van Heeringen (eds.) *The International Handbook of Suicide and Attempted Suicide*. John Wiley & Sons, Chichester. pp. 249–60.

Dean K *et al*. (2007). Predictors of violent victimization amongst those with psychosis. *Acta Psychiatrica Scandinavica*, **116**, 345–53.

Deary IJ, Johnson W and Houlihan LM (2009). Genetic foundations of human intelligence. *Human Genetics*, **126**, 215–32.

Deb S, Thomas M and Bright C (2001). Mental disorder in adults with intellectual disability: 2. The rate of behaviour disorder among a community-based population aged between 16–64 years. *Journal of Intellectual Disability Research*, **45**, 506–14.

Debast I *et al*. (2014). Personality traits and personality disorders in late middle and old age: do they remain stable? A literature review. *Clinical Gerontologist*, **37**, 253–71.

De Hert M *et al*. (2015). The use of continuous treatment versus placebo or intermittent treatment strategies in stabilized patients with schizophrenia: a systematic review and meta-analysis of randomized controlled trials with first- and second-generation antipsychotics. *CNS Drugs*, **29**, 637–58.

De J and Wand APF (2015). Delirium screening: a systematic review of delirium screening tools in hospitalized patients. *Gerontologist*, **55**, 1079–99.

DeLong MR and Wichmann T (2007). Circuits and circuit disorders of the basal ganglia. *Archives of Neurology*, **64**, 20–4.

Demirkan A *et al*. (2013). Genetic risk profiles for depression and anxiety in adult and elderly cohorts. *Molecular Psychiatry*, **16**, 773–83.

Dempster E *et al*. (2013). Epigenetic studies of schizophrenia: progress, predicaments, and promise for the future. *Schizophrenia Bulletin*, **39**, 11–16.

Dening T (2013). Principles of service provision in old age psychiatry. In: T Dening, A Thomas (eds). *Oxford Textbook of Old Age Psychiatry*, 2nd edn. Oxford University Press, Oxford.

Denollet J *et al*. (2010). A general propensity to psychological distress affects cardiovascular outcomes: evidence from research on the Type D (Distressed) personality profile. *Circulation: Cardiovascular Quality and Outcome*, **3**, 546–57.

Department of Health (1990). *The Care Programme Approach for People with a Mental Illness Referred to the Special Psychiatric Services*. Department of Health, London.

Department of Health (1999). *National Service Framework for Mental Health: Modern standards and service models*. Department of Health, London.

Department of Health (2000). *The NHS Plan: A plan for investment, a plan for reform*. Department of Health, London.

Department of Health (2009). *Living Well with Dementia: a National Dementia Strategy*. www.dh.gov.uk/en/Publicationsandstatistics/Publications/PublicationsPolicyAndGuidance/DH_094058.

Derby IM (1933). Manic-depressive 'exhaustion' deaths. *Psychiatric Quarterly*, **7**, 435–9.

Dervic K *et al*. (2004). Religious affiliation and suicide attempt. *American Journal of Psychiatry*, **161**, 2303–8.

Detering KM *et al*. (2010) The impact of advance care planning on end of life care in elderly patients: randomised controlled trial. *British Medical Journal*, **340**, c1345.

Devenand DP (2002). Comorbid psychiatric disorders in late life depression. *Biological Psychiatry*, **52**, 236–46.

Devenand DP *et al*. (2015). Olfactory deficits predict cognitive decline and Alzheimer dementia in an urban community. *Neurology*, **84**, 182–9.

Devereaux PJ *et al*. (2002). Double Blind, you have been voted off the Island! *Evidence Based Medicine Health Notebook*, **5**, 36–7.

de Vos J *et al*. (2014). Meta-analysis on the efficacy of pharmacotherapy versus placebo on anorexia nervosa. *Journal of Eating Disorders*, **2**, 27.

Dhejne C *et al*. (2014). An analysis of all applications for sex reassignment surgery in Sweden, 1960–2010: prevalence, incidence, and regrets. *Archives of Sexual Behavior*, **43**, 1535–45.

Dickens CM *et al*. (2006). Contribution of depression and anxiety to impaired health-related quality of life following first myocardial infarction. *British Journal of Psychiatry*, **189**, 367–72.

Dickey CC, McCarley RW and Shenton ME (2002). The brain in schizotypal personality disorder: a review of structural MRI and CT findings. *Harvard Review of Psychiatry*, **10**, 1–15.

Dilley MD and Fleminger S (2009). Intracranial infections. In: David A, Fleminger S, Kopelman M *et al*. (eds.) *Lishman's Organic Psychiatry*. Wiley-Blackwell, Oxford. pp. 397–472.

Diniz BS *et al*. (2013). Late-life depression and risk of vascular dementia and Alzheimer's disease: systematic review and meta-analysis of community-based cohort studies. *British Journal of Psychiatry*, **202**, 329–35.

Dixon LB and Stroup ST (2015). Medications for schizophrenia: making a good start. *American Journal of Psychiatry*, **172**, 209–11.

Doherty JL and Owen MJ (2014). Genomic insights into the overlap between psychiatric disorders: Implications for research and clinical practice. *Genomic Medicine*, **6**, 29.

Dolan M and Bishay N (1996). The effectiveness of cognitive therapy in the treatment of non-psychotic morbid jealousy. *British Journal of Psychiatry*, **168**, 588–93.

Dolan M *et al*. (2002). Serotonergic and cognitive impairment in impulsive aggressive personality disordered offenders: are there implications for treatment? *Psychological Medicine*, **32**, 105–17.

Dold M *et al*. (2013). Benzodiazepine augmentation of antipsychotic drugs in schizophrenia: A meta-analysis and Cochrane review of randomized controlled trials. *European Neuropsychopharmacology*, **23**, 1023–33.

Done DJ *et al*. (1994). Childhood antecedents of schizophrenia and affective illness: social adjustment at ages 7 and 11. *British Medical Journal*, **309**, 699–703.

Dorahy MJ *et al.* (2014). Dissociative identity disorder: an empirical overview. *Australian and New Zealand Journal of Psychiatry,* **48**, 402–17.

D'Orban PT (1979). Women who kill their children. *British Journal of Psychiatry,* **134**, 560–71.

Dorph-Petersen K-A and Lewis DA (2011). Stereological approaches to identifying neuropathology in psychosis. *Biological Psychiatry,* **69**, 113–26.

Dosen A (2009). Psychiatric and behaviour disorders among adult persons with intellectual disability. In: Gelder MG, Andreasen NC, López-Ibor JJJr, and Geddes JR (eds.) *The New Oxford Textbook of Psychiatry,* 2nd edn. Oxford University Press, Oxford. pp. 1854–60.

Doty RL (2012). Olfactory dysfunction in Parkinson disease. *Nature Reviews Neurology,* **8**, 329–39.

Dougherty DD *et al.* (2002). Prospective long-term follow-up of 44 patients who received cingulotomy for treatment-refractory obsessive-compulsive disorder. *American Journal of Psychiatry,* **159**, 269–75.

Dowden C, Antonowiez D and Andrews DA (2003). The effectiveness of relapse prevention with offenders: a meta-analysis. *International Journal of Offender Therapy and Comparative Criminology,* **47**, 516–28.

Drake RE, Mueser KT and Brunette MF (2007). Management of persons with co-occurring severe mental illness and substance use disorder: program implications. *World Psychiatry,* **6**, 131–6.

Drescher J *et al.* (2012). Minding the body: Situating gender identity diagnoses in the ICD-11. *International Review of Psychiatry,* **24**, 568–77.

Drescher J *et al.* (2016). Gender incongruence of childhood in the ICD-11: controversies, proposal, and rationale. *Lancet Psychiatry,* **3**, 297–304.

Dressing H, Kuehner C and Gass P (2006). The epidemiology and characteristics of stalking. *Current Opinion in Psychiatry,* **19**, 395–9.

Driessen E *et al.* (2010). Does pre-treatment severity moderate the efficacy of psychological treatment of adult outpatient depression? A meta-analysis. *Journal of Consulting and Clinical Psychology,* **78**, 668–80.

Driessen E *et al.* (2015). The efficacy of short-term psychodynamic psychotherapy for depression: A meta-analysis update. *Clinical Psychology Review,* **42**, 1–15.

Driver DI, Gogtay N and Rapoport JL (2013) Childhood onset schizophrenia and early onset schizophrenia spectrum disorders. *Child and Adolescent Psychiatric Clinics of North America,* **22**(4), 539–5.

Druss BG *et al.* (2014). Randomized trial of an electronic personal health record for patients with serious mental illnesses. *American Journal of Psychiatry,* **171**, 360–8.

Ducat L *et al.* (2014). The mental health comorbidities of diabetes. *Journal of the American Medical Association,* **312**, 691–2.

Duffy RM and Kelly BD (2015). Psychiatric assessment and treatment of survivors of torture. *Advances in Psychiatric Treatment,* **21**, 106–15.

Dugbartey AT (1998). Neurocognitive aspects of hypothyroidism. *Archives of Internal Medicine,* **158**, 1413–18.

Duman RS (eds.) (2009). *Neurochemical Theories of Depression.* Oxford University Press, New York.

Dunbar HF (1954). *Emotions and Bodily Changes.* Columbia University Press, New York.

Dunn M *et al.* (2014). The use of leverage in community mental health: Ethical guidance for practitioners. *International Journal of Social Psychiatry,* **60**, 759–65.

Duric V and Duman RS (2013). Depression and treatment response: Dynamic interplay of signaling pathways and altered neural processes. *Cellular and Molecular Life Sciences,* **70**, 39–53.

Durkheim E (1951). *Suicide: A study in sociology* (transl. JA Spaulding and G Simpson). Free Press, Glencoe, IL.

Duyckaerts C *et al.* (2009). Classification and basic pathology of Alzheimer disease. *Acta Neuropathologica,* **118**, 5–36.

Dwyer J and Reid S (2004). Ganser's syndrome. *Lancet,* **364**, 471–3.

Eastwood S and Bisson JI (2008). Management of factitious disorders: a systematic review. *Psychotherapy and Psychosomatics,* **77**, 209–18.

Eaton J *et al.* (2011). Scale up of services for mental health in low-income and middle-income countries. *Lancet,* **378**, 1592–603.

Ecker C *et al.* (2015). Neuroimaging in autism spectrum disorder: Brain structure and function across the lifespan. *Lancet Neurology,* **14**, 1121–34.

Edelstyn NMJ and Oyebode F (1999). A review of the phenomenology and cognitive neuropsychological origins of the Capgras syndrome. *International Journal of Geriatric Psychiatry,* **14**, 48–59.

Edwards G (1977). Alcoholism: a controlled trial of 'treatment' and 'advice'. *Journal of Studies on Alcohol,* **38**, 1004–31.

Edwards J, McGorry PD and Pennell K (2000). Models of early intervention in psychosis: an analysis of service approaches. In: Birchwood M, Fowler D and Jackson C (eds.) *Early Intervention in Psychosis: a guide to concepts, evidence and interventions.* John Wiley & Sons, New York. pp. 281–314.

Egan MF *et al.* (2001). Effect of COMT Val108–158 Met genotype on frontal lobe function and risk for schizophrenia. *Proceedings of the National Academy of Sciences of the United States of America,* **98**, 6917–22.

Egger HL and Angold A (2006). Common emotional and behavioral disorders in preschool children: presentation, nosology, and epidemiology. *Journal of Child Psychology and Psychiatry,* **47**(3-4), 313–37.

Ehlers A (2009). Post-traumatic stress disorder. In: MG Geder *et al.* (eds). *New Oxford Textbook of Psychiatry,* OUP, Oxford, pp. 700–13.

Ehlers A, Harvey AG and Bryant RA (2009). Stress-related and adjustment disorders. In: MG Gelder *et al.* (eds). *New Oxford Textbook of Psychiatry,* OUP, Oxford, pp. 693–700.

Ehlers A, Ehring T and Kleim B (2012). Information processing in posttraumatic stress disorder. *The Oxford Handbook of Traumatic Stress Disorders,* OUP, New York, pp. 191–218.

Einfeld SL, Ellis LA and Emerson E (2011). Comorbidity of intellectual disability and mental disorder in children and adolescents: A systematic review. *Journal of Intellectual and Developmental Disability,* **36**(2), 137–43.

Eisenberg L (1986). Mindlessness and brainlessness in psychiatry. *British Journal of Psychiatry,* **148**, 497–508.

Eisler I *et al.* (2015). Family interventions. In: A. Thapar *et al.* (eds). *Rutter's Child and Adolescent Psychiatry.* John Wiley & Sons, Chichester, pp. 510–20.

Ekers D *et al.* (2014). Behavioural activation for depression: An update of meta-analysis of effectiveness and sub group analysis. *PLoS One, 9*, e100100.

Ellison-Wright I, Bullmore E (2010). Anatomy of bipolar disorder and schizophrenia: a meta-analysis. *Schizophrenia Research,* **117**, 1–12.

Ellison-Wright Z and Boardman C (2015). Diagnosis and management of ASD in children and adolescents. *Progress in Neurology and Psychiatry,* **19**, 28–32.

Eng B *et al.* (2013). A guide to intellectual disability psychiatry assessments in the community. *Advances in Psychiatric Treatment,* **19**, 429–36.

Engel GL (1977). The need for a new medical model: a challenge for biomedicine. *Science, 196*, 129–96.

Engels *et al.* (2014). Clinical pain in schizophrenia. A systematic review. *Journal of Pain,* **15**, 457–67.

Ennis L *et al.* (2014). Collaborative development of an electronic Personal Health Record for people with severe and enduring mental health problems. *BMC Psychiatry,* **14**, 305.

Epping EA *et al.* (2016). Longitudinal psychiatric symptoms in prodromal Huntington's disease: a decade of data. *American Journal of Psychiatry,* **173**, 184–92.

Eranti SV *et al.* (2013). Gender difference in age of onset of schizophrenia: a meta-analysis. *Psychological Medicine,* **43**, 155–67.

Ernst C, Mechawar N and Turecki G (2009). Suicide neurobiology. *Progress in Neurobiology*, **89**, 315–33.

Eronen M, Hakola P and Tiihonen J (1996). Mental disorders and homicidal behaviour in Finland. *Archives of General Psychiatry,* **53**, 497–501.

Erskine HE *et al.* (2013). Research review: Epidemiological modelling of attention-deficit/hyperactivity disorder and conduct disorder for the Global Burden of Disease Study 2010. *Journal of Child Psychology and Psychiatry,* **54**, 1263–74.

Escriba PV, Ozaita A and Garcia-Sevilla JA (2004). Increased mRNA expressions of alpha2A-adrenoceptors, serotonin receptors and mu-opioid receptors in the brains of suicide victims. *Neuropsychopharmacology,* **29**, 1512–21.

Espie CA and Kyle SD (2009). Primary insomnia: an overview of practical management using cognitive behavioural techniques. *Sleep Medicine Clinics,* **4**, 559–69.

Essen-Møller E (1971). Suggestions for further improvement of the international classification of mental disorders. *Psychological Medicine, 1*, 308–11.

Essex B, Doig R and Renshaw J (1990). Pilot study of records of shared care for people with mental illnesses. *British Medical Journal*, **300**, 1442.

Eysenck HJ (1970a). *The Structure of Human Personality*. Methuen, London.

Eysenck HJ (1970b). A dimensional system of psychodiagnosis. In: AR Mahrer (ed.) *New Approaches to Personality Classification*. Columbia University Press, New York. pp. 169–207.

Eysenck HJ and Eysenck SBG (1976). *Psychoticism as a Dimension of Personality*. Hodder and Stoughton, London.

Fabrega H (2000). Culture, spirituality and psychiatry. *Current Opinion in Psychiatry,* **13**, 525–53.

Fairburn C (1999). Risk factors for anorexia nervosa: three integrated case-control comparisons. *Archives of General Psychiatry,* **56**, 468–76.

Fairburn CG (2013). *Overcoming Binge Eating,* 2nd edn. Guilford Press, New York, NY.

Fairburn CG and Harrison PJ (2003). Eating disorders. *Lancet,* **361**, 407–16.

Fairburn CG *et al.* (1999). A cognitive-behavioural theory of anorexia nervosa. *Behaviour Research and Therapy,* **37**, 1–13.

Fairburn CG *et al.* (2009a). Transdiagnostic cognitive-behavioural therapy for patients with eating disorders: a two-site trial with 60-week follow-up. *American Journal of Psychiatry,* **166**, 311–19.

Fairburn CG *et al.* (2009b). Bulimia nervosa. In: Gelder MG, Andreasen NC, Lopez-Ibor JJJr and Geddes JR (eds.) *New Oxford Textbook of Psychiatry*, 2nd edn. Oxford Univesity Press, Oxford, pp. 800–11.

Fairburn CG *et al.* (2013) Enhanced cognitive behaviour therapy for adults with anorexia nervosa. *Behaviour Research and Therapy,* **51**, 2–8.

Fairburn CG *et al.* (2015). A transdiagnostic comparison of enhanced cognitive behaviour therapy (CBT-E) and interpersonal psychotherapy in the treatment of eating disorders. *Behaviour Research and Therapy,* **70**, 64–71.

Falkai P and Bogerts B. Neuropathology (2009). In: MG Gelder, NC Andreasen, JJ Lopez-Ibor, JR Geddes (eds). *New Oxford Textbook of Psychiatry*. OUP, Oxford, pp. 177–85.

Fanous AH and Kendler KS (2004). The genetic relationship of personality to major depression and schizophrenia. *Neurotoxicity Research,* **6**, 43–50.

Faris REL and Dunham HW (1939). *Mental Disorders in Urban Areas*. Chicago University Press, Chicago, IL.

Farrington DP (2002). Key results from the first forty years of the Cambridge study in delinquent development. In: TP Thornberry and MD Kern (eds.) *Taking Stock of Delinquency: An overview of findings from contemporary longitudinal studies*. Kluwer/Plenum, New York.

Farrington DP (2009). Psychosocial causes of offending. In: MG Gelder, NC Andreasen, JJ Lopez-Ibor, and J Geddes (eds.) *The New Oxford Textbook of Psychiatry*. Oxford University Press, Oxford, pp.1908–16.

Farrington DP and Welsh BC (2008). *Saving Children from a Life of Crime: Early risk factors and effective interventions*. Oxford University Press, New York.

Farrington DP *et al.* (1988). Are there any successful men from criminogenic backgrounds? *Psychiatry,* **51**, 116–30.

Fazel M (2015). Methylphenidate for ADHD. *British Medical Journal,* **351**, h5875.

Fazel M, Wheeler J and Danesh J (2005). Prevalence of serious mental disorder in 7000 refugees resettled in western countries: a systematic review. *Lancet*, **365**, 1309–14.

Fazel M *et al.* (2012a). Mental health of displaced and refugee children resettled in high-income countries: risk and protective factors. *Lancet,* **379**, 266–82.

Fazel M *et al.* (2014a). Mental health interventions in schools 1: Mental health interventions in schools in high-income countries. *Lancet Psychiatry,* **1**, 377–87.

Fazel M *et al.* (2014b). Mental health interventions in schools in low-income and middle-income countries. *Lancet Psychiatry,* **1**, 388–98.

Fazel M *et al.* (2015). Refugee, asylum-seeking and internally displaced children and adolescents. In: M Rutter *et al.* (eds.)

Child and Adolescent Psychiatry, 6th edn. Blackwell, Oxford. pp. 573–85.

Fazel S and Danesh J (2002). Serious mental disorder in 23,000 prisoners: a systematic review of 62 surveys. *Lancet*, 359, 545–50.

Fazel S and Grann M (2004). Psychiatric morbidity among homicide offenders: a Swedish population study. *American Journal of Psychiatry*, 161, 2129–31.

Fazel S and Grann M (2006) The population impact of severe mental illness on violent crime. *American Journal of Psychiatry*, 163, 1397–1403.

Fazel S *et al.* (2001). Hidden psychiatric morbidity in elderly prisoners. *British Journal of Psychiatry*, 179, 535–9.

Fxazel S, Vassos E and Danesh J (2002). Prevalence of epilepsy in prisoners: systematic review. *British Medical Journal*, 324, 1495.

Fazel S *et al.* (2005). Suicides in male prisoners in England and Wales, 1978–2003. *Lancet*, 366, 1301–2.

Fazel S *et al.* (2007). Severe mental illness and risk of sexual offending in men: a case-control study based on Swedish national registers. *Journal of Clinical Psychiatry*, 68, 588–96.

Fazel S *et al.* (2009a). Schizophrenia and violence: systematic review and meta-analysis. *PloS Med* 6(8): e1000120.

Fazel S *et al.* (2009b). Neurological disorders and violence: a systematic review and meta-analysis with a focus on epilepsy and traumatic brain injury. *Journal of Neurology*, 256, 1591–602.

Fazel S *et al.* (2011a). Risk of violent crime in individuals with epilepsy and traumatic brain injury: A 35-year Swedish population study. *PLoS Medicine*, 8, e1001150.

Fazel S *et al.* (2011b). Prison suicide in 12 countries: an ecological study of 861 suicides during 2003–2007. *Social Psychiatry and Psychiatric Epidemiology*, 46, 191–5.

Fazel S *et al.* (2011c). Use of risk assessment instruments to predict violence and antisocial behaviour in 73 samples involving 24 827 people: systematic review and meta-analysis. *British Medical Journal*, 345, e4692.

Fazel S *et al.* (2012). Use of risk assessment instruments to predict violence and antisocial behaviour in 73 samples involving 24 827 people: systematic review and meta-analysis. *British Medical Journal*, 345, e4692.

Fazel S *et al.* (2013). Premature mortality in epilepsy and the role of psychiatric comorbidity: a total population study. *Lancet*, 382, 1646–54.

Fazel S *et al.* (2014a). Violent crime, suicide, and premature mortality in patients with schizophrenia and related disorders: a 38-year total population study in Sweden. *Lancet Psychiatry*, 1, 44–54.

Fazel S *et al.* (2014b). Suicide, fatal injuries, and other causes of premature mortality in patients with traumatic brain injury: a 41-year Swedish population study. *JAMA Psychiatry*, 71, 326–33.

Fazel S *et al.* (2014c). The health of the homeless in high-income countries: descriptive epidemiology and risk factors. *Lancet*, 384, 1529–40.

Fearon P *et al.* (2006). Incidence of schizophrenia and other psychoses in ethnic minority groups in three English cities: results from the MRC ÆSOP study. *Psychological Medicine*, 36, 1541–50.

Feighner *et al.* (1972). Diagnostic criteria for use in psychiatric research. *Archives of General Psychiatry*, 26, 57–63.

Feinstein A *et al.* (2014). The link between multiple sclerosis and depression. *Nature Reviews Neurology*, 10, 507–17.

Fergusson DM, Horwood LJ and Lynskey MT (1993). Prevalence and comorbidity of DSM-III-R diagnoses in a birth cohort of 15-year-olds. *Journal of the American Academy of Child and Adolescent Psychiatry*, 32, 1127–34.

Fergusson DM, Horwood LJ and Boden JM (2009). Reactions to abortion and subsequent mental health. *British Journal of Psychiatry*, 195, 420–6.

Fergusson DM *et al.* (2012). Life stress, 5-HTTLPR and mental disorder. *British Journal of Psychiatry*, 198, 129–35.

Fersum K *et al.* (2013). Efficacy of classification-based cognitive functional therapy in patients with non-specific chronic low back pain: a randomized controlled trial. *European Journal of Pain*, 17, 916–28.

Fiedorowicz JG *et al.* (2011). Subthreshold hypomanic symptoms in progression from unipolar major depression to bipolar depression. *American Journal of Psychiatry*, 168, 40–8.

Fiest KM *et al.* (2013). Depression in epilepsy. A systematic review and meta-analysis. *Neurology*, 80, 590–9.

Fineberg NA *et al.* (2014). New developments in human neuro-cognition: Clinical, genetic, and brain imaging correlates of impulsivity and compulsivity. *CNS Spectrums*, 19, 69–89.

Fink M, Shorter E and Taylor MA (2010). Catatonia is not schizophrenia: Kraepelin's error and the need to recognize catatonia as an independent syndrome in medical nomenclature. *Schizophrenia Bulletin*, 36, 314–20.

Finnerup NB *et al.* (2015). Pharmacotherapy for neuropathic pain in adults: a systematic review and meta-analysis. *Lancet Neurology*, 14, 162–73.

Finney GR (2009). Normal pressure hydrocephalus. *International Review of Neurobiology*, 84, 263–81.

Fioritti A, Lo RL and Melega V (1997). Reform said or done? The case of Emilia-Romagna within the Italian psychiatric context. *American Journal of Psychiatry*, 154, 94–8.

Firn M *et al.* (2012). A dismantling study of assertive outreach services: comparing activity and outcomes following replacement with the FACT model. *Social Psychiatry and Psychiatric Epidemiology*, 48, 997–1003.

First MB *et al.* (1997). *Structured Clinical Interview for DSM-IV Axis II Personality Disorders (SCID-II)*. American Psychiatric Association, Washington, DC.

Fish FJ (1962). *Schizophrenia*. John Wright, Bristol.

Fiske A *et al.* (2009). Depression in older adults. *Annual Review of Clinical Psychology*, 5, 363–89.

Flament MF and Robaey P. (2009). Obsessive-compulsive disorder and tics in children and adolescents. In: MG Gelder, NC Andreasen, JJ Lopez-Ibor, JR Geddes (eds.) *New Oxford Textbook of Psychiatry*. Oxford University Press, Oxford. pp. 1680–93.

Fleminger S (2009). Head injury. In: AS David, S Fleminger, MD Kopelman, S Lovestone, JDC Mellers (eds) *Lishman's Organic Psychiatry*, 4th edn. Wiley-Blackwell, Oxford. pp. 167–279.

Fleminger S (2009). Cerebrovascular disorders. In: David AS, Fleminger S, Kopelman M *et al.* (eds.) *Lishman's Organic Psychiatry*, 4th edn. Wiley Blackwell, Oxford. pp. 473–542.

Foley K-R *et al.* (2014). Relationship between family quality of life and day occupations of young people with Down syndrome. *Social Psychiatry and Psychiatric Epidemiology*, 49, 1455–65.

Folstein MF, Folstein SE and McHugh PR (1975). 'Mini-mental state'. A practical method for grading the cognitive state of patients for the clinician. *Journal of Psychiatric Research*, **12**, 189–98.

Fombonne E (2009). Epidemiology of pervasive developmental disorders. *Pediatric Research*, **65**(6), 591–98.

Fonagy P and Kächele H (2009). Psychoanalysis and other long-term dynamic psychotherapies. In: Gelder M, Andreasen N, Lopez-Ibor J, Geddes J (eds.) *New Oxford Textbook of Psychiatry*. Oxford University Press, Oxford. pp. 1337–50.

Fonagy P and Target M (2009). Psychodynamic child psychotherapy. In: MG Gelder, NC Andreasen, JJ Lopez-Ibor, JR Geddes (eds.) *New Oxford Textbook of Psychiatry*. Oxford University Press, Oxford. pp. 1769–77.

Forneris CA *et al.* (2013). Interventions to prevent post-traumatic stress disorder: A systematic review. *American Journal of Preventive Medicine*, **44**, 635–50.

Forti-Buratti MA *et al.* (2016). Psychological treatments for depression in pre-adolescent children (12 years and younger): systematic review and meta-analysis of randomised controlled trials. *European Child and Adolescent Psychiatry*, **25**, 1045–54.

Fossey J *et al.* (2006). Effect of enhanced psychosocial care on antipsychotic use in nursing home residents with severe dementia: cluster randomized trial. *British Medical Journal*, **332**, 756–758A.

Foster T, Gillespie K and McClelland R (1997). Mental disorders and suicide in Northern Ireland. *British Journal of Psychiatry*, **170**, 447–52.

Foulkes SH and Lewis E (1944). Group analysis: a study in the treatment of groups on psychoanalytic lines. *British Journal of Medical Psychology*, **20**, 175–82.

Fraguas D *et al.* (2014). Duration of untreated psychosis predicts functional and clinical outcome in children and adolescents with first-episode psychosis: A 2-year longitudinal study. *Schizophrenia Research*, **152**, 130–8.

Frances AJ and Nardo JM (2013). ICD-11 should not repeat the mistakes made by DSM-5. *Br J Psychiatry*, **1**, 1–2.

Frank E, Kupfer DJ and Perel JM (1990). Three-year outcomes of maintenance therapies in recurrent depression. *Archives of General Psychiatry*, **48**, 1053–9.

Frank JD (1967). *Persuasion and Healing*. Johns Hopkins Press, Baltimore, MD.

Franko DL *et al.* (2013). A longitudinal investigation of mortality in anorexia nervosa and bulimia nervosa. *American Journal of Psychiatry*, **170**, 917–25.

Fraser LM, O'Carroll RE and Ebmeier KP (2008). The effect of electroconvulsive therapy on autobiographical memory: a systematic review. *The Journal of ECT*, **24**, 10–17.

Frazer KA, Murrasy SS, Schork NJ and Topol EJ (2009) Human genetic variation and its contribution to complex traits. *Nature Reviews Genetics*, **10**, 241–51.

Freeman CP (2013). Cognitive adverse effects of ECT. In: J Waite, A Eaton (eds.) *The ECT Handbook*. RCPsych Publications, London. pp. 76–86.

Freeman D and Garety P (2014). Advances in understanding and treating persecutory delusions: a review. *Social Psychiatry and Psychiatric Epidemiology*, **49**, 1179–89.

Freeman W and Watts JW (1942). *Psychosurgery*. Thomas, Springfield, IL.

Freemantle N (2004). Is NICE delivering the goods? *British Medical Journal*, **329**, 1003.

Freud S (1917). Mourning and melancholia. In: *The Standard Edition of the Complete Psychological Works*, Vol. 14. Hogarth Press, London. pp. 243–58.

Friedman JI *et al.* (2014). Pharmacological treatments of non-substance-withdrawal delirium: a systematic review of prospective trials. *American Journal of Psychiatry*, **171**, 151–9.

Friedman M and Rosenman RH (1959). Association of specific behaviour pattern with blood and cardiovascular findings. *Journal of the American Medical Association*, **169**, 1286–96.

Frisell T *et al.* (2011). Violent crime runs in families: a total population study of 12.5 million individuals. *Psychological Medicine*, **41**, 97–105.

Frith C (1996). Neuropsychology of schizophrenia: what are the implications of intellectual and experiential abnormalities for the neurobiology of schizophrenia? *British Medical Bulletin*, **52**, 618–26.

Fromm-Reichmann F (1948). Notes on the development of treatment of schizophrenia by psychoanalytic psychotherapy. *Psychiatry*, **11**, 263–73.

Frühauf S *et al.* (2013). Efficacy of psychological interventions for sexual dysfunction: a systematic review and meta-analysis. *Archives of Sexual Behavior*, **42**, 915–33.

Fukuda K *et al.* (1994). Chronic fatigue syndrome: a comprehensive approach to its definition and management. *Annals of Internal Medicine*, **121**, 953–9.

Fuhrmann D *et al.* (2015). Adolescence as a sensitive period of brain development. *Trends in Cognitive Sciences*, **19**, 558–66.

Fulford K, Peile E and Caroll H (2012). *Essential Values-Based Practice*. Cambridge University Press, Cambridge.

Fulford KWM (1989). *Moral Theory and Medical Practice*. Cambridge University Press, Cambridge.

Fulton M and Winokur G (1993). A comparative study of paranoid and schizoid personality disorders. *British Journal of Psychiatry*, **150**, 1363–7.

Furukawa TA (2004). Meta-analyses and mega-trials: neither is the infallible, universal standard. *Evidence Based Medicine Health Notebook*, **7**, 34–5.

Fusar-Poli P *et al.* (2013a). The psychosis high-risk state. A comprehensive state-of-the-art review. *JAMA Psychiatry*, **70**, 107–20.

Fusar-Poli P *et al.* (2013b). Progressive brain changes in schizophrenia related to antipsychotic treatment? A meta-analysis of longitudinal MRI studies. *Neuroscience and Biobehavioral Reviews*, **37**, 1680–91.

Fusar-Poli *et al.* (2015). Treatments of negative symptoms in schizophrenia: meta-analysis of 168 randomized placebo-controlled trials. *Schizophrenia Bulletin*, **41**, 892–9.

Fusar-Poli P *et al.* (2016). Prognosis of brief psychotic episodes. A meta-analysis. *JAMA Psychiatry*, **73**, 211–20.

Fyer AJ *et al.* (1995). Specificity in familial aggregation of phobic disorders. *Archives of General Psychiatry*, **52**, 564–73.

Fyer MR *et al.* (1988). Co-morbidity of borderline personality disorder. *Archives of General Psychiatry*, **45**, 348–52.

Gabbard G (2007). *Personality Disorders. Gabbard's treatment of psychiatric disorders*, 4th edn. APPI, Washington DC.

Gage S *et al.* (2015). Association between cannabis and psychosis: epidemiologic evidence. *Biological Psychiatry, 79*, 549–56.

Gajalakshmi V and Peto R (2007). Suicide rates in rural Tamil Nadu, South India: verbal autopsy of 39 000 deaths in 1997–98. *International Journal of Epidemiology, 36*, 203–7.

Galappathie N and Khan ST (2016). End-of-life care in psychiatry: 'one chance to get it right.' *BJPsych Bulletin 40*, 38–40.

Galimbeti D *et al.* (2015). Psychiatric symptoms in frontotemporal dementia: epidemiology, phenotypes, and differential diagnosis. *Biological Psychiatry, 78*, 684–92.

Galletly C *et al.* (2016). Royal Australian and New Zealand College of Psychiatrists clinical practice guidelines for the management of schizophrenia and related disorders. *Australian and New Zealand Journal of Psychiatry, 50*, 410–72.

Games D *et al.* (1995). Alzheimer-type neuropathology in transgenic mice overexpressing V717F beta-amyloid precursor protein. *Nature, 373*, 523–7.

Gandaglia G *et al.* (2014). A systematic review of the association between erectile dysfunction and cardiovascular disease. *European Urology, 65*, 968–78.

Gannon TA and Rose MR (2008). Female child sexual offenders: towards integrating theory and practice. *Aggression and Violent Behavior, 13*, 442–61.

Garber HL (1988). *The Milwaukee Project: Preventing mental retardation in children at risk.* American Association on Mental Retardation, Washington, DC.

Gardner W *et al.* (1993). Two scales for measuring patients perceptions for coercion during mental-hospital admission. *Behavioral Sciences & the Law, 11*, 307–21.

Garety PA and Freeman D (2013). The past and future of delusions research: from the inexplicable to the treatable. *British Journal of Psychiatry, 203*, 327–33.

Garner M *et al.* (2009). Research in anxiety disorders: from the bench to the bedside. *European Neuropsychopharmacolgy, 19*, 381–90.

Garralda ME *et al.* (2015). Somatoform and related disorders. In: A. Thapar *et al.* (eds). *Rutter's Child and Adolescent Psychiatry.* John Wiley & Sons, Chichester, pp. 1035–54.

Gartlehner G *et al.* (2008). Comparative benefits and harms of second-generation antidepressants: background paper for the American College of Physicians. *Annals of Internal Medicine, 149*, 734–50.

Gath A (1978). *Down's Syndrome and the Family.* Academic Press, London.

Gath A and McCarthy J (2009). Families with a member with intellectual disability and their needs. In: MG Gelder, NC Andreasen, JJ López-IborJr and JR Geddes (eds.) *The New Oxford Textbook of Psychiatry,* 2nd edn. Oxford University Press, Oxford. pp. 1883–6.

Gath D, Cooper P and Day A (1982). Hysterectomy and psychiatric disorder: 1. Levels of psychiatric morbidity before and after hysterectomy. *British Journal of Psychiatry, 140*, 335–42.

Gaugler JE *et al.* (2009). Predictors of change in caregiver burden and depressive symptoms following nursing home admission. *Psychology and Aging, 24*(20), 385–96.

Gaupp R (1974). The scientific significance of the case of Ernst Wagner. In: SR Hirsch and M Shepherd (eds.) *Themes and Variations in European Psychiatry.* John Wright and Sons, Bristol.

Gauron EF and Dickinson JK (1966). Diagnostic decision making in psychiatry. *Archives of General Psychiatry, 14*, 225–32.

Gavin NI *et al.* (2005). Perinatal depression: a systematic review of prevalence and incidence. *Obstetrics and Gynaecology, 106*, 1071–83.

Gazzaniga MS (2000). Cerebral specialization and interhemispheric communication. Does the corpus callosum enable the human condition? *Brain, 123*, 1293–326.

Geddes J (1999). Asking structured and focused clinical questions: essential first step of evidence-based practice. *Evidence Based Mental Health, 2*, 35–6.

Geddes JR *et al.* (2003). Relapse prevention with antidepressant drug treatment in depressive disorders: a systematic review. *Lancet, 361*, 653–61.

Geddes JR *et al.* (2004). Long-term lithium therapy for bipolar disorder: systematic review and meta-analysis of randomized controlled trials. *American Journal of Psychiatry, 161*, 217–22.

Geddes JR and Miklowitz DJ (2013). Treatment of bipolar disorder. *The Lancet, 381*, 1672–82.

Geddes JR *et al.* (2009). Lamotrigine for treatment of bipolar depression: independent meta-analysis and meta-regression of individual patient data from five randomized trials. *British Journal of Psychiatry, 194*, 4–9.

Geddes JR *et al.* (2016). Comparative evaluation of quetiapine plus lamotrigine combination versus quetiapine monotherapy (and folic acid versus placebo) in bipolar depression (CEQUEL): a 2 × 2 factorial randomized trial. *Lancet Psychiatry, 3*, 31–9.

Gelauff J *et al.* (2014). The prognosis of functional (psychogenic) motor symptoms. *Journal of Neurology, Neurosurgery and Psychiatry, 85*, 220–6.

Gelder MG (1986). Neurosis: another tough old word. *British Medical Journal, 292*, 972–3.

Gelder MG, Marks IM and Wolff H (1978). Desensitization and psychotherapy in phobic states: a controlled enquiry. *British Journal of Psychiatry, 113*, 53–73.

Gelder MG, Andreasen NC, López-Ibor JJJr and Geddes JR (eds.) (2009). *The New Oxford Textbook of Psychiatry.* Oxford University Press, Oxford.

Gelder MG, Andreasen NC, López-Ibor JJ Jr, and Geddes JR (eds) (2009). Section 9: Child and Adolescent Psychiatry. In: *New Oxford Textbook of Psychiatry.* Oxford University Press, Oxford.

General Medical Council (2009a). *Confidentiality.* General Medical Council, London.

General Medical Council (2009b). *Tomorrow's Doctors. Outcomes and Standards for Undergraduate Medical Education.* General Medical Council, London, pp.104.

George N *et al.* (2016). The current treatment of non-cardiac chest pain. *Alimentary Pharmacology, 43*, 213–39.

Gerger H, Munder T, Barth J (2014). Specific and nonspecific psychological interventions for PTSD symptoms: A meta-analysis with problem complexity as a moderator. *Journal of Clinical Psychology, 70*(7), 601–15.

Gerger H *et al.* (2015). Does it matter who provides psychological interventions for medically unexplained symptoms? A meta-analysis. *Psychotherapy and Psychosomatics, 84*, 217–26.

Gershon ES and Alliey-Rodriguez N (2013). New ethical issues for genetic counseling in common mental disorders. *American Journal of Psychiatry, 170*, 968–76.

Ghodse H *et al*. (2010). *Trends in UK Deaths Associated with Abuse of Volatile Substances, 1971–2008*. Volatile Substance Abuse (VSA) Mortality Project International Centre for Drug Policy (ICDP), St Georges, University of London, London.

Gibbons R *et al*. (2007). Early evidence on the effects of regulators' suicidality warnings on SSRI prescriptions and suicide in children and adolescents. *American Journal of Psychiatry*, **164**, 1356–63.

Gigante AD *et al*. (2012). Brain glutamate levels measured by magnetic resonance spectroscopy in patients with bipolar disorder: a meta-analysis. *Bipolar Disorders*, **14**, 478–87.

Gilbody SM, House AO and Sheldon T (2002). Routine administration of Health Quality of Life (HRQoL) and needs assessment instruments to improve psychological outcome—a systematic review. *Psychological Medicine*, **32**, 1345–56.

Gill B *et al*. (1996). *Psychiatric Morbidity among Homeless People*. HMSO, London.

Gill ON *et al*. (2013). Prevalent abnormal prion protein in human appendixes after bovine spongiform encephalopathy epizootic: large scale survey. *British Medical Journal*, **347**, f5675.

Gillam SJ *et al*. (1989). Ethnic differences in consultation rates in urban general practice. *British Medical Journal*, **299**, 958–60.

Gillies D, Taylor F, Gray C, O'Brien L and D'Abrew N (2013). Psychological therapies for the treatment of post-traumatic stress disorder in children and adolescents (Review). *Evidence-Based Child Health: A Cochrane Review Journal*, **8**(3), 1004–116.

Gillman K and Whyte I (2004). *Adverse Syndromes and Psychiatric Drugs*. Oxford University Press, Oxford.

Gilman JM *et al*. (2012). Subjective and neural responses to intravenous alcohol in young adults with light and heavy drinking patterns. *Neuropsychopharmacology*, **37**, 467–77.

Giordano S. (2013). *Children with Gender Identity Disorder: A Clinical, Ethical, and Legal Analysis* (Vol. 9): Routledge, Abingdon.

Gitlin DF, Levenson JL and Lyketsos CG (2004). Psychosomatic medicine: a new psychiatric subspecialty. *Academic Psychiatry*, **28**, 4–11.

Glenn AL and Raine A (2014). Neurocriminology: implications for the punishment, prediction and prevention of criminal behavior. *Nature Reviews Neuroscience*, **15**, 54–63.

Glaser D et al. (2015) Child sexual abuse. In: A Thapar et al. (eds). *Rutter's Child and Adolescent Psychiatry*, 6th edition. Wiley, Chichester, pp. 376–88.

Glenn T and Monteith S (2014). New measures of mental state and behaviour based on data collected from sensors, smartphones, and the Internet. *Current Psychiatry Reports*, **16**, 523.

Glover G, Arts G and Babu KS (2006). Crisis resolution/home treatment teams and psychiatric admission rates in England. *British Journal of Psychiatry*, **189**, 441–45.

Goate A *et al*. (1991). Segregation of a missense mutation in the amyloid precursor protein gene with familial Alzheimer's disease. *Nature*, **349**, 704–6.

Goffman E (1961). *Asylums: Essays on the social situation of mental patients and other inmates*. Doubleday, New York.

Gold PW. (2015). The organization of the stress system and its dysregulation in depressive illness. *Molecular Psychiatry*, **20**, 32–47.

Goldberg D (1972). *The Detection of Psychiatric Illness by Questionnaire*. Maudsley Monograph No. 21. Oxford University Press, London.

Goldberg D (2010). The classification of mental disorder: a simpler system for DSM-V and ICD-11. *Advances in Psychiatric Treatment*, **16**, 14–19.

Goldberg D (ed.) (1997). *The Maudsley Handbook of Practical Psychiatry*. Oxford Medical Publications, Oxford.

Goldberg D and Hillier VP (1979). A scaled version of the General Health Questionnaire. *Psychological Medicine*, **9**, 139–45.

Goldberg D and Huxley P (1980). *Mental Illness in the Community*. Tavistock Publications, London.

Goldberg D *et al*. (1976). A comparison of two psychiatric screening tests. *British Journal of Psychiatry*, **129**, 61–7.

Goldberg D, Steele J and Smith J (1980). Teaching psychiatric interview techniques to family doctors. *Acta Psychiatrica Scandinavica*, **62**, 41–7.

Goldberg D, Tylee A and Walters P (2009). Psychiatry in primary care. In: Gelder MG, Andreasen NC, López-Ibor JJJr and Geddes JR (eds.) *New Oxford Textbook of Psychiatry*, 2nd edn. Oxford University Press, Oxford. pp. 1480–9.

Goldberg EM and Morrison SL (1963). Schizophrenia and social class. *British Journal of Psychiatry*, **109**, 785–802.

Goldman H and Morrissey JP (1985). The alchemy of mental health policy: homelessness and the fourth cycle of reform. *American Journal of Public Health*, **75**, 727–31.

Goldstein RB *et al*. (1991). The prediction of suicide: sensitivity, specificity, and predictive value of a multivariate model applied to suicide among 1906 patients with affective disorders. *Archives of General Psychiatry*, **48**, 418–22.

Goncalves DC and Byrne GJ (2012). Interventions for generalized anxiety disorder in older adults: systematic review and meta-analysis. *Journal of Anxiety Disorders*, **26**, 1–11.

Gonzalez A *et al*. (2014). Subtypes of exposure to intimate partner violence within a Canadian child welfare sample: Associated risks and child maladjustment. *Child Abuse & Neglect*, **38**, 1934–44.

Gonzalez-Burgos G *et al*. (2015). Alterations in cortical network oscillations and parvalbumin neurons in schizophrenia. *Biological Psychiatry*, **77**, 1031–40.

Goodkind M *et al*. (2013). Functional neurocircuitry and neuroimaging studies of anxiety disorders. In: DS Charney, JD Buxbaum, P Sklaar, EJ Nestler (eds). *Neurobiology of Mental Illness*. Oxford University Press, Oxford, pp. 606–20.

Goodman R, Simonoff E and Stevenson J (1995). The impact of child IQ, parent IQ and sibling IQ on child behavioural deviance scores. *Journal of Child Psychology and Psychiatry*, **36**(3), 409–425.

Goodman JH *et al*. (2014). Anxiety disorders during pregnancy: a systematic review. *Journal of Clinical Psychiatry*, **75**, e1153–84.

Goodman SH *et al*. (2011). Maternal depression and child psychopathology: a meta-analytic review. *Clinical Child and Family Psychology Review*, **14**, 1–27.

Goodwin FK and Jamison KR (2007). *Manic-depressive Illness: Bipolar disorders and recurrent depression*, 2nd edn. New York: Oxford University Press.

Goodwin GM *et al*. (2016). Evidence-based guidelines for treating bipolar disorder: revised third edition recommendations from the British Association for Psychopharmacology. *Journal of Psychopharmacology*, 30, 495–553.

Gordon H and Grubin D (2004). Psychiatric aspects of the assessment and treatment of sex offenders. *Advances in Psychiatric Treatment*, 10, 73–80.

Gore FM *et al.* (2011). Global burden of disease in young people aged 10-24 years: a systematic analysis. *Lancet*, 377, 2093–102.

Gorin-Lazard A *et al.* (2012). Is hormonal therapy associated with better quality of life in transsexuals? A cross-sectional study. *Journal of Sexual Medicine*, 9, 531–41.

Gottesman I (1991). *Schizophrenia Genesis: The origins of madness.* W. H. Freeman, New York.

Gottesman II and Gould TD (2003). The endophenotype concept in psychiatry: etymology and strategic intentions. *American Journal of Psychiatry*, 160, 636–45.

Gottesman I and Shields J (1967). A polygenic theory of schizophrenia. *Proceedings of the National Academy of Sciences USA*, 58, 199–205.

Goudriaan AE *et al.* (2004). Pathological gambling: a comprehensive review of biobehavioral findings. *Neurosciences and Biobehavioral Reviews*, 28, 123–41.

Gould MS *et al.* (2005). Evaluating iatrogenic risk of youth suicide screening programs: a randomized controlled trial. *JAMA*, 293, 1635–43.

Gournellis R *et al.* (2014). Psychotic major depression in older people: a systematic review. *International Journal of Geriatric Psychiatry*, 29, 784–96.

Graham P (2009). Cognitive behaviour therapies for children and families. In: MG Gelder, NC Andreasen, JJ Lopez-Ibor and JR Geddes (eds.) *New Oxford Textbook of Psychiatry*. Oxford University Press, Oxford. pp. 1777–86.

Graham SA and Fisher SE (2013). Decoding the genetics of speech and language. *Current Opinion in Neurobiology*, 23, 43–51.

Grandhe R *et al.* (2016). New chronic pain treatments in the outpatient setting. *Current Pain and Headache Reports*, 20, 33.

Grann M and Fazel S (2004). Substance misuse and violent crime: Swedish population study. *British Medical Journal*, 328, 1233–4.

Grant BF *et al.* (2004). Prevalence, correlates, and disability of personality disorders in the United States: results from the national epidemiologic survey on alcohol and related conditions. *Journal of Clinical Psychiatry*, 65, 948–58.

Grant BF *et al.* (2015). Epidemiology of DSM-5 alcohol use disorder: results from the National Epidemiologic Survey on Alcohol and Related Conditions III. *JAMA Psychiatry*, 72, 757–66.

Grant JE *et al.* (2010). Introduction to behavioral addictions. *American Journal of Drug and Alcohol Abuse*, 36, 233–41.

Gratten J *et al.* (2014). Large-scale genomics unveils the genetic architecture of psychiatric disorders. *Nature Neuroscience*, 17, 782–90.

Gray J *et al.* (1991). The neuropsychology of schizophrenia. *Behavioral and Brain Sciences*, 14, 1–84.

Gray R *et al.* (2016). Is adherence therapy an effective adjunct treatment for patients with schizophrenia spectrum disorders? A systematic review and meta-analysis. *BMC Psychiatry*, 16, 90.

Gray SL *et al.* (2015). Cumulative use of strong anticholinergics and incident dementia: a prospective cohort study. *JAMA Internal Medicine*, 175, 401–7.

Green EK *et al.* (2016). Copy number variation in bipolar disorder. *Molecular Psychiatry*, 21, 89–93.

Green JG *et al.* (2010). Childhood adversities and adult psychiatric disorders in the national comorbidity survey replication I: Associations with first onset of DSM-IV disorders. *Archives of General Psychiatry*, 67, 113–23.

Green MF (2006). Cognitive impairment and functional outcome in schizophrenia and bipolar disorder. *Journal of Clinical Psychiatry*, 67 (Suppl. 9), 3–8.

Green MF (2015). Social cognition in schizophrenia. *Nature Reviews Neuroscience*, 16, 620–31.

Greenberg MT *et al.* (2015). Prevention of mental disorders and promotion of competence. In: A. Thapar *et al.* (eds). *Rutter's Child and Adolescent Psychiatry*. John Wiley & Sons, Chichester, pp. 215–26.

Greenfield SF *et al.* (2010). Substance abuse in women. *Psychiatric Clinics of North America*, 33, 339–55.

Greenhalgh T (2010). *How to Read a Paper*. Wiley Blackwell, Oxford.

Greeven A *et al.* (2014). Personality predicts time to remission and clinical status in hypochondriasis during a 6-year follow-up. *Journal of Nervous and Mental Disease*, 202, 402–7.

Gressier F *et al.* (2015). Post-partum depressive symptoms and medically assisted conception: a systematic review and meta-analysis. *Human Reproduction*, 30, 2575–86.

Griebel G and Holsboer F (2012). Neuropeptide receptor ligands as drugs for psychiatric diseases: the end of the beginning? *Nature Reviews Drug Discovery*, 11, 462–78.

Griesinger W (1867). *Mental Pathology and Therapeutics*, 2nd edn. (transl. CL Robertson and J Rutherford). New Sydenham Society, London. p. 130.

Griffiths KM *et al.* (2014). Effectiveness of programs for reducing the stigma associated with mental disorders. A meta-analysis of randomized controlled trials. *World Psychiatry*, 2, 161–75.

Grote NK *et al.* (2010). A meta-analysis of depression during pregnancy and the risk of preterm birth, low birth weight and intrauterine growth restriction. *Archives of General Psychiatry*, 67, 1012–24.

Groves JO (2007). Is it time to reassess the BNDF hypothesis of depression? *Molecular Psychiatry*, 12, 1079–88.

Gudjonsson GH (1992). *The Psychology of Interrogations, Confessions and Testimony*. John Wiley & Sons, Chichester.

Gunderson JG and Links PL (2014). *Handbook of Good Psychiatric Management (GPM) for Borderline Patients*. American Psychiatric Press, Washington DC.

Gunillo P *et al.* (2015). Does tobacco use cause psychosis? Systematic review and meta-analysis. *Lancet Psychiatry*, 2, 718–25.

Gunn J and Taylor P (2014). *Forensic Psychiatry*, 2nd edn. Hodder Arnold, London.

Gunnell D *et al.* (1995). Relation between parasuicide, suicide, psychiatric admissions, and socioeconomic deprivation. *British Medical Journal*, 311, 226–30.

Gunnell D, Saperia J and Ashby D (2005). Selective serotonin reuptake inhibitors (SSRIs) and suicide in adults: meta-analysis of drug company data from placebo-controlled, randomized controlled trials submitted to the MHRRA's safety review. *British Medical Journal*, 330, 385.

Guralnick MJ (2005). Early intervention for children with intellectual disabilities: Current knowledge and future prospects. *Journal of Applied Research in Intellectual Disabilities*, **18**, 313–24.

Guralnick MJ (2016). Early intervention for children with intellectual disabilities: An update. *Journal of Applied Research in Intellectual Disabilities*. doi:10.1111/jar.12233.

Gureje O *et al.* (1997). Somatization in cross-cultural perspective: a World Health Organization study in primary care. *American Journal of Psychiatry*, **154**, 989–95.

Gureje O *et al.* (1998). Persistent pain and well-being: a World Health Organization Study in Primary Care. *Journal of the American Medical Association*, **280**, 147–51.

Guthrie E (2008). Medically unexplained symptoms in primary care. *Advances in Psychiatric Treatment*, **14**, 432–40.

Guthrie E *et al.* (2001). Randomised controlled trial of brief psychological intervention after deliberate self-poisoning. *British Medical Journal*, **323**, 135–8.

Guy W (1976). *Clinical Global Impressions (CGI). ECDEU Assessment Manual for Psychopharmacology (revised)*. US Department of Health, Education and Welfare, NIMH, Rockville, MD.

Guze S (1989). Biological psychiatry: is there any other kind? *Psychological Medicine*, **19**, 315–23.

Guzzetta F and de Girolamo G (2009). Epidemiology of personality disorders. In: M Gelder *et al.* (eds.) *New Oxford Textbook of Psychiatry*, 2nd edn. Oxford University Press, Oxford. pp. 881–6.

Hachinski V, Lassen NA and Marshall J (1974). Multi-infarct dementia. *Lancet*, **ii**, 207–9.

Hackman A *et al.* (2011). *Oxford Guide to Imagery in Cognitive Therapy*. Oxford University Press, Oxford.

Haddad PM and Anderson IM (2007). Recognising and managing antidepressant discontinuation symptoms. *Advances in Psychiatric Treatment*, **13**, 44–57.

Haggarty SJ and Perlis RH (2014). Translation: Screening for novel therapeutics with disease-relevant cell types derived from human stem cell models. *Biological Psychiatry*, **75**, 952–60.

Hajima SV *et al.* (2013). Brain volumes in schizophrenia: a meta-analysis in over 18,000 subjects. *Schizophrenia Bulletin*, **39**, 1129–38.

Hale B *et al.* (2015). Legal issues in the care and treatment of children with mental health problems. In: A. Thapar *et al.* (eds). *Rutter's Child and Adolescent Psychiatry*. John Wiley & Sons, Chichester, pp. 239–49.

Hales SA, Abbey SE and Rodin GM (2009). Psychiatric aspects of surgery (including transplantation). In: MG Gelder, NC Andreasen, JJ López-IborJr and JR Geddes (eds.) *New Oxford Textbook of Psychiatry*. Oxford University Press, Oxford. pp. 1096–9.

Halford J and Brown T (2009). Cognitive behavioural therapy as an adjunctive treatment in chronic physical illness. *Advances in Psychiatric Treatment*, **15**, 306–17.

Hall J *et al.* (2015). Genetic risk for schizophrenia: convergence on synaptic pathways involved in plasticity. *Biological Psychiatry*, **77**, 52–8.

Hall W (2015). What has research over the past two decades revealed about the adverse health effects of recreational cannabis use? *Addiction*, **110**, 19–35.

Hall W and Degenhardt L (2011). Cannabis and the increased incidence and persistence of psychosis. *British Medical Journal*, **342**, 511–12.

Hallahan B *et al.* (2011). Structural magnetic resonance imaging in bipolar disorder: An international collaborative mega-analysis of individual adult patient data. *Biological Psychiatry*, **69**, 326–35.

Hamburg DA *et al.* (1953). Clinical importance of emotional problems in the care of patients with burns. *New England Journal of Medicine*, **248**, 355–9.

Hamilton CE, Falshaw L and Browne KD (2002). The link between recurrent maltreatment and offending behaviour. *International Journal of Offender Therapy and Comparative Criminology*, **46**, 75–94.

Hamilton M (1959). The assessment of anxiety states by rating. *British Journal of Medical Psychology*, **32**, 50–5.

Hamilton M (1967). Development of a rating scale for primary depressive illness. *British Journal of Social and Clinical Psychology*, **6**, 278–96.

Hanlon C *et al.* (2015). District mental healthcare plans for five low- and middle-income countries: commonalities, variations and evidence gaps. *British Journal of Psychiatry*, s1–s8. doi: 10.1192/bjp.bp.114.153767.

Hanly JG (2014). Diagnosis and management of neuropsychiatric SLE. *Nature Reviews Immunology*, **10**, 338–47.

Hardy J and Revesz T (2012). The spread of neurodegenerative disease. *New England Journal of Medicine*, **366**, 2126–8.

Hardy JA and Higgins GA (1992). Alzheimer's disease: the amyloid cascade hypothesis. *Science*, **256**, 184–5.

Hare EH (1973). A short note on pseudo-hallucinations. *British Journal of Psychiatry*, **122**, 469–73.

Hare RD (1983). Diagnosis of antisocial personality in two prison populations. *American Journal of Psychiatry*, **140**, 887–90.

Hare RD (1991). *The Psychopathy Checklist-Revised (PCL-R)*. Multi-Health Systems, Toronto.

Harmer CJ *et al.* (2009). Why do antidepressants take so long to work? A cognitive neuropsychological model of antidepressant drug action. *British Journal of Psychiatry*, **195**, 102–8.

Harris AM *et al.* (2009). Somatization increases disability independent of comorbidity. *Journal of General Internal Medicine*, **24**(2), 155–61.

Harris EC and Barraclough B (1997). Suicide as an outcome for mental disorders: a meta-analysis. *British Journal of Psychiatry*, **170**, 205–28.

Harris EC and Barraclough B (1998). Excess mortality of mental disorder. *British Journal of Psychiatry*, **173**, 11–53.

Harris JC (2014). New classification for neurodevelopmental disorders in DSM-5. *Current Opinion in Psychiatry*, **27**, 95–7.

Harrison G *et al.* (2001). Recovery from psychotic illness: a 15- and 25-year international follow-up study. *British Journal of Psychiatry*, **178**, 506–17.

Harrison G *et al.* (1994). Residence of incident cohort of psychotic patients after 13 years of follow-up. *British Medical Journal*, **308**, 813–19.

Harrison JR and Owen MJ (2016). Alzheimer's disease: the amyloid hypothesis on trial. *British Journal of Psychiatry*, **208**, 1–3.

Harrison NA and Kopelman MD (2009). Endocrine diseases and metabolic disorders. In: David A, Fleminger S and Kopelman M *et al.* (eds.) *Lishman's Organic Psychiatry*. Wiley Blackwell, Oxford. pp. 617–88.

Harrison PJ (1999). The neuropathology of schizophrenia. A criticial review of the data and their interpretation. *Brain*, **122**, 593–624.

Harrison PJ (2004). The hippocampus in schizophrenia: a review of the neuropathological evidence and its pathophysiological implications. *Psychopharmacology,* **174**, 151–62.

Harrison PJ (2015a). Recent genetic findings in schizophrenia and their therapeutic relevance. *Journal of Psychopharmacology,* **29**, 85–96.

Harrison PJ (2015b). The current and potential impact of genetics and genomics on neuropsychopharmacgoloy. *European Neuropsychopharmacology,* **25**, 671–81.

Harrison PJ (2016). Molecular neurobiological clues to the pathogenesis of bipolar disorder. *Current Opinion in Neurobiology,* **36**, 1–6.

Harrison PL and Oakland T (2000). *Adaptive Behavior Assessment System*. San Antonio, TX, The Psychological Corporation.

Hart AB and Kranzler HR (2015). Alcohol dependence genetics: lessons learned from genome-wide association studies (GWAS) and post-GWAS analyses. *Alcoholism: Clinical and Experimental Research,* **39**, 1312–27.

Hart H *et al.* (2014). Pattern classification of response inhibition in ADHD: Toward the development of neurobiological markers for ADHD. *Human Brain Mapping,* **35**, 3083–94.

Harvey AG *et al.* (2015). Sleep interventions: a developmental perspective. In: A. Thapar *et al.* (eds). *Rutter's Child and Adolescent Psychiatry.* John Wiley & Sons, Chichester, pp. 999–1015.

Harvey SB and Wessely S (2009). Chronic fatigue syndrome: identifying zebras amongst the horses. *BMC Medicine,* **7**, 58.

Harwood D and Jacoby R (2000). Suicidal behaviour among the elderly. In: K Hawton and K van Heeringen (eds.) *The International Handbook of Suicide and Attempted Suicide*. John Wiley & Sons, Chichester. pp. 275–92.

Harwood D *et al.* (2000). Suicide in older people: mode of death, demographic factors, and medical contact before death. *International Journal of Geriatric Psychiatry,* **15**, 736–43.

Harwood D *et al.* (2001). Psychiatric disorder and personality factors associated with suicide in older people: a descriptive and case-control study. *International Journal of Geriatric Psychiatry,* **16**, 155–65.

Harwood D *et al.* (2006). Life problems and physical illness as risk factors for suicide in older people: a descriptive and case-control study. *Psychological Medicine,* **36**, 1265–74.

Hasler G *et al.* (2008). Altered cerebral γ-aminobutyric acid type a-benzodiazepine receptor binding in panic disorder determined by [^{11}C]flumazenil positron emission tomography. *Archives of General Psychiatry,* **65**, 1166–75.

Hassan L *et al.* (2011). Prospective cohort study of mental health during imprisonment. *British Journal of Psychiatry,* **198**, 37–42.

Haw C *et al.* (2001). Psychiatric and personality disorders in deliberate self-harm patients. *British Journal of Psychiatry,* **178**, 48–54.

Hawton K (2000). General hospital management of suicide attempters. In: K Hawton and K van Heeringen (eds.) *The International Handbook of Suicide and Attempted Suicide*. John Wiley & Sons, Chichester. pp. 519–38.

Hawton K (ed.) (2005). *Prevention and Treatment of Suicidal Behaviour: From science to practice*. Oxford University Press, Oxford.

Hawton K (2012). Self-harm and suicide in adolescents. *Lancet,* **379**, 2373–82.

Hawton K and van Heeringen K (2009). Suicide. *Lancet,* **373**, 1372–81.

Hawton K, Houston K and Shepherd R (1999). Suicide in young people: study of 174 cases, aged under 25 years, based on coroner's and medical records. *British Journal of Psychiatry,* **175**, 271–4.

Hawton K *et al.* (2000). Doctors who kill themselves: a study of the methods used for suicide. *Quarterly Journal of Medicine,* **93**, 351–7.

Hawton K *et al.* (2001). Suicide in doctors: a study of risk according to gender, seniority and specialty in medical practitioners in England and Wales, 1979–1995. *Journal of Epidemiology & Community Health,* **55**, 296–300.

Hawton K *et al.* (2001). The influence of economic and social environment on deliberate self-harm and suicide: an ecological and person-based study. *Psychological Medicine,* **31**, 827–36.

Hawton K *et al.* (2002). Deliberate self-harm among adolescents: self-report survey in schools in England. *British Medical Journal,* **325**, 1207–11.

Hawton K, Zahl D and Weatherall R (2003a). Suicide following deliberate self-harm; long-term follow-up of patients who presented to a general hospital. *British Journal of Psychiatry,* **182**, 537–42.

Hawton K *et al.* (2003b). Deliberate self-harm in Oxford, 1990–2000: a time of change in patient characteristics. *Psychological Medicine,* **33**, 987–95.

Hawton K *et al.* (2003c). Deliberate self-harm in adolescents: a study of characteristics and trends in Oxford, 1990–2000. *Journal of Child Psychology and Psychiatry,* **44**, 1191–8.

Hawton K, Malmberg A and Simkin S (2004a). Suicide in doctors: a psychological autopsy study. *Journal of Psychosomatic Research,* **57**, 1–4.

Hawton K *et al.* (2004b). UK legislation on analgesic packs: before and after study of long-term effects on poisonings. *British Medical Journal,* **329**, 1076–9.

Hawton K *et al.* (2004c). Self-cutting: patient characteristics compared with self-poisoners. *Suicide and Life-Threatening Behaviour,* **34**, 199–207.

Hawton K *et al.* (2007). Self-harm in England: a tale of three cities. Multicentre study of self-harm. *Social Psychiatry and Psychiatric Epidemiology,* **42**, 513–21.

Hawton K, Bergen H and Simkin S (2010). Toxicity of antidepressants: rates of suicide relative to prescribing and non-fatal overdose. *British Journal of Psychiatry,* **196**, 354–8.

Hawton K *et al.* (2012). Self-harm and suicide in adolescents. *Lancet,* **379**, 2373–82.

Hay P *et al.* (2014). Royal Australian and New Zealand College of Psychiatrists clinical practice guidelines for the treatment of eating disorders. *Australian and New Zealand Journal of Psychiatry,* **48**, 977–1008.

Hay PJ (2009). Post-partum psychosis: Which women are at highest risk? *PLoS Medicine,* **6**, e1000027, 130–1.

Hay PJ *et al.* (1993). Treatment of obsessive-compulsive disorder by psychosurgery. *Acta Psychiatrica Scandinavica,* **87**, 197–207.

Hay P *et al.* (2012). Treatment for severe and enduring anorexia nervosa: a review. *Australian and New Zealand Journal of Psychiatry,* **46**, 1136–44.

Hay P (2013). A systematic review of evidence for psychological treatments in eating disorders 2005–2012. *International Journal of Eating Disorders,* **46**, 46–69.

Haynes B (1999). Can it work? Does it work? Is it worth it? *British Medical Journal*, **319**, 652–3.

Health and Social Care Information Centre (2015). Statistics on alcohol. http://www.hscic.gov.uk/catalogue/PUB17712/alc-eng-2015-rep.pdf

Hecker E (1871). Die Hebephrenie. *Virchows Archiv für Pathologie and Anatomie*, **52**, 394–429.

Hegarty JD *et al.* (1994). One hundred years of schizophrenia: a meta-analysis of the outcome literature. *American Journal of Psychiatry*, **151**, 1409–16.

Hegeman JM *et al.* (2012). Phenomenology of depression in older compared with younger adults: meta-analysis. *British Journal of Psychiatry*, **200**, 275–81.

Heijnen WT *et al.* (2010). Antidepressant pharmacotherapy failure and response to subsequent electroconvulsive therapy: a meta-analysis. *Journal of Clinical Psychopharmacology*, **30**, 616–19.

Heiman JR (2002). Psychological treatments for female sexual dysfunction: are they effective and do we need them? *Archives of Sexual Behavior*, **31**, 445–50.

Heinrich TW and Marcangelo M (2009). Psychiatric issues in solid organ transplantation. *Harvard Review of Psychiatry*, **17**, 398–496.

Hejl A, Hogh P and Waldemar G (2002). Potentially reversible conditions in 1000 consecutive memory clinic patients. *Journal of Neurology, Neurosurgery and Psychiatry*, **73**, 390–4.

Helbig-Lang S *et al.* (2014). The role of safety behaviors in exposure-based treatment for panic disorder and agoraphobia: Associations to symptom severity, treatment course, and outcome. *Journal of Anxiety Disorders*, **28**, 836–44.

Helfer B *et al.* (2016). Efficacy and safety of antidepressants added to antipsychotics for schizophrenia: a systematic review and meta-analysis. *American Journal of Psychiatry*, **173**, 876–86.

Hem E *et al.* (2004). Suicide risk in cancer patients from 1960 to 1999. *Journal of Clinical Oncology*, **22**, 4209–16.

Hemmeter UM, Hemmeter-Spernal J and Krieg JC (2010). Sleep deprivation in depression. *Expert Review in Neurotherapeutics*, **10**, 1101–15.

Henderson C, Evans-Lacko S and Thornicroft G (2013). Mental illness stigma, help seeking, and public health programs. *American Journal of Public Health*, **103**, 777–80.

Henderson M and Mellers JDC (2009). Movement disorders. In: David A *et al.* (eds.) *Lishman's Organic Psychiatry*. Wiley Blackwell, Oxford. pp. 745–816.

Henderson S and Fratiglioni L (2009). The ageing population and the epidemiology of mental disorders among the elderly. In: Gelder MG, Andreasen NC, Lopez-Ibor JJ and Geddes JR (eds.) *New Oxford Textbook of Psychiatry*. Oxford University Press, Oxford. pp. 1517–23.

Hennegan JM *et al.* (2015). Contact with the baby following stillbirth and parental mental health and wellbeing: a systematic review. *BMJ Open*, **5**, e008616.

Heppner FL *et al.* (2015). Immune attack: the role of inflammation in Alzheimer disease. *Nature Reviews Neuroscience*, **16**, 358–72.

Hermans D *et al.* (2008). Autobiographical memory specificity and affect regulation: coping with a negative life event. *Depression and Anxiety*, **25**, 787–92

Heslop P *et al.* (2014). The Confidential Inquiry into premature deaths of people with intellectual disabilities in the UK: a population-based study. *Lancet*, **383**, 889–95.

Heston LL (1966). Psychiatric disorders in foster home reared children of schizophrenic mothers. *British Journal of Psychiatry*, **112**, 819–25.

Hettema JM (2008). What is the genetic relationship between anxiety and depression? *American Journal of Medical Genetics*, **148C**, 140–6.

Hettema JM *et al.* (2003). A twin study of the genetics of fear conditioning. *Archives of General Psychiatry*, **60**, 702–8.

Hettema JM, Prescott CA and Kendler KS (2004). Genetic and environmental sources of covariation between generalized anxiety disorder and neuroticism. *American Journal of Psychiatry*, **161**, 1581–7.

Hettema JM *et al.* (2005). The structure of genetic and environmental risk factors for anxiety disorders in men and women. *Archives of General Psychiatry*, **62**, 182–9.

Heussler HS (2016). Management of sleep disorders in neurodevelopmental disorders and genetic syndromes. *Current Opinion in Psychiatry*, **29**, 138–43.

Heylens G *et al.* (2012). Gender identity disorder in twins: A review of the case report literature. *Journal of Sexual Medicine*, **9**, 751–7.

Heylens G *et al.* (2014). Effects of different steps in gender reassignment therapy on psychopathology: a prospective study of persons with a gender identity disorder. *Journal of Sexual Medicine*, **11**, 119–26.

Heyman I *et al.* (2015). Brain disorders and psychopathology. In: A. Thapar *et al.* (eds). *Rutter's Child and Adolescent Psychiatry*. John Wiley & Sons, Chichester, pp. 389–402.

Hill J (2003). Early identification of individuals at risk for antisocial personality. *British Journal of Psychiatry*, **44**, S11–14.

Hill J *et al.* (2001). Child sexual abuse, poor parental care and adult depression: evidence for different mechanisms. *British Journal of Psychiatry*, **179**, 104–9.

Hill K *et al.* (2004). Hypofrontality in schizophrenia: a meta-analysis of functional imaging studies. *Acta Psychiatrica Scandinavica*, **110**, 243–56.

Hjelmeland H *et al.* (2002). Why people engage in parasuicide: a cross-cultural study of intentions. *Suicide and Life-Threatening Behaviour*, **32**, 380–93.

Hjorthoj C *et al.* (2015). Association between alcohol and substance use disorders and all-cause and cause-specific mortality in schizophrenia, bipolar disorder, and unipolar depression: a nationwide, prospective, register-based study. *Lancet Psychiatry*, **2**, 801–8.

Ho RCM *et al.* (2012). Neuropsychiatric aspects of carbon monoxide poisoning: diagnosis and management. *Advances in Psychiatric Treatment*, **18**, 94–101.

Hobbs M (2005). Brief dynamic psychotherapy. In: Bloch S (ed.) *An Introduction to the Psychotherapies*, 4th edn. Oxford University Press, Oxford.

Hodes GE *et al.* (2015). Neuroimmune mechanisms of depression. *Nature Neuroscience*, **18**, 1386–93.

Hodgins D C *et al.* (2011). Gambling disorders. *The Lancet*, **378**, 1874–84.

Holland AJ (2009). Classification, diagnosis, psychiatric assessment, and needs assessment. In: Gelder MG, Andreasen NC,

López-Ibor JJJr, and Geddes JR (eds.) *The New Oxford Textbook of Psychiatry*, 2nd edn. Oxford University Press, Oxford. pp. 1819–24.

Holland T, Clare IC and Mukhopadhyay T (2002). Prevalence of criminal offending by men and women with intellectual disability and the characteristics of offenders: implications for research and service development. *Journal of Intellectual Disability Research*, **46**, 6–20.

Hollingshead AB and Redlich FC (1958). *Social Class and Mental Illness: A community study*. John Wiley & Sons, New York.

Hollis C (2015). Schizophrenia in children and adolescents. *BJPsych Advances*, **21**, 333–41.

Holloway F, Oliver N, Collins E and Carson J (1995). Case management: a critical review of the outcome literature. *European Psychiatry*, **10**, 113–28.

Holmes J (2000). Object relations, attachment theory, self-psychology, and interpersonal psychoanalysis. In: MG Gelder, JJ López-IborJr and NC Andreasen (eds.) *The New Oxford Textbook of Psychiatry*. Oxford University Press, Oxford. pp. 306–12.

Holmes J *et al.* (2014). Effects of minimum unit pricing for alcohol on different income and socioeconomic groups: a modelling study. *The Lancet*, **383**, 1655–64.

Holmes T and Rahe RH (1967). The social adjustment rating scale. *Journal of Psychosomatic Research*, **11**, 213–18.

Holoyda BJ and Kellaher DC. (2016). The biological treatment of paraphilic disorders: an updated review. *Current Psychiatry Reports*, **18**, 1–7.

Holt RIG and Mitchell AJ (2015). Diabetes mellitus and severe mental illness: mechanisms and clinical implications. *Nature Reviews Endocrinology*, **11**, 79–89.

Holt RIG *et al.* (2014). NIDDK International Conference Report on Diabetes and Depression: current understanding and future directions. *Diabetes Care*, **37**, 2067–77.

Hookway C *et al.* (2015). Irritable bowel syndrome in adults in primary care: summary of updated NICE guidance. *British Medical Journal*, **350**, h701.

Hope T *et al.* (1999). Natural history of behavioural changes and psychiatric symptoms in Alzheimer's disease. A longitudinal study. *British Journal of Psychiatry*, **174**, 39–44.

Hope T, Savelescu J and Hendrick J (2008) *Medical Ethics and Law: The core curriculum*, 2nd edn. Churchill Livingstone, Edinburgh.

Hoppe C and Elger CE (2011). Depression in epilepsy: a critical review from a clinical perspective. *Nature Reviews Neurology*, **7**, 462–72.

Horwood J, Thomas K, Duffy L, Gunnell D, Hollis C, Lewis G, Thompson A, Wolke D, Zammitt S and Harrison G, (2008). 108–Frequency of psychosis-like symptoms in a non-clinical population of 12 year olds: Results from the Alspac Birth Cohort. *Schizophrenia Research*, **98**, 77–78.

Hotopf M (2004). Preventing somatization. *Psychological Medicine*, **34**, 195–8.

Hotopf MH, Noah N and Wessely S (1996). Chronic fatigue and psychiatric morbidity following viral meningitis: a controlled study. *Journal of Neurology, Neurosurgery and Psychiatry*, **60**, 504–9.

Hou RH *et al.* (2012). When a minor head injury results in enduring symptoms: a prospective investigation of risk factors for postconcussional syndrome after mild traumatic

brain injury. *Journal of Neurology, Neurosurgery and Psychiatry*, **83**, 217–23.

Hoult J (1986). Community care of the acutely mentally ill. *British Journal of Psychiatry*, **149**, 137–44.

Houston K, Hawton K and Shepperd R (2001). Suicide in young people aged 15–24: a psychological autopsy study. *Journal of Affective Disorders*, **63**, 159–70.

Howard LM *et al.* (2014a). Non-psychotic mental disorders in the perinatal period. *Lancet*, **384**, 1775–88.

Howard LM *et al.* (2014b). No health without perinatal mental health. *Lancet*, **384**, 1723–24.

Howard R *et al.* (1995). Magnetic resonance imaging volumetric measurements of the superior temporal gyrus, hippocampus, parahippocampal gyrus, frontal and temporal lobes in late paraphrenia. *Psychological Medicine*, **25**, 495–503.

Howard R *et al.* (2012). Donepezil and memantine for moderate-to-severe Alzheimer's disease. *New England Journal of Medicine*, **366**, 893–903.

Howe AS *et al.* (2016). Candidate genes in panic disorder: Meta-analyses of 23 common variants in major anxiogenic pathways. *Molecular Psychiatry*, **21**, 665–79.

Howell MJ (2012). Parasomnias: an updated review. *Neurotherapeutics*, **9**, 753–75.

Howes OD, Murray RM (2014). Schizophrenia: an integrated sociodevelopmental-cognitive model. *Lancet*, **383**, 1677–87.

Howes OD *et al.* (2012). The nature of dopamine dysfunction in schizophrenia and what this means for treatment. Meta-analysis of imaging studies. *Archives of General Psychiatry*, **69**, 776–86.

Howes OD *et al.* (2015). Glutamate and dopamine in schizophrenia: an update for the 21st century. *Journal of Psychopharmacology*, **29**, 97–115.

Howes OD *et al.* (2017) Treatment-resistant schizophrenia: treatment response and resistance in psychosis (TRRIP) working group consensus guidelines on diagnosis and terminology. *American Journal of Psychiatry* **174**, 216–229.

Howlett JR and Stein MB (2016). Prevention of trauma and stressor-related disorders: A review. *Neuropsychopharmacology*, **41**, 357–69.

Howlin P (2008). Special education. In: M Rutter *et al.* (eds.) *Child and Adolescent Psychiatry*, 5th edn. Blackwell, Oxford. pp. 1189–206.

Hoyer J *et al.* (2009). Worry exposure versus applied relaxation in the treatment of generalized anxiety disorder. *Psychotherapy and Psychosomatics*, **78**, 106–15.

Huang B *et al.* (2006). Race-ethnicity and the prevalence and co-occurrence of Diagnostic and Statistical Manual of Mental Disorders, Fourth Edition, alcohol and drug use disorders and Axis I and II disorders: United States, 2001 to 2002. *Comprehensive Psychiatry*, **47**, 252–7.

Huang Y *et al.* (2009). DSM-IV personality disorders in the WHO world mental health surveys. *British Journal of Psychiatry*, **195**, 46–53.

Huang CQ *et al.* (2010). Chronic diseases and risk of depression in old age: a meta-analysis of published literature. *Ageing Research Reviews*, **9**, 131–41.

Hubert J and Hollins S (2006). Men with severe learning disabilities and challenging behaviour in long-stay hospital care. *The British Journal of Psychiatry*, **188**(1), 70–4.

Hucker S (2009). Child molesters and other sex offenders. In: MG Gelder, NC Andreasen, JJ Lopez-Ibor, and J Geddes (eds.) *The New Oxford Textbook of Psychiatry*. Oxford University Press, Oxford, pp. 1960–5.

Hughes N (2012). Nobody made the connection: The prevalence of neurodisability in young people who offend. The Office of the Children's Commissioner, London. https://www.childrenscommissioner.gov.uk/sites/default/files/publications/Nobody%20made%20the%20connection.pdf

Huline-Dickens S (2013). The mental state examination. *Advances in Psychiatric Treatment*, **19**, 97–8.

Hulme C *et al.* (2015). Educational interventions for children's learning difficulties. In: A. Thapar *et al.* (eds). *Rutter's Child and Adolescent Psychiatry*. John Wiley & Sons, Chichester, pp. 533–44.

Hunt IM *et al.* (2009). Suicide in recently discharged psychiatric patients. *Psychological Medicine*, **39**, 443–9.

Hunter R and MacAlpine I (eds.) (1963). *Three Hundred Years of Psychiatry*. Oxford University Press, London.

Hurley TD and Edenberg HJ (2012). Genes encoding enzymes involved in ethanol metabolism. *Alcohol Research*, **34**, 339–44.

Huybrechts KF *et al.* (2014). Antidepressant use in pregnancy and the risk of cardiac defects. *New England Journal of Medicine*, **370**, 2397–407.

Huybrechts KF *et al.* (2015). Antidepressant use late in pregnancy and risk of persistent pulmonary hypertension of the newborn. *JAMA*, **313**, 2142–51.

Hwang SW and Burns T (2014). Health interventions for people who are homeless. *Lancet*, **384**, 1541–7.

Hyde TM and Ron MA (2011). The secondary schizophrenias. In: D Weinberger and PJ Harrison (eds.) *Schizophrenia*, 3rd edn. Wiley Blackwell, Oxford, pp. 165–84.

Hyman S (2007). Can neuroscience be integrated into the DSM-V? *Nature Reviews Neuroscience*, **8**, 725–32.

Iadecola C (2013). The pathobiology of vascular dementia. *Neuron*, **80**, 844–66.

Iivanainen M (2009). Epilepsy and epilepsy-related behavior disorders among people with intellectual disability. In: Gelder MG, Andreasen NC, López-Ibor JJJr, and Geddes JR (eds.) *The New Oxford Textbook of Psychiatry*, 2nd edn. Oxford University Press, Oxford. pp. 1860–70.

Ijzendoorn MH *et al.* (2015). Residential and foster care. In: A. Thapar *et al.* (eds). *Rutter's Child and Adolescent Psychiatry*. John Wiley & Sons, Chichester, pp. 261–72.

Imboden JB, Canter A and Cluff LE (1961). Convalescence from influenza: a study of the psychological and clinical determinants. *Archives of Internal Medicine*, **108**, 393–9.

Ingvar DH and Franzen G (1974). Anomalies of cerebral blood flow distribution in patients with chronic schizophrenia. *Acta Psychiatrica Scandinavica*, **50**, 425–62.

Inouye SK *et al.* (2014a). Delirium in elderly people. *Lancet*, **383**, 911–22.

Inouye SK *et al.* (2014b). Doing damage in delirium: the hazards of antipsychotic prescribing in elderly people. *Lancet Psychiatry*, **1**, 312–14.

Inskip HM, Harris EC and Barraclough B (1998). Lifetime risk of suicide for affective disorder, alcoholism and schizophrenia. *British Journal of Psychiatry*, **172**, 35–7.

Inter-Agency Standing Committee (2007). *IASC Guidelines on Mental Health and Psychosocial Support in Emergency Settings, 2007*. Geneva: IASC.

International League Against Epilepsy (1989). Commission on Classification and Terminology: proposal for revised classification of epilepsies and epileptic syndromes. *Epilepsia*, **30**, 389–99.

Iqbal K *et al.* (2016). Tau and neurodegenerative disease: the story so far. *Nature Reviews Neurology*, **12**, 15–27.

Irwin DJ *et al.* (2013). Parkinson's disease dementia: convergence of α-synuclein, tau and amyloid-β pathologies. *Nature Reviews Neuroscience*, **14**, 626–36.

Isaac MI and Paauw DS (2014). Medically unexplained symptoms. *Medical Clinics of North America*, **98**, 663–72.

Isacsson G *et al.* (2010). The increased use of antidepressants has contributed to the worldwide reduction in suicide rates. *British Journal of Psychiatry*, **196**, 429–33.

IsHak WW and Tobia G. (2013). DSM-5 changes in diagnostic criteria of sexual dysfunctions. *Reproductive System & Sexual Disorders*, **2**, 122.

Isomura K *et al.* (2015). Population-based, multi-generational family clustering study of social anxiety disorder and avoidant personality disorder. *Psychological Medicine*, **45**, 1581–9.

Ives R (2009). Disorders relating the use of volatile substances. In: Gelder MG, Andreason NC, Lopez-Ibor JJ, Geddes JR (eds.) *New Oxford Textbook of Psychiatry*. Oxford University Press, Oxford. pp. 502–6.

Iyegbe C *et al.* (2014). The emerging molecular architecture of schizophrenia, polygenic risk scores and the clinical implications for GxE research. *Social Psychiatry and Psychiatric Epidemiology*, **49**, 169–82.

Jaaskelainen E *et al.* (2013). A systematic review and meta-analysis of recovery in schizophrenia. *Schizophrenia Bulletin*, **39**, 1296–306.

Jablensky A (2016). Psychiatric classifications: validity and utility. *World Psychiatry*, **15**, 26–31.

Jablensky A *et al.* (1992). Schizophrenia: manifestations, incidence and course in different cultures: a World Health Organization 10-Country study. *Psychological Medicine. Monograph Supplement*, **20**, 1–97.

Jablensky A, Kirkbride JB and Jones PB (2011). Schizophrenia: the epidemiological horizon. In: D Weinberger and PJ Harrison (eds.) *Schizophrenia*, 3rd edn. Wiley Blackwell, Oxford. pp. 185–225.

Jack CR *et al.* (2013). Tracking pathophysiological processes in Alzheimer's disease: an updated hypothetical model of dynamic biomarkers. *Lancet Neurology*, **12**, 207–16.

Jacob A *et al.* (2004). Charles Bonnet syndrome—elderly people and visual hallucinations. *British Medical Journal*, **328**, 1552–4.

Jacobi F *et al.* (2004). Prevalence, co-morbidity and correlates of mental health disorders in the general population: results from the German Health Interview and Examination Survey (GHS). *Psychological Medicine*, **34**, 597–611.

Jacobs R and Barrenho E (2011). Impact of crisis resolution and home treatment teams on psychiatric admissions in England. *British Journal of Psychiatry*, **199**, 71–6.

Jacobson E (1938). *Progressive Relaxation*. Chicago University Press, Chicago.

Jacoby R (2009). Assessment of mental disorder in older patients. In: MG Gelder, NC Andreasen, JJ Lopez-Ibor and JR Geddes (eds.) *The New Oxford Textbook of Psychiatry*, 2nd edn. Oxford University Press, Oxford. pp. 1524–9.

Jaffee SR and Price TS (2007). Gene–environment correlations: a review of the evidence and implications for prevention of mental illness. *Molecular Psychiatry*, 12, 432–42.

Jäger M and Rössler W (2010). Enhancement of outpatient treatment adherence: Patients' perceptions of coercion, fairness and effectiveness. *Psychiatry Research*, 180, 48–53.

Jakubovski E et al. (2015). Systematic review and meta-analysis: dose-response relationship of selective serotonin re-uptake inhibitors in major depressive disorder. *American Journal of Psychiatry*, 173, 174–83.

James A et al. (2004). Attention deficit hyperactivity disorder and suicide: a review of possible associations. *Acta Psychiatrica Scandinavica*, 110, 408–15.

James A et al. (2015). Provision of intensive treatment: intensive outreach, day units, and in-patient units. In: A. Thapar et al. (eds). *Rutter's Child and Adolescent Psychiatry*. John Wiley & Sons, Chichester, pp. 648–60.

James AC et al. (2013). Cognitive behavioural therapy for anxiety disorders in children and adolescents. *Cochrane Database Systematic Reviews*, 6.

Janakiraman R and Benning T (2010). Attention-deficit hyperactivity disorder in adults. *Advances in Psychiatric Treatment*, 16(2),.96–104.

Jansen WJ et al. (2015). Prevalence of cerebral amyloid pathology in persons without dementia. A meta-analysis. *JAMA*, 313, 1924–38.

Jarde A et al. (2016). Neonatal outcomes in women with untreated antenatal depression compared with women without depression. A systematic review and meta-analysis. *JAMA Psychiatry*, 73, 826–37.

Jardri R et al. (2011). Cortical activations during auditory verbal hallucinations in schizophrenia. A coordinate-based meta-analysis. *American Journal of Psychiatry*, 168, 73–81.

Jaspers K (1913). *Allgemeine Psychopathologie*. Springer, Berlin.

Jaspers K (1963). *General Psychopathology* (translated from the 7th German edition by J Hoenig and MW Hamilton). Manchester University Press, Manchester.

Jaspers K (1968). The phenomenological approach in psychopathology. *British Journal of Psychiatry*, 114, 1313–23.

Jauhar S et al. (2014a). Cognitive-behavioural therapy for the symptoms of schizophrenia: systematic review and meta-analysis with examination of potential bias. *British Journal of Psychiatry*, 204, 20–9.

Jauhar S et al. (2014b). Alcohol and cognitive impairment. *Advances in Psychiatric Treatment*, 20, 304–13.

Javitt DC and Zukin SR (1991). Recent advances in the phencyclidine model of schizophrenia. *American Journal of Psychiatry*, 148, 1301–8.

Jay EL et al. (2014). Testing a neurobiological model of depersonalization disorder using repetitive transcranial magnetic stimulation. *Brain Stimulation*, 7, 252–9.

Jenkins J et al. (2015). Psychosocial adversity. In: A. Thapar et al. (eds). *Rutter's Child and Adolescent Psychiatry*. John Wiley & Sons, Chichester, pp. 330–40.

Jenkins R et al. (2005). Psychiatric and social aspects of suicidal behaviour in prisons. *Psychological Medicine*, 35, 257–69.

Ji WY et al. (2006). A twin study of personality disorder heritability. *Chinese Journal of Epidemiology*, 27, 137–41.

Jick H, Kaye JA and Jick SS (2004). Antidepressants and the risk of suicidal behaviours. *Journal of the American Medical Association*, 292, 338–43.

Jilek WG (2000). Traditional non-Western folk healing as relevant to psychiatry. In: MG Gelder, JJ López-IborJr and NC Andreasen (eds.) *The New Oxford Textbook of Psychiatry*. Oxford University Press, Oxford.

Johns A (2009). Offending, substance misuse, and mental disorder. In: MG Gelder, NC Andreasen, JJ Lopez-Ibor, and J Geddes (eds.) *The New Oxford Textbook of Psychiatry*. Oxford University Press, Oxford, pp. 1926–8.

Johnson AR et al. (2015). Postnatal depression among women availing maternal health services in a rural hospital in South India. *Pakistan Journal of Medical Sciences*, 31, 408.

Johnson J et al. (1999). Childhood maltreatment increases risk for personality disorders during early adulthood. *Archives of General Psychiatry*, 56, 600–6.

Johnson LA et al. (2013). Current 'legal highs'. *Journal of Emergency Medicine*, 44, 1108–15.

Johnson S et al. (2005). Randomised controlled trial of acute mental health care by a crisis resolution team: the north Islington crisis study. *British Medical Journal*, 331, 599.

Johnstone EC et al. (1976). Cerebral ventricular size and cognitive impairment in chronic schizophrenia. *Lancet*, ii, 924–6.

Johnstone EC, Macmillan JF and Crow TJ (1987). The occurrence of organic disease of possible or probable aetiological significance in a population of 268 cases of first episode schizophrenia. *Psychological Medicine*, 17, 371–9.

Joinson C et al. (2011). Timing of menarche and depressive symptoms in adolescent girls from a UK cohort. *British Journal of Psychiatry*, 198, 17–23.

Joinson C et al. (2015). Early childhood psychological factors and risk for bedwetting at school age in a UK cohort. *European Child & Adolescent Psychiatry*, 25, 519–28.

Jokinen J (2011). CSF 5-HIAA and exposure to and expression of interpersonal violence in suicide attempters. *Journal of Affective Disorders*, 132, 173–8.

Jonas DE et al. (2014). Pharmacotherapy for adults with alcohol use disorders in outpatient settings: a systematic review and meta-analysis. *JAMA*, 311, 1889–900.

Jonas RK et al. (2014). The 22q11.2 deletion syndrome as a window into complex neuropsychiatric disorders over the lifespan. *Biological Psychiatry*, 75, 351–60.

Jones DPH (2009). Assessment of parenting for the family court. *Psychiatry*, 8, 38–42.

Jones E and Wessely S (2003). "Forward psychiatry" in the military: Its origins and effectiveness. *Journal of Traumatic Stress*, 16, 411–19.

Jones, E and Wessely S (2014). "Battle for the mind: World War 1 and the birth of military psychiatry." *The Lancet*, 384, 1708–14.

Jones I et al. (2014). Bipolar disorder, affective psychosis, and schizophrenia in pregnancy and the post-partum period. *Lancet*, 384, 1789–99.

Jones K (1992). *A History of the Mental Health Services*. Routledge & Kegan Paul, London.

Jones M (1968). *Social Psychiatry in Practice*. Penguin Books, Harmondsworth.

Jones P et al. (1994). Child development risk factors for adult schizophrenia in the British 1946 birth cohort. *Lancet,* **344,** 1398–402.

Jones WR et al. (2012). Eating disorders: clinical features and the role of the general psychiatrist. *Advances in Psychiatric Treatment,* **18,** 34–43.

Josephs KA (2007). Capgras syndrome and its relationship to neurodegenerative disease. *Archives of Neurology,* **64,** 1762–6.

Joyce PR (2009). Epidemiology of mood disorders. In: MG Gelder, NC Andreasen, JJ Lopez-Ibor and JR Geddes (eds.) *New Oxford Textbook of Psychiatry.* Oxford University Press, Oxford. pp. 645–50.

Judd LL et al. (2002). The long-term natural history of the weekly symptomatic status of bipolar I disorder. *Archives of General Psychiatry,* **59,** 530–7.

Julian MM (2013). Age at adoption from institutional care as a window into the lasting effects of early experiences. *Clinical Child and Family Psychology Review,* **16**(2), 101–145.

Judge C et al. (2015). Gender dysphoria–prevalence and co-morbidities in an Irish adult population. *Neurological and Psychiatric Disorders in Endocrine Diseases,* **17,** 24.

Juruena FM et al. (2015). Early life stress in depressive patients: Role of glucocorticoid and mineralocorticoid receptors and of hypothalamic-pituitary-adrenal axis activity. *Current Pharmaceutical Design,* **21,** 1369–78.

Kader L and Pantelis C (2009). Ethical aspects of drug treatment. In: Bloch S and Green S (eds.) *Psychiatric Ethics.* Oxford University Press, Oxford. pp. 339–400.

Kahlbaum K (1863). *Die Gruppierung der Psychischen Krankheiten.* Kafemann, Danzig.

Kahn E (1928). Die psychopathischen Personlichkeiten. In: *Handbuch der Geisteskrankheiten,* Springer, Berlin. p. 227.

Kahn RS and Keefe RSE (2013). Schizophrenia is a cognitive illness. Time for a change in focus. *JAMA Psychiatry,* **70,** 1107–12.

Kahn RS and Sommer I (2015). The neurobiology and treatment of first-episode schizophrenia. *Molecular Psychiatry,* **20,** 84–97.

Kahn RS et al. (2015). Schizophrenia. *Nature Reviews Disease Primers,* **1,** 1–23.

Kaiser RH et al. (2015). Large-scale network dysfunction in major depressive disorder: A meta-analysis of resting-state functional connectivity. *JAMA Psychiatry,* **72,** 603–11.

Kakuma R et al. (2011). Human resources for mental health care: current situation and strategies for action. *Lancet,* **378,** 1654–63.

Kales HC et al. (2011) Trends in antipsychotic use in dementia 1999–2007. *Archives of General Psychiatry,* **68,** 190–7.

Kales HC et al. (2015). Assessment and management of behavioral and psychological symptoms of dementia. *British Medical Journal,* **250,** h369.

Kalia LV and Lang AE (2015). Parkinson's disease. *Lancet,* **386,** 896–912.

Kaltiala-Heino R (2009). Involuntary psychiatric treatment. *Nordic Journal of Psychiatry,* 50, 27–34 http://dx.doi.org/10.3109/08039489609081385

Kambeitz JP and Howes OD (2015). The serotonin transporter in depression: Meta-analysis of in vivo and post mortem findings and implications for understanding and treating depression. *Journal of Affective Disorders,* **186,** 358–66.

Kanaan RAA, Lepine JP and Wessely SC (2007). The association or otherwise of the functional somatic syndromes. *Psychosomatic Medicine,* **69,** 855–9.

Kandel DB et al. (2013). Epidemiology of substance use disorders. In: DS Charney, JD Buxbaum, P Sklaar, EJ Nestler (eds), *Neurobiology of Mental Illness,* Oxford University Press, Oxford, pp. 772–87.

Kandel ER (1998). A new intellectual framework for psychiatry. *American Journal of Psychiatry,* **155,** 457–69.

Kane J et al. (1988). Clozapine for the treatment-resistant schizophrenic. A double-blind comparison with chlorpromazine. *Archives of General Psychiatry,* **45,** 789–96.

Kane JC et al. (2014). Mental, neurological, and substance use problems among refugees in primary health care: analysis of the Health Information System in 90 refugee camps. *BMC Medicine,* **12,** 1.

Kane JM and Correll CU (2016). The role of clozapine in treatment-resistant schizophrenia. *JAMA Psychiatry,* **73,** 187–8.

Kanner AM (2016). Management of psychiatric and neurological comorbidities in epilepsy. *Nature Reviews Neurology,* **12,** 106–16.

Kanner L (1943). Autistic disturbance of affective contact. *Nervous Child,* **2,** 217–50.

Kapil V et al. (2014). Misuse of the γ-aminobutyric acid analogues baclofen, gabapentin and pregabalin in the UK. *British Journal of Clinical Pharmacology,* **78,** 190–1.

Kapur N and House A (1998). Against a high-risk strategy in the prevention of suicide. *Psychiatric Bulletin,* **22,** 534–6.

Kapur S (2003). Psychosis as a state of aberrant salience: a framework linking biology, phenomenology, and pharmacology in schizophrenia. *American Journal of Psychiatry,* **160,** 13–23.

Kapur S, Zipursky RB and Remington G (1999). Clinical and theoretical implications of 5-HT$_2$ and D$_2$ receptor occupancy of clozapine, risperidone, and olanzapine in schizophrenia. *American Journal of Psychiatry,* **156,** 286–93.

Kapur S et al. (2005). Evidence for onset of antipsychotic effects within the first 24 hours of treatment. *American Journal of Psychiatry,* **162,** 939–46.

Karch CM and Goate AM (2015). Alzheimer's disease risk genes and mechanisms of disease pathogenesis. *Biological Psychiatry,* **77,** 43–51.

Karg K et al. (2011). The serotonin transporter promoter variant (5-HTTLPR), stress, and depression meta-analysis revisited. *Archives of General Psychiatry,* **68,** 444–54.

Kasanin J (1994). The acute schizoaffective psychoses. 1933. *American Journal of Psychiatry,* **151,** 144–54.

Kaski M (2009). Aetiology of intellectual disability: general issues and prevention. In: Gelder MG, Andreasen NC, López-Ibor JJJr and Geddes JR (eds.) *The New Oxford Textbook of Psychiatry,* 2nd edn. Oxford University Press, Oxford. pp. 1830–7.

Katerndahl DA (1993). Lifetime prevalence of panic states. *American Journal of Psychiatry,* **150,** 246–9.

Katon W et al. (1990). Distressed high utilizers of medical care: DSM-III-R diagnoses and treatment needs. *General Hospital Psychiatry,* **12,** 355–62.

Katon W, Lin EHB and Kroenke K (2007). The association of depression and anxiety with medical symptom burden in patients with chronic medical illness. *General Hospital Psychiatry,* **29,** 147–55.

Katon WJ (2003). Clinical and health services relationships between major depression, depressive symptoms, and general medical illness. *Biological Psychiatry*, **54**, 216–26.

Katsakou C *et al.* (2011). Why do some voluntary patients feel coerced into hospitalization? A mixed-methods study. *Psychiatry Research*, **187**, 275–82.

Kaufman DM, Milstein MJ (2017). *Kaufman's Clinical Neurology for Psychiatrists*, 8th edn. Elsevier, Amsterdam.

Kay DW *et al.* (1976). The differentiation of paranoid from affective psychoses by patients' premorbid characteristics. *British Journal of Psychiatry*, **129**, 207–15.

Kay DWK and Roth M (1961). Environmental and hereditary factors in the schizophrenias of old age ('late paraphrenia') and their bearing on the general problem of causation in schizophrenia. *Journal of Mental Science*, **107**, 649–86.

Kay DWK, Beamish P and Roth M (1964). Old age mental disorders in Newcastle-upon-Tyne: 1: a study in prevalence. *British Journal of Psychiatry*, **110**, 146–58.

Kay SR, Fiszbein A and Opler LA (1987). The Positive and Negative Syndrome Scale (PANSS) for schizophrenia. *Schizophrenia Bulletin*, **13**, 261–76.

Kaye C and Lingiah T (2000). *Culture and Ethnicity in Secure Psychiatric Practice: Working with difference.* Jessica Kingsley, London.

Kaye WH *et al.* (2013). Nothing tastes as good as skinny feels: the neurobiology of anorexia nervosa. *Trends in Neurosciences*, **36**, 110–20.

Keel P and Forney KJ (2013). Psychosocial risk factors for eating disorder. *International Journal of Eating Disorders*, **46**, 433–9.

Kehagia AA, Barker RA and Robbins TW (2010). Neuropsychological and clinical heterogeneity of cognitive impairment and dementia in patients with Parkinson's disease. *Lancet Neurology*, **9**, 1200–13.

Kelleher I *et al.* (2012). Prevalence of psychotic symptoms in childhood and adolescence: a systematic review and meta-analysis of population-based studies. *Psychological Medicine*, **42**, 1857–63.

Kellner CH *et al.* (2006). Continuation electroconvulsive therapy vs pharmacotherapy for relapse prevention in major depression: a multisite study from the Consortium for Research in Electroconvulsive Therapy (CORE). *Archives of General Psychiatry*, **63**, 1337–44.

Kellner CH *et al.* (2010). Bifrontal, bitemporal and right unilateral electrode placement in ECT: randomised trial. *British Journal of Psychiatry*, **196**, 226–34.

Kelly BD (2015). Best interests, mental capacity legislation and the UN Convention on the Rights of Persons with Disabilities. *BJPsych Advances*, **21**, 188–95.

Kelly C (2008). Memory clinics. *Psychiatry*, **7**, 61–3.

Kemner SM *et al.* (2015). The role of life events and psychological factors in the onset of first and recurrent mood episodes in bipolar offspring: Results from the Dutch Bipolar Offspring Study. *Psychological Medicine*, **45**, 2571–81.

Kendall T *et al.* (2013). Management of autism in children and young people: summary of NICE and SCIE guidance. *British Medical Journal*, **347**, f4865.

Kendell L *et al.* (2014). Crime and psychiatric disorders among youth in the US population: an analysis of the national comorbidity survey—adolescent supplement. *Journal of the American Academy of Child & Adolescent Psychiatry*, **53**, 888–98.

Kendell RE (1975). *The Role of Diagnosis in Psychiatry.* Blackwell, Oxford.

Kendler KS (1982). Demography of paranoid psychosis (delusional disorder). *Archives of General Psychiatry*, **39**, 890–902.

Kendler KS (1997). The diagnostic validity of melancholic major depression in a population-based sample of female twins. *Archives of General Psychiatry*, **54**, 299–304.

Kendler KS (2001). Twin studies of psychiatric illness—an update. *Archives of General Psychiatry*, **58**, 1005–14.

Kendler KS (2005). 'A gene for...': the nature of gene action in psyhiatric disorders. *American Journal of Psychiatry*, **162**, 1243–52.

Kendler KS and Walsh D (1995). Schizophreniform disorder, delusional disorder and psychotic disorder not otherwise specified: clinical features, outcome and familial psychopathology. *Acta Psychiatrica Scandinavica*, **91**, 370–8.

Kendler KS, Gruenberg AM and Strauss JS (1981). An independent analysis of the Copenhagen sample for the Danish adoption study of schizophrenia. The relationship between schizotypal personality disorder and schizophrenia. *Archives of General Psychiatry*, **38**, 982–7.

Kendler KS, Masterson CC and Davis KL (1985). Psychiatric illness in first-degree relatives of patients with paranoid psychosis, schizophrenia and medical illness. *British Journal of Psychiatry*, **47**, 524–31.

Kendler KS, Neale MC and Walsh D (1995). Evaluating the spectrum concept of schizophrenia in the Roscommon Family Study. *American Journal of Psychiatry*, **152**, 749–54.

Kendler KS *et al.* (2001). The genetic epidemiology of irrational fears and phobias in men. *Archives of General Psychiatry*, **58**, 257–65.

Kendler KS, Gardner CO and Prescott CA (2002). Toward a comprehensive developmental model for major depression in women. *American Journal of Psychiatry*, **159**, 1133–45.

Kendler KS *et al.* (2003). Life event dimensions of loss, humiliation, entrapment and danger in the prediction of onsets of major depression and generalized anxiety. *Archives of General Psychiatry*, **60**, 789–96.

Kendler KS, Kuhn J and Prescott CA (2004). The interrelationship of neuroticism, sex, and stressful life events in the prediction of episodes of major depression. *American Journal of Psychiatry*, **161**, 631–6.

Kendler KS *et al.* (2006). Dimensional representations of DSM-IV cluster A personality disorders in a population-based sample of Norwegian twins: a multivariate study. *Psychological Medicine*, **36**, 1583–91.

Kendler KS *et al.* (2007). The heritability of cluster A personality disorders assessed by both personal interview and questionnaire. *Psychological Medicine*, **37**, 655–65.

Kendler KS *et al.* (2013). Familial influences on conduct disorder reflect 2 genetic factors and 1 shared environmental factor. *JAMA Psychiatry*, **70**, 78–86.

Kendrick T, Burns T and Freeling P (1995). Randomised controlled trial of teaching general practitioners to carry out structured assessments of their long-term mentally ill patients. *British Medical Journal*, **311**, 93–8.

Kennedy N *et al.* (2004). Ethnic differences in first clinical presentation of bipolar disorder: Results from an epidemiological study. *Journal of Affective Disorders*, **83**, 161–8.

Kennedy Bergen R, Edleson JL and Renzetti CM (2005). *Violence against Women: Classic papers*. Pearson Education, Inc., Boston, MA.

Kenworthy T *et al.* (2004). *Psychological Interventions for those who have Sexually Offended or are at risk of Offending (Review)*. The Cochrane Collaboration, John Wiley & Sons, Chichester.

Keown P *et al.* (2011). Association between provision of mental illness beds and rate of involuntary admissions in the NHS in England 1988–2008: ecological study. *British Medical Journal*, **343**, d3736.

Kerkhof A (2000). Attempted suicide; patterns and trends. In: K Hawton and K van Heeringen (eds.) *The International Handbook of Suicide and Attempted Suicide*. John Wiley & Sons, Chichester. pp. 49–64.

Kernberg OF (1975). *Borderline Conditions and Pathological Narcissism*. Jason Aronson, New York.

Keshavan MS *et al.* (2014). Changes in the adolescent brain and the pathophysiology of psychotic disorders. *Lancet Psychiatry*, **1**, 549–58.

Kessing LV *et al.* (2015). Use of lithium and anticonvulsants and the rate of chronic kidney disease: a nationwide population-based study. *JAMA Psychiatry*, **72**, 1182–191.

Kessing LV *et al.* (2015). Causes of decreased life expectancy over the life span in bipolar disorder. *Journal of Affective Disorders*, **180**, 142–7.

Kessler RC, Zhao S and Katz SJ (1999). Past-year use of outpatient services for psychiatric problems in the National Comorbidity Survey. *American Journal of Psychiatry*, **156**, 115–23.

Kessler RC (2004). The epidemiology of dual diagnosis. *Biological Psychiatry*, **56**, 730–7.

Kessler RC *et al.* (2005a). Lifetime prevalence and age-of-onset distributions of DSM-IV disorders in the National Comorbidity Survey Replication. *Archives of General Psychiatry*, **62**, 593–602.

Kessler RC *et al.* (2005b). Prevalence, severity and comorbidity of 12-month DSM-IV disorders in the National Comorbidity Survey Replication. *Archives of General Psychiatry*, **62**, 617–27.

Kessler RC *et al.* (2005c) Lifetime prevalence and age-of-onset distributions of DSM-IV disorders in the National Comorbidity Survey replication. *Archives of General Psychiatry*, **62**, 593–602.

Kessler RC *et al.* (2012). Twelve-month and lifetime prevalence and lifetime morbid risk of anxiety and mood disorders in the United States. *International Journal of Methods in Psychiatric Research*, **21**, 169–84.

Kessler RC *et al.* (2013) The prevalence and correlates of binge eating disorder in the World Health Organization World Mental Health Surveys. *Biological Psychiatry*, **73**, 904–14.

Kety SS *et al.* (1994). Mental illness in the biological and adoptive relatives of schizophrenic adoptees. Replication of the Copenhagen Study in the rest of Denmark. *Archives of General Psychiatry*, **51**, 442–55.

Khandaker GM *et al.* (2011). A quantitative meta-analysis of population-based studies of premorbid intelligence and schizophrenia. *Schizophrenia Research*, **132**, 220–7.

Khandaker GM *et al.* (2013). Prenatal maternal infection, neurodevelopment and adult schizophrenia: a systematic review of population-based studies. *Psychological Medicine*, **43**, 239–57.

Khasraw M and Posner JB (2010). Neurological complications of systemic cancer. *Lancet Neurology*, **9**, 1214–27.

Kieling C *et al.* (2011). Child and adolescent mental health worldwide: evidence for action. *Lancet*, **378**, 1515–25.

Kilbourne EM *et al.* (1996). Tryptophan produced by Showa Denko and epidemic eosinophilic-myalgia syndrome. *Journal of Rheumatology*, **23**, 81–8.

Killaspy H *et al.* (2006). The REACT study: randomised evaluation of assertive community treatment in north London. *British Medical Journal*, **332**, 815–18.

Kiloh LG, Smith JS and Johnson GF (1988). *Physical Treatments in Psychiatry*. Blackwell Scientific Publications, Oxford.

Kilpatrick DG and Acierno R (2003). Mental health needs of crime victims: epidemiology and outcomes. *Journal of Traumatic Stress*, **16**, 119–32.

King-Hele S *et al.* (2009). Risk of stillbirth and neonatal death linked with maternal mental illness: a national cohort study. *Archives of Disease in Childhood*, **94**, F105–10.

Kipps CM and Hodges JR (2005). Cognitive assessment for clinicians. *Journal of Neurology, Neurosurgery and Psychiatry*, **76** (Suppl. 1), i22–30.

Kirkbride J *et al.* (2012a). Incidence of schizophrenia and other psychoses in England, 1950–2009: A systematic review and meta-analyses. *PLoS One*, **7**, e31660.

Kirkbride J *et al.* (2012b). Prenatal nutrition, epigenetics and schizophrenia risk: can we test causal effects? *Epigenomics*, **4**, 303–15.

Kirov G *et al.* (2015). What a psychiatrist needs to know about copy number variants. *Advances in Psychiatric Treatment*, **21**, 157–63.

Kisely SR and Goldberg DP (1996). Physical and psychiatric comorbidity in general practice. *British Journal of Psychiatry*, **169**, 236–42.

Kiser DP *et al.* (2015). Annual Research Review: The (epi) genetics of neurodevelopmental disorders in the era of whole-genome sequencing–unveiling the dark matter. *Journal of Child Psychology and Psychiatry*, **56**, 278–95.

Kishi T *et al.* (2012). Are antipsychotics effective for the treatment of anorexia nervosa? Results from a systematic review and meta-analysis. *Journal of Clinical Psychiatry*, **73**, 757–66.

Klein M (1952). Notes on some schizoid mechanisms. In: J Jacobs and J Riviere (eds.) *Developments in Psychoanalysis*. Hogarth Press, London. pp. 292–320.

Klein M (1964). Delineation of two drug-responsive anxiety syndromes. *Psychopharmacologia*, **5**, 397–408.

Klein RG *et al.* (2012). Clinical and functional outcome of childhood attention-deficit/hyperactivity disorder 33 years later. *Archives of General Psychiatry*, **69**, 1295–303.

Kleinman A (2009). Global mental health: a failure of humanity. *Lancet*, **374**, 603–4.

Kleinridders A *et al.* (2014). Insulin action in brain regulates systemic metabolism and brain function. *Diabetes*, **63**, 2232–43.

Klerman GL *et al.* (1984). *Interpersonal Psychotherapy of Depression*. Basic Books, New York.

Klerman GL *et al.* (1987). Efficacy of a brief psychosocial intervention for symptoms of stress and distress among patients in primary care. *Medical Care*, **25**, 1078–88.

Kliegman RM *et al.* (eds.)(2016). *Nelson Textbook of Pediatrics*, 20th edn. Elsevier, Philadelphia.

Knapp M *et al.* (1999). Private, voluntary or public? Comparative cost-effectiveness in community mental health care. *Policy and Politics*, **27**, 25–41.

Knappe S *et al.* (2012). Re-examining the differential familial liability of agoraphobia and panic disorder. *Depression and Anxiety*, **29**, 931–8.

Knight T *et al.* (2012). Prevalence of tic disorders: a systematic review and meta-analysis. *Pediatric Neurology*, **47**, 77–90.

Knott CS *et al.* (2015). All cause mortality and the case for age specific alcohol consumption guidelines: pooled analyses of up to 10 population based cohorts. *British Medical Journal*, **350**, h384.

Koch H *et al.* (2007). Demographic characteristics and quality of life of patients with unexplained complaints: a descriptive study in general practice. *Quality of Life Research*, **16**, 1483–9.

Koch JLA (1891). *Die Psychopathischen Minderwertigkeiter*. Dorn, Ravensburg.

Koenig HG and Blazer DG (1992). Epidemiology of geriatric affective disorders. *Clinics in Geriatric Medicine*, **8**, 235–51.

Koesters M *et al.* (2013). Agomelatine efficacy and acceptability revisited: systematic review and meta-analysis of published and unpublished randomised trials. *British Journal of Psychiatry*, **203**, 179–87.

Koning JPF *et al.* (2010). Dyskinesia and parkinsonism in antipsychotic-naive patients with schizophrenia, first-degree relatives and healthy controls: a meta-analysis. *Schizophrenia Bulletin*, **36**, 723–31.

Konrad N *et al.* (2015). Paraphilias. *Current Opinion in Psychiatry*, **28**, 440–4.

Koopmans GT, Donker MCH and Rutten FHH (2005). Length of hospital stay and health services use of medical inpatients with comorbid noncognitive mental disorders: a review of the literature. *General Hospital Psychiatry*, **27**, 44–56.

Kooyman I and Walsh E (2011). Societal outcomes in schizophrenia. In: D Weinberger and PJ Harrison (eds.) *Schizophrenia*, 3rd edn. Wiley Blackwell, Oxford. pp. 644–65.

Kotov R *et al.* (2013). Boundaries of schizoaffective disorder. Revisiting Kraepelin. *JAMA Psychiatry*, **70**, 1276–86.

Kowalski RM *et al.* (2014). Bullying in the digital age: A critical review and meta-analysis of cyberbullying research among youth. *Psychological Bulletin*, **140**, 1073.

Kozma A, Mansell J and Beadle-Brown J (2009). Outcomes in different residential settings for people with intellectual disability: a systematic review. *American Journal on Intellectual and Developmental Disabilities*, **114**, 193–222.

Kraepelin E (1904). *Clinical Psychiatry: A textbook for students and physicians*. Macmillan, New York.

Kraepelin E (1919). *Dementia Praecox and Paraphrenia*. Livingstone, Edinburgh.

Kraepelin E (1921). *Manic Depressive Insanity and Paranoia*. Livingstone, Edinburgh.

Kreitman N (1961). The reliability of psychiatric diagnosis. *Journal of Mental Science*, **107**, 876–86.

Kreitman N (1976). The coal gas story. United Kingdom suicide rates, 1960–71. *British Journal of Preventative and Social Medicine*, **30**, 86–93.

Kreitman N (ed.) (1977). *Parasuicide*. John Wiley & Sons, London.

Kretschmer E (1927). Der sensitive Beziehungswahn. Reprinted and translated as Chapter 8 in *Themes and Variations in European Psychiatry* (eds. SR Hirsch and M Shepherd). Wright, Bristol (1974).

Kril JJ and Harper CG (2012). Neuroanatomy and neuropathology associated with Korsakoff's syndrome. *Neuropsychology Review*, **22**, 72–80.

Kroenke K, Spitzer MD and Williams DSW (2001). The PHQ-9: validity of a brief depression severity measure. *Journal of General Internal Medicine*, **16**, 606–13.

Krstic D and Knuesel I (2013). Deciphering the mechanism underlying late-onset Alzheimer disease. *Nature Reviews Neurology*, **9**, 25–34.

Krupa T *et al.* (2005). How do people who receive assertive community treatment experience this service? *Psychiatric Rehabilitation Journal*, **29**, 18–24.

Kubler-Ross E (1969). *On Death and Dying*. Macmillan, New York.

Kuhn S and Gallinat J (2013). Resting-state brain activity in schizophrenia and major depression: a quantitative meta-analysis. *Schizophrenia Bulletin*, **39**, 358–65.

Kumari V and Postma P (2005). Nicotine use in schizophrenia: the self-medication hypotheses. *Neuroscience and Biobehavioral Reviews*, **29**, 1021–34.

Kumsta R, Kreppner J, Kennedy M, Knights N, Rutter M and Sonuga-Barke E (2015). Psychological consequences of early global deprivation. *European Psychologist*.

Kuyken W *et al.* (2015). Effectiveness and cost-effectiveness of mindfulness based cognitive therapy compared with maintenance antidepressant treatment in the prevention of depressive relapse of recurrence (PREVENT): A randomised controlled trial. *The Lancet*, **386**, 63–73.

Kvale G, Berggren U and Milgrom P (2004). Dental fear in adults: a meta-analysis of behavioural interventions. *Community Dentistry and Oral Epidemiology*, **32**, 250–64.

Lachs MS and Pillemer KA (2015). Elder abuse. *New England Journal of Medicine*, **373**, 1947–56.

Lally J *et al.* (2016). Augmentation of clozapine with electroconvulsive therapy in treatment resistant schizophrenia: A systematic review and meta-analysis. *Schizophrenia Research*, **171**, 215–24.

Lamontagne Y *et al.* (2000). Anxiety, significant losses, depression and irrational beliefs in first-offence shop-lifters. *Canadian Journal of Psychiatry*, **45**, 63–9.

Landi P *et al.* (2016). Insight in psychiatry and neurology: state of the art, and hypotheses. *Harvard Review of Psychiatry*, **24**, 214–28.

Landsberger SA *et al.* (2013). Assessment and treatment of deaf adults with psychiatric disorders: a review of the literature for practitioners. *Journal of Psychiatric Practice*, **19**, 87–97.

Langa KM and Levine DA (2014). The diagnosis and management of mild cognitive impairment. A clinical review. *JAMA*, **312**, 2551–61.

Langbaum JB *et al.* (2013). Ushering in the study and treatment of preclinical Alzheimer disease. *Nature Reviews Neurology*, **9**, 371–81.

Langdon R *et al.* (2014). The Fregoli delusion: A disorder of person identification and tracking. *Topics in Cognitive Science*, **6**, 615–31.

Lange J (1931). *Crime as Destiny* (transl. C Haldane). George Allen, London.

Langfeldt G (1961). The erotic jealousy syndrome. A clinical study. *Acta Psychiatrica Scandinavica*, **36** (Suppl. 151), 7–68.

Langguth B *et al.* (2013). Tinnitus: causes and management. *Lancet Neurology*, **12**, 920–30.

Långström *et al.* (2015). Sexual offending runs in families: A 37-year nationwide study. *International Journal of Epidemiology*, **44**, 713–20.

Large M *et al.* (2008). Homicide due to mental disorder in England and Wales over 50 years. *British Journal of Psychiatry*, **193**, 130–3.

Large M *et al.* (2011). Cannabis use and earlier onset of psychosis. *Archives of General Psychiatry*, **68**, 555–61.

Larsen ER *et al.* (2015). Use of psychotropic drugs during pregnancy and breast-feeding. *Acta Psychiatrica Scandinavica*, **445**, 1–28.

Lasègue C (1877). Les exhibitionnistes. *Union Medicale*, **23**, 709–14.

Lau JYF and Eley TC (2010). The genetics of mood disorders. *Annual Review of Clinical Psychology*, **6**, 313–37.

Laursen TM *et al.* (2014). Excess early mortality in schizophrenia. *Annual Review of Clinical Psychology*, **10**, 425–48.

Lawrence AA. (2010). Sexual orientation versus age of onset as bases for typologies (subtypes) for gender identity disorder in adolescents and adults. *Archives of Sexual Behavior*, **39**, 514–45.

Lawrie S *et al.* (2016a). Improving classification of psychoses. *Lancet Psychiatry*, **3**, 367–74.

Lawrie S *et al.* (2016b). Towards diagnostic markers for the psychoses. *Lancet Psychiatry*, **3**, 375–85.

Lazare A (1973). Hidden conceptual models in clinical psychiatry. *New England Journal of Medicine*, **288**, 345–51.

Leadership Alliance for the Care of Dying People (2014). *One Chance to get it Right: Improving people's experience of care in the last few days and hours of life.* LACDP.

Leckman JF *et al.* (2015). Clinical assessment and diagnostic formulation. In: A. Thapar *et al.* (eds). *Rutter's Child and Adolescent Psychiatry.* John Wiley & Sons, Chichester, pp. 403–18.

Le Couteur A *et al.* (2015). Autism spectrum disorder. In: A. Thapar *et al.* (eds). *Rutter's Child and Adolescent Psychiatry.* John Wiley & Sons, Chichester, pp. 661–82.

Lecrubier Y *et al.* (1997). The Mini International Neuropsychiatric Interview (MINI). A short diagnostic structured interview: Reliability and validity according to the CIDI. *European Psychiatry*, **12**, 224–31.

LeDoux J (1998). *The Emotional Brain.* Weidenfeld & Nicolson, London.

Lee RS *et al.* (2014). A meta-analysis of neuropsychological functioning in first-episode bipolar disorders. *Journal of Psychiatric Research*, **57**, 1–11.

Leentjens AFG *et al.* (2011). Psychosomatic medicine and consultation-liaison psychiatry: scope of practice, processes, and competencies for psychiatrists or psychosomatic medicine specialists: a consensus statement of the European Association of Consultation-Liaison Psychiatry and the Academy of Psychosomatic Medicine. *Psychosomatics*, **52**, 19–25.

Leff J (1993). All the homeless people—where do they all come from? *British Medical Journal*, **306**, 669–70.

Leff J *et al.* (1982). A controlled trial of social intervention in the families of schizophrenic patients. *British Journal of Psychiatry*, **141**, 121–34.

Leff J *et al.* (1985). A controlled trial of social intervention in the families of schizophrenic patients: two-year follow-up. *British Journal of Psychiatry*, **146**, 594–600.

Leggio L *et al.* (2009). Typologies of alcohol dependence: from Jellinek to genetics and beyond. *Neuropsychology Review*, **19**, 115–29.

Le Grange D *et al.* (2015). Randomized clinical trial of family-based treatment and cognitive-behavioral therapy for adolescent bulimia nervosa. *Journal of the American Academy of Child and Adolescent Psychiatry*, **54**, 886–94.

Lehmann SW (2003). Psychiatric disorders in older women. *International Review of Psychiatry*, **15**, 269–79.

Lehn A *et al.* (2016). Functional neurological disorders: mechanisms and treatment. *Journal of Neurology*, **263**, 611–20.

Lehrke R (1972). A theory of X-linkage of major intellectual traits. *American Journal of Mental Deficiency*, **76**, 611–19.

Leibenluft E *et al.* (2015). Bipolar disorder in childhood. In: A. Thapar *et al.* (eds). *Rutter's Child and Adolescent Psychiatry.* John Wiley & Sons, Chichester, pp. 858–73.

Lemoine P and Nava Z (2012). Prolonged-release formulation of melatonin (Circadin) for the treatment of insomnia. *Expert Opinion on Pharmacotherapy*, **13**, 895–905.

Lemoine P and Zisapel N (2012). Prolonged-release formulation of melatonin (Circadin) for the treatment of insomnia. *Expert Opinion on Pharmacotherapy*, **13**(6), 895–905.

Lennox B, Coles A and Vincent A (2012). Antibody-mediated encephalitis: a treatable cause of schizophrenia. *British Journal of Psychiatry*, **200**, 92–4.

Lennox B *et al.* (2017) Prevalence and clinical associations of neuronal cell surface antibodies in acute first episode psychosis: a cohort study. *Lancet Psychiatry*, **4**, 42–48.

Leonhard K (1957). *The Classification of Endogenous Psychoses*, 8th edn. (transl. R Berman). Irvington, New York.

Leonhard K, Korff I and Schultz H (1962). Die Temperamente und den Familien der monopolaren und bipolaren phasishen Psychosen. *Psychiatrie und Neurologie*, **143**, 416–34.

Lepping P, Russell I and Freudenmann RW (2007). Antipsychotic treatment of primary delusional parasitosis—systematic review. *British Journal of Psychiatry*, **191**, 198–205.

Lepping P, Baker C and Freudenmann RW (2010). Delusional infestation in dermatology in the UK: prevalence, treatment strategies, and feasibility of a randomized controlled trial. *Clinical and Experimental Dermatology*, **35**, 841–84.

Lesca G *et al.* (2013). GRIN2A mutations in acquired epileptic aphasia and related childhood focal epilepsies and encephalopathies with speech and language dysfunction. *Nature Genetics*, **45**, 1061–6.

Lesch KP *et al.* (1996). Association of anxiety-related traits with a polymorphism in the serotonin transporter gene regulatory region. *Science*, **274**, 1527–31.

Lester G *et al.* (2004). Unusually persistent complainants. *British Journal of Psychiatry*, **184**, 352–6.

Leucht S, Kissling W and McGrath J (2004). Lithium for schizophrenia revisited: a systematic review and meta-analysis of randomized controlled trials. *Journal of Clinical Psychiatry*, **65**, 177–86.

Leucht S *et al.* (2009). Second-generation versus first-generation antipsychotic drugs for schizophrenia: a meta-analysis. *Lancet*, **373**, 31–41.

Leucht S *et al.* (2012a). Putting the efficacy of psychiatric and general medicine medication into perspective: Review of meta-analyses. *British Journal of Psychiatry*, **200**, 97–106.

Leucht S *et al.* (2012b). Antipsychotic drugs versus placebo for relapse prevention in schizophrenia: a systematic review and meta-analysis. *Lancet, 379*, 2063–71.

Leucht S *et al.* (2013). Comparative efficacy and tolerability of 15 antipsychotic drugs in schizophrenia: a multiple-treatments meta-analysis. *Lancet, 382*, 951–62.

Leung CM, Chung WS and So EP (2002). Burning charcoal: an indigenous method of suicide in Hong Kong. *Journal of Clinical Psychiatry, 63*, 447–50.

Levin E (1997). Carers. In: R Jacoby and C Oppenheimer (eds.) *Psychiatry in the Elderly*. Oxford University Press, Oxford. pp. 392–402.

Levkovitz Y *et al.* (2011). Efficacy of antidepressant for dysthymia: A meta-analysis of placebo-controlled randomized trials. *Journal of Clinical Psychiatry, 72*, 509–14.

Lewis AJ (1934). Melancholia: a clinical survey of depressive states. *Journal of Mental Science, 80*, 277–8.

Lewis AJ (1936). Problems of obsessional neurosis. *Proceedings of the Royal Society of Medicine, 29*, 352–36.

Lewis AJ (1953). Health as a social concept. *British Journal of Sociology, 4*, 109–24.

Lewis AJ (1970). Paranoia and paranoid: a historical perspective. *Psychological Medicine, 1*, 2–12.

Lewis EO (1929). *Report on an Investigation into the Incidence of Mental Deficiency in Six Areas 1925–27*. HMSO, London.

Lewis G and Appleby L (1988). Personality disorder: the patients psychiatrists dislike. *British Journal of Psychiatry, 153*, 44–9.

Lewis G, Hawton K and Jones P (1997). Strategies for preventing suicide. *British Journal of Psychiatry, 171*, 351–4.

Lezak MD *et al.* (2012). *Neuropsychological Assessment*. 5th edn. Oxford University Press, New York.

Li M *et al.* (2016). Maltreatment in childhood substantially increases the risk of adult depression and anxiety in prospective cohort studies: Systematic review, meta-analysis, and proportional attributable fractions. *Psychological Medicine, 46*, 717–30.

Lichtenstein P *et al.* (2009). Common genetic determinants of schizophrenia and bipolar disorder in Swedish families: a population-based study. *Lancet, 373*, 234–9.

Licinio J and Wong M-L (2016). Serotonergic neurons derived from induced pluripotent stem cells (iPSCs): A new pathway for research on the biology and pharmacology of major depression. *Molecular Psychiatry, 21*, 1–2.

Liddle PF (1987). The symptoms of chronic schizophrenia. A re-examination of the positive–negative dichotomy. *British Journal of Psychiatry, 151*, 145–51.

Liddle PF (2013). Tardive dyskinesia in schizophrenia. *British Journal of Psychiatry, 203*, 6–7.

Liddle PF *et al.* (1992). Patterns of cerebral blood flow in schizophrenia. *British Journal of Psychiatry, 160*, 179–86.

Lieb K *et al.* (2004). Borderline personality disorder. *Lancet, 364*, 453–61.

Lieb K *et al.* (2010). Pharmacotherapy for borderline personality disorder. *British Journal of Psychiatry, 196*, 4–12.

Lievesley K *et al.* (2014). A review of the predisposing, precipitating and perpetuating factors in chronic fatigue syndrome in children and adolescents. *Clinical Psychology Review, 34*, 233–48.

Lin JJ *et al.* (2012). Uncovering the neurobehavioural comorbidities of epilepsy across the lifespan. *Lancet, 380*, 1180–92.

Linde K (2009). St John's Wort. *Forschende Komplementarmedizin, 16*, 146–55.

Linde K *et al.* (2005). St John's Wort for depression: meta-analysis of randomised controlled trials. *British Journal of Psychiatry, 186*, 99–107.

Lindesay J (2008) Neurotic disorders. In: R Jacoby, C Oppenheimer, T Dening and A Thomas (eds.) *The Oxford Textbook of Old Age Psychiatry*. Oxford University Press, Oxford. pp. 573–90.

Linehan MM (1993). *Cognitive-Behavioral Treatment of Borderline Personality Disorder*. Guilford, New York.

Linehan MM *et al.* (1991). Cognitive-behavioral treatment of chronically parasuicidal borderline patients. *Archives of General Psychiatry, 48*, 1060–4.

Linehan MM *et al.* (1994). Interpersonal outcome of cognitive behavioural treatment for chronically suicidal borderline patients. *American Journal of Psychiatry, 151*, 1771–6.

Lingford-Hughes A *et al.* (2010). Neuropharmacology of addiction and how it informs treatment. *British Medical Bulletin, 96*, 93–110.

Lingford-Hughes AR *et al.* (2012). BAP updated guidelines: evidence-based guidelines for the pharmacological management of substance abuse, harmful use, addiction and comorbidity: recommendations from BAP. *Journal of Psychopharmacology, 26*, 899–52.

Linnoila MI and Virkkunen M (1992). Aggression, suicidality and serotonin. *Journal of Clinical Psychiatry, 53*, 46–51.

Linschoten M *et al.* (2016). Sensate focus: a critical literature review. *Sexual and Relationship Therapy, 31*, 230–47.

Linscott RJ and van Os J (2013). An updated and conservative systematic review and meta-analysis of epidemiological evidence on psychotic experiences in children and adults: on the pathway from proneness to persistence to dimensional expression across mental disorders. *Psychological Medicine, 43*, 1133–49.

Linton SJ (2000). A review of psychological risk factors in back and neck pain. *Spine, 25*, 1148–56.

Lipowski ZJ (1988). Somatization: the concept and its clinical application. *American Journal of Psychiatry, 145*, 1358–68.

Litt MD *et al.* (2009). Momentary pain and coping in temporomandibular disorder pain: exploring mechanisms of cognitive behavioural treatment for chronic pain. *Pain, 145*, 160–8.

Littlewood R and Lipsedge M (1997). *Aliens and Alienists*, 3rd edn. Routledge, London.

Liu CC *et al.* (2013). Apolipoprotein E and Alzheimer disease: risk, mechanisms and therapy. *Nature Reviews Neurology, 9*, 106–18.

Livingston G *et al.* (2014a). Long-term clinical and cost-effectiveness of psychological intervention for family carers of people with dementia: a single-blind, randomised, controlled trial. *Lancet Psychiatry, 1*, 539–48.

Livingston G *et al.* (2014b). Non-pharmacological interventions for agitation in dementia: systematic review of randomized controlled trials. *British Journal of Psychiatry, 205*, 436–42.

Llaneza P *et al.* (2012). Depressive symptoms and the menopause transition. *Maturitas, 71*, 120–30.

Lock J (2015). An update on evidence-based psychosocial treatments for eating disorders in children and adolescents. *Journal of Clinical Child and Adolescent Psychology, 44*, 707–21.

Lodhi S and Agrawal N (2012). Neurocognitive problems in epilepsy. *Advances in Psychiatric Treatment,* **18**, 232–40.

Logue MW *et al.* (2015). The Psychiatric Genomics Consortium Posttraumatic Stress Disorder Workgroup: Posttraumatic stress disorder enters the age of large-scale genomic collaboration. *Neuropsychopharmacology,* **40**, 2287–97.

Lopresti AL and Drummond PD (2013). Obesity and psychiatric disorders: commonalities in dysregulated biological pathways and their implications for treatment. *Progress in Neuropsychopharmacology and Biological Psychiatry,* **45**, 92–9.

Loranger AW, Janca A and Sartorius N (eds.) (1997). *Assessment and Diagnosis of Personality Disorders: the ICD-10 International Personality Disorder Examination (IPDE).* Cambridge University Press, Cambridge.

Lovestone S (2009a). Dementia: Alzheimer's disease. In: Gelder MG, Andreasen NC, Lopez-Ibor JJJr and Geddes JR (eds) *New Oxford Textbook of Psychiatry.* Oxford University Press, Oxford. pp. 333–43.

Lovestone S (2009b). Other disorders of the nervous system. In: David A *et al.* (eds.) *Lishman's Organic Psychiatry.* Wiley Blackwell, Oxford. pp. 845–905.

Loy CT *et al.* (2014). Genetics of dementia. *Lancet,* **383**, 828–40.

Lu H, Yang Y, Liu P (2013). Brain imaging methodologies, 4th edn. In: Charney DS, Sklar P, Buxbaum JD and Nester EJ (eds.) *Neurobiology of Mental Illness.* Open University Press, New York. Ch. 15.

Lu H-C and Mackie K (2016). An introduction to the endogenous cannabinoid system. *Biological Psychiatry,* **79**, 516–25.

Lubke GH *et al.* (2014). Genome-wide analyses of borderline personality features. *Molecular Psychiatry,* **19**, 923–9.

Lubs HA *et al.* (2012). Fragile X and X-linked intellectual disability: four decades of discovery. *The American Journal of Human Genetics,* **90**, 579–90.

Luby JL *et al.* (2003). The clinical picture of depression in preschool children. *Journal of the American Academy of Child and Adolescent Psychiatry,* **42**, 340–8.

Luciano M (2014). Proposals for ICD-11: a report for WPA membership. *World Psychiatry,* **13**, 206–8.

Lund C *et al.* (2011). Poverty and mental disorders: breaking the cycle in low-income and middle-income countries. *Lancet,* **378**, 1502–14.

Lund C *et al.* (2016). Integration of mental health into primary care in low- and middle-income countries: the PRIME mental healthcare plans. *British Journal of Psychiatry,* **208**, s1–s3.

Luppa M *et al.* (2012). Age- and gender-specific prevalence of depression in latest-life—systematic review and meta-analysis. *Journal of Affective Disorders,* **136**, 212–21.

Lustyk MKB *et al.* (2009). Cognitive-behavioural therapy for premenstrual syndrome and premenstrual dysphoric disorder: a systematic review. *Archives of Women's Mental Health,* **12**, 85–96.

Luty J (2014). Drug and alcohol addiction: new challenges. *Advances in Psychiatric Treatment,* **20**, 413–21.

Luty J (2015a). Drug and alcohol addiction: do psychosocial treatments work? *Advances in Psychiatric Treatment,* **21**, 132–43.

Luty J (2015b). Drug and alcohol addiction: new pharmacotherapies. *Advances in Psychiatric Treatment,* **21**, 33–41.

Lyons MJ *et al.* (1995). Differential heritability of adult and juvenile antisocial traits. *Archives of General Psychiatry,* **52**, 906–15.

Lyst MJ and Bird A (2015). Rett syndrome: a complex disorder with simple roots. *Nature Reviews Genetics,* **16**, 261–75.

Mace C (2001). All in the mind? The history of hysterical conversion as a clinical concept. In: PW Halligan, C Bass and JC Marshall (eds.) *Contemporary Approaches to the Study of Hysteria: Clinical and theoretical perspectives.* Oxford University Press, Oxford.

Mackenzie IR *et al.* (2010). Nomenclature and nosology for neuropathologic subtypes of frontotemporal lobar degeneration: an update. *Acta Neuropathologica,* **119**, 1–4.

MacLeod R *et al.* (2013). Recommendations for the predictive genetic test in Huntington's disease. *Clinical Genetics,* **83**, 221–31.

Macritchie KA and Young AH (2004). Adverse syndromes associated with lithium. In: P Haddad, S Dursun and B Deakin (eds.) *Adverse Syndromes and Psychiatric Drugs.* Oxford University Press, New York. pp. 90–124.

Maden A (2007). Dangerous and severe personality disorder: antecedents and origins. *British Journal of Psychiatry,* **190**, 8–11.

Maercker A *et al.* (2008). Adjustment disorders, posttraumatic stress disorder and depressive disorders in old age: findings from a community survey. *Comprehensive Psychiatry,* **49**, 113–20.

Maes M *et al.* (2011). The new '5-HT' hypothesis of depression: cell-mediated immune activation induces indoleamine 2, 3-dioxygenase which leads to lower plasma tryptophan and an increased synthesis of detrimental tryptophan catabolites (TRYCATs), both of which contribute to the onset of depression. *Progress in Neuro-Psychopharmacology and Biological Psychiatry,* **35**, 702–21.

Maguire M *et al.* (2012). *The Oxford Handbook of Criminology,* 5th edn. Oxford University Press, Oxford.

Maher B (2008). The case of the missing heritability. *Nature,* **456**, 18–21.

Mahlios *et al.* (2013). The autoimmune basis of narcolepsy. *Current Opinion in Neurobiology,* **23**, 767–73.

Maiden NL *et al.* (2003). Quantifying the burden of emotional ill-health amongst patients referred to a specialist rheumatology service. *Rheumatology,* **42**, 750–7.

Maina G, Forner F and Bogetto F (2005). Randomized controlled trial comparing brief dynamic and supportive therapy with waiting list condition in minor depressive disorders. *Psychotherapy and Psychosomatics,* **74**, 43–50.

Maj M (2005). 'Psychiatric comorbidity': an artefact of current diagnostic systems? *British Journal of Psychiatry,* **186**, 182–4.

Malhi GS (2015). Antidepressants in bipolar depression: yes, no, maybe? Evidence-based. *Mental Health,* **18**, 100–2.

Malmberg A, Simkin S and Hawton K (1999). Suicide in farmers. *British Journal of Psychiatry,* **175**, 103–5.

Malt UF (2009). Psychiatric aspects of accidents, burns and other trauma. In: MG Gelder, NC Andreasen, JJ López-IborJr and JR Geddes (eds.) *The New Oxford Textbook of Psychiatry,* 2nd edn. Oxford University Press, Oxford, pp.1105–13.

Mandy W and Lai MC (2016). Annual Research Review: The role of the environment in the developmental psychopathology of autism spectrum condition. *Journal of Child Psychology and Psychiatry and Allied Disciplines,* **57**, 271–92.

Maniglio R. (2013). Prevalence of child sexual abuse among adults and youths with bipolar disorder: A systematic review. *Clinical Psychology Review,* **33**, 561–73.

Mann J *et al.* (2005). Suicide prevention strategies: a systematic review. *Journal of the American Medical Association, 294*, 2064–76.

Mann KF and Kiefer F (2009). Alcohol and psychiatric and physical disorders. In: Gelder MG, Andreason NC, Lopez-Ibor JJJr and Geddes JR (eds.) *New Oxford Textbook of Psychiatry*, 2nd edn. Oxford University Press, Oxford. pp. 442–7.

Manoranjitham SD *et al.* (2010). Risk factors for suicide in rural south India. *British Journal of Psychiatry, 196*, 26–30.

Manschreck TC and Khan NL (2006). Recent advances in the treatment of delusional disorder. *Canadian Journal of Psychiatry, 51*, 114–19.

Manu P *et al.* (2014). Markers of inflammation in schizophrenia: association vs. causation. *World Psychiatry, 13*, 189–92.

March JS and Vitiello B (2009). Clinical messages from the Treatment for Adolescents with Depression Study (TADS). *American Journal of Psychiatry, 166*, 1118–23.

Marcks BA *et al.* (2011). Longitudinal course of obsessive-compulsive disorder in patients with anxiety disorders: A 15-year prospective follow-up study. *Comprehensive Psychiatry, 52*, 670–7.

Marcus MD and Wildes JE (2009). Obesity: is it a mental disorder? *International Journal of Eating Disorders, 42*, 739–53.

Marder SR and Galderisi S (2017). The current conceptualization of negative symptoms in schizophrenia. *World Psychiatry, 16*, 14–24.

Margoshes BG and Webster BS (2000). Why do occupational injuries have different health outcomes? In: TG Mayer, RJ Gatchel and PB Polatin (eds.) *Occupational Musculoskeletal Disorders*. Lippincott, Williams & Wilkins, Philadelphia, PA.

Markowitsch HJ and Staniloiu A (2012). Amnesic disorders. *Lancet, 380*, 1429–40.

Markowitz JC (2003). Interpersonal psychotherapy for chronic depression. *Journal of Clinical Psychology, 59*, 847–58.

Marneros A *et al.* (2012). Delusional disorders—are they simply paranoid schizophrenia? *Schizophrenia Bulletin, 38*, 561–8.

Marques JK *et al.* (2005). Effects of a relapse prevention program on sexual recidivism: final results from California's Sex Offender Treatment and Evaluation Project (SOTEP). *Sexual Abuse: a Journal of Research and Treatment, 17*(1), 79–107.

Marshall EJ (2008). Doctors' health and fitness to practice: treating addicted doctors. *Occupational Medicine, 58*, 334–40.

Marshall M (2003). Acute psychiatric day hospitals. *British Medical Journal, 327*, 116–17.

Marshall M and Lockwood A (1998). Assertive community treatment for people with severe mental disorders. *Cochrane Database of Systematic Reviews*, Issue 2, CD001089.

Marshall M *et al.* (2003). Day hospital versus admission for acute psychiatric disorders. *Cochrane Database of Systematic Reviews*, Issue 1, CD004026. doi: 10.1002/14651858.CD004026.

Marshall WL and Marshall LE. (2015). Psychological treatment of the paraphilias: a review and an appraisal of effectiveness. *Current Psychiatry Reports, 17*, 1–6.

Marshall M, Gray A, Lockwood A and Green R (1997). Case management for severe mental disorders. *The Cochrane Collaboration*. doi: 10.1002/14651858.CD000050.

Marteau TM *et al.* (2009). Changing behaviour through state intervention. *British Medical Journal, 338*, b1415.

Mårtensson B *et al.* (2015). Bright white light therapy in depression: a critical review of the evidence. *Journal of Affective Disorders, 182*, 1–7.

Martin G *et al.* (2004). Correlates of firesetting in a community sample of young adolescents. *Australian and New Zealand Journal of Psychiatry, 38*, 148–54.

Martin J *et al.* (2015). The relative contribution of common and rare genetic variants to ADHD. *Translational Psychiatry, 5*, e506.

Masters WH and Johnson VE (1970). *Human Sexual Inadequacy*. Churchill, London.

Mataix-Cols D *et al.* (2010). Hoarding disorder: a new diagnosis for DSM-V? *Depression and Anxiety, 27*(6), 556–72.

Matson JL and Williams LW. (2013). Differential diagnosis and comorbidity: distinguishing autism from other mental health issues. *Neuropsychiatry, 3*, 233–43.

Matsunaga S *et al.* (2015a). Memantine monotherapy for Alzheimer's disease: a systematic review and meta-analysis. *PLoS One, 10*, 30123289.

Matsunaga S *et al.* (2015b). Combination therapy with cholinesterase inhibitors and memantine for Alzheimer's disease: a systematic review and meta-analysis. *International Journal of Neuropsychopharmacology, 18*, 5.

Mattheisen M *et al.* (2015). Genome-wide association study in obsessive-compulsive disorder: Results from the OCGAS. *Molecular Psychiatry, 20*, 337–44.

Matthews FE *et al.* (2013). A two-decade comparison of prevalence of dementia in individuals aged 65 years and older from three geographical areas of England: results of the Cognitive Function and Ageing Study I and II. *Lancet, 382*, 1405–12.

Matthews G and Deary IJ (2009). *Personality Traits*, 3rd edn. Cambridge University Press, Cambridge.

Maudsley H (1879). *The Pathology of the Mind*. Macmillan, London.

Maudsley H (1885). *Responsibility in Mental Disease*. Kegan Paul and Trench, London.

Maurer K, Volk S and Gerbaldo H (1997). Auguste D and Alzheimer's disease. *Lancet, 349*, 1546–9.

Maust DT *et al.* (2015). Antipsychotics, other psychotropics, and the risk of death in patients with dementia: number needed to harm. *JAMA Psychiatry, 72*, 438–45.

Mavridis D *et al.* (2015). A primer on network meta-analysis with emphasis on mental health. *Evidence Based Mental Health, 18*, 40–6.

May PA *et al.* (2014). Prevalence and characteristics of fetal alcohol spectrum disorders. *Pediatrics, 134*, 855–66.

Maynard BR *et al.* (2015). Treatment for school refusal among children and adolescents: A systematic review and meta-analysis. *Research on Social Work Practice*, doi: 10.1177/1049731515598619.

Mayou R (2014). Is the DSM-5 chapter on somatic symptom disorder any better than DSM-IV somatoform disorder? *British Journal of Psychiatry, 204*, 418–19.

Mayou R and Farmer A (2002). ABC of psychological medicine: functional somatic symptoms and syndromes. *British Medical Journal, 325*, 265–8.

Mayou RA, Ehlers A and Hobbs M (2000). Psychological debriefing for road traffic accident victims: three-year follow-up of a randomized controlled trial. *British Journal of Psychiatry, 176*, 589–93.

Mazure CM and Maciejewski PK (2003). A model of risk for major depression: effects of life stress and cognitive style vary by age. *Depression and Anxiety, 17*, 26–33.

McCartt AT, Hellinga LA and Kirley B (2010). The effects of minimum legal drinking age 21 laws on alcohol-related driving in the United States. *Journal of Safety Research*, **41**, 173–81.

McClellan J and Stock S. (2013). Practice parameter for the assessment and treatment of children and adolescents with schizophrenia. *Journal of the American Academy of Child & Adolescent Psychiatry*, **52**, 976–90.

McClure GMG (2000). Changes in suicide in England and Wales 1960–1997. *British Journal of Psychiatry*, **176**, 64–7.

McConnell D *et al.* (2014). Resilience in families raising children with disabilities and behavior problems. *Research in Developmental Disabilities*, **35**, 833–48.

McCool ME *et al.* (2016). Prevalence of female sexual dysfunction among premenopausal women: A systematic review and meta-analysis of observational studies. *Sexual Medicine Reviews*, **4**, 197–212.

McCutcheon P *et al.* (2015). Treatment resistant or resistant to treatment? Antipsychotic plasma levels in patients with poorly controlled psychotic symptoms. *Journal of Psychopharmacology*, **29**, 892–7.

McElroy S *et al.* (2012). Current pharmacotherapy options for bulimia nervosa and binge eating disorder. *Expert Opinion on Pharmacotherapy*, **13**, 2015–26.

McElroy S *et al.* (2015). Overview of the treatment of binge eating disorder. *CNS Spectrums*, **20**, 546–56.

McElroy SL and Keck PE (2009). Habit and impulse control disorder. In: MG Geder, NC Andreasen, JJ Lopez-Ibor, JR Geddes (eds). *New Oxford Textbook of Psychiatry*. Oxford University Press, Oxford, pp. 911–19.

McEvoy J (2016). *Supporting People with Intellectual Disabilities Experiencing Loss and Bereavement: Theory and Compassionate Practice*. Sue Read (ed.). Jessica Kingsley Publishers, London, 2014.

McGirr A *et al.* (2015). A systematic review and meta-analysis of randomized, double-blind placebo-controlled trials of ketamine in the rapid treatment of major depressive episodes. *Psychological Medicine*, **45**, 693–704.

McGorry PD (2015). Early intervention in psychosis: obvious, effective, overdue. *Journal of Nervous and Mental Disease*, **203**, 310–18.

McGrath J *et al.* (2008). Schizophrenia: a concise overview of incidence, prevalence, and mortality. *Epidemiologic Reviews*, **30**, 67–76.

McGrath JJ and Murray RM (2011). Environmental risk factors in schizophrenia. In: D Weinberger and PJ Harrison (eds.) *Schizophrenia*, 3rd edn. Wiley-Blackwell, Oxford. pp. 226–44.

McGuffin P and Thapar A (1992). The genetics of personality disorder. *British Journal of Psychiatry*, **160**, 12–23.

McGuire J (2008). A review of effective interventions for reducing aggression and violence. *Philosophical Transactions of the Royal Society B*, **363**, 2577–97.

McKeith IG *et al.* (2017). Diagnosis and management of dementia with Lewy bodies: fourth consensus report of the DLB Consortium. *Neurology*, **89**, 88–110.

McKenna PJ (1984). Disorders with overvalued ideas. *British Journal of Psychiatry*, **145**, 579–85.

McLaughlin KA *et al.* (2012). Childhood adversities and first onset of psychiatric disorders in a national sample of US adolescents. *Archives of General Psychiatry*, **69**, 1151–60.

McManus MA *et al.* (2013). Paraphilias: definition, diagnosis and treatment. *F1000prime Reports*, **5**, 36.

McManus S *et al.* (2009). *Adult Psychiatric Morbidity in England, 2007*. NHS Information Centre for Health and Social Care, Leeds.

McNally MR and Fremouw WJ. (2014). Examining risk of escalation: A critical review of the exhibitionistic behavior literature. *Aggression and Violent Behavior*, **19**, 474–85.

McShane R *et al.* (1997). Do neuroleptic drugs hasten cognitive decline in dementia? Prospective study with necropsy follow-up. *British Medical Journal*, **314**, 266–70.

Meadow R (1985). Management of Munchausen syndrome by proxy. *Archives of Disease in Childhood*, **60**, 385–93.

Mechanic D (1978). *Medical Sociology*, 2nd edn. Free Press, Glencoe, IL.

Medalia A, Saperstein AM (2013). Does cognitive remediation for schizophrenia improve functional outcomes? *Current Opinion in Psychiatry*, **26**, 151–7.

Medic G *et al.* (2013). Dosing frequency and adherence in chronic psychiatric disease: systematic review and meta-analysis. *Neuropsychiatric Disease and Treatment*, **9**, 1119–31.

Mefford HC *et al.* (2012). Genomics, intellectual disability, and autism. *New England Journal of Medicine*, **366**, 733–43.

Mehlum L *et al.* (1991). Personality disorders 2–5 years after treatment: a prospective follow-up study. *Acta Psychiatrica Scandinavica*, **84**, 72–7.

Mehta S *et al.* (2010). Risk of cerebrovascular adverse events in older adults using antipsychotic agents: a propensity-matched retrospective cohort study. *Journal of Clinical Psychiatry*, **71**, 689–98.

Meichenbaum DH (1977). *Cognitive-Behaviour Modification*. Plenum, New York.

Meijer A *et al.* (2011). Prognostic association of depression following myocardial infarction with mortality and cardiovascular events: a meta-analysis of 25 years of research. *General Hospital Psychiatry*, **33**, 203–16.

Meijer A *et al.* (2013). Adjusted prognostic association of depression following myocardial infarction with mortality and cardiovascular events: individual patient data meta-analysis. *British Journal of Psychiatry*, **203**, 90–102.

Meltzer H, Gatward R, Goodman R and Ford T (2000). *The Mental Health of Children and Adolescents in Great Britain*. HM Stationery Office.

Mellado-Calvo N and Fleminger S (2009). Cerebral tumours. In: David AS *et al.* (eds.) *Lishman's Organic Psychiatry*, 4th edn. Wiley Blackwell, Oxford. pp. 281–308.

Mellers JD (2009). Epilepsy. In: David AS *et al.* (eds.) *Lishman's Organic Psychiatry*, 4th edn. Wiley Blackwell, Oxford. pp. 309–95.

Meltzer H *et al.* (2008). Patterns of suicide by occupation in England and Wales: 2001–2005. *British Journal of Psychiatry*, **193**, 73–6.

Meltzer HY (2004). What's atypical about atypical antipsychotic drugs? *Current Opinion in Pharmacology*, **1**, 53–7.

Meltzer HY *et al.* (2003). Clozapine treatment for suicidality in schizophrenia: International Suicide Prevention Trial (InterSePT). *Archives of General Psychiatry*, **60**, 82–91.

Menon V (2011). Large-scale brain networks and psychopathology: a unifying triple network model. *Trends in Cognitive Sciences*, **15**, 483–506.

Mercer CH *et al.* (2003). Sexual function problems and help seeking behaviour in Britain: national probability sample survey. *British Medical Journal*, **327**, 426–7.

Merikangas KR *et al.* (2010). Lifetime prevalence of mental disorders in U.S. adolescents: results from the National Comorbidity Survey Replication—Adolescent Supplement (NCS-A). *Journal of the American Academy of Child & Adolescent Psychiatry*, **49**, 980–9.

Mersfelder TL and Nichols WH (2016). Gabapentin abuse, dependence, and withdrawal. *Annals of Pharmacotherapy*, **50**, 229–23.

Merskey H (2000). Conversion and dissociation. In: MG Gelder, JJ Lopez-IborJr and NC Andreasen (eds.) *The New Oxford Textbook of Psychiatry*. Oxford University Press, Oxford.

Merritt K *et al.* (2016). Nature of glutamate alterations in schizophrenia. A meta-analysis of proton magnetic resonance spectroscopy studies. *JAMA Psychiatry*, **73**, 665–74.

Mesholam-Gately R and Giuliano AJ (2009). Neurocognition in first-episode schizophrenia. A meta-analytic review. *Neuropsychology*, **23**, 315–36.

Mesulam MM (1998). From sensation to cognition. *Brain*, **121**, 1013–52.

Meyer IH (2013). Prejudice, social stress, and mental health in lesbian, gay, and bisexual populations: Conceptual issues and research evidence. *Psychological Bulletin*, **1**, 3–26.

Meyer JH (2013). Neurochemical imaging and depressive behaviours. In: Cowen PJ, Sharp T, Lau JYF (eds.) *Behavioral Neurobiology of Depression and Its Treatment*. Springer Berlin Heidelberg, pp. 101–34.

Meyer-Lindenberg A (2010). From maps to mechanisms through neuroimaging of schizophrenia. *Nature*, **468**, 194–202.

Mezey GC and Robbins I (2009). The impact of criminal victimization. In: Gelder M, Andreasen N, López-Ibor JJr and Geddes J (eds.) *The New Oxford Textbook of Psychiatry*, 2nd edn. Oxford University Press, Oxford. pp. 1984–90.

Miglis MG and Guilleminault C (2014). Kleine–Levin syndrome: a review. *Nature and Science of Sleep*, **6**, 19–26.

Milad MR and Rauch SL (2012). Obsessive-compulsive disorder: Beyond segregated cortico-striatal pathways. *Trends in Cognitive Sciences*, **16**, 43–51.

Miller B *et al.* (2011). Meta-analysis of paternal age and schizophrenia risk in male versus female offspring. *Schizophrenia Bulletin*, **37**, 1039–47.

Ministry of Justice (2015). *Youth Justice Statistics 2013/14, England and Wales*. London, UK.

Minuchin S, Rosman B and Baker L (1978). *Psychosomatic Families: Anorexia nervosa in context*. Harvard University Press, Cambridge, MA.

Minzenberg MJ *et al.* (2009). Meta-analysis of 41 functional neuroimaging studies of executive function in schizophrenia. *Archives of General Psychiatry*, **66**, 811–22.

Miresco MJ and Kirmayer LJ (2006). The persistence of mind–brain dualism in psychiatric reasoning about clinical scenarios. *American Journal of Psychiatry*, **163**, 913–18.

Mirra SS *et al.* (1991). The Consortium to Establish a Registry for Alzheimer's Disease (CERAD). Part II. Standardization of the neuropathologic assessment of Alzheimer's disease. *Neurology*, **41**, 479–86.

Mishara BL (2007). Prevention of deaths from intentional pesticide poisoning. *Crisis*, **28**, 10–20.

Mitchell AJ (2009). A meta-analysis of the accuracy of the Mini-Mental State Examination in the detection of dementia and mild cognitive impairment. *Journal of Psychiatric Research*, **43**, 411–31.

Mitchell AJ *et al.* (2011). Clinical recognition of dementia and cognitive impairment in primary care: a meta-analysis of physician accuracy. *Acta Psychiatrica Scandinavica*, **124**, 165–83.

Mitchell AJ *et al.* (2013). Is the prevalence of metabolic syndrome and metabolic abnormalities increased in early schizophrenia? A comparative meta-analysis of first episode, untreated and treated patients. *Schizophrenia Bulletin*, **39**, 295–305.

Mitchell AJ *et al.* (2014). Accuracy of one or two simple questions to identify alcohol-use disorder in primary care: a meta-analysis. *British Journal of General Practice*, **64**, e408–18.

Mitchell JE and Crow S (2006). Medical complications of anorexia nervosa and bulimia nervosa. *Current Opinion in Psychiatry*, **19**, 438–43.

Mitchell PB *et al.* (2011). Comparison of depressive episodes in bipolar disorder and in major depressive disorder within bipolar disorder pedigrees. *The British Journal of Psychiatry*, **199**, 303–9.

Mitchell SL *et al.* (2009). The clinical course of advanced dementia. *New England Journal of Medicine*, **361**, 1529–38.

Mittan RJ (2009). Psychosocial treatment programs in epilepsy: a review. *Epilepsy and Behavior*, **16**, 371–80.

Miura T *et al.* (2014). Comparative efficacy and tolerability of pharmacological treatments in the maintenance treatment of bipolar disorder: a systematic review and network meta-analysis. *Lancet Psychiatry*, **1**, 351–9.

Miyamoto S *et al.* (2015). Schizophrenia: when clozapine fails. *Current Opinion in Psychiatry*, **28**, 243–48.

Moberg PJ *et al.* (2014). Meta-analysis of olfactory function in schizophrenia, first-degree family members, and youths at-risk for psychosis. *Schizophrenia Bulletin*, **40**, 50–9.

Moberg T *et al.* (2011). CSF 5-HIAA and exposure to and expression of interpersonal violence in suicide attempters. *Journal of Affective Disorders*, **132**(1), 173–8.

Modrego PJ (2010) Depression in Alzheimer's disease. Pathophysiology, diagnosis, and treatment. *Journal of Alzheimer's Disease*, **21**, 1077–87.

Moeschler JB *et al.* (2014). Comprehensive evaluation of the child with intellectual disability or global developmental delays. *Pediatrics*, **134**, e903–e918.

Moestrup L and Hansen HP (2015). Existential concerns about death: A qualitative study of dying patients in a Danish hospice. *American Journal of Hospice and Palliative Medicine*, **32**, 427–36.

Mohatt J *et al.* (2014). Treatment of separation, generalized, and social anxiety disorders in youths. *American Journal of Psychiatry*, **171**, 741–8.

Moher D *et al.* (2009). Preferred reporting items for systematic reviews and meta-analyses: The PRISMA statement. *Annals of Internal Medicine*, **151**, 264–9.

Mollica RF, Culhane MA and Hovelson DH (2009). The special psychiatric problems of refugees. In: Gelder MG, Andreasen NC, López-Ibor JJJr and Geddes JR (eds.) *New Oxford Textbook of Psychiatry*, 2nd edn. Oxford University Press, Oxford. pp. 1493–549.

Monahan J (1997). Clinical and actuarial predictions of violence. In: D Faigman, D Kaye, M Saks and J Sanders (eds.) *Modern Scientific Evidence: the law and science of expert testimony*. West Publishing, St Paul, MN. pp. 309.

Monahan J *et al.* (2005). Use of leverage to improve adherence to psychiatric treatment in the community. *Psychiatric Services*, 56, 37–44.

Moncrieff J (2015). Antipsychotic maintenance treatment: time to rethink? *PLoS Medicine*, 8, e1001861.

Montgomery SA and Asberg M (1979). A new depression rating scale designed to be sensitive to change. *British Journal of Psychiatry*, 134, 382–9.

Montgomery SA *et al.* (2014). A randomised, double-blind study in adults with major depressive disorder with an inadequate response to a single course of selective serotonin reuptake inhibitor or serotonin–noradrenaline reuptake inhibitor treatment switched to vortioxetine or agomelatine. *Human Psychopharmacology: Clinical and Experimental*, 29(5), 470–82.

Moran P (2002). The epidemiology of personality disorders. *Psychiatry*, 1, 8–11.

Moran P *et al.* (2000). The prevalence of personality disorder among UK primary care attenders. *Acta Psychiatrica Scandinavica*, 102, 52–7.

Morgan C and Gayer-Anderson C (2016). Childhood adversities and psychosis: evidence, challenges, implications. *World Psychiatry*, 15, 93–102.

Morgan C *et al.* (2005). Pathways to care and ethnicity. 1: Sample characteristics and compulsory admission. *British Journal of Psychiatry*, 186, 281–9.

Morgan C *et al.* (2010). Migration, ethnicity, and psychosis: toward a sociodevelopmental model. *Schizophrenia Bulletin*, 36, 655–64.

Morgan C *et al.* (2014). Reappraising the long-term course and outcome of psychotic disorders: the AESOP-10 study. *Psychological Medicine*, 44, 2713–26.

Morgan C *et al.* (2005). Pathways to care and ethnicity. 1: Sample characteristics and compulsory admission. Report from the AESOP study. *British Journal of Psychiatry*, 186, 281–9.

Morgan VA *et al.* (2008). Intellectual disability co-occurring with schizophrenia and other psychiatric illness: population-based study. *British Journal of Psychiatry*, 193, 364–72.

Morgenthaler TI *et al.* (2007). Practice parameters for the clinical evaluation and treatment of circadian rhythm sleep disorders. *Sleep*, 30, 1445–59.

Morley S *et al.* (2013). Examining the evidence about psychological treatment for chronic pain. Time for a paradigm shift? *Pain*, 154, 1929–31.

Morris J *et al.* (2011). Treated prevalence of and mental health services received by children and adolescents in 42 low and middle income countries. *Journal of Child Psychology and Psychiatry*, 52, 1239–46.

Morris JB and Beck AT (1974). The efficacy of antidepressant drugs. A review of research (1958–1972). *Archives of General Psychiatry*, 30, 667–74.

Morris JK and Alberman E. (2009). Trends in Down's syndrome live births and antenatal diagnoses in England and Wales from 1989 to 2008: analysis of data from the National Down Syndrome Cytogenetic Register. *BMJ*, 339, b3794.

Morris K *et al.* (2012). Psychiatrists and termination of pregnancy. Clinical, legal and ethical aspects. *Australian and New Zealand Journal of Psychiatry*, 46, 18–27.

Morrison AP *et al.* (2014). Cognitive therapy for people with schizophrenia spectrum disorders not taking antipsychotic drugs: a single-blind randomised controlled trial. *Lancet*, 383, 1395–403.

Mortimer AM (2011). Using clozapine in clinical practice. *Advances in Psychiatric Treatment*, 17, 256–63.

Moscovitch DA (2009). What is the core fear in social phobia? A new model to facilitate individualized case conceptualization and treatment. *Cognitive and Behavioural Practice*, 16, 123–34.

Moshe SL *et al.* (2015). Epilepsy: new advances. *Lancet*, 385, 884–98.

Moussavi S *et al.* (2007). Depression, chronic diseases, and decrements in health: results from the World Health Surveys. *The Lancet*, 370, 851–8.

Mufson L *et al.* (2004). A randomised effectiveness trial of interpersonal psychotherapy for depressed adolescents. *Archives of General Psychiatry*, 61, 577–84.

Mukherjee S, Sackheim HA and Lee C (1988). Electroconvulsive therapy of acute manic episodes: a review of fifty years experience. *Convulsive Therapy*, 4, 74–80.

Mullen PE (2004). The autogenic (self-generated) massacre. *Behaviour Sciences and the Law*, 22, 311–23.

Mullen PE and Maack LH (1985). Jealousy, pathological jealousy and aggression. In: DP Farington and J Gunn (eds.) *Aggression and Dangerousness*. John Wiley & Sons, Chichester.

Mullen PE and Ogloff JRP (2009). Assessing and managing the risk of violence towards others. In: MG Gelder, NC Andreasen, JJ Lopez-Ibor JJ and JR Geddes (eds.) *The New Oxford Textbook of Psychiatry*, 2nd edn. Oxford University Press, Oxford. pp. 1991–2002.

Mullen PE *et al.* (2006). Assessing and managing the risks in the stalking situation. *Journal of the American Academy of Psychiatry and the Law*, 34, 439–50.

Mullen PE, Pathé M and Purcell R (2009). *Stalkers and their Victims*, 2nd edn. Cambridge University Press, Cambridge.

Muller A *et al.* (2013). Psychiatric aspects of bariatric surgery. *Current Psychiatry Reports*, 15, 397.

Muller N *et al.* (2015). The role of inflammation in schizophrenia. *Frontiers in Neuroscience*, 9, 372.

Munro A (2009). Persistent delusional symptoms and disorders. In: MG Gelder, NC Andreasen, JJ Lopez-Ibor and JR Geddes (eds.) *New Oxford Textbook of Psychiatry*, 2nd edn. Oxford University Press, Oxford, pp. 609–28.

Murad MH *et al.* (2010). Hormonal therapy and sex reassignment: A systematic review and meta-analysis of quality of life and psychosocial outcomes. *Clinical Endocrinology*, 72, 214–31.

Murphy BP and Brewer W (2011). Early intervention in psychosis: clinical aspects of treatment. *Advances in Psychiatric Treatment*, 17, 408–18.

Murphy SE *et al.* (2013). The effect of the serotonin transporter polymorphism (5-HTTLPR) on amygdala function: A meta-analysis. *Molecular Psychiatry*, 18, 512–20.

Murray J and Williams P (1986). Self–reported illness and general practice consultations in Asian born and British born residents of West London. *Social Psychiatry*, 21, 139–45.

Murray L et al. (2009). The development of anxiety disorders in childhood: an integrative review. *Psychological Medicine*, **39**, 1413–23.

Murray LK et al. (2014). A common elements treatment approach for adult mental health problems in low- and middle-income countries. *Cognitive and Behavioral Practice*, **21**, 111–23.

Murray RM and Lewis SW (1987). Is schizophrenia a neurodevelopmental disorder? *British Medical Journal*, **295**, 681–2.

Murray RM and Reveley A (1981). The genetic contribution to the neuroses. *British Journal of Hospital Medicine*, **25**, 185–90.

Musiek ES and Holtzman DM (2015). Three dimensions of the amyloid hypothesis: time, space and 'wingmen'. *Nature Reviews Neuroscience*, **18**, 800–6.

Mynors-Wallis LM et al. (1995). Randomized controlled trial comparing problem solving treatment with amitriptyline and placebo for major depression in primary care. *British Medical Journal*, **310**, 441–5.

Nair A et al. (2014). Relationship between cognition, clinical and cognitive insight in psychotic disorders: a review and meta-analysis. *Schizophrenia Research*, **152**, 191–200.

Naito A (2007). Internet suicide in Japan: implications for child and adolescent mental health. *Clinical Child Psychology Psychiatry*, **12**, 583–97.

Nanni V, Uher R, Danese A (2012). Childhood maltreatment predicts unfavorable course of illness and treatment outcome in depression: a meta-analysis. *American Journal of Psychiatry*, **169**(2), 141–51.

Napier AD et al. (2014). Culture and health. *Lancet*, **384**, 1607–39.

Narrow WE et al. (2002). Revised prevalence estimates in mental disorders in the United States: using a clinical significance criterion to reconcile two surveys' estimates. *Archives of General Psychiatry*, **59**, 115–23.

Nash JR et al. (2008). Serotonin 5-HT$_{1A}$ receptor binding in people with panic disorder. Positron emission tomography study. *British Journal of Psychiatry*, **193**, 229–34.

National Center for Juvenile Justice (2014). *Juvenile Offenders and Victims: 2014 National Report*. Pittsburgh, USA.

National Confidential Inquiry into Suicide and Homicide (2015). *National Confidential Inquiry into Suicide and Homicide by People with Mental Illness: Annual Report: England and Wales*. University of Manchester, Manchester.

National Institute for Clinical Excellence (2003). *Guidance on the Use of Electroconvulsive Therapy*. Technology Appraisal 59. National Institute for Clinical Excellence, London.

National Institute for Clinical Excellence (2004a). *Eating Disorders: Core interventions in the treatment and management of anorexia nervosa, bulimia nervosa and eating disorders*. Clinical Guideline 9. National Institute for Clinical Excellence, London.

National Institute for Clinical Excellence (2004b). *Self-Harm: the short-term physical and psychological management and secondary prevention of self-harm in primary and secondary care*. Clinical Guideline 16. National Institute for Clinical Excellence, London.

National Institute for Health and Clinical Excellence (2005a). *Obsessive–Compulsive Disorder: Core interventions in the treatment of obsessive–compulsive disorder and body dysmorphic disorder*. Clinical Guideline 31. National Institute for Health and Clinical Excellence, London.

National Institute for Health and Clinical Excellence (2005c). *Violence. The short-term management of disturbed/violent behaviour in psychiatric in-patient settings and emergency departments*. Clinical Guideline 25. National Institute for Health and Clinical Excellence, London.

National Institute for Health and Clinical Excellence (2005d). *Depression in Children and Young People: Identification and management in primary, community and secondary care*. National Institute for Health and Clinical Excellence, London.

National Institute for Health and Clinical Excellence (2007). *Drug Misuse: Psychosocial interventions*. Clinical Guideline 51. National Institute for Health and Clinical Excellence, London.

National Institute for Health and Clinical Excellence (2009a). *Depression: the treatment and management of depression in adults*. Clinical Guideline 90. National Institute for Health and Clinical Excellence, London.

National Institute for Health and Clinical Excellence (2009b). *Borderline Personality Disorder (BPD)*. Clinical Guideline 78. National Institute for Health and Clinical Excellence, London.

National Institute for Health and Clinical Excellence (2010). *Anxiety: Management of anxiety (panic disorder, with and without agoraphobia, and generalized anxiety disorder) in adults in primary, secondary and community care*. Clinical Guideline 22. National Institute for Health and Clinical Excellence, London.

National Institute for Health and Clinical Excellence (2011a). *Alcohol-Use Disorders: Diagnosis, assessment and management of harmful drinking and alcohol dependence*. Clinical Guideline 115. National Institute for Health and Clinical Excellence, London.

National Institute for Health and Clinical Excellence (2011b). *Psychosis with Coexisting Substance Misuse*. Clinical Guideline 120. National Institute for Health and Clinical Excellence, London.

National Institute for Health and Care Excellence. (2013a). *Post-traumatic stress disorder (PTSD). Evidence Update 49*. A summary of selected new evidence relevant to NICE clinical guideline 26 'The management of PTSD in adults and children in primary and secondary care' (2005). NICE, Manchester.

National Institute for Health and Clinical Excellence (2013b). *Psychosis and Schizophrenia in Children and Young People: Recognition and management*. Clinical Guideline 155. National Institute for Health and Clinical Excellence, London.

National Institute for Health and Clinical Excellence (2014a). *Psychosis and Schizophrenia in Adults: Treatment and management*. Clinical Guideline 178. National Institute for Health and Clinical Excellence, London.

National Institute for Care and Health Excellence (2013c). *Antisocial behaviour and conduct disorders in children and young people: recognition and management*. Clinical Guideline CG158. NICE, London.

National Institute for Care and Health Excellence (2014b). Bipolar disorder: the assessment and management of bipolar disorder in adults, children and young people in primary and secondary care. National Clinical Guideline, 185. NICE, London.

National Institute for Health and Care Excellence (2014c). *Antenatal and Postnatal Mental Health: Clinical management and service guidance*. NICE guidelines [CG192], London.

National Institute for Health and Care Excellence (2015a). *Hypnotics*. NICE advice [KTT6], London.

National Institute for Health and Care Excellence (NICE) (2015b). Guideline NG10: *Violence and Aggression: short-term management in mental health, health and community settings.* NICE, London.

National Institute for Health and Care Excellence (2016). *Attention Deficit Hyperactivity Disorder: Diagnosis and Management of ADHD in Children, Young People and Adults.* NICE Clinical Guidelines, No. 72. 2016 update. National Collaborating Centre for Mental Health (UK).

National Institute for Mental Health in England (NIMHE) (2003). *Personality Disorder: No longer a diagnosis of exclusion. Policy implementation guidance for the development of services for people with personality disorder.* Department of Health, London.

Neeleman J and Wessely S (1997). Changes in classification of suicide in England and Wales: time trends and associations with coroners' professional backgrounds. *Psychological Medicine,* 21, 467–72.

Nelson JC and Papakostas GI (2009). Atypical antipsychotic augmentation in major depressive disorder: a meta-analysis of placebo-controlled randomized trials. *American Journal of Psychiatry,* 166, 980–91.

Nelson JC *et al.* (2014) A systematic review and meta-analysis of lithium augmentation of tricyclic and second generation antidepressants in major depression. *Journal of Affective Disorders,* 168, 269–75.

Nemeroff CB and Goldschmidt-Clermont PJ (2012). Heartache and heartbreak—the link between depression and cardiovascular disease. *Nature Reviews Cardiology,* 9, 526–39.

Nemeth G *et al.* (2017). Cariprazine versus risperidone monotherapy for the treatment of predominant negative symptoms in patients with schizophrenia: a randomised, double-blind, controlled trial. *Lancet,* 389, 1103–13.

Neuropathology Group of the Medical Research Council Cognitive Function and Ageing Study (2001). Pathological correlates of late-onset dementia in a multicentre, community-based population in England and Wales. *Lancet,* 357, 169–75.

New AS *et al.* (2004). Low prolactin response to fenfluramine in impulsive aggression. *Journal of Psychiatric Research,* 38, 223–30.

New AS *et al.* (2008). Recent advances in the biological study of personality disorders. *Psychiatric Clinics of North America,* 31, 441–61.

Newton-Howes G *et al.* (2010). The prevalence of personality disorder, its comorbidity with mental state disorders and its clinical significance in community mental health teams. *Social Psychiatry and Psychiatric Epidemiology,* 45, 453–60.

Newton-Howes G *et al.* (2015). Personality disorder across the life course. *Lancet,* 385, 727–34.

Ng B and Atkins M (2012). Home assessment in old age psychiatry: a practical guide. *Advances in Psychiatric Treatment,* 18, 400–7.

Nicholls D and Barrett E (2015). Eating disorders in children and adolescents. *BJPsych Advances,* 21, 206–16.

Nickerson A *et al.* (2011). A critical review of psychological treatments of posttraumatic stress disorder in refugees. *Clinical Psychology Review,* 31, 399–417.

Nicodemus KK *et al.* (2008). Serious obstetric complications interact with hypoxia-regulated/vascular-expression genes to influence schizophrenia risk. *Molecular Psychiatry,* 13, 873–7.

Nicodemus KK *et al.* (2010). Biological validation of increased schizophrenia risk with NRG1, ERBB4, and AKT1 epistasis via functional neuroimaging in healthy controls. *Archives of General Psychiatry,* 67, 991–1001.

Niculescu AB *et al.* (2015) Understanding and predicting suicidality using a combined genomic and clinical risk assessment approach. *Molecular Psychiatry,* 20, 1266–1285.

Niederkrotenthaler T *et al.* (2010). Role of media reports in completed and prevented suicide: Werther v. Papageno effects. *British Journal of Psychiatry,* 197, 234–43.

Nielsen RE *et al.* (2015). Second-generation antipsychotic effect on cognition in patients with schizophrenia—a meta-analysis of randomized clinical trials. *Acta Psychiatrica Scandinavica,* 131, 185–96.

Nolen WA, Van de Putte JJ and Dijken WA (1988). Treatment strategy in depression. 2. MAO inhibitors in depression resistant tricyclic antidepressants: two controlled cross-over studies with tranylcypromine versus 1,5-hydroxytryptophan and nomifensine. *Acta Psychiatrica Scandinavica,* 78, 676–83.

Norbury CF *et al.* (2015). Disorders of speech, language, and communication. In: A. Thapar *et al.* (eds). *Rutter's Child and Adolescent Psychiatry.* John Wiley & Sons, Chichester, pp. 683–701.

Nord M and Farde L (2011). Antipsychotic occupancy of dopamine receptors in schizophrenia. *CNS Neuroscience and Therapeutics,* 17, 97– 103.

Nordentoft M, Mortensen PB and Pedersen CB. (2011). Absolute risk of suicide after first hospital contact in mental disorder. *Archives of General Psychiatry,* 68, 1058–64.

Norton S *et al.* (2014). Potential for primary prevention of Alzheimer's disease: an analysis of population data. *Lancet Neurology,* 13, 788–94.

Novak B *et al.* (2007). Sex offenders and insanity: an examination of 42 individuals found not guilty by reason of insanity. *Journal of the American Academy of Psychiatry and the Law,* 35, 444–5.

Nowell PD *et al.* (1997). Benzodiazepines and zolpidem for chronic insomnia: a meta-analysis of treatment efficacy. *Journal of the American Medical Association,* 278, 2170–7.

Noyes R (2009). Hypochondriasis (health anxiety). In: MG Gelder, NC Andreasen, JJ López-IborJr and JR Geddes (eds.) *The New Oxford Textbook of Psychiatry,* 2nd edn. Oxford University Press, Oxford. pp. 1021–8.

Nuechterlein KH *et al.* (2008). The MATRICS Consensus Cognitive Battery, Part 1: Test selection, reliability, and validity. *American Journal of Psychiatry,* 165, 203–13.

Nuesch E *et al.* (2013). Comparative efficacy of pharmacological and non-pharmacological interventions in fibromyalgia syndrome: network meta-analysis. *Annals of the Rheumatic Diseases,* 72, 955–62.

Nutt DJ *et al.* (2015). The dopamine theory of addiction: 40 years of highs and lows. *Nature Reviews Neuroscience,* 16, 305–12.

Oberlander JG and Henderson LP (2012). The Sturm und Drang of anabolic steroid use: angst, anxiety, and aggression. *Trends in Neurosciences,* 35, 382–92.

O'Brien JT and Thomas A (2015). Vascular dementia. *Lancet,* 386, 1698–706.

O'Brien JT et al (2017) Clinical practice with anti-dementia drugs: a revised (third) consensus statement from the British Association for Psychopharmacology, *Journal of Psychopharmacology*, **31**, 147–68.

O'Brien S *et al.* (2011). Diagnosis and management of premenstrual disorders. *British Medical Journal*, **342**, d2994.

O'Connell H *et al.* (2014). Managing delirium in everyday practice: towards cognitive-friendly hospitals. *Advances in Psychiatric Treatment*, **20**, 380–9.

O'Connor E *et al.* (2016). Primary care screening and treatment of depression in pregnant and postpartum women. Evidence report and systematic review for the US Preventive Services Task Force. *JAMA*, **315**, 388–406.

O'Connor N (1968). Psychology and intelligence. In: M Shepherd and DL Davis (eds.) *Studies in Psychiatry*. Oxford University Press, London.

O'Connor TG *et al.* (2016). Maternal affective illness in the perinatal period and child development: findings on developmental timing, mechanisms, and intervention. *Current Psychiatry Reports*, **18**, 1–5.

Ødegaard Ø (1932). Emigration and insanity. *Acta Psychiatrica Scandinavica*, Suppl. 4.

Ogloff JRP (2009). Mental disorders among offenders in correctional settings. In: MG Gelder, NC Andreasen, JJ Lopez-Ibor, and J Geddes (eds.) *The New Oxford Textbook of Psychiatry*. Oxford University Press, Oxford, pp. 1933–7.

O'Grady J (2009). The expert witness in the Criminal Court: assessment, reports and testimony. In: MG Gelder, NC Andreasen, JJ Lopez-Ibor, and J Geddes (eds.) *The New Oxford Textbook of Psychiatry*. Oxford University Press, Oxford, pp. 2003–9.

Ohi K *et al.* (2012). Personality traits and schizophrenia: evidence from a case-control study and meta-analysis. *Psychiatry Research*, **198**, 7–11.

O'Keefe JH *et al.* (2014). Alcohol and cardiovascular health: the dose makes the poison … or the remedy. *Mayo Clinic Proceedings*, **89**, 382–93.

Okkels N *et al.* (2013). Changes in the diagnosed incidence of early onset schizophrenia over four decades. *Acta Psychiatrica Scandinavica*, **127**, 62–8.

Olatunji BO, Cisler JM and Deacon BJ (2010. Efficacy of cognitive behavioral therapy for anxiety disorders: a review of meta-analytic findings. *Psychiatric Clinics of North America*, **33**, 557–77.

Olde Hartman TC *et al.* (2009). Medically unexplained symptoms, somatisation disorder and hypochondriasis: course and prognosis. A systematic review. *Journal of Psychosomatic Research*, **66**, 363–77.

Olden KW and Chepyala P (2008). Functional nausea and vomiting. *Nature Clinical Practice Gastroenterology and Hepatology*, **5**, 202–8.

Olfson M *et al.* (2015). Trends in mental health care among children and adolescents. *New England Journal of Medicine*, **373**, 1079.

Olney JW and Farber NB (1995). Glutamate receptor dysfunction and schizophrenia. *Archives of General Psychiatry*, **52**, 998–1007.

Olweus D (2013). School bullying: Development and some important challenges. *Annual Review of Clinical Psychology*, **9**, 751–80.

Opjordsmoen S (2014). Delusional disorder as a partial psychosis. *Schizophrenia Bulletin*, **40**, 244–7.

Oppenheimer C (2009). Special features of psychiatric treatment for the elderly. In: Gelder MG, Andreasen NC, Lopez-Ibor JJ and Geddes JR (eds.) *New Oxford Textbook of Psychiatry*, 2nd edn. Oxford University Press, Oxford. pp. 1571–8.

Oppenheimer C (2013). Personality in later life: personality disorder and the effects of illness on personality. In: Dening T and Thomas A (eds.) *Oxford Textbook of Old Age Psychiatry*, 2nd edn. Oxford University Press, Oxford, Chapter 53.

Oro AB *et al.* (2014). *Autistic Behavior Checklist (ABC) and Its Applications: Comprehensive Guide to Autism*. Springer, New York, pp. 2787–98.

Öst LG and Breitholtz E (2000). Applied relaxation vs. cognitive therapy in the treatment of generalized anxiety disorder. *Behaviour Research and Therapy*, **38**, 777–90.

Öst LG *et al.* (2001). One versus five sessions of exposure and five sessions of cognitive therapy in the treatment of claustrophobia. *Behaviour Research and Therapy*, **39**, 167–81.

Overall JE and Gorham DR (1962). The Brief Psychiatric Rating Scale. *Psychological Reports*, **10**, 799–812.

Owen MJ (2014). New approaches to psychiatric diagnostic classification. *Neuron*, **84**, 564–71.

Owen MJ *et al.* (2016). Schizophrenia. *Lancet*,**388**, 86–97.

Owens D, Horrocks J and House A (2002). Fatal and non-fatal repetition of self-harm: systematic review. *British Journal of Psychiatry*, **181**, 193–9.

Oyebode F (2014). *Sims' Symptoms in the Mind: an introduction to descriptive psychopathology*, 5th edn. Saunders, London.

Palazzoli M *et al.* (1978). *Paradox and Counterparadox*. Aronson, New York.

Palmer BW *et al.* (2009). What do we know about neuropsychological aspects of schizophrenia? *Neuropsychology Review*, **19**, 365–84.

Palmu R *et al.* (2011). Mental disorders after burn injury: a prospective study. *Burns*, **37**(4), 601–9.

Palpacuer C *et al.* (2015). Risks and benefits of nalmefene in the treatment of adult alcohol dependence: A systematic literature review and meta-analysis of published and unpublished double-blind randomized controlled trials. *PLoS Medicine*, **12**, e1001924.

Papakostas GI *et al.* (2008). Treatment of SSRI-resistant depression: a meta-analysis comparing within- versus across-class switches. *Biological Psychiatry*, **63**, 699–704.

Paris J and Black DW. (2015). Borderline personality disorder and bipolar disorder: What is the difference and why does it matter? *Journal of Nervous and Mental Disease*, **203**, 3–7.

Park M and Unutzer J (2011). Geriatric depression in primary care. *Psychiatric Clinics of North America*, **34**, 469-87.

Park RJ *et al.* (2017). Deep brain stimulation in anorexia nervosa: hope for the hopeless or explotation of the vulnerable? The Oxford Neuroethics Gold Standard Framework. *Frontiers in Psychiatry*. Doi.org/10.3389/fpsyt.2017.00044.

Parker C, Coupland C and Hippisley-Cox J (2010). Antipsychotic drugs and risk of venomous thromboembolism: nested case–control study. *British Medical Journal*, **641**, c4245.

Parker G and Hadzi-Pavlovic D (1992). Parental representations of melancholic and non-melancholic depressives: examining for specificity to depressive type and for evidence of additive effects. *Psychological Medicine*, **22**, 657–65.

Parker G *et al.* (2015). Melancholia and catatonia: disorders or specifiers? *Current Psychiatry Reports*, **17**, 536.

Parkes CM, Benjamin B and Fitzgerald RG (1969). Broken heart: a statistical study of increased mortality among widowers. *British Medical Journal,* i, 740–3.

Parnas J *et al.* (1982). Perinatal complications and clinical outcome within the schizophrenia spectrum. *British Journal of Psychiatry,* 140, 416–20.

Parrott AC (2013). Human psychobiology of MDMA or 'Ecstasy': an overview of 25 years of empirical research. *Human Psychopharmacology: Clinical and Experimental,* 28, 289–307.

Parry-Jones WL (1972). *The Trade in Lunacy.* Routledge & Kegan Paul, London.

Parsons T (1951). *The Social System.* Free Press, Glencoe, IL.

Paschou P (2013). The genetic basis of Gilles de la Tourette syndrome. *Neuroscience and Biobehavioral Reviews,* 37, 1026–39.

Pasmanick B, Scarpitti FR and Lefton M (1964). Home versus hospital care for schizophrenics. *Journal of the American Medical Association,* 187, 177–81.

Patel B *et al.* (2014) Psychosocial interventions for dementia: from evidence to practice. *Advances in Psychiatric Treatment,* 20, 340–9.

Patel V and Prince M (2010). Global mental health: a new global health field comes of age. *Journal of the American Medical Association,* 303, 1976–7.

Patel V *et al.* (2010). Effectiveness of an intervention led by lay health counsellors for depressive and anxiety disorders in primary care in Goa, India (MANAS): a cluster randomised controlled trial. *Lancet,* 376, 2086–95.

Patel V *et al.* (2011). A renewed agenda for global mental health. *Lancet,* 378, 1441–2.

Pathé M, Mullen PE and Purcell R (1999). Stalking: false claims of victimisation. *British Journal of Psychiatry,* 174, 170–2.

Patton GC *et al.* (2016). Our future: a *Lancet* commission on adolescent health and wellbeing. *Lancet,* 387, 2423–78.

Pavlou MP and Lachs MS (2006). Could self-neglect in adults be a geriatric syndrome? *Journal of the American Geriatrics Society,* 54, 831–42.

Paykel ES (1978). Contribution of life events to causation of psychiatric illness. *Psychological Medicine,* 8, 245–53.

Paykel ES *et al.* (1999). Prevention of relapse in residual depression by cognitive therapy. *Archives of General Psychiatry,* 56, 829–35.

Pearce JB (2009). Counselling and psychotherapy for children. In: MG Gelder, Andreasen NC, López-Ibor JJJr, and Geddes JR (eds.) *The New Oxford Textbook of Psychiatry.* Oxford University Press, Oxford. pp. 1764–69.

Pearson CM *et al.* (2015). A risk and maintenance model for bulimia nervosa: from impulsive action to compulsive behavior. *Psychological Review,* 122, 516–35.

Pedersen CB and Mortensen PB (2001). Family history, place and season of birth as risk factors for schizophrenia in Denmark: a replication and reanalysis. *British Journal of Psychiatry,* 179, 46–52.

Pederson LH, Henrikson TB and Olsen J (2010). Fetal exposure to antidepressants and normal milestone development at 6 and 19 months of age. *Pediatrics* 125, e600–8.

Pediatric OCD Treatment Study Team (2004). Cognitive behaviour therapy, sertraline, and their combination for children and adolescents with obsessive-compulsive disorder: the Pediatric OCD Treatment Study (POTS) randomized controlled trial. *Journal of the American Medical Association,* 292, 1969–76.

Peen J and Dekker J (2004). Is urbanicity an environmental risk factor for psychiatric disorders? *Lancet,* 363, 2012–13.

Pendlebury ST and Rothwell PM (2009). Prevalence, incidence, and factors associated with post-stroke dementia: a systematic review and meta-analysis. *Lancet Neurology,* 8, 1006–18.

Pennant ME *et al.* (2015). Computerised therapies for anxiety and depression in children and young people: A systematic review and meta-analysis. *Behaviour Research and Therapy,* 67, 1–18.

Penninx BW *et al.* (1999). Minor and major depression and the risk of death in older persons. *Archives of General Psychiatry,* 56, 889–95.

Penrose L (1938). *A Clinical and Genetic Study of 1280 Cases of Mental Deficiency.* HMSO, London.

Penttilä M *et al.* (2014). Duration of untreated psychosis as predictor of long-term outcome in schizophrenia: systematic review and meta-analysis. *British Journal of Psychiatry,* 28, 88–94.

Pepper J, Hariz M and Zrinzo L (2015). Deep brain stimulation versus anterior capsulotomy for obsessive-compulsive disorder: a review of the literature. *Journal of Neurosurgery,* 122, 1028–37.

Peraala J *et al.* (2007). Lifetime prevalence of psychotic and bipolar I disorders in a general population. *Archives of General Psychiatry,* 64, 19–28

Peralta V, Cuesta MJ (2016). Delusional disorder and schizophrenia: a comparative study across multiple domains. *Psychological Medicine,* 46, 2829–39.

Perez JA *et al.* (2013). Genetics of anxiety disorders. In: DS Charney, JD Buxbaum, P Sklaar, EJ Nestler (eds). *Neurobiology of Mental Illness.* Oxford University Press, Oxford, pp. 537–48.

Perley MJ and Guze SB (1962). Hysteria—the stability and usefulness of clinical criteria. *New England Journal of Medicine,* 266, 421–6.

Perrin JS *et al.* (2012). Electroconvulsive therapy reduces frontal cortical connectivity in severe depressive disorder. *Proceedings of the National Academy of Sciences,* 109, 5464–8.

Perry DW *et al.* (2002). Mental impairment in the West Midlands: 10 years on. *Medicine, Science and the Law,* 42, 325–33.

Pertusa A *et al.* (2010). Refining the diagnostic boundaries of compulsive hoarding: A critical review. *Clinical Psychology Review,* 30, 371–86.

Perugi G *et al.* (2015). Mixed features in patients with a major depressive episode: The BRIDGE-II-MIX study. *Journal of Clinical Psychiatry,* 76, 351–8.

Petersen L and Sorensen TIA (2011). Studies based on the Danish Adoption Register: schizophrenia, BMI, smoking, and mortality in perspective. *Scandinavian Journal of Public Health,* 39 (suppl. 7), 191–5.

Petersen L, Mortensen PB and Pedersen CB (2011). Paternal age at birth of first child and risk of schizophrenia. *American Journal of Psychiatry,* 168, 82–8.

Peterson RL and Pennington BF (2015). Developmental dyslexia. *Annual Review of Clinical Psychology,* 11, 283–307.

Peterson ZD *et al.* (2011). Prevalence and consequences of adult sexual assault of men: review of empirical findings and state of the literature. *Clinical Psychology Review,* 31, 1–24.

Petrides G *et al.* (2015). Electroconvulsive therapy augmentation in clozapine-resistant schizophrenia: a prospective, randomized study. *American Journal of Psychiatry,* 172, 52–8.

Petronis A (2010). Epigenetics as a unifying principle in the aetiology of complex traits and diseases. *Nature, 465*, 721–7.

Petry N (2010). Pathological gambling and the DSM-V. *International Gambling Studies, 10*, 113–15.

Pezawas L *et al.* (2003). Recurrent brief depressive disorder reinvestigated: a community sample of adolescents and young adults. *Archives of General Psychiatry, 33*, 407–18.

Pharoah F *et al.* (2010). Family intervention for schizophrenia. *Cochrane Database of Systematic Reviews, 12*, CD000088.

Phelan M and Blair G (2008). Medical history taking in psychiatry. *Advances in Psychiatric Treatment, 14*, 229–34.

Phelan M, Wykes T and Goldman H (1994). Global functioning scales: A review. *Social Psychiatry and Epidemiology, 29*, 205–11.

Phelan M *et al.* (1995). The Camberwell Assessment of Need: the validity and reliability of an instrument to assess the needs of people with severe mental illness. *British Journal of Psychiatry, 167*, 589–95.

Phillips KA *et al.* (2006). Delusional versus non-delusional body dysmorphic disorder: clinical features and course of illness. *Journal of Psychiatric Research, 40*, 95–104.

Phillips ML and Kupfer DJ (2013). Bipolar disorder diagnosis: challenges and future directions. *The Lancet, 381*, 1654–62.

Phillips ML and Swartz HA (2014). A critical appraisal of neuroimaging studies of bipolar disorder: Toward a new conceptualization of underlying neural circuitry and a road map for future research. *American Journal of Psychiatry, 171*, 829–43.

Phillips PC (2008). Epistasis—the essential role of gene interactions in the structure and evolution of genetic systems. *Nature Reviews Genetics, 9*, 855–67.

Pichot P (1994). Nosological models in psychiatry. *British Journal of Psychiatry, 164*, 232–40.

Pickles A *et al.* (2001). Child psychiatric symptoms and psychosocial impairment: relationship and prognostic significance. *British Journal of Psychiatry, 179*, 230–5.

Pilling S *et al.* (2011). Diagnosis, assessment, and management of harmful drinking and alcohol dependence: summary of NICE guidance. *British Medical Journal, 342*, d700.

Pilling S *et al.* (2013). Recognition, assessment and treatment of social anxiety disorder: Summary of NICE guidance. *British Medical Journal, 346*, f2541.

Pine DS *et al.* (2015). Anxiety disorders. In: A. Thapar *et al.* (eds). *Rutter's Child and Adolescent Psychiatry.* John Wiley & Sons, Chichester, pp. 822–40.

Pinquart M and Sörensen S (2003). Differences between caregivers and noncaregivers in psychological health and physical health: a meta-analysis. *Psychology and Aging, 18*, 250–67.

Pinsky E *et al.* (2015). Pediatric consultation and psychiatric aspects of somatic disease. In: A. Thapar *et al.* (eds). *Rutter's Child and Adolescent Psychiatry.* John Wiley & Sons, Chichester, pp. 586–98.

Pirkis J and Burgess P (1998). Suicide and recency of health care contacts: a systematic review. *British Journal of Psychiatry, 173*, 462–74.

Pivonello R *et al.* (2015). Neuropsychiatric disorders in Cushing's syndrome. *Frontiers in Neuroscience, 9*, 129.

Plack K, Herpertz S and Petrak F (2010). Behavioral medicine interventions in diabetes. *Current Opinion in Psychiatry, 23*, 131–8.

Platt B *et al.* (2010a). Systematic review of the prevalence of suicide in veterinary surgeons. *Occupational Medicine, 60*, 436–46.

Polanczyk G *et al.* (2010). Etiological and clinical features of childhood psychotic symptoms: results from a birth cohort. *Archives of General Psychiatry, 67*, 328–38.

Polanczyk GV *et al.* (2015). Annual research review: A meta-analysis of the worldwide prevalence of mental disorders in children and adolescents. *Journal of Child Psychology and Psychiatry, 56*, 345–65.

Pollock VE *et al.* (1990). Childhood antecedents of antisocial behavior: parental alcoholism and physical abusiveness. *American Journal of Psychiatry, 147*, 1290–3.

Pompili M *et al.* (2013). Indications for electroconvulsive treatment in schizophrenia: a systematic review. *Schizophrenia Research, 146*, 1–9.

Ponniah K *et al.* (2013). An update on the efficacy of psychological treatments for obsessive–compulsive disorder in adults. *Journal of Obsessive-Compulsive and Related Disorders, 2*, 207–18.

Poole R (2010). Illness deception and work: incidence, manifestations and detection. *Occupational Medicine, 60*(2), 127–32.

Popovic D *et al.* (2014). Risk factors for suicide in schizophrenia: systematic review and clinical recommendations. *Acta Psychiatrica Scandinavica, 130*, 418–26.

Porsteinsson AP *et al.* (2014). Effect of citalopram on agitation in Alzheimer disease: the CitAD randomized clinical trial. *JAMA, 311*, 682–91.

Porteous DJ *et al.* (2014). DISC1 as a genetic risk factor for schizophrenia and related major mental illness: response to Sullivan. *Molecular Psychiatry, 19*, 141–3.

Posener HD and Jacoby R (2008). Testamentary capacity. In: R Jacoby, C Oppenheimer, T Dening and A Thomas (eds.) *The Oxford Textbook of Old Age Psychiatry*. Oxford University Press, Oxford. pp. 753–60.

Post F (1972). The management and nature of depressive illnesses in late life: a follow-through study. *British Journal of Psychiatry, 121*, 393–404.

Poulsen S *et al.* (2014). A randomized controlled trial of psychoanalytic psychotherapy or cognitive-behavioral therapy for bulimia nervosa. *American Journal of Psychiatry, 171*, 109–16.

Poulton R *et al.* (2015). The Dunedin Multidisciplinary Health and Development Study: overview of the first 40 years, with an eye to the future. *Social Psychiatry and Psychiatric Epidemiology, 50*, 679–93.

Powell GE (2009). Cognitive assessment. In: MG Gelder, NC Andreasen, JJ Lopez-Ibor and JR Geddes (eds.) *The New Oxford Textbook of Psychiatry*, 2nd edn. Oxford University Press, Oxford.

Pratt JH (1908). Results obtained in treatment of pulmonary tuberculosis by the class method. *British Medical Journal*, ii, 1070–1.

Prentky R and Righthand S (2003). *Juvenile Sex Offender Assessment Protocol-II (J-SOAP-II) Manual*. US Department of Justice, Office of Justice Programs, Office of Juvenile Justice and Delinquency Prevention Washington, DC.

Press Complaints Commission (2007). *Newspaper and Magazine Publishing in the UK: Editors' code of practice*. Press Complaints Commission, London.

Price JL and Drevets WC. (2012). Neural circuits underlying the pathophysiology of mood disorders. *Trends in Cognitive Sciences*, **16**, 61–71.

Prichard JC (1835). *A Treatise on Insanity*. Sherwood Gilbert and Piper, London.

Priebe S *et al.* (2005). Reinstitutionalisation in mental health care: comparison of data on service provision from six European countries. *British Medical Journal*, **330**, 123–6.

Priebe S *et al.* (2013). Effectiveness of financial incentives to improve adherence to maintenance treatment with antipsychotics: cluster randomised controlled trial. *British Medical Journal*, **347**, f5847.

Prime Minister's Strategy Unit (2003). *Alcohol Harm Reduction Strategy for England*. Cabinet Office, London.

Prince M *et al.* (2013). The global prevalence of dementia. A systematic review and meta-analysis. *Alzheimers and Dementia*, **9**, 63–75.

Prins JB, Van der Meer JW and Bleijenberg G (2006). Chronic fatigue syndrome. *The Lancet*, **367**, 346–55.

Prins H (2009). Arson (fire-raising). In: MG Gelder, NC Andreasen, JJ Lopez-Ibor, and J Geddes (eds.) *The New Oxford Textbook of Psychiatry*. Oxford University Press, Oxford, pp. 1965–70.

Prochaska JO and DiClemente CC (1986). Towards a comprehensive model of change. In: WR Miller and N Heather (eds.) *Treating Addictive Behaviours: Processes of change*. Plenum Press, New York. pp. 3–27.

Project MATCH Research Group (1997). Matching alcoholism treatments to client heterogeneity: Project MATCH post-treatment drinking outcomes. *Journal of Studies on Alcohol*, **58**(1), 7–29.

Prossin AR *et al.* (2010). Dysregulation of regional endogenous opioid function in borderline personality disorder. *American Journal of Psychiatry*, **167**, 925–33.

Prusiner SB (2013). Biology and genetics of prions causing neurodegeneration. *Annual Review of Genetics*, **47**, 601–23.

Psychological Corporation (2004). *Wechsler Abbreviated Scales of Intelligence (WASI)*. Harcourt Assessment Co., London.

Qin P *et al.* (2003). Suicide risk in relation to socioeconomic, demographic, psychiatric, and familial factors: a national register-based study of all suicides in Denmark, 1981–1997. *American Journal of Psychiatry*, **160**, 765–72.

Qizilibash N *et al.* (2015). BMI and risk of dementia in two million people over two decades: a retrospective cohort study. *Lancet Diabetes and Endocrinology*, **3**, 431–6.

Rahkonen T *et al.* (2001) Systematic intervention for supporting community care of elderly people after a delirium episode. *International Psychogeriatrics*, **13**, 37–49.

Rahman A *et al.* (2008). Cognitive behaviour therapy-based intervention by community health workers for mothers with depression and their infants in rural Pakistan: a cluster-randomised controlled trial. *Lancet*, **372**, 902–9.

Rahman A *et al.* (2015). Global psychiatry. In: M Rutter *et al.* (eds.) *Child and Adolescent Psychiatry*, 6th edn. Blackwell, Oxford. pp. 201–14.

Rai D *et al.* (2013). Country-and individual-level socioeconomic determinants of depression: Multilevel cross-national comparison. *The British Journal of Psychiatry*, **202**, 195–203.

Raine A *et al.* (2000). Reduced prefrontal grey matter and reduced autonomic activity in antisocial personality disorder. *Archives of General Psychiatry*, **57**, 119–27.

Raine A *et al.* (2005). Neurocognitive impairments in boys on the life-course persistent antisocial path. *Journal of Abnormal Psychology*, **114**(1), 38–49.

Rajaraman D *et al.* (2012). The acceptability, feasibility and impact of a lay health counsellor delivered health promoting schools programme in India: a case study evaluation. *BMC Health Services Research*, **12**, 1.

Ramchandani P *et al.* (2009). Effect of parental psychiatric and physical illness on child development. In: MG Gelder, NC Andreasen, JJ Lopez-Ibor, JR Geddes (eds). *New Oxford Textbook of Psychiatry*. OUP, Oxford, pp. 1752–8.

Rametti G *et al.* (2011). White matter microstructure in female to male transsexuals before cross-sex hormonal treatment. A diffusion tensor imaging study. *Journal of Psychiatric Research*, **45**, 199–204.

Ramtekkar U and Ivanenko A (2015). Sleep in children with psychiatric disorders. *Seminars in Pediatric Neurology*, **22**, 148–55.

Rang HP *et al.* (2015). *Rang & Dale's Pharmacology*. Elsevier Health Sciences.

Ranganath C and Ritchey M (2012). Two cortical systems for memory-guided behaviour. *Nature Reviews Neuroscience*, **13**, 713–26.

Raphael B and Wilson J (2000). *Psychological Debriefing. Theory, practice and evidence*. Cambridge University Press, Cambridge.

Rapoport JL *et al.* (2015). Obsessive compulsive disorder. In: A. Thapar *et al.* (eds). *Rutter's Child and Adolescent Psychiatry*. John Wiley & Sons, Chichester, pp. 841–57.

Rapoport MJ (2012). Depression following traumatic brain injury: epidemiology, risk factors and management. *CNS Drugs*, **26**, 111–21.

Rapoport RN (1960). *Community as Doctor*. Tavistock Publications, London.

Ray WA *et al.* (2009). Atypical antipsychotic drugs and the risk of sudden cardiac death. *New England Journal of Medicine*, **360**, 225–35.

Reardon JM and Nathan NL (2007). The specificity of cognitive vulnerabilities to emotional disorders: anxiety sensitivity, looming vulnerability and explanatory style. *Journal of Anxiety Disorders*, **21**, 625–43.

Reed G *et al.* (2016). Disorders related to sexuality and gender identity in the ICD-11: revising the ICD-10 classification based on current scientific evidence, best clinical practices, and human rights considerations. *World Psychiatry*, **15**, 205–21.

Reed RV *et al.* (2012). Mental health of displaced and refugee children resettled in low-income and middle-income countries: risk and protective factors. *Lancet*, **379**, 250–65.

Rees E *et al.* (2014). Analysis of copy number variations at 15 schizophrenia-associated loci. *British Journal of Psychiatry*, **204**, 108–14.

Rees PM, Fowler CJ and Maas CP (2007). Sexual dysfunction 2: sexual function in men and women with neurological disorders. *Lancet*, **369**, 512–25.

Rees S *et al.* (2014). Onset of common mental disorders and suicidal behavior following women's first exposure to gender based violence: A retrospective, population-based study. *BMC Psychiatry*, **14**, 312.

Reichenberg A *et al.* (2016). Discontinuity in the genetic and environmental causes of the intellectual disability spectrum. *Proceedings of the National Academy of Sciences*, 113(4), 1098–103.

Reichenpfader U *et al.* (2014). Sexual dysfunction associated with second-generation antidepressants in patients with major depressive disorder: results from a systematic review with network meta-analysis. *Drug Safety,* 37, 19–31.

Regier DA *et al.* (1990). Comorbidity of mental disorders with alcohol and other drug abuse. Results from the Epidemiologic Catchment Area (ECA) Study. *Journal of the American Medical Association,* 264, 2511–18.

Reid AH and Ballinger BR (1987). Personality disorder in mental handicap. *Psychological Medicine,* 17, 983–7.

Reiss S and Szyszko J (1983). Diagnostic overshadowing and professional experience with the mentally retarded person. *American Journal of Mental Deficiency,* 87, 396–402.

Remington G *et al.* (2014). The neurobiology of relapse in schizophrenia. *Schizophrenia Research,* 152, 381–90.

Reutens S, Nielsen O and Sachdev P (2010). Depersonalization disorder. *Current Opinion in Psychiatry*, 23, 278–83.

Reynolds CF III *et al.* (2006). Maintenance treatment of major depression in old age. *New England Journal of Medicine,* 354, 1130–8.

Reynolds GP and Kirk SL (2010). Metabolic side effects of antipsychotic drug treatment—pharmacological mechanisms. *Pharmacology and Therapeutics,* 125, 169–79.

Reynolds S *et al.* (2012). Effects of psychotherapy for anxiety in children and adolescents: A meta-analytic review. *Clinical Psychology Review,* 32, 251–62.

Rhebergen D *et al.* (2015). Older age is associated with rapid remission of depression after electroconvulsive therapy: a latent class growth analysis. *American Journal of Geriatric Psychiatry,* 23, 274–82.

Ribe AR *et al.* (2015). Long-term risk of dementia in persons with schizophrenia. A Danish population-based cohort study. *JAMA Psychiatry,* 72, 1095–101.

Richards F and Curtice M (2011). Mania in late life. *Advances in Psychiatric Treatment,* 17, 357–64.

Richman N, Stevenson J and Graham PJ (1982). Pre-school to school: a behavioural study. *Behavioural Development: A Series of Monographs.*

Ridley NJ *et al.* (2013). Alcohol-related dementia: an update of the evidence. *Alzheimers Research and Therapy,* 5, 3.

Rieckmann N *et al.* (2006). Course of depressive symptoms and medication adherence after acute coronary syndromes: an electronic medication monitoring study. *Journal of the American College of Cardiology,* 48, 2218–22.

Riemann D *et al.* (2015). The neurobiology, investigation and treatment of chronic insomnia. *Lancet Neurology,* 14, 547–58.

Rihmer Z *et al.* (2010). Current research on affective temperaments. *Current Opinion in Psychiatry,* 23, 12–18.

Riisgaard A *et al.* (2015). Long-term risk of dementia in persons with schizophrenia. A Danish population-based cohort study. *JAMA Psychiatry,* 72, 1095–101.

Riley RD, Lambert PC and Abo-Zaid, G (2010). Meta-analysis of individual participant data: Rationale, conduct, and reporting. *British Medical Journal,* 340, c221.

Ring A *et al.* (2004). Do patients with unexplained physical symptoms pressurise general practitioners for somatic treatment? A qualitative study. *British Medical Journal,* 328, 1057.

Ritchie K *et al.* (2004). Prevalence of DSM-IV psychiatric disorder in the French elderly population. *British Journal of Psychiatry,* 184, 147–52.

Ritson B (2005). Treatment for alcohol-related problems. *British Medical Journal,* 330, 139–41.

Roberts AH (1969). *Brain Damage in Boxers.* Pitman, London.

Roberts E *et al.* (2016). Mortality of people with chronic fatigue syndrome: a retrospective cohort study in England and Wales from the South London and Maudsley NHS Foundation Trust Biomedical Research Centre (SLaMBRC) Clinical Record Interactive Search (CRIS) Register. *Lancet,* 387, 1638–43.

Robertson J *et al.* (2007). Person-centred planning: factors associated with successful outcomes for people with intellectual disabilities. *Journal of Intellectual Disability Research,* 51, 232–43.

Robertson J *et al.* (2015). Prevalence of epilepsy among people with intellectual disabilities: A systematic review. *Seizure,* 29, 46–62.

Robins LN (1966). *Deviant Children Grown Up, A Sociological and Psychiatric Study of Sociopathic Personality.* Baltimore: Williams and Wilkins.

Robins LN (1993). Vietnam veterans' rapid recovery from heroin addiction: a fluke or normal expectation? *Addiction,* 88, 1041–54.

Robins LN and Regier DA (1991). *Psychiatric Disorder in America: the epidemiological catchment area study.* Free Press, New York.

Robins LN *et al.* (1988). The Composite International Diagnostic Interview. An epidemiologic instrument suitable for use in conjunction with different diagnostic systems and in different cultures. *Archives of General Psychiatry,* 45, 1069–77.

Robinson L *et al.* (2010) Primary care and dementia: 2. Long-term care at home: psychosocial interventions, information provision, carer support and case management. *International Journal of Psychogeriatrics,* 25, 657–64.

Robinson P (2014). Severe and enduring eating disorders: recognition and management. *Advances in Psychiatric Treatment,* 20, 392–401.

Robinson RG and Jorge RE (2016). Post-stroke depression: a review. *American Journal of Psychiatry,* 173, 221–31.

Robjant K and Fazel M (2010). The emerging evidence for narrative exposure therapy: A review. *Clinical Psychology Review,* 30, 1030–9.

Robson P (2009). *Forbidden Drugs.* Oxford University Press, Oxford.

Rockliff HE *et al.* (2014). A systematic review of psychosocial factors associated with emotional adjustment in in vitro fertilization patients. *Human Reproduction Update,* 20, 594–613.

Rodda J, Morgan S and Walker Z (2009) Are cholinesterase inhibitors effective in the management of behavioural and psychological symptoms of dementia in Alzheimer's disease? *International Psychogeriatrics,* 21, 821–34.

Rodrigues H *et al.* (2014). Does D-cycloserine enhance exposure therapy for anxiety disorders in humans? A meta-analysis. *PloS One,* 9, p.e93519.

Roessner V *et al.* (2013). Pharmacological treatment of tic disorders and Tourette Syndrome. *Neuropharmacology,* 68, 143–9.

Rogers A *et al.* (2003). Patients' understanding and participation in a trial designed to improve the management of antipsychotic medication: a qualitive study. *Social Psychiatry and Psychiatric Epidemiology,* 38, 720–7.

Rohde P *et al.* (2013). Key characteristics of major depressive disorder occurring in childhood, adolescence, emerging adulthood, and adulthood. *Clinical Psychological Science,* 1, 41–53.

Rohrer JD *et al.* (2015). C9orf72 expansions in frontotemporal dementia and amyotrophic lateral sclerosis. *Lancet Neurology,* 14, 291–301.

Rosanoff AJ, Handy LM and Rosanoff IA (1934). Criminality and delinquency in twins. *Journal of Criminal Law and Criminology,* 24, 923–34.

Rosell DR *et al.* (2010). Increased serotonin 2A receptor availability in the orbitofrontal cortex of physically aggressive personality disordered patients. *Biological Psychiatry,* 67, 1154–62.

Rosenhan DL (1973). On being sane in insane places. *Science,* 179, 250–8.

Rosenthal NE, Sack DA and Gillin JC (1984). Seasonal affective disorder: a description of the syndrome and preliminary findings wih light therapy. *Archives of General Psychiatry,* 41, 24–30.

Ross CA *et al.* (2014). Huntington disease: natural history, biomarkers and prospects for therapeutics. *Nature Reviews Neurology,* 10, 204–16.

Rossignol D *et al.* (2014). Environmental toxicants and autism spectrum disorders: a systematic review. *Translational Psychiatry,* 4, e360.

Rössler W *et al.* (2016). Does menopausal transition really influence mental health? Findings from the prospective long-term Zurich study. *World Psychiatry,* 15, 146–54.

Rossor MN *et al.* (2010). The diagnosis of young-onset dementia. *Lancet Neurology,* 9, 793–806.

Roth M (1955). The natural history of mental disorder in old age. *Journal of Mental Science,* 101, 281–301.

Roth T *et al.* (2011). Prevalence and perceived health associated with insomnia based on DSM-IV-TR; International Statistical Classification of Diseases and Related Health Problems, Tenth Revision; and Research Diagnostic Criteria/International Classification of Sleep Disorders, Second Edition Criteria: Results from the America Insomnia survey. *Biological Psychiatry,* 69, 592–600.

Rothman D (1971). *The Discovery of the Asylum.* Little Brown, Boston, MA.

Routley V (2007). Motor vehicle exhaust gas suicide: review of countermeasures. *Crisis,* 28, 28–35.

Roy A *et al.* (2000). The genetics of suicidal behaviour. In: K Hawton and K van Heeringen (eds.) *The International Handbook of Suicide and Attempted Suicide.* John Wiley & Sons, Chichester. pp. 209–22.

Royal College of Psychiatrists (2000). *Good Psychiatric Practice.* Royal College of Psychiatrists, London.

Royal College of Psychiatrists (2001). *Diagnostic Criteria for Psychiatric Disorders for Use with Adults with LD [DC-LD].* Royal College of Psychiatrists, London.

Royal College of Psychiatrists (2005). *The Third Report of the Royal College of Psychiatrists Special Committee on ECT.* Gaskell Press, London.

Royal College of Psychiatrists (2010). *College Report CR160 Good Psychiatric Practice: Confidentiality and Information Sharing.* 2nd edn. RCP, London.

Rubia K (2012). ADHD: what have we learned from neuroimaging? *Cutting Edge Psychiatry in Practice,* 2, 16–21.

Rudolf MCJ and Logan S (2005). What is the long-term outcome for children who fail to thrive? A systematic review. *Community Child Health, Public Health, and Epidemiology,* 90, 925–31.

Ruhe HG, Mason NS and Schene AH (2007). Mood is indirectly related to serotonin, norepinephrine and dopamine levels in humans: a meta-analysis of monoamine depletion studies. *Molecular Psychiatry,* 12, 331–59.

Ruocco AC *et al.* (2013). Neural correlates of negative emotionality in borderline personality disorder: an activation-likelihood-estimation meta-analysis. *Biological Psychiatry,* 73, 153–60.

Ruschena D *et al.* (2003). Choking deaths: the role of antipsychotic medication. *British Journal of Psychiatry,* 183, 446–50.

Ruscio AM *et al.* (2010). The epidemiology of obsessive-compulsive disorder in the National Comorbidity Survey Replication. *Molecular Psychiatry,* 15, 53–63.

Rush AJ *et al.* (2003). The 16-item Quick Inventory of Depressive Symptomatology (QIDS) Clinician Rating (QIDS-C) and Self-Report (QIDS-SR): A psychometric evaluation in patients with chronic major depression. *Biological Psychiatry,* 54, 573–83.

Rush AJ *et al.* (2008). *Handbook of Psychiatric Measures.* American Psychiatric Publishing, Washington DC.

Russell G and Burns A (2014). Charles Bonnet syndrome and cognitive impairment: a systematic review. *International Psychogeriatrics,* 26, 1431–43.

Russell GFM (1979). Bulimia nervosa: an ominous variant of of anorexia nervosa. *Psychological Medicine,* 9, 429–48.

Russell MC (2008). Scientific resistance to research, training and utilization of eye movement desensitization and reprocessing (EMDR) therapy in treating post-war disorders. *Social Science and Medicine,* 67, 1737–46.

Rutter M (1972). Relationships between child and adult psychiatric disorders. *Acta Psychiatrica Scandinavica,* 48, 3–21.

Rutter M (1991). *Maternal Deprivation Reassessed.* Penguin, London.

Rutter M (2005). Environmentally mediated risks for psychopathology: research strategies and findings. *Journal of the American Academy of Child and Adolescent Psychiatry,* 44, 3–18.

Rutter M (2006). *Genes and Behaviour: Nature–nurture interplay explained.* Blackwell, Oxford.

Rutter M (2011). Child psychiatric diagnosis and classification: concepts, findings, challenges and potential. *Journal of Child Psychology and Psychiatry,* 52, 647–60.

Rutter M and Rutter M (1993). *Developing Minds: Challenge and continuity across the life span.* Basic Books, New York.

Rutter M, Graham P and Birch HG (1970a). *A Neuropsychiatric Study of Childhood.* Heinemann, London.

Rutter M et al. (1976b). Isle of Wight Studies 1964–1974. *Psychological Medicine,* 6, 313–32.

Rutter M *et al.* (1975). Attainment and adjustment in two geographical areas III: some factors accounting for area differences. *British Journal of Psychiatry,* 126, 520–33.

Rutter M *et al.* (1976). Isle of Wight Studies 1964–1974. *Psychological Medicine,* 6, 313–32.

Rutter M *et al.* (eds.) (2008). *Rutter's Child and Adolescent Psychiatry,* 5th edn. Blackwell, Oxford.

Rutz W, von Knorring L and Walinder J (1992). Long-term effects of an educational program for general practitioners given by the Swedish Committee for the prevention and treatment of depression. *Acta Psychiatrica Scandinavica,* 85, 83–8.

Ryan R (1994). Post-traumatic stress disorder in persons with developmental disabilities. *Community Mental Health Journal,* **30**, 45–54.

Ryle A and Kerr IB (2016) *Introducing Cognitive Analytic Therapy: Principles and practice,* 2nd edn. Wiley–Blackwell, Oxford.

Ryu A and Kim TH (2015). Premenstrual syndrome: a mini-review. *Maturitas,* **82**, 436–40.

Sabah M *et al.* (2012). Herpes simplex encephalitis. *BMJ,* **344**, e3166.

Sachdev *et al.* (2014). Classifying neurocognitive disorders: the DSM-5 approach. *Nature Reviews Neurology,* **10**, 634–42.

Sachs K and Mehler PS (2016). Medical complications of bulimia nervosa and their treatments. *Eating and Weight Disorders,* **21**, 13–18.

Sackett DL (1996). Evaluation of clinical method. In: DJ Weatherall, JGG Ledingham and DA Warrell (eds.) *Oxford Textbook of Medicine,* 3rd edn. Oxford University Press, Oxford. pp. 15–21.

Sackheim HA *et al.* (2009). Effect of concomitant pharmacotherapy on electroconvulsive therapy outcomes. Short-term efficacy and adverse effects. *Archives of General Psychiatry,* **66**, 729–37.

Saez-Fonseca JA, Lee L and Walker Z (2007). Long-term outcome of depressive pseudodementia in the elderly. *Journal of Affective Disorders,* **101**, 123–9.

Saha S, Chant D and McGrath J (2007). A systematic review of mortality in schizophrenia—is the differential mortality gap worsening over time? *Archives of General Psychiatry,* **64**, 1123–31.

Sahin M and Sur M (2015). Genes, circuits, and precision therapies for autism and related neurodevelopmental disorders. *Science,* **350**, aab3897.

Sainsbury P and Barraclough B (1968). Differences between suicide rates. *Nature,* **220**, 1252–3.

Saito S and Ihara M (2016). Interaction between cerebrovascular disease and Alzheimer pathology. *Current Opinion in Psychiatry,* **29**, 168–73.

Sajatovic M *et al.* (2015). A report on older-age bipolar disorder from the International Society for Bipolar Disorders Task Force. *Bipolar Disorders,* **17**, 689–704.

Samara MT *et al.* (2016). Early improvement as a predictor of later response to antipsychotics in schizophrenia: a diagnostic test review. *American Journal of Psychiatry,* **172**, 617–29.

Samartzis L *et al.* (2014). White matter alterations in early stages of schizophrenia: a systematic review of diffusion tensor imaging studies. *Journal of Neuroimaging,* **24**, 101–10.

Sameroff A *et al.* (1987). IQ scores of 4-year-old children: social-environmental risk factors. *Pediatrics,* **79**, 343–50.

Samuels JF *et al.* (2008). Prevalence and correlates of hoarding behavior in a community-based sample. *Behaviour Research and Therapy,* **46**, 836–44.

Sanacora G (2010). Cortical inhibition, gamma-aminobutyric acid and major depression: there is plenty of smoke but is there fire? *Biological Psychiatry,* **67**, 397–8.

Santiago PN *et al.* (2013). A systematic review of PTSD prevalence and trajectories in DSM-5 defined trauma exposed populations: Intentional and non-intentional traumatic events. *PloS One,* **8**, e59236.

Saravanan B *et al.* (2004). Culture and insight revisited. *British Journal of Psychiatry,* **184**, 107–9.

Sareen J (2014) Posttraumatic stress disorder in adults: Impact, comorbidity, risk factors, and treatment. *Canadian Journal of Psychiatry,* **59**, 460–7.

Sargant W and Slater E (1963). *An Introduction to Physical Methods of Treatment in Psychiatry.* Livingstone, Edinburgh.

Sariaslan A *et al.* (2016). Schizophrenia and subsequent neighborhood deprivation: revisiting the social drift hypothesis using population, twin and molecular genetic data. *Translational Psychiatry,* **6**, e796.

Sartorius N *et al.* (2010). WPA guidance on how to combat stigmatization of psychiatry and psychiatrists. *World Psychiatry,* **9**, 131–44.

Satizabal CL *et al.* (2016). Incidence of dementia over three decades in the Framingham Heart Study. *New England Journal of Medicine,* **374**, 523–32.

Savitz JB, Price JL and Drevets WC. (2014). Neuropathological and neuromorphometric abnormalities in bipolar disorder: View from the medial prefrontal cortical network. *Neuroscience and Biobehavioral Reviews,* **42**, 132–47.

Saxena S and Lawler D (2009). Delirium in the elderly: a clinical review. *Postgraduate Medical Journal,* **85**, 405–13.

Saxena S *et al.* (2006). World Health Organization's Mental Health Atlas 2005:implications for policy development. *World Psychiatry,* **5**, 179–84.

Saxena S *et al.* (2007). Resources for mental health: scarcity, inequity, and inefficiency. *Lancet,* **370**, 878–89.

Saylor D *et al.* (2016). HIV-associated neurocognitive disorder—pathogenesis and prospects for treatment. *Nature Reviews Neurology,* **12**, 234–43.

Scadding JG (1967). Diagnosis: the clinician and the computer. *Lancet,* **ii**, 877–82.

Scaglia F (ed.) (2014). *Inborn Errors of Metabolism: From neonatal screening to metabolic pathways.* Oxford University Press, Oxford.

Scalzo SJ *et al.* (2015). Wernicke–Korsakoff syndrome not related to alcohol use: a systematic review. *Journal of Neurology, Neurosurgery and Psychiatry,* **86**, 1362–8.

Scammell TE (2015). Narcolepsy. *New England Journal of Medicine,* **373**, 2654–62.

Schaefer J *et al.* (2013). The global cognitive impairment in schizophrenia: Consistent over decades and around the world. *Schizophrenia Research,* **150**, 42–50.

Schanda H *et al.* (2004). Homicide and major mental disorders: a 25-year study. *Acta Psychiatrica Scandinavica,* **110**, 98–107.

Schapira K *et al.* (2001). Relationship of suicide rates to social factors and availability of lethal methods: comparison of suicide in Newcastle upon Tyne, 1961–1994. *British Journal of Psychiatry,* **178**, 458–64.

Schapiro AHV *et al.* (2014). Slowing of neurodegeneration in Parkinson's disease and Huntington's disease: future therapeutic prospects. *Lancet,* **384**, 545–55.

Schapira AHV et al. (2017). Non-motor features of Parkinson disease. *Nature Reviews Neuroscience* (AOL 8 June 2017).

Scheltens P *et al.* (2016). Alzheimer's disease. *Lancet,* **388**, 505–517.

Schiffman J *et al.* (2004). Childhood videotaped social and neuromotor precursors of schizophrenia: a prospective investigation. *American Journal of Psychiatry,* **161**, 2021–7.

Schimming C and Harvey PD (2004). Disability reduction in elderly patients with schizophrenia. *Journal of Psychiatric Practice*, 10, 283–95.

Schizophrenia Working Group of the Psychiatric Genomics Consortium (2014). Biological insights from 108 schizophrenia-associated genomic loci. *Nature*, 511, 421–7.

Schlapobersky J and Pines M (2009). Group methods in adult psychiatry. In: MG Gelder, Andreasen NC, López-Ibor JJJr, and Geddes JR (eds.) *The New Oxford Textbook of Psychiatry*. Oxford University Press, Oxford. pp. 1350–69.

Schmahmann JD and Pandya DN (2008). Disconnection syndromes of basal ganglia, thalamus, and cerebrocerebellar systems. *Cortex*, 44, 1037–66.

Schmahmann JD *et al.* (2008). Cerebral white matter neuroanatomy, clinical neurology, and neurobehavioral correlates. *Annals of the New York Academy of Sciences*, 1142, 266–309.

Schmidtke A *et al.* (1996). Attempted suicide in Europe: rates, trends and sociodemographic characteristics of suicide attempters during the period 1989–1992. Results of the WHO/EURO Multicentre Study on Parasuicide. *Acta Psychiatrica Scandinavica*, 93, 327–38.

Schmucker M and Lösel F (2008). Does sexual offender treatment work? A systematic review of outcome evaluations. *Psicothema*, 20, 10–19.

Schneider K (1959). *Clinical Psychopathology*. Grune and Stratton, New York.

Schneider LS, Dagerman K and Insel PS (2006). Efficacy and adverse effects of atypical antipsychotics for dementia: meta-analysis of randomized, placebo-controlled trials. *American Journal of Geriatric Psychiatry*, 14, 191–210.

Schoeler T *et al.* (2016). Continued versus discontinued cannabis use in patients with psychosis: a systematic review and meta-analysis. *Lancet Psychiatry*, 3, 215–25.

Schoeyen HK *et al.* (2014). Treatment-resistant bipolar depression: A randomized controlled trial of electroconvulsive therapy versus algorithm-based pharmacological treatment. *American Journal of Psychiatry*, 172, 41–51.

Schubert CR *et al.* (2014). Translating human genetics into novel treatment targets for schizophrenia. *Neuron*, 84, 537–41.

Schwartz MA and Wiggins OP (1987). Typifications. The first step for clinical diagnosis in psychiatry. *Journal of Nervous and Mental Disorders*, 175, 65–77.

Scott A (2005). College Guidelines on electroconvulsive therapy: an update for prescribers. *Advances in Psychiatric Treatment*, 11, 150–6.

Scott AI and Waite J (2013). Monitoring a course of ECT. In: J Waite, A Eaton (eds.) *The ECT Handbook*. RCPsych Publications, London. pp. 60–70.

Scott J *et al.* (2006). Cognitive-behavioural therapy for severe and recurrent bipolar disorders: randomised controlled trial. *British Journal of Psychiatry*, 188, 313–20.

Scott PD (1960). The treatment of psychopaths. *British Medical Journal*, i, 1641–6.

Scott S (2009a). Developmental psychopathology and classification in childhood and adolescence. In: MG Gelder, NC Andreasen, JJ Lopez–Ibor and JR Geddes (eds.) *New Oxford Textbook of Psychiatry*, 2nd edn. Oxford University Press, Oxford. pp. 1589–94.

Scott S *et al.* (2015a). Parenting programs. In: A. Thapar *et al.* (eds). *Rutter's Child and Adolescent Psychiatry*. John Wiley & Sons, Chichester, pp. 483–95.

Scott S *et al.* (2015b). Oppositional and conduct disorders. In: A. Thapar *et al.* (eds). *Rutter's Child and Adolescent Psychiatry*. John Wiley & Sons, Chichester, pp. 911–30.

Scottish Executive Central Research Unit (2002). *The 2000 Scottish Crime Survey Overview Report*. Scottish Executive, Edinburgh.

Scottish Intercollegiate Guidelines Network (SIGN) (2013). *Management of Schizophrenia*. Edinburgh: SIGN; 2013 (SIGN publication no. 131).

Sedman G (1970). Theories of depersonalization: a reappraisal. *British Journal of Psychiatry*, 117, 1–14.

Seeman MV (2016). Erotomania and recommendations for treatment. *Psychiatric Quarterly*, 87, 355–64.

Segal H (1963). *Introduction to the Work of Melanie Klein*. Heinemann Medical, London.

Segal M *et al.* (2016). Intellectual disability is associated with increased risk for obesity in a nationally representative sample of US children. *Disability and Health Journal*, 9, 392–8.

Segal T and Ranjith G (2016). Psychiatric assessment on medical wards: a guide for general psychiatrists. *Advances in Psychiatric Treatment*, 22, 8–15.

Segal ZV *et al.* (2012). *Mindfulness-Based Cognitive Therapy for Depression*. Guildford Press, New York, NY.

Seitz DP *et al.* (2013). Pharmacological treatments for neuropsychiatric symptoms of dementia in long-term care: a systematic review. *International Psychogeriatrics*, 25, 185–203.

Sekar A *et al.* (2016). Schizophrenia risk from complex variation of complement component 4. *Nature*, 530, 177–83.

Selten JP *et al.* (2010). Schizophrenia and 1957 pandemic of influenza: meta-analysis. *Schizophrenia Bulletin*, 36, 219–28.

Semkovska M and McLoughlin DM (2010). Objective cognitive performance associated with electroconvulsive therapy for depression: a systematic review and meta-analysis. *Biological Psychiatry*, 68, 568–77.

Sen A (7 A.D.) *What Theory of Justice?* Sheldonian Theatre, Oxford: OPHI Conference http://ophi.org.uk/subindex.php?id=video0.

Sendt KV *et al.* (2015). A systematic review of factors influencing adherence to antipsychotic medication in schizophrenia-spectrum disorders. *Psychiatry Research*, 225, 14–30.

Series H and Esiri M (2012). Vascular dementia: a pragmatic review. *Advances in Psychiatric Treatment*, 18, 372–80.

Severus WE *et al.* (2008). What is the optimal serum lithium level in the long-term treatment of bipolar disorder? A review. *Bipolar Disorders*, 10, 231–7.

Sexton CE, Mackay C and Ebmeier K (2009). A systematic review of diffusion tensor imaging studies in affective disorders. *Biological Psychiatry*, 66, 814–23.

Shaffer D (1974). Suicide in childhood and early adolescence. *Journal of Child Psychology and Psychiatry*, 15, 275–91.

Shafran R *et al.* (2013). Advances in the cognitive behavioural treatment of obsessive compulsive disorder. *Cognitive Behaviour Therapy*, 42, 265–74.

Shah N *et al.* (2015). Update in diagnosis and treatment of chronic pelvic pain syndromes. *Current Bladder Dysfunction Reports*, 10, 198–206.

Shah SM *et al.* (2011). Antipsychotic prescribing to older people living in care homes and the community in England and Wales. *International Journal of Geriatric Psychiatry, 26,* 423–34.

Shamloul R and Ghanem H. (2013). Erectile dysfunction. *Lancet, 381,* 153–65.

Shapiro PA (2015). Management of depression after myocardial infarction. *Current Cardiology Reports, 17,* 80.

Sharp T and Cowen PJ (2011). 5-HT and depression: is the glass half-full? *Current Opinion in Pharmacology, 11,* 45–51.

Sharpe M (2013). Somatic symptoms: beyond 'medically unexplained'. *British Journal of Psychiatry, 203,* 320–1.

Sharpe M (2014). Psychological medicine and the future of psychiatry. *British Journal of Psychiatry, 204,* 91–2.

Sharpe M and Carson AJ (2001). 'Unexplained' somatic symptoms, functional syndromes, and somatisation: do we need a paradigm shift? *Annals of Internal Medicine, 134,* 926–30.

Sharpe M and Mayou R (2004). Somatoform disorders: a help or a hindrance to good patient care? *British Journal of Psychiatry, 184,* 465–7.

Sharpe M *et al.* (2014). Integrated collaborative care for comorbid major depression in patients with cancer (SMaRT Oncology-2): A multicentre randomised controlled effectiveness trial. *The Lancet, 384,* 1099–108.

Sharpe M *et al.* (2015). Rehabilitative treatments for chronic fatigue syndrome: long-term follow-up from the PACE trial. *Lancet Psychiatry, 2,* 1067–74.

Shaw JM *et al.* (2016). Developing a clinical pathway for the identification and management of anxiety and depression in adult cancer patients: an online Delphi consensus process. *Supportive Care in Cancer, 24,* 22–41.

Shaw RJ *et al.* (2012). Impact of ethnic density on adult mental disorders: narrative review. *British Journal of Psychiatry, 201,* 11–19.

Shear MK *et al.* (2011). Complicated grief and related bereavement issues for DSM-5. *Depression and Anxiety, 28,* 103–17.

Sheehan B (2012). Assessment scales in dementia. *Therapeutic Advances in Neurological Disorders, 5,* 349–58.

Sheldon WH *et al.* (1940). *The Varieties of Human Physique.* Harper, London.

Shepherd M (1961). Morbid jealousy: some clinical and social aspects of a psychiatric symptom. *Journal of Mental Science, 107,* 687–753.

Shepherd M *et al.* (1966). *Psychiatric Illness in General Practice.* Oxford University Press, Oxford.

Shepherd MK *et al.* (2014). Orofacial pain: a guide for the headache physician. *Headache: The Journal of Head and Face Pain, 54,* 22–39.

Shiers D *et al.* (2015). Health inequalities and psychosis: time for action. *British Journal of Psychiatry, 207,* 471–3.

Shimada-Sugimoto M *et al.* (2015). Genetics of anxiety disorders: Genetic epidemiological and molecular studies in humans. *Psychiatry and Clinical Neurosciences, 69,* 388–401.

Shin SH *et al.* (2015). Childhood emotional neglect, negative emotion-driven impulsivity and alcohol use in young adulthood. *Child Abuse and Neglect, 50,* 94–103.

Shore JH, Vollmer WM and Tatum EL (1989). Community patterns of post-traumatic stress disorder. *Journal of Nervous and Mental Disease, 177,* 681–5.

Shorter E (1992). *From Paralysis to Fatigue. A history of psychosomatic illness in the modern era.* The Free Press, New York.

Sibbald B *et al.* (1996). Investigation of whether on-site general practice counsellors have an impact on psychotropic drug prescribing rates and costs. *British Journal of General Practice, 46,* 63–7.

Siegel JM (2009). The neurobiology of sleep. *Seminars in Neurology, 29,* 277–96.

Sierra M and David AS (2011). Depersonalisation: a selective impairment of self-awareness. *Consciousness and Cognition, 1,* 99–108.

Sierra M *et al.* (2012). Depersonalization disorder and anxiety: a special relationship? *Psychiatry Research, 197,* 123–7.

Siever LJ *et al.* (2002). The borderline diagnosis III: identifying endophenotypes for genetic studies. *Biological Psychiatry, 51,* 964–8.

Silberberg D *et al.* (2015). Brain and other nervous system disorders across the lifespan—global challenges and opportunities. *Nature, 527,* S151–4.

Silva AJ *et al.* (1998). The dangerousness of persons with delusional jealousy. *Journal of the American Academy of Psychiatry and the Law, 26,* 607–23.

Silveira JM and Seeman MV (1995). Shared psychotic disorder: a critical review of the literature. *Canadian Journal of Psychiatry, 40,* 389–95.

Silver SM, Rogers S and Russell M (2008). Eye movement desensitization and reprocessing (EMDR) in the treatment of war veterans. *Journal of Clinical Psychology, 64,* 947–57.

Simeone JC *et al.* (2015). An evaluation of variation in published estimates of schizophrenia prevalence from 1990–2013: a systematic literature review. *BMC Psychiatry, 15,* 193.

Simon GE and Savarino J (2007). Suicide attempts among patients starting depression treatment with medications or psychotherapy. *American Journal of Psychiatry, 164,* 1029–34.

Simon GE *et al.* (1999). An international study of the relation between somatic symptoms and depression. *New England Journal of Medicine, 341,* 1329–35.

Simon GE *et al.* (2006). Suicide risk during antidepressant treatment. *American Journal of Psychiatry, 163,* 41–7.

Simon L *et al.* (2013). Regional grey matter structure differences between transsexuals and healthy controls—a voxel based morphometry study. *PLoS ONE, 8,* e83947.

Simon NM (2013). Treating complicated grief. *Journal of the American Medical Association, 310,* 416–23.

Simon SS *et al.* (2015). Cognitive behavioral therapies in older adults with depression and cognitive deficits: a systematic review. *International Journal of Geriatric Psychiatry, 30,* 223–33.

Simonoff E *et al.* (2007). ADHD symptoms in children with mild intellectual disability. *Journal of the American Association of Child and Adolescent Psychiatry, 46,* 591–600.

Simonoff E *et al.* (2015). Intellectual disability. In: Thapar A *et al.* (eds.) *Rutter's Child and Adolescent Psychiatry.* John Wiley & Sons, Ltd, Chichester, pp. 719–37.

Sin J and Norman I (2013). Psychoeducational interventions for family members of people with schizophrenia: a mixed-methods systematic review. *Journal of Clinical Psychiatry, 74,* E1145–U56.

Sinclair J and Green J (2005). Understanding resolution of deliberate self harm: qualitative interview study of patients' experiences. *British Medical Journal, 330,* 1112–15.

Singer HS *et al.* (2012). Moving from PANDAS to CANS. *The Journal of Pediatrics, 160*(5):725–31.

Singh SP and Burns T (2006). Race and mental health: there is more to race than racism. *British Medical Journal*, 333, 648–51.

Singh T *et al.* (2016). Rare loss-of-function variants in SETD1A are associated with schizophrenia and developmental disorders. *Nature Neuroscience*, 19, 571–7.

Singleton N *et al.* (2003). Substance misuse among prisoners in England and Wales. *International Review of Psychiatry*, 15, 150–2.

Skegg K (2005). Self-harm. *Lancet*, 366, 1471–83.

Skegg K *et al.* (2003). Sexual orientation and self-harm in men and women. *American Journal of Psychiatry*, 160, 541–6.

Skillback T *et al.* (2015). Cerebrospinal fluid tau and amyloid-β1-42 in patients with dementia. *Brain*, 138, 2716–31.

Skinner BF (1953). *Science and Human Behaviour*. Macmillan, New York.

Skodol A (2008). Longitudinal course and outcome of personality disorders. *Psychiatric Clinics of North America*, 31, 495–503.

Skodol AE *et al.* (2002). The borderline diagnosis I: psychopathology, comorbidity, and personality structure. *Biological Psychiatry*, 51, 936–50.

Skodol AE *et al.* (2005). The collaborative longitudinal personality disorders study (CLPS): overview and implications. *Journal of Personality Disorders*, 19(5), 487–504.

Skodol AE *et al.* (2005). Two-year prevalence and stability of individual DSM-IV criteria for schizotypal, borderline, avoidant, and obsessive-compulsive personality disorders: toward a hybrid model of Axis II disorders. *American Journal of Psychiatry*, 162, 883–9.

Skoog I (2004). Psychiatric epidemiology of old age: the H70 study—the NAPE lecture 2003. *Acta Psychiatrica Scandinavica*, 109, 4–18.

Slade M *et al.* (2000). Threshold Assessment Grid (TAG): the development of a valid and brief scale to assess the severity of mental illness. *Social Psychiatry and Psychiatric Epidemiology*, 35, 78–85.

Slade M *et al.* (2014). Uses and abuses of recovery: implementing recovery-oriented practices in mental health systems. *World Psychiatry*, 13, 12–20.

Slater E (1965). The diagnosis of hysteria. *British Medical Journal*, i, 1395–9.

Slater E and Shields J (1969). Genetical aspects of anxiety. In MH Lader (ed.) *Studies of anxiety*. British Journal of Psychiatry Special Publication, London.

Slater E, Beard AW and Glithero E (1963). The schizophrenia-like psychoses of epilepsy. *British Journal of Psychiatry*, 109, 95–150.

Slatkin M (2008). Linkage disequilibrium—understanding the evolutionary past and mapping the medical future. *Nature Reviews Genetics*, 9, 477–85.

Slifstein M *et al.* (2015). Deficits in prefrontal cortical and extrastriatal dopamine release in schizophrenia. A positron emission tomographic functional magnetic resonance imaging study. *JAMA Psychiatry*, 72, 316–24.

Slikboer R *et al.* (2016). A systematic review and meta-analysis of behaviourally based psychological interventions and pharmacological interventions for trichotillomania. *Clinical Psychologist* 21, 20–32.

Small JG, Klapper MH and Kellams JJ (1988). Electroconvulsive treatment compared with lithium in the management of manic states. *Archives of General Psychiatry*, 45, 727–32.

Smink F *et al.* (2012). Epidemiology of eating disorders: incidence, prevalence and mortality rates. *Current Psychiatry Reports*, 14, 406–14.

Smith DG and Robbins TW (2013). The neurobiological underpinnings of obesity and binge eating: a rationale for adopting the food addiction model. *Biological Psychiatry*, 73, 804–10.

Smith DH *et al.* (2013). Chronic neuropathologies of single and repetitive TBI: substrates of dementia? *Nature Reviews Neurology*, 9, 211–21.

Smith YL *et al.* (2005). Sex reassignment: Outcomes and predictors of treatment for adolescent and adult transsexuals. *Psychological Medicine*, 35, 89–99.

Smyth MG and Hoult J (2000). The home treatment enigma. *British Medical Journal*, 29, 305–9.

Snowling M *et al.* (2015). Disorders of reading, mathematical and motor development. In: A. Thapar *et al.* (eds). *Rutter's Child and Adolescent Psychiatry*. John Wiley & Sons, Chichester, pp. 702–18.

Snyder PJ *et al.* (2016). Effects of testosterone treatment in older men. *New England Journal of Medicine*, 374, 611–24.

Solla P *et al.* (2015). Paraphilias and paraphilic disorders in Parkinson's disease: a systematic review of the literature. *Movement Disorders*, 30, 604–13.

Somashekar B *et al.* (2013). Psychopharmacotherapy of somatic symptom disorders. *International Review of Psychiatry*, 25, 107–15.

Sonuga-Barke EJS *et al.* (2015). ADHD and hyperkinetic disorder. In: A. Thapar *et al.* (eds). *Rutter's Child and Adolescent Psychiatry*. John Wiley & Sons, Chichester, pp. 738–56.

Soothill K, Ackerley E and Francis B (2004). The criminal careers of arsonists. *Medicine, Science and the Law*, 44, 27–40.

Sørensen P *et al.* (2011). A randomized clinical trial of cognitive behavioural therapy versus short-term psychodynamic psychotherapy versus no intervention for patients with hypochondriasis. *Psychological Medicine*, 41, 431–41.

Sovner R and Hurley AD (1989). Ten diagnostic principles for recognizing psychiatric disorders in mentally retarded persons. *Psychiatric Aspects of Mental Retardation*, 8, 9–15.

Spiegel D *et al.* (2013). Dissociative disorders in DSM-5. *Annual Review of Clinical Psychology*, 9, 299–326.

Spielberger CD *et al.* (1983). *Manual for the State-Trait Anxiety Inventory*. Consulting Psychologists' Press, Palo Alto, CA.

Spielmans GI *et al.* (2013). Adjunctive atypical antipsychotic treatment for major depressive disorder: A meta-analysis of depression, quality of life, and safety outcomes. *PLoS Medicine*, 10, e1001403.

Spina E and Scordo MG (2002). Clinically significant drug interactions with antidepressants in the elderly. *Drugs and Aging*, 19, 299–320.

Spinelli M (2009). Postpartum psychosis: detection of risk and management. *American Journal of Psychiatry*, 166, 405–8.

Spitzer M (1990). On defining delusions. *Comprehensive Psychiatry*, 31, 377–97.

Spitzer R, First MB and Williams JBW (1992). Now is the time to retire the term 'organic mental disorders'. *American Journal of Psychiatry*, 149, 240–4.

Spitzer R *et al.* (2006). A brief measure for assessing generalized anxiety disorder. The GAD-7. *Archives of Internal Medicine*, 166, 1092–7.

Spitzer RL, Williams JBD and Gibbon M (1987). *Structured Clinical Interview for DSMIV (SCID)*. New York State Psychiatric Institute, New York.

Spitzer RL *et al.* (1994). Utility of a new procedure for diagnosing mental disorders in primary care. The PRIME-MD 1000 study. *Journal of the American Medical Association, 272*, 1749–56.

Stack S (2000). Suicide: a 15-year review of the sociological literature. Part I: cultural and economic factors. *Suicide Life Threatening Behaviour, 30*, 145–62.

Stack S (2003). Media coverage as a risk factor in suicide. *Journal of Epidemiology Community Health, 57*, 238–40.

Stafford MR *et al.* (2015). Efficacy and safety of pharmacological and psychological interventions for the treatment of psychosis and schizophrenia in children, adolescents and young adults: A systematic review and meta-analysis. *PLoS One, 10*, e0117166.

Stalker K and McArthur K. (2012). Child abuse, child protection and disabled children: A review of recent research. *Child Abuse Review, 21*, 24–40.

Stanek G *et al.* (2012) Lyme borreliosis. *Lancet, 379*, 461-473.

Stanghellini G and Broome MR (2014). Psychopathology as the basic science of psychiatry. *British Journal of Psychiatry, 205*, 169–70.

Staniloiu A and Markowitsch HJ (2014). Dissociative amnesia. *Lancet Psychiatry, 1*, 226–41.

Starcevic V (2015). Hypochondriasis: treatment options for a diagnostic quagmire. *Australasian Psychiatry, 23*, 369–73.

Statham DJ *et al.* (1998). Suicidal behaviour: an epidemiological and genetic study. *Psychological Medicine, 28*, 839–55.

Steadman HJ, Gounis K, Denis D *et al.* (2001). Assessing the New York City involuntary outpatient commitment pilot program. *Psychiatric Services, 52*(3), 330–6.

Steege JF and Zolnoun DA (2009). Evaluation and treatment of dyspareunia. *Obstetrics and Gynecology, 113*, 1124–36.

Steensma TD *et al.* (2013). Gender identity development in adolescence. *Hormones and Behavior, 64*, 288–97.

Steiger A and Kimura M (2010). Wake and sleep EEG provide biomarkers in depression. *Journal of Psychiatric Research, 44*, 242–52.

Stein A *et al.* (2014). Effects of perinatal mental disorders on the fetus and child. *The Lancet, 384*, 1800–19.

Stein LJ and Test MA (1980). Alternative to mental hospital treatment. 1. Conceptual model, treatment program and clinical evaluation. *Archives of General Psychiatry, 37*, 392–7.

Stein MB and Stein DJ (2008). Social anxiety disorder. *Lancet, 371*, 1115–25.

Steinbrecher N *et al.* (2011). The prevalence of medically unexplained symptoms in primary care. *Psychosomatics, 52*(3), 263–71

Steinhausen HC (2002). The outcome of anorexia nervosa in the 20th century. *American Journal of Psychiatry, 159*, 1284–93.

Stenager EN and Stenager E (2000). Physical illness and suicidal behaviour. In: K Hawton and K van Heeringen (eds.) *The International Handbook of Suicide and Attempted Suicide*. John Wiley & Sons, Chichester.

Stengel E (1952). Enquiries into attempted sucide. *Proceedings of the Royal Society of Medicine, 45*, 613–20.

Stengel E (1959). Classification of mental disorders. *Bulletin of the World Health Organization, 21*, 601–3.

Stengel E and Cook NG (1958). *Attempted Suicide: Its social significance and effects*. Chapman & Hall, London.

Stephan KE, Friston KJ and Frith CD (2009). Dysconnection in schizophrenia. From abnormal synaptic plasticity to failures of self-monitoring. *Schizophrenia Bulletin, 35*, 509–27.

Stevens H *et al.* (2015). Post-illness-onset risk of offending across the full spectrum of psychiatric disorders. *Psychological Medicine, 45*, 2447–57.

Stinton C *et al.* (2015). Pharmacological management of Lewy body dementia: a systematic review and meta-analysis. *American Journal of Psychiatry, 172*, 731–42.

Stockings E *et al.* (2016). Prevention, early intervention, harm reduction and treatment of substance misuse in young people. *Lancet Psychiatry, 3*, 280–96.

Stockmeier CA (2003). Involvement of serotonin in depression: evidence from post-mortem and imaging studies of serotonin receptors and the serotonin transporter. *Journal of Psychiatric Research, 37*, 357–73.

Stolte M *et al.* (2016). A critical review of outcome measures used to evaluate the effectiveness of comprehensive, community based treatment for young children with ASD. *Research in Autism Spectrum Disorders, 23*, 221–34.

Stone J *et al.* (2005). Systematic review of misdiagnosis of conversion symptoms and 'hysteria'. *British Medical Journal*, doi:10.1136/bmj.38628.466898.55.

Stone MH, Hurt SW and Stone DK (1987). The PI-500: long-term follow-up of borderline inpatients meeting DSM III criteria. I: global outcome. *Journal of Personality Disorders, 1*, 291–8.

Stores G (2015). Sleep disorders in children and adolescents. *BJPsych Advances, 21*, 124–31.

Storr A (2000). Analytical psychology (Jung). In: MG Gelder, JJ López-IborJr and NC Andreasen (eds.) *The New Oxford Textbook of Psychiatry*, Chapter 3.3.1. Oxford University Press, Oxford.

Strain JJ, Klipstein K and Newcorm J (2009) Adjustment disorders. In: MG Gelder, NC Andreasen, JJ Lopez–Ibor and JR Geddes (eds.) *New Oxford Textbook of Psychiatry*, 2nd edn. Oxford University Press, Oxford. pp. 716–24.

Strang J *et al.* (2010). Impact of supervision of methadone consumption on deaths related to methadone overdose (1993–2008): analyses using OD4 index in England and Scotland. *British Medical Journal, 341*, 640.

Stroebe M, Schut H and Stroebe W (2007). Health outcomes of bereavement. Lancet, 370, 1960–73.

Strömgren E (1985). World-wide issues in psychiatric diagnosis and classification and the Scandinavian point of view. *Mental Disorders, Alcohol and Drug Related Problems*. Excerpta Medica, Amsterdam.

Strydom A *et al.* (2009). The relationship of dementia prevalence in older adults with intellectual disability (ID) to age and severity of ID. *Psychological Medicine, 39*, 13–21.

Substance Abuse and Mental Health Services Administration (2010). Overview of findings from the 2009 National Survey on Drug Use and Health. Office of Applied Studies, Substance Abuse and Mental Health Administration, Rockville, MD.

Sullivan PF (2013). Questions about DISC1 as a genetic risk factor for schizophrenia. *Molecular Psychiatry, 18*, 1050–2.

Sullivan PF, Neale MC, Kendler KS (2000). Genetic epidemiology of major depression: review and meta-analysis. *American Journal of Psychiatry, 157*(10), 1552–62.

Sullivan PF, Kendler KS and Neale MC (2003). Schizophrenia as a complex trait—evidence from a meta-analysis of twin studies. *Archives of General Psychiatry*, 60, 1187–92.

Suominen K *et al.* (1996). Mental disorders and comorbidity in attempted suicide. *Acta Psychiatrica Scandinavica*, 94, 234–40.

Surtees PD *et al.* (2008). Depression and ischemic heart disease mortality: evidence from the EPIC-Norfolk United Kingdom Prospective Cohort Study. *American Journal of Psychiatry*, 165, 515–23.

Swaab DF (2009). Sexual differentiation of the human brain in relation to gender identity and sexual orientation. *Functional Neurology*, 24, 17.

Swanson JW *et al.* (2000). Involuntary outpatient commitment and reduction of violent behaviour in persons with severe mental illness. *British Journal of Psychiatry*, 176, 324–31.

Swartz MS *et al.* (1999). Can involuntary outpatient commitment reduce hospital recidivism?: Findings from a randomized trial with severely mentally ill individuals. *American Journal of Psychiatry*, 156, 1968–75.

Swendsen J *et al.* (2012). Use and abuse of alcohol and illicit drugs in US adolescents: Results of the National Comorbidity Survey–Adolescent Supplement. *Archives of General Psychiatry*, 69, 390–8.

Szanto K *et al.* (2007). A suicide prevention program in a region with a very high suicide rate. *Archives of General Psychiatry*, 64, 914–20.

Szasz TS (1960). The myth of mental illness. *American Psychology*, 15, 113–18.

Szmukler G (2001). Violence risk prediction in practice. *British Journal of Psychiatry*, 178, 84–5.

Szmukler G and Appelbaum P (2008). Treatment pressures, leverage, coercion and compulsion in mental health care. *Journal of Mental Health*, 17 (3), 233–44.

Talbot P *et al.* (2010). *Key Concepts in Learning Disabilities*. Sage, Los Angeles.

Talbott JA, Jefferies M and Arana JD (1987). CMHCs: relationships with academia and the state. *Community Mental Health Journal*, 23, 271–81.

Tan MS *et al.* (2015). Efficacy and adverse effects of *Ginkgo biloba* for cognitive impairment and dementia: a systematic review and meta-analysis. *Journal of Alzheimer's Disease*, 43, 589–603.

Tandon R *et al.* (2013). Definition and description of schizophrenia in the DSM-5. *Schizophrenia Research*, 150, 3–10.

Tansella M (2002). The scientific evaluation of mental health treatments: an historical perspective. *Evidence Based Mental Health*, 5, 4–5.

Tarrier N *et al.* (1998). Randomised controlled trial of intensive cognitive behaviour therapy for patients with chronic schizophrenia. *British Medical Journal*, 317, 303–7.

Taylor D (2008). Psychoanalytic and psychodynamic therapies for depression: the evidence base. *Advances in Psychiatric Treatment*, 14, 401–13.

Taylor D *et al.* (2011). Pharmacological interventions for people with depression and chronic physical health problems: systematic review and meta-analyses of safety and efficacy. *British Journal of Psychiatry*, 198, 179–88.

Taylor D, Paton C, Kapur S (2015). *The Maudsley Prescribing Guidelines in Psychiatry*, 12th edn. John Wiley, Chichester.

Taylor FK (1981). On pseudo-hallucinations. *Psychological Medicine*, 11, 265–72.

Taylor JE and Harvey ST (2010). A meta-analysis of the effects of psychotherapy with adults sexually abused in childhood. *Clinical Psychology Review*, 30, 749–67.

Taylor JL *et al.* (2002). Evaluation of a group intervention for convicted arsonists with mild and borderline intellectual disabilities. *Criminal Behavior and Mental Health*, 12, 282–93.

Taylor M and Perera U (2015). NICE CG178 Psychosis and Schizophrenia in Adults: Treatment and Management—an evidence-based guideline? *British Journal of Psychiatry*, 206, 357–9.

Taylor PJ and Dunn E (2009). Management of offenders with mental disorder in specialist forensic mental health services. In: MG Gelder, NC Andreasen, JJ Lopez-Ibor, and J Geddes (eds.) *The New Oxford Textbook of Psychiatry*. Oxford University Press, Oxford, pp. 2015–21.

Taylor PJ, Mahandra B and Gunn J (1983). Erotomania in males. *Psychological Medicine*, 13, 645–50.

Taylor WD *et al.* (2013). The vascular depression hypothesis: mechanisms linking vascular disease with depression. *Molecular Psychiatry*, 18, 963–74.

Teicher MH and Samson JA (2016). Annual research review: Enduring neurobiological effects of childhood abuse and neglect. *Journal of Child Psychology and Psychiatry and Allied Disciplines*, 57, 241–66.

Tess AV and Smetana GW (2009). Medical evaluation of patients undergoing electroconvulsive therapy. *New England Journal of Medicine*, 360, 1437–44.

Thapar A (2012). Depression in adolescence. *The Lancet*, 379, 1056–67.

The European School Survey Project on Alcohol and Other Drugs 2011). http://www.espad.org/en/Reports--Documents/ESPAD-Reports/

Thibaut F *et al.* (2010). The World Federation of Societies of Biological Psychiatry (WFSBP) guidelines for the biological treatment of paraphilias. *World Journal of Biological Psychiatry*, 11, 604–55.

Thomas A, Chess S and Birch HG (1968). *Temperament and Behaviour Disorders in Children*. University Press, New York.

Thomas D (2010). Methods for investigating gene–environment interactions in candidate pathway and genome-wide association studies. *Annual Review of Public Health*, 31, 21–36.

Thompson A *et al.* (2014). Behavioral and psychiatric symptoms in prion disease. *American Journal of Psychiatry*, 171, 265–74.

Thompson A *et al.* (2016). At-risk mental state for psychosis: identification and current treatment approaches. *BJPsych Advances*, 22, 186–93.

Thompson AE and Pearce JB (2009). The child as witness. In: MG Gelder, NC Andreasen, JJ Lopez-Ibor, JR Geddes (eds.) *New Oxford Textbook of Psychiatry*. Oxford University Press, Oxford. pp. 1761–3.

Thomson L and Darjee R (2009). Associations between psychiatric disorder and offending. In: MG Gelder, NC Andreasen, JJ Lopez-Ibor and J Geddes (eds.) *The New Oxford Textbook of Psychiatry*. Oxford University Press, Oxford, pp. 1917–26.

Thomson M (1998). *The Problem of Mental Deficiency. Eugenics, democracy, and social policy in Britain, c.1870–1959*. Oxford University Press, Oxford.

Thornicroft G (2006). *Shunned: Discrimination against people with mental illness*. Oxford University Press, Oxford.

Thornicroft G and Tansella M (2013). The balanced care model: the case for both hospital- and community-based mental healthcare. *British Journal of Psychiatry*, **202**, 246–8.

Thornicroft G *et al*. (2013). Clinical outcomes of Joint Crisis Plans to reduce compulsory treatment for people with psychosis: a randomised controlled trial. *The Lancet*, **381**, 1634–41.

Tienari P *et al*. (2003). Genetic boundaries of the schizophrenia spectrum: evidence form the Finnish adoptive family study of schizophrenia. *American Journal of Psychiatry*, **160**, 1587–94.

Tienari P *et al*. (2004). Genotype–environment interaction in schizophrenia-spectrum disorder. Long-term follow-up study of Finnish adoptees. *British Journal of Psychiatry*, **184**, 216–22.

Tiihonen J *et al*. (2006). Effectiveness of antipsychotic treatments in a nationwide cohort of patients in community care after first hospitalisation due to schizophrenia and schizoaffective disorder: observational follow-up study. *British Medical Journal*, **333**, 224.

Tiihonen J *et al*. (2012). Polypharmacy with antipsychotics, antidepressants, or benzodiazepine and mortality in schizophrenia. *Archives of General Psychiatry*, **69**, 476–83.

Tizard J (1964). *Community Services for the Mentally Handicapped*. Oxford University Press, London.

Tol WA *et al*. (2011). Mental health and psychosocial support in humanitarian settings: linking practice and research. *Lancet*, **378**, 1581–91.

Toledo JB *et al*. (2013). Contribution of cerebrovascular disease in autopsy confirmed neurodegenerative disease cases in the National Alzheimer's Coordinating Centre. *Brain*, **136**, 2697–706.

Tondo L *et al*. (1997). Effectiveness of restarting lithium treatment after its discontinuation in bipolar I and bipolar II disorders. *American Journal of Psychiatry*, **154**, 548–50.

Tong Y and Phillips MR (2010). Cohort-specific risk of suicide for different mental disorders in China. *British Journal of Psychiatry*, **196**, 467–73.

Tonge BJ *et al*. (2014). A review of evidence-based early intervention for behavioural problems in children with autism spectrum disorder: the core components of effective programs, child-focused interventions and comprehensive treatment models. *Current Opinion in Psychiatry*, **27**, 158–65.

Torgersen S *et al*. (2000). A twin study of personality disorders. *Comprehensive Psychiatry*, **41**(6), 416–25.

Torgesen S *et al*. (2001). The prevalence of personality disorders in a community sample. *Archives of General Psychiatry*, **58**, 590–6.

Torniainen M *et al*. (2015). Antipsychotic treatment and mortality in schizophrenia. *Schizophrenia Bulletin*, **41**, 656–63.

Torrey EF and Yolken RH (2010). Psychiatric genocide: Nazi attempts to eradicate schizophrenia. *Schizophrenia Bulletin*, **36**, 26–32.

Tortelli A *et al*. (2015). Schizophrenia and other psychotic disorders in Caribbean-born migrants and their descendants in England: systematic review and meta-analysis of incidence rates, 1950–2013. *Social Psychiatry and Psychiatric Epidemiology*, **50**, 1039–55.

Toth M (2015). Mechanisms of non-genetic inheritance and psychiatric disorders. *Neuropsychopharmacology*, **40**, 129–40.

Tracy DK and David AS (2015). Clinical neuromodulation in psychiatry: the state of the art or an art in a state? *BJPsych Advances*, **21**(6), 396–404.

Treasure J (2004). Motivational interviewing. *Advances in Psychiatric Treatment*, **10**, 331–7.

Treasure J *et al*. (2015). Has the time come for a staging model to map the course of eating disorders from high risk to severe enduring illness? An examination of the evidence. *Early Intervention in Psychiatry*, **9**, 173–84.

Treiman DM (1999). Violence and the epilepsy defense. *Neurologic Clinics*, **17**, 245–55.

Triebwasser J *et al*. (2013). Paranoid personality disorder. *Journal of Personality Disorders* **27**, 795–805.

Trim RS *et al*. (2013). Predictors of initial and sustained remission from alcohol use disorders: Findings from the 30-year follow-up of the San Diego prospective study. *Alcoholism: Clinical and Experimental Research*, **37**, 1424–31.

True WR *et al*. (1993). A twin study of genetic and environmental contributions to liability of posttraumatic stress symptoms. *Archives of General Psychiatry*, **50**, 257.

Tseng W-S (2006). From peculiar psychiatric disorders through culture bound syndromes to culture-related specific syndromes. *Transcultural Psychiatry*, **43**, 554–76.

Tsertsvadze A *et al*. (2009). Oral phosphodiesterase-5 inhibitors and hormonal treatments for erectile dysfunction: a systematic review and meta-analysis. *Annals of Internal Medicine*, **151**, 650–W218.

Tunbridge EM, Harrison PJ and Weinberger DR (2006). Catechol-o-methyltransferase, cognition and psychosis: Val[158]Met and beyond. *Biological Psychiatry*, **60**, 141–52

Turkington D, Martindale B and Bloch-Thorseen GR (2005). Schizophrenia. In: GO Gabbard, JS Beck and J Holmes (eds.) *Oxford Textbook of Psychotherapy*, Chapter 14. Oxford University Press, Oxford.

Turner DT *et al*. (2014). Psychological interventions for psychosis: a meta-analysis of comparative outcome studies. *American Journal of Psychiatry*, **171**, 523–38.

Turner MA *et al*. (2002). Subcortical dementia. *British Journal of Psychiatry*, **180**, 148–51.

Turton P *et al*. (2009). Long-term psychosocial sequelae of stillbirth: phase II of a nested case-control cohort study. *Archives of Women's Mental Health*, **12**, 35–41.

Tyrer P (2013). *Models for Mental Disorder*. 5th edn. Wiley-Blackwell, Oxford.

Tyrer P (2014). A comparison of DSM and ICD classifications of mental disorder. *Advances in Psychiatric Treatment*, **20**, 280–5.

Tyrer P and Baldwin D (2006). Generalized anxiety disorder. *Lancet*, **368**, 2156–66.

Tyrer P and Methuen C (2007). *Rating Scales in Psychiatry*. RCPsych Publications, London.

Tyrer P, Seivewright H and Johnson T (2004a). The Nottingham study of neurotic disorder *Psychological Medicine*, **34**, 1385–94.

Tyrer P, Reed GM and Crawford MJ (2015) Classification, assessment, prevalence, and effect of personality disorder. *Lancet*, **385**, 717–25.

Tyrer RA and Fazel M (2014). School and community-based interventions for refugee and asylum seeking children: A systematic review. *PloS One*, **9**, e89359.

Uchida H *et al.* (2009) Increased antipsychotic sensitivity in elderly patients: evidence and mechanisms. *Journal of Clinical Psychiatry,* **70**, 397–405.

Uher R and Rutter M (2012). Classification of feeding and eating disorders: review of evidence and proposals for ICD-11. *World Psychiatry,* **11**, 80–92.

UK Alcohol Treatment Trial Research Team (2005). Effectiveness of treatment for alcohol problems. Findings of the randomised UK Alcohol Treatment Trial (UKATT). *British Medical Journal,* **331**, 54.

UK ECT Review Group (2003). Efficacy and safety of electroconvulsive therapy in depressive disorders: a systematic review and meta-analysis. *Lancet,* **361**, 799–808.

Ungar M (2015). Practitioner review: Diagnosing childhood resilience—a systemic approach to the diagnosis of adaptation in adverse social and physical ecologies. *Journal of Child Psychology and Psychiatry and Allied Disciplines,* **56**, 4–17.

United Nations (2010). *World Population Ageing 2009.* Department of Economic and Social Affairs, Population Division. New York.

United Nations Office on Drugs and Crime (2010). International Statistics on Crime and Justice, Harrendorf, Heiskanen & Malby (eds.). *HEUNI Publication Series No. 64,* Helsinki.

UN Population Division (2015). *World Urbanization Prospects: The 2014 Revision.* New York: United Nations Department of Economics and Social Affairs, Population Division.

Unutzer J (2007). Late-life depression. *New England Journal of Medicine,* **357**, 2269–76.

Upthegrove R *et al.* (2015). Adverse childhood events and psychosis in bipolar affective disorder. *The British Journal of Psychiatry,* **206**, 191–7.

US Office of Surgeon General (2012). *2012 National Strategy for Suicide Prevention: Goals and Objectives for Action: A Report of the U.S. Surgeon General and of the National Action Alliance for Suicide Prevention.* Washington (DC): US Department of Health & Human Services (US).

Vaillant GE (2003). A 60-year follow-up of alcoholic men. *Addiction,* **98**, 1043–51.

Valenti M *et al.* (2008). Electroconvulsive therapy in the treatment of mixed states in bipolar disorder. *European Psychiatry,* **23**, 53–6.

Valenti E *et al.* (2015). Informal coercion in psychiatry: a focus group study of attitudes and experiences of mental health professionals in ten countries. *Social Psychiatry and Psychiatric Epidemiology,* **50**, 1297–308.

Valkanova V and Ebmeier KP (2013). Vascular risk factors and depression in later life: a systematic review and meta-analysis. *Biological Psychiatry,* **73**, 406–13.

Vancampfort D *et al.* (2015). Risk of metabolic syndrome and its components in people with schizophrenia and related psychotic disorders, bipolar disorder and major depressive disorder: a systematic review and meta-analysis. *World Psychiatry,* **14**, 339–47.

van de Wouw E *et al.* (2012). Prevalence, associated factors and treatment of sleep problems in adults with intellectual disability: A systematic review. *Research in Developmental Disabilities,* **33**, 1310–32.

van Ijzendoorn M (1995). Adult attachment representations, parental responsiveness, and infant attachment: A meta-analysis on the predictive validity of the Adult Attachment Interview. *Psychological Bulletin,* **117**, 387–403.

Van Kessel K *et al.* (2008). A randomized controlled trial of cognitive behavior therapy for multiple sclerosis fatigue. *Psychosomatic Medicine,* **7**, 205–13.

van Kesteren CFMG *et al.* (2017). Immune involvement in the pathogenesis of schizophrenia: a meta-analysis on postmortem brain studies. *Translational Psychiatry,* **7**, e1075.

van Os J (2016). 'Schizophrenia' does not exist. *British Medical Journal,* **352**, i375.

Van Os J *et al.* (2003). Do urbanicity and familial liability coparticipate in causing psychosis. *American Journal of Psychiatry,* **160**, 477–82.

Van Os J, Kenis G and Rutten BPF (2010). The environment and schizophrenia. *Nature,* **468**, 203–12.

Van Soest T *et al.* (2009). The effects of cosmetic surgery on body image, self-esteem, and psychological problems. *Journal of Plastic, Reconstructive & Aesthetic Surgery,* **62**, 1238–44.

Vaughn CE and Leff JP (1976). The influence of family and social factors on the course of psychiatric illness. A comparison of schizophrenic and depressed neurotic patients. *British Journal of Psychiatry,* **129**, 125–37.

Vaughn MG *et al.* (2015). Deliberate self-harm and the nexus of violence, victimization, and mental health problems in the United States. *Psychiatry Research,* **225**, 588–95.

Vauhkonen K (1968). On the pathogenesis of morbid jealousy with special reference to the personality traits of an interaction between jealous patients and their spouses. *Acta Psychiatrica Scandinavica Supplement,* **202**, 2–261.

Vázquez GH *et al.* (2013). Overview of antidepressant treatment of bipolar depression. *International Journal of Neuropsychopharmacology,* **16**, 1673–85.

Vázquez GH *et al.* (2014). Pharmacological treatment of bipolar depression. *Advances in Psychiatric Treatment,* **20**, 193–201.

Veale D (2007). Cognitive behavioural therapy for obsessive compulsive disorder. *Advances in Psychiatric Treatment,* **13**, 438–46.

Veale D and Roberts A (2014). Obsessive-compulsive disorder. *British Medical Journal,* **348**, g2183.

Veale D *et al.* (2014). Atypical antipsychotic augmentation in SSRI treatment refractory obsessive-compulsive disorder: A systematic review and meta-analysis. *BMC Psychiatry,* **14**, 317.

Velayudhan L *et al.* (2014). Review of brief cognitive tests for patients with suspected dementia. *International Psychogeriatrics,* **26**, 1247–62.

Ventriglio A *et al.* (2016). Relevance of culture-bound syndromes in the 21st century. *Psychiatry and Clinical Neurosciences,* **70**, 3–6.

Verdel BM *et al.* (2010). Use of antidepressant drugs and risk of osteoporotic and non-osteoporotic fractures. *Bone,* **47**, 604–9.

Vergani F *et al.* (2010). Surgical, medical and hardware adverse events in a series of 141 patients undergoing subthalmic deep brain stimulation for Parkinson disease. *World Neurosurgery,* **73**, 338–44.

Verghese PB, Castellano JM and Holtzman DM (2011). Apolipoprotein E in Alzheimer's disease and other neurological disorders. *Lancet Neurology,* **10**, 241–52.

Verkuijl N *et al.* (2015). Childhood attention-deficit/hyperactivity disorder. *BMJ,* **350**, h2168.

Vicens V *et al.* (2016). Structural and functional brain changes in delusional disorder. *British Journal of Psychiatry*, **208**, 153–9.

Vickerman KA and Margolin G (2009). Rape treatment outcome research: empirical findings and state of the literature. *Clinical Psychology Review*, **29**, 431–48.

Victor M *et al.* (1971). *The Wernicke-Korsakoff Syndrome*. Blackwell, Oxford.

Victor TA *et al.* (2010). Relationship between amygdala responses to masked faces and mood state and treatment in major depressive disorder. *Archives of General Psychiatry*, **67**, 1128–38.

Victoroff J *et al.* (2014). Pharmacological management of persistent hostility and aggression in persons with schizophrenia spectrum disorders: a systematic review. *Journal of Neuropsychiatry and Clinical Neurosciences*, **26**, 283–312.

Videnovic A (2013). Treatment of Huntington disease. *Current Treatment Options in Neurology*, **15**, 424–38.

Viens M *et al.* (2003). Trait anxiety and sleep-onset insomnia: evaluation of treatment using anxiety management training. *Journal of Psychosomatic Research*, **54**, 31–7.

Vieta E *et al.* (2008). Efficacy and safety of quetiapine in combination with lithium or divalproex for maintenance of patients with bipolar I disorder (International trial 126). *Journal of Affective Disorders*, **109**, 251–63.

Vigod SN *et al.* (2015). Antipsychotic drug use in pregnancy: high dimensional, propensity matched, population based cohort study. *British Medical Journal*, **350**, h2298.

Vigod SN *et al.* (2016). Depression in pregnancy. *British Medical Journal*, **352**, i1547.

Vincent A *et al.* (2011). Autoantibodies associated with diseases of the CNS: new developments and future challenges. *Lancet Neurology*, **10**, 759–72.

Visscher PM, Hill WG and Wray NR (2008). Heritability in the genomics era—concepts and misconceptions. *Nature Reviews Genetics*, **9**, 255–66.

Vissers LE *et al.* (2016). Genetic studies in intellectual disability and related disorders. *Nature Reviews Genetics*, **17**, 9–18.

Volkmar F *et al.* (2014). Practice parameter for the assessment and treatment of children and adolescents with autism spectrum disorder. *Journal of the American Academy of Child & Adolescent Psychiatry*, **53**(2), 237–57.

Vreeker A *et al.* (2015). Cognitive enhancing agents in schizophrenia and bipolar disorder. *European Neuropsychopharmacology*, **25**, 969–1002.

Waern M *et al.* (2002). Mental disorder in elderly suicides: a case-control study. *American Journal of Psychiatry*, **159**, 450–5.

Wagenaar AC, Tobler AL and Komro KA (2010). Effects of alcohol tax and price policies on morbidity and mortality. A systematic review. *Research and Practice*, **100**, 2270–8.

Waite J (2013). Patients' and carers perspectives on ECT. In: J Waite, A Eaton (eds.) *The ECT Handbook*. RCPsych Publications, London. pp. 224–9.

Wakefield JC (1992). The concept of mental disorder. On the boundary between biological facts and social values. *American Psychology*, **47**, 373–88.

Walker A *et al.* (2013a). Treatment of depression in adults with cancer: a systematic review of randomized controlled trials. *Psychological Medicine*, **44**, 897–907.

Walker J *et al.* (2013b). Prevalence of depression in adults with cancer: a systematic review. *Annals of Oncology*, **24**, 895–900.

Walker Z *et al.* (2015). Lewy body dementias. *Lancet*, **386**, 1683–97.

Walle JV *et al.* (2012). Practical consensus guidelines for the management of enuresis. *European Journal of Pediatrics*, **171**, 971–83.

Walters JTR and Owen MJ (2016). Genome-wide significant associations for cannabis dependence severity: relevance to psychiatric disorders. *JAMA Psychiatry*, **73**, 443–4.

Wang HF *et al.* (2015). Efficacy and safety of cholinesterase inhibitors and memantine in cognitive impairment in Parkinson's disease, Parkinson's disease dementia, and dementia with Lewy bodies: systematic review with meta-analysis and trial sequential analysis. *Journal of Neurology, Neurosurgery and Psychiatry*, **86**, 135–43.

Ward CH *et al.* (1962). The psychiatric nomenclature. *Archives of General Psychiatry*, **7**, 198–205.

Warrell DA, Cox TM and Firth JD (2010). *Oxford Textbook of Medicine*. Oxford University Press, New York.

Wasserman D and Wasserman C (eds.) (2009). *Oxford Textbook of Suicidology and Suicide Prevention*. Oxford University Press, New York.

Watson JB and Rayner R (1920). Conditioned emotional reactions. *Journal of Experimental Psychology*, **3**, 1–14.

Watson HJ and Bulik CM (2013). Update on the treatment of anorexia nervosa: review of clinical trials, practice guidelines and emerging interventions. *Psychological Medicine*, **43**, 2477–500.

Watts J and Priebe S (2002). A phenomenological account of users' experiences of assertive community treatment. *Bioethics*, **16**, 439–54.

Webb RT *et al.* (2012). Suicide risk in primary care patients with major physical disease: a case-control study. *Archives of General Psychiatry*, **69**, 256–64.

Weinberger DR (1987). Implications of normal brain development for the pathogenesis of schizophrenia. *Archives of General Psychiatry*, **44**, 660–9.

Weinberger DR and Levitt P (2011). Neurodevelopmental origins of schizophrenia. In: Weinberger DR and Harrison PJ (eds.) *Schizophrenia*, 3rd edn. Wiley Blackwell, Oxford. pp. 393–412.

Weinberger DR and Radulescu E (2016). Finding the elusive pychiatric "lesion" with 21st-century neuroanatomy: A note of caution. *American Journal of Psychiatry*, **173**, 27–33.

Weissman AM *et al.* (2004). Pooled analysis of antidepressant levels in lactating mothers, breast milk, and nursing infants. *American Psychiatric Association*, **161**, 1066–78.

Wells A (2013). Advances in metacognitive therapy. *International Journal of Cognitive Therapy*, **6**, 186–201.

Wertheimer A (2001). *A Special Scar: The experiences of people bereaved by suicide*. Brunner-Routledge, Hove.

Wertheimer J (1997). Psychiatry of the elderly: a consensus statement. *International Journal of Geriatric Psychiatry*, **12**, 432–5.

Wesseloo R *et al.* (2016). Risk of postpartum relapse in bipolar disorder and post-partum psychosis: A systematic review and meta-analysis. *American Journal of Psychiatry*, **173**, 117–27.

Westbrook D *et al.* (2011). *An Introduction to Cognitive Behaviour Therapy: Skills and applications*. Sage Publications, London.

While *et al.* (2012). Implementation of mental health service recommendations in England and Wales and suicide rates, 1997–2006: a cross-sectional and before-and-after observational study. *Lancet*, **379**, 1005–12.

White PD *et al.* (2011). Comparison of adaptive pacing therapy, cognitive behaviour therapy, graded exercise therapy, and specialist medical care for chronic fatigue syndrome (PACE): a randomized trial. *Lancet*, **377**, 823–36.

White PD, Rickards H and Zeman AZJ (2012). Time to end the distinction between mental and neurological illnesses. *British Medical Journal*, **344**, e3454.

Whiteford HA *et al.* (2013). Global burden of disease attributable to mental and substance use disorders: findings from the Global Burden of Disease Study 2010. *Lancet*, **382**, 1575–86.

Whiting D and Cowen PJ (2013). Drug information update: Agomelatine. *The Psychiatrist*, **37**, 356–8.

Whitley E *et al.* (1999). Ecological study of social fragmentation, poverty, and suicide. *British Medical Journal*, **319**, 1037.

Whitney I, Smith PK and Thompson D (1994). Bullying and children with special needs. In: PK Smith and S Sharp (eds.) *School Bullying: Insights and perspectives*. Routledge, London. pp. 213–40.

Whittington CJ *et al.* (2004). Selective serotonin reuptake inhibitors in childhood depression: systematic review of 363,published versus unpublished data. *Lancet*, **363**, 1341–5.

Wichstrøm L *et al.* (2012). Prevalence of psychiatric disorders in preschoolers. *Journal of Child Psychology and Psychiatry*, **53**, 695–705.

Wieck A and Haddad PM (2004). Hyperprolactinaemia. In: PM Haddad, S Dursun and B Deakin (eds.) *Adverse Syndromes and Psychiatric Drugs. A clinical guide*. Oxford University Press, Oxford. pp. 69–88.

Wijkstra J *et al.* (2010). Treatment of unipolar psychotic depression: a randomized double blind study comparing imipramine, venlafaxine and venlafaxine plus quetiapine. *Acta Psychiatrica Scandinavica*, **121**, 190–200.

Wilcox HC (2004). Association of alcohol and drug use disorders and completed suicide: an empirical review of cohort studies. *Drug and Alcohol Dependence*, **76** (Suppl.), S11–S19.

Wiles N *et al.* (2013). Cognitive behavioural therapy as an adjunct to pharmacotherapy for primary care based patients with treatment resistant depression: Results of the CoBalt randomised controlled trial. *The Lancet*, **381**, 375–84.

Wilhelm S *et al.* (2014). Modular cognitive-behavioral therapy for body dysmorphic disorder: a randomized controlled trial. *Behavior Therapy*, **45**, 314–27.

Wilkinson D and Andersen HF (2007). Analysis of the effect of memantine in reducing the worsening of clinical symptoms in patients with moderate to severe Alzheimer's disease. *Dementia and Geriatric Cognitive Disorders*, **24**, 138–45.

Wilkinson D *et al.* (2009). Effectiveness of donepezil in reducing clinical worsening of patients with mild to moderate Alzheimer's disease. *Dementia and Geriatric Cognitive Disorders*, **28**, 244–51.

Wilkinson P (2013). Psychological treatments. In: T Dening and A Thomas (eds.) *Oxford Textbook of Old Age Psychiatry*, 2nd edn. Oxford University Press, Oxford.

Williams JMG and Pollock LR (2000). The psychology of suicidal behaviour. In: K Hawton and K van Heeringen (eds.) *The International Handbook of Suicide and Attempted Suicide*. John Wiley & Sons, Chichester.

Williams M and Viscusi JA (2016). Hoarding disorder and a systematic review of treatment with cognitive behavioral therapy. *Cognitive Behaviour Therapy*, 45, 93–110.

Williams JMG *et al.* (2014). Mindfulness-based cognitive therapy for preventing relapse in recurrent depression: A randomized dismantling trial. *Journal of Consulting and Clinical Psychology*, **82**, 275–86.

Williams MJ *et al.* (2011). Mindfulness-based cognitive therapy for severe health anxiety (hypochondriasis): an interpretative phenomenological analysis of patients' experiences. *British Journal of Clinical Psychology*, **50**, 379–97.

Williamson OD *et al.* (2014). Antidepressants in the treatment for chronic low back pain: questioning the validity of meta-analyses. *Pain Practice*, **14**, E33–E41.

Willner P *et al.* (2013). Group-based cognitive-behavioural anger management for people with mild to moderate intellectual disabilities: cluster randomised controlled trial. *British Journal of Psychiatry*, bjp. bp. 112.124529.

Wilson RP and Bhattacharyya S (2016). Antipsychotic efficacy in psychosis with co-morbid cannabis misuse: a systematic review. *Journal of Psychopharmacology*, **30**, 99–111.

Wilson S and Pinner G (2013). Driving and dementia: a clinician's guide. *Advances in Psychiatric Treatment*, **19**, 89–96.

Wilson S *et al.* (2004). Prevalence of irritable bowel syndrome: a community survey. *British Journal of General Practice*, **54**, 495–502.

Wilson S *et al.* (2014). A systematic review of interventions to promote social support and parenting skills in parents with an intellectual disability. *Child: Care, Health and Development*, **40**, 7–19.

Wilson SJ *et al.* (2010). British Association for Psychopharmacology consensus statement on evidence-based treatment of insomnia, parasomnias and circadian rhythm disorders. *Journal of Psychopharmacology*, **24**, 1577–600.

Wincze JP and Weisberg RB (2015). *Sexual Dysfunction: A guide for assessment and treatment*. Guilford Publications, New York.

Wing JK and Brown GW (1970). *Institutionalism and Schizophrenia*. Cambridge University Press, London.

Wing JK and Furlong R (1986). A haven for the severely disabled within the context of a comprehensive psychiatric community service. *British Journal of Psychiatry*, **149**, 449–57.

Wing JK, Cooper JE and Sartorius N (1974). *Measurement and Classification of Psychiatric Symptoms; an instruction manual for the PSE and the CATEGO programme*. Cambridge University Press, Cambridge.

Wing JK *et al.* (1998). Health of the Nation Outcome Scales (HoNOS). Research and development. *British Journal of Psychiatry*, **172**, 11–18.

Winkelman JW (2015). Insomnia disorder. *New England Journal of Medicine*, **373**, 1437–44.

Winstock AR and Schifano F (2009). Disorders relating the use of ecstasy and other 'party drugs'. In: Gelder MG, Andreasen NC, Lopez-Ibor JJ, Geddes JR (eds.) *New Oxford Textbook of Psychiatry*, 2nd edn. Oxford: Oxford University Press. pp. 494–502.

Winstock AR, Ford C and Witton J (2010). Assessment and management of cannabis use disorders in primary care. *British Medical Journal*, **340**, 800–4.

Winter S *et al.* (2016). Transgender people: health at the margins of society. *Lancet*, **388**, 390–400.

Winterer G and McCarley RW (2011). Electrophysiology of schizophrenia. In: D Weinberger and PJ Harrison (eds.) *Schizophrenia*. Wiley-Blackwell, Oxford, pp. 311–33.

Winterer G and Weinberger DR (2004). Genes, dopamine and cortical signal-to-noise ratio in schizophrenia. *Trends in Neurosciences*, **27**, 683–90.

Wisniewski SR *et al.* (2009). Can phase III trial results of antidepressant medications be generalized to clinical practice? A STAR* D report. *American Journal of Psychiatry*, **166**, 599–607.

Witlox J *et al.* (2010). Delirium in elderly patients and the risk of postdischarge mortality, institutionalization, and dementia. A meta-analysis. *Journal of the American Medical Association*, **304**, 443–51.

Wittchen H-U *et al.* (2010). Agoraphobia: a review of the diagnostic classificatory position and criteria. *Depression and Anxiety*, **27**, 113–33.

Wittchen HU *et al.* (2011). The size and burden of mental disorders and other disorders of the brain in Europe 2010. *European Neuropsychopharmacology*, **21**, 655–79.

Wium-Andersen MK *et al.* (2016). Elevated C-reactive protein and late-onset bipolar disorder in 78 809 individuals from the general population. *British Journal of Psychiatry*, **208**, 138–45.

Wolff HG (1962). A concept of disease in man. *Psychosomatic Medicine*, **24**, 25–30.

Wolitzky-Taylor KB *et al.* (2008). Psychological approaches in the treatment of specific phobias: A meta-analysis. *Clinical Psychology Review*, **28**, 1021–37.

Wolpe J (1958). *Psychotherapy by Reciprocal Inhibition*. Stanford University Press, Stanford, CA.

Wolpert L (1999). *Malignant Sadness: the anatomy of depression*, 2nd edn. Faber, London.

Wolpert M (2009). Organization of services for children and adolescents with mental health problems. In: Gelder MG, Andreasen NC, Lopez-Ibor JJ, Geddes JR (eds.) *New Oxford Textbook of Psychiatry*, 2nd edn. Oxford: Oxford University Press. pp. 1807–11.

Wong EKO *et al.* (2013a). The interface between neurology and psychiatry: the case of multiple sclerosis. *Advances in Psychiatric Treatment*, **19**, 370–7.

Wong WB *et al.* (2013b). Statins in the prevention of dementia and Alzheimer's disease: A meta-analysis of observational studies and an assessment of confounding. *Pharmacoepidemiology and Drug Safety*, **22**, 345–58.

Wooden MDG *et al.* (2009). Frequent attenders with mental disorders at a general hospital emergency department. *Emergency Medicine Australasia*, **21**(3), 191–5.

Wooff K and Goldberg DP (1988). Further observations on the practice of community care in Salford. Differences between community psychiatric nurses and mental health social workers. *British Journal of Psychiatry*, **153**, 30–7.

Woolfenden S *et al.* (2012). A systematic review of the diagnostic stability of autism spectrum disorder. *Research in Autism Spectrum Disorders*, **6**, 345–54.

World Health Organization (1973). *Report of the International Pilot Study of Schizophrenia*. Vol. 1, World Health Organization, Geneva.

World Health Organization (1984). *Mental Health Care in Developing Countries: A critical appraisal of research findings*. World Health Organization, Geneva.

World Health Organization (1992a). *Glossary: Differential definitions of SCAN items and commentary on the SCAN text*. World Health Organization, Geneva.

World Health Organization (1992b). *The ICD-10 Classification of Mental and Behavioural Disorders: Clinical descriptions and diagnostic guidelines*. World Health Organization, Geneva.

World Health Organization (2010). Suicide rates per 100,000 by country, year and sex. http://www.who.int/mental_health/prevention/suicide_rates/en/index.html

World Health Organization (2010). *mhGAP Intervention Guide for Mental, Neurological and Substance Use Disorders in Non-specialized Health Settings*. WHO Press, Geneva.

World Health Organization (2012). *Public Health Action for the Prevention of Suicide: A framework*. WHO, Geneva.

World Health Organization (2014). *Preventing Suicide: A global imperative*. WHO, Geneva.

World Medical Association (2000). *Declaration of Geneva: Ethical principles for medical research involving human subjects*. World Medical Association, Edinburgh.

Wright C *et al.* (2004). A systematic review of home treatment services. Classification and sustainability. *Social Psychiatry & Psychiatric Epidemiology*, **39**, 789–96.

Wright D, Ost J and French CC (2006). Recovered and false memories. *The Psychologist*, **19**, 352–5.

Wulff K *et al.* (2010). Sleep and circadian rhythms disruption in psychiatric and neurodegenerative disease. *Nature Reviews Neuroscience*, **11**, 589–90.

Wylie K *et al.* (2016). Serving transgender people: clinical care considerations and service delivery models in transgender health. *Lancet*, **388**, 401–11.

Yalom I and Leszcz M (2005). *The Theory and Practice of Group Psychotherapy*, 5th edn. Basic Books, New York.

Yang YH *et al.* (2015). Statins reduce the risk of dementia in patients with late-onset depression: a retrospective cohort study. *PLoS One*, **10**, e0137914.

Yankner BA, Lu T and Loerch P (2008). The aging brain. *Annual Review of Pathology—Mechanisms of Disease*, **3**, 41–66.

Yeh P *et al.* (2012). Restless legs syndrome: a comprehensive overview on its epidemiology, risk factors, and treatment. *Sleep and Breathing*, **16**, 987–1007.

Yesufu-Udechuku A *et al.* (2015). Interventions to improve the experience of caring for people with severe mental illness: systematic review and meta-analysis. *British Journal of Psychiatry*, **206**, 268–74.

Yilmaz Z *et al.* (2015). Genetics and epigenetics of eating disorders. *Advances in Genomics and Genetics*, **5**, 131–50.

Yokoi F *et al.* (2002). Dopamine D_2 and D_3 receptor occupancy in normal humans treated with the antipsychotic drug aripiprazole (OPC 14597): a study using positron emission tomography and [^{11}C]raclopride. *Neuropsychopharmacology*, **27**, 248–59.

Yonkers KA *et al.* (1996). Phenomenology and course of generalized anxiety disorder. *British Journal of Psychiatry*, **168**, 308–13.

Yonkers KA *et al.* (2011). Does antidepressant use attenuate the risk of a major depressive episode in pregnancy? *Epidemiology*, **22**, 848–54.

Young AH (2014). The effects of HPA axis function on cognition and its implications for the pathophysiology of bipolar disorder. *Harvard Review of Psychiatry*, **6**, 331–3.

Young AH *et al.* (2010). A double blind placebo-controlled study of quetiapine and lithium in adults in the acute phase of bipolar depression (EMBOLDEN I). *Journal of Clinical Psychiatry*, **71**, 150–62.

Young JW and Geyer MA (2010). Action of modafinil-increased motivation via the dopamine transporter inhibition and D1 receptors? *Biological Psychiatry, 67*, 784–7.

Young RC *et al.* (1978). A rating scale for mania: reliability, validity and sensitivity. *British Journal of Psychiatry, 133*, 429–35.

Young S *et al.* (2015). Forensic psychiatry. In: A. Thapar *et al.* (eds). *Rutter's Child and Adolescent Psychiatry.* John Wiley & Sons, Chichester, pp. 636–47.

Youth Justice Board (2011). *Youth Justice Statistics 2009/10.* www. justice.gov.uk/publications/youth-justice-statistics.htm

Yule W *et al.* (2015). Post traumatic stress disorder. In: A. Thapar *et al.* (eds). *Rutter's Child and Adolescent Psychiatry.* John Wiley & Sons, Chichester, pp. 806–21.

Yung AR and McGorry PD (1996). The initial prodrome in psychosis: descriptive and qualitative aspects. *Australian and New Zealand Journal of Psychiatry, 30*, 587–99.

Yung PM and Keltner AA (1996). A controlled comparison on the effect of muscle and cognitive relaxation procedures on blood pressure: implications for the behavioural treatment of borderline hypertensives. *Behaviour Research and Therapy, 43*, 821–6.

Zachar P and Kendler KS (2007). Psychiatric disorders: a conceptual taxonomy. *American Journal of Psychiatry, 164*, 557–65.

Zanarini MC *et al.* (2006). Prediction of the 10-year course of borderline personality disorder. *American Journal of Psychiatry, 163*, 827–32.

Zeanah CH *et al.* (2015). Disorders of attachment and social engagement related to deprivation. In: A. Thapar *et al.* (eds). *Rutter's Child and Adolescent Psychiatry.* John Wiley & Sons, Chichester, pp. 793–805.

Zeman A *et al.* (2004). Narcolepsy and excessive daytime sleepiness. *British Medical Journal, 329*, 724–8.

Zhao GF *et al.* (2008). A cross-sectional study on the mental status of 780 survivors after Wenchuan earthquake. *Chinese Journal of Evidence-Based Medicine, 8*(10), 815–19.

Zhou X *et al.* (2015). Comparative efficacy and acceptability of psychotherapies for depression in children and adolescents: A systematic review and network meta-analysis. *World Psychiatry, 14*, 207–22.

Zigman WB. (2013). Atypical aging in down syndrome. *Developmental Disabilities Research Reviews, 18*, 51–67.

Zigmond AS and Snaith RP (1983). The hospital anxiety and depression scale. *Acta Psychiatrica Scandinavica, 67*, 361–70.

Zimbron J *et al.* (2013). Pre-morbid fertility in psychosis: findings from the AESOP first episode study. *Schizophrenia Research, 156*, 168–73.

Zimmerman M *et al.* (2008). The frequency of personality disorders in psychiatric patients. *Psychiatric Clinics of North America, 31*, 405–20.

Zipfel S *et al.* (2015). Anorexia nervosa: aetiology, assessment, and treatment. *Lancet Psychiatry, 2*, 1099–111.

Zipursky RB *et al.* (2013). The myth of schizophrenia as a progressive brain disease. *Schizophrenia Bulletin, 39*, 1363–72.

Zipursky RB *et al.* (2014). Risk of symptom recurrence with medication discontinuation in first-episode psychosis: a systematic review. *Schizophrenia Research, 152*, 408–14.

Zohar J, Fostick L and Juven-Wetzler J (2009). Obsessive compulsive disorder. In: Gelder MG, Andreasen NC, Lopez-Ibor JJ, Geddes JR (eds.) *New Oxford Textbook of Psychiatry*, 2nd edn. Oxford: Oxford University Press. pp. 767–73.

Zubiaurre-Elorza *et al.* (2013). Cortical thickness in untreated transsexuals. *Cerebral Cortex, 23*, 2855–62.

Zucker KJ and Lawrence A (2009). Epidemiology of gender identity disorder: Recommendations for the standards of care of The World Professional Association for Transgender Health. *International Journal of Transgenderism, 11*, 8–18.

Zucker KJ *et al.* (2015). Gender dysphoria and paraphilic sexual disorders. In: A. Thapar *et al.* (eds). *Rutter's Child and Adolescent Psychiatry.* John Wiley & Sons, Chichester, pp. 983–98.

Zucker KJ *et al.* (2016). Gender dysphoria in adults. *Annual Review of Clinical Psychology, 12*, 217–47.

Zuckerman M (2005). *Psychobiology of Personality.* Cambridge University Press, New York.

Index

Notes: Tables, boxes and figures are indicated by an italic *t, b* and *f* following the page number.

vs. indicates a comparison or differential diagnosis